FLUID, ELECTROLYTE, AND ACID-BASE DISORDERS

in Small Animal Practice

FLUID, ELECTROLYTE, AND ACID-BASE DISORDERS

IN SMALL ANIMAL PRACTICE

THIRD EDITION

STEPHEN P. DIBARTOLA, DVM, DACVIM

PROFESSOR OF MEDICINE
DEPARTMENT OF VETERINARY CLINICAL SCIENCES
COLLEGE OF VETERINARY MEDICINE
THE OHIO STATE UNIVERSITY
COLUMBUS, OH

With 36 Contributing Authors

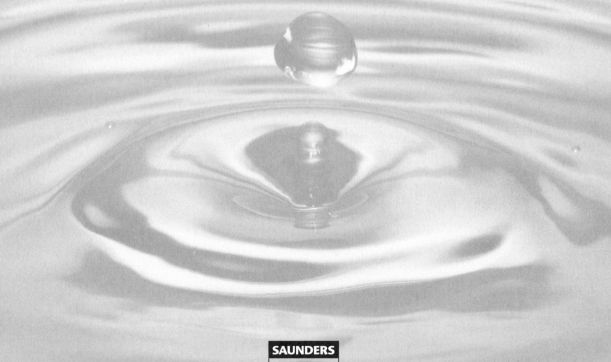

SAUNDERS

ELSEVIER

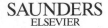

11830 Westline Industrial Drive
St. Louis, Missouri 63146

FLUID, ELECTROLYTE, AND ACID-BASE DISORDERS
IN SMALL ANIMAL PRACTICE

ISBN 13 978-0-7216-3949-9
ISBN 10 0-7216-3949-6

Notice

Previous editions copyrighted 2000, 1992.

ISBN: 13 978-0-7216-3949-9
ISBN: 10 0-7216-3949-6

Publishing Director: Linda Duncan
Acquisitions Editor: Liz Fathman
Developmental Editor: Shelly Stringer
Publishing Services Manager: Pat Joiner
Project Manager: David Stein
Design Direction: Jyotika Shroff
Editorial Assistant: Jennifer Hong

Printed in the United States of America

Last digit is the print number: 9 8 7 6 5 4 3 2 1

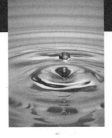

CONTRIBUTORS

Sarah K. Abood, DVM, PhD
Assistant Professor
Department of Small Animal Clinical Sciences
College of Veterinary Medicine
Michigan State University
East Lansing, MI, USA
Enteral Nutrition

Shane Bateman, DVM, DVSc, DACVECC
Clinical Associate Professor
Department of Veterinary Clinical Sciences
College of Veterinary Medicine
The Ohio State University
Columbus, OH, USA
*Disorders of Magnesium: Magnesium Deficit and
Excess*
Introduction to Fluid Therapy
Shock Syndromes

Alexander W. Biondo, DVM, MSC, PhD
Associate Professor
Departmento de Medicina Veterinaria
Universidade Federal do Parana
Curitiba, Parana, Brazil;
Visiting Professor
Department of Pathobiology
College of Veterinary Medicine
University of Illinois
Urbana, IL, USA
*Disorders of Chloride: Hyperchloremia and
Hypochloremia*

**Nichole Birnbaum, DVM, DACVIM (Small Animal
Internal Medicine)**
Staff Internist
Veterinary Internal Medicine of Northern Virginia
Manassas, VA, USA
*Fluid and Electrolyte Disturbances in Gastrointestinal
and Pancreatic Disease*

**Amanda K. Boag, MA, VetMB, MRCVS, DACVIM
(Small Animal Internal Medicine)**
Lecturer in Emergency and Critical Care/Internal
Medicine
Department of Veterinary Clinical Science
Royal Veterinary College
North Mymms, Hertfordshire, UK
*Fluid Therapy with Macromolecular Plasma Volume
Expanders*

**John D. Bonagura, DVM, MS, DACVIM (Cardiology
and Small Animal Internal Medicine)**
Professor of Medicine
Department of Veterinary Clinical Sciences
College of Veterinary Medicine
The Ohio State University
Columbus, OH, USA;
Cardiology Service Head
The Ohio State University Veterinary Teaching
Hospital
The Ohio State University
Columbus, OH, USA;
Member
Davis Heart and Lung Research Institute
The Ohio State University
Columbus, OH, USA
Fluid and Diuretic Therapy in Heart Failure

C.A. Tony Buffington, DVM, PhD, DACVN
Professor
Department of Veterinary Clinical Sciences
College of Veterinary Medicine
The Ohio State University
Columbus, OH, USA
Enteral Nutrition

Sharon A. Center, DVM, DACVIM (Small Animal Internal Medicine)
Professor of Medicine
Department of Clinical Sciences
College of Veterinary Medicine
Cornell University
Ithaca, NY, USA
Fluid, Electrolyte, and Acid-Base Disturbances in Liver Disease

Daniel L. Chan, DVM, DACVECC, DACVN, MRCVS
Lecturer, Veterinary Emergency and Critical Care
Department of Veterinary Clinical Sciences
The Royal Veterinary College
Hertfordshire, UK
Total Parenteral Nutrition

Dennis J. Chew, DVM, DACVIM (Small Animal Internal Medicine)
Professor of Medicine
Department of Veterinary Clinical Sciences
College of Veterinary Medicine
The Ohio State University
Columbus, OH, USA;
Attending Clinician
Veterinary Medical Teaching Hospital
College of Veterinary Medicine
The Ohio State University
Columbus, OH, USA
Disorders of Calcium: Hypercalcemia and Hypocalcemia
Fluid Therapy During Intrinsic Renal Failure

Peter D. Constable, BVSc, MS, PhD, DACVIM (Large Animal Internal Medicine)
Professor of Medicine
Department of Veterinary Clinical Medicine
College of Veterinary Medicine
University of Illinois
Urbana, IL, USA
Strong Ion Approach to Acid-Base Disorders

Larry D. Cowgill, DVM, PhD, DACVIM (Small Animal Internal Medicine)
Professor of Medicine
Department of Medicine and Epidemiology
School of Veterinary Medicine
University of California
Davis, CA, USA
Hemodialysis

Thomas K. Day, DVM, MS, DACVA, DACVECC
Director of Emergency and Critical Care
Louisville Veterinary Specialty and Emergency Services
Louisville, KY, USA
Shock Syndromes

Helio Autran de Morais, DVM, PhD, DACVIM (Small Animal Internal Medicine and Cardiology)
Clinical Associate Professor
Department of Medical Sciences
School of Veterinary Medicine
University of Wisconsin
Madison, WI, USA;
Section Head
Small Animal Medicine
University of Wisconsin Veterinary Medical Teaching Hospital
Madison, WI, USA
Disorders of Chloride: Hyperchloremia and Hypochloremia
Disorders of Potassium: Hypokalemia and Hyperkalemia
Respiratory Acid-Base Disorders
Mixed Acid-Base Disorders
Strong Ion Approach to Acid-Base Disorders
Fluid and Diuretic Therapy in Heart Failure

Thierry Francey, Dr. med. vet., DACVIM (Small Animal Internal Medicine)
Lecturer Small Animal Internal Medicine and Nephrology
Department of Medicine and Epidemiology
School of Veterinary Medicine
University of California
Davis, CA, USA
Hemodialysis

Lisa M. Freeman, DVM, PhD, DACVN
Associate Professor
Department of Clinical Sciences
School of Veterinary Medicine
Tufts University
North Grafton, MA, USA
Total Parenteral Nutrition

Jennifer A. Gieg, DVM
Resident, Small Animal Internal Medicine
Department of Veterinary Clinical Sciences
College of Veterinary Medicine
The Ohio State University
Columbus, OH, USA
Fluid Therapy During Intrinsic Renal Failure

Bernard D. Hansen, DVM, MS, DACVIM (Small Animal Internal Medicine), DACVECC
Associate Professor
Department of Clinical Sciences
College of Veterinary Medicine
North Carolina State University
Raleigh, NC, USA
Technical Aspects of Fluid Therapy

Ann E. Hohenhaus, DVM, DACVIM (Oncology and Small Animal Internal Medicine)
Chairman
Department of Medicine
The Bobst Hospital of The Animal Medical Center
New York, NY, USA;
Head
George Jaqua Transfusion Medicine Service
The Bobst Hospital of The Animal Medical Center
New York, NY, USA
Blood Transfusion and Blood Substitutes

Dez Hughes, BVSc, MRCVS, DACVECC
Senior Lecturer
Veterinary Clinical Sciences
Royal Veterinary College
London, UK;
Section Chief, Emergency and Critical Care
Veterinary Clinical Sciences
Royal Veterinary College
London, UK
Fluid Therapy with Macromolecular Plasma Volume Expanders

Rebecca A. Johnson, DVM, PhD, DACVA
Clinical Instructor
Department of Surgical Sciences
School of Veterinary Medicine
University of Wisconsin
Madison, WI, USA
Respiratory Acid-Base Disorders

Catherine W. Kohn, VMD, DACVIM (Large Animal Internal Medicine)
Professor of Medicine
Department of Veterinary Clinical Sciences
College of Veterinary Medicine
The Ohio State University
Columbus, OH, USA
Applied Physiology of Body Fluids in Dogs and Cats

Mary Anna Labato, DVM, DACVIM (Small Animal Internal Medicine)
Clinical Associate Professor
Department of Clinical Sciences
School of Veterinary Medicine
Tufts University
North Grafton, MA, USA
Peritoneal Dialysis

Linda B. Lehmkuhl, DVM, MS, DACVIM (Cardiology)
Staff Cardiologist
MedVet Medical Center for Pets
Worthington, OH, USA
Fluid and Diuretic Therapy in Heart Failure

Andrew L. Leisewitz, BVSc(Hons), MMedVet(Med), DECVIM-CA
Associate Professor
Veterinary Topical Diseases
Faculty of Veterinary Science
University of Pretoria
Pretoria, South Africa
Mixed Acid-Base Disorders

Karol A. Mathews, DVM, DVSc, DACVECC
Professor
Department of Clinical Studies
Ontario Veterinary College
University of Guelph
Guelph, Ontario, Canada
Monitoring Fluid Therapy and Complications of Fluid Therapy

Mary A. McLoughlin, DVM, MS, DACVS
Associate Professor of Small Animal Surgery
Department of Veterinary Clinical Sciences
College of Veterinary Medicine
The Ohio State University
Columbus, OH, USA
Enteral Nutrition

Larry Allen Nagode, DVM, MS, PhD
Associate Professor of Pathology
Department of Veterinary Biosciences
College of Veterinary Medicine
The Ohio State University
Columbus, OH, USA
Disorders of Calcium: Hypercalcemia and Hypocalcemia

David L. Panciera, DVM, MS, DACVIM (Small Animal Internal Medicine)
Professor of Medicine
Department of Small Animal Clinical Sciences
Virginia-Maryland Regional College of Veterinary Medicine
Virginia Tech
Blacksburg, VA, USA
Fluid Therapy in Endocrine and Metabolic Disorders

Peter J. Pascoe, BVSc., DACVA, DVA, DECVA, MRCVS
Professor
Department of Surgical and Radiological Sciences
School of Veterinary Medicine
University of California
Davis, CA, USA;
Professor
Veterinary Medical Teaching Hospital
School of Veterinary Medicine
University of California-Davis
Davis, CA, USA
Perioperative Management of Fluid Therapy

Thomas J. Rosol, DVM, PhD, DACVP
Dean and the Ruth Stanton Chair for Veterinary
    Medicine, Professor
Department of Veterinary Biosciences
College of Veterinary Medicine
Ohio State University
Columbus, OH, USA
*Disorders of Calcium: Hypercalcemia and
    Hypocalcemia*

**Linda A. Ross, DVM, MS, DACVIM (Small Animal
Internal Medicine)**
Associate Professor of Medicine
Department of Clinical Sciences
School of Veterinary Medicine
Tufts University
North Grafton, MA, USA;
Associate Professor
Clinical Sciences
Foster Hospital for Small Animals
Tufts University School of Veterinary Medicine
North Grafton, MA, USA
Peritoneal Dialysis

Patricia A. Schenck, DVM, PhD
Assistant Professor
Endocrinology Section
Diagnostic Center for Population and Animal Health
College of Veterinary Medicine
Michigan State University
Lansing, MI, USA
*Disorders of Calcium: Hypercalcemia and
    Hypocalcemia*

**Kenneth W. Simpson, BVM&S, PhD, DACVIM
(Small Animal Internal Medicine), DECVIM**
Associate Professor of Medicine
Department of Clinical Sciences
College of Veterinary Medicine
Cornell University
Ithaca, NY, USA
*Fluid and Electrolyte Disturbances in Gastrointestinal
    and Pancreatic Disease*

**Maxey L. Wellman, DVM, PhD, DACVP (Clinical
Pathology)**
Associate Professor of Pathology
Department of Veterinary Biosciences
College of Veterinary Medicine
The Ohio State University
Columbus, OH, USA
Applied Physiology of Body Fluids in Dogs and Cats

**Michael D. Willard, DVM, MS, DACVIM (Small
Animal Internal Medicine)**
Professor of Medicine
Department of Small Animal Medicine and Surgery
College of Veterinary Medicine
Texas A&M University
College Station, TX, USA
*Disorders of Phosphorus: Hypophosphatemia
    and Hyperphosphatemia*

To my family and friends
for all they have taught me about life and to Mr. Charles Donovan who taught me the simple
joy of perpetual intellectual curiosity—*eruditio gratia eruditionis.*

DEDICATION TO THE SECOND EDITION
To my parents, Martha Weimann and Philip DiBartola,
for insisting that I acquire the formal education they could not;

To my wife, Maxey Wellman,
for standing by me despite my imperfections;

To my children, Matthew, Michael, Alex, and Stephanie,
for teaching me about unconditional love;

To my childhood friend, Pudge Albao,
For teaching me about loyalty; and,

To my colleague, Dennis Chew,
for teaching me enthusiasm for clinical medicine and compassion for pet owners.

DEDICATION TO THE FIRST EDITION
To my wife Maxey and our three sons, Matthew, Michael and Alex.

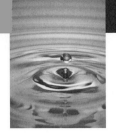

PREFACE

The name of "Fluid Therapy in Small Animal Practice" has been changed to "Fluid, Electrolyte, and Acid-Base Disorders in Small Animal Practice" to more accurately reflect the content of the book. The purpose of the third edition remains the same as that of previous editions, namely "to bring together in one place information about fluid, electrolyte, and acid-base physiology and fluid therapy as they apply to small animal practice." I remain convinced that a good foundation in physiology and pathophysiology is an essential part of veterinary education and enhances the clinician's approach to the patient. Thoughtful evaluation of laboratory results provides valuable insight into the fluid, electrolyte, and acid-base status of the animal and can only improve the veterinary care provided.

The in-depth approach of the previous editions has been retained in the third edition. The book is divided into five sections: applied physiology, electrolyte disorders, acid-base disorders, fluid therapy, and special therapy. The first sections of the book on fluid, electrolyte, and acid-base physiology and disorders have been changed and updated. Many of the figures in these sections have been re-drawn for clarity and visual appeal, and several new figures have been created by Mr. Tim Vojt, artist and computer graphics specialist in our Biomedical Media section at the College of Veterinary Medicine at Ohio State University. The initial chapter on the physiology of body fluids has been extensively revised by Dr. Maxey Wellman for simplification and clarification. Chapter 6 on Disorders of Calcium once again has been thoroughly revised and the material on hypocalcemia expanded. A full chapter by Drs. Helio de Morais and Peter Constable has been devoted to the nontraditional approach to acid-base chemistry to emphasize recent contributions to that topic by veterinary authors. I have enlisted the help of Dr. Shane Bateman, one of our critical care specialists at Ohio State University, with Chapters 8, 14, and 23. His contributions bring the material in Chapter 14 closer in line with our current approach to fluid therapy at the Ohio State University Veterinary Teaching Hospital. A chapter on monitoring and complications of fluid therapy by Dr. Karol Mathews has been added, also reflecting the critical care specialist's perspective. The material on liver disease has been afforded a separate chapter as has material on the gastrointestinal tract. This edition welcomes Dr. David Panciera as an author in the area of endocrine and metabolic disease. Drs. Lisa Freeman and Daniel Chan of Tufts University have contributed their expertise on parenteral nutrition, and a chapter on enteral nutrition by Drs. Sarah Abood, Mary McLoughlin, and Tony Buffington has been added to the third edition. Drs. Mary Ann Labato and Linda Ross have contributed their approach to peritoneal dialysis in Chapter 28 and Drs. Larry Cowgill and Thierry Francey have extensively revised and updated their authoritative chapter on hemodialysis. The appendix has been omitted to allow space for expansion of other chapters and addition of new material.

As in previous editions, I encourage those who read and use this book to write or e-mail me (dibartola.1@osu.edu) about errors, controversial issues, and suggestions for improvement. The use of textbooks should be supplemented by reading the veterinary and human medical literature. Such an approach allows clinicians to maintain both the historical perspective and a contemporary view of medicine. In keeping with this belief, the use of extensive references has been retained and expanded in this edition. Considerable effort has been expended to ensure the accuracy of information provided here, but drug dosages always should be verified.

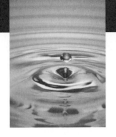

ACKNOWLEDGMENTS

I am grateful to many people for help in completing the third edition of this book. The concept of a book on disturbances of fluid, electrolyte, and acid-base balance for veterinarians originated in discussions with Dr. Dennis Chew, and this book represents the evolution of material taught to second-year veterinary students at the College of Veterinary Medicine and the approach to fluid therapy used in small animal patients at the Ohio State University Veterinary Teaching Hospital. I am indebted to Dr. Helio de Morais for encouraging me to undertake revisions of the book, and for his support throughout the process. I also thank Dr. Shane Bateman for helping me to more fully develop the critical care specialist's perspective in the third edition. Warm thanks and sincere appreciation go to all contributors who have shared their expertise in specific areas and provided comprehensive chapters on clinically relevant topics. As in previous editions, Tim Vojt of our Biomedical Media Department continues to provide original artwork. Tim has a natural talent for taking a clinician's scribbled ideas and turning them into logical and visually pleasing line drawings. Thanks also go to editors and staff members at Elsevier, including Tony Winkel, Shelly Stringer, and David Stein. I thank all of them for their contributions. Lastly, I must once again thank my family for putting up with me as I try to juggle all aspects of my personal and professional life.

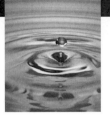

CONTENTS

SECTION III • ACID-BASE DISORDERS

SECTION IV • FLUID THERAPY

SECTION V • SPECIAL THERAPY

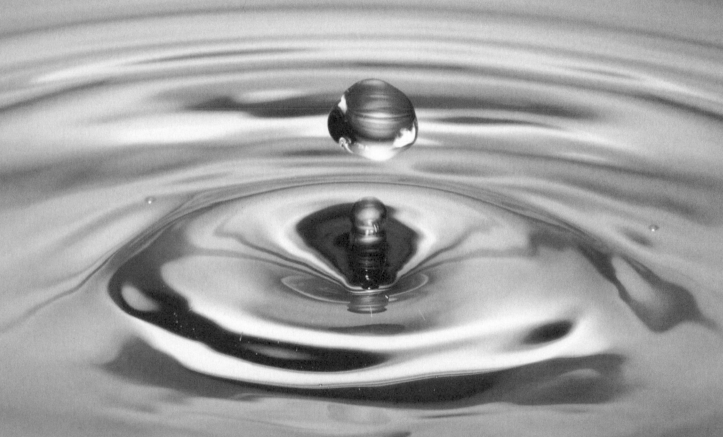

APPLIED PHYSIOLOGY

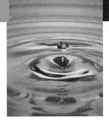

CHAPTER · I

APPLIED PHYSIOLOGY OF BODY FLUIDS IN DOGS AND CATS

Maxey L. Wellman, Stephen P. DiBartola, and Catherine W. Kohn

Appropriate treatment of fluid and electrolyte abnormalities requires a basic understanding of the physiology of fluid balance. The purpose of this chapter is to provide an overview of the principles of body fluid homeostasis, beginning with a brief review of body fluid compartments. This is followed by a discussion of measurement of solutes in body fluids and the concepts of anion gap, osmolal gap, and zero balance.

DISTRIBUTION OF BODY FLUIDS

In health, approximately 60% of an adult animal's body weight is water. Estimates of total body water in adult dogs that are neither very thin nor obese are 534 to 660 mL/kg.[25] There are some species and individual variations in total body water, likely related to age, gender, and body composition. In humans, total body water declines with age and is lower in women than in men.[12] Similarly, an age-related decrease in total body water has been described in puppies and kittens during the first 6 months of life.[33] Because fat has a lower water content than lean tissue, fluid needs should be estimated on the basis of lean body mass to avoid overhydration, especially in patients with cardiac or renal insufficiency or in those with hypoproteinemia. Formulas for estimating lean body mass are based on the assumptions that (1) in normal small animal patients, approximately 20% of body weight is due to fat, (2) morbid obesity increases body fat to approximately 30% of body weight, and (3) body weight is a reasonable estimate of lean body mass in thin patients:

Normal body weight × 0.8 = Lean body mass

Obese body weight × 0.7 = Lean body mass

Thin body weight × 1.0 = Lean body mass

Water is the major component of all body fluids, which are distributed into several physically distinct compartments. Body fluids in each compartment equilibrate with fluids in other compartments via multiple mechanisms across a wide variety of membranes to maintain homeostasis. The volume of fluid in each of these compartments has been estimated using various isotope or dye dilution techniques and calculating their volume of distribution. Results are expressed either as a percentage of body weight, which is easy to measure when calculating fluid therapy needs, or as a percentage of total body water, which is a useful conceptualization of body fluid compartments. Studies of body fluid compartments often are performed in experimental animals that have been anesthetized, splenectomized, or nephrectomized. Data from these kinds of studies vary with the protocol used and thus provide only approximations of fluid compartment sizes in healthy awake animals. The second edition of this book contains a more detailed discussion of the techniques involved in determination of total body water and the amount of fluid in the various compartments.

As shown in Fig. 1-1, the largest volume of fluid in the body is inside cells. The **intracellular fluid (ICF) compartment** comprises approximately 40% of body weight (approximately two thirds of total body water). The composition of ICF is very different from extracellular fluid (ECF; Fig. 1-2). Intracellular homeostasis is maintained by shifts in water, solutes, and numerous other substances across the cell membrane.

Any fluid not contained inside a cell is in the **extracellular fluid compartment** (approximately one third of total body water). Fluid shifts that occur during changes in hydration can have a marked effect on the ECF, and in most disease states, loss of fluids occurs initially from the ECF. For example, in diarrhea, a large volume of gastrointestinal fluid is lost; in renal failure, a large volume of ECF may be excreted. Fluid losses often are treated using parenteral fluids, which initially enter the ECF. Therefore it is important to be able to estimate the volume of the ECF compartment and the volume of fluid lost to initiate appropriate fluid replacement and monitor fluid therapy.

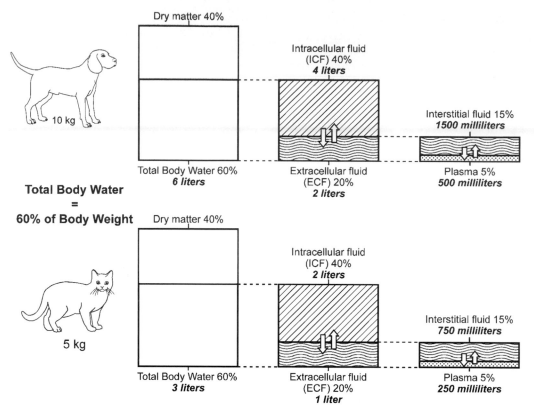

Fig. 1-1 Compartments of total body water expressed as percentage of body weight and total body water for a 10-kg dog and a 5-kg cat.

Unfortunately, data from dye dilution studies of ECF volume are difficult to interpret because no indicator is truly confined to the ECF space. Estimates of ECF vary dramatically with the indicator used. ECF volumes reported for adult, healthy dogs and cats vary between 15% and 30% of body weight. The wide range in estimates of ECF volume likely results from the variety of techniques used to measure this space and the heterogeneity of ECFs, which include interstitial fluid (ISF), plasma, and transcellular fluids. Dense connective tissue, cartilage, and bone also contain a small amount of ECF. From a physiologic perspective and based on multiple studies using various indicators, the most accurate estimate of the ECF in adult small animals is 27% of lean body weight. However, an easier distribution of body fluids to remember is the 60:40:20 rule: 60% of body weight is water, 40% of body weight is ICF, and 20% of body weight is ECF (see Fig. 1-1). Many clinicians use 20% as an estimate for ECF when calculating fluid therapy needs for their patients.

As mentioned above and as shown in Fig. 1-1, ECF is distributed among several different subcompartments. Most ECF (about three fourths) is in spaces surrounding cells and is called **interstitial fluid**. Although accurate studies of the size of the ISF compartment in dogs and cats have not been reported, estimates derived from measurement of fluids in other compartments indicate that the ISF comprises approximately 15% of body weight (approximately 24% of total body water). About one fourth of the ECF is within blood vessels and is called the **intravascular compartment** (plasma). Intravascular fluids are approximately 5% of body weight (approximately 8% to 10% of total body water). Most of the intravascular fluid is plasma. Plasma volume estimates range from 42 to 58 mL/kg in adult dogs that are neither very thin nor obese.[25] Few data for cats are available. Estimates for plasma volume in cats are 37 to 49 mL/kg.[25] Jain noted that blood volume, which includes erythrocytes, is a function of lean body mass and estimated blood volume in the cat as 62 to 66 mL/kg (6% to 7% of body weight) and in the dog as 77 to 78 mL/kg (8% to 9% of body weight).[23]

Fluids produced by specialized cells to form cerebrospinal fluid, gastrointestinal fluid, bile, glandular secretions, respiratory secretions, and synovial fluid are in the **transcellular fluid compartment,** which is estimated as approximately 1% of body weight (approximately 2% of total body water). Dense connective tissues, bone, and cartilage contain approximately 15% of total body water. However, these tissues exchange fluids slowly with other compartments. Because this fluid usually is not taken into account for routine fluid therapy, this compartment is not shown in Fig. 1-1. Thus a more

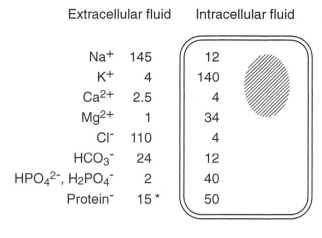

Extracellular fluid		Intracellular fluid
Na$^+$	145	12
K$^+$	4	140
Ca^{2+}	2.5	4
Mg^{2+}	1	34
Cl$^-$	110	4
HCO$_3^-$	24	12
HPO$_4^{2-}$, H$_2$PO$_4^-$	2	40
Protein$^-$	15 *	50

mEq/L

*0 in interstitial fluid, 15 in plasma

Fig. 1-2 Average values for electrolyte concentrations in extracellular and intracellular fluid. Note marked concentration differences for many electrolytes.

simplified distribution of total body water often used for fluid therapy is:

ICF is approximately ⅔ of total body water

ECF is approximately ⅓ of total body water

ISF is approximately ¾ of ECF

Intravascular fluid is approximately ¼ of ECF

Although body fluids traditionally are conceptualized anatomically within these various compartments, water and solutes in these spaces are in dynamic equilibrium across the cell membrane, capillary endothelium, and specialized lining cells. Fluids and electrolytes shift among compartments to maintain homeostasis within each compartment. In health, the concentration of a particular substance may be similar or very different among the various fluid compartments. During disease, fluid volumes and solute concentrations may change dramatically. Loss or gain of fluid or electrolytes from one compartment likely will alter the volume and solute concentration of other compartments.

DISTRIBUTION OF BODY SOLUTES

In addition to water, body fluids contain various concentrations of solutes. Total body content of solutes may be measured by cadaver analysis (desiccation) or by isotope dilution studies. Every solute has a space or apparent volume of distribution. Dilution studies of body solute content yield variable results depending on the volume of distribution of the particular tracer used to estimate the solute space. There are limited data in the literature from cadaver and isotope dilution studies of body solute content in small animals, and most of the following discussion is based on data from studies in humans.[12,46]

Solutes are not distributed homogeneously throughout body fluids. Vascular endothelium and cell membranes have different permeabilities for various solutes. Healthy vascular endothelium is relatively impermeable to the cellular components of blood and to plasma proteins. Consequently, the volume of distribution of cells and proteins is the plasma space itself. However, the vascular endothelium is freely permeable to ionic solutes, and the concentration of these ions is almost the same in ISF as in plasma. Cell membranes maintain intracellular solutes at very different concentrations from that of the ECF. The composition of solutes in the ECF and ICF is compared in Fig. 1-2, and concentrations of solutes in plasma and in ISF and ICF are listed in Table 1-1.

The slightly increased concentration of anions and decreased concentration of cations in ISF as compared with plasma occur primarily because of the presence of negatively charged plasma proteins in plasma. The equilibrium concentrations of permeable anions and cations across the vascular endothelium are determined by the Gibbs-Donnan equilibrium, which occurs because negatively charged, nondiffusible proteins affect the distribution of other small charged solutes. In clinical practice, the difference in concentrations of anions and cations across the vascular endothelium is negligible, and the effects of the Gibbs-Donnan equilibrium are usually ignored. Thus in clinical practice, plasma concentrations of solutes are considered to reflect solute concentrations throughout the ECF. Average values for ECF concentrations of important solutes in dogs and cats are given in Table 1-2. Normal values may vary among laboratories.

Table 1-1 shows that although the solute composition of ECF and ICF is quite different, the total numbers of cations and anions in all body fluids are equal to maintain electroneutrality. The most abundant cation in the ECF is sodium (Na$^+$). Most of the body Na$^+$ is in the extracellular space. Approximately 70% of body Na$^+$ in humans is exchangeable, and 30% is fixed as insoluble salts in bone.[46] The percentage of exchangeable sodium is important because only exchangeable solutes are osmotically active. Cell membranes are permeable to Na$^+$, which tends to diffuse into cells. In health, however, cell membrane sodium, potassium-adenosinetriphosphatase (Na$^+$, K$^+$-ATPase) actively removes Na$^+$ from cells, thus maintaining a steep extracellular-to-intracellular concentration gradient for Na$^+$.

The most abundant anions in ECF are chloride (Cl$^-$) and bicarbonate (HCO$_3^-$). The volume of distribution of Cl$^-$ is primarily the ECF volume. Bicarbonate is present in all body fluids and can be generated from CO$_2$ and H$_2$O in the presence of carbonic anhydrase. The ECF also

TABLE 1-1   Approximate Ionic Composition of the Body Water Compartments

Ion	Plasma (mEq/L)	Plasma Water* (mEq/L)	Interstitial Fluid† (mEq/L)	Skeletal Muscle Cell (mEq/L)
Cations				
Na^+	142	152.7	145.1	12.0
K^+	4.3	4.6	4.4	140
Ca^{2+} (ionized)	2.5	2.7	2.4	4.0
Mg^{2+} (ionized)	1.1	1.2	1.1	34
Total	149.9	161.2	153	190
Anions				
Cl^-	104	111.9	117.4	4
HCO_3^-	24	25.8	27.1	12
HPO_4^{2-}, $H_2PO_4^{1-}$	2	2.2	2.3	40
Proteins	14	15	0	50
Other	5.9	6.3	6.2	84‡
Total	149.9	161.2	153	190

Source: Adapted from Woodbury DM. In Ruch TC and Patton HD (eds): Physiology and Biophysics, 20th ed. Philadelphia, WB Saunders, 1974; from Rose BD: Clinical Physiology of Acid-Base and Electrolytes, 3rd ed. New York, McGraw-Hill Book Co., 1989, with permission of the McGraw-Hill Companies.
*Plasma water content is assumed to be 93% of plasma volume.
†Gibbs-Donnan factors used as multipliers are 0.95 for univalent cations, 0.90 for divalent cations, 1.05 for univalent anions, and 1.10 for divalent anions.
‡This largely represents organic phosphates such as ATP.

contains a small but physiologically important concentration of K^+. For example, alterations in ECF K^+ concentrations may result in muscle weakness (hypokalemia) or cardiotoxicity (hyperkalemia).

In contrast to ECF, the primary cations in ICF are K^+ and magnesium (Mg^{2+}). Most of the body K^+ is in the ICF, where K^+ is the most abundant cation. Cell membranes are permeable to K^+. The K^+ concentration gradient between ICF and ECF is maintained by cell membrane Na^+, K^+-ATPase, which moves K^+ into cells against a concentration gradient. The ratio of intracellular

to extracellular K^+ concentration is important in generating and maintaining the cell membrane potential at approximately -70 mV (see Appendix). Almost 100% of body K^+ in humans is exchangeable.[46] Unfortunately, a reliable, practical method for measuring the intracellular K^+ concentration is not available, and changes in serum K^+ concentration may not reflect changes in total body K^+ stores (see Chapter 5). The predominant anions in the ICF are organic phosphates and proteins.

ICFs are not homogeneous. Concentrations of solutes vary in different cell types and in different subcellular compartments. From a clinical perspective, these differences usually are ignored. However, it is important to remember that the heterogeneity of the solute distribution in ICF or ECF may play a very important role in some disease processes.

Transcellular fluids include cerebrospinal fluid, gastrointestinal fluid, bile, glandular secretions, and joint fluid. Transcellular fluids usually are not simply transudates of plasma. Transcellular fluid composition varies according to the cells that form the fluid. Concentrations of solutes in transcellular fluids will be discussed in later chapters, related to alterations in fluid balance involving specific transcellular fluids, such as loss of enteric fluids in diarrhea.

UNITS OF MEASURE

Definitions can be tedious, but familiarity with a few may help with understanding subsequent sections in this

TABLE 1-2   Average Plasma Concentrations of Electrolytes in Dogs and Cats

Substance	Units	Dog	Cat
Sodium	mEq/L	145	155
Potassium	mEq/L	4	4
Ionized calcium	mg/dL	5.4	5.1
Total calcium	mg/dL	10	9
Total magnesium	mg/dL	3	2.5
Chloride	mEq/L	110	120
Bicarbonate	mEq/L	21	20
Phosphate	mg/dL	4	4
Proteins	g/dL	7	7
Lactate	mg/dL	15	15

chapter. The definitions are presented in sequence of discussion, not alphabetically.

ATOMIC MASS (ALSO REFERRED TO AS RELATIVE ATOMIC MASS OR ATOMIC WEIGHT)

Most naturally occurring elements consist of one or more isotopes of that element, each of which has a different mass. For example, carbon in the environment consists of approximately 99% ^{12}C and 1% ^{13}C. The atomic mass of an element is an average mass based on the distribution of stable isotopes for that element. The atomic mass of an element is the weight of that element relative to the weight of the ^{12}C isotope of carbon, which is defined as 12.000. Atomic mass usually is reported with no units or as atomic mass units. The atomic mass is shown in most periodic tables of the elements. The atomic weights of some biologically important elements and the molecular weights of important compounds in body fluids are listed in Table 1-3.

The atomic mass of elements is of less physiologic importance than the molecular mass (molecular weight or formula weight) of the compounds they form.

TABLE 1-3 Atomic and Molecular Weights of Physiologically Important Substances

Substance	Symbol or Formula	Atomic or Molecular Weight	Valence
Calcium ion	Ca	40.1	+2
Carbon	C	12.0	0
Chloride ion	Cl	35.5	−1
Hydrogen ion	H	1.0	+1
Magnesium ion	Mg	24.3	+2
Nitrogen	N	14.0	0
Oxygen	O	16.0	0
Phosphorus	P	31.0	0
Potassium ion	K	39.1	+1
Sodium ion	Na	23.0	+1
Sulfur	S	32.1	0
Ammonia	NH_3	17.0	0
Ammonium ion	NH_4	18.0	+1
Bicarbonate ion	HCO_3	61.0	−1
Carbon dioxide	CO_2	44.0	0
Glucose	$C_6H_{12}O_6$	180.0	0
Lactate ion	$C_3H_5O_3$	89.0	−1
Phosphate ion	PO_4	95.0	−3
	HPO_4	96.0	−2
	H_2PO_4	97.0	−1
Sulfate ion	SO_4	96.1	−2
Urea	NH_2CONH_2	60.0	0
Water	H_2O	18.0	0

Source: Adapted from Rose BD: Clinical Physiology of Acid-Base and Electrolyte Disorders, ed 3, New York, 1989, McGraw-Hill, with permission of the McGraw-Hill Companies.

MOLECULAR MASS (MOLECULAR WEIGHT)

Many elements combine to form physiologically important compounds. The molecular mass of a compound is the sum of the atomic masses of the atoms that form the compound. For example, the molecular mass of water (H_2O) is 18 and represents two times the atomic mass of hydrogen (2×1) plus the atomic mass of oxygen (16).

FORMULA WEIGHT

Ionic compounds do not really form molecules, and a more appropriate term for the mass of these substances is formula weight. For example, the formula weight of $CaCl_2$ is the atomic mass of Ca^{2+} (40) plus two times the atomic mass of Cl^- (2×35.5) = 111.

MOLE

A mole is defined as 6.023×10^{23} particles. Some physiology texts define a mole as the molecular (or atomic) weight of a substance in grams, but a mole really just describes 6.023×10^{23} (Avogadro's number) particles. It is defined as the number of atoms in exactly 12 g of ^{12}C. One mole of a substance weighs its molecular weight in grams (see section on Molecular Mass).

MOLAR MASS

The molar mass is the mass in grams of 1 mol of a substance. By definition, 1 mol of carbon has a mass of 12 g. Molar masses are numerically equivalent to atomic or molecular weights but are reported in grams. For example, 1 mol Na weighs 23 g. Molar mass and gram molecular weight often are used interchangeably.

MOLALITY

The number of moles of solute per kilogram of solvent.

MOLARITY

The number of moles of solute per liter of solution.

Note: The molarity and molality of most biologic solutions are approximately equal because the density of water is 1 kg/L. The slight difference between molarity and molality of a substance in plasma is because of nonaqueous proteins and lipids, which make up about 6% of the total volume. Usually this difference is unimportant, and the terms molality and molarity often are used interchangeably.

MILLIMOLE AND MILLIGRAM

The prefix "milli" refers to 1 one-thousandth. A millimole is 1×10^{-3} mol; a milligram is 1×10^{-3} g. Many biologic substances in body fluids are measured in millimoles or milligrams.

CONCENTRATION

Concentration refers to the amount of a substance that is present in a specified volume. The amount of a substance can be expressed as mass (grams or milligrams), moles (or millimoles), or equivalents (or milliequivalents). Volume usually is expressed as liters (L), deciliters (dL), or milliliters (mL). A **deciliter** is one tenth of a liter (i.e., 100 mL).

Many solutions used for fluid therapy are **percent solutions**. Percent concentration refers to a number of parts in 100 parts of solution. This may be used to express concentration in terms of weight per unit weight, weight per unit volume, or volume per unit volume. For example, a 0.9% solution of NaCl contains 0.9 g of NaCl per 100 mL of solution because 100 mL H_2O is equal to 100 g H_2O (0.9 g NaCl/100 g H_2O). Because a gram is equal to 1000 mg and a deciliter is equal to 100 mL of solution, a 0.9% solution of NaCl contains 900 mg NaCl per deciliter (9000 mg NaCl/L). Similarly, a 10% solution of $CaCl_2$ contains 10 g of $CaCl_2$ per 100 mL of solution, or 10 g of $CaCl_2$ per deciliter (100 g/L), and 5% dextrose contains 5 g of dextrose per deciliter (50 g/L).

CATION

A cation is an atom or molecule with a positive charge. A monovalent cation has one positive charge (e.g., Na^+), and a divalent cation has two positive charges (e.g., Ca^{2+}).

ANION

An anion is an atom or molecule with a negative charge. A monovalent anion has one negative charge (e.g., Cl^-), and a divalent anion has two negative charges (e.g., SO_4^{2-}).

VALENCE

Ions in body fluids combine according to ionic charge (valence) rather than weight. The number of cations (positively charged ions) in solution always equals the number of anions (negatively charged ions) to maintain electroneutrality. A univalent anion has a charge of negative one (e.g., Cl^-); a divalent cation has a charge of positive two (Ca^{2+}). One atom of Ca^{2+} combines with two atoms of Cl^- to form $CaCl_2$. It is useful to express concentrations of solutes in body fluids in equivalents per liter (Eq/L) or milliequivalents per liter (mEq/L) to reflect the charge or valence of the solute. The equivalent weight of a substance is the atomic, molecular, or formula weight of a substance divided by the valance.

ELECTROCHEMICAL EQUIVALENCE

Rose[47] defines electrochemical equivalence as follows:

One equivalent is defined as the weight in grams of an element that combines with or replaces 1 gram of hydrogen ion (H^+). Since 1 g of H^+ is equal to 1 mol of H^+ (containing approximately 6.02 10^{23} particles), 1 mol of any univalent anion (charge equals 1^-) will combine with this H^+ and is equal to 1 equivalent (Eq).

For example, 1 mol (1 equivalent) of Cl^- combines with 1 mol of H^+; 1 mol (1 equivalent) of Na^+ could replace 1 mol of H^+; one atom of Ca^{2+} combines with two atoms of Cl^- to form $CaCl_2$. Therefore it is useful to

express concentrations of solutes in body fluids in equivalents per liter (Eq/L), thus reflecting the charge or valence of the solute.

EQUIVALENT WEIGHT

The equivalent weight of a substance is the atomic, molecular, or formula weight divided by the valence. The milliequivalent (mEq) weight is 10^{-3} times the equivalent weight. For an element like sodium, which has a valence of +1, the milliequivalent weight is equal to its atomic weight. Therefore each millimole of Na^+ provides 1 mEq. In contrast, the milliequivalent weight of Ca^{2+} is one half its atomic weight because its valence is +2. Each millimole of Ca^{+2} provides 2 mEq (0.5 mmol provides 1 mEq). These relationships may be summarized as:

Millimolecular weight/valence = milliequivalent weight

Millimoles × valence = milliequivalents (mEq)

To convert concentrations:

$$mEq/L = mmol/L \times valence$$

$$mEq/L = \frac{mg/dL \times 10}{molecular\,weight} \times valence$$

Note: The multiplication by 10 in the numerator converts mg/dL to mg/L. The denominator converts milligrams to millimoles. Multiplying by the valence converts to milliequivalents.

Phosphate can exist in body fluids in three different ionic forms: $H_2PO_4^{1-}$, HPO_4^{2-}, and PO_4^{3-} (see Chapter 7). At the normal pH of ECF, approximately 80% of phosphate is in the HPO_4^{2-} form and 20% is in the $H_2PO_4^{1-}$ form. Therefore the average valence of phosphate in ECF is $0.8 \times (-2) + 0.2 \times (-1) = -1.8$. At a normal plasma phosphate concentration of 4 mg/dL,

$$\frac{4 \times 10}{31} \times 1.8 = 2.3\,mEq/L$$

OSMOLALITY AND OSMOLARITY

Regardless of its weight, 1 mol of any substance contains the same number of particles (6.023×10^{23}; Avogadro's law). Solutes exert an osmotic effect in solution that is dependent only on the number of particles in solution, not their chemical formula, weight, size, or valence. One osmole (Osm) is defined as 1 g molecular weight of any nondissociable substance; therefore each osmole also contains 6.023×10^{23} molecules.

If a substance does not dissociate in solution (e.g., glucose), 1 mol equals 1 Osm. If a substance dissociates in solution, the number of osmoles equals the number of dissociated particles. For example, assuming that NaCl completely dissociates into Na^+ and Cl^- in solution, each millimole of NaCl provides 2 milliosmoles (mOsm): 1 mOsm of Na^+ and 1 mOsm of Cl^-. If a compound in solution dissociates into two or three particles, the number of osmoles in solution is increased two or three times, respectively (e.g., $CaCl_2$).

The milliosmolar concentration of a solution may be expressed as the solution's milliosmolarity or milliosmolality.

Osmolality refers to the number of osmoles per kilogram of solvent. An aqueous solution with an osmolality of 1.0 results when 1 Osm of a solute is added to 1 kg of water. The volume of the resulting solution exceeds 1 L by the relatively small volume of the solute. In clinical veterinary medicine, osmolality is expressed as mOsm/kg.

Osmolarity refers to the number of osmoles per liter of solution. If 1 Osm of a solute is placed in a beaker and enough water is added to make the total volume 1 L, the osmolarity of the resulting solution is 1. In biologic fluids, there is a negligible difference between osmolality and osmolarity, and the term osmolality is used in this discussion. In clinical veterinary medicine, osmolarity is expressed as mOsm/L.

In clinical medicine, osmolality is measured in serum because the addition of anticoagulants for plasma samples would increase solute in the sample. Serum osmolality usually is measured by freezing-point depression, which is more precise and accurate than vapor pressure determinations. One osmole of a solute in 1 kg of water depresses the freezing point of the water by 1.86° C.[53] Average values for measured serum osmolality in the dog and cat are 300 and 310 mOsm/kg, respectively.[7,17] Measured osmolality may not be the same as calculated osmolality (see below).

Effective and Ineffective Osmoles

In any fluid compartment, the osmotic effect of a solute is in part dependent on the permeability of the solute across the membranes separating the compartment. Consider the two fluid compartments in a rigid box in Fig. 1-3. Assume that the membrane dividing the two compartments is freely permeable to urea and water but is impermeable to glucose. When urea is added to the left compartment (top), it moves down its concentration gradient from left to right, and water moves down its concentration gradient from right to left until there are equal concentrations of urea and water on both sides of the membrane. No fluid rises in the column attached to the left fluid compartment because urea is an **ineffective osmole** and does not generate osmotic pressure. In biologic fluids, urea is a small molecule that freely diffuses across most cell membranes and therefore does not contribute to effective osmolality.

When glucose is added to the left compartment (bottom), water moves down its concentration gradient from right to left, but glucose cannot move across the membrane. This movement of water from a solution of lesser solute concentration across a semipermeable membrane to a solution of greater solute concentration is called

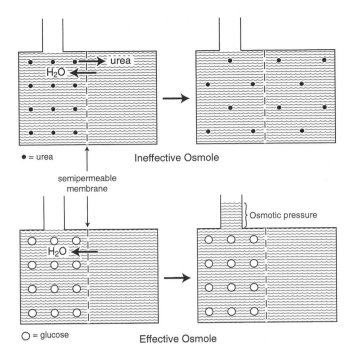

Fig. 1-3 Effective and ineffective osmoles. *Top,* Effect of adding a permeable solute such as urea (small closed circles) to the fluid on one side of a membrane. In this setting, equilibrium is reached by urea equilibration across the membrane rather than water movement into the urea compartment. Consequently, no osmotic pressure is generated. *Bottom,* Effect of adding an impermeable solute such as glucose (large open circles) to the fluid on one side of a membrane. As water moves into the glucose compartment, hydraulic pressure is generated (measured by the height of the column of water above the glucose compartment), which at equilibrium equals the osmotic pressure of the solution.

osmosis. The fluid in the left compartment cannot expand in size, and the influx of water resulting from the osmotic effect of glucose causes the solution to rise in the column. The height of fluid in the column is proportional to the osmotic pressure generated by glucose. In this example, glucose is an **effective osmole** because it generates osmotic pressure by causing a shift of water across the boundary membrane. Glucose is an effective osmole in this setting because the boundary membrane is impermeable to glucose but permeable to water. In biologic fluids, glucose can contribute to osmolality because it is not freely diffusible.

Tonicity

The effective osmolality of a solution is referred to as the **tonicity** of the solution. A freezing-point depression osmometer measures all osmotically active particles in the solution. Thus the measured osmolality of a solution includes both effective and ineffective osmoles. The tonicity of a solution may be less than the measured osmolality if both effective and ineffective osmoles are present. Thus the tonicity and osmolality of a solution are not necessarily equal—a circumstance that often is true in biologic solutions.

Measured Osmolality

The osmolality determined with an osmometer is the measured osmolality, which typically is not the same as the calculated osmolality estimated using various formulas (see discussion below).

Calculated Osmolality

The calculated osmolality is an estimate of serum osmolality using various formulas. The formulas include solutes that have a major contribution to total osmolality. Calculated osmolality often is less than measured osmolality because the formulas either exclude some osmotically active particles or estimate their contribution (see discussion below).

Osmolal Gap

Osmolal gap is the difference between measured osmolality and calculated osmolality (see discussion below).

Colloid Osmotic Pressure (oncotic pressure)

Colloids are large molecular weight (MW, 30,000) particles present in a solution. The component of the total osmotic pressure in plasma contributed by colloids is called the colloid osmotic pressure (oncotic pressure). The plasma proteins are the major colloids present in normal plasma. Although colloid osmotic pressure is only about 0.5% of the total osmotic pressure, oncotic pressure is extremely important in transcapillary fluid dynamics. Oncotic pressure can be measured using an oncometer.

Several examples related to fluid therapy are included here to illustrate how these definitions may be used in clinical veterinary medicine.

Example 1. Determine how many millimoles, milliequivalents, and milliosmoles of sodium and chloride there are in 0.9% NaCl.

Concentration of 0.9% NaCl: (See definition above)	0.9 g NaCl/100 mL of solution = 900 mg NaCl/dL
Formula weight of NaCL = (See definition above; use atomic weight from Table 1-3 or periodic table)	atomic mass of Na + atomic mass of Cl 23 + 35.5 = 58.5
Molar mass of NaCl = (See definition above)	58.5 g
Convert grams to moles: (See definition above)	$9 \text{ g NaCl} \times \dfrac{1 \text{ mol}}{58.5 \text{ g}} = 0.154 \text{ mol NaCl}$
Convert moles to millimoles: (See definition above)	$0.154 \text{ mol} \times \dfrac{1000 \text{ mmol}}{\text{mol}} = 154 \text{ mmol NaCl}$
Determine millimoles of Na^+ and Cl^-:	NaCl in solution dissociates into Na^+ and Cl^- yielding 154 mmol/L of Na^+ and 154 mmol/L of Cl^-
Determine milliequivalent of Na^+ and Cl^-:	Millimoles × valence = Milliequivalents Na^+ and Cl^- each have a valence of 1 154 mmol × 1 = 154 mEq of Na^+ 154 mmol × 1 = 154 mEq of Cl^-

Note: Because Na^+ and Cl^- each have a valence of 1, the number of milliequivalents equals the number of millimoles. There are 154 mEq/L of Na^+ and 154 mEq/L of Cl^- in 0.9% NaCl.

Determine milliosmole of Na^+ and Cl^-:	NaCl in solution dissociates into Na^+ and Cl^-, so the mOsm/L in 0.9% NaCl is the sum of the mOsm for each component 154 mEq/L Na^+ + 154 mEq/L Cl^- 154 mOsm/L Na^+ + 154 mOsm/L Cl^- = 308 mOsm/L

Example 2. Determine how many millimoles, milliequivalents, and milliosmoles of calcium and chloride there are in 1 L of a 10% solution of $CaCl_2$.

Concentration of 10% $CaCl_2$: (See definition above)	10 g $CaCl_2$/100 mL of solution = 10 g $CaCl_2$/dL
To convert deciliters to liters:	10 g $CaCl_2$/dL × 10 dL/L = 100 g $CaCl_2$/L
Formula weight of 10% $CaCl_2$ = (See definition above; use atomic weight from Table 1-3 or periodic table)	atomic mass of Ca^{+2} + 2(atomic mass of Cl^-) 40.1 + 2(35.5) = 111.1
Molar mass: (See definition above)	111.1 g
Convert grams to moles: (See definition above)	$100 \text{ g CaCl}_2 \times \dfrac{1 \text{ mol}}{111.1 \text{ g}} = 0.9 \text{ mol CaCl}_2$

Continued

Example 2.—cont'd

Convert moles to millimoles: (See definition above)	$0.9 \text{ mol} \times \dfrac{1000 \text{ mmol}}{\text{mol}} = 900 \text{ mmol CaCl}_2$
Determine millimoles of Ca^{+2} and Cl^-:	$CaCl_2$ in solution dissociates into $Ca^{+2} + 2Cl^-$ yielding 900 mmol/L of Ca^+ and $2 \times 900 = 1800$ mmol/L of Cl^-
Determine milliequivalent of Ca^{+2} and Cl^-:	Millimoles $\times$ valence = Milliequivalents Ca^{+2} has a valence of 2 Cl^- has a valence of 1 900 mmol $Ca^{+2} \times 2 = 1800$ mEq of Ca^{+2} 900 mmol $Cl^- \times 1 = 900$ mEq of Cl^-

Note: Because Ca^{+2} has a valence of 2 and Cl^- has a valence of 1, the number of milliequivalents equals two times the number of millimoles for Ca^{+2} and one times the number of millimoles for Cl^-.

Determine milliosmole of Ca^{+2} and Cl^-:	$CaCl_2$ in solution dissociates into $Ca^{+2} + 2Cl^-$ mOsm/L in 10% $CaCl_2$ is the sum of the milliosmole for each component 1800 mEq/L Ca^{+2} + 900 mEq/L Cl^- 1800 mOsm/L Ca^{+2} + 900 mOsm/L Cl^- = 2700 Osm/L

EXCHANGE OF WATER BETWEEN INTRACELLULAR AND EXTRACELLULAR FLUID SPACES

The number of osmotically active particles in each space determines the volume of fluid in the ICF and ECF compartments. The osmolality of physiologic fluids is dominated by small solutes that are present in high concentrations. In serum, sodium, potassium, chloride, bicarbonate, urea, and glucose are present in high enough concentrations to individually affect osmolality. Together these make up more than 95% of the total osmolality of serum. Larger molecules like albumin contribute little to the osmolality.

As mentioned above, osmotic activity depends on the solute and its permeability across the membrane. Sodium is the most abundant cation in the ECF. Although there is variation among different types of cells, many cell membranes are impermeable to sodium. Sodium movement across most cell membranes occurs by active transport. Consequently, Na^+ and its associated anions account for most of the osmotically active particles in the ECF and as such are considered effective osmoles.

Glucose and urea are two other substances with potential osmotic activity. Many cell membranes are not freely permeable to glucose, in which case glucose would be osmotically active. Urea is a small molecule that is freely diffusible across most cell membranes. Urea does not have a major contribution to effective osmolality in the ECF. Urea may have an impact on serum osmolality if it is increased.

Osmolality of the ECF may be estimated using various formulas. This is called the calculated osmolality because it is based on estimating the contribution of osmotically active substances. Calculated osmolality by itself is not very useful because it is simply an estimate based on the concentration of commonly measured solutes. Calculated osmolality, which is an estimate, may not be the same as measured osmolality, which is determined by an osmometer.

The formulas for calculated osmolality include various combinations of the most osmotically active solutes, but none include all osmotically active solutes because not all solutes are measured on routine biochemical profiles. The formulas also assume complete dissociation of some solutes, which may not be true in serum.

One of the most commonly used formulas for calculating the osmolality of serum is[46]:

ECF osmolality (mOsm/kg) =

$$2\left([Na^+] + [K^+]\right) + \frac{[glucose]}{18} + \frac{[BUN]}{2.8}$$

In all formulas, Na^+ and K^+ are measured in mmol/L or mEq/L. In this formula, the contribution of Cl^- and HCO^{3-} is estimated by multiplying the major cations by 2, assuming the serum must remain electrically neutral. The concentrations of glucose and blood urea nitrogen (BUN) are divided by 18 and 2.8, respectively, to convert mg/dL to mmol/L (The molecular weight of glucose is 180 and the molecular weight of urea is 28, and there are 10 dL/L).

Several other formulas have been suggested for estimation (calculated osmolality) of the true serum osmolality (measured osmolality). These formulas vary based on which major solutes are included and whether constants are added to estimate the effects of other solutes. Including K^+ is a more accurate estimate of measured osmolality. Remember, in all formulas, Na^+ and K^+ are measured in mmol/L or mEq/L. If glucose and BUN are measured in mg/dL, the conversion factor is included in the formula. If glucose and BUN are measured in mmol/L, delete the conversion factor (see below). Alternate formulas are listed in the second edition of this book.

Not all potentially osmotic substances are osmotically active in body fluids. Cell membranes are permeable to urea and K^+; therefore these solutes are ineffective osmoles. Effective osmolality is calculated as[46]:

$$\text{Effective ECF osmolality} = 2 \times Na^+ + \frac{[\text{glucose}]}{18}$$

In healthy dogs and cats, the contribution of glucose to the effective osmolality of the ECF is small (about 4 to 6 mOsm/kg) based on blood glucose concentrations of 70 to 110 mg/dL. Therefore $2 \times [Na^+]$ is a good approximation of the ECF effective osmolality.

All body fluid spaces are isotonic with one another. Thus the effective osmolality of the ICF also may be estimated by doubling the ECF Na^+ concentration, $[Na^+]$, even though the Na^+ concentration in ICF is small. Because all body fluid spaces are isotonic, the tonicity of

total body water also may be approximated by doubling the plasma $[Na^+]$. The tonicity of total body water also may be expressed as the ratio of the sum of all exchangeable cations and all exchangeable anions to the volume of total body water. Exchangeable ions are able to move throughout the fluid compartment. The total number of milliosmoles of exchangeable cations and anions may be estimated from the expression:

$$2[Na^+]_e + 2[K^+]_e$$

Therefore:

$$2 \times \text{plasma}[Na^+] \approx \frac{2[Na^+]_e + 2[K^+]_e}{\text{TBW}}$$

and

$$\text{Plasma}[Na^+] \approx \frac{[Na^+]_e + [K^+]_e}{\text{TBW}}$$

This relationship is represented graphically in Fig. 1-4.[13,47] Examination of Fig. 1-4 shows that when total exchangeable Na^+ increases, serum sodium concentration also increases,[47] and these changes are usually associated with body fluid hypertonicity. A decrease in total exchangeable Na^+ or K^+ is associated with hyponatremia, a decrease in

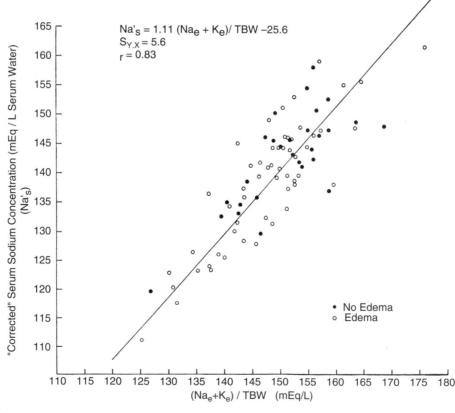

Fig. 1-4 Relationship of plasma $[Na^+]$ to $([Na^+]_e + [K^+]_e)/$TBW. $[Na^+]_e$, Total exchangeable Na^+; $[K^+]_e$, total exchangeable K^+; *TBW*, total body water. (From Edelman IS, Leibman J, O'Meara MP, et al: Interrelations between serum sodium concentration, serum osmolarity and total exchangeable sodium, total exchangeable potassium, and total body water, *J Clin Invest* 37:1236-1256, 1958.)

plasma osmolality, and hypotonicity. The effect of a decrease in total exchangeable K^+ on serum $[Na^+]$ is not intuitively obvious but is clinically important.[47] Rose explained that a decrease in serum $[K^+]$ results in a shift of K^+ out of cells. To maintain electroneutrality, Na^+ shifts into cells, thus causing hyponatremia.

Serum (and therefore ECF) osmolality in dogs is approximately 300 mOsm/kg, and fluids with effective osmolalities greater than 300 mOsm/kg are hypertonic to plasma, whereas those with effective osmolalities less than 300 mOsm/kg are hypotonic to plasma. Those with effective osmolalities of 300 mOsm/kg are isotonic to plasma. In health, addition or loss of fluid or solute to or from the body results in alterations in body fluid space volumes and tonicity. These alterations elicit homeostatic shifts of fluid between compartments so that fluid spaces return to isotonicity (see Chapter 3).

In most disease states, fluid and solutes initially are lost from the ECF. Three basic types of fluid and solute loss may occur: solute in excess of water (loss of hypertonic fluids), isotonic loss (loss of isotonic fluids), or water in excess of solute (loss of hypotonic fluids) (Table 1-4).[27] Solute and water losses theoretically may occur in any proportion along the continuum between solute loss with no water loss (e.g., peritoneal dialysis with a salt-poor solution) and water loss with no solute loss (e.g., water deprivation).

When solute is lost in excess of water (hypertonic fluid loss), the osmolality of the ECF decreases relative to that of the ICF. This could be seen in oozing of serum from the skin of burn patients, which occurs much more commonly in human medicine than in veterinary medicine. Water passes from the ECF through the cell membrane to the ICF, thus diluting ICF solute until the effective osmolalities of ECF and ICF are again equal. The osmolalities of both ICF and ECF decrease. This homeostatic fluid shift decreases ECF volume. When hypertonic fluid is lost from the ECF and volume depletion occurs, homeostatic water shifts further compromise the ECF volume and effective circulating blood volume, thus compounding fluid losses.

During water deprivation, the tonicity of ECF increases relative to that of the ICF. Water shifts out of cells and into ECF until the osmolalities of the two compartments are equal. The osmolalities of both ICF

TABLE 1-4 Effect of Water and Solute Losses from Body Fluids

Loss	ECF	Theoretical Replacement Fluid
Hypotonic	Hypertonic	Hypotonic
Isotonic	Isotonic	Isotonic
Hypertonic	Hypotonic	Isotonic/hypertonic

TABLE 1-5 Clinical Signs of Water versus Salt Depletion

Clinical Features	Salt Depletion	Water Lack
Physical findings		
Thirst	Normal	Increased
Skin turgor	Decreased	Normal
Pulse	Rapid	Normal
Blood pressure	Low	Normal
Laboratory findings		
Urine volume	Normal	Decreased
Urine concentration	Normal	Increased
Serum proteins	Increased	Normal
Hemoglobin and hematocrit	Increased	Normal
Blood urea nitrogen	Increased	High normal
Serum sodium and chloride	Decreased	Increased
Treatment	Salt	Water

and ECF are greater than during the state of normal hydration. This water shift augments the ECF volume, thus helping to preserve the effective circulating blood volume and protecting against the development of shock.

Loss or gain of isotonic fluid from the ECF results in no change in ECF osmolality, and no osmotically mediated water shifts between the ICF and ECF occur. Loss of isotonic fluid results in a decrease in ECF volume, whereas gain of isotonic fluid increases the ECF volume. Isotonic fluid loss, if of sufficient magnitude, results in hypovolemia and shock. Clinical signs of salt depletion (hypertonic fluid loss) are compared with those in water deprivation (hypotonic fluid loss) in Table 1-5. These concepts are discussed further in Chapter 3.

EXCHANGE OF WATER BETWEEN PLASMA AND INTERSTITIAL SPACES

Most of the ECF is in either the interstitial compartment (approximately three quarters of the ECF) or the intravascular compartment, most of which is plasma (approximately one quarter of the ECF). The partitioning of fluid between plasma and ISF spaces is critically important for maintenance of the effective circulating blood volume. The effective blood volume has been defined as "the component of blood volume to which the volume-regulatory system responds by causing renal sodium and water retention in the setting of cardiac and hepatic failure even though measured total blood and plasma volume may be increased."[40,49]

Exchange of solutes and fluid between plasma and interstitial spaces occurs at the capillary level. The volume of the vascular space is controlled by a balance between forces that favor filtration of fluid through the vascular endothelium into the interstitial space (capillary hydrostatic pressure and tissue oncotic pressure) and forces that tend to retain fluid within the vascular space (plasma oncotic pressure and tissue hydrostatic pressure). **Oncotic pressure** is the osmotic pressure generated by plasma proteins in the vascular space. Starling's law describes these relationships (Fig. 1-5):

$$\text{Net filtration} = K_f\left[(P_{cap} - P_{if}) - (\pi_p - \pi_{if})\right]$$

where K_f represents the net permeability of the capillary wall, P represents the hydrostatic pressure generated by the heart (P_{cap}) or tissues (P_{if}), and π represents the oncotic pressure generated by plasma proteins (π_p) or filtered proteins and mucopolysaccharides in the interstitium (π_{if}).

The net filtration pressure in healthy capillaries is about 0.3 to 0.5 mm Hg at the proximal (arteriolar) end of the capillary.[47] Near the venule, the forces favoring filtration are less than the forces favoring reabsorption of fluid into the vascular space because capillary hydrostatic pressure decreases along the length of the capillary, but capillary oncotic pressure remains approximately the same.[47] Some of the fluid that is filtered into the interstitium at the proximal end of the capillary is reabsorbed distally; the remainder of the filtered fluid is transported by lymphatics in the interstitium. The hydrostatic pressure transferred from arterioles to the capillaries is controlled by autoregulation of the precapillary sphincter. Autoregulation protects the capillary from increases in hydrostatic pressure caused by systemic hypertension, which may cause a dangerous loss of vascular fluid into the ISF by filtration.

During water depletion, capillary oncotic pressure increases and hydrostatic pressure may decrease if depletion is severe enough to cause hypovolemia. These alterations in Starling's forces favor a decrease in net filtration of fluid into the interstitium at the level of the capillary. Increased reabsorption of ISF augments effective circulating blood volume, thus decreasing plasma protein concentration and increasing hydrostatic pressure. Conversely, loss of plasma protein decreases plasma

oncotic pressure and increases the net force favoring filtration of fluid out of the capillary. Loss of intravascular fluid increases plasma oncotic pressure, but filtration of fluid into the interstitium produces the edema observed in hypoproteinemic states. Thus in the healthy animal, maintenance of plasma volume depends on a fine balance between the forces favoring filtration and those favoring reabsorption in the capillary.

ELECTRONEUTRALITY AND THE ANION GAP

In body fluids, the sum of all cations must equal the sum of all anions to fulfill the law of electroneutrality. In the clinical setting, however, all anions and cations in body fluids are not routinely measured. Fig. 1-6 compares the concentrations of the commonly measured anions and the commonly measured cations in a gamblegram. The commonly measured cations are Na^+ and K^+, and the commonly measured anions are Cl^- and HCO_3^-. The sum of the concentrations of commonly measured anions is less than the sum of the concentrations of commonly measured cations. In other words, there are more unmeasured anions (UAs) than unmeasured cations (UCs). From this observation, the concept of the anion gap was developed. It is important to remember that there is no real difference between the total number of anions and the total number of cations in the body. In the clinical setting, the anion gap is used to predict changes in the UAs or less commonly in the UCs.

The anion gap is defined as the difference between the UAs and the UCs. According to the law of electroneutrality,

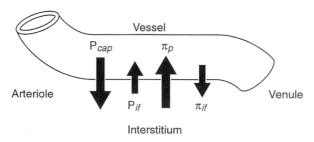

Fig. I-5 Factors affecting fluid movement at the level of the capillary. P_{cap}, Capillary hydrostatic pressure; P_{if}, interstitial hydrostatic pressure; π_p, capillary oncotic pressure; π_{if}, interstitial oncotic pressure.

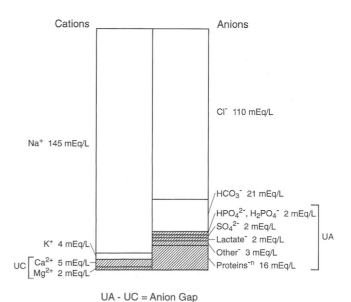

UA – UC = Anion Gap

Fig. I-6 Relative concentrations of unmeasured anions (UAs) and cations (UCs) in extracellular fluid (ECF).

$$Na^+ + K^+ + UC = Cl^- + HCO_3^- + UA$$

Rearranging this equation,

$$(Na^+ + K^+) - (Cl^- + HCO_3^-) = UA - UC = anion\ gap$$

The range for the normal anion gap varies by species and is approximately 12 to 24 mEq/L in dogs and 13 to 27 mEq/L in cats (see Chapter 9). The average anion gap in cats is approximately 24 mEq/L[30] and in dogs is 18 to 19 mEq/L.[10] The higher average anion gap in cats suggests a higher net charge on proteins in this species. Younger animals may have a lower anion gap. For example, foals with relative hyperphosphatemia and hypocalcemia may have a lower anion gap.[14] Little information on variations in anion gap in pediatric small animal patients is available. In 3-day-old puppies, however, anion gap values were reported to be approximately 16 mEq/L in one study,[35] suggesting that anion gaps in neonatal puppies are within the reference ranges for adults.

The primary usefulness of the anion gap is to detect an increase in UAs as an aid in the diagnosis of metabolic acidosis. Clinically relevant changes in the anion gap usually are from changes in UAs, and most of these changes are caused by increases in UAs associated with organic acids. For example, the ketoacidosis that occurs in some diabetic patients causes an increase in UAs, resulting in an increase in the anion gap. Similarly, the increased UAs that occur with ethylene glycol intoxication result in an increased anion gap. The derivation and clinical application of the principle of the anion gap are discussed further in Chapters 9 and 10.

THE OSMOLAL GAP

The **osmolal gap** is defined as the difference between the measured and the calculated serum osmolalities:

$$Osmolal\ gap = Osm_m - Osm_c$$

Reference values for osmolal gaps in dogs are given in Table 1-6. Data for osmolal gaps in cats are not reported in the literature. Attempts to derive osmolal gaps from published data on measured serum osmolalities and electrolyte concentrations in cats yield confusing results (see footnote to Table 1-6). Values for the osmolal gap vary with the formula used to calculate osmolality. Numerous formulas have been derived to calculate serum osmolality (see earlier section on exchange of water between ICF and ECF spaces, above).

One of the most commonly used formulas to estimate osmolality is:

$$2(Na^+ + K^+) + \frac{glucose}{18} + \frac{BUN}{2.8}$$

Some laboratories report a calculated osmolality based on these various formulas because it is easy to program

TABLE 1-6 Reference Ranges for Osmolal Gap

Species	Osmolal Gap (mOsm/kg)	Reference
Dog	10 ± 6	Grauer[15]
Dog	10.1 ± 5.9	Hauptman[20]
Dog	0-10	Shull[51]

Serum osmolality values in normal cats were reported to be approximately 308 ± 5 mOsm/kg (Chew et al[7]). When mean values for serum Na (155 mEq/L), K (4 mEq/L), glucose (120 mg/dL), and blood urea nitrogen (BUN; 24 mg/dL) are substituted into the equation 2(Na + K) + glucose/18 + BUN/2.8, a value of 333 mOsm/kg is obtained for cats. Calculated plasma osmolality values greater than measured values have generally been attributed to laboratory error. Why calculated plasma osmolality exceeds measured plasma osmolality using mean values from normal cats is unclear.

the analyzer to perform the calculation. It is important to remember that these are estimates of the actual osmolality, which must be measured using an osmometer. Serum osmolality most frequently is measured by freezing-point depression. Measured osmolality is higher than calculated osmolality because Osm_m measures all osmotically active solutes, whereas the formulas used for Osm_c do not account for all osmotically active solutes in serum. The difference (gap) between the measured (actual) and calculated (estimated) osmolality is called the osmolal gap.

Calculation of the osmolal gap is most helpful when unsuspected osmoles are present in ECF, thus increasing the osmolal gap as a result of an increase in the measured but not the calculated osmolality (e.g., ethylene glycol poisoning), and when assessing the significance of the serum Na^+ concentration (see Chapter 3). During the acute stage (6 to 12 hours after exposure) of ethylene glycol toxicity, the osmolal gap is increased. This increased osmolal gap could be helpful in the diagnosis of ethylene glycol toxicity if a measured osmolality is requested. Hyponatremia with a normal osmolal gap suggests dilutional hyponatremia (e.g., overhydration). This rules out the presence of abnormal osmotically active particles that could cause a shift of water from ICF to ECF, thus decreasing the serum sodium concentration. The osmolal gap is discussed further in Chapter 3.

HOMEOSTASIS: ZERO BALANCE

In the healthy adult animal at rest in a thermoneutral environment, daily intake of water, nutrients, and minerals is balanced by daily excretion of these substances or their metabolic by-products. Thus in this homeostatic state, the animal does not experience a net gain or loss of water, nutrients, or minerals and is said to be in **zero balance**. In a sedentary dog or cat in a thermoneutral environment, obligatory daily losses of water occur (Fig. 1-7). Input is

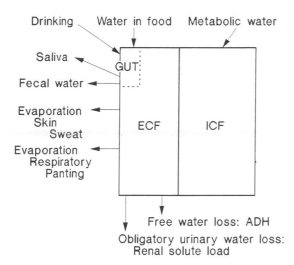

Fig. 1-7 Total body water: daily input and obligatory losses. (Adapted from Chew RW: Water metabolism of mammals. In Mayer WW, Van Gelder RG, editors: *Physiologic mammalogy: vol II, Mammalian reaction to stressful environments,* New York, 1965, Academic Press, pp. 43-177.)

equal to output in zero balance, and the volume of water added to body fluids by food and water consumption and by metabolism is equal to the volume of water lost in urine, feces, and saliva (i.e., sensible water loss) and evaporation from cutaneous and respiratory epithelia (i.e., insensible water loss).[29] Although the classical definition of insensible water loss in healthy animals is water lost via the skin or lungs, in clinical veterinary medicine water lost in the feces and saliva also is included in insensible losses. This approach is used because it usually is impractical to measure fecal and salivary water losses, which are small under normal conditions. This chapter uses the clinical definition of insensible water loss. Although evaporative losses may be great in heat-stressed, exercising, or active animals, the most important and predictable obligatory daily loss of water in healthy, sedentary dogs and cats in a thermoneutral environment occurs via the urine. Values for water input by drinking and water loss via urine, feces, or total insensible avenues in healthy dogs and cats have been variously estimated in the literature (Table 1-7).

Maintenance fluid need may be defined as the volume of fluid required daily to maintain the animal in zero fluid balance. Maintenance needs thus are determined by daily sensible and insensible losses, by ambient temperature and humidity, by the animal's voluntary or forced activity, and by disease. A high ambient temperature, especially with low humidity, results in increased insensible evaporative losses and therefore in increased maintenance fluid requirements. Similarly, fever and increased metabolic rate associated with disease may increase fluid requirements. Estimates of maintenance fluid needs during thermal stress or disease usually are based on empirical adjustments of the estimated basal fluid requirements. Maintenance fluid requirements also are determined partially by composition of the diet. In dogs and cats, most absorbed dietary nitrogen and minerals not required to maintain zero balance or to provide for growth or tissue repair are excreted daily in the urine. The volume of urine required for solute excretion thus is a function of both the amount of solute in the diet and the osmolality of the urine. Diets with higher solute contents require greater total water intake than do diets of relatively lower solute content. Most small animals have free access to water and therefore ingest sufficient water to support urinary excretion of dietary solutes. Sick animals often are inactive and have a poor appetite or are anorexic. Water requirements to replace insensible losses

TABLE 1-7 Measurements of Daily Water Intake and Output in Sedentary Dogs and Cats

Measurement	Species	mL/kg/day*	Condition or Diet	Reference
Input				
Water drunk	Feline	71.3		Chew 1965
	Feline	50.6		Thrall and Miller 1976
	Canine	56.1–70.8		Chew 1965
	Canine	38.9 (19.5–84)		O'Connor 1969
Output				
Urine volume	Canine	13.3 (10.5–17.9)	Caged	O'Connor 1969
Fecal water	Feline	25–29 g/day	Caged	Jackson and Tovey 1977
	Feline	56 g/day	Caged	Thrall 1976
Insensible loss	Canine	20.5	69% H_2O diet	Smith et al. 1964
	Feline	12.42	70% H_2O diet	Hamlin and Tashjian 1964
	Feline	29.0	Dry ration	Thrall and Miller 1976
	Canine	26.2 (8.1–70.7)	Beef and biscuit	O'Connor 1969

*Except as noted in table.

related to activity and to support renal solute excretion thus are decreased, and maintenance water requirements presumably are lower than in healthy individuals. Increased insensible water losses caused by fever or increased metabolic rate during disease may offset this decrease in water requirement. Basal needs must be defined accurately if water requirements during disease are to be estimated using increments of basal requirements. To address this issue, the following discussion focuses on the relationship between basal water requirements and dietary solute in sedentary small animals in a thermoneutral environment.

WATER LOSSES

URINARY AND FECAL WATER LOSS

Daily urinary water losses may be divided into obligatory water loss (i.e., water needed to excrete the daily renal solute load) and free water loss (i.e., water excreted unaccompanied by solute under the control of antidiuretic hormone [ADH]). Clearance of free water increases during relative water excess, thus protecting the animal from the overhydration and hypotonicity that would result from retention of water in excess of solutes. Obligatory renal water loss must occur even in states of relative water deficit so that solute may be eliminated from the body. Similarly, a small daily, obligatory fecal water loss is required for fecal excretion of solute. Obligatory fecal water loss may increase if fecal solute increases (e.g., addition of $CaCl_2$ or $MgCl_2$ to the diet). These ions increase fecal solute because Ca^{2+} and Mg^{2+} are poorly absorbed from the gastrointestinal tract. Maintenance water requirements must include at least enough water to allow renal and fecal solute excretion.

OBLIGATORY URINARY AND FECAL WATER LOSSES

The amount of water required for elimination of the urinary solute load in theory depends on the maximal urine osmolality that can be achieved by the animal (Table 1-8). However, solute usually is not excreted at maximal urine osmolality, especially when water is readily available for vol-

untary consumption. Urinary osmolalities from experimental dogs at rest and in water balance ranged from 1000 to 2000 mOsm/kg.[17] In a study of client-owned dogs, urine osmolality ranged from 161 to 2830 mOsm/kg, and urine osmolality was greater in the morning (mean, 1541 ± 527 mOsm/kg; range, 273 to 2620 mOsm/kg) than in the evening (mean, 1400 ± 586 mOsm/kg; range, 161 to 2830 mOsm/kg).[55] There was no effect of gender on urine osmolality, but urine osmolality decreased significantly with age.

Fig. 1-8 depicts urine volume and urine osmolality plotted as a function of urine solute in a dog fed varying quantities of food.[38] Increased intake produced increased renal solute and increased urine volume; however, urine osmolality remained approximately 1600 mOsm/kg (1200 to 2000 mOsm/kg).[39] Urine osmolalities did not, as might be expected, increase toward the maximum attainable (2400 to 2800 mOsm/kg) in water-deprived dogs.[8,17] Thus urine osmolality is conserved in the presence of increased urine solute load by an increase in urine volume. The physiologic mechanisms that conserve urine osmolality as renal solute load varies are not well defined.

The renal solute load is derived from dietary sources of protein and minerals and comprises urea, Na^+, K^+, Ca^{2+}, Mg^{2+}, NH_4^+, and other cations and PO_4^{3-}, Cl^-, SO_4^{2-}, and other anions. When estimating solute load from diet for an animal in zero balance, all nitrogen is assumed to form urea. Urea constitutes two thirds of the urinary solute load in dogs.[38] The amount of solute in the diet is determined by the composition and the quantity of food and minerals ingested. Increasing dietary

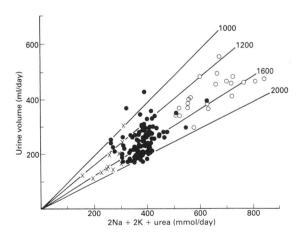

Fig. 1-8 Urine volume of a dog plotted against urinary excretion of solute (2Na + 2K + urea) during consumption of 320 (×), 385 (●), and 770 (○) grams of food. Each symbol represents data from 1 day. The lines labeled 1000, 1200, 1600, and 2000 indicate urine osmolality (mOsm/kg). (From O'Connor WJ, Potts DJ: Kidneys and drinking in dogs. In Michell AR, editor: *Renal disease in dogs and cats: comparative and clinical aspects,* Oxford, 1988, Blackwell Scientific, p. 35.)

TABLE 1-8 Maximal Urine Osmolalities (mOsm/kg)

Species	mOsm/kg	Reference
Dog	2425	Chew[8]
Dog	2791	Hardy and Osborne[17*]
Cat	3200	Chew[8]
Cat	3420–4980	Thrall and Miller[54]
Cat	2984	Ross and Finco[48*]

*Values obtained after dehydration resulting in 5% body weight loss.

protein results in increased urea production. Metabolism of carbohydrates and fats yields only CO_2 and H_2O and does not produce urea or other solutes that must be excreted in the urine. Diets high in minerals that are well absorbed from the gut (usually NaCl) provide more solute for excretion.

Not all solute produced by metabolism of ingested and absorbed food is necessarily excreted in the urine. Fecal excretion of solutes does occur. In most healthy dogs, however, daily fecal Na^+, K^+, and Cl^- excretion is substantially lower than urinary mineral excretion. The daily renal solute load is thus a function of the quantity of food ingested and of diet composition. Assuming a range of urine osmolalities in healthy dogs between 1000 and 2000 mOsm/kg and a urine solute load of approximately 400 mOsm in a 10-kg dog, the range of urine output would be 200 to 400 mL or 20 to 40 mL/kg/day. Urine volume is thus a function of renal solute load. Another important factor that determines urine volume is the total quantity of water ingested per day. Total water consumption depends both on water in the diet and on water voluntarily consumed by drinking.

URINARY FREE WATER

Excretion of urinary free water is controlled by stimulation or inhibition of secretion of ADH and by thirst. Urinary free water increases when enough water has been ingested to dilute body solute and result in hypotonicity. A 1% to 2% decrease in serum osmolality inhibits secretion of ADH and abolishes thirst in humans.[43,44] During water depletion, body water osmolality increases and ADH secretion is stimulated. An increase in serum osmolality of 1% to 2% is sufficient to provoke maximal ADH secretion in humans.[43,44] In dogs, osmolality increases of 1% to 3% stimulate thirst.[37,39] A water loss of 5 mL/kg of body weight provoked drinking in experimental dogs.[45] Therefore daily urinary free water losses are very small during water deficiency in otherwise healthy dogs and cats.

RESPIRATORY AND CUTANEOUS EVAPORATIVE LOSSES

Cutaneous evaporative water losses usually are small in dogs and cats. Cats in hot environments are reported to lick themselves with saliva to promote evaporative cooling.[8] This phenomenon is rarely observed in clinical practice, but if it occurs, salivary water losses could significantly increase water need. Evaporative water loss from the skin is minimal in dogs and cats because eccrine sweat glands (which are limited in distribution to the foot pads) do not participate in thermoregulation in these species. Evaporative water losses usually are less in healthy, sedentary cats in a thermoneutral environment compared with dogs (see Table 1-7), probably because cats rarely pant. Evaporative losses in caged, sedentary laboratory dogs are quite variable from dog to dog, and

some individuals experience significant daily losses via this route (Table 1-9). Dogs in the study summarized in Table 1-9 fell into two categories: those that remained quiet in their cages all of the time and those that ran in circles, barking for several hours each day. The mean evaporative loss for all dogs was 27 mL/kg/day. This value overestimates evaporative loss in quiet dogs. For dogs at rest, evaporative losses usually were less than 1 mL/kg/hr. During periods of activity, evaporative losses were estimated at almost 7 mL/kg/hr.[38]

The total water intake per day of the dogs in Table 1-9 was quite variable from dog to dog, ranging from approximately 20 to 91 mL/kg/day. If insensible loss (primarily composed of respiratory evaporative loss) for each dog is subtracted from total daily water intake, the range of water intake unrelated to insensible losses is narrower (11 to 20 mL/kg/day) than the range for total water intake. This emphasizes the profound effect that insensible losses may have on daily water balance in dogs.

Increases in ambient temperature, especially in association with low relative humidity, may result in marked increases in respiratory water evaporation in dogs. The panting response to heat is more efficient in dogs than in cats. At an ambient temperature of 40° C, cats increase their respiratory rate 4.5 times, whereas dogs can increase their respiratory rate 12 to 20 times.[8] The estimated respiratory water loss in a panting dog at 41° C was 469 mL/day, whereas that for a cat under the same conditions was 41 mL/day (Table 1-10).

WATER INTAKE

WATER IN FOOD

The percentage of water in pet foods is variable. In general, canned foods are more than 70% water, semimoist foods 20% to 40% water, and dry foods less than 10% water.[28] Two representative cat diets are described in Table 1-11. Therefore water in food makes up a variable proportion of total daily water consumption, depending on what type of diet is fed (Figs. 1-9 and 1-10). Cats can exist without drinking water if fed a diet of cod, salmon, or beefsteak.[41] If the beefsteak or salmon was partially desiccated, cats became hydropenic (increased serum osmolality and serum sodium concentration), anorexic, and cachectic. Thus cats may meet their water needs solely from the water in some foods.

DRINKING

The volume of water voluntarily ingested each day by healthy, sedentary dogs and cats in a thermoneutral environment depends on the composition and the quantity of the diet ingested. Water intake decreases in experimental dogs if food intake is limited (Fig. 1-11).[8,9,31,32] After a 1-day fast, drinking decreased to 25% to 50% of the normal volume in dogs. After a 14- to 18-day fast,

TABLE 1-9 Water Intake and Urinary Losses of Solute and Water in Six Sedentary Experimental Dogs Receiving the Same Diet

Dog	Average Wt. (kg)	Water Intake				Water Loss							
		Food and Metabolic (mL/day)	Drunk (mL/day)	Average Total Water		Evaporation		Urine			Urine (mOsm/ kg)	Urine Solute/ Day (mOsm)
				(mL/day)	(mL/kg/day)	(mL/day)	Average (mL/kg/ day)	(mL/day)	Average (mL/kg/ day)	Total H$_2$O Evaporated (mL/kg/day)		
Titch	12.7	300	854 ± 465	1154	90.9	961 ± 358	75.7	243 ± 41	19.1	15.2	1706 ± 441	415
Lassie	15.2	300	291 ± 102	691	45.5	386 ± 115	25.4	204 ± 71	13.4	20.1	1836 ± 139	375
Kim	20.5	363	482 ± 188	842	41.1	545 ± 176	26.6	292 ± 50	14.2	14.5	1519 ± 211	444
Gina	10.7	187	135 ± 53	322	30.1	209 ± 49	19.5	123 ± 16	11.5	10.6	2016 ± 216	248
Blackie	20.7	250	153 ± 80	403	19.5	167 ± 54	8.1	217 ± 29	10.5	11.4	1652 ± 305	359
Sandy	19.8	250	151 ± 62	401	20.3	165 ± 50	8.3	258 ± 31	13	12	1079 ± 124	278
Mean		275	344.3	635.5	41.2	405.5	27.3	222.8	13.6	14	1634.7	353

Adapted from O'Connor WJ, Potts DJ: The external water exchanges of normal laboratory dogs. QJ Exp Physiol 54:244–265, 1969.

TABLE 1-10 Respiratory Water Losses of Panting Mammals[*]

Species	Weight (kg)	Respiratory Water Loss (g/min)	Respiratory Water Loss (g/day)	Percentage Heat Production Lost
Dog	16	0.326	469	57
Cat	3.5	0.029	41.2	9.4

Data from Chew RM: Water metabolism of mammals. In Mayer WW, Van Gelder RG, editors: Physiologic mammalogy, vol II, Mammalian reaction to stressful environments, New York, 1965, Academic Press, pp. 43-177.
[*]*Temperature, 41° C; relative humidity, 32%.*

drinking was 45% of the normal volume in dogs.[8] Conversely, if water intake is limited, food intake decreases in dogs and cats.[41] As mentioned earlier, cats continue to eat and survive on some diets without drinking water. In dogs that are chronically deprived of food, a basal level of drinking is maintained.[2] In sick, anorexic small animal patients, drinking may decrease, and because they do not have access to water from food, total water intake may decrease drastically. However, the water requirement of such animals is probably quite low. In quiet, sick animals, the major obligatory water loss occurs via the urine (assuming no other major contemporary fluid loss such as in diarrhea or vomitus). The renal solute load and obligatory renal water loss decrease because the animal is not eating. However, animals in a catabolic state obviously do produce urea and ions for excretion as a result of catabolism of lean body mass. Figures for renal solute loads generated from endogenous sources are not readily available in the literature. Water requirements of a sick animal may be increased if the animal is febrile, having seizures, or experiencing abnormal losses, such as in vomitus or diarrhea. These contemporary water needs are in addition to the **maintenance** water required to maintain zero balance during inanition and inactivity in the presence of diminished but still present obligatory urinary water losses.

The volume of water drunk increases as the water in the diet decreases (see Table 1-11). Dogs maintain a uniform total water intake when food water is decreased by commensurately increasing drinking (see Fig. 1-9). However, cats may not increase drinking enough to maintain total water intake when consuming a diet low in water (see Fig. 1-10). Cats receiving dry food diets may ingest insufficient water. This issue has been investigated extensively as a contributing factor in the development of lower urinary tract disease in cats. Some investigators believe that a low ratio of total water intake to dry matter in the diet predisposes a cat to lower urinary tract disease. Diets with a ratio of total water to dry matter greater than 3 have been suggested as an aid in prevention of lower urinary tract disease.[4,21] The ratio of total water to dry matter is an index of the moisture content of the food and of the cat's drinking response to that diet. As predicted, canned foods have higher ratios than do dry foods (Table 1-12). Although cats drink more when consuming dry instead of canned foods, their total water intakes are usually lower with dry than with canned foods.

The solute load of the diet also influences drinking water. Approximately two thirds of the renal solute load is urea, an end product of protein metabolism, and increasing the protein content of the diet increases the renal solute load. Diets higher in protein also are associated with greater total water intake. The ions Na^+, K^+, Ca^{2+}, Mg^{2+}, PO_4^{3-}, Cl^-, and SO_4^{2-} also contribute to dietary solute. Increasing percentages of salt in foods are associated with increased water intake in both cats and dogs.[6,21] This principle has been exploited to increase voluntary water consumption in cats that are fed dry food diets and are at risk for developing lower urinary tract disease. The protein content of the diet may significantly affect renal solute load and urine volume. Increased renal solute load supplied by a higher protein diet may provoke increased water consumption.

METABOLIC WATER

Metabolic water contributes approximately 10% to 15% of total water intake in dogs and cats, depending on diet.[4] Nutrients differ in their yield of metabolic water

TABLE 1-11 Effect of Diet on Water Intake in Cats

Food	Dry Matter Intake (g/day)	Food Water[*] (g/day)	Water Drunk[†] (mL/day)	Total Water Intake (mL/day)	Ratio of Total Water to Dry Matter
Dry	76.9 ± 17.4	7.4 ± 1.7 (8.8)	167.2 ± 40.1 (>90)	174.6 ± 41.6	2.3 ± 0.2
Canned	35.2 ± 7.2	116 ± 23.6 (76.8)	22.8 ± 12.8 (14)	139.0 ± 31.4	3.9 ± 0.3

Data from Seefeldt SL, Chapman TE: Body water content and turnover in cats fed dry and canned rations, Am J Vet Res 40:183-185, 1979.
[*]*Figures in parentheses represent approximate percentage of diet that was water.*
[†]*Figures in parentheses represent approximate percentage of total water intake that was drunk.*

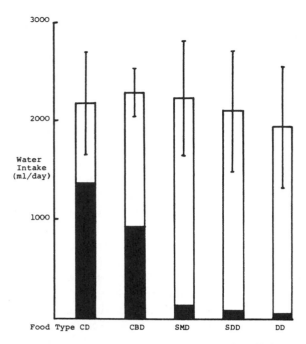

Fig. 1-9 Effect of food type on water intake in dogs. Each column represents the total daily water intake (mean ± SD) for four dogs fed different diets. The solid area shows the amount of endogenous food water; the clear area shows water drunk. *CD,* Canned; *CBD,* canned meat and biscuit mixture; *SMD, SDD,* intermediate moisture foods; *DD,* = dry. (From Burger IH, Anderson RS, Holme DW: Nutritional factors affecting water balance in the dog and cat. In Anderson RS, editor: *Nutrition of the dog and cat,* Oxford, 1980, Pergamon Press, p. 149.)

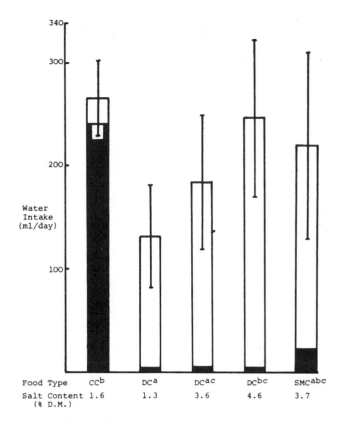

Fig. 1-10 Effect of food type and salt content on water intake in cats. Each column represents the total daily water intake (mean ± SD) for cats on various diets. The same group of 6 cats was used for all foods except DC diet 4.6% salt, data for which were obtained from a different experiment using another group of 12 cats. The solid area shows food water, and the clear area shows water drunk. Total water intake for foods bearing different superscript letters is significantly different ($P < 0.05$, Student's *t* test). *CC,* Canned; *DC,* dry; *SMC,* intermediate moisture food. (From Burger IH, Anderson RS, Holme DW: Nutritional factors affecting water balance in the dog and cat. In Anderson RS, editor: *Nutrition of the dog and cat,* Oxford, 1980, Pergamon Press, p. 151.)

(Table 1-13). Although fats provide the most water per gram, carbohydrates provide the most water per calorie and per liter of oxygen.[3,8] Therefore high-carbohydrate diets spare the water requirement by providing more metabolic water per calorie. Carbohydrates and fats also spare water loss because they do not generate renal solute.[3] The volume of metabolic water generated per day in humans, and by inference in dogs and cats, is relatively small compared with the total daily water intake.[11] Metabolic water is difficult to quantitate in the clinical setting, and many studies ignore its contribution to water homeostasis. Definitive water balance studies should include evaluation of metabolic water.[50]

WATER REQUIREMENTS

MAINTENANCE

Water balance is complex, and there is no single maintenance water requirement for each animal. In healthy, sedentary dogs and cats in a thermoneutral environment, water intake is largely dependent on diet. Water requirement is a function of the renal solute load in the diet and the associated obligatory renal water losses for urinary solute excretion. In clinical practice, maintenance

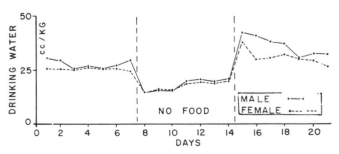

Fig. 1-11 Comparison of composite drinking curves of male and female dogs during alimentation and food deprivation. Each curve is the composite of 10 experiments. (From Cizek LJ: Long-term observations on the relationship between food and water consumption in the dog, *Am J Physiol* 197:342-346, 1959.)

TABLE 1-12 Ratios of Total Water to Dry Matter in Cat Foods

Investigator	Canned Cat Foods	Semimoist Cat Foods	Dry Cat Foods
Thrall and Miller[54]	3.7		2.0-2.4
Jackson and Tovey[22]	3.2		2.8,* 2.3†
Holme[21]	5.6	2.8	2.4
Seefeldt and Chapman[50]	3.9		2.3
Jenkins and Coulter	2.9	1.8	1.8

Data from DiBartola SP, Buffington CA: Feline urologic syndrome. In Slatter D, editor: Textbook of small animal surgery, Philadelphia, 1993, WB Saunders, pp. 1473-1487.
*Expanded.
†Nonexpanded.

fluid needs in small animal patients are often empirically defined as 60 mL/kg/day for smaller dogs and 40 mL/kg/day for larger dogs.[34] Alternatively, maintenance needs have been assessed on the basis of caloric needs: 1 mL of water per kilocalorie of energy required.[18,19] Early studies of water balance in healthy, caged dogs documented that mean water intake was approximately 1 mL/kcal ingested.[2] Normal maintenance energy requirement is defined as the number of calories required to sustain the basal metabolic rate; to provide energy for digestion, absorption, and assimilation of nutrients (thermal effect of feeding); to maintain body temperature in a nonthermoneutral environment; and for normal activity.[24] Maintenance energy expenditure may be calculated from the following formula[5]:

$$140 \text{ kcal} \times \text{body weight}^{0.73}$$

A 10-kg dog would require 750 kcal of energy per day or 75 kcal/kg/day. Following the rule of 1 mL/kcal, the water requirement would be 75 mL/kg/day.

Opinions vary on the formula for calculating maintenance caloric needs.[36] Basal energy requirements may be calculated and then multiplied by a factor of approximately two[36] to obtain maintenance needs. The basal energy

TABLE 1-13 Metabolic Water per Gram of Nutrient

Nutrient	Grams Metabolic Water per Gram of Nutrient
Carbohydrate	0.6
Protein	0.41
Fat	1.07

Data from Davidson S, Passmore R, Brock JR, et al: Water and electrolytes. In Davidson S, editor: Human nutrition and dietetics, Edinburgh, 1979, Churchill Livingstone, pp. 81-89.

requirement is defined as the caloric need of a resting, healthy dog in a postabsorptive state (i.e., renal solute load has been excreted) about 18 hours after feeding[24] and in a thermoneutral environment. Basal energy requirement has been variously calculated from the following formulas[1,5]:

(a) Basal energy requirement = $70 \times$ body weight $(\text{kg})^{0.73}$

(b) Basal energy requirement = $97 \times$ body weight $(\text{kg})^{0.655}$

There has been considerable debate over the most appropriate exponent to use to relate body weight to metabolic size in the dog.[1,26,42] We prefer the exponent 0.655 and use formula (b), which has been supported in the veterinary literature.[26,42]

Maintenance energy requirements are higher than basal needs primarily to provide calories for the normal activity of a healthy dog. Based on formula (b), a 10-kg dog has a basal energy requirement of 44 kcal/kg/day and a maintenance requirement of 88 kcal/kg/day. Assuming 1 mL of water required per kilocalorie of energy need, the maintenance water requirement for this dog would be approximately 88 mL/kg/day. A 50-kg dog would require 25 mL/kg/day for basal water needs and 50 mL/kg/day for maintenance. If basal water requirements were estimated from formula (a), a 10-kg dog would have a basal daily water requirement of 38 mL/kg and a maintenance requirement of 76 mL/kg.

Estimates of maintenance water needs based on caloric requirements are similar to the empirical values for maintenance needs used by some clinicians. However, it is important to remember that caloric needs are a logarithmic function of body weight, and larger dogs require less fluid per kilogram of body weight than do smaller dogs.

The physiologic reason for the correlation between caloric and water needs is not well documented. The relationship may, in fact, be indirect. Water requirements and caloric needs may be related because water intake is in part a function of renal solute load, which is related to diet: both to the quantity of food ingested and to the composition of the food. However, the renal solute load per calorie in the diet varies with the composition of the diet. Diets vary in water content (dry versus canned) and in nutrient composition and hence in renal solute load per calorie. Fats provide more kilocalories per gram (9 kcal/g) than do carbohydrates or proteins (4 kcal/g). Fats provide more milliliters of water per gram (1.07) than do carbohydrates (0.56) or proteins (0.40).[3] High-protein diets increase renal solute load, whereas fats and carbohydrates do not contribute to it. The mineral content of diets also varies. Therefore the animal's water requirement may be viewed more accurately as a function of total water content and renal solute load of the diet rather than strictly as a function of calories ingested.

Thus the relationship 1 mL of water per 1 kcal of energy may be fortuitous.

BASAL

Fluid requirements for sick, inappetent small animals have not been well documented. Decreased food intake or anorexia reduces renal solute load and hence water requirements. However, clinicians frequently base estimates of water requirements for patients on tables derived from the formula for maintenance energy requirements: $140 \times$ body weight $(kg)^{0.73}$.[19] Haskins[19] commented that the use of tables for water intake based on this formula might overestimate the water requirements of sick patients. In fact, the water requirement of an inappetent, sedentary sick animal in a thermoneutral environment may approach basal water need. The basal water requirement for a healthy animal may be defined, analogously to the basal energy need, as water required when the animal is resting, is in a postabsorptive state (i.e., the renal solute load has been excreted), and is not exposed to thermal stress.

Basal water needs of dogs and cats have not been well studied. Water intake of healthy dogs and cats in a thermoneutral environment and deprived of food has been measured in a few experiments (Table 1-14). Two investigators found that quiet, food-deprived dogs (body weights 8 to 15 kg) or cats (approximately 3.5 kg) confined to metabolism cages drank about 5 mL/kg of water daily. A third investigator found that intake was considerably higher (17.6 ± 2.2 mL/kg/day) in dogs of about the same body weight. The dogs in the latter experiment may have been more active and may have had larger evaporative losses and greater compensatory drinking than dogs or cats in the previous experiments. If basal water need is estimated by determining the basal energy requirement, using the preceding formula,[1] the water requirement of a 10-kg dog would be 40 mL/kg/day, assuming 1 mL of water per kilocalorie of

energy required. Data for dogs deprived of food suggest that basal water requirements may be much lower. This fact is not surprising if we consider that when water intakes of dogs in the study by O'Connor and Potts[38] (see Table 1-9) were corrected for water intake that balanced evaporative losses, total water intakes were 11 to 20 mL/kg/day. This value approximates the accepted general range for daily urine production in dogs. Thus if dogs are deprived of food and urine volumes decrease substantially (renal solute load decreases), the water need may be small.

Water requirements of sick animals may be increased over basal requirements owing to increased contemporary fluid losses with such causes as evaporation (through panting), diarrhea, vomiting, or dilute urine. Clinicians must estimate how much water needs increase by assessing the volume of these additional fluid losses. However, fluid needs still may not approach 40 to 60 mL/kg/day.

Assessing the basal water need of dogs and cats from the basal energy requirement provides a high estimate for water compared with the minimal requirement documented in experiments with dogs and cats deprived of food. This disparity makes estimating basal water needs of inappetent, quiet dogs problematic. Data on basal water needs of small animals would help clinicians to devise appropriate strategies for fluid therapy in inappetent, sick animals by providing a baseline assessment from which maintenance or replacement fluid needs may be estimated by use of a multiplication factor (i.e., maintenance = 2 × basal water need). Current methods for assessing fluid needs may overestimate the patient's actual requirements because sick patients are inappetent and inactive. Administration of an excessive volume of fluid could be detrimental, especially to patients with heart failure or oliguric renal failure. Most patients respond satisfactorily to currently used standard fluid-replacement regimens because the kidneys readily excrete excess fluid and solute. When calculating water needs, however, it would be

TABLE 1-14 Water Consumption in Food-Deprived Dogs and Cats

Number	Body Weight (kg)	Days Starvation	Average Water Consumption (mL/kg)	Reference
10 dogs*	NR†	7	17.6 ± 2.2	Cizek[9]
5 dogs	8-11	15	4.0	Morris and Collins[31]
2 dogs	9.47	4	4.1 (3.2-5.0)	Prentiss et al[41]
	11.71			
2 dogs	11.71	9	5.4 (3.0-7.7)	Prentiss et al[41]
	9.47			
2 cats	3.59	7	5.2 (3.7-6.7)	Prentiss et al[41]

*Beagle or hound type of dogs.
†NR, Not reported.

prudent to consider that inactive, sick animals with decreased or no food intake may require less water than usual empirical estimates may indicate.

REFERENCES

1. Abrams JT: The nutrition of the dog. In Rechcigl M, editor: *CRC handbook series in nutrition and food. Section G: diets, culture media, and food supplements,* Boca Raton, FL, 1977, CRC Press, p. 1.
2. Adolph EF: Measurements of water drinking in dogs, *Am J Physiol* 125:75, 1939.
3. Anderson RS: Water balance in the dog and cat, *J Small Anim Pract* 23:588, 1982.
4. Anderson RS: Fluid balance and diet. Proceedings of the Seventh Kal Kan Symposium, Columbus, OH, 1983, p. 19.
5. Brody S, Proctor RC, Ashworth US: *Growth and development with special reference to domestic animals. XXXIV. Basal metabolism, endogenous nitrogen, creatinine and neutral sulphur excretions as functions of body weights,* Columbia, MO, 1934, University of Missouri.
6. Burger IH, Anderson RS, Holme DW: Nutritional factors affecting water balance in the dog and cat. In Anderson RS, editor: *Nutrition of the dog and cat,* Oxford, 1980, Pergamon Press, p. 145.
7. Chew DJ, Leonard M, Muir WW: Effect of sodium bicarbonate infusion on serum osmolality, electrolyte concentrations, and blood gas tensions in cats, *Am J Vet Res* 52:12, 1991.
8. Chew RM: Water metabolism of mammals. In Mayer WW and Van Gelder RG, editors: *Physiologic mammalogy, vol II: Mammalian reaction to stressful environments,* New York, 1965, Academic Press, p. 43.
9. Cizek LJ: Longterm observations on relationship between food and water ingestion in the dog, *Am J Physiol* 197:342, 1959.
10. Constable PD, Stämpfli HR: Experimental determination of net protein charge and A_{tot} and K_a of nonvolatile buffers in canine plasma, *J Vet Intern Med* 2005 (in press).
11. Davidson S, Passmore R, Brock JF, et al: Water and electrolytes. In Davidson S, editor: *Human nutrition and dietetics,* Edinburgh, 1979, Churchill Livingstone, p. 81.
12. Edelman IS, Leibman J: Review: anatomy of body water and electrolytes, *Am J Med* 27:256, 1959.
13. Edelman IS, Leibman J, O'Meara MP, et al: Interrelations between serum sodium concentration, serum osmolarity and total exchangeable sodium, total exchangeable potassium and total body water, *J Clin Invest* 37:1236, 1958.
14. Gossett KA: Effect of age on anion gap in clinically healthy normal Quarter Horses, *Am J Vet Res* 44:1744, 1983.
15. Grauer GF, Thrall MA, Henre BA, et al: Early clinicopathologic findings in dogs ingesting ethylene glycol, *Am J Vet Res* 45:2299-2303, 1984.
16. Hamlin R, Tashjian R: Water and electrolyte intake and output and quantity of feces in healthy cats, *Vet Med/Small Animal Clin* 59:746, 1964.
17. Hardy RM, Osborne CA: Water deprivation test in the dog: maximal normal values, *J Am Vet Med Assoc* 174:479, 1979.
18. Harrison JB, Sussman HH, Pickering DE: Fluid and electrolyte therapy in small animals, *J Am Vet Med Assoc* 137:637, 1960.
19. Haskins SC: Fluid and electrolyte therapy, *Compend Contin Educ Pract Vet* 6:244, 1984.
20. Hauptman JG, Tvedten H: Osmolal and anion gaps in dogs with acute endotoxic shock, *Am J Vet Res* 47:1617-1619, 1986.
21. Holme DW: Research into the feline urological syndrome. Proceedings of the Kal Kan Symposium for Treatment of Dog and Cat Diseases, Columbus, OH, 1977, p. 40.
22. Jackson OF, Tovey JD: Water balance studies in domestic cats, *Feline Pract* 7:30, 1977.
23. Jain NC: *Schalm's veterinary hematology,* Philadelphia, 1986, Lea & Febiger.
24. Kleiber M: *The fire of life,* Huntington, NY, 1975, Robert E. Krieger Publishing.
25. Kohn K, DiBartola S: Composition and distribution of body fluids in dogs and cats. In DiBartola S, editor: *Fluid therapy in small animal practice,* ed 2, Philadelphia, 2000, WB Saunders, p. 6.
26. Kronfeld DS: Protein and energy estimates for hospitalized dogs and cats. Proceedings of Purina International Nutrition Symposium, Orlando, FL, 1991, p. 5.
27. Leaf A: The clinical and physiologic significance of the serum sodium concentration, *N Engl J Med* 267:24, 1962.
28. Lewis LD, Morris ML: *Small animal clinical nutrition,* Topeka, KS, 1987, Mark Morris Associates.
29. Maxwell MH, Kleeman CR, Narins RG: *Clinical disorders of fluid and electrolyte metabolism,* New York, 1987, McGraw-Hill.
30. McCullough SM, Constable PS: Calculation of the total plasma concentration of nonvolatile weak acids and the effective dissociation constant of nonvolatile buffers in plasma for use in the strong ion approach to acid-base balance in cats, *Am J Vet Res* 64:1047-51, 2003.
31. Morris ML, Collins DR: Anorexia in the dog, *Vet Med Small Anim Clin* 62:753, 1967.
32. Morris ML, Collins DR: A new solution to the problem of anorexia, *Vet Med Small Anim Clin* 62:1075, 1967.
33. Moulton CR: Age and chemical development in mammals, *J Biol Chem* 57:79, 1923.
34. Muir WW, DiBartola SP: Fluid therapy. In Kirk RW, editor: *Current veterinary therapy, VIII,* Philadelphia, 1983, WB Saunders, p. 28.
35. Nattie EE, Edwards WH, Marin-Padilla M: Newborn puppy cerebral acid-base regulation in experimental asphyxia and recovery, *J Appl Physiol* 56:1178, 1984.
36. *Nutrient requirements of dogs,* Washington, DC, 1985, National Academy Press.
37. O'Connor WJ: Drinking by dogs during and after running, *J Physiol* 250:247, 1975.
38. O'Connor WJ, Potts DJ: The external water exchanges of normal laboratory dogs, *Q J Exp Physiol* 54:244, 1969.
39. O'Connor WJ, Potts DJ: Kidneys and drinking in dogs. In Michell AR, editor: *Renal disease in dogs and cats: comparative and clinical aspects,* Oxford, 1988, Blackwell Scientific, p. 30.
40. Peters JP: The role of sodium in the production of edema, *N Engl J Med* 239:353, 1948.
41. Prentiss PG, Wolf AV, Eddy HA: Hydropenia in cat and dog. Ability of the cat to meet its water requirements solely from a diet of fish or meat, *Am J Physiol* 196:625, 1959.
42. Rivers JPW, Burger LH: Allometry in dog nutrition. In *Nutrition of the dog and cat, Waltham Symposium No. 7.* Cambridge, 1989, Cambridge University Press, p. 67.
43. Robertson GL: Thirst and vasopressin function in normal and disordered states of water balance, *J Lab Clin Med* 101:351, 1983.

44. Robertson GL, Shelton RL, Athar S: The osmoregulation of vasopressin, *Kidney Int* 10:25, 1976.
45. Robinson EA, Adolph EF: Pattern of normal water drinking in dogs, *Am J Physiol* 139:39, 1943.
46. Rose BD: *Clinical physiology of acid-base and electrolytes,* New York, 1984, McGraw-Hill.
47. Rose BD: *Clinical physiology of acid-base and electrolyte disorders,* New York, 1989, McGraw-Hill, p. 5.
48. Ross LA, Finco DR: Relationship of selected clinical renal function tests to glomerular filtration rate and renal blood flow in cats, *Am J Vet Res* 42:1704, 1981.
49. Schrier RW: Pathogenesis of sodium and water retention in high-output and low-output cardiac failure, nephrotic syndrome, cirrhosis, and pregnancy, *N Engl J Med* 319:1065, 1988.
50. Seefeldt SL, Chapman TE: Body water content and turnover in cats fed dry and canned rations, *Am J Vet Res* 40:183, 1979.
51. Shull RM: The value of anion gap and osmolal gap determinations in veterinary medicine, *Vet Clin Pathol* 7:12-14, 1978.
52. Smith RC, Haschen T, Hamlin RL, et al: Water and electrolyte intake and output and quantity of feces in the healthy dog, *Vet Med* 59:743, 1964.
53. Smithline N, Gardner KD: Gaps—anionic and osmolal, *JAMA* 236:1594, 1976.
54. Thrall BE, Miller LG: Water turnover in cats fed dry rations, *Feline Pract* 6:10, 1976.
55. van Vonderen IK, Kooistra HS, Rijnberk A: Intra- and interindividual variation in urine osmolality and urine specific gravity in healthy pet dogs of various ages, *J Vet Intern Med* 11:30, 1997.

APPENDIX TO CHAPTER I

The cell membrane is composed of a hydrophobic lipid bilayer with embedded protein molecules that play structural and functional roles. This configuration allows the cell membrane to act as an electrical capacitor that stores energy. Some of the embedded proteins act as hydrophilic pores in the membrane. One embedded functional protein is Na$^+$, K$^+$-ATPase, which pumps sodium out of and potassium into the cell in an Na/K ratio of 3:2. In this model, the cell membrane acts as a capacitor; the hydrophilic protein pores provide resistance; and the Na$^+$, K$^+$-ATPase provides energy.

The intracellular concentration of potassium (140 mEq/L) is much higher than its extracellular concentration (4 mEq/L). Consequently, potassium diffuses out of the cell down its concentration gradient. However, the cell membrane is impermeable to most intracellular anions (e.g., proteins and organic phosphates). A net negative charge develops inside the cell as potassium ions diffuse out of the cell, and a net positive charge accumulates outside the cell. As a result, a potential difference is generated across the cell membrane. The principal extracellular cation is sodium, which enters the cell relatively slowly down its concentration and electrical gradients because the cell membrane is much less permeable to sodium than to potassium. Diffusion of potassium from the cell continues until the ECF acquires sufficient positive charge to prevent further diffusion of potassium ions out of the cell.

The ratio of intracellular and extracellular concentrations of potassium ($[K^+]_I/[K^+]_O$) is the major determinant of the resting cell membrane potential difference. This potential difference is demonstrated by the Nernst equation, which is derived from the general equation for free-energy change (ΔG^C):

$$\Delta G^C = RT \times \ln\left(\frac{[c^+]_I}{[c^+]_O}\right) + zFE_m \tag{1}$$

where R is the gas constant (8.314 J/K/mol), T is the absolute temperature in K ($^\circ$C + 273), $[c^+]_I$ is the concentration of cation inside the cell, $[c^+]_O$ is the concentration of cation outside the cell, z is the valence, F is the Faraday constant (96,484 C/Eq), and E_m is the membrane potential in volts.

The first term on the right side of this equation represents the osmotic work required to transport 1 mol of particles across the membrane against a concentration gradient of $[c^+]_I/[c^+]_O$, and the second term represents the electrical work required to transport the same number of particles across the membrane against an electrical gradient.

At equilibrium, $\Delta G^C = 0$, and solving the equation for E_m yields:

$$E_m = -\left(\frac{RT}{zF}\right)\ln\left(\frac{[c^+]_I}{[c^+]_O}\right) \tag{2}$$

At 37° C and with a monovalent ion (e.g., K$^+$), the term $RT/zF = 26.67$ mV. Converting to the base 10 logarithm and specifying potassium as the cation:

$$E_m = -26.67(2.303)\log_{10}\left(\frac{[K^+]_I}{[K^+]_O}\right)$$

$$E_m = -61\log_{10}\left(\frac{[K^+]_I}{[K^+]_O}\right) \tag{3}$$

The Nernst equation is valid only when there is no net current flow.

The Goldman-Hodgkin-Katz constant-field equation is a modification of the Nernst equation used to calculate the membrane potential based on the membrane permeability ratio for sodium and potassium (P_{Na}/P_K). This equation allows determination of the individual ionic contributions to E_m by summing the individual concentrations and permeability effects:

$$E_m = -61 \log_{10} \frac{P_K[K^+]_I + P_{Na}[Na^+]_I}{P_K[K^+]_O + P_{Na}[Na^+]_O} \qquad (4)$$

where P_{Na} and P_K are the membrane permeabilities for sodium and potassium.

A term r is included in the constant-field equation to take into account the effect of the electrogenic Na$^+$, K$^+$-ATPase pump under steady-state conditions. This term is usually assigned the Na/K transport ratio of the Na$^+$,K$^+$-ATPase ($r = 3/2 = 1.5$). If the membrane permeability of potassium is assigned a value of 1.0 and the cell membrane is known to be 100 times more permeable to potassium than to sodium,

$$E_m = -61 \log_{10} \frac{rP_K[K^+]_I + P_{Na}[Na^+]_I}{rP_K[K^+]_O + P_{Na}[Na^+]_O}$$

$$E_m = -61 \log_{10} \frac{1.5P_K[K^+]_I + 0.01P_{Na}[Na^+]_I}{1.5P_K[K^+]_O + 0.01P_{Na}[Na^+]_O} \qquad (5)$$

Any ion that is not actively transported across the membrane cannot contribute to the membrane potential, and the transmembrane distribution of such an ion must follow the resting potential. Chloride is not considered in the Goldman-Hodgkin-Katz equation because chloride is usually passively distributed across the cell membrane according to the prevailing E_m.

CHAPTER · 2

APPLIED RENAL PHYSIOLOGY

Stephen P. DiBartola

"Superficially it might be said that the function of the kidneys is to make urine; but in a more considered view one can say that the kidneys make the stuff of philosophy itself."
—*Homer W. Smith*

Each day the glomeruli of the kidneys filter an enormous volume of plasma water, and the tubules must reabsorb most of this water along with vital solutes so that only a small volume of water and unneeded solutes are excreted as urine. For example, a normal 10-kg dog may have a glomerular filtration rate (GFR) of 4 mL/min/kg. In the course of 1 day, this dog would filter 57.6 L of plasma water in its kidneys. If 60% of body weight is water, this volume represents almost 10 times the dog's total body water.

The same dog may have a urine output of 33 mL/kg/day. Thus more than 99% of plasma water filtered by the glomeruli is reabsorbed by the tubules. The proximal tubules and loops of Henle reabsorb approximately 85% of the filtered water and solutes, whereas the collecting ducts adjust the final composition of urine to compensate for fluctuations in intake and prevent changes in the volume and composition of body fluids. The major functions of the various segments of the nephron are depicted in Fig. 2-1.

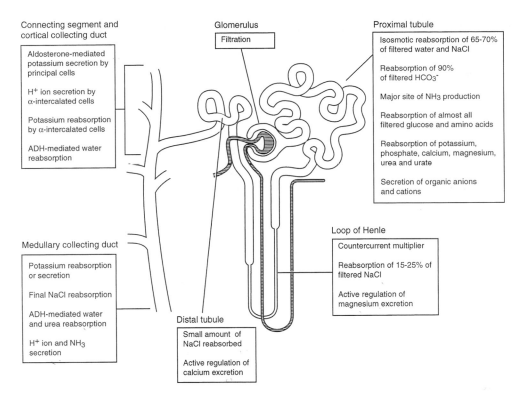

Fig. 2-1 Major functions of each portion of the nephron. (Drawing by Tim Vojt.)

CONCEPT OF RENAL CLEARANCE

An appreciation of the concept of clearance is crucial to understanding how renal function is evaluated clinically. The renal clearance of a substance is the volume of plasma that contains the amount of the substance excreted in the urine in 1 minute. It is the volume of plasma that must be filtered each minute to account for the amount of the substance appearing in the urine each minute under steady-state conditions. If the concentration of the substance in urine is U_x and the urine flow rate is V, the amount of the substance excreted in the urine per minute is $U_x V$. If the concentration of the substance in plasma is P_x, the volume of plasma that contains the same quantity of that substance or the volume of plasma that must be filtered per minute to account for that amount in the urine is $U_x V/P_x$, the standard clearance formula. The clearance of any substance may be calculated, but the clearance of certain substances (e.g., inulin, p-aminohippuric acid [PAH], and creatinine) provides important information about renal function (see measurement of glomerular filtration rate and measurement of renal blood flow and renal plasma flow below).

GLOMERULAR FILTRATION

GLOMERULAR MORPHOLOGY

The glomerular capillary wall or filtration barrier consists of three components: the capillary endothelium, basement membrane, and visceral epithelium (Fig. 2-2). The glomerulus is a unique vascular structure consisting of a capillary bed interposed between two arterioles, the afferent and efferent arterioles. The glomerular capillary divides into several branches, each of which forms a lobule of the glomerulus. The **capillary endothelium** of the glomerulus is fenestrated by openings 50 to 100 nm in diameter. These openings exclude cells from the ultrafiltrate, but macromolecules are not restricted based on size. The luminal surface of the endothelium is covered by negatively charged sialoglycoproteins that contribute to the charge selectivity of the filtration barrier.

The **glomerular basement membrane** is composed of the lamina rara interna on the endothelial side, the central lamina densa, and the lamina rara externa on the epithelial side. The lamina rara interna and lamina rara externa contain polar noncollagenous proteins that contribute to the negative charge of the filtration barrier. The lamina densa contains nonpolar collagenous proteins that

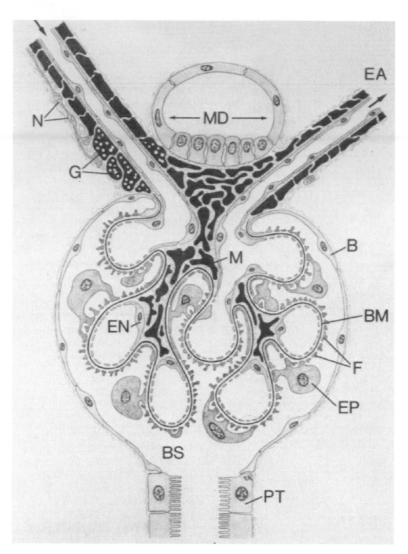

Fig. 2-2 Schematic representation of the glomerulus demonstrating the afferent and efferent arterioles, juxtaglomerular apparatus, and glomerular capillary loops. At the vascular pole, an afferent arteriole (AA) enters and an efferent arteriole (EA) leaves the glomerulus. At the urinary pole, Bowman's space (BS) becomes the tubular lumen of the proximal tubule (PT). The epithelial cells composing Bowman's capsule (B) enclose Bowman's space. Smooth muscle cells proper of the arterioles and all cells derived from smooth muscle are shown in black, including the granular cells (G). The afferent arteriole is innervated by sympathetic nerve terminals (N). The extraglomerular mesangial cells are located at the angle between AA and EA and continue into the mesangial cells (M) of the glomerular tuft. The glomerular capillaries are outlined by fenestrated endothelial cells (EN) and covered from the outside by the epithelial cells (EP) with foot processes (F). The glomerular basement membrane (BM) is continuous throughout the glomerulus. At the vascular pole, the thick ascending limb touches with the macula densa (MD), the extraglomerular mesangium.[27]

contribute primarily to the size selectivity of the filtration barrier. The filtration barrier is permeable to molecules with effective molecular radii less than 2 nm and impermeable to those with radii greater than 4 nm.

The **visceral epithelial cells** or **podocytes** constitute the outermost portion of the filtration barrier. They cover the glomerular basement membrane and glomerular capillaries on the urinary side of the barrier with their primary and interdigitating secondary foot processes. Filtration slits, 10 to 30 nm in width, are located between the secondary foot processes. The podocytes are phagocytic and may engulf macromolecules trapped by the filtration slits. They are invested with a negatively charged sialoglycoprotein coat that contributes to the charge selectivity of the filtration barrier. It is believed that the visceral epithelial cells synthesize the glomerular basement membrane.

The **mesangium** is not a part of the filtration barrier but a stabilizing core of tissue forming an anchor for the glomerulus at the vascular pole and along the axes of the capillary lobules. The mesangial cells are in contact with the basement membrane in areas where there is no capillary endothelium. The extraglomerular mesangium fills the space between the macula densa and the glomerular arterioles and constitutes part of the juxtaglomerular apparatus (JGA). The mesangial cells contain microfilaments and can contract in response to specific hormones (e.g., angiotensin II), thus altering the surface area available for filtration. They also synthesize prostaglandins that contribute to renal vasodilatation. The mesangium also contains macrophages that can clear filtration residues from the mesangial space by phagocytosis.

The glomerular capillary wall is a size- and a charge-selective barrier to filtration. Its **size selectivity** resides primarily in the lamina densa of the glomerular basement membrane. The glomerulus generally excludes molecules with radii greater than 4 nm. Inulin, with a molecular mass of 5200 daltons and radius of 1.4 nm, permeates freely, whereas serum albumin, with a molecular mass of 69,000 daltons and radius of 3.6 nm, permeates minimally.

The **charge selectivity** of the glomerulus resides in the negatively charged sialoglycoproteins (e.g., laminin and fibronectin) and peptidoglycans (e.g., heparan sulfate) of the capillary endothelium, lamina rara interna, lamina rara externa, and visceral epithelium. At any given effective molecular radius, negatively charged macromolecules experience greater restriction to filtration than do neutral ones. Positively charged macromolecules experience less restriction to filtration than do neutral ones of the same size (Fig. 2-3).

DETERMINANTS OF GLOMERULAR FILTRATION

The term **glomerular filtration rate** refers to the total filtration rate of both kidneys and represents the sum of the

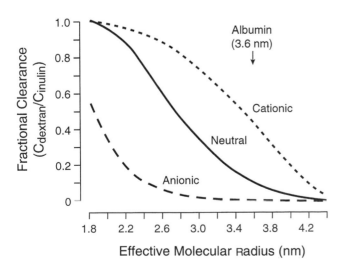

Fig. 2-3 Effect of electrostatic charge on filtration of macromolecules across the glomerular capillary wall. (Drawing by Tim Vojt.)

single-nephron glomerular filtration rates (SNGFRs) of all nephrons. The number of nephrons per kidney reflects the size of the animal. The feline kidney has approximately 200,000 nephrons, the canine kidney approximately 400,000, and the human kidney approximately 1,200,000 nephrons. SNGFR may differ among some groups of nephrons under normal conditions, and additional changes may occur in response to such factors as water deprivation, increased water intake, increased salt intake, or increased protein intake. Superficial cortical nephrons have short loops of Henle with little or no penetration into the renal medulla. These nephrons tend to excrete relatively more solute and water. Juxtamedullary nephrons have long loops of Henle that penetrate the inner medulla, and these nephrons tend to conserve solute and water. All of the nephrons in the canine and feline kidney are thought to have long loops of Henle.

The glomerular ultrafiltrate is a protein-free ultrafiltrate of plasma containing water and all of the crystalloids of plasma in concentrations similar to those in plasma. The concentrations are not exactly the same because of the Gibbs-Donnan effect. The same Starling forces that govern the movement of fluid across other capillaries in the body determine SNGFR, but there are some important differences in the glomerulus that account for the relatively high rate of filtration:

$$\text{SNGFR} = K_f[(P_{GC} - P_T) - (\pi_{GC} - \pi_T)]$$

where P_{GC} is the hydrostatic pressure in the glomerular capillary, which falls slightly along the length of the glomerular capillary, averaging 55 mm Hg; P_T is the hydrostatic pressure in Bowman's space, which is higher than systemic interstitial pressure, averaging 20 mm Hg; π_{GC} is the oncotic pressure in the glomerular capillary, which increases along the length of the capillary because of loss of protein-free ultrafiltrate into Bowman's space, averaging 20 mm Hg; and π_T is the oncotic pressure in Bowman's space and is negligible because the ultrafiltrate is nearly protein free. If π_T is neglected, the formula for SNGFR simplifies to:

$$\text{SNGFR} = K_f(P_{GC} - P_T - \pi_{GC})$$

These relationships are depicted in Fig. 2-4, in which average pressure values are those reported for dogs[32] and cats.[5] If the average pressures just described are considered alone, it can be seen that the net filtration pressure in the glomerulus is approximately 15 mm Hg, which is similar to values obtained for systemic capillaries. The fact that GFR is so much higher than the movement of fluid across systemic capillaries is explained by different values for K_f.

The ultrafiltration constant, K_f, is dependent on the surface area available for filtration and the permeability per unit area of capillary to crystalloids and water. The morphology of the glomerulus is such that the surface

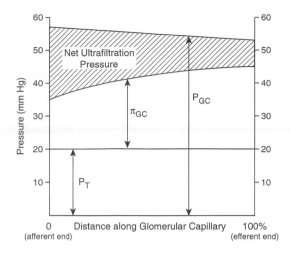

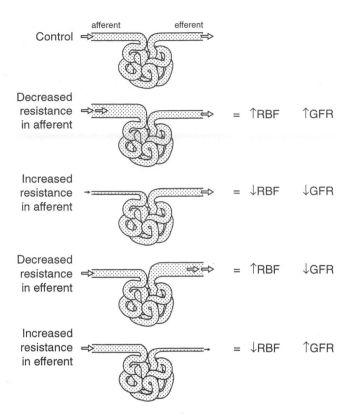

		Mean values for Dog and Cat	
P_{GC}	Hydrostatic pressure in glomerular capillary	52	58
π_{GC}	Plasma oncotic pressure in glomerular capillary	20	22
P_T	Hydrostatic pressure in Bowman's Space	20	18
π_T	Oncotic pressure in Bowman's Space	0	0
	Net ultrafiltration pressure	12	18

Fig. 2-4 Graphic representation of the generation of net filtration pressure in the glomerulus as governed by Starling forces. (Drawing by Tim Vojt.)

Fig. 2-5 Effects of alterations in afferent and efferent arteriolar tone on renal blood flow and glomerular filtration rate. (Drawing by Tim Vojt.)

area available for filtration is much greater than that found in the capillary beds of skeletal muscle, and the unit permeability of the glomerular endothelium is more than 100 times that of skeletal muscle capillaries. This much higher value for K_f in glomerular capillaries than in systemic capillaries accounts for the much higher rate of filtration. The ultrafiltration coefficient, K_f, is not constant and can change as a result of disease and in response to hormones that cause mesangial cells to contract (e.g., angiotensin II).

Changes in the resistance of the afferent (preglomerular) and efferent (postglomerular) arterioles may have a marked effect on GFR. Alterations in resistance in the afferent arterioles lead to parallel changes in GFR and renal blood flow (RBF), but changes in resistance in the efferent arterioles lead to divergent changes in GFR and RBF (Fig. 2-5). The interplay of the effects of neural and hormonal factors on vascular tone in the kidney is complex, but the main purpose of these effects is to minimize even slight changes in GFR that could have drastic adverse effects on the volume and composition of the extracellular fluid.

The resistance of these arterioles is regulated by the autonomic nervous system and by numerous vasoactive mediators (Table 2-1). Stimulation of the sympathetic nervous system results in release of norepinephrine from nerves terminating on the afferent and efferent arterioles. Norepinephrine can cause afferent and efferent vasocon-

TABLE 2-1 Effects of Selected Vasoactive Mediators on Glomerular Hemodynamics

Substance	Afferent Arteriole	Efferent Arteriole
Vasodilators		
Acetylcholine	Relax	Relax
Nitric oxide	Relax	Relax
Dopamine	Relax	Relax
Bradykinin	Relax	Relax
Prostacyclin	Relax	Relax
Prostaglandin E_2	Relax	No effect
Prostaglandin I_2	Relax	Relax
Vasoconstrictors		
Norepinephrine	Constrict	Constrict
Angiotensin II	Constrict	Constrict
Endothelin	Constrict	Constrict
Thromboxane	Constrict	Constrict
Vasopressin	No effect	Constrict

From Valtin H, Schafer JA: Renal function, *Boston, 1995, Little, Brown and Company, p. 107.*

striction, but efferent arteriolar constriction usually predominates. As a result, RBF decreases with minimal changes in GFR (i.e., filtration fraction [FF] increases). Angiotensin II also causes efferent more than afferent vasoconstriction and has similar effects on RBF and GFR. Stimulation of dopaminergic receptors causes afferent and efferent vasodilatation and increased RBF with little change in GFR at low concentrations of dopamine. Norepinephrine, angiotensin II, and antidiuretic hormone (ADH, vasopressin) cause vasoconstriction while at the same time promoting the production of prostaglandins that cause vasodilatation. These prostaglandins (PGE_2 and PGI_2) play an important role in maintaining RBF in hypovolemic states when angiotensin II and norepinephrine concentrations are increased. The effects of these prostaglandins are limited to the kidney because they are rapidly metabolized in the pulmonary circulation. Nonsteroidal antiinflammatory drugs that inhibit generation of prostaglandins by the cyclooxygenase pathway may cause renal ischemia and acute renal insufficiency in hypovolemic patients.[8,10] Locally produced kinins also cause vasodilatation and favor redistribution of RBF to inner cortical nephrons. Mediators produced locally by the vascular endothelium also contribute to afferent and efferent vasoconstriction (e.g., endothelin and thromboxane) and vasodilatation (e.g., nitric oxide and prostacyclin).

MEASUREMENT OF GLOMERULAR FILTRATION RATE

Consider a substance that is filtered by the glomeruli but neither reabsorbed nor secreted by the tubules. Under steady-state conditions, the following mass balance equation may be written:

$$\text{Amount filtered} = \text{amount excreted}$$

$$P_x \times \text{GFR} = U_x \times V$$

where P_x is the plasma concentration of x (mg/mL), U_x is the urine concentration of x (mg/mL), V is the urine flow rate (mL/min), and GFR is the glomerular filtration rate (mL/min). Dividing both sides of the equation by P_x:

$$\text{GFR} = U_x V / P_x$$

Note that this equation is the same as the formula for clearance presented before. Thus the renal clearance of a substance that is neither reabsorbed nor secreted is equal to GFR. Inulin is a polymer of fructose with a molecular mass of 5200 daltons. It is not bound to plasma proteins and is freely filtered by the glomeruli. It is neither reabsorbed nor secreted by the tubules. It is not metabolized by the kidney or any other organ. It is uncharged and not subject to the Gibbs-Donnan effect. In summary, inulin is an ideal substance for the measurement of GFR, and inulin clearance is the laboratory standard for GFR determination. Normal values for GFR as measured by inulin clearance are 3 to 5 mL/min/kg in the dog[13,18] and 2.5 to 3.5 mL/min/kg in the cat.[13,40]

Inulin clearance is not used clinically because it requires intravenous infusion of inulin and an assay that is not routinely available in most clinical pathology laboratories. Creatinine is produced endogenously in the body and excreted primarily by glomerular filtration, so its clearance can be used to estimate GFR in the steady state. The only requirements for determination of **endogenous** creatinine clearance are an accurately timed urine sample (usually 24 hours), determination of the patient's body weight, and measurement of serum and urine creatinine concentrations.

In the dog and cat, creatinine is filtered by the glomeruli and is neither reabsorbed nor secreted by the tubules.[15-17,19] In most clinical pathology laboratories, creatinine is measured by the alkaline picrate reaction. This reaction is not entirely specific for creatinine and measures another group of substances collectively known as noncreatinine chromagens. These substances are found in plasma, where they may constitute up to 50% of the measured creatinine at normal serum creatinine concentrations, but only small amounts appear in urine.[18,19] When the creatinine concentration is determined using the alkaline picrate reaction, the presence of noncreatinine chromagens causes endogenous creatinine clearance to underestimate GFR. This problem may be avoided by using more accurate methods (e.g., peroxidase-antiperoxidase) to measure the creatinine concentration.[19] Values for endogenous creatinine clearance in the dog and cat are approximately 2 to 5 mL/min/kg.[4,14,19]

To circumvent the problem of noncreatinine chromagens and to improve accuracy, some investigators have advocated determination of **exogenous** creatinine clearance. In this test, which is somewhat more cumbersome, creatinine is administered subcutaneously to the animal to increase the serum creatinine concentration and reduce the relative effect of the noncreatinine chromagens. For example, a normal dog may have a serum creatinine concentration of 1.0 mg/dL, of which 0.5 mg/dL represents noncreatinine chromagens. This measurement represents a 50% error. If, however, the dog's serum creatinine concentration is increased to 10 mg/dL by subcutaneous administration of creatinine, the noncreatinine chromagens still represent only 0.5 mg/dL, and the error is reduced to 5%. Exogenous creatinine clearance exceeds endogenous creatinine clearance and more closely approximates inulin clearance in the dog.[17]

The amount of any substance excreted by the kidneys is the algebraic sum of the amount filtered and the amount handled by the tubules:

$$U_x V = P_x \text{GFR} + T_x$$

where T_x is the amount handled by tubules (mg/min).

The term T_x is a positive number if the substance experiences net secretion and a negative number if it experiences net reabsorption. Dividing both sides of the equation by P_x yields the familiar clearance formula:

$$C_x = \text{GFR} + T_x/P_x$$

Thus the clearance of a substance experiencing net reabsorption is less than GFR (T_x is negative), and the clearance of a substance experiencing net secretion is greater than GFR (T_x is positive). The ratio of the clearance of a substance to inulin clearance gives an indication of the net handling of that substance by the kidney. If the ratio is less than 1.0, the substance experiences net reabsorption; if it is greater than 1.0, it experiences net secretion.

RENAL BLOOD FLOW AND RENAL PLASMA FLOW

The kidneys receive 25% or more of cardiac output. The major sites of resistance within the kidney are the afferent and efferent arterioles, with an approximately 80% to 90% decrease in perfusion pressure across this region of the renal vasculature (Fig. 2-6). Blood flow is not uniform throughout the kidney. In dogs, more than 90% of RBF is normally directed to the renal cortex, less than 10% to the outer medulla, and only 2% to 3% to the inner medulla.[45] The actual rate of flow to the renal cortex is approximately 100 times that of resting muscle and is required for glomerular filtration. Blood flow to the medulla is similar to that of resting muscle, and this reduced flow is necessary for normal function of the urinary concentrating mechanism.

AUTOREGULATION

Autoregulation refers to the intrinsic ability of an organ to maintain blood flow at a nearly constant rate despite changes in arterial perfusion pressure. In the kidney, between perfusion pressures of 80 and 180 mm Hg, GFR and RBF vary less than 10% (Fig. 2-7). Flow (Q) is equal to pressure (P) divided by resistance (R). As pressure increases, flow can remain constant only if resistance increases proportionately. The site of this resistance change in the kidney is the afferent arteriole. Autoregulation is intrinsic to the kidney and occurs in the isolated, denervated kidney and in the adrenalectomized animal. However, it is impaired by anesthesia in proportion to the depth of anesthesia. The afferent arterioles are maximally dilated at mean arterial pressures of 70 to 80 mm Hg, and at lower pressures, GFR declines linearly with RBF (i.e., autoregulation is lost). It is likely that autoregulation of RBF is a consequence of the need to regulate GFR closely and thus maintain tight control over water and salt balance.

Two physiologic mechanisms contribute to autoregulation. The **myogenic mechanism** is based on the principle that smooth muscle tends to contract when stretched and relax when shortened. As the afferent arteriole is stretched by increased perfusion pressure, it constricts, thus limiting transmission of this increased pressure to the glomerulus and minimizing any change in glomerular capillary hydrostatic pressure and SNGFR. The myogenic mechanism represents a coarse control that operates with a delay of 1 to 2 seconds.

Tubuloglomerular feedback represents a local intrarenal negative feedback mechanism for individual nephrons. The morphologic basis for this physiologic mechanism is the JGA. Increased sodium chloride concentration or transport in the distal tubule is sensed by the extraglomerular mesangial cells of the JGA as they monitor sodium chloride transport across the tubular cells of the macula densa. This results in afferent arteriolar constriction and possibly decreased capillary permeability in the parent glomerulus. The local mediator of this afferent arteriolar constriction is unknown. It may be adenosine, or it may result from increased inter-

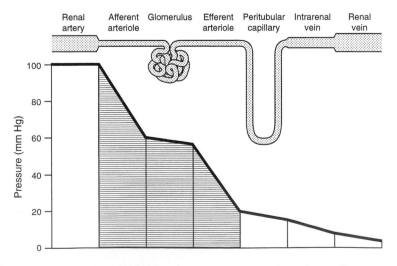

Fig. 2-6 Pattern of hydrostatic pressure and vascular resistance in the renal circulation. (Drawing by Tim Vojt.)

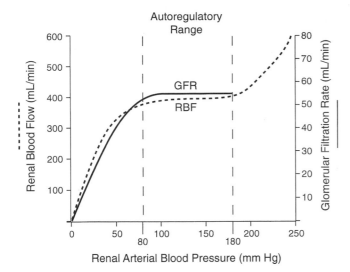

Fig. 2-7 Autoregulation of renal blood flow and glomerular filtration rate. (Drawing by Tim Vojt.)

stitial chloride concentration or osmolality in the region of the JGA. Whatever the cause of the afferent arteriolar constriction, SNGFR is decreased, thus reducing filtration and minimizing NaCl loss in that nephron. Tubuloglomerular feedback represents a fine control that operates with a 10- to 12-second delay.

MEASUREMENT OF RENAL BLOOD FLOW AND RENAL PLASMA FLOW

Consider the following mass balance equation[46]:

Amount entering the kidney = amount leaving the kidney

$$P_{AX} \times RPF_A = P_{VX} \times RPF_V + U_X V$$

$$P_{AX} \times RPF_A - P_{VX} \times RPF_V = U_X V$$

where P_{AX} is the renal arterial plasma concentration of x, RPF_A is the arterial renal plasma flow (RPF), P_{VX} is the renal venous plasma concentration of x, RPF_V is the venous RPF, U_X is the urine concentration of x, and V is the urine flow.

If we ignore the slight difference between renal arterial and venous plasma flow (with probably less than 1% error), the equation simplifies to:

$$(P_{AX} - P_{VX})RPF = U_X V$$

$$RPF = U_X V/(P_{AX} - P_{VX})$$

If we choose a substance that is completely removed from the blood in one pass through the kidney, P_{VX} is zero and $RPF = U_X V/P_{AX}$. If the substance x is not metabolized and is not excreted by any organ other than the kidney, its concentration in any peripheral vessel equals P_{AX}. Thus $RPF = U_X V/P_X$.

PAH is filtered by the glomeruli and secreted by the peritubular capillaries into the tubules so that approxi-

mately 90% of it is removed in one pass through the kidney. It is not metabolized or excreted by any other organ. Thus it approximately meets the preceding assumptions and $RPF = U_{PAH}V/P_{PAH}$. Now it can be seen that the clearance of PAH is an estimate of RPF. When PAH is infused during a clearance study, it is essential that P_{PAH} be maintained at a concentration much below the tubular transport maximum (T_{max}) for PAH. If not, P_{VX} cannot be neglected.

Some blood flows through regions of the kidney that do not remove PAH (e.g., renal capsule, perirenal fat, and renal pelvis), and as a result, P_{VX} is not really zero. Thus the term **effective** RPF is more appropriately used when speaking of PAH clearance. Furthermore, only 90% of PAH is removed from the blood during a single pass through the kidney. This also contributes to the fact that P_{VX} for PAH is not really zero. A closer approximation of RPF can be determined by sampling renal arterial and venous blood and measuring their respective PAH concentrations. The **extraction ratio** for PAH is then determined:

$$E_X = (P_{AX} - P_{VX})/P_{AX}$$

A more accurate calculation of RPF is then:

$$RPF = C_{PAH}/E_{PAH}$$

$$RPF = U_{PAH}V/P_{PAH}E_{PAH}$$

The extraction ratio for PAH is 0.9 because approximately 90% of it is removed from the blood in a single pass through the kidney. Notice that if we substitute the equation for E_X into the preceding equation, we get $RPF = U_X V/(P_{AX} - P_{VX})$, which is the same equation as derived before for RPF.

Another way to determine RPF is by use of the Fick principle, which states that the amount of a substance (V) removed by an organ is equal to the blood flow to the organ (Q) times the arteriovenous concentration difference of the substance in question ($C_A - C_V$):

$$V = Q(C_A - C_V)$$

$$Q = V/(C_A - C_V)$$

Using the kidney as an example and equating the amount of the substance removed to the amount excreted ($U_X V$):

$$RPF = U_X V/(P_{AX} - P_{VX})$$

Note that this equation is identical to that derived before using the mass balance principle.

If the hematocrit is known, RBF can be calculated from the RPF by using the following equation:

$$RBF = \frac{RPF}{(1 - \text{hematocrit})}$$

In the dog and cat, normal values for RPF are 7 to 20 mL/min/kg and 8 to 22 mL/min/kg, respectively.[34,35,40]

If all of the plasma were filtered in one pass of blood through the glomeruli, an immovable mass of red blood cells would be all that remained behind at the efferent arteriole of the glomerular capillary. This does not occur because π_{GC} increases along the length of the capillary and, in conjunction with P_T, effectively opposes further filtration. The **filtration fraction** is the fraction of plasma flowing through the kidneys that is filtered into Bowman's space. It is determined by the following equation:

$$FF = GFR/RPF$$

In the dog and cat, values for FF are 0.32 to 0.36 and 0.33 to 0.41, respectively. These values are higher than those observed in humans, in whom FF is approximately 0.20.

RENAL TUBULAR FUNCTION

The terms reabsorption and secretion refer to the direction of transport across an epithelium. In the kidney, **reabsorption** refers to movement of water and solutes from the tubular lumen to the peritubular interstitium. **Secretion** refers to movement of water and solutes from the peritubular interstitium to the tubular lumen. Some substances experience reabsorption in one part of the nephron and secretion in another part (e.g., urate and potassium). The term reabsorption often is used to denote net reabsorption, which is the algebraic sum of the fluxes in both directions across the renal tubular epithelium.

The **luminal** membranes separate the cytoplasm of the tubular cell from the tubular fluid. The **basolateral** membranes separate the cytoplasm of the tubular cell from the lateral intercellular spaces and the peritubular interstitium. The **transmembrane** potential difference (PD) refers to the electrical PD between the outside and inside of the cell. The **transepithelial** or **transtubular** PD is the electrical PD between the tubular lumen and the peritubular interstitium and is the algebraic sum of the transmembrane PD between the tubular lumen and cell cytoplasm and the transmembrane PD between the peritubular interstitium and cell cytoplasm. These relationships are depicted in Fig. 2-8. Transmembrane PD usually is −60 to −70 mV (cell interior negative), whereas transepithelial PD is only a few millivolts. In the early proximal tubule, the tubular lumen is a few millivolts

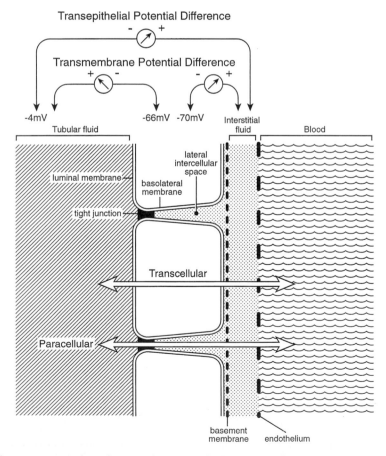

Fig. 2-8 Diagram demonstrating selected terminology as applied to the renal tubular epithelium: luminal versus basolateral membranes, transmembrane versus transepithelial potential difference, and transcellular versus paracellular transport. (Drawing by Tim Vojt.)

negative relative to the peritubular interstitium, whereas in the later proximal tubule, the tubular lumen is a few millivolts positive relative to the peritubular interstitium. In the thick ascending limb of Henle's loop, the transepithelial PD is lumen positive, but in the distal tubule, the transepithelial PD is lumen negative. The transepithelial PD affects movement of charged solutes across the renal tubular epithelium and contributes to the electrochemical gradient for such solutes.

The **paracellular** route refers to movement of solutes and water between cells (i.e., from the tubular lumen to the lateral intercellular space across tight junctions connecting epithelial cells). The **transcellular** route refers to movement of solutes and water through the cytoplasm of the tubular cells. The junctions between renal epithelial cells at the luminal surface are classified as **leaky** (proximal tubules) or **tight** (distal convoluted tubules, collecting ducts). Leaky epithelia do not generate large transepithelial concentration gradients, exhibit a small transepithelial PD, and have high water permeability, whereas tight epithelia can generate large transepithelial concentration gradients, exhibit a large transepithelial PD, and have low basal water permeability. The paracellular route allows movement of ions (e.g., potassium, chloride) and large, nonpolar solutes by passive diffusion and solvent drag. Electrochemical, hydrostatic, and oncotic gradients are important driving forces for reabsorption by the paracellular route. The paracellular route accounts for only 1% of the surface area available for reabsorption and 5% to 10% of water transport, whereas the transcellular route accounts for 99% of the available surface area and 90% to 95% of water transport. Both passive and active transport processes occur by the transcellular route, and all active transport processes must occur by this route.

That renal tubular reabsorption occurs may be recognized intuitively by considering the composition of normal urine. Many low-molecular-weight solutes essential to normal physiological function (e.g., glucose, amino acids, bicarbonate) are freely filtered at the glomerulus but do not normally appear in urine. Thus they must have been reabsorbed along the course of the renal tubule. In the proximal tubule, water follows solute reabsorption osmotically, and solute reabsorption is said to occur isosmotically (i.e., the reabsorbed fluid has the same osmolality as extracellular fluid). Approximately two thirds of all water and solute reabsorption occurs in the proximal tubules. Almost 99% of glucose and amino acids and 90% or more of bicarbonate are reabsorbed in the early proximal tubules (Fig. 2-9). The reabsorption of bicarbonate occurs as a consequence of the tubular secretion of hydrogen ions and is crucial to renal regulation of acid-base balance (see Chapter 9).

RENAL TRANSPORT PROCESSES

Four types of transport processes contribute to renal tubular reabsorption: passive diffusion, facilitated diffu-

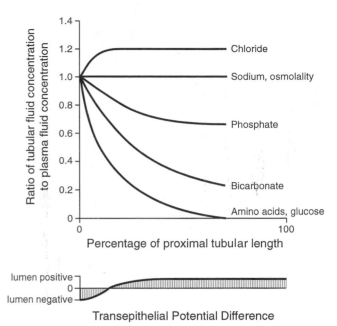

Fig. 2-9 Changes in the solute composition and transepithelial potential difference along the length of the proximal nephron. (Drawing by Tim Vojt.)

sion, primary active transport, and secondary active transport.

Passive diffusion is the movement of a substance across a membrane as a result of random molecular motion. Simple diffusion can take place directly through the lipid bilayer of the cell membrane, which occurs for substances with high lipid solubility. Simple diffusion can also occur through hydrophilic protein channels embedded in the cell membrane. Simple diffusion requires no expenditure of metabolic energy. The rate of transfer of solute is dependent on the permeability characteristics of the membrane, the electrochemical gradient (i.e., the combination of the electrical PD and chemical concentration difference across the membrane), and the hydrostatic pressure across the membrane. The rate of diffusion is linearly related to the concentration of the diffusing solute, and there is no maximal rate of transfer (V_{max}). Passive diffusion is not a saturable process because a carrier is not involved.

Facilitated diffusion is the movement of a substance across a membrane down its electrochemical gradient after binding with a specific carrier protein in the membrane. The carrier protein binds the substance to be transported at one side of the cell membrane. The occupied carrier then undergoes a conformational change that causes translocation of the substance across the cell membrane. The substance is then released from the carrier on the other side of the membrane. Unlike simple diffusion, facilitated diffusion is a saturable process characterized by a maximal rate of transfer (V_{max}) because a carrier is involved. The carrier has structural specificity and affinity for the substance transported, and the process is subject to competitive inhibition. Facilitated diffusion does not directly require metabolic energy, and transfer may occur in either direction across the membrane, depending on the prevailing electrochemical gradient. Examples of facilitated diffusion in the proximal tubule include the transport of glucose and amino acids at the basolateral membrane.

Primary active transport is the movement of a substance across a membrane in combination with a carrier protein but against an electrochemical gradient. Active transport requires metabolic energy, which is supplied by the hydrolysis of adenosine triphosphate (ATP). It is a saturable process characterized by a V_{max} and is subject to metabolic (e.g., cellular oxidative poisons) and competitive (e.g., competition for the carrier by a structurally similar compound) inhibition. Examples of primary active transporters include Na^+,K^+-adenosinetriphosphatase (Na^+,K^+-ATPase) in basolateral membranes of tubular cells throughout the nephron, H^+-ATPase in luminal membranes of tubular cells throughout the nephron, and H^+,K^+-ATPase in luminal membranes of α-intercalated cells in the collecting ducts.

Secondary active transport is the movement of two substances across a membrane after combination with a single carrier protein. The process is called **cotransport** if the transported substances are moving in the same direction across the membrane (e.g., glucose, amino acids, or phosphate with sodium at the luminal membrane of the proximal tubular cell) and **countertransport** if the transported substances are moving in opposite directions across the membrane (e.g., sodium and hydrogen ions at the luminal membrane of the proximal tubular cell). The "uphill" (i.e., against a concentration gradient) transport of one substance (e.g., glucose) is linked to the "downhill" (i.e., down an electrochemical gradient) transport of another substance (e.g., sodium). When the carrier is occupied by only one of the substances, it is not mobile in the cell membrane, whereas an unoccupied carrier or one that is occupied by both of the substances is mobile in the membrane. This process is saturable, demonstrates structural specificity and affinity of the carrier for the substances transported, and may be competitively inhibited. The uphill transport occurs without direct input of metabolic energy, and the substance transported uphill is said to experience secondary active transport. The metabolic energy for secondary active transport at the luminal membranes comes from the primary active transport of sodium out of the tubular cell at the basolateral membrane by Na^+,K^+-ATPase, a process that maintains a low intracellular sodium concentration.

Pinocytosis refers to the uptake by cells of particles too large to diffuse through the cell membrane. Filtered proteins are reabsorbed in the proximal tubule by this mechanism.

Solvent drag refers to the process whereby water (the solvent) moving across an epithelium by osmosis can drag dissolved solutes along with it.

MORPHOLOGY OF THE PROXIMAL TUBULE

Several morphologic features of proximal tubular cells suggest their primary role in the reabsorption of solutes and water. The brush border of the luminal surface of the proximal tubular cells consists of microvilli, which increase surface area, and lateral cellular interdigitations, which increase the surface area of the basolateral membranes (Fig. 2-10). Abundant mitochondria supply energy in the form of ATP required for active transport.

The proximal tubule exhibits intrasegmental axial heterogeneity with the most proximal segments being ultrastructurally the most complex and suited for the mechanisms of solute transport described earlier.[27] This morphologic complexity decreases along the length of the proximal tubule. In the first segment of the proximal tubule (P1 or S1), sodium, water, bicarbonate, amino acids, glucose, and phosphate are transported. In the second segment (P2 or S2), sodium, water, and chloride are reabsorbed, and organic acids and bases may be transported.[38] Organic acids and bases may also be secreted in the third segment (P3 or S3).[27] The low-specificity transport system for organic anions and cations in the proximal tubule allows elimination of many drugs and other foreign organic compounds from the body.

SODIUM TRANSPORT

Sodium may enter tubular cells at their luminal surface by several different mechanisms. In the proximal tubule, sodium may be cotransported across the luminal membranes of the cell with glucose, amino acids, or phosphate or may experience countertransport with hydrogen ions secreted into the tubular lumen by the Na^+-H^+ antiporter that facilitates bicarbonate reabsorption. In the loop of Henle, sodium enters via an Na^+-K^+-$2Cl^-$ carrier that is competitively inhibited by furosemide,[33] and in the distal

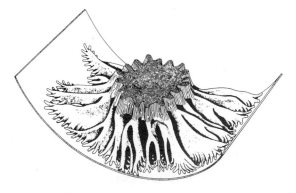

Fig. 2-10 Three-dimensional model of a proximal tubular cell showing microvilli and lateral cellular interdigitations.[27]

convoluted tubule, sodium enters via an Na^+-Cl^- cotransporter that is inhibited by thiazide diuretics. In the collecting duct, sodium enters via a luminal sodium channel that generates a lumen-negative PD favoring chloride reabsorption.

Thus in most segments of the nephron, sodium enters the tubular cell at the luminal membrane down an electrochemical gradient that favors sodium entry into the cell (i.e., the interior of the cell has a low sodium concentration and is negative with respect to the exterior). Sodium then experiences primary active transport out of the cell and into the lateral intercellular spaces and peritubular interstitium by the Na^+,K^+-ATPase located in the basolateral cell membranes. This enzyme hydrolyzes ATP and translocates two potassium ions into the cell and three sodium ions out of the cell.[1] It is located only in the basolateral membranes and functions to maintain a favorable electrochemical gradient for the passive entry of sodium into the tubular cells across their luminal membranes. Thus sodium is reabsorbed in conjunction with glucose, amino acids, phosphate, and bicarbonate in the proximal tubule and with chloride in the loop of Henle and distal tubule. The different mechanisms for sodium reabsorption in the nephron and the regulation of sodium reabsorption in the kidney are discussed in Chapter 3.

GLUCOSE TRANSPORT

Sodium attaches to a carrier in the luminal membrane of the proximal tubular cell, and this step is followed by attachment of glucose to the carrier. Translocation of the carrier occurs, and glucose is released to the interior of the cell while sodium enters down its electrochemical gradient (the interior of the cell is negative and its sodium concentration is low). As the intracellular glucose concentration increases, glucose leaves the cell by facilitated diffusion across the basolateral cell membranes. The Na^+,K^+-ATPase in the basolateral membranes continues to remove sodium from the cell, thus maintaining a favorable electrochemical gradient for sodium entry and expending the metabolic energy required for glucose transport.

Glucose transport meets the criteria for carrier-mediated transport in that it is a saturable process. Plotting the amount filtered ($P_x \times$ GFR), the amount excreted ($U_x \times V$), and the amount handled by the tubules (T_x) for a substance against the plasma concentration of that substance (P_x) yields a renal titration curve and allows determination of the **renal threshold** (plasma concentration at which the substance first appears in the urine) and **tubular transport maximum** (maximal amount of the substance that can be transported by the tubules, T_{max} or T_M). A renal titration curve for glucose is depicted in Fig. 2-11. The T_{max} for glucose is constant and relatively high, so it is usually not exceeded in health. Consequently, the kidney does not regulate plasma glucose concentration. In humans, the T_{max} for glucose is approximately 375 mg/min. In the dog, it is approximately 100 mg/min,[23,41] and in the cat,

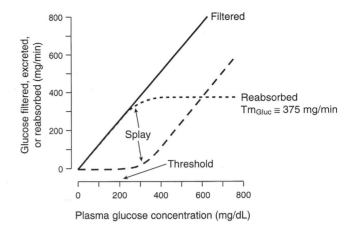

Fig. 2-11 Glucose titration curve showing filtration, reabsorption, and urinary excretion of glucose at increasing plasma glucose concentrations. Tm_{Gluc} refers to the maximal amount of glucose that can be transported per minute. (Drawing by Tim Vojt.)

50 mg/min.[28] In the renal titration curve, the T_{max} for glucose is approached somewhat gradually. This characteristic is called **splay** and is thought to result from nephron heterogeneity. Some nephrons excrete glucose before the average T_{max} is reached, whereas others continue to reabsorb glucose after the average T_{max} has been reached (i.e., the T_{max} for glucose differs slightly among nephrons).

PHOSPHATE

The uptake of phosphate into the proximal tubular cell is similar to that of glucose in that it is coupled to sodium entry at the luminal membrane. An important distinction from glucose transport, however, is that the T_{max} for phosphate is low and readily exceeded as plasma phosphate concentration increases. Hormones also alter the T_{max} for phosphate, notably parathyroid hormone (PTH). PTH decreases the T_{max} for phosphate and increases renal phosphate excretion. Thus the kidney, acting in concert with PTH, serves as a regulator of the plasma phosphate concentration.

AMINO ACIDS

The proximal tubular reabsorption of amino acids is also coupled to luminal sodium uptake. The T_{max} values for the different groups of amino acids are very high, and 99% of the filtered load of amino acids is reabsorbed in the proximal tubule. Thus the kidney is not a regulator of plasma amino acid concentrations. There are at least four carrier systems for amino acids: one each for neutral, basic, acidic, and the iminoglycine (i.e., proline and hydroxyproline) amino acids.

PINOCYTOSIS

Low-molecular-weight proteins (including several hormones and immunoglobulin light chains) are filtered at the glomerulus and reabsorbed by the proximal tubular cells, where they are hydrolyzed to their constituent amino acids, and these are returned to the circulation. Filtered proteins of small molecular mass may be hydrolyzed to amino acids by brush border enzymes at the luminal surface of the proximal tubular cell and their amino acids taken into the cell by cotransport with sodium. Alternatively, filtered proteins of larger molecular mass may attach to endocytic sites on the luminal cell membrane. These sites invaginate to form endosomes, which then fuse with lysosomes to form endolysosomes, in which digestion of the proteins occurs. The amino acids leave the endolysosomes and cross the basolateral membranes of the tubular cells by facilitated diffusion. This endocytic mechanism has a very high capacity, which is not normally exceeded in health.

UREA

Urea may experience passive reabsorption in the proximal tubules, depending on tubular flow rate. Increased tubular flow, as occurs during diuresis, is the result of decreased reabsorption of water from the tubular fluid. This decreases the tubular fluid urea concentration and decreases the concentration gradient of urea across the tubular epithelium. Thus less urea is reabsorbed at higher tubular flow rates. With decreased tubular flow, as occurs during dehydration, there is increased reabsorption of water from the tubular fluid. This increases the concentration gradient of urea across the tubular epithelium and increases passive urea reabsorption. In dehydrated patients, increased reabsorption of urea may lead to an increase in blood urea nitrogen (BUN) even before GFR is decreased. This contributes to the observation that the BUN/creatinine ratio tends to be higher in patients with prerenal azotemia than in hydrated patients with primary renal azotemia.

The tubular handling of urea in some segments of the nephron plays an important role in the urinary concentrating mechanism (see role of urea under The Urinary Concentrating Mechanism below). At least three urea transporters (UT1, UT2, and UT3) have been identified in the kidney.[43] UT1 is a vasopressin-responsive luminal urea transporter located in the inner medullary collecting ducts. It is involved in the majority of urea reabsorption in this segment of the nephron, and urea permeability can be increased approximately fourfold by attachment of vasopressin to basolateral V2 receptors. UT2 is found in the descending thin limbs of Henle's loops and allows urea to reenter the descending thin limbs, thus preventing its escape from the renal medulla (so-called urea recycling). UT3 is found in the descending vasa recta and participates in countercurrent exchange between ascending and descending vasa recta. The UT2 transporters are up-regulated during water deprivation, thus promoting inner medullary hypertonicity and conservation of water. UT1 is up-regulated by feeding a low protein diet and may serve to limit nitrogen loss. UT3 seems to be constitutively expressed in the kidney.

THE URINARY CONCENTRATING MECHANISM

Urinary concentration is a function of the juxtamedullary nephrons with long loops of Henle that penetrate deep into the renal medulla. There are two main steps in this process. First, transport of sodium chloride without water from the ascending limb of Henle's loop renders the medullary interstitium hyperosmotic. Second, vasopressin (ADH) increases the water permeability of the collecting duct, and tubular fluid traversing this segment of the nephron equilibrates osmotically with the hyperosmotic interstitium.

Strikingly different transport properties of various portions of the nephron form the basis for understanding the urinary concentrating mechanism (Table 2-2).

TABLE 2-2   Differential Permeability Characteristics of Nephron Segments

Portion of Nephron	NaCl	Urea	Water (ADH)	Water (No ADH)
Descending limb of Henle's loop*	Passive	Passive†	Passive	Passive
Thin ascending limb of Henle's loop*	Passive	Passive†	0	0
Thick ascending limb of Henle's loop	Active	0	0	0
Distal convoluted tubule	Active	0	0	0
Cortical collecting duct	Active‡	0	Passive	0
Outer medullary collecting duct	0	0	Passive	0
Inner medullary collecting duct	Active	Passive	Passive§	0

Modified from Rose BD: Clinical physiology of acid-base and electrolyte disorders, *New York, 1994, McGraw-Hill, p. 112, with permission of the McGraw-Hill Companies.*
*Permeability to NaCl exceeds permeability to urea in these segments.
†Passive reabsorption in these segments constitutes urea recycling.
‡Responsive to aldosterone.
§Permeable to urea in the basal state and permeability increased by ADH.

The hairpin configuration of Henle's loop is the anatomic basis for countercurrent multiplication and allows a single osmotic effect to be multiplied over the length of the loop. The vessels accompanying the loops of Henle into the medulla are called vasa recta. They prevent dissipation of the medullary osmotic gradient by a process called countercurrent exchange (see Role of the Vasa Recta below). The countercurrent multiplier concept was first applied to urine concentration by W. Kuhn, a physical chemist, in 1942.[2,21] As early as 1909, however, K. Peter had noted a correlation between the length of the Henle's loop and the ability of a given species to concentrate its urine.

ROLE OF THE ASCENDING LIMB OF HENLE'S LOOP

The ascending limb of Henle's loop is impermeable to water. Sodium chloride is actively transported from the thick portion of the ascending limb without accompanying water so that an osmotic gradient of approximately 200 mOsm/kg is generated. This active transport of sodium chloride is the primary energy-requiring step of the urinary concentrating mechanism.

Active sodium transport is accomplished by the Na+, K+-ATPase located in the basolateral membranes of the tubular cells. This enzyme maintains a low intracellular concentration of sodium and promotes passive entry of sodium at the luminal membrane down a concentration gradient. The luminal carrier binds one sodium ion, one potassium ion, and two chloride ions.[33] Chloride delivery is the rate-limiting step in this transport process, and loop diuretics such as furosemide impair distal sodium reabsorption by competing with chloride for the luminal carrier.[33]

Fluid reaching the distal convoluted tubule is hyposmotic (100 mOsm/kg) compared with the fluid entering the descending limb of Henle's loop (300 mOsm/kg). If fluid in the loops were stationary, the active transport of sodium chloride out of the thick ascending limb without water would increase the interstitial osmolality to 400 mOsm/kg and decrease the osmolality of the fluid within the ascending limb to 200 mOsm/kg. The descending limb of Henle's loop is highly permeable to water, and water would be extracted from this site, increasing the osmolality of the tubular fluid in this segment of the nephron to 400 mOsm/kg.

However, the fluid within Henle's loops is not stationary. New tubular fluid with an osmolality of 300 mOsm/kg is constantly entering the descending limb of Henle's loop from the proximal tubule. As fluid continues to move through the loops and an osmotic gradient of 200 mOsm/kg is generated, this single osmotic effect is multiplied over the length of Henle's loop (Fig. 2-12). The magnitude of the gradient from the beginning of the loop to its hairpin turn is a function of the length of the loop itself. Thus the vertical osmotic gradient greatly exceeds the horizontal gradient at any given level. This is the countercurrent multiplier concept of urinary concentration.

ROLE OF THE COLLECTING DUCTS AND ANTIDIURETIC HORMONE

The collecting duct is divided into three segments: the cortical collecting duct, outer medullary collecting duct, and inner medullary collecting duct. These segments differ in their permeability to sodium and urea (see Table 2-2). The main role of the cortical collecting duct is delivery of fluid with a very high urea concentration to the outer medullary collecting duct. This occurs because sodium chloride and water are removed from this segment of the nephron, but urea is not. The main functions of the inner medullary collecting duct are to add urea to the inner medullary interstitium and to produce maximally concentrated urine by osmotic equilibration of tubular fluid with the hyperosmotic interstitium under the influence of ADH.[7,25] This segment of the nephron is permeable to urea, and its urea permeability is increased by ADH (see section on urea above).

As just described, fluid entering the distal tubule is hyposmotic to plasma (approximately 100 mOsm/kg). Without the collecting duct, the so-called countercurrent multiplier would dilute tubular fluid. In the presence of ADH, this hyposmotic fluid equilibrates osmotically with the cortical interstitium (osmolality, 300 mOsm/kg) as the tubular fluid flows through the cortical collecting duct. By this process, approximately two thirds of the tubular water is removed before delivery to the medullary collecting duct. For example, 100 mOsm of solute in 1 L of tubular fluid is reduced to 100 mOsm of solute in 0.33 L of tubular fluid (300 mOsm/kg) with 0.67 L of water reabsorbed. Even more water can be reabsorbed, depending on how much active sodium reabsorption occurs in the cortical collecting duct in response to aldosterone stimulation. These effects markedly reduce fluid delivery to the medullary collecting duct. Tubular fluid entering the medullary collecting duct is thus isosmotic with plasma but much reduced in volume. It is in the medullary collecting duct that the final concentration of urine occurs.

The water permeability of the epithelium of the collecting duct is dependent on the action of ADH. In the presence of ADH, water is removed from the collecting duct as the fluid osmotically equilibrates with a progressively hyperosmotic medullary interstitium, and the final osmolality of the urine may approximate that of the papillary interstitium. In humans, this maximal urine osmolality is 900 to 1400 mOsm/kg.[39] In dogs and cats, however, urine osmolality can approach 2800 and 3000 mOsm/kg, respectively.[20,40] Water reabsorption in the distal convoluted tubule and connecting tubule is minimal because of their relative impermeability to water, regardless of the presence or absence of ADH. Thus

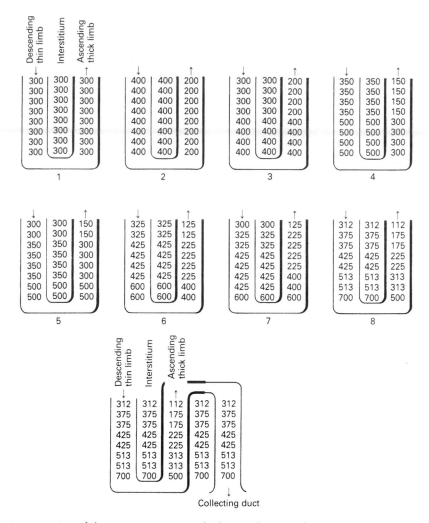

Fig. 2-12 Stepwise operation of the countercurrent multiplier mechanism of urinary concentration. Numbers refer to osmolalities (mOsm/kg H_2O) of tubular fluid and interstitium. (Reprinted with permission from Valtin H: *Renal function: mechanisms preserving fluid and solute balance in health,* ed 2, Boston, 1983, Little, Brown, and Company, p. 166.)

water reabsorption in the cortical collecting duct under the influence of ADH is important in reducing the fluid load delivered to the medullary collecting duct.

In the absence of ADH, the collecting duct is impermeable to water. The fluid entering this portion of the nephron has an osmolality of approximately 100 mOsm/kg. Under these conditions, additional sodium chloride without water is removed from the tubular fluid during its course through the cortical collecting duct and inner medullary collecting duct so that the final urine osmolality can be as low as 50 mOsm/kg. However, the outer medullary collecting duct is impermeable to sodium.

Even in the absence of ADH, urine osmolality may be greater than 50 mOsm/kg if the animal is dehydrated. The GFR is decreased by dehydration, and there is an increase in the proximal tubular reabsorption of

sodium chloride and water. Less tubular fluid reaches the distal nephron, and urine osmolality can approach 400 mOsm/kg.[44]

ROLE OF THE VASA RECTA

If the water removed from the medullary collecting duct in the presence of ADH were allowed to remain in the medullary interstitium, the hyperosmotic gradient would dissipate rapidly. However, this does not occur because of the countercurrent exchange function of the vasa recta. Plasma in the vasa recta entering the medulla from the cortex encounters an increasingly hyperosmotic medullary interstitium. As a result, water is removed from the vessels, and solutes (e.g., sodium chloride and urea) enter the vessels. After passing the hairpin turn of the loop, the vasa recta climb back toward the renal cortex. Now they encounter a medullary interstitium of progressively decreasing osmolality so that water enters the vessels and solutes are removed. In this way, water is removed from and solutes are recycled back into the medullary interstitium, thus preventing dissipation of the osmotic gradient. This process is known as countercurrent exchange. That the vasa recta can effectively remove water and recycle solute may be appreciated by considering the different flow rates in the vasa recta and medullary collecting duct. Although only 5% of RPF goes to the renal medulla, this flow is much greater than the approximately 3% of GFR that enters the medullary collecting ducts. Consider, for example, a 10-kg dog with a GFR of 4 mL/min/kg and an RPF of 12 mL/min/kg. RPF in the medulla would be 6 mL/min (5% of 120), and tubular fluid flow in the renal medulla would be 1.2 mL/min (3% of 40), a fivefold difference. These factors contribute to the effective removal of water from the medullary interstitium and prevent dissipation of the osmotic gradient in this region of the kidney.

ROLE OF UREA

Although there is evidence for active transport of sodium chloride from the thick ascending limb of Henle's loop, active transport has not been demonstrated in the thin descending and ascending limbs. A two-solute model of the urinary concentrating mechanism was developed simultaneously in 1972 by Stephenson and by Kokko and Rector.[22,26,42] This model requires an important contribution by urea as the second solute.

The thin descending limb of Henle's loop has a low passive permeability for sodium chloride and an even lower permeability for urea, but it is highly permeable to water. The resting permeability of the inner medullary collecting duct to urea is enhanced by ADH. The distal convoluted tubule, cortical collecting duct, and outer medullary collecting duct are relatively impermeable to urea, even in the presence of ADH. Thus the urea concentration of tubular fluid increases markedly in this portion of the nephron.

During a state of water conservation (i.e., antidiuresis), the plasma ADH concentration is high. More urea is passively removed from the inner medullary collecting duct and enters the medullary interstitium. In dogs, urea constitutes more than 40% of the total medullary solute concentration during antidiuresis (after 24 hours of water deprivation) but less than 10% during water diuresis.[6,29]

Urea increases medullary interstitial osmolality without a change in the sodium concentration in this region. Thus water is removed osmotically from the thin descending limb of Henle's loop by the high concentration of urea in the medullary interstitium. The sodium concentration of the tubular fluid in the descending limb of Henle's loop eventually exceeds the medullary interstitial sodium concentration because the thin descending limb of Henle's loop has a low permeability for sodium. The sodium permeability of the thin ascending limb of Henle's loop is high, and as the tubular fluid rounds the hairpin turn and enters this portion of the nephron, sodium can be removed passively into the medullary interstitium down a concentration gradient (Fig. 2-13).

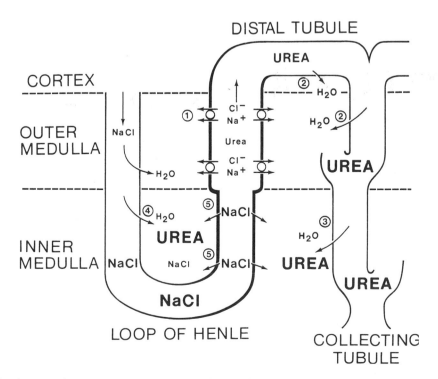

Fig. 2-13 Role of urea in the urinary concentrating mechanism. (Reprinted by permission of the *N Engl J Med* 295:1059-1067, 1976.)

ENDOCRINE FUNCTIONS OF THE KIDNEY

The kidney is responsible for endocrine functions that play essential roles in the regulation of red cell production by the bone marrow, defense of the extracellular fluid volume (ECFV), and maintenance of calcium homeostasis. Gradual loss of these endocrine functions occurs during the progression of chronic renal disease and contributes to specific manifestations of the uremic syndrome, such as nonregenerative anemia, systemic hypertension, and renal secondary hyperparathyroidism.

ERYTHROPOIETIN PRODUCTION

Erythropoietin (EPO) is glycoprotein hormone with a molecular mass of 35,000 daltons that stimulates red blood cell production by the bone marrow. In the fetus, EPO is produced in the liver, but shortly after birth production switches to the kidneys, which become the major source of EPO in the adult animal. Decreased oxygen delivery to the kidney is the major stimulus for EPO production. An oxygen sensor (thought to be a heme protein) detects decreased oxygen tension and activates transcriptional factors that increase transcription of the EPO gene. Peritubular interstitial fibroblasts in the renal cortex and outer medulla are the primary site of EPO synthesis in the kidney.[31] EPO binds to receptors on erythroid progenitor cells in the bone marrow promoting their viability, proliferation, and terminal differentiation into erythrocytes.[11]

Absolute or relative deficiency of EPO is the primary cause of the anemia of chronic renal failure.[24] Recombinant human EPO has been used successfully to correct the anemia of chronic renal failure in human patients.[12] Although initially effective in correcting the anemia of renal failure in dogs and cats, use of recombinant human EPO is associated with antibody formation in up to 50% of treated dogs and cats after 1 to 3 months of treatment.[9] The resulting anemia can be more severe than that present before treatment because the induced antibodies can cross-react with the animal's native EPO. The canine EPO gene has been isolated,[30] and recombinant canine EPO has been used to stimulate erythropoiesis in normal dogs[37] and in those with naturally occurring chronic renal failure.[36] It is not as effective when used in dogs that have developed red cell aplasia from previous treatment with recombinant human EPO.

RENIN-ANGIOTENSIN SYSTEM

The main role of the renin-angiotensin system (RAS) is defense of the ECFV via sodium homeostasis. The role of the kidney in maintenance of sodium balance is discussed further in Chapter 3.

Renin is an enzyme synthesized and stored in the granular cells of the JGA (specialized smooth muscle cells in the afferent arterioles). The kidney is the most important source of renin, but renin is also found in many other tissues (e.g., vascular endothelium, adrenal gland, and brain). Local production of angiotensin II in some tissues may be important in the regulation of local processes without having a systemic effect. The RAS of the brain may be involved in control of systemic blood pressure, secretion of ADH, catecholamine release, and thirst.

There are three major stimuli for renin release. Decreased renal perfusion pressure caused by systemic hypotension (pressure below 80 to 90 mm Hg) or ECFV depletion is sensed in the afferent arterioles by the granular cells, which increase their secretion of renin. Stimulation of cardiac and arterial baroreceptors by systemic hypotension leads to increased sympathetic neural activity and increased concentrations of circulating catecholamines, which in turn stimulate renin release via β_1-adrenergic receptors on granular cells. Lastly, changes in distal tubular flow and delivery of chloride affect renin release. Decreased ECFV or chronic NaCl depletion decreases distal tubular flow and delivery of chloride to the macula densa (partly as a consequence of enhanced proximal reabsorption of water and NaCl), which in turn stimulates renin release. Expansion of the ECFV or NaCl loading increases distal tubular flow and delivery of chloride to the macula densa, which inhibits renin release. The release of renin is inhibited by a direct effect of angiotensin II on the granular cells, which constitutes a negative feedback loop.

Renin converts the α_2-globulin angiotensinogen (which is synthesized and released by the liver) to angiotensin I, and this is the rate-limiting step of the RAS cascade. Angiotensin-converting enzyme is found in vascular endothelium and cleaves the carboxyl-terminal (C-terminal) two amino acids from the inactive decapeptide angiotensin I to yield the active octapeptide angiotensin II. This step in the RAS cascade is not rate limiting, and most of the angiotensin I is rapidly converted to angiotensin II.

The effects of angiotensin II restore ECFV. Angiotensin II causes arteriolar vasoconstriction in many organs (renal, splanchnic, and cutaneous vascular beds are most sensitive), which increases systemic blood pressure. It enhances the sensitivity of vascular smooth muscle to and facilitates the release of norepinephrine from the adrenal medulla and sympathetic nerve terminals, thus secondarily affecting systemic blood pressure. Angiotensin II causes increased proximal tubular reabsorption of sodium by stimulating the Na^+-H^+ antiporter in luminal membranes of proximal tubular cells. It causes increased secretion of aldosterone from the zona glomerulosa of the adrenal cortex, and aldosterone in turn causes increased reabsorption of sodium chloride in the cortical collecting duct. Lastly, angiotensin II causes alterations in glomerular and postglomerular hemodynamics that enhance sodium and water reabsorption. Angiotensin II causes constriction of the efferent and afferent arterioles, an effect thought to be mediated by thromboxane A_2. The efferent arteriole constricts more than the afferent so that the FF increases (i.e., RPF decreases more than GFR). Renal hemodynamic changes favoring salt and water reabsorption occur in the postglomerular capillary beds secondary to these glomerular hemodynamic changes. These changes include decreased peritubular capillary hydrostatic pressure and increased peritubular capillary oncotic pressure. Angiotensin II can cause glomerular mesangial cells to contract, potentially reducing the surface area for filtration and decreasing the ultrafiltration coefficient, K_f. Angiotensin II stimulates release of vasodilator prostaglandins (e.g., PGE_2 and PGI_2) from glomeruli. By this mechanism, the potentially harmful vasoconstrictive effects of angiotensin II on the kidney are minimized.

ACTIVATION OF VITAMIN D

Vitamin D_3 (cholecalciferol) is obtained in the diet or by ultraviolet irradiation of the compound 7-dehydrocholesterol in skin. The liver hydroxylates cholecalciferol to 25-hydroxycholecalciferol, which is the predominant form of vitamin D_3 in plasma. In the kidney, 25-hydroxycholecalciferol is converted to the active form of vitamin D_3, 1,25-dihydroxycholecalciferol (calcitriol), by the enzyme 25-hydroxycholecalciferol-1α-hydroxylase, which is found in the mitochondria of the proximal tubular cells. Calcitriol interacts with its high-affinity receptor (the vitamin D receptor [VDR]) in target tissues forming a ligand-activated transcription factor that travels to the nucleus of the cell and interacts with specific DNA sequences in vitamin D-responsive genes.

The activity of the 1α-hydroxylase system is closely regulated by PTH, calcium, phosphate, and calcitriol itself, which exerts negative feedback inhibition on 1α-hydroxylase. Hypocalcemia and PTH stimulate calcitriol synthesis. There is an inverse relationship between calcium concentrations and the activity of the 1α-hydroxylase enzyme system that may arise directly or may be secondary to changes in the secretion of PTH in response to alterations in serum calcium concentration. Some evidence exists to support a direct suppressive effect of calcium on 1α-hydroxylase activity in proximal tubular cells.[3] The 1α-hydroxylase enzyme system is stimulated by hypophosphatemia and inhibited by hyperphosphatemia.

The major effects of 1,25-dihydroxycholecalciferol (calcitriol) are increased intestinal absorption of calcium and phosphate, a permissive effect on PTH-mediated bone resorption of calcium and phosphate, and negative feedback control on PTH synthesis and secretion by the parathyroid glands. The actions of vitamin D are discussed in more detail in Chapter 6.

REFERENCES

1. Avison MJ, Gullans SR, Ogino T, et al: Measurement of Na-K coupling ratio of Na-K ATPase in rabbit proximal tubules, *Am J Physiol* 253:C126, 1987.
2. Berliner RW: Mechanisms of urine concentration. *Kidney Int* 22:202, 1982.
3. Bland R, Walker EA, Hughes SV, et al: Constitutive expression of 25-hydroxyvitamin D3-1alpha-hydroxylase in a transformed human proximal tubule cell line: evidence for direct regulation of vitamin D metabolism by calcium, *Endocrinology* 140:2027-2034, 1999.
4. Bovee KC, Joyce T: Clinical evaluation of glomerular function: 24-hour creatinine clearance in dogs, *J Am Vet Med Assoc* 174:488, 1979.
5. Brown SA: Determinants of glomerular ultrafiltration in cats, *Am J Vet Res* 54:970, 1993.
6. Bulger RE: Composition of renal medullary tissue, *Kidney Int* 31:557, 1987.
7. Chandhoke PS, Saidel CM, Knepper MA: Role of inner medullary collecting duct NaCl transport in urinary concentration, *Am J Physiol* 249:F688, 1985.
8. Clive DM, Stoff JS: Renal syndromes associated with nonsteroidal antiinflammatory drugs, *N Engl J Med* 310:563, 1984.
9. Cowgill LD, James KM, Levy JK, et al: Use of recombinant human erythropoietin for the management of anemia in dogs and cats with renal failure, *J Am Vet Med Assoc* 212:521-528, 1998.
10. Dunn MJ: Nonsteroidal antiinflammatory drugs and renal function, *Annu Rev Med* 35:411, 1984.
11. Ebert BL, Bunn HF: Regulation of the erythropoietin gene. *Blood* 94:1864-1877, 1999.
12. Eschbach JW, Egrie J, Downing M, et al: Correction of anemia of end-stage renal disease with recombinant human erythropoietin, *N Engl J Med* 316:73-78, 1987.
13. Fettman MJ, Allen TA, Wilke WL, et al: Single-injection method for evaluation of renal function with ^{14}C-inulin and ^{3}H-tetraethylammonium bromide in dogs and cats, *Am J Vet Res* 46:482, 1985.
14. Finco DR: Simultaneous determination of phenolsulfonphthalein excretion and endogenous creatinine clearance in the normal dog, *J Am Vet Med Assoc* 159:336, 1971.
15. Finco DR, Barsanti JA: Mechanism of urinary excretion of creatinine by the cat, *Am J Vet Res* 43:2207, 1982.
16. Finco DR, Brown SA, Crowell WA, et al: Exogenous creatinine clearance as a measure of glomerular filtration rate in dogs with reduced renal mass, *Am J Vet Res* 52:1029, 1991.
17. Finco DR, Coulter DB, Barsanti JA: Simple, accurate method for clinical estimation of glomerular filtration rate in the dog, *Am J Vet Res* 42:1874, 1981.
18. Finco DR, Duncan JR: Evaluation of blood urea nitrogen and serum creatinine concentrations as indicators of renal dysfunction: a study of 111 cases and a review of related literature, *J Am Vet Med Assoc* 168:593, 1976.
19. Finco DR, Tabaru H, Brown SA, et al: Endogenous creatinine clearance measurement of glomerular filtration rate in dogs, *Am J Vet Res* 54:1575, 1993.
20. Hardy RM, Osborne CA: Water deprivation test in the dog: Maximal normal values, *J Am Vet Med Assoc* 174:479, 1979.
21. Jamison RJ: The renal concentrating mechanism, *Kidney Int* 32(suppl 21):S43, 1987.
22. Jamison RL, Maffly RH: The urinary concentrating mechanism, *N Engl J Med* 295:1059, 1976.
23. Keyes JL, Swanson RE: Dependence of glucose Tm on GFR and tubular volume, *Am J Physiol* 221:1, 1971.

24. King LG, Giger U, Diserens D, et al: Anemia of chronic renal failure in dogs, *J Vet Int Med* 6:264-270, 1992.

25. Kokko JP: The role of the collecting duct in urinary concentration, *Kidney Int* 31:606, 1987.

26. Kokko JP, Rector FC Jr: Countercurrent multiplication system without active transport in inner medulla, *Kidney Int* 2:214, 1972.

27. Koushanpour E, Kriz W: *Renal physiology: principles, structure, and function,* New York, 1986, Springer-Verlag.

28. Kruth SA, Cowgill LD: Renal glucose transport in the cat (abstract), *Proc Am Coll Vet Intern Med* 78: 1982.

29. Levitin H, Goodman A, Pigeon G, et al: Composition of the renal medulla during water diuresis, *J Clin Invest* 41:1145, 1962.

30. MacLeod JN, Tetreault JW, Lorschy KAS, et al: Expression and bioactivity of recombinant canine erythropoietin, *Am J Vet Res* 59:1144-1148, 1998.

31. Maxwell PH, Ferguson DJP, Nicholls LG, et al: Sites of erythropoietin production, *Kidney Int* 51:393, 1997.

32. Navar LG, Bell PD, Crowell WA, et al: Evaluation of the single nephron glomerular filtration coefficient in the dog, *Kidney Int* 12:137, 1977.

33. O'Grady SM, Palfrey HC, Field M: Characteristics and function of Na-K-2Cl cotransport in epithelial tissues, *Am J Physiol* 253:C177, 1987.

34. Osbaldiston GW, Fuhrman W: The clearance of creatinine, inulin, **para**-aminohippurate and phenolsulfonphthalein in the cat, *Can J Comp Med* 34:138, 1970.

35. Powers TE, Powers JD, Garg RC: Study of the double isotope single-injection method for estimating renal function in purebred beagle dogs, *Am J Vet Res* 38:1933, 1977.

36. Randolph JF, Scarlett J, Stokol T, et al: Clinical efficacy and safety of recombinant canine erythropoietin in dogs with anemia of chronic renal failure and dogs with recombinant human erythropoietin-induced red cell aplasia, *J Vet Int Med* 18:81-91, 2004.

37. Randolph JF, Stokol T, Scarlett JM, et al: Comparison of biological activity and safety of recombinant canine erythropoietin with that of recombinant human erythropoietin in clinically normal dogs, *Am J Vet Res* 60:636-642, 1999.

38. Rose BD: *Clinical physiology of acid-base and electrolyte disorders,* New York, 1994, McGraw-Hill, p. 94.

39. Rose BD: *Clinical physiology of acid-base and electrolyte disorders,* New York, 1994, McGraw-Hill, p. 115.

40. Ross LA, Finco DR: Relationship of selected clinical renal function tests to glomerular filtration rate and renal blood flow in cats, *Am J Vet Res* 42:1704, 1981.

41. Shannon J, Farber S, Troast L: The measurement of glucose Tm in the normal dog, *Am J Physiol* 133:752, 1941.

42. Stephenson JL: Concentration of urine in a central core model of the renal counterflow system, *Kidney Int* 2:85, 1972.

43. Tsukaguchi H, Shayakul C, Berger UV, et al: Urea transporters in kidney: molecular analysis and contribution to the urinary concentrating process, *Am J Physiol* 275:F319-F324, 1998.

44. Valtin H, Edwards BR: GFR and the concentration of urine in the absence of vasopressin, Berliner-Davidson re-explored, *Kidney Int* 31:634, 1987.

45. Valtin H, Schafer JA: *Renal function,* Boston, 1995, Little, Brown and Company, p. 98.46. Valtin H, Schafer JA: *Renal function,* Boston, 1995, Little, Brown and Company, p. 90.

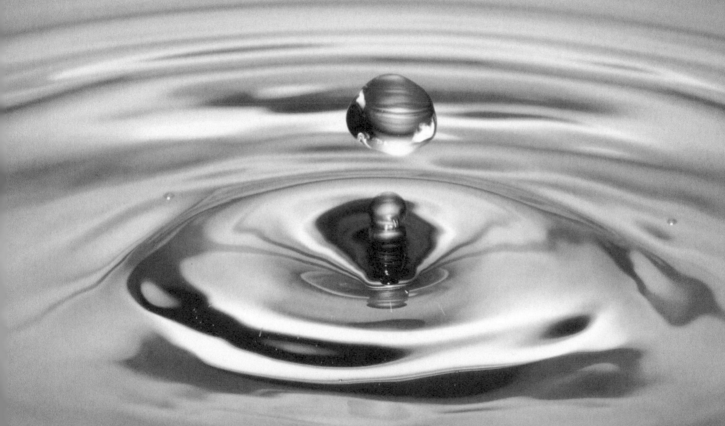

ELECTROLYTE DISORDERS

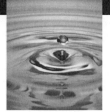

CHAPTER · 3

DISORDERS OF SODIUM AND WATER: HYPERNATREMIA AND HYPONATREMIA

Stephen P. DiBartola

The volume and tonicity of body fluids are maintained within a narrow normal range by regulation of sodium and water balance. The volume of extracellular fluid (ECF) is determined by the total body sodium content, whereas the osmolality and sodium concentration of ECF are determined by water balance. The kidney plays a crucial role in these processes by balancing the excretion of salt and water with their intake and by avidly conserving them when intake is restricted (Table 3-1).

TERMINOLOGY

OSMOLALITY

The **osmolality** of a solution refers to the concentration of osmotically active particles in that solution. Osmolality is a function only of the number of particles and is not related to their molecular weight, size, shape, or charge. One mole of a nondissociating substance (e.g., glucose or urea) dissolved in 1 kg of water decreases the freezing point of the resultant solution by 1.86° C. Such a solution has an osmolality of 1 Osm/kg or 1000 mOsm/kg.

The term **osmolarity** refers to the number of particles of solute per liter of solution, whereas the term **osmolality** refers to the number of particles of solute per kilogram of solvent. When considering the physiology of body fluids, the difference between osmolality and osmolarity is negligible because body fluids typically are dilute aqueous solutions. In clinical medicine, the term osmolality is used, and the osmolality of body fluids usually is measured by freezing-point depression osmometry. A solution is said to be **hyperosmotic** if its osmolality is greater than that of the reference solution (often plasma) and **hyposmotic** if its osmolality is less than that of the reference solution. An **isosmotic** solution has an osmolality identical to that of the reference solution.

The normal plasma osmolality of dogs and cats is slightly higher than that of humans and ranges from 290 to 310 mOsm/kg in dogs and from 290 to 330 mOsm/kg in

TABLE 3-1 Renal Regulation of Sodium and Water Balance

	Osmoregulation	Volume Regulation
What is sensed	Plasma osmolality	Effective circulating volume
Sensors	Hypothalamic osmoreceptors	Carotid sinus
		Aortic arch
		Glomerular afferent arterioles
		Cardiac atria
		Large pulmonary vessels
Effectors	Vasopressin	Renin-angiotensin-aldosterone system
	Thirst	Sympathetic nervous system
		Atrial natriuretic peptide
		"Pressure natriuresis"
		Antidiuretic hormone
What is affected	Water excretion	Urine sodium excretion
	Water intake	

Modified from Rose BD: Clinical physiology of acid base and electrolyte disorders, ed 4, New York, 1994, McGraw-Hill, p. 256, with permission of the McGraw-Hill Companies.

cats. In one study, 20 dogs under resting conditions had plasma osmolality values of 292 to 308 mOsm/kg with a mean value of 301 mOsm/kg.[55] In a study of the effects of sodium bicarbonate infusion in cats, baseline serum osmolality ranged from 290 to 330 mOsm/kg.[19] Plasma osmolality can be estimated from the equation:

$$\text{Calculated plasma osmolality} = 2\text{Na} + \frac{\text{BUN}}{2.8} + \frac{\text{glucose}}{18}$$

where BUN is blood urea nitrogen. In this equation, the concentrations of urea and glucose in milligrams per deciliter are converted to millimoles per liter by the conversion factors 2.8 and 18. The **measured** osmolality should not exceed the **calculated** osmolality by more than 10 mOsm/kg.[36,117] If it does, an abnormal **osmolal gap** is said to be present. This occurs when an unmeasured solute (i.e., one not accounted for in the equation) is present in large quantity in plasma (e.g., mannitol or metabolites of ethylene glycol) or when hyperlipemia or hyperproteinemia results in pseudohyponatremia (see section on hyponatremia with normal plasma osmolality).[36,43,46]

SPECIFIC GRAVITY

The term **specific gravity** refers to the ratio of the weight of a volume of liquid to the weight of an equal volume of distilled water. Specific gravity depends not only on the number of particles present in the solution but also on their molecular weight. The clinician can easily measure specific gravity with a handheld refractometer. Multiplying the last two digits of the urine specific gravity (USG) by 36 gives a rough estimate of urine osmolality in dogs.[59] This rule may be misleading if the urine sample contains a large amount of high-molecular-weight solute because substances with high molecular weights have a greater effect on specific gravity than on osmolality. The effects on urine osmolality of some solutes are shown in Table 3-2.

TONICITY OR EFFECTIVE OSMOLALITY

Changes in the osmolality of ECF may or may not initiate movement of water between the intracellular and extracellular compartments. A change in the concentration of **permeant** solutes (e.g., urea, ethanol) does not cause movement of water because these solutes are distributed equally throughout total body water (TBW). A change in the concentration of **impermeant** solutes (e.g., glucose, sodium) does cause movement of water because such solutes do not readily cross cell membranes. **Tonicity** refers to the ability of a solution to initiate water movement and is dependent on the presence of impermeant solutes in the solution.[35] Thus tonicity may be thought of as **effective osmolality**. A solution is **hypertonic** to a reference solution from which it is separated by a semipermeable membrane if its concentration of impermeant solutes is greater than that of the reference solution. A solution is **hypotonic** to the reference solution if its concentration of impermeant solutes is less than that of the reference solution. A solution is **isotonic** to the reference solution if its concentration of impermeant solutes equals that of the reference solution.

Tonicity or effective osmolality may be estimated as $P_{osm} - \text{BUN}/2.8$. Consider a dog with the following laboratory values: serum sodium, 125 mEq/L; BUN, 280 mg/dL; and glucose, 90 mg/dL. This patient is hyponatremic and azotemic and has plasma hyperosmolality (calculated plasma osmolality = 355 mOsm/kg) but hypotonicity (effective plasma osmolality = 255 mOsm/kg). Clinical measurement of osmolality by freezing-point depression osmometry does not distinguish between permeant and impermeant solutes and thus does not provide direct information about the tonicity of a solution.

DIURESIS

The term **diuresis** refers to urine flow that is greater than normal (i.e., >1 to 2 mL/kg/hr in dogs and cats). The term **solute**, or **osmotic**, diuresis refers to increased urine flow caused by excessive amounts of nonreabsorbed solute within the renal tubules (e.g., polyuria associated with diabetes mellitus, administration of mannitol). During osmotic diuresis, urine osmolality approaches plasma osmolality. The term **water** diuresis refers to increased urine flow caused by decreased reabsorption of solute-free water in the collecting ducts (e.g., polyuria associated with psychogenic polydipsia or diabetes insipidus). During water diuresis, urine osmolality is less than plasma osmolality.

The term **isosthenuria** refers to urine with an osmolality equal to that of plasma, and **hyposthenuria** refers to urine with an osmolality less than that of plasma. The term **hypersthenuria**, or **baruria**, refers to urine with an osmolality greater than that of plasma, but this term is rarely used and only to describe urine that is very concentrated.

TYPES OF DEHYDRATION

Dehydration occurs when fluid loss from the body exceeds fluid intake. Dehydration may be classified according to the type of fluid lost from the body and the

TABLE 3-2 Effect of Selected Solutes on Urine Osmolality*

Substance	Molecular Mass (daltons)	Contribution to Osmolality (mOsm/kg)
Albumin	69,000	0.144
Diatrizoate ion	613	16.313
Glucose	180	55.555

*1.0 g/dL of each of the listed solutes added to distilled water would increase specific gravity by 0.010 but would have the effects on osmolality shown in the table.

tonicity of the remaining body fluids. Pure water loss and loss of hypotonic fluid result in **hypertonic** dehydration because the tonicity of the remaining body fluids is increased. Loss of fluid with the same osmolality as that of ECF results in **isotonic** dehydration because there is no osmotic stimulus for water movement and the remaining body fluids are unchanged in tonicity. Loss of hypertonic fluid or loss of isotonic fluid with water replacement results in **hypotonic** dehydration because the remaining body fluids become hypotonic. The types of dehydration and their relative effects on the volume and tonicity of the intracellular and extracellular compartments are shown in Fig. 3-1.

SERUM SODIUM CONCENTRATION

The serum sodium concentration is an indication of the amount of sodium relative to the amount of water in the ECF and provides no direct information about total body sodium content. Patients with hyponatremia or hypernatremia may have decreased, normal, or increased total body sodium content. An increased serum sodium concentration (hypernatremia; >155 mEq/L in dogs or >162 mEq/L in cats) implies hyperosmolality, whereas a decreased serum sodium concentration (hyponatremia; <140 mEq/L in dogs or <149 mEq/L in cats) usually, but not always, implies hyposmolality. Hyponatremia develops when the patient is unable to excrete ingested water or when urinary and insensible fluid losses have a combined osmolality greater than that of ingested or parenterally administered fluids. Hypernatremia develops when water intake has been inadequate, when the lost fluid is hypotonic to ECF, or when an excessive amount of sodium has been ingested or administered parenterally.

NORMAL PHYSIOLOGY

RENAL HANDLING OF SODIUM

Sodium is filtered by the glomeruli and reabsorbed by the renal tubules. The metabolic energy (i.e., adenosine triphosphate [ATP]) for sodium transport in the kidney is required by Na^+, K^+-adenosinetriphosphatase (Na^+, K^+-ATPase) in the basolateral membranes of the tubular cells. This enzyme translocates sodium from the cytoplasm of the tubular cells to the peritubular interstitium and maintains a low intracellular concentration of sodium, which promotes sodium entry into the cell at the luminal surface.

Approximately 67% of the filtered load of sodium is reabsorbed isosmotically with water in the proximal tubules. In the early proximal tubule, sodium crosses the luminal membrane by cotransport with glucose, amino acids, and phosphate and in exchange for H^+ ions via the luminal Na^+-H^+ antiporter (during the latter process HCO_3^- is reabsorbed). Reabsorption of water and sodium with HCO_3^- and other solutes in this segment of the nephron increases the Cl^- concentration in tubular fluid and facilitates Cl^- reabsorption later in the proximal tubule. In the late proximal tubule, sodium is reabsorbed primarily with Cl^-. In this region, the luminal Na^+-H^+ antiporter works in parallel with a luminal Cl^--$anion^-$ antiporter, and the net effect is NaCl reabsorption (H^+ $anion^-$ is recycled back and forth across the membrane).

Approximately 25% of the filtered load of sodium is reabsorbed in the loop of Henle, primarily in the thick ascending limb. In the thin descending and ascending limbs of Henle's loop, sodium and Cl^- are passively reabsorbed. In the thick ascending limb, sodium crosses the

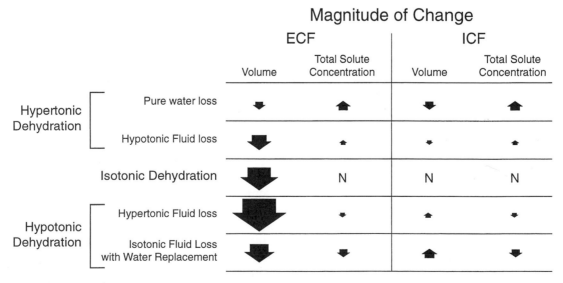

Fig. 3-I Types of dehydration. *ECF,* Extracellular fluid; *ICF,* intracellular fluid; *N,* normal. (Drawing by Tim Vojt.)

luminal membranes via the Na^+-H^+ antiporter and by an Na^+-K^+-$2Cl^-$ cotransporter.[99] This Na^+-K^+-$2Cl^-$ cotransporter is the site of action of the loop diuretics **furosemide** and **bumetanide**. There is a strong electrochemical gradient for Na^+ entry across the luminal membrane in this region (i.e., strongly lumen-positive transepithelial potential difference and high luminal sodium concentration).

Approximately 5% of the filtered load of sodium is reabsorbed in the distal convoluted tubule and connecting segment. In the early distal tubule (up to the connecting segment), sodium crosses the luminal membrane by means of an Na^+-Cl^- cotransporter. This cotransporter is inhibited by the **thiazide** diuretics.[33]

Approximately 3% of the filtered load of sodium is reabsorbed in the collecting ducts, and this segment of the nephron is responsible for altering sodium reabsorption in response to dietary fluctuations. In the late distal tubule (so-called connecting segment) and collecting ducts, sodium enters passively through Na^+ channels in the luminal membranes of the principal cells.[100,116] This movement of Na^+ generates a lumen-negative transepithelial potential difference that facilitates Cl^- reabsorption. The Na^+ channel in the principal cells is blocked by the diuretics **amiloride** and **triamterene**. One of the main effects of aldosterone is to increase the number of open luminal Na^+ channels in the cortical collecting ducts, thus altering sodium reabsorption in response to changes in dietary sodium intake. The renal tubular mechanisms for sodium reabsorption are summarized in Fig. 3-2.

RENAL REGULATION OF SODIUM BALANCE

ECF volume is directly dependent on body sodium content. The body is able to sense and respond to very small changes in sodium content. The adequacy of body sodium content is perceived as the fullness of the circulating blood volume. The term **effective circulating volume** has been used to refer to the relative fullness of the circulating portion of the extracellular compartment as perceived by the body. There are several sensors in the afferent limb of the body's regulatory system for control of sodium balance (see Table 3-1). Low-pressure mechanoreceptors (i.e., volume receptors) in the cardiac atria and pulmonary vessels and high-pressure baroreceptors (i.e., pressure receptors) in the aortic arch and carotid sinus play a primary role in the body's ability to sense the adequacy of the circulating volume. Within the kidney, the juxtaglomerular apparatus responds to changes in perfusion pressure with changes in renin production and release. Less well characterized are receptors in the liver and the central nervous system that may contribute to sodium homeostasis.

The kidney constitutes the primary efferent limb of sodium control and regulates sodium balance by excreting an amount of sodium each day equal to that ingested. There are several overlapping control mechanisms for reg-

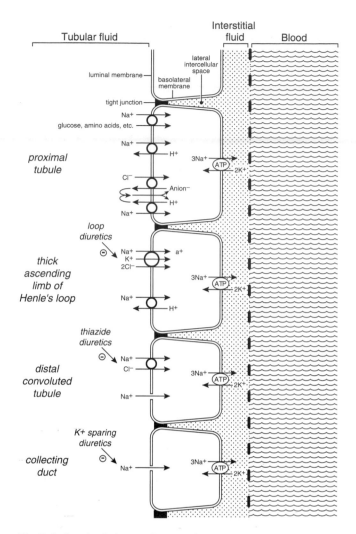

Fig. 3-2 Renal tubular mechanisms for the reabsorption of sodium along the length of the nephron. (Drawing by Tim Vojt.)

ulation of renal handling of sodium. This redundancy of controls serves to protect against sodium imbalance should one control mechanism fail. The two points of control for sodium balance in the kidney are glomerular filtration and tubular reabsorption. Autoregulation maintains renal blood flow and glomerular filtration rate (GFR) relatively constant despite fluctuations in systemic arterial pressure; thus the filtered load of sodium is also kept relatively constant (see Chapter 2).

Glomerulotubular Balance

Even slight changes in GFR have the potential to have drastic effects on sodium balance if the absolute amount of sodium reabsorbed by the tubules remains constant. Consider a normal 10-kg dog in sodium balance with a serum sodium concentration of 145 mEq/L and a GFR of 4 mL/min/kg. The daily filtered load of sodium in this dog would be 57.6 L/day × 145 mEq/L = 8352 mEq/day. If the kidneys reabsorb 99.5% of the filtered load of sodium (8310 mEq/day), the amount excreted in the urine is 42 mEq/day. Consider what would happen if there was a **primary** (i.e., **spontaneous**) increase in GFR of only 1% but the absolute amount of sodium reabsorbed remained unchanged. The filtered load of sodium would be 58.2 L/day × 145 mEq/L = 8439 mEq/day, but the amount reabsorbed would remain 8310 mEq/day. This would result in the excretion of 129 mEq/day, an amount three times that normally excreted. Under these conditions, the dog would develop negative sodium balance. Glomerulotubular balance prevents this scheme of events from occurring.

If spontaneous (primary) fluctuations in GFR occur, the absolute tubular reabsorption of filtered solutes changes in a similar direction. Thus the fraction of the filtered load that is reabsorbed remains relatively constant despite spontaneous changes in GFR. This principle is called **glomerulotubular balance**, and its mechanisms are incompletely understood.

One mechanism is related to the fact that much of the sodium in the proximal tubules is reabsorbed along with several other solutes (e.g., glucose, amino acids, phosphate, and bicarbonate). A spontaneous increase in GFR increases the filtered load of all of these solutes, and their increased concentration in the proximal tubule enhances sodium reabsorption. Changes in peritubular capillary hydrostatic and oncotic pressures probably also play an important role in glomerulotubular balance. If GFR spontaneously increases without a change in renal plasma flow (RPF) (i.e., the filtration fraction increases), the blood leaving the efferent arterioles has lower hydrostatic and higher oncotic pressures, thus favoring water and solute reabsorption in the proximal tubules (Fig. 3-3). Autoregulation (see Chapter 2) also contributes to glomerulotubular balance. When renal perfusion pressure is increased, afferent arteriolar constriction prevents transmission of the increased hydrostatic pressure to the glomerular capillaries and minimizes any increase in GFR and filtered solute load.

Ingestion of a sodium load causes thirst, water consumption, and expansion of ECF volume. These events lead to a **compensatory (secondary)** increase in GFR by increasing hydrostatic pressure and decreasing oncotic pressure in the glomerular capillaries. Increased stretching of the afferent arterioles decreases renin secretion (and ultimately angiotensin II production). Volume expansion also causes increased atrial stretch, release of atrial natriuretic peptide, and natriuresis.

There is a paradox here. How can an increase in GFR in one situation cause an increase in the tubular reabsorption of sodium and in another situation cause a decrease in the tubular reabsorption of sodium? The answer to the paradox lies in the fundamental difference between the kidney's reaction to a spontaneous (primary) increase and its reaction to a compensatory (secondary) increase in GFR. Glomerulotubular balance is evoked in the former but not the latter situation.

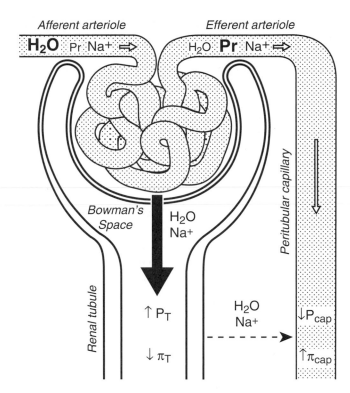

Fig. 3-3 Effects of changes in Starling forces on tubular reabsorption of water and sodium. If glomerular filtration rate (GFR) increases without a change in renal plasma flow (RPF) (or if RPF decreases more than GFR as may occur in dehydration), the filtration fraction (GFR/RPF) will increase (i.e., more water and sodium will be filtered from the glomeruli into Bowman's space). This sequence of events will result in lower hydrostatic pressure (P_{cap}) and higher oncotic pressure (π_{cap}) in the peritubular capillaries (downstream from the glomerular capillaries) and higher hydrostatic pressure (P_T) and lower oncotic pressure (π_T) in the renal tubules (downstream from Bowman's space). These changes in Starling forces will facilitate water and sodium reabsorption from the tubular fluid into the peritubular capillaries, thus minimizing loss of water and sodium in the urine. (Drawing by Tim Vojt.)

Aldosterone

Changes in renal reabsorption of sodium in response to dietary fluctuations in sodium intake are mediated by the hormone aldosterone, which is synthesized in the zona glomerulosa of the adrenal cortex. The production and release of aldosterone are stimulated by angiotensin II, hyperkalemia, and adrenocorticotropic hormone (ACTH). Its release is inhibited by dopamine and atrial natriuretic peptide. Aldosterone increases sodium reabsorption by increasing the number and activity of open sodium channels in the luminal membranes of the principal cells in the collecting ducts.

Peritubular Capillary Factors (Starling Forces)

Increased sodium intake leads to expansion of the ECF volume and compensatory increases in both GFR and RPF (i.e., the filtration fraction remains unchanged).

This increases hydrostatic pressure and decreases oncotic pressure in the peritubular capillaries, thus reducing sodium and water reabsorption in the proximal tubules. Decreased sodium intake leads to volume contraction. In this setting, RPF decreases more than GFR (i.e., the filtration fraction increases). This results in decreased hydrostatic and increased oncotic pressures in the peritubular capillaries and enhanced proximal tubular reabsorption of sodium and water (see Fig. 3-3).

Catecholamines

Catecholamine-induced vasoconstriction usually affects the efferent more than the afferent arterioles. The resultant increase in filtration fraction alters peritubular capillary hemodynamics so as to favor water and sodium reabsorption (i.e., decreased hydrostatic pressure and increased oncotic pressure). Catecholamines also directly stimulate proximal tubular sodium reabsorption through an α_1-adrenergic effect and stimulate renin release from the granular cells of the juxtaglomerular apparatus through a β_1-adrenergic effect. The angiotensin II ultimately produced also stimulates proximal tubular sodium reabsorption. The direct effects of catecholamines on proximal tubular sodium reabsorption are important because they offset the tendency of the increase in systemic arterial pressure to cause pressure natriuresis (see Pressure Natriuresis).

Angiotensin II

Decreased perfusion pressure in the afferent arterioles increases renin release from the granular cells of the juxtaglomerular apparatus and initiates the cascade of events leading to production of angiotensin II. Angiotensin II–induced vasoconstriction causes efferent more than afferent arteriolar constriction, which results in an increase in filtration fraction and changes in peritubular capillary Starling forces (decreased hydrostatic pressure and increased oncotic pressure) that facilitate proximal tubular reabsorption of sodium and water (see Fig. 3-3). Angiotensin II also directly stimulates the Na^+-H^+ antiporter in the proximal tubules, which facilitates sodium reabsorption and stimulates secretion of aldosterone from the adrenal gland.

Atrial Natriuretic Peptide

Atrial natriuretic peptide is one member of a family of natriuretic proteins that also includes brain natriuretic peptide (which ironically predominates in the cardiac ventricles) and C-type natriuretic peptide in the central nervous system.[82] Atrial natriuretic peptide is synthesized and stored in atrial myocytes until it is released in response to atrial distention caused by volume expansion. It has a number of effects that facilitate renal excretion of sodium. Atrial natriuretic peptide causes dilatation of the afferent arterioles and constriction of the efferent arterioles, leading to a primary increase in GFR. It relaxes mesangial cells, resulting in an increase in the glomerular

surface area available for filtration. Atrial natriuretic peptide also inhibits sodium reabsorption in the cortical and inner medullary collecting ducts and inhibits renin secretion, thereby decreasing production of angiotensin II and limiting the effects of angiotensin II on proximal tubular sodium reabsorption. Finally, it inhibits aldosterone secretion by adrenal zona glomerulosa.

Pressure Natriuresis

Renal sodium excretion and water excretion are markedly increased when renal arterial pressure increases even slightly without a change in GFR. The mechanism for pressure natriuresis appears to be entirely intrarenal and does not require neural or endocrine input (i.e., it occurs in the isolated denervated kidney). The effectors of sodium balance are summarized in Table 3-3.

REGULATION OF WATER BALANCE

The osmolality of ECF and serum sodium concentration are regulated by adjusting water balance. Osmoreceptors in the hypothalamus constitute the afferent limb (sensors) for regulation of water balance. Vasopressin release is stimulated when the osmoreceptors shrink in response to plasma hyperosmolality and is inhibited when they swell in response to plasma hypoosmolality. Vasopressin (water output) and thirst (water input) constitute the efferent limb (effectors) for the regulation of water balance (see Table 3-1).

Vasopressin (Antidiuretic Hormone)

Vasopressin (antidiuretic hormone [ADH]) is a nine-amino-acid peptide synthesized in neurons of the supraoptic and paraventricular nuclei in the hypothalamus (Fig. 3-4). It travels down the axons of these neurons and is released into the circulation at the level of the neurohypophysis.

Vasopressin increases the reabsorption of water in the collecting ducts of the kidney and increases the permeability of the medullary collecting ducts to urea.[1] Vasopressin attaches to V_2 receptors on the basolateral membranes of the principal cells of the cortical and medullary collecting ducts. The hormone-receptor complex activates a guanine nucleotide regulatory protein (G_s), resulting in replacement of guanosine diphosphate (GDP) with guanosine triphosphate (GTP) and stimulation of adenyl cyclase in the cell membrane. Formation of cyclic adenosine monophosphate (cAMP) results in activation of protein kinase A, which in turn phosphorylates a specific serine residue on subunits of the tetrameric aquaporin 2 (AQP2) proteins found in membranes of subapical vesicles in the cytoplasm of the principal cells. Phosphorylation results in trafficking and insertion of AQP2 water channels into the luminal membranes of the principal cells.[97,130] When vasopressin is absent or in low concentration, AQP2 channels are removed from the luminal membrane by endocytosis. Aquaporin 3 (AQP3) and 4 (AQP4) channels are found in

TABLE 3-3 Effectors of Sodium Balance

Effector	Stimuli for Release	Inhibitors of Release	Major Effects
Aldosterone	Angiotensin II Hyperkalemia Adrenocorticotropic hormone	Dopamine ANP	Increased number and activity of luminal Na^+ channels and basolateral Na^+, K^+ ATPase in principal cells of cortical collecting ducts
Angiotensin II	↓ Renal perfusion pressure*	↑ Renal perfusion pressure*	Systemic vasoconstriction Glomerular arteriolar vasoconstriction (efferent > afferent) Stimulates proximal Na^+ reabsorption Stimulates aldosterone secretion
Atrial natriuretic peptide (ANP)	↑ Atrial stretch	↓ Atrial stretch	Inhibits Na^+ reabsorption in parts of collecting duct Directly increases glomerular filtration rate
Catecholamines	↓ Effective circulating volume	↑ Effective circulating volume	Vasoconstriction Glomerular arteriolar vasoconstriction (efferent > afferent) Increase proximal tubular Na^+ reabsorption (α_1 effect) Stimulate renin release (β_1 effect)
Renin	↓ Perfusion pressure in juxtaglomerular apparatus Sympathetic nervous system activity Decreased Cl^- delivery to macula densa	Angiotensin II ANP Antidiuretic hormone	Not an "effector"—an enzyme that converts angiotensinogen to angiotensin I

Via release and action of renin.

the basolateral membranes of the principals cells and represent exit pathways for water that enters the cells via the luminal AQP2 channels. The AQP3 channel is found in the cortical and outer medullary collecting ducts, whereas AQP4 is located primarily in the inner medullary collecting

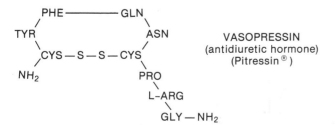

Fig. 3-4 Comparison of the chemical structures of desmopressin and vasopressin. *PHE*, Phenylalanine; *TYR*, tyrosine; *GLN*, glutamine; *ASN*, asparagine; *CYS*, cysteine; *PRO*, proline; *ARG*, arginine; *GLY*, glycine.

ducts. In the absence of vasopressin, urine osmolality can be decreased to as low as 50 mOsm/kg by continued reabsorption of sodium without water as tubular fluid passes down the collecting ducts.

The effect of vasopressin on urea reabsorption may be important in the pathogenesis of medullary washout of solute in chronic polyuric states. Chronic diuresis can lead to depletion of urea from the medullary interstitium by suppression of vasopressin release and impaired urea reabsorption in the medullary collecting ducts. During antidiuresis, urea may constitute more than 40% of the medullary solute. During diuresis, however, it may constitute less than 10% of the medullary solute.[15,83] The urinary concentrating mechanism is discussed in Chapter 2.

Stimuli for Vasopressin Release

The major stimulus for vasopressin release is hypertonicity of plasma reaching the osmoreceptors of the hypothalamus. The threshold for vasopressin release in humans corresponds to a plasma osmolality of 280 mOsm/kg, and similar or slightly higher threshold values have been observed in healthy experimental dogs.[28,107,109] Below this osmolality, vasopressin release is suppressed, and urine is maximally diluted. One hour after oral administration of water at 40 mL/kg, normal dogs developed a mean urine osmolality of 132 mOsm/kg (range, 68 to 244 mOsm/kg).[55] In humans, the release of vasopressin is maximal at a plasma osmolality of 294 mOsm/kg, and at this plasma osmolality the thirst mechanism becomes operative.[109] Thus changes in plasma osmolality as small as 1% to 2% above normal lead to maximal vasopressin release. The gain of the system is such that a 1-mOsm/kg increase in plasma osmolality leads to an almost 100-mOsm/kg increase in urine osmolality. The vasopressin system curtails water excretion, but further defense against hypertonicity requires a normal thirst mechanism and access to water. The thirst mechanism has both osmoreceptors and volume receptors. The volume receptors for the thirst mechanism are stimulated by angiotensin II and may be under control of the renin-angiotensin system.[93]

The next most important stimulus for vasopressin release is volume depletion sensed by baroreceptors in the left atrium, aortic sinus, and carotid sinuses. A decrease in blood volume of 5% to 10% lowers the threshold for vasopressin release and increases the sensitivity of the osmoregulatory mechanism (Fig. 3-5).[49,109] Nonosmotic stimulation of vasopressin by actual or perceived volume depletion plays a major role in the generation and perpetuation of hyponatremia in states of true volume depletion and in edematous states associated with hypervolemia (see Hyponatremia With Volume Depletion and Hyponatremia With Volume Excess below).

Other stimuli for vasopressin release include nausea, pain, and emotional anxiety. Many drugs and some electrolyte disturbances affect the release and renal action of vasopressin. The effects of some of these are depicted in Fig. 3-6.

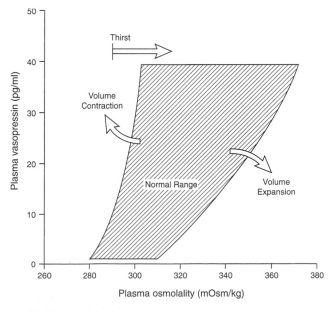

Fig. 3-5 Relationship between plasma osmolality and plasma vasopressin concentration. Volume depletion lowers the threshold for vasopressin release and increases the sensitivity of the osmoregulatory system, whereas volume expansion has the opposite effect. (Drawing by Tim Vojt.)

Role of the Kidney in Water Balance

Three conditions must be met for the kidneys to excrete a water load normally. First, there must be adequate delivery of tubular fluid to distal diluting sites (ascending limb of Henle's loop) where NaCl is removed without water, rendering the tubular fluid hypotonic to the medullary interstitium. Adequate distal delivery requires normal RPF, normal GFR, and normal isosmotic reabsorption of sodium and water from the proximal tubules mediated by aquaporin 1 (AQP1) channels in the luminal and basolateral membranes of these cells. In the presence of volume depletion, RPF is usually decreased more than GFR, and enhanced proximal tubular reabsorption of sodium and water may result from changes in postglomerular hemodynamics (see Fig. 3-3). These factors may prevent adequate distal delivery of tubular fluid for dilution.

Second, the ascending limb of Henle's loop must function normally. That is, NaCl must be removed from this segment of the nephron without water. Loop diuretics (e.g., furosemide and ethacrynic acid) impair NaCl removal from this portion of the nephron, and some interstitial renal diseases may disrupt the normal architecture of this region, leading to impaired dilution of tubular fluid in the ascending limbs of Henle's loops.

Last, in the absence of vasopressin, the collecting ducts must remain impermeable to water throughout their course. If any of these conditions is not met, a disorder of water excretion and a state of ECF hypotonicity and hyponatremia may result.

In the absence of vasopressin, the collecting ducts remain impermeable to water, the urine becomes maximally dilute, and polyuria develops. Hypertonicity and hypernatremia occur if the animal is unable to drink enough water to balance the tremendous loss of water in the urine. Hypertonicity and hypernatremia also may develop in states of osmotic diuresis (e.g., diabetes mellitus, mannitol administration, chronic renal failure, postobstructive diuresis). Urine osmolality approaches plasma osmolality during osmotic diuresis, and the solute responsible for the diuresis displaces sodium and other electrolytes in the urine.[44] Hypertonicity develops to the extent that displaced sodium remains in the ECF.

Defense Against Hypotonicity

It is crucial to the survival of the animal that the brain be protected against changes in plasma tonicity because an increase in brain water content of more than 10% is incompatible with life.[118] The fact that animals with chronic hyponatremia may have serum sodium concentrations 10% or more below normal attests to the brain's ability to adapt to hypotonicity. For example, based on osmotic considerations alone, a decrease in serum sodium concentration from 145 to 132 mEq/L would correspond to an increase in intracellular water of 10%. During acute hypotonicity, water moves into the brain. The

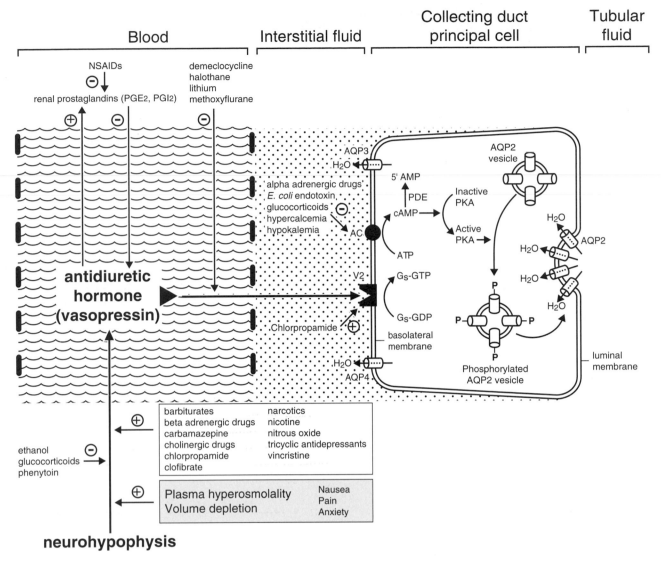

Fig. 3-6 Effects of selected drugs and electrolytes on vasopressin release and action. *AC,* Adenyl cyclase; *5'-AMP,* 5'-adenosine monophosphate; *AQP,* aquaporin; *ATP,* adenosine triphosphate; *cAMP,* cyclic adenosine monophosphate; *G_s,* stimulatory guanine nucleotide regulatory protein; *GDP,* guanosine diphosphate; *GTP,* guanosine triphosphate; *NSAIDs,* nonsteroidal antiinflammatory drugs; *PDE,* phosphodiesterase; *PGE,* prostaglandin E; *PGI,* prostacyclin; *PKA,* protein kinase A. (Drawing by Tim Vojt.)

increase in hydrostatic pressure in the interstitial compartment of the brain immediately forces sodium-containing ECF into the cerebrospinal fluid. This movement of fluid out of the brain occurs within minutes and limits the change in brain water content to much less than would be anticipated based on osmotic considerations alone.[118] During the first 24 hours of hypotonicity, movement of potassium out of cells also contributes substantially to the protection of the brain from an acute decrease in plasma osmolality. After 24 to 48 hours, a reduction in the cellular content of organic solutes contributes to the brain's

defense against hypotonicity. These organic osmolytes are substances that can be used by cells to maintain intracellular tonicity without having adverse effects on cellular metabolism and include amino acids (e.g., taurine, glutamate, and glutamine), methylamines (e.g., phosphocreatine), and polyols (e.g., *myo*-inositol). The very devices that protect the brain against plasma hypotonicity predispose it to injury when hyponatremia is corrected. Solutes lost during adaptation must be recovered, and this process requires several days. If correction of hyponatremia proceeds more quickly than recovery of lost solutes can occur, a devastating complication of treatment called osmotic demyelination syndrome (myelinolysis) may occur (see Treatment of Hyponatremia).

CLINICAL APPROACH TO THE PATIENT WITH HYPERNATREMIA

All clinical conditions associated with hypernatremia reflect hyperosmolality and hypertonicity of the ECF if the solute in question is impermeant. A deficit of pure water, loss of hypotonic fluids, or gain of sodium can cause hypertonicity of the ECF and hypernatremia. The causes of hypernatremia are listed in Box 3-1, and the clinical approach to the patient with hypernatremia is outlined in Fig. 3-7.

Box 3-1	**Causes of Hypernatremia**

Pure Water Deficit
  Primary hypodipsia (e.g., in miniature schnauzers)
  Diabetes insipidus
    Central
    Nephrogenic
  High environmental temperature
  Fever
  Inadequate access to water

Hypotonic Fluid Loss
  Extrarenal
    Gastrointestinal
      Vomiting
      Diarrhea
      Small intestinal obstruction
    Third-space loss
      Peritonitis
      Pancreatitis
    Cutaneous
      Burns
  Renal
    Osmotic diuresis
      Diabetes mellitus
      Mannitol infusion
    Chemical diuretics
    Chronic renal failure
    Nonoliguric acute renal failure
    Postobstructive diuresis

Impermeant Solute Gain
  Salt poisoning
  Hypertonic fluid administration
    Hypertonic saline
    Sodium bicarbonate
    Parenteral nutrition
    Sodium phosphate enema
  Hyperaldosteronism
  Hyperadrenocorticism

PURE WATER LOSS

When a deficit of pure water develops, the ECF becomes hypertonic in relation to the intracellular fluid (ICF), and osmotic forces cause movement of water from the intracellular to the extracellular compartment. The result is that the volume loss is shared proportionately between the extracellular and intracellular compartments. Approximately two thirds of the volume loss comes from the intracellular compartment and one third from the extracellular compartment. Plasma volume is one fourth of the ECF, and thus one twelfth of the volume loss ($\frac{1}{4} \times \frac{1}{3}$) is derived from the intravascular space. The oncotic pressure generated by plasma proteins favors retention of water within vessels, and the plasma compartment may not share proportionately in the volume loss.[35] As a result of these factors, volume depletion is usually not a clinical feature of pure water loss. It is almost impossible for a conscious animal with an intact thirst mechanism and access to water to develop hypertonicity caused by pure water loss. Thus hypertonicity associated with pure water loss usually implies that water intake has been defective.

Consider a normal 10-kg dog with a serum osmolality of 300 mOsm/kg. We assume that TBW is 60% of body weight, with 40% being intracellular and 20% extracellular, and that the major extracellular (i.e., NaCl) and intracellular (i.e., KCl) solutes are impermeant. The number of osmoles of solute in ECF would be 2 L × 300 mOsm/kg = 600 mOsm, and the number in ICF would be 4 L × 300 mOsm/kg = 1200 mOsm. Without access to drinking water, a loss of 1 L of pure water from ECF would cause water to move from ICF to ECF so as to equalize osmolality between the compartments according to the following equation:

$$\text{New ECF osmolality} = \text{new ICF osmolality}$$
$$600 \text{ mOsm}/(1 + x)\text{ L} = 1200 \text{ mOsm}/(4 - x)\text{ L}$$

where x is the volume of water moving between compartments:

$$600(4 - x) = 1200(1 + x)$$
$$x = 0.67 \text{ L}$$

The new volumes and osmolalities are:

ECF: 600 mOsm/1.67 L = 360 mOsm/kg
ICF: 1200 mOsm/3.33 L = 360 mOsm/kg

Note that the intracellular compartment has lost an amount equal to two thirds of the water deficit (0.67 L) and that the final ECF volume (1.67 L) is lower than the original volume (2 L) by an amount equal to one third of the total water deficit (0.33 L). Thus the two compartments have shared proportionately in the water loss. These changes are depicted in Fig. 3-8.

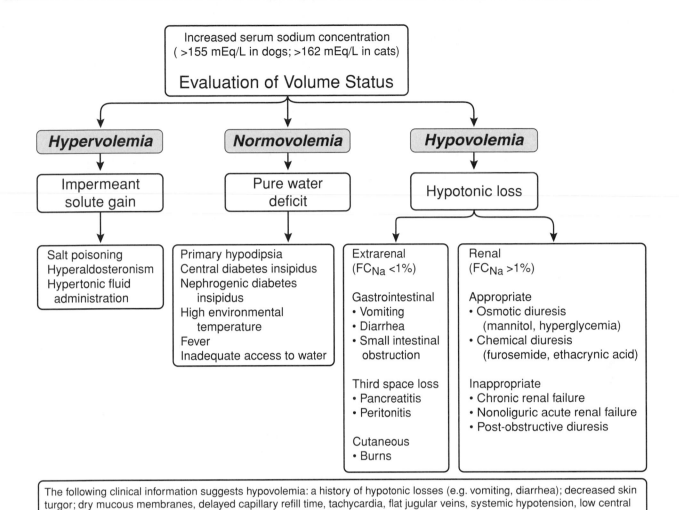

Fig. 3-7 Clinical approach to the patient with hypernatremia. FC_{Na}, Fractional clearance of sodium.

Development of a pure water deficit is uncommon in small animal medicine. The main causes of hypertonicity related to pure water deficit are hypodipsia caused by neurologic disease, and diabetes insipidus, which represents abnormal renal loss of water. Other causes of pure water deficit include respiratory losses during exposure to high environmental temperature (e.g., panting), fever, and inadequate access to water (e.g., frozen water bowl, inattentive owner).

Rarely, chronic hypernatremia may occur in fully conscious animals that have access to water. In these cases, abnormal osmoregulation of ADH release caused by underlying hypothalamic lesions results in hypodipsia. Animals that are unable to obtain water because central nervous system disease has resulted in an altered sensorium may also be hypernatremic, but in these instances, the hypernatremia is simply a result of water deprivation. Hypodipsic hypernatremia related to defective osmoregulation of ADH has been reported in a dog with hydrocephalus and normal pituitary function.[28] In normal individuals, administration of hypertonic saline increases plasma osmolality and simultaneously causes volume expansion. Osmoreceptors are stimulated by hyperosmolality but inhibited by volume expansion. Normally the response to hyperosmolality takes precedence, and ADH secretion increases, resulting in decreased urine volume and increased urine osmolality. The affected dog experienced increased urine volume and decreased urine osmolality in response to an infusion of hypertonic saline, indicating defective osmoreceptor function as observed in human patients with hypodipsic hypernatremia. Similarly, destruction of osmoreceptors in the hypothalamus was thought to be responsible for adipsia and hypernatremia in a dog with focal granulomatous meningoencephalitis.[89] Weakness and polymyopathy have been reported in a young cat with hypodipsia, hypernatremia, and hypertonicity associated with hydrocephalus and hypopituitarism, and hypernatremia, adipsia, and diabetes insipidus have been observed in a young dalmatian dog with dysplasia of the rostral diencephalon.[5,30]

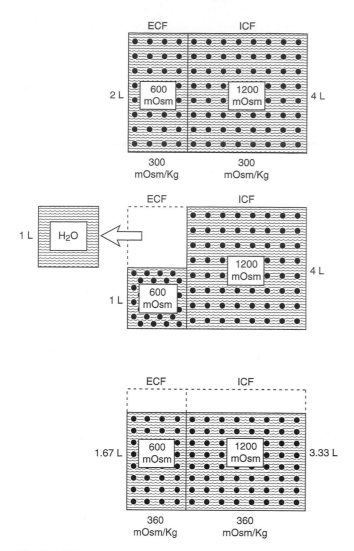

Fig. 3-8 Effect of loss of 1 L of water on volume and tonicity of extracellular fluid (ECF) and intracellular fluid (ICF). (Drawing by Tim Vojt.)

Hypodipsia, hypernatremia, and hypertonicity caused by an abnormal thirst mechanism have been reported in young female miniature schnauzers and in a young Great Dane.[24,58,64,125] One miniature schnauzer with hypodipsic hypernatremia had severe behavioral disturbances, and holoprosencephaly was found at necropsy.[120] However, grossly visible neuroanatomic abnormalities were not identified in a previous report.[24] Whether a spectrum of neuroanatomic abnormalities exists in these dogs (which appear to have a form of congenital adipsic hypernatremia) is not known. Infusion of hypertonic saline has been shown to lead to an increase in urine volume and a decrease in urine osmolality compatible with defective osmoregulation of ADH.[24] Clinical signs in affected dogs are associated with hypertonicity and include anorexia, lethargy, weakness, disorientation, ataxia, and seizures. Affected dogs can be managed clinically by addition of water to their food, but hypernatremia and neurologic

dysfunction recur whenever water supplementation is discontinued. In a Norwegian elkhound with adipsic hypernatremia, the adipsia resolved spontaneously at 2 years of age.[51]

Central or pituitary diabetes insipidus (CDI) is caused by a partial or complete lack of vasopressin production and release from the neurohypophysis.[53] It may result from trauma or neoplasia or may be idiopathic in dogs and cats.* Visceral larva migrans has also been reported to cause CDI in a dog.[84] In one dog with hypernatremia, hypertonicity, and gastric dilatation-volvulus, CDI was present and caused by neurohypophyseal atrophy secondary to a cystic craniopharyngeal duct.[32] Congenital CDI is rare[48,73,129] but has been reported in two sibling Afghan pups.[104] Traumatic CDI may be transient in nature. Hypophysectomy for treatment of hyperadrenocorticism results in transient CDI that may take several weeks to resolve.[87] Marked hypernatremia occurs in dogs in the first 24 hours after hypophysectomy and can be prevented by prophylactic treatment with desmopressin (DDAVP).[52] In the month after surgery, serum sodium concentrations in control dogs were not markedly different from those observed in the DDAVP-treated group, suggesting that the dogs with untreated CDI drank sufficient water to maintain relatively normal plasma osmolality. The transient nature of CDI after hypophysectomy may result from the fact that some of the vasopressin-producing neurons from the hypothalamus terminate in the median eminence.

Animals with CDI have severe polydipsia and polyuria. Their urine typically is hyposthenuric (urine osmolality, 60 to 200 mOsm/kg), but urine osmolality may approach 400 to 500 mOsm/kg in the presence of dehydration. Variability in USG and urine osmolality values at the time of presentation in dogs and cats with diabetes insipidus presumably is related to hydration status and severity of vasopressin deficiency. In one study, dogs were classified as having complete or partial CDI based on the magnitude of increase in their USG and urine osmolality after induction of 5% dehydration.[53] Dogs with complete CDI had USG values of 1.001 to 1.007 that did not change substantially after induction of 5% dehydration, whereas dogs with partial CDI has USG values of 1.002 to 1.016 that increased to 1.010 to 1.018 after induction of 5% dehydration. In both groups, there was a substantial (>50%) increase in USG 2 hours after administration of 1 to 5 U of aqueous arginine vasopressin. Affected dogs responded well to administration of DDAVP acetate (1 to 2 drops in both eyes every 12 to 24 hours), but the prognosis was dependent on the underlying cause of CDI. Many older dogs with CDI had tumors in the region of the pituitary gland and developed neurologic signs.

*References 4,16,26,39,47,48,60,91,96,103,106,111.

Increased plasma osmolality and hypernatremia may occur in dogs and cats with CDI. These results suggest that some affected dogs and cats do not obtain enough water to maintain water balance and are presented in a hypertonic state. Severe hypernatremia and neurologic dysfunction may occur if the animal cannot maintain adequate water intake.[32,106] In contrast, with psychogenic polydipsia, plasma osmolality and serum sodium concentration may be lower than normal at presentation.[77] Administration of vasopressin leads to an increase in urine osmolality or specific gravity in dogs and cats with CDI, but the initial response may be less than expected because of renal medullary washout of solute. In one study, USG values increased to 1.018 to 1.022 after vasopressin administration in dogs with complete CDI and to 1.018 to 1.036 in dogs with partial CDI.[53]

Treatment with vasopressin restores medullary hypertonicity and normal urinary concentrating ability. Historically, vasopressin tannate in oil (pitressin tannate) has been used to treat CDI in small animal practice. The dosage is 3 to 5 U for dogs or 1 to 2 U for cats given intramuscularly or subcutaneously every 24 to 72 hours as needed to control polyuria and polydipsia. To avoid the possibility of water intoxication, it is recommended that the treatment interval be determined by recurrence of polyuria. This product is no longer commercially available.

DDAVP is a structural analog of vasopressin (see Fig. 3-4) that has a more potent antidiuretic effect than vasopressin but minimal vasopressive effect and is relatively resistant to metabolic degradation. DDAVP is available as a nasal spray (0.1 mg/mL), injectable solution (4 µg/mL), or tablet for oral administration (0.1 and 0.2 mg). The injectable solution is much more expensive than the nasal spray, and the nasal spray has been used subcutaneously in dogs and in a cat with CDI at a dosage of 1 µg/kg without adverse effects.[73,74] Polyuria and polydipsia in a cat with CDI were controlled with 1 µg/kg administered subcutaneously every 12 hours or 1.5 µg/kg administered conjunctivally every 8 hours. One drop of the nasal spray contains 1.5 to 4 µg of DDAVP, and the duration of effect varies from 8 to 24 hours.[37] In humans, the bioavailability of DDAVP after oral administration was 0.1% as compared with 3% to 5% after intranasal administration, and gastrointestinal absorption was improved when it was given in a fasted state.[40,108] In dogs, an antidiuretic effect was observed even after orally administered doses as low as 50 µg.[126]

Chlorpropamide is a sulfonylurea hypoglycemic agent that potentiates the renal tubular effects of small amounts of vasopressin and may be useful in management of animals with partial CDI. Its effect may occur by up-regulation of ADH receptors in the kidney.[31] The recommended dosage of chlorpropamide is 10 to 40 mg/kg/day orally, and hypoglycemia is a potential adverse effect. It has been useful in the management of CDI (up to 50% reduction in urine output) in some reports but not in others, possibly because some animals have partial and some have complete CDI.[73,111]

In the broadest sense, the term nephrogenic diabetes insipidus (NDI) may be used to describe a diverse group of disorders in which structural or functional abnormalities interfere with the ability of the kidneys to concentrate urine (Box 3-2).[11,76] Congenital NDI is a rare disorder in small animal medicine.[11,68,76] Affected animals are presented at a very young age for severe polyuria and polydipsia. In reported cases, urine osmolality and specific gravity have been in the hyposthenuric range. Affected animals show no response to water deprivation testing, exogenous vasopressin administration, or hypertonic saline infusion. In one case report, the plasma vasopressin concentration was markedly increased.[68] Congential NDI in human patients can arise from mutations in the V2 receptor (X-linked recessive inheritance) or from mutations in the AQP2 channel (autosomal recessive inheritance). Low affinity V2 receptors were thought to be responsible for congenital NDI in a family of Siberian huskies.[88]

Thiazide diuretics (chlorothiazide 20 to 40 mg/kg every 12 hours or hydrochlorothiazide 2.5 to 5.0 mg/kg twice a day) have been used to treat animals with CDI and

---

Box 3-2 Causes of Nephrogenic Diabetes Insipidus

Congenital (primary)
Acquired (secondary)
  Functional
    Drugs
      Glucocorticoids
      Lithium
      Demeclocycline
      Methoxyflurane
      Escherichia coli endotoxin (e.g., pyelonephritis, pyometra)
      Diuretics
    Electrolyte disturbances
      Hypokalemia
      Hypercalcemia
    Altered medullary hypertonicity
      Hypoadrenocorticism
    Multifactorial or unknown mechanism
      Hepatic insufficiency
      Hyperthyroidism
      Hyperadrenocorticism
    Postobstructive diuresis
    Acromegaly
  Structural
    Medullary interstitial amyloidosis (e.g., in cats, shar-pei dog)
    Polycystic kidney disease
    Chronic pyelonephritis
    Chronic interstitial nephritis

NDI. Diuretic administration results in mild dehydration, enhanced proximal renal tubular reabsorption of sodium, decreased delivery of tubular fluid to the distal nephron, and reduced urine output. Thiazides have been reported to result in a 20% to 50% reduction in urine output in dogs with NDI and in cats with CDI.[11,16,73,76,121] In other reports, thiazides were reported to be ineffective in reducing urine output in a dog and a cat with CDI.[47,60] Restriction of dietary sodium and protein reduces the amount of solute that must be excreted in the urine each day and thus further reduces obligatory water loss and polyuria. A low-salt diet and hydrochlorothiazide (2 mg/kg orally twice a day) were used successfully to manage a dog with congenital NDI for 2 years.[121] The dog's water consumption decreased from an average of approximately 900 mL/kg/day to 200 mL/kg/day with treatment.

HYPOTONIC FLUID LOSS

When hypotonic fluid is lost from the extracellular compartment, the osmotic stimulus for water to move from the intracellular to the extracellular compartment is less than the stimulus for water movement created by pure water loss. Thus hypotonic losses cause a greater reduction in the ECF volume, and the animal is more likely to show clinical signs of volume depletion (e.g., tachycardia, weak pulses, and delayed capillary refill time). As the tonicity of the fluid lost increases toward the normal tonicity of ECF, the volume deficit of the extracellular compartment becomes progressively more severe (Fig. 3-9). In the case of isotonic losses, no osmotic stimulus for water movement is present. The entire loss is borne by the extracellular compartment, and hypovolemic shock may occur if the loss has been of sufficient magnitude (e.g., severe hemorrhage).

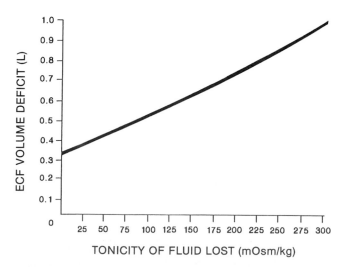

Fig. 3-9 Magnitude of extracellular fluid (ECF) volume deficit caused by loss of 1 L of fluid of varying tonicity.

Consider what would occur in the previous example if our 10-kg dog suffered a loss from the extracellular compartment of 1 L of fluid with an osmolality of 150 mOsm/kg. Such a loss would leave 450 mOsm of solute and 1 L of water in the extracellular compartment. Once again, water moves from the intracellular to the extracellular compartment until the osmolality has been equalized. Thus:

$$\text{New ECF osmolality} = \text{new ICF osmolality}$$
$$450 \text{ mOsm}/(1 + x) \text{ L} = 1200 \text{ mOsm}/(4 - x) \text{ L}$$

where x is the volume of water moving between compartments:

$$450(4 - x) = 1200(1 + x)$$
$$x = 0.36 \text{ L}$$

The new volumes and osmolalities are:

ECF: 450 mOsm/1.36 L   = 330 mOsm/kg
ICF: 1200 mOsm/3.64 L = 330 mOsm/kg

Note that the extracellular volume deficit is more severe than in the previous example of pure water loss (0.64 L versus 0.33 L). These changes are depicted in Fig. 3-10. The more closely the fluid lost approximates ECF in tonicity, the greater the volume loss from the ECF compartment.

For simplicity, these examples are based on many assumptions that in reality may not be true. For example, TBW is not 60% of body weight in all individuals, the number of osmoles in the ECF may have been altered by electrolyte losses not detected clinically, the effects of hydrostatic forces resulting from extracellular volume depletion have not been considered, some solutes may not be strictly impermeant, and compensatory physiologic responses have not been considered. Nonetheless, such calculations are helpful in understanding the pathophysiology of hypertonic states, and they provide useful clinical approximations.

Hypotonic fluid losses are the most common type encountered in small animal medicine. They may be classified as extrarenal (e.g., gastrointestinal, third-space loss, and cutaneous) or renal. Causes of gastrointestinal losses include vomiting, diarrhea, and small intestinal obstruction; causes of third-space losses include pancreatitis and peritonitis. Cutaneous losses are usually not clinically important in dogs and cats. Eccrine sweat glands are limited to the foot pads and serve no thermoregulatory function, and burns are encountered uncommonly in small animal practice. Renal losses may result from osmotically (e.g., diabetes mellitus, mannitol) or chemically (e.g., furosemide, corticosteroids) induced diuresis or from defective urinary concentrating ability related to intrinsic renal disease (e.g., chronic

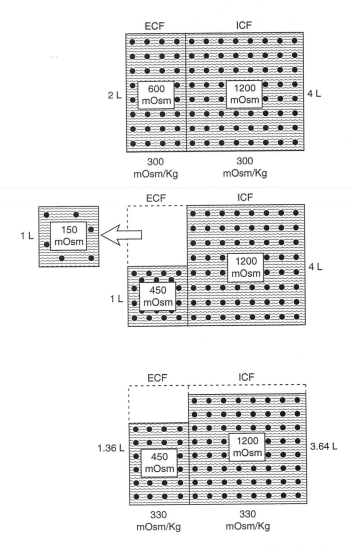

Fig. 3-10 Effect of loss of 1 L of hypotonic fluid (150 mOsm/kg) on volume and tonicity of extracellular fluid (ECF) and intracellular fluid (ICF). (Drawing by Tim Vojt.)

renal failure, nonoliguric acute renal failure, postobstructive diuresis).

GAIN OF IMPERMEANT SOLUTE

Gain of impermeant solute is uncommon in small animal medicine. The addition of a sodium salt to ECF causes hypernatremia, whereas gain of an impermeant solute that does not contain sodium (e.g., glucose and mannitol) initially causes hyponatremia because water is drawn into ECF. However, hypernatremia occurs as osmotic diuresis develops because urine osmolality approaches plasma osmolality and the sodium-free solute replaces sodium in urine. The sodium displaced from the urine remains in the ECF and contributes to hypernatremia.

The development of hypertonicity as a result of excessive salt ingestion is unlikely if the animal in question has an intact thirst mechanism and access to water. The addition of impermeant solute without water expands the extracellular compartment at the expense of the intracellular compartment as water moves from ICF to ECF to equalize osmolality. This volume overload may lead to pulmonary edema if the patient has underlying cardiac disease. Consider again our example of the 10-kg dog. The addition of 200 mOsm of solute to the ECF without any water would be equivalent to ingestion of 5.85 g of sodium chloride (5.85 g NaCl = 100 mmol Na and 100 mmol Cl). The addition of this impermeant solute to ECF causes movement of water from the intracellular to extracellular compartments until osmolality has been equalized. Thus:

$$\text{New ECF osmolality} = \text{new ICF osmolality}$$
$$800 \text{ mOsm}/(2 + x)\text{ L} = 1200 \text{ mOsm}/(4 - x)\text{ L}$$

where x is the volume of water moving between compartments:

$$800(4 - x) = 1200(z + x)$$
$$x = 0.4 \text{ L}$$

The new volumes and osmolalities are:

ECF: 800 mOsm/2.4 L   = 333 mOsm/kg
ICF: 1200 mOsm/3.6 L   = 333 mOsm/kg

Note that ECF volume has been expanded by 0.4 L and that this volume has been derived from ICF. In the normal animal, this expansion of the extracellular compartment leads to natriuresis, and the volume deficit is repaired by ingestion of water in response to plasma hyperosmolality. These changes are depicted in Fig. 3-11.

In one report of salt poisoning in dogs, a defective water softener resulted in delivery of drinking water containing 10% sodium chloride as compared with normal tap water containing less than 0.1%.[66] The affected dogs developed progressive ataxia, seizures, prostration, and death. Their serum sodium concentrations ranged from 185 to 190 mEq/L. Histopathology showed focal areas of perivascular hemorrhage and edema in the midbrain. In another case report, presumptive salt poisoning resulted from ingestion of seawater and subsequent restriction of fresh drinking water.[20] Another dog developed fatal hypernatremia after it ingested a large amount of a salt-flour mix.[71] After ingestion of a salt-flour figurine, the dog began vomiting and developed polyuria and polydipsia. The owner removed the dog's water source, and it ingested more of the salt-flour mix. Seizures, pyrexia, and sinus tachycardia developed, and the serum sodium concentration reached 211 mEq/L.

Therapeutic administration of hyperosmolar solutions containing large amounts of sodium during cardiac resuscitation can cause hypernatremia and hypertonicity (e.g., hypertonic saline, sodium bicarbonate). For example,

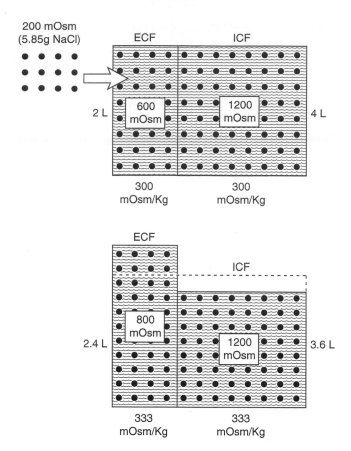

200 mOsm
(5.85g NaCl)

ECF — ICF

600 mOsm — 1200 mOsm

2 L — 4 L

300 mOsm/Kg — 300 mOsm/Kg

ECF

ICF

800 mOsm — 1200 mOsm

2.4 L — 3.6 L

333 mOsm/Kg — 333 mOsm/Kg

Fig. 3-11 Effect of addition of 200 mOsm solute (5.85 g NaCl) on volume and tonicity of extracellular fluid (ECF) and intracellular fluid (ICF). (Drawing by Tim Vojt.)

serum sodium concentration reached 174 mEq/L within 15 minutes after beginning infusion of 7.2% NaCl at a rate of 15 mL/kg in normal beagles.[2] Sodium phosphate enemas may also result in mild hypernatremia.[3] Primary hyperaldosteronism is rare in dogs, but several cases have been reported in cats (see Chapter 5 for more information). Mild hypernatremia also may occur in dogs with hyperadrenocorticism.[86,101]

CLINICAL SIGNS OF HYPERNATREMIA

The clinical signs of hypernatremia primarily are neurologic and related to osmotic movement of water out of brain cells. A rapid decrease in brain volume may cause rupture of cerebral vessels and focal hemorrhage. The severity of clinical signs is related more to the rapidity of onset of hypernatremia than to the magnitude of hypernatremia. In dogs and cats, clinical signs of hypernatremia are observed when the serum sodium concentration exceeds 170 mEq/L.[54,66,71,106] If hypernatremia develops slowly, the brain has time to adapt to the hypertonic state by production of intracellular solutes (e.g., inositol and amino acids) called **osmolytes** or **idiogenic osmoles**. These substances prevent dehydration of the brain and

allow patients with chronic hypernatremia to be relatively asymptomatic.

Where described in dogs and cats, clinical signs of hypernatremia and hypertonicity have included anorexia, lethargy, vomiting, muscular weakness, behavioral change, disorientation, ataxia, seizures, coma, and death.* If hypotonic losses are the cause of hypernatremia, clinical signs of volume depletion (e.g., tachycardia, weak pulses, and delayed capillary refill time) may be observed on physical examination. If hypernatremia has developed as a result of gain of sodium, signs of volume overload (e.g., pulmonary edema) may be observed, especially in patients with underlying cardiac disease. Patients with CDI or NDI typically are presented for evaluation of severe polydipsia and polyuria.

TREATMENT OF HYPERNATREMIA

The main goals in treating patients with hypernatremia are to replace the water and electrolytes that have been lost and, if necessary, to facilitate renal excretion of excess sodium. The first priority in treatment should be to restore the ECF volume to normal. The next priority is to diagnose and treat the underlying disease responsible for the water and electrolyte deficits.

PURE WATER LOSS

Total body solute (TBS) is the product of TBW and plasma osmolality (P_{osm}). If a patient's fluid loss has been limited to pure water, the following relationship is true:

$$\text{TBS (present)} = \text{TBS (previous)}$$
$$\text{TBW (present)} \times P_{osm} \text{ (present)} = \text{TBW (previous)} \times P_{osm} \text{ (previous)}$$

If we assume that body water (TBW) is 60% of body weight measured in kilograms (Wt) and that $2.1 \times P_{Na}$ is an estimate of P_{osm}:

$$2.1 \times P_{Na} \text{ (present)} \times 0.6 \times \text{Wt (present)}$$
$$= 2.1 \times P_{Na} \text{ (previous)} \times 0.6 \, \text{Wt (previous)}$$

This equation reduces to:

$$P_{Na} \text{ (present)} \times \text{Wt (present)} =$$
$$P_{Na} \text{ (previous)} \times \text{Wt (previous)}$$

$$\text{Wt (previous)} = \frac{P_{Na} \text{ (present)} \times \text{Wt (present)}}{P_{Na} \text{ (previous)}}$$

The water deficit is the difference between the previous and present body weights:

$$\text{Wt (previous)} - \text{Wt (present)} =$$
$$\frac{P_{Na} \text{ (present)} \times \text{Wt (present)}}{P_{Na} \text{ (previous)}} - \text{Wt (present)}$$

*References 5,20,24,28,30,66,71,106,125.

or

$$Wt\,(present) \times \left(\frac{P_{Na}\,(present)}{P_{Na}\,(previous)} - 1 \right)$$

Consider a previously normal dog that has been deprived of water for several days. The dog weighs 10 kg at presentation, and its serum sodium concentration is 170 mEq/L. Assuming a previously normal serum sodium concentration of 145 mEq/L, the dog's water deficit can be calculated:

$$Water\,deficit = Wt\,(present) \times \left(\frac{P_{Na}\,(present)}{P_{Na}\,(previous)} - 1 \right)$$

$$Water\,deficit = 10 \left[\left(\frac{170}{145} - 1 \right) \right] = 1.72\,L$$

The original estimates of TBW and serum sodium concentration may be modified based on information available to the clinician at presentation. For example, if the dog's normal serum sodium concentration is known from a previous admission, this value can be substituted in place of 145 mEq/L. If the dog's previous normal body weight is known, the water deficit may simply be estimated as the difference between the previous and present body weights. The assumption inherent in the latter calculation is that the patient has not gained or lost tissue mass. For a short period, this is a reasonable assumption because loss of 1 kg of tissue mass requires an expenditure of approximately 1600 kcal. This caloric expenditure would require fasting for 2 to 3 days in a normal 10-kg dog with a basal energy requirement of approximately 700 kcal.

A pure water deficit can be replaced by giving 5% dextrose in water intravenously. This solution technically is only slightly hypotonic to plasma (278 mOsm/kg), but the glucose ultimately enters cells and is metabolized so that administration of 5% dextrose is equivalent to administration of water. The water deficit must be replaced and hypernatremia corrected slowly over 48 hours. The brain adapts to hypertonicity by the production of osmolytes or idiogenic osmoles that prevent cellular dehydration. Excessively rapid lowering of the serum sodium concentration may result in movement of water into brain cells and development of cerebral edema. In human patients, correction of the serum sodium concentration at a rate of less than 0.5 mEq/L/hr minimizes the risk of neurologic complications related to water intoxication.[119] The animal's serum sodium concentration should be monitored serially during replacement of the water deficit.

HYPOTONIC LOSS

As described earlier, hypotonic losses cause more severe extracellular volume contraction than do losses of pure water. As the tonicity of the fluid lost approaches the tonicity of ECF, the extracellular volume deficit becomes greater (see Fig. 3-9). As a result, signs of volume deple-tion are more likely with hypotonic losses, and the original replacement fluid should be isotonic so that extracellular volume repletion proceeds rapidly.

In the presence of hemorrhagic shock, whole blood, plasma, or a colloid solution is the ideal fluid to administer. The hemoglobin in whole blood improves oxygen-carrying capacity. The plasma proteins in whole blood and plasma or the dextrans in a colloid solution increase and maintain intravascular volume by increasing oncotic pressure. In many animals that have experienced severe hypotonic losses over an extended time period, replacement of the ECF volume with an isotonic crystalloid solution (e.g., 0.9% NaCl and lactated Ringer's solution) is adequate. A volume up to four times the suspected intravascular deficit may be required because the isotonic crystalloid solution distributes rapidly throughout the ECF compartment (ECF volume is four times intravascular volume). After the extracellular volume has been expanded, hypotonic fluids (e.g., 0.45% NaCl and half-strength lactated Ringer's solution) can be administered to provide fluids for maintenance needs and ongoing losses (see Chapter 14).

GAIN OF IMPERMEANT SOLUTE

The patient with an excess of sodium-containing impermeant solute in the ECF can be treated by administration of 5% dextrose intravenously. The main disadvantage of this approach is that it causes further expansion of the extracellular compartment in a patient already suffering from ECF volume expansion. In an animal with normal cardiac and renal function, this volume expansion leads to diuresis and natriuresis, and ECF volume returns to normal. In an animal with underlying cardiac disease or oliguria related to primary renal disease, this approach may lead to development of pulmonary edema. Administration of a loop diuretic (e.g., furosemide and ethacrynic acid) promotes excretion of the existing sodium load and hastens return of ECF volume to normal. As in the case of pure water deficit, it is essential that fluid administration proceeds slowly and that serum sodium concentration be lowered gradually over 48 hours to avoid neurologic complications.

CLINICAL APPROACH TO THE PATIENT WITH HYPONATREMIA

The presence of hyponatremia usually, but not always, implies hypoosmolality. Thus the first step in the approach to the patient with hyponatremia is to determine whether hypoosmolality of the ECF is present. This can be determined by measurement of plasma osmolality. The evaluation of hyponatremia then may be approached using the patient's plasma osmolality as a guide. This approach is outlined in Fig. 3-12, and the causes of hyponatremia are listed in Box 3-3.

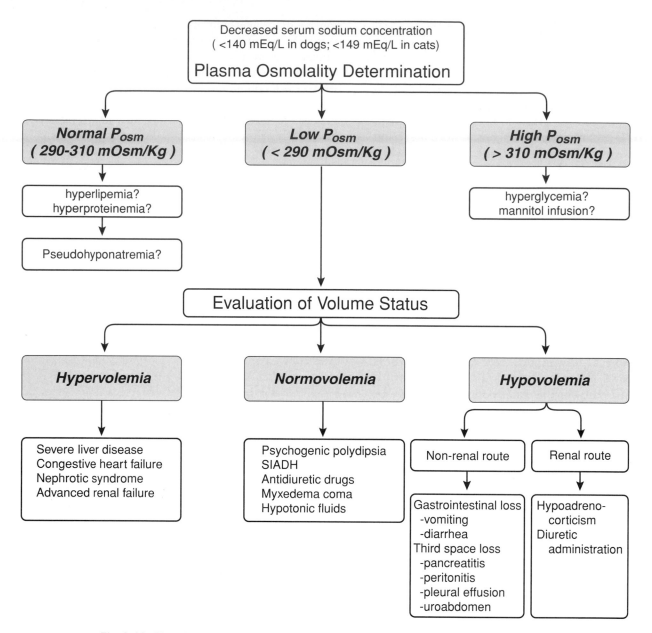

Fig. 3-12 Clinical approach to the patient with hyponatremia. P_{osm}, Plasma osmolality; *SIADH,* syndrome of inappropriate antidiuretic hormone. (From DiBartola SP: Hyponatremia, *Vet Clin North Am Small Anim Pract* 28:515-532, 1998.)

HYPONATREMIA WITH NORMAL PLASMA OSMOLALITY

Sodium is present as charged particles in the aqueous phase of body fluids. Approximately 93% of plasma volume is occupied by water, and the remaining 7% consists largely of proteins and lipids. Historically, serum sodium concentration has been measured by flame photometry. Flame photometry measures the number of sodium ions in a specific volume of plasma or serum. Thus the sodium concentration is measured as if the sodium ions were present throughout the entire sample volume, whereas actually they are active only in the aqueous phase. Normally this error is small. In plasma or serum samples containing a large amount of lipid or protein, however, the error may be larger, and the decrease in measured serum sodium concentration could be misleading to the clinician (Fig. 3-13). When serum sodium concentration is measured by direct potentiometry using ion-selective electrodes, large amounts of lipid or protein in the sample should not affect the measured serum sodium concentration. However, if the serum sample is diluted before measurement, large amounts of lipid or protein may still affect the measured serum sodium concentration.[75] Therefore the clinician must be familiar with the laboratory method used so as to interpret serum sodium concentrations properly. The occurrence of a decreased serum sodium concentra-

Box 3-3	Causes of Hyponatremia

With Normal Plasma Osmolality
Hyperlipemia
Hyperproteinemia

With High Plasma Osmolality
Hyperglycemia
Mannitol infusion

With Low Plasma Osmolality
And hypervolemia
  Severe liver disease
  Congestive heart failure
  Nephrotic syndrome
  Advanced renal failure
And normovolemia
  Psychogenic polydipsia
  Syndrome of inappropriate antidiuretic hormone secretion
  Antidiuretic drugs (see Fig. 3-6)
  Myxedema coma of hypothyroidism
  Hypotonic fluid infusion
And hypovolemia
  Gastrointestinal loss
    Vomiting
    Diarrhea
  Third-space loss
    Pancreatitis
    Peritonitis
    Uroabdomen
    Pleural effusion (e.g., chylothorax)
    Peritoneal effusion
  Cutaneous loss
    Burns
  Hypoadrenocorticism
  Diuretic administration

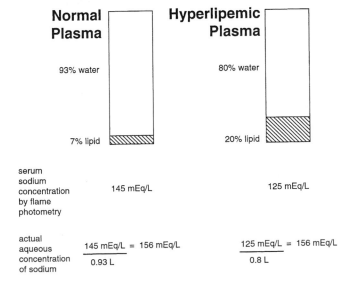

Fig. 3-13 Effect of increased plasma lipids on serum sodium concentration (pseudohyponatremia or factitious hyponatremia). (From DiBartola SP: Hyponatremia, *Vet Clin North Am Small Anim Pract* 28:515-532, 1998.)

tion as a result of laboratory methodology in the presence of normal plasma osmolality is called **pseudohyponatremia** or **factitious hyponatremia**. Pseudohyponatremia occurs in conditions associated with hyperlipidemia or severe hyperproteinemia.

Plasma osmolality in patients with pseudohyponatremia is normal because lipids and proteins are very large molecules that contribute very little to plasma osmolality. If pseudohyponatremia is present, the calculated plasma osmolality is low because of a spuriously low serum sodium concentration, whereas the measured osmolality is normal. Thus when an abnormal osmolal gap is present and the measured osmolality is normal, pseudohyponatremia should be suspected. The diagnosis of pseudohyponatremia can be made by visual inspection of plasma for lipemia and by measurement of the total plasma protein concentration. Hyperlipemia severe enough to cause pseudohyponatremia is visible to the naked eye as lactescent plasma. Each milligram per deciliter of lipid in serum reduces the sodium concentration by 0.002 mEq/L (e.g., a serum triglyceride concentration of 1000 mg/dL would be expected to reduce the serum sodium concentration by 2 mEq/L).[95] In the case of hyperproteinemia, each gram per deciliter of protein above a concentration of 8 g/dL reduces the serum sodium concentration by approximately 0.25 mEq/L (e.g., the serum sodium concentration of a patient with a serum protein concentration of 12 g/dL would be expected to be reduced by 1 mEq/L).[118] At such protein concentrations the plasma may be viscous, and this is likely to occur mainly in patients with plasma cell dyscrasias. Thus whereas pseudohyponatremia may be intellectually interesting, it is unlikely to be of clinical relevance in most instances. Furthermore, pseudohyponatremia itself has no consequences for the health of the patient. Its importance lies in the ability of the clinician to recognize it and refrain from treating the patient for hyponatremia. Treatment should be directed at the underlying disorder causing hyperproteinemia or hyperlipidemia.

HYPONATREMIA WITH INCREASED PLASMA OSMOLALITY

If an impermeant solute is added to ECF, water moves from ICF to ECF, and the osmolality of both compartments increases (see Fig. 3-11).[35] If the added solute is something other than sodium, the serum sodium concentration is reduced by the translocation of water, but the plasma osmolality is higher than normal.

Hyponatremia with hyperosmolality is usually caused by hyperglycemia in diabetes mellitus, wherein each 100-mg/dL increase in glucose may decrease the serum sodium concentration by 1.6 mEq/L.[69] This correction factor worked well up to a blood glucose concentration of 440 mg/dL in a study in normal humans made transiently hyperglycemic by infusion of somatostatin, but the correction factor was much greater at higher blood glucose concentrations.[61] The authors concluded that an overall correction factor of a 2.4-mEq/L decrement in sodium for each 100-mg/dL increment in glucose would be preferable. In the diabetic patient, both hyperlipidemia and hyperglycemia may contribute to decreased serum sodium concentration. Administration of the osmotic diuretic mannitol also can cause hyponatremia with plasma hyperosmolality. The calculated osmolality is normal, the measured osmolality is high, and the osmolal gap is increased in the presence of mannitol, which is an unmeasured osmole. Hyperglycemia does not affect the osmolal gap because the plasma glucose concentration is part of the equation used to calculate plasma osmolality (i.e., it is a measured osmole).

Initially, TBW content is not altered in the setting of hyponatremia with hyperosmolality. Rather, there is an altered distribution of water between intracellular and extracellular compartments. However, a reduction in TBW content develops to the extent that these substances cause an osmotic diuresis.

HYPONATREMIA WITH DECREASED PLASMA OSMOLALITY

The total body sodium content and ECF volume of patients with hyponatremia and hypoosmolality may be normal, decreased, or increased. Therefore the second step in the evaluation of the patient with hyponatremia is to estimate total body sodium content and ECF volume status. This is best done by clinical assessment of the patient based on history, physical examination, and a few ancillary tests. A good history often indicates a source of fluid loss (e.g., vomiting, diarrhea, or diuretic administration), and the physical examination provides important clues to the patient's volume status. The following physical findings should be assessed: skin turgor, moistness of the mucous membranes, capillary refill time, pulse rate and character, appearance of the jugular veins (distended or flat), and presence or absence of ascites or edema. Measurements of hematocrit and total plasma protein concentration, as well as systemic blood pressure and central venous pressure determinations, if available, further clarify the patient's ECF volume status.

Hyponatremia with Volume Depletion

For a patient with volume depletion (hypovolemia) to develop hyponatremia, the total body deficit of sodium must exceed that of water. Hyponatremic patients with volume depletion have lost fluid by renal or nonrenal routes. Gastrointestinal losses (e.g., vomiting, diarrhea) and third-space losses, such as pleural effusion or peritoneal effusion caused by peritonitis, pancreatitis, or uroabdomen, are the most important nonrenal losses of fluid and NaCl.[17,128] Gastrointestinal losses are often hypotonic in nature. The question thus arises, "If the losses are hypotonic, how does the patient become hyponatremic?" The answer follows from three physiologic events and reflects the body's tendency to preserve volume at the expense of tonicity. First, volume depletion decreases GFR, enhances isosmotic reabsorption of sodium and water in the proximal tubules, and decreases delivery of tubular fluid to distal diluting sites. These events impair excretion of water. Second, volume depletion is a strong nonosmotic stimulus for vasopressin release, and the increased plasma vasopressin concentration further impairs water excretion. Third, the patient is thirsty because of volume depletion and continues to drink water if it is available. All of these factors have a dilutional effect on the remaining body fluids.

Recall the previous example of the loss of 1 L of fluid with an osmolality of 150 mOsm/kg and consider what would happen if the animal in question drinks 1 L of pure water after sustaining the hypotonic loss. The added water increases the ECF volume from 1.36 to 2.36 L, and the resulting hypotonicity rapidly drives water into cells to equalize osmolality:

$$\text{New ECF osmolality} = \text{new ICF osmolality}$$
$$\frac{450 \text{ mOsm}}{(2.36 - x) \text{ L}} = \frac{1200 \text{ mOsm}}{(3.64 + x) \text{ L}}$$

where x is the volume of water moving between compartments:

$$450(3.64 + x) = 1200(2.36 - x)$$
$$x = 0.72 \text{ L}$$

The new volumes and osmolalities are:

$$\text{ECF}: \frac{450 \text{ mOsm}}{1.64 \text{ L}} = 275 \text{ mOsm/kg}$$
$$\text{ICF}: \frac{1200 \text{ mOsm}}{4.36 \text{ L}} = 275 \text{ mOsm/kg}$$

Note that in this example the intracellular compartment is expanded (4.36 L). The volume of the extracellular compartment (1.64 L) is greater than it was when the same hypotonic loss was not replaced (1.36 L) but still less than the previous normal value (2 L). Thus hypotonic (or isotonic) losses replaced by pure water lead to expansion of the ICF space. These changes are depicted in Fig. 3-14.

Renal fluid and NaCl losses resulting in hyponatremia are usually caused by hypoadrenocorticism or diuretic administration. In one study, 81% of 225 dogs with hypoadrenocorticism were hyponatremic at presentation.[102] Mineralocorticoid deficiency in hypoadrenocorticism results in urinary loss of NaCl and depletion of ECF volume. Volume depletion is a strong nonosmotic stimulus for vasopressin release and impairs water excretion. Hyperkalemia typically accompanies hyponatremia in hypoadrenocorticism.[102,105,114,127] However, some dogs with hypoadrenocorticism have only glucocorticoid deficiency at the time of presentation and thus have normal serum potassium concentrations.[85,110] Glucocorticoids are necessary for complete suppression of vasopressin release,

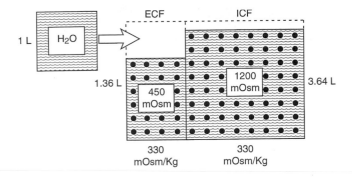

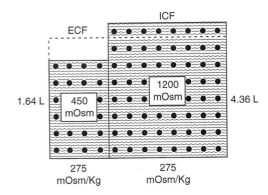

Fig. 3-14 Effect of drinking 1 L of water after a loss of 1 L of hypotonic fluid (150 mOsm/kg) on volume and tonicity of extracellular fluid (ECF) and intracellular fluid (ICF). (Drawing by Tim Vojt.)

and in their absence impaired water excretion and hyponatremia can occur.[25] Occasionally, dogs with gastrointestinal fluid losses develop electrolyte disturbances that mimic hypoadrenocorticism.[27,92] Hyponatremia associated with third-space loss of fluid has been reported with pleural effusion related to chylothorax, lung lobe torsion, and neoplasia.[79,122,128,131] In these reports, hyponatremia was attributed at least in part to removal of sodium-rich fluid by thoracocentesis. However, many of these animals had evidence of volume depletion, and it is likely that nonosmotic vasopressin secretion also played a role in the development of hyponatremia. Affected dogs also had mild hyperkalemia attributed to decreased renal excretion of potassium caused by volume depletion and decreased distal renal tubular flow. Similar findings have been observed in dogs and cats with peritoneal effusion and in dogs in late pregnancy.[8,72,115] The pathogenesis of hyponatremia and mild hyperkalemia in dogs with gastrointestinal losses is probably similar to that described for dogs with pleural and peritoneal effusions, but the explanation for the rare occurrence of similar electrolyte abnormalities in dogs in late pregnancy is unknown. When the cause of hyponatremia and hyperkalemia is unclear, an ACTH stimulation test should be performed to rule out hypoadrenocorticism.

Diuretics contribute to impaired water excretion and dilution of sodium in the ECF by decreased distal delivery of tubular fluid and nonosmotic stimulation of vasopressin release, which occur in response to volume depletion. Furthermore, potassium depletion caused by diuretics can contribute to hyponatremia because shifting of intracellular potassium into the extracellular compartment in exchange for sodium may occur. Hyponatremia has been associated with chronic blood loss in dogs.[124] It was thought that defective urinary concentrating ability in these dogs was caused by impaired vasopressin release in response to plasma hypoosmolality and loss of NaCl from the renal medullary interstitium. Some of these dogs had hypoadrenocorticism and gastrointestinal fluid losses that might have contributed to their hyponatremia. Normal concentrating ability returned after resolution of hyponatremia.

Hyponatremia with Volume Excess

Hyponatremia may occur despite the presence of increased total body sodium and expansion of the ECF compartment in patients with ascites or edema. Some of the pathophysiologic events in these patients impair the excretion of ingested water and exert a dilutional effect on the serum sodium concentration. Hyponatremia with volume excess (hypervolemia) is observed in three clinical conditions: congestive heart failure, severe liver disease, and nephrotic syndrome. In these disorders, there is a perception of circulating volume depletion by the body, and the regulatory mechanisms invoked result in volume expansion. This perceived volume deficit has been referred to as **decreased effective circulating volume** or **decreased effective arterial blood volume**.

Three major pathophysiologic mechanisms are operative in the pathogenesis of sodium retention and impaired water excretion in these clinical conditions. The renin-angiotensin system is activated by reduced renal perfusion and causes increased sodium retention by the kidneys. Decreased renal perfusion, decreased GFR, and increased proximal tubular reabsorption of sodium and water result in decreased delivery of tubular fluid to distal diluting sites and impairment of free water excretion. A decrease in effective arterial blood volume results in nonosmotic stimulation of vasopressin release and further impairment of water excretion. Impaired free water excretion causes dilution of retained sodium and results in hyponatremia despite the presence of increased total body sodium content and expansion of the ECF compartment. In addition, a primary intrarenal mechanism for sodium retention is thought to be operative in patients with the nephrotic syndrome.

In cirrhosis and the nephrotic syndrome, intravascular volume may be reduced as a result of decreased oncotic pressure caused by hypoalbuminemia. This volume depletion causes nonosmotic stimulation of vasopressin release and impaired water excretion. Reduction of cardiac output has also been observed to increase plasma concentrations of vasopressin. In congestive heart failure, decreased cardiac output is sensed by baroreceptors in the carotid and aortic sinuses, resulting in nonosmotic release of vasopressin. With chronic left atrial distention, the sensitivity of baroreceptors located in this site is presumably blunted, explaining the relative lack of vasopressin suppression that would be expected in acute left atrial distention.

The pathophysiology of sodium retention in the nephrotic syndrome appears to be complex. In some nephrotic patients with hypervolemia, the renin-angiotensin system appears to be suppressed. This conclusion is based on decreased plasma concentrations of renin and aldosterone and suggests a primary intrarenal mechanism for sodium retention.[13] The site of this intrarenal mechanism of sodium retention is not clear. In one experimental study, a distal site was implicated, whereas some investigators have suggested that alterations in filtration fraction and the glomerular ultrafiltration coefficient may be responsible.[29,67]

In severe liver disease, arteriovenous shunting, splanchnic venous pooling, ascites caused by portal hypertension, and decreased oncotic pressure caused by hypoalbuminemia all may lead to decreased effective circulating volume resulting in nonosmotic stimulation of vasopressin release and activation of the renin-angiotensin system.[34] Sodium retention and impairment of water excretion result.

Hyponatremia with hypervolemia may also be seen in advanced renal failure. Positive water balance may occur in the presence of continued polydipsia if there are an insufficient number of functional nephrons to excrete the required amount of free water. Approximately 70% of filtered water is reabsorbed isosmotically in the proximal tubules. If GFR is very low, the amount of water that can be excreted even with complete suppression of vasopressin release may be insufficient to prevent positive water balance in the presence of continued water intake. For example, consider a 10-kg dog with advanced renal failure and a GFR of 2 mL/min (approximately 5% of normal). The daily filtered load of water would be 2.88 L, and if 2.02 L (70%) is reabsorbed in the proximal tubules, the maximum volume of water that could be excreted is 860 mL. In the presence of polydipsia, it is conceivable that water intake would exceed this volume and dilutional hyponatremia would develop.

Hyponatremia with Normal Volume

Hyponatremia with normal volume (normovolemia) may occur as a result of psychogenic polydipsia, clinical conditions characterized by inappropriate secretion of vasopressin, administration of hypotonic fluids or drugs with antidiuretic effects, and myxedema coma of severe hypothyroidism. Approximately 67% of TBW is located within cells. Therefore only 33% of the water retained in these disorders is distributed to the extracellular compartment, and only 8% is located in the plasma compartment. However, this mild volume expansion does increase GFR and decrease proximal tubular reabsorption of sodium and water, thus leading to natriuresis. If excessive water intake or inappropriate vasopressin release continues, a new steady state is achieved with a slightly expanded ECF volume and plasma hypoosmolality. Overt signs of hypervolemia are usually not present because the majority of retained water is distributed to the intracellular compartment.

Psychogenic polydipsia usually occurs in large-breed dogs. The owner may report that the dog has a nervous disposition or that polydipsia seemed to begin after some stressful event. Some hyperactive dogs placed in an exercise-restricted environment have developed psychogenic polydipsia, and some dogs with this disorder may have developed it as a learned behavior to gain attention from the owner.[38] Some dogs with psychogenic polydipsia lower their water intake dramatically as a result of the stress of hospitalization, and this is sometimes a useful diagnostic observation. In one study, dogs with psychogenic polydipsia had daily water consumption of 150 to 250 mL/kg, USG of 1.001 to 1.003, urine osmolality of 102 to 112 mOsm/kg, plasma osmolality of 285 to 295 mOsm/kg, and serum sodium concentration of 131 to 140 mEq/L.[77] Hyponatremia with plasma hypoosmolality was thus documented in this study. Approximately 67% of affected dogs had a normal response to water deprivation, whereas others had some degree of medullary washout but responded to gradual water deprivation. Psychogenic polydipsia has not yet been reported in cats.

The syndrome of inappropriate ADH secretion (SIADH) refers to vasopressin release in the absence of normal osmotic or nonosmotic stimuli. This syndrome occurs in human patients and may be drug induced or associated with various types of malignancies, pulmonary diseases, and central nervous system disorders.[132] Several patterns of vasopressin secretion have been observed in human patients with SIADH: erratic changes in secretion unrelated to plasma osmolality, a normal increase in vasopressin secretion in response to changes in plasma osmolality but occurring at a lower threshold ("reset osmostat"), normal vasopressin secretion when plasma osmolality is normal or increased but inability to reduce vasopressin secretion appropriately after a water load ("vasopressin leak"), and low basal vasopressin concentration that fails to increase as plasma osmolality increases, suggesting increased renal sensitivity to vasopressin or presence of another antidiuretic substance.

SIADH is rare in dogs. It has been reported in association with dirofilariasis, undifferentiated carcinoma, neoplasia in the region of the hypothalamus, and granulomatous amebic meningoencephalitis.[10,12,45,65] Inappropriate vasopressin secretion may have played a role in the pathogenesis of hyponatremia in a dog with glucocorticoid deficiency.[25] Idiopathic SIADH also has been characterized in dogs.[41,107] Two of the dogs with idiopathic SIADH had hyponatremia, hypoosmolality, and inappropriately high vasopressin concentrations (7 to 30 pmol/L). Urine osmolality was inappropriately high (213 to 535 mOsm/kg) in one dog in the presence of plasma hypoosmolality. The threshold and sensitivity of vasopressin secretion were studied by infusion of hypertonic saline. One dog demonstrated a pattern of reset osmostat and the other a pattern consistent with vasopressin leak.[107] The vasopressin receptor antagonist OPC-31260, used at a dosage of 3 mg/kg orally twice a day for a 3-year period, successfully increased urine output and decreased USG in a dog with idiopathic SIADH, but serum sodium concentration was not normalized.[41]

The diagnosis of SIADH must be made by excluding other causes of hyponatremia. The following criteria should be met before establishing a diagnosis of SIADH:

1. Hyponatremia with plasma hypoosmolality.
2. Inappropriately high urine osmolality in the presence of plasma hypoosmolality. (Urine osmolality is often >300 mOsm/kg in human patients with SIADH. A urine osmolality >100 mOsm/kg should be considered abnormal in a patient with hyponatremia and plasma hypoosmolality. A urine osmolality <100 mOsm/kg would normally be expected as a result of complete suppression of vasopressin release. Urine osmolality is important in distinguishing psychogenic polydipsia and SIADH. Urine is maximally diluted in psychogenic polydipsia but not in SIADH.)
3. Normal renal, adrenal, and thyroid function.
4. Presence of natriuresis despite hyponatremia and plasma hypoosmolality as a result of mild volume expansion (urine sodium concentration usually >20 mEq/L in human patients).
5. No evidence of hypovolemia, which could result in nonosmotic stimulation of vasopressin release.
6. No evidence of ascites or edema, which could result in hyponatremia with hypervolemia (i.e., no evidence of severe liver disease, congestive heart failure, or nephrotic syndrome).
7. Correction of hyponatremia by fluid restriction.

Impaired osmoregulation of vasopressin release was observed in 11 dogs with liver disease (7 of which had large congenital portosystemic shunts).[113] Either the threshold for vasopressin release was increased or the magnitude of response decreased in these dogs, but plasma vasopressin and sodium concentrations were within the normal reference range. Affected dogs had evidence of excessive glucocorticoid secretion, and their response was similar to that previously described for dogs with spontaneous hyperadrenocorticism.[7]

A syndrome of cerebral salt wasting is thought to be responsible for hyponatremia in some human patients after subarachnoid hemorrhage or transsphenoidal surgery for pituitary tumors.[6,23] Hyponatremia resulting from cerebral salt wasting must be differentiated from that caused by SIADH because patients with the former disorder are volume depleted and require NaCl and water replacement, whereas those with SIADH require water restriction. Atrial and brain natriuretic factors may be responsible for the urinary loss of sodium in affected patients. Recognition of volume depletion depends on clinical findings such as changes in skin turgor, systemic blood pressure, central venous pressure, heart rate, and character of peripheral pulses. Hyponatremia must be corrected slowly (see Treatment of Hyponatremia), and SIADH should be suspected if hyponatremia worsens after saline infusion. Fludrocortisone also has been used in human patients with cerebral salt wasting to facilitate sodium retention.

Severe hypothyroidism with myxedema in humans can result in hyponatremia, possibly because of decreased distal delivery of tubular fluid and nonosmotic stimulation of vasopressin release. Hyponatremia in this setting is corrected by thyroid hormone replacement. In four reported cases of myxedema coma in dogs, hyponatremia was found in two of three dogs in which the serum sodium concentration was measured.[18,70]

Total body exchangeable cation content (sodium and potassium) decreases during long-distance exercise in Alaskan sled dogs despite no apparent change in TBW, and consequently hyponatremia develops.[62] A large urine volume is mandated by high dietary protein intake, and apparently excessive urinary sodium losses occur despite a physiologic response (i.e., activation of the renin-angiotensin-aldosterone system) aimed at sodium conservation.[63]

Drugs that stimulate the release of vasopressin or potentiate its renal effects may lead to hyponatremia with normovolemia. Nitrous oxide, barbiturates, isoproterenol, and narcotics are drugs used during anesthesia and surgery that stimulate vasopressin release from the neurohypophysis and may contribute to impaired water excretion in the postoperative period. Chlorpropamide potentiates the action of vasopressin possibly by inhibiting vasopressin-stimulated production of prostaglandin E_2 or by up-regulating vasopressin receptors in the kidney.[31] Nonsteroidal antiinflammatory drugs have a similar effect because of their inhibition of prostaglandin production. The antineoplastic drugs vincristine and cyclophosphamide also impair water excretion. Fig. 3-6 shows the effects of various drugs on the release and action of vasopressin.

CLINICAL SIGNS OF HYPONATREMIA

The clinical signs of hyponatremia are related more to the rapidity of onset than to the severity of the associated plasma hypoosmolality. In human patients, deaths and severe complications of hyponatremia were most common when the serum sodium concentration acutely decreased to less than 120 mEq/L or at a rate greater than 0.5 mEq/L/hr.[22] Cerebral edema and water intoxication occur if hyponatremia develops faster than the brain's defense mechanisms can be called into play. Reduction in plasma osmolality and influx of water into the central nervous system cause the clinical signs observed in acute hyponatremia. A 30- to 35-mOsm/kg gradient can result in translocation of water between plasma and the brain in dogs.[50] Clinical signs are often absent in chronic disorders characterized by slower decreases in serum sodium concentration and plasma osmolality. During hyponatremia of chronic onset, brain volume is adjusted toward normal by loss of potassium and organic osmolytes from cells.

Acute water intoxication is likely only if the patient has some underlying cause of impaired water excretion at the time a water load occurs. For example, water-loaded dogs given repositol vasopressin developed signs of acute water intoxication.[57] Early signs were mild lethargy, nausea, and slight weight gain; more severe signs included vomiting, coma, and a marked increase in body weight. One dog in this study died from pulmonary and cerebral edema. Weakness, incoordination, and seizures may also result from acute water intoxication. In one clinical report, a Labrador retriever developed acute hyponatremia (125 mEq/L) and severe neurologic signs (i.e., coma) after swimming for many hours in a lake.[123] The dog spontaneously underwent marked diuresis and recovered with supportive care, suggesting that it was capable of suppressing vasopressin release in response to the water load.

TREATMENT OF HYPONATREMIA

The two main goals of treatment in hyponatremia are to diagnose and manage the underlying disease and, *if necessary,* increase serum sodium concentration and plasma osmolality. Severe, symptomatic hyponatremia of acute onset (<24 to 48 hours' duration) may result in seizures, cerebral edema, or death and requires prompt treatment. In human patients with acute hyponatremia, correction of serum sodium concentration may be required at rates up to 12 mEq/L/day.[118] However, severe, symptomatic hyponatremia of rapid onset is rare in small animal practice. Because of inexperience with the management of acute hyponatremia in dogs and cats and the known risks of overly rapid correction of hyponatremia, only use of conventional crystalloid solutions (e.g., lactated Ringer's solution and 0.9% saline) is recommended. Use of 3% NaCl is not recommended.

Patients with chronic hyponatremia often have few or no clinical signs directly attributable to their hypoosmolality. This is probably because the brain has had sufficient time to adapt to plasma hypotonicity. In fact, treatment of chronic hyponatremia can be more dangerous than the disorder itself. In human patients, complications of treatment may occur when chronic (>48 hours' duration) hyponatremia is corrected too rapidly

(i.e., when the serum sodium concentration is increased by >10 to 12 mEq/L in 24 hours).[81,118]

When hyponatremia and hypoosmolality are corrected, potassium and organic osmolytes lost during adaptation must be restored to the cells of the brain. If replacement of these solutes does not keep pace with the increase in serum sodium concentration that occurs as a result of treatment, brain dehydration and injury—called osmotic demyelination or myelinolysis—may result.[81,118] Experimental studies have confirmed that this syndrome is a result of a rapid and large increase in serum sodium concentration and is not a consequence of hyponatremia and hypoosmolality. Human patients with hyponatremia of more than 72 hours' duration are more susceptible than those with hyponatremia of less than 24 hours' duration.[118] The neural lesions of myelinolysis develop several days after correction of hyponatremia and consist of myelin loss and injury to oligodendroglial cells in the pons and other sites in the brain (e.g., thalamus, subcortical white matter, and cerebellum). Lesions may take several days to develop, but on magnetic resonance imaging they are hyperintense on T2-weighted images, hypointense on T1-weighted images, and are not enhanced after gadolinium injection.[81]

Similar lesions have been reported in experimental dogs with hyponatremia with correction rates of 15 mEq/L/day even without overcorrection to hypernatremia.[80] In veterinary medicine, myelinolysis first was reported in two dogs after correction of hyponatremia associated with trichuriasis.[98] In one dog, a serum sodium concentration of 101 mEq/L had been corrected to 136 mEq/L in less than 38 hours (correction rate, >22 mEq/L/day), and in the other, a serum sodium concentration of 108 mEq/L had been corrected to 134 mEq/L in less than 38 hours (correction rate, >16 mEq/L/day). Clinical signs developed 3 to 4 days after correction of hyponatremia and consisted of lethargy, weakness, and ataxia progressing to hypermetria and quadriparesis. Lesions were detected by magnetic resonance imaging and were located in the thalamus as compared with the more typical pontine location in affected human patients. From this experience, it was recommended that dogs with asymptomatic chronic hyponatremia be treated by mild water restriction and monitoring of serum sodium concentration. Symptomatic dogs with chronic hyponatremia should be treated conservatively at correction rates less than 10 to 12 mEq/L/day (0.5 mEq/L/hr). Serial monitoring of serum sodium concentration is necessary because the actual rate of correction may not correspond to the calculated rate of correction. Correction should be carried out with conventional crystalloid solutions (e.g., lactated Ringer's solution and 0.9% NaCl) in a volume calculated specifically to replace the patient's volume deficit. The clinician must remember that volume repletion in hypovolemic patients abolishes the nonosmotic stimulus for vasopressin release and allows the animal to excrete solute-free water via the kidneys. This in itself tends to correct the hyponatremia. Thus caution should be exercised even when using conventional crystalloid fluid therapy.

Three additional cases of suspected myelinolysis in dogs with chronic hyponatremia caused by hypoadrenocorticism or trichuriasis have been reported.[9,21,90] The rates of correction of hyponatremia in these dogs were 22 mEq/L on day 1 and 17 mEq/L on day 2, 32 mEq/L over 2 days, and 17 mEq/L in 9 hours.[9,21,90] The neurologic signs that developed (e.g., spastic tetraparesis, loss of postural and proprioceptive responses, dysphagia, trismus, and decreased menace response) were similar to those originally described by O'Brien.[98] The dogs of these reports gradually recovered over several weeks.

Water intake should be carefully restricted to a volume less than urine output in normovolemic patients with hyponatremia (e.g., psychogenic polydipsia), or drugs causing an antidiuretic effect should be discontinued if possible. Demeclocycline and lithium inhibit vasopressin release and have been used to treat SIADH in humans, but water restriction is probably the safest approach.[42]

In edematous patients, dietary sodium restriction and diuretic therapy should be considered. A 0.9% NaCl solution can be administered concurrently with loop diuretics (e.g., furosemide) to effect more rapid correction of hyponatremia in overhydrated symptomatic patients. The occurrence of chronic hyponatremia in patients with congestive heart failure is often a sign of advanced disease and responds poorly to treatment. Administration of furosemide and an angiotensin-converting enzyme inhibitor (e.g., enalapril) may improve stroke volume and cardiac output by reducing preload and afterload and may decrease vasopressin secretion and enhance water excretion, which in turn may facilitate resolution of hyponatremia.

CLINICAL APPROACH TO POLYURIA AND POLYDIPSIA

Normal daily water intake and urine output in dogs and cats are influenced by the nutrient, mineral, and water content of the diet. Normal water intake should not exceed 90 mL/kg/day in dogs and 45 mL/kg/day in cats. Normal urine output ranges from 20 to 45 mL/kg/day in dogs and cats. Dogs with disorders such as psychogenic polydipsia, CDI, and NDI may have water consumption as much as five times normal.

Dogs and cats with polyuria and polydipsia are encountered frequently in small animal practice. The causes of polyuria and polydipsia, their pathophysiologic mechanisms, and the necessary confirmatory laboratory tests are presented in the Table 3-4. The most common

TABLE 3-4   Causes of Polyuria and Polydipsia in Small Animal Practice

Disease	Mechanism of Polyuria and Polydipsia	Confirmatory Tests
Chronic renal disease* (S)	Osmotic diuresis in remnant nephrons Disruption of medullary architecture by structural disease	ECC CBC Profile Urinalysis Radiography Ultrasonography
Hyperadrenocorticism* (W)	Defective ADH release and action Psychogenic	LDDST, HDDST Plasma ACTH Ultrasonography
Diabetes mellitus* (S)	Osmotic diuresis caused by glucosuria	Blood glucose Urinalysis
Hyperthyroidism* (W)	Increased medullary blood flow and MSW Psychogenic Hypercalciuria	T_4 Technetium scan
Pyometra (W)	*Escherichia coli* endotoxin Immune complex glomerulonephritis	History Physical CBC Abdominal radiographs
Postobstructive diuresis (S)	Elimination of retained solutes Defective response to ADH Defective sodium reabsorption	History Physical examination Urinalysis
Hypercalcemia (W)	Defective ADH action Increased medullary blood flow Impaired NaCl transport in loop of Henle Hypercalcemic nephropathy Direct stimulation of thirst center	Serum calcium

Continued

TABLE 3-4 Causes of Polyuria and Polydipsia in Small Animal Practice—cont'd

Disease	Mechanism of Polyuria and Polydipsia	Confirmatory Tests
Liver disease (W)	Decreased urea synthesis with loss of medullary solute Decreased metabolism of endogenous hormones (e.g., cortisol, aldosterone) Psychogenic (hepatic encephalopathy) Hypokalemia	Liver enzymes Serum bile acids Blood ammonia Liver biopsy
Pyelonephritis (W)	E. coli endotoxin Increased renal blood flow MSW Renal parenchymal damage	Urinalysis Urine culture CBC Excretory urography Abdominal ultrasonography
Hypoadrenocorticism (W)	Renal sodium loss with MSW	Serum sodium and potassium ACTH stimulation
Hypokalemia (W)	Defective ADH action Increased medullary blood flow and loss of medullary solute	Serum potassium
Diuretic phase of oliguric ARF (S)	Elimination of retained solutes Defective sodium reabsorption	History CBC Profile Urinalysis Abdominal ultrasonography Renal biopsy
Partial urinary tract obstruction (S)	Redistribution of renal blood flow Defective sodium reabsorption Renal parenchymal damage	History Physical examination
Drugs (W)	Various mechanisms depending on drug	History
Salt administration (S)	Osmotic diuresis caused by excess sodium administered	History
Excessive parenteral fluid administration (W) (polyuria only)	Water diuresis caused by excess water administered	History
Central diabetes insipidus (CDI) (W)	Congenital lack of ADH (rare) Acquired lack of ADH (idiopathic, tumor, trauma)	Water deprivation test Exogenous ADH test ADH assay
Nephrogenic diabetes insipidus (NDI) (W)	Congenital lack of renal response to ADH (very rare) Acquired lack of renal response to ADH (see Table 3–5)	Water deprivation test Exogenous ADH test ADH assay ECC
Psychogenic polydipsia (PP) (W)	Neurobehavioral disorder (anxiety?) Increased renal blood flow MSW	Water deprivation test Exogenous ADH test Behavioral history
Renal glucosuria (S)	Solute diuresis caused by gluosuria	Blood glucose Urinalysis
Primary hypoparathyroidism (W)	Unknown (psychogenic?)	Serum calcium Serum phosphorus Serum PTH
Acromegaly (W, S)	Insulin antagonism Glucose intolerance Diabetes mellitus in affected cats	Neuroradiography Growth hormone assay
Polycythemia (W)	Unknown (increased blood viscosity?)	CBC
Multiple myeloma (W)	Unknown (increased blood viscosity?)	Serum protein electrophoresis
Renal MSW (W)	Depletion of medullary interstitial solute (urea, sodium, potassium)	Gradual water deprivation (3–5 days) Hickey-Hare test

Adapted from Bruyette DS, Nelson RW: How to approach the problems of polyuria and polydipsia, Vet Med 81:112, 1986.
*Most common causes of polyuria and polydipsia.
Abbreviations: (W), water diuresis; (S), solute diuresis; ACTH, adrenocorticotropic hormone; ADH, antidiuretic hormone; ARF, acute renal failure; CBC, complete blood count; PTH, parathyroid hormone; ECC, endogenous creatinine clearance; MSW, medullary washout of solute; LDDST, low-dose dexamethasone suppression test; HDDST, high-dose dexamethasone suppression test.

causes are chronic renal failure in dogs and cats, diabetes mellitus in dogs and cats, hyperadrenocorticism in dogs, and hyperthyroidism in cats. These common causes must always be ruled out before beginning an exhaustive diagnostic evaluation of the animal.

Determination of the specific gravity of a random urine sample from the animal is a logical starting point for evaluation of polyuria and polydipsia. If a random USG is greater than 1.030 to 1.035, the clinician should obtain additional history to rule out other disorders that may have been confused with polyuria (e.g., urinary incontinence and dysuria). If a random USG is less than 1.025 to 1.030, an initial diagnostic evaluation is warranted.

Many causes of polyuria and polydipsia can be ruled out by an initial database consisting of a complete history and physical examination, complete blood count, biochemical profile (including electrolytes), urinalysis, urine culture, and abdominal radiographs. If the animal is otherwise healthy, it is helpful to instruct the owner to quantitate and record the animal's daily water consumption at home over a 3- to 5-day period. Determination of water intake at home prevents potential reduction in water intake precipitated by the stress of hospitalization.

With some exceptions (e.g., psychogenic polydipsia), polydipsia usually occurs as a consequence of polyuria. If polydipsia occurs without polyuria, the clinician must consider causes such as high ambient temperature (i.e., increased insensible water losses), regular prolonged exercise, water consumption to replace a previous hydration deficit, and third-space distribution of consumed water. Excessive administration of parenteral fluids causes polyuria without polydipsia. The diagnostic approach to polyuria and polydipsia is summarized in Table 3-4 and Fig. 3-15.

LABORATORY EVALUATION OF POLYURIA AND POLYDIPSIA

ENDOGENOUS CREATININE CLEARANCE

In chronic progressive renal disease, urinary concentrating ability is impaired after two thirds of the nephron population has become nonfunctional, whereas azotemia does not develop until three quarters of the nephrons have become nonfunctional. Thus the main indication for determination of endogenous creatinine clearance is the clinical suspicion of renal disease in a patient with polyuria and polydipsia but normal BUN and serum creatinine concentrations. The only requirements for determination of endogenous creatinine clearance are an accurately timed collection of urine (usually 24 hours), determination of the patient's body weight, and measurement of serum and urine creatinine concentrations. Failure to collect all urine produced results in an erro-

neously reduced calculated clearance value. Use of creatinine clearance as an estimate of GFR is discussed further in Chapter 2.

WATER DEPRIVATION TEST

The water deprivation test is indicated in evaluation of animals with confirmed polydipsia and polyuria, the cause of which remains undetermined after the initial diagnostic evaluation. It is usually performed in animals with hyposthenuria (USG <1.007) that are suspected to have CDI, NDI, or psychogenic polydipsia. An animal that is dehydrated but has dilute urine has already failed the test and should not be subjected to water deprivation. In such an animal, failure to concentrate urine is probably caused by structural or functional renal dysfunction or administration of drugs that interfere with urinary concentrating ability. The water deprivation test is also contraindicated in animals that are azotemic. The test should be performed with extreme caution in animals with severe polyuria because such patients may rapidly become dehydrated during water deprivation if they have defective urinary concentrating ability.

At the beginning of the water deprivation test, the bladder must be emptied and baseline data collected (body weight, hematocrit, total plasma proteins, skin turgor, serum osmolality, urine osmolality, and USG). Water is then withheld, and these parameters are monitored every 2 to 4 hours. Urine and serum osmolalities are the best parameters to follow, but osmolality results are often not immediately available to the clinician. Thus USG and body weight assume great importance for decision making during performance of the test. An increase in total plasma protein concentration is a relatively reliable indicator of progressive dehydration, but increases in hematocrit and changes in skin turgor are less reliable.[55] Serum creatinine and BUN concentrations should not increase during a properly conducted water deprivation test.

The bladder should be emptied at the time of each urine collection. Maximal stimulation of ADH release is present after loss of 5% of body weight. The test is concluded when the patient either demonstrates adequate concentrating ability or becomes dehydrated as evidenced by loss of 5% or more of its original body weight. It is important when weighing the animal to use the same scale each time and to empty the bladder at each evaluation.

In normal dogs, dehydration becomes evident after a mean of 42 hours but occasionally may not occur until after 96 hours.[55] The time required for dehydration to develop during water deprivation testing in dogs with disorders characterized by polyuria and polydipsia may be as short as a few hours or up to 12 hours. By the time dehydration is evident, normal dogs develop a USG of 1.050 to 1.076, urine osmolality of 1787 to 2791 mOsm/kg, and a urine/plasma osmolality ratio of 5.7 to 8.9.[55] Normal cats developed USG values of 1.047 to 1.087 and

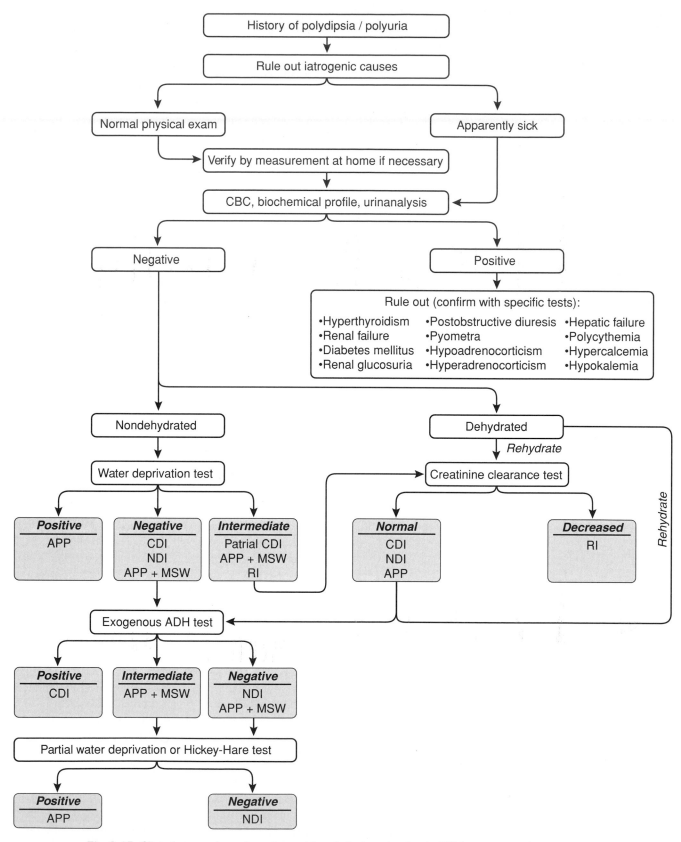

Fig. 3-15 Clinical approach to the patient with polydipsia and polyuria. *APP,* Apparent psychogenic polydipsia; *CBC,* complete blood count; *CDI,* central diabetes insipidus; *MSW,* medullary solute washout; *NDI,* nephrogenic diabetes insipidus; *RI,* renal insufficiency with solute diuresis. (From Fenner WR: *Quick reference to veterinary medicine,* ed 2, Philadelphia, 1991, JB Lippincott, p. 110.)

urine osmolalities of 1581 to 2984 mOsm/kg after water deprivation of sufficient duration (approximately 40 hours) to induce 5% loss of body weight.[112] Failure to achieve maximal urinary solute concentration does not localize the level of the malfunction, but a structural or functional defect may be present anywhere along the hypothalamic-pituitary-renal axis. Furthermore, animals with renal medullary solute washout may have impaired concentrating capacity regardless of the underlying cause of polyuria and polydipsia.

If there has been less than 5% increase in urine osmolality or less than 10% change in USG for three consecutive determinations or if the animal has lost 5% or more of its original weight, 0.25 to 0.5 U/kg aqueous vasopressin (pitressin) (up to a total dose of 5 U) or 5 μg of DDAVP may be given subcutaneously and parameters of urinary concentrating ability monitored at 30, 60, and 120 minutes after ADH injection. Normal dogs and those with psychogenic polydipsia should show no additional response to ADH administration in this setting. The expected responses to water deprivation for dogs with various disorders of water balance are shown in Fig. 3-16.

MODIFIED WATER DEPRIVATION TEST

A modified water deprivation test has been described for the diagnosis of polyuric disorders in dogs. Water is removed from the animal's cage and the urinary bladder emptied, after which urine osmolality or specific gravity is measured and the bladder emptied on an hourly basis. Maximal urine solute concentration is defined as occurring whenever less than 5% increase in urine osmolality occurs on sequential determinations. This maximal concentration occurred at a mean urine osmolality of 1414 mOsm/kg in normal dogs after 24 hours of water deprivation.[94] At this time, 2 to 3 U of aqueous vasopressin was administered subcutaneously and the urine osmolality determined at 1 and 2 hours after injection. Further increase in urine osmolality after administration of vasopressin should not exceed 10% in normal dogs. In this study, dogs with CDI showed an average 292% increase in urine osmolality after aqueous ADH, dogs with partial

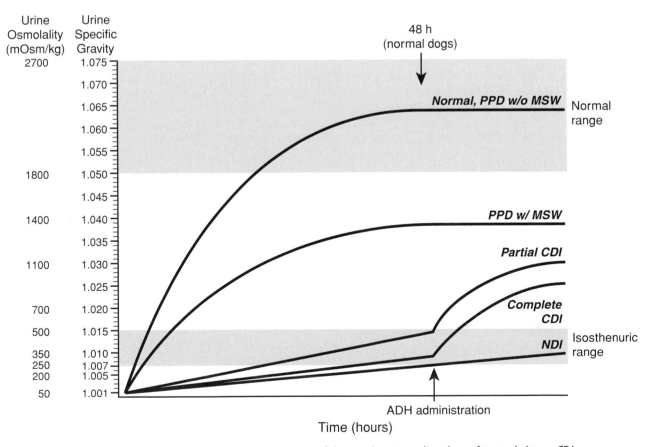

Fig. 3-16 Idealized response to water deprivation of dogs with various disorders of water balance, *CDI,* Central diabetes insipidus; *NDI,* nephrogenic diabetes insipidus; *MSW,* medullary solute washout; *ADH,* antidiuretic hormone.

CDI an average 28% increase, and dogs with hyperadrenocorticism an average 20% increase. The time required to develop dehydration ranged from 3 to 11.5 hours in dogs with psychogenic polydipsia, complete or partial CDI, and hyperadrenocorticism.

GRADUAL WATER DEPRIVATION

Gradual water deprivation can be performed to eliminate diagnostic confusion caused by renal medullary solute washout. The owner can be instructed to restrict water consumption to 120 mL/kg/day 72 hours before, to 90 mL/kg/day 48 hours before, and to 60 mL/kg/day 24 hours before the scheduled water deprivation test. In dogs with psychogenic polydipsia, this promotes release of endogenous vasopressin, increased permeability of the inner medullary collecting ducts to urea, and restoration of the normal gradient of medullary hypertonicity. An alternative approach is to instruct the owner to reduce water consumption by approximately 10% per day over a 3- to 5-day period (but not to less than 60 mL/kg/day). This approach should be used only in animals that are otherwise healthy on initial clinical evaluation, and the owner should provide dry food ad libitum and weigh the dog daily to monitor for loss of body weight.

HICKEY-HARE TEST

In the Hickey-Hare test, water (20 mL/kg) is administered by stomach tube, an indwelling urinary catheter is placed, and urine flow (mL/min) is determined.[78] Hypertonic saline (2.5%) is administered intravenously at a rate of 0.25 mL/min/kg for 45 minutes. Urine volume is recorded every 15 minutes during the infusion and for 45 minutes afterward. The normal response to this procedure is a decrease in the rate of urine production caused by stimulation of ADH release by plasma hyperosmolality. It is useful in the differentiation of psychogenic polydipsia with renal medullary solute washout from NDI after negative water deprivation and exogenous ADH test results. In NDI, there should be no change or an actual increase in urine flow, whereas in psychogenic polydipsia with renal medullary solute washout, repletion of solute (e.g., NaCl) should have occurred, and the response to hypertonic saline should be normal (decreased urine volume). This test is cumbersome, is contraindicated for patients with congestive heart failure, and may lead to signs of hypernatremia in patients that cannot excrete a sodium load. It has largely been replaced by gradual water deprivation as described previously.

EXOGENOUS ANTIDIURETIC HORMONE TESTING

The exogenous vasopressin test may be used for debilitated patients in which water deprivation is considered hazardous or to further characterize a concentrating defect detected by the routine water deprivation test. In the **aqueous vasopressin test**, an intravenous infusion of aqueous vasopressin (pitressin) at 10 mU/kg is given over 60 minutes. The bladder is emptied at the start of the study, and parameters of urinary concentrating ability are measured before and at 30-minute intervals for 3 hours after beginning the infusion. The bladder is emptied at each measurement. In one report, maximal reponse to aqueous vasopressin in water-loaded dogs usually occurred at 60 minutes (range, 30 to 90 minutes) and consisted of USG values of 1.012 to 1.033, urine osmolalities of 429 to 1437 mOsm/kg, and urine/plasma osmolality ratios of 1.5 to 5.1.[56] Water should be provided ad libitum during testing, but water loading should not be performed in clinical patients.

In the **repositol vasopressin test**, 3 to 5 U of vasopressin tannate in oil (pitressin tannate) is given intramuscularly, and the bladder is emptied 3 to 6 hours after injection. Parameters of urinary concentrating ability are measured before and at 6, 9, 12, and 24 hours after injection. Oral water loading must be avoided because of the danger of potentially lethal water intoxication.[57] Maximal response to repositol vasopressin occurred 8 to 12 hours after injection and consisted of USG values of 1.028 to 1.057, urine osmolalities of 1052 to 1850 mOsm/kg, and urine/plasma osmolality ratios of 3.9 to 6.7.[57]

The standard or modified water deprivation test is the preferred initial test of urinary concentrating ability because mean maximal values are usually higher with this test and results are easier to interpret (Table 3-5). Why higher values for parameters of urinary concentrating ability are achieved with this test as compared with the exogenous vasopressin tests is unknown. Possible explanations include the actions of antidiuretic substances other than ADH that may be present in hydropenic individuals, the effect of slower renal medullary blood flow in dehydrated patients, and intensification of the medullary interstitial gradient in dehydrated individuals.

TABLE 3-5 Mean Maximal Values for Parameters of Total Urine Solute Concentration*

	WDT	RVPT	AVPT
U_{osm} (mOsm/kg)	2199	1518	933
Urine specific gravity	1.063	1.042	1.021
U_{osm}/P_{osm}	7.2	5.6	3.3

From Hardy RM, Osborne CA: Water deprivation test in the dog: maximal normal values, J Am Vet Med Assoc 174:479, 1979; Hardy RM, Osborne CA: Aqueous vasopressin response test in clinically normal dogs undergoing water diuresis: technique and results, Am J Vet Res 43:1987, 1982; and Hardy RM, Osborne CA: Repositol vasopressin response test in clinically normal dogs undergoing water diuresis: technique and results, Am J Vet Res 43:1991, 1982.

*Normal dogs undergoing routine water deprivation testing (WDT), repositol vasopressin testing (RVPT), and aqueous vasopressin testing (AVPT).

REFERENCES

1. Abramov M, Beauwens R, Cogan E: Cellular events in vasopressin action, *Kidney Int* 32(suppl 21):S56, 1987.
2. Ajito T, Suzuki K, Iwabuchi S: Effect of intravenous infusion of 7.2% hypertonic saline solution on serum electrolytes and osmotic pressure in healthy beagles, *J Vet Med Sci* 61:637, 1999.
3. Atkins CE, Tyler R, Greenlee P: Clinical, biochemical, acid-base, and electrolyte abnormalities in cats after hypertonic sodium phosphate enema administration, *Am J Vet Res* 46:980, 1985.
4. Authement JM, Boudrieau RJ, Kaplan PM: Transient traumatically induced central diabetes insipidus in a dog, *J Am Vet Med Assoc* 194:683, 1989.
5. Bagley RS, de Lahunta A, Randolph JF, et al: Hypernatremia, adipsia, and diabetes insipidus in a dog with hypothalamic dysplasia, *J Am Anim Hosp Assoc* 29:267, 1993.
6. Betjes MGH: Hyponatremia in acute brain disease: the cerebral salt wasting syndrome, *Eur J Int Med* 13:9, 2002.
7. Biewenga WJ, Rijnberk A, Mol JA: Osmoregulation of systemic vasopressin release during long-term glucocorticoid excess: a study in dogs with hyperadrenocorticism, *Acta Endocrinol* 124:583, 1991.
8. Bissett SA, Lamb M, Ward CR: Hyponatremia and hyperkalemia associated with peritoneal effusion in four cats, *J Am Vet Med Assoc* 218:1590, 2001.
9. Brady CA, Vite CE, Drobatz KJ: Severe neurological sequelae in a dog after treatment of hypoadrenal crisis, *J Am Vet Med Assoc* 215:222, 1999.
10. Breitschwerdt EB, Root CR: Inappropriate secretion of antidiuretic hormone in a dog, *J Am Vet Med Assoc* 175:181, 1979.
11. Breitschwerdt EB, Verlander JW, Bribernik TN: Nephrogenic diabetes insipidus in three dogs, *J Am Vet Med Assoc* 179:235, 1981.
12. Brofman PJ, Knostman KA, DiBartola SP: Granulomatous amebic meningoencephalitis causing the syndrome of inappropriate secretion of antidiuretic hormone in a dog, *J Vet Int Med* 17:230, 2003.
13. Brown E, Markandu ND, Roulston JE, et al: Is the renin-angiotensin-aldosterone system involved in the sodium retention of the nephrotic syndrome? *Nephron* 32:102, 1982.
14. Bruyette DS, Nelson RW: How to approach the problems of polyuria and polydipsia, *Vet Med* 81:112, 1986.
15. Bulger RE: Composition of renal medullary tissue, *Kidney Int* 31:557, 1987.
16. Burnie AG, Dunn JK: A case of central diabetes insipidus in the cat: diagnosis and treatment, *J Small Anim Pract* 23:237, 1979.
17. Burrows CF, Bovee KC: Metabolic changes due to experimentally induced rupture of the canine urinary bladder, *Am J Vet Res* 35:1083, 1974.
18. Chastain CB, Graham CL, Riley MG: Myxedema coma in two dogs, *Canine Pract* 9:20, 1982.
19. Chew DJ, Leonard M, Muir WW: Effect of sodium bicarbonate infusion on serum osmolality, electrolyte concentrations, and blood gas tensions in cats, *Am J Vet Res* 52:12, 1991.
20. Chew M: Salt poisoning in a boxer bitch. *Vet Rec* 85:685, 1969.
21. Churcher RK, Watson ADJ, Eaton A: Suspected myelinolysis following rapid correction of hyponatremia in a dog, *J Am Anim Hosp Assoc* 35:493, 1999.
22. Cluitmans FH, Meinders AE: Management of severe hyponatremia: rapid or slow correction? *Am J Med* 88:161, 1990.
23. Coenraad MJ, Meinders AE, Taal JC, et al: Hyponatremia in intracranial disorders, *Neth J Med* 58:123, 2001.
24. Crawford MA, Kittleson MD, Fink GD: Hypernatremia and adipsia in a dog, *J Am Vet Med Assoc* 184:818, 1984.
25. Crow SE, Stockham SL: Profound hyponatremia associated with glucocorticoid deficiency in a dog, *J Am Anim Hosp Assoc* 21:393, 1985.
26. Davenport DJ, Chew DJ, Johnson GC: Diabetes insipidus associated with metastatic pancreatic carcinoma in a dog, *J Am Vet Med Assoc* 189:204, 1986.
27. DiBartola SP, Johnson SE, Davenport DJ, et al: Clinicopathologic findings resembling hypoadrenocorticism in dogs with primary gastrointestinal disease, *J Am Vet Med Assoc* 187:60, 1985.
28. DiBartola SP, Johnson SE, Johnson GC, et al: Hypodipsic hypernatremia in a dog with defective osmoregulation of antidiuretic hormone, *J Am Vet Med Assoc* 204:922, 1994.
29. Dorhout Mees EJ: Edema formation in the nephrotic syndrome, *Contrib Nephrol* 43:64, 1984.
30. Dow SW, Fettman MJ, LeCouteur RA, et al: Hypodipsic hypernatremia and associated myopathy in a hydrocephalic cat with transient hypopituitarism, *J Am Vet Med Assoc* 191:212, 1987.
31. Durr JA, Hensen J, Ehnis T, et al: Chlorpropamide upregulates antidiuretic hormone receptors and unmasks constitutive receptor signaling, *Am J Physiol* 278:F799, 2000.
32. Edwards DF, Richardson DC, Russell RG: Hypernatremic, hypertonic dehydration in a dog with diabetes insipidus and gastric dilatation-volvulus, *J Am Vet Med Assoc* 182:973, 1983.
33. Ellison DH, Velazquez H: Thiazide-sensitive sodium chloride cotransport in early distal tubule, *Am J Physiol* 253:F546, 1987.
34. Epstein M: Derangements of renal water handling in liver disease, *Gastroenterology* 89:1415, 1985.
35. Feig PU, McCurdy DK: The hypertonic state, *N Engl J Med* 297:1444, 1977.
36. Feldman BF, Rosenberg DP: Clinical use of anion and osmolal gaps in veterinary medicine, *J Am Vet Med Assoc* 178:396, 1981.
37. Feldman EC, Nelson RW: Water metabolism and diabetes insipidus. In Feldman EC, Nelson RW, editors: *Canine and feline endocrinology and reproduction*, ed 3, Philadelphia, 2004, WB Saunders, p. 37.
38. Feldman EC, Nelson RW: Water metabolism and diabetes insipidus. In Feldman EC, Nelson RW, editors: *Canine and feline endocrinology and reproduction*, ed 3, Philadelphia, 2004, WB Saunders, p. 18.
39. Ferguson DC, Biery DN: Diabetes insipidus and hyperadrenocorticism associated with high plasma adrenocorticotropin concentration and a hypothalamic/pituitary mass in a dog, *J Am Vet Med Assoc* 193:835, 1988.
40. Fjellestad-Paulsen A, Hoglund P, Lundin S, et al: Pharmacokinetics of 1-deamino-8-D-arginine vasopressin after various routes of administration in healthy volunteers, *Clin Endocrinol* 38:177, 1993.
41. Fleeman LM, Irwin PJ, Phillips PA, et al: Effects of an oral vasopressin receptor antagonist (OPC-31260) in a dog with syndrome of inappropriate secretion of antidiuretic hormone, *Aust Vet J* 78:825, 2000.
42. Forrest JN, Cox M, Hong C, et al: Superiority of demeclocycline over lithium in the treatment of chronic syndrome

of inappropriate secretion of antidiuretic hormone, *N Engl J Med* 298:173, 1978.

43. Gennari FJ: Serum osmolality: uses and limitations, *N Engl J Med* 310:102, 1984.

44. Gennari FJ, Kassirer JP: Osmotic diuresis, *N Engl J Med* 291:714, 1974.

45. Giger U, Gorman NT: Oncologic emergencies in small animals. Part II. Metabolic and endocrine emergencies, *Compend Contin Educ Pract Vet* 6:805, 1984.

46. Grauer GF, Grauer RM: Veterinary clinical osmometry, *Compend Contin Educ Pract Vet* 5:539, 1983.

47. Green RA, Farrow CS: Diabetes insipidus in a cat, *J Am Vet Med Assoc* 164:524, 1974.

48. Greene CE, Wong PL, Finco DR: Diagnosis and treatment of diabetes insipidus in two dogs using two synthetic analogs of antidiuretic hormone, *J Am Anim Hosp Assoc* 15:371, 1979.

49. Gross PA, Ketteler M, Hausmann C, et al: The charted and uncharted waters of hyponatremia, *Kidney Int* 32(suppl 21):S67, 1987.

50. Guisado R, Arieff AI, Massry SG: Effects of glycerol infusions on brain water and electrolytes, *Am J Physiol* 227:865, 1974.

51. Hall EF: Hypernatremia and adipsia in a dog (letter), *J Am Vet Med Assoc* 185:4, 1984.

52. Hara Y, Masuda H, Taoda T, et al: Prophylactic efficacy of desmopressin acetate for diabetes insipidus after hypophysectomy in the dog, *J Vet Med Sci* 65:17, 2003.

53. Harb MF, Nelson RW, Feldman EC, et al: Central diabetes insipidus in dogs: 20 cases (1986-1995), *J Am Vet Med Assoc* 209:1884, 1996.

54. Hardy RM: Hypernatremia, *Vet Clin North Am Small Anim Pract* 19:231, 1989.

55. Hardy RM, Osborne CA: Water deprivation test in the dog: maximal normal values, *J Am Vet Med Assoc* 174:479, 1979.

56. Hardy RM, Osborne CA: Aqueous vasopressin response test in clinically normal dogs undergoing water diuresis: technique and results, *Am J Vet Res* 43:1987, 1982.

57. Hardy RM, Osborne CA: Repositol vasopressin response test in clinically normal dogs undergoing water diuresis: technique and results, *Am J Vet Res* 43:1991, 1982.

58. Hawks D, Giger U, Miselis R, et al: Essential hypernatremia in a young dog, *J Small Anim Pract* 32:420, 1991.

59. Hendriks HJ, de Bruijne JJ, Van den Brom WE: The clinical refractometer: a useful tool for the determination of specific gravity and osmolality of canine urine, *Tijdschr Diergeneeskd* 103:1065, 1978.

60. Henry WB, Sieber SE: Traumatic diabetes insipidus in a dog, *J Am Vet Med Assoc* 146:1317, 1965.

61. Hillier TA, Abbott RD, Barrett EJ: Hyponatremia: evaluating the correction factor for hyperglycemia, *Am J Med* 106:399, 1999.

62. Hinchcliff KW, Reinhart GA, Burr JR, et al: Effect of racing on serum sodium and potassium concentrations and acid-base status of Alaskan sled dogs, *J Am Vet Med Assoc* 210:1615, 1997.

63. Hinchcliff KW, Reinhart GA, Burr JR, et al: Exercise-associated hyponatremia in Alaskan sled dogs: urinary and hormonal responses, *J Appl Physiol* 83:824, 1997.

64. Hoskins JD, Rothschmitt J: Hypernatremic thirst deficiency in a dog, *Vet Med* 79:489, 1984.

65. Houston DM, Allen DG, Kruth SA, et al: Syndrome of inappropriate antidiuretic hormone secretion in a dog, *Can Vet J* 30:423, 1989.

66. Hughes DE, Sokolowski JH: Sodium chloride poisoning in the dog, *Canine Pract* 5:28, 1978.

67. Ichikawa I, Rennke HG, Hoyer JR, et al: Role for intrarenal mechanism in the impaired salt excretion of experimental nephrotic syndrome, *J Clin Invest* 71:91, 1983.

68. Joles JA, Gruys E: Nephrogenic diabetes insipidus in a dog with renal medullary lesions, *J Am Vet Med Assoc* 174:830, 1979.

69. Katz MA: Hyperglycemia-induced hyponatremia, *N Engl J Med* 289:843, 1973.

70. Kelly MJ, Hill JR: Canine myxedema stupor and coma, *Compend Contin Educ Pract Vet* 6:1049, 1984.

71. Khanna C, Boermans HJ, Wilcock B: Fatal hypernatremia in a dog from salt ingestion, *J Am Anim Hosp Assoc* 33:113, 1997.

72. Kitchell BE, Fan TM, Kordick D, et al: Peliosis hepatitis in a dog infected with *Bartonella henselae*, *J Am Vet Med Assoc* 216:519, 2000.

73. Kraus KH: The use of desmopressin in diagnosis and treatment of diabetes insipidus in cats, *Compend Contin Educ Pract Vet* 9:752, 1987.

74. Kraus KH, Turrentine MA, Jergens AE, et al: Effect of desmopressin acetate on bleeding times and plasma von Willebrand factor in Doberman pinscher dogs with von Willebrand's disease, *Vet Surg* 18:103, 1989.

75. Ladenson JH, Apple FS, Koch DD: Misleading hyponatremia due to hyperlipemia: a method-dependent error, *Ann Intern Med* 95:707, 1981.

76. Lage AL: Nephrogenic diabetes insipidus in a dog, *J Am Vet Med Assoc* 163:251, 1973.

77. Lage AL: Apparent psychogenic polydipsia. In Kirk RW, editor: *Current veterinary therapy VI*, Philadelphia, 1977, WB Saunders, p. 1098.

78. Lage AL: Nephrogenic diabetes insipidus. In Kirk RW, editor: *Current veterinary therapy VI*, Philadelphia, 1977, WB Saunders, p. 1102.

79. Lamb WA, Muir P: Lymphangiosarcoma associated with hyponatremia and hyperkalemia in a dog, *J Small Anim Pract* 35:374, 1994.

80. Laureno R: Central pontine myelinolysis following rapid correction of hyponatremia, *Ann Neurol* 13:232, 1983.

81. Laureno R, Karp BI: Myelinolysis after correction of hyponatremia, *Ann Int Med* 126:57, 1997.

82. Levin ER, Gardner DG, Samson WK: Natriuretic peptides, *N Engl J Med* 339:321, 1998.

83. Levitin H, Goodman A, Pigeon G, et al: Composition of the renal medulla during water diuresis, *J Clin Invest* 41:1145, 1962.

84. Lieberman LL, Kircher CH, Lein DH: Polyuria and polydipsia associated with pituitary visceral larval migrans in a dog, *J Am Anim Hosp Assoc* 15:237, 1979.

85. Lifton SJ, King LG, Zerbe CA: Glucocorticoid deficient hypoadrenocorticism in dogs: 18 cases (1986-1995), *J Am Vet Med Assoc* 209:2076, 1996.

86. Ling GV, Stabenfeldt GH, Comer KM, et al: Canine hyperadrenocorticism: pretreatment clinical and laboratory evaluation of 117 cases, *J Am Vet Med Assoc* 174:1211, 1979.

87. Lubberink AA: Therapy for spontaneous hyperadrenocorticism. In Kirk RW, editor: *Current veterinary therapy VII*, Philadelphia, 1980, WB Saunders, p. 979.

88. Luzius H, Jans DA, Grunbaum EG, et al: A low affinity vasopressin V2-receptor in inherited nephrogenic diabetes insipidus, *J Recept Res* 12:351, 1992.

89. MacKay BM, Curtis N: Adipsia and hypernatraemia in a dog with focal hypothalamic granulomatous meningoencephalitis, *Aust Vet J* 77:14, 1999.

90. MacMillan KL: Neurologic complications following treatment of canine hypoadrenocorticism, *Can Vet J* 44:490, 2003.

91. Madewell BR, Osborne CA, Norrdin RA, et al: Clinicopathologic aspects of diabetes insipidus in the dog, *J Am Anim Hosp Assoc* 11:497, 1975.

92. Malik R, Hunt GB, Hinchliffe JM, et al: Severe whipworm infection in the dog, *J Small Anim Pract* 31:185, 1990.

93. Mann JFE, Johnson AK, Ganten D, et al: Thirst and the renin angiotensin system, *Kidney Int* 32(suppl 21):S27, 1987.

94. Mulnix JA, Rijnberk A, Hendriks HJ: Evaluation of a modified water-deprivation test for diagnosis of polyuric disorders in dogs, *J Am Vet Med Assoc* 169:1327, 1976.

95. Narins RG, Jones ER, Stom MC, et al: Diagnostic strategies in disorders of fluid, electrolyte and acid base homeostasis, *Am J Med* 72:496, 1982.

96. Neer TM, Reavis DU: Craniopharyngioma and associated central diabetes insipidus and hypothyroidism in a dog, *J Am Vet Med Assoc* 182:519, 1983.

97. Neilsen S, Frokiaer J, Marples D, et al: Aquaporins in the kidney: from molecules to medicine, *Physiol Rev* 82:205, 2002.

98. O'Brien DP, Kroll RA, Johnson GC, et al: Myelinolysis after correction of hyponatremia in two dogs, *J Vet Intern Med* 8:40, 1994.

99. O'Grady SM, Palfrey HC, Field M: Characteristics and function of Na-K-2Cl cotransport in epithelial tissues, *Am J Physiol* 253:C177, 1987.

100. Palmer LG, Frindt G: Amiloride sensitive Na^+ channels from the apical membrane of rat cortical collecting tubule, *Proc Natl Acad Sci USA* 83:2767, 1986.

101. Peterson M: Hyperadrenocorticism, *Vet Clin North Am Small Anim Pract* 14:731, 1984.

102. Peterson ME, Kintzer PP, Kass PH: Pretreatment clinical and laboratory findings in dogs with hypoadrenocorticism—225 cases (1979-1993), *J Am Vet Med Assoc* 208:85, 1996.

103. Pittari JM: Central diabetes insipidus in a cat, *Feline Pract* 24:18, 1996.

104. Post K, McNeill JRJ, Clark EG, et al: Congenital central diabetes insipidus in two sibling Afghan hound pups, *J Am Vet Med Assoc* 194:1086, 1989.

105. Rakich PM, Lorenz MD: Clinical signs and laboratory abnormalities in 23 dogs with spontaneous hypoadrenocorticism, *J Am Anim Hosp Assoc* 20:647, 1984.

106. Reidarson TH, Weis DJ, Hardy RM: Extreme hypernatremia in a dog with central diabetes insipidus: a case report, *J Am Anim Hosp Assoc* 26:89, 1990.

107. Rijnberk A, Biewenga WJ, Mol JA: Inappropriate vasopressin secretion in two dogs, *Acta Endocrinol* 117:59, 1988.

108. Rittig S, Jensen AR, Jensen KT, et al: Effect of food intake on the pharmacokinetics and antidiuretic activity of oral desmopressin (DDAVP) in hydrated normal subjects, *Clin Endocrinol* 48:235, 1998.

109. Robertson GL: Thirst and vasopressin function in normal and disordered states of water balance, *J Lab Clin Med* 101:351, 1983.

110. Rogers W, Straus J, Chew D: A typical hypoadrenocorticism in three dogs, *J Am Vet Med Assoc* 179:155, 1981.

111. Rogers WA, Valdez H, Anderson BC, et al: Partial deficiency of antidiuretic hormone in a cat, *J Am Vet Med Assoc* 170:545, 1977.

112. Ross LA, Finco DR: Relationship of selected clinical renal function tests to glomerular filtration rate and renal blood flow in cats, *Am J Vet Res* 42:1704, 1981.

113. Rothuizen J, Biewenga WJ, Mol JA: Chronic glucocorticoid excess and impaired osmoregulation of vasopressin release in dogs with hepatic encephalopathy, *Domest Anim Endocrinol* 12:13, 1995.

114. Schaer M, Chen CL: A clinical survey of 48 dogs with adrenocortical hypofunction, *J Am Anim Hosp Assoc* 19:443, 1983.

115. Schaer M, Halling KB, Collins KE, et al: Combined hyponatremia and hyperkalemia mimicking acute hypoadrenocorticism in three pregnant dogs, *J Am Vet Med Assoc* 218:897, 2001.

116. Schuster VL, Stokes JB: Chloride transport by the cortical and outer medullary collecting duct, *Am J Physiol* 253:F203, 1987.

117. Shull RM: The value of anion gap and osmolal gap determinations in veterinary medicine, *Vet Clin Pathol* 7:12, 1978.

118. Sterns RH, Ocdol H, Schrier RW, et al: Hyponatremia: pathophysiology, diagnosis and therapy. In Narins RG, editor: *Maxwell and Kleeman's clinical disorders of fluid and electrolyte metabolism,* New York, 1994, McGraw-Hill, p. 583.

119. Sterns RH, Spital A, Clark EC: Disorders of water balance. In Kokko JP, Tannen RL, editors: *Fluids and electrolytes,* Philadelphia, 1996, WB Saunders, p. 63.

120. Sullivan SA, Harmon BG, Purinton PT, et al: Lobar holoprosencephaly in a Miniature Schnauzer with hypodipsic hypernatremia, *J Am Vet Med Assoc* 223:1783, 2003.

121. Takemura N: Successful long-term treatment of congenital nephrogenic diabetes insipidus in a dog, *J Small Anim Pract* 39:592, 1998.

122. Thompson MD, Carr AP: Hyponatremia and hyperkalemia associated with chylous pleural and peritoneal effusion in a cat, *Can Vet J* 43:610, 2002.

123. Toll J, Barr SC, Hickford FH: Acute water intoxication in a dog, *J Vet Emerg Crit Care* 9:19, 1999.

124. Tyler RD, Qualls CW, Heald RD, et al: Renal concentrating ability in dehydrated hyponatremic dogs, *J Am Vet Med Assoc* 191:1095, 1987.

125. Van Heerden J, Geel J, Moore DJ: Hypodipsic hypernatremia in a miniature schnauzer, *J S Afr Vet Assoc* 63:39, 1992.

126. Vilhardt H, Bie P: Antidiuretic response in conscious dogs following peroral administration of arginine vasopressin and its analogs, *Eur J Pharmacol* 93:201, 1983.

127. Willard MD, Schall WD, McCaw DE, et al: Canine hypoadrenocorticism: report of 37 cases and review of 39 previously reported cases, *J Am Vet Med Assoc* 180:59, 1982.

128. Willard MD, Fossum TW, Torrance A, et al: Hyponatremia and hyperkalemia associated with idiopathic or experimentally induced chylothorax in four dogs, *J Am Vet Med Assoc* 199:353, 1991.

129. Winterbotham J, Mason K: Congenital diabetes insipidus in a kitten, *J Small Anim Pract* 24:569, 1983.

130. Yamamoto T, Sasaki S: Aquaporins in the kidney: emerging new aspects, *Kidney Int* 54:1041, 1998.

131. Zenger E: Persistent hyperkalemia associated with nonchylous pleural effusion in a dog, *J Am Anim Hosp Assoc* 28:411, 1992.

132. Zerbe R, Stropes L, Robertson G: Vasopressin function in the syndrome of inappropriate antidiuresis, *Annu Rev Med* 31:315, 1980.

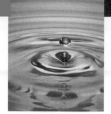

CHAPTER • 4

DISORDERS OF CHLORIDE: HYPERCHLOREMIA AND HYPOCHLOREMIA

Helio Autran de Morais and Alexander W. Biondo

Whereas for a long time it was assumed that chloride ions were reabsorbed entirely passively with sodium—the "mendicant" role of chloride—more recent studies suggest that several distinctive reabsorptive transport mechanisms operate in parallel.[76]

Chloride constitutes approximately two thirds of the anions in plasma and the remainder of extracellular fluid (ECF). It also is the major anion filtered by the glomeruli and reabsorbed in the renal tubules. Chloride is important not only for maintaining osmolality but also actively participates in acid-base regulation.

Chloride is present in plasma at a mean concentration of approximately 110 mEq/L in dogs and 120 mEq/L in cats.[13] Chloride concentration in venous samples is 3 to 4 mEq/L lower than in arterial samples when cells are separated from plasma anaerobically.[80] The intracellular concentration of chloride is much lower than its plasma concentration and is dependent on the resting membrane potential of the cell. Muscle cells, for example, have a resting membrane potential of approximately −68 mV and an average chloride concentration ($[Cl^-]$) of 2 to 4 mEq/L, whereas red blood cells have a resting membrane potential of approximately −15 mV and an average $[Cl^-]$ of 60 mEq/L.[50] This higher intracellular concentration of chloride ions in erythrocytes allows chloride to move in and out of the red blood cells very effectively, as dictated by electrical charges on either side of the cell membrane. This is an important difference from other cells and is the basis of the so-called "chloride-shift" in the red cell membrane.[50] The chloride ion distribution in various body fluids is summarized in Box 4-1.

CHLORIDE METABOLISM

GASTROINTESTINAL TRACT

Under normal conditions, humans produce 1 to 2 L of gastric juice daily. The sodium concentration ($[Na^+]$) and $[Cl^-]$ of gastric juice are quite variable, ranging from 20 to

---

Box 4-1	**Chloride Ion in Various Body Fluids**

Extracellular (ECF) and Intracellular Fluid (ICF)

Most prevalent anion in ECF

Polyvalent anions (e.g., DNA, RNA, proteins, organic phosphates) replace chloride ion in ICF

Chloride concentration in the ECF is dependent on cell resting membrane potential:
Muscle cells: 2-4 mEq/L
Epithelial cells: 20 mEq/L
Red blood cells: 60 mEq/L

Stomach

Most prevalent anion in gastric juice

Chloride concentration is greater than sodium and potassium concentrations whenever gastric juice pH is <4.0

Intestine

Most prevalent anion in small and large intestinal fluids

Highest chloride concentration is found in the ileum, whereas colonic fluids have the lowest chloride concentration

Kidneys

Most prevalent anion in glomerular ultrafiltrate

80% of filtered sodium is reabsorbed accompanied by chloride

Chloride transport in cortical collecting tubules is associated with regulation of acid-base balance

From de Morais HSA: Chloride ion in small animal practice: the forgotten ion, J Vet Emerg Crit Care 2:11-24, 1992.

100 mEq/L and 120 to 160 mEq/L, respectively.[69] In the **jejunum,** sodium is absorbed actively against small electrochemical gradients and also through relatively large mucosal "pores" in the proximal bowel. Chloride absorption in the jejunum generally follows sodium to maintain electroneutrality. It is believed that chloride reabsorption in the jejunum occurs via the paracellular route in response to the transepithelial potential generated by active sodium transport.[20] The **ileum** is less permeable to ions than is the jejunum. Absorption of chloride and secretion of bicarbonate in the ileum are coupled by processes that may involve active transport of one or both ions. Highly efficient absorption of sodium and chloride occurs in the **colon,** where 90% of the sodium and chloride entering is reabsorbed. There appears to be no direct or indirect coupling between sodium and chloride or bicarbonate reabsorption in the distal colon. Active chloride reabsorption and bicarbonate secretion occur in the distal colon. Chloride also can be secreted in the jejunum, ileum, and colon.[20,69] **Pancreatic juice** usually is not rich in chloride ions. However, there is a reciprocal relationship between chloride and bicarbonate concentration in pancreatic fluid that is dependent on flow rate, with chloride being the major anion at lower rates of secretion.[20]

KIDNEYS

The kidneys play an important role in the regulation of plasma chloride concentration. After sodium, chloride is the most prevalent ion in the glomerular ultrafiltrate. Most of the chloride filtered is reabsorbed in the renal tubules. The traditional view of epithelial transport in the kidney represents the chloride ion as an obedient passive partner that follows the actively transported sodium ion. This view does not apply to many epithelia, including specific nephron segments. Chloride transport is intimately related to sodium and fluid transport and to cellular acid-base metabolism.[76]

Chloride reabsorption in the proximal tubule is actively and passively linked to active sodium reabsorption. A formate-chloride exchange mechanism exists in the luminal membrane of proximal tubular cells and is responsible for active chloride reabsorption.[72] Reabsorbed chloride returns to the systemic circulation at the basolateral membrane primarily by a potassium chloride (K^+-Cl^-) cotransporter. Of filtered chloride, approximately 50% to 60% is reabsorbed by the proximal convoluted and straight tubules. Chloride reabsorption occurs transcellularly in the thick ascending limb of Henle's loop, leading to the generation of a lumen-positive transepithelial voltage. Sodium is reabsorbed transcellularly or paracellularly, and the transepithelial voltage drives the latter process. Chloride ion delivery is the rate-limiting step in this process, and net sodium chloride (NaCl) transport increases directly with fluid [Cl^-] concentration. Loop diuretics such as furosemide and bumetanide act in the loop of Henle by competing for the chloride site on the Na^+-K^+-$2Cl^-$ carrier.[20,42,72,76]

A comprehensive model explaining sodium chloride transport in the distal tubule is not yet available. This is because of, in part, the cellular heterogeneity of this nephron segment and differences among species and because a portion of this nephron segment is not accessible to micropuncture techniques in rats, the most extensively studied species. Thiazide diuretics act by inhibiting the Na^+-Cl^- carrier in the early distal tubule, apparently at the chloride site.[42] Conversely, loop diuretics do not block NaCl reabsorption at this site. Chloride ion transport in the collecting tubule is closely related to bicarbonate transport.[72] Little is known about chloride transport in the medullary collecting tubules. In the cortical collecting tubules, however, the paracellular pathway, which is highly conductive for chloride ions, is an important route for reabsorption of chloride by diffusion down an electrochemical gradient. An increase in the lumen-positive transepithelial potential difference (TPD) decreases net chloride reabsorption, whereas a decrease in TPD increases chloride reabsorption. Therefore hormones that change TPD in the cortical collecting tubule can affect chloride reabsorption. Experimentally, administration of deoxycorticosterone acetate (DOCA) twice daily resulted in a mild increase in [Na^+] and no change in [Cl^-].[49] The resulting increase in strong ion difference (SID; the difference between all strong cations and all strong anions in plasma; see Chapter 13) was associated with a mild increase in bicarbonate ion concentration ([HCO_3^-]). Administration of DOCA in sodium-supplemented dogs caused a significant increase in plasma [Na^+] and [HCO_3^-] with no change in plasma [Cl^-].[59] When $NaHCO_3$ instead of NaCl was added to the diet, [Na^+] and [HCO_3^-] increased significantly, whereas [Cl^-] decreased. Increased urinary loss of chloride is believed to be associated with hyperadrenocorticism. In a study of 117 dogs with hyperadrenocorticism, only 12 had [Cl^-] below 105 mEq/L.[56] However, 25 of these dogs had hypernatremia, and the [Cl^-] could have been low relative to the [Na^+]. The mean [Na^+] was 149.9 mEq/L, and the mean [Cl^-] was 108 mEq/L (mean [Cl^-] after correcting for changes in free water was 105 mEq/L). The cortical collecting duct is the main site of action for mineralocorticoids and glucocorticoids.[15] Administration of DOCA increases TPD in rats and rabbits, increasing sodium reabsorption in the cortical collecting tubules. Such an effect could explain the observed changes in chloride and sodium concentrations in dogs with hyperadrenocorticism.

CHLORIDE AND ACID-BASE BALANCE

METABOLIC ACIDOSIS

Metabolic acidoses are traditionally divided into hyperchloremic (normal anion gap [AG]) and normochloremic (high AG) based on the AG and [Cl^-]. The AG is the difference between measured cations (sodium and potassium) and measured anions (chloride and bicarbonate) (see Chapters 9 and 10). Physiologically, there is no AG because electroneutrality must be maintained and the AG is the difference between the unmeasured anions (UA^-) and unmeasured cations (UC^+). The AG is a simplification that is helpful clinically. Metabolic acidosis usually results from an increase in the concentration of a strong anion. Strong anions are anions that are completely dissociated at body pH (e.g., Cl^-, lactate, ketoanions). If the strong anion added is chloride, the sum of the measured anions ($[Cl^-] + [HCO_3^-]$) will remain the same, and the AG will not change (so-called hyperchloremic or normal AG acidosis). If the strong anion added is an unmeasured anion (e.g., lactate), $[Cl^-]$ will remain normal, whereas $[HCO_3^-]$ will decrease. The sum of the measured anions will decrease, thus increasing the AG (so-called normochloremic or high AG acidosis).

The acid-base status of plasma is regulated by changing Pco_2 in the lungs and SID in the kidneys, the latter being accomplished mainly by differential reabsorption of sodium and chloride ions in the renal tubules. Chloride is the most prevalent strong anion in the ECF. At a constant $[Na^+]$, a decrease in $[Cl^-]$ increases SID causing hypochloremic alkalosis, whereas an increase in $[Cl^-]$ decreases SID causing hyperchloremic acidosis. The effects of increasing $[Cl^-]$ without changing $[Na^+]$ can be understood when considering a fluid with an SID = 0 (e.g., 0.9% NaCl where $[Na^+]$ = $[Cl^-]$ and thus SID = $[Na^+] - [Cl^-]$ = 0). It is known that 0.9% NaCl administration leads to metabolic acidosis. The classical explanation is that infusion of a fluid without bicarbonate dilutes $[HCO_3^-]$ in plasma and leads to acidosis. However, the degree of acidosis after normal saline infusion correlates best with the amount of chloride given and with the increase in serum $[Cl^-]$.[85] There was a weaker correlation with the volume administered and no increase in plasma volume, calling into question the traditional concept of dilutional acidosis.

CHLORIDE IN METABOLIC ALKALOSIS

Chloride participates in the genesis, maintenance, and correction of metabolic alkalosis because decreases in $[Cl^-]$ increase SID, causing metabolic alkalosis. The role of chloride is supported by the inverse relationship between chloride and bicarbonate in metabolic alkalosis,[4] the fact that chloride depletion is accompanied by increased plasma $[HCO_3^-]$,[67] and the fact that chronic metabolic alkalosis cannot be produced experimentally if chloride is available in the diet.[54] In addition, during recovery from chronic hypercapnia, the compensatory increase in $[HCO_3^-]$ will not normalize if dietary chloride is restricted.[78]

Chloride was first linked to metabolic alkalosis in dogs when MacCallum et al[58] observed hypochloremia

and an increase in "alkali reserve" in dogs with loss of gastric fluid caused by pyloric obstruction. The classical hypothesis associates the genesis and maintenance of metabolic alkalosis primarily with volume contraction. According to this hypothesis, volume depletion accompanying alkalosis augments fluid reabsorption in the proximal tubules. Alkalosis is maintained because bicarbonate ions are preferentially reabsorbed in this segment.[36] Volume expansion suppresses fluid and bicarbonate reabsorption, and more bicarbonate and chloride ions are delivered to distal nephron segments, which possess greater capacity to reabsorb chloride than bicarbonate. Chloride then is retained, bicarbonate is excreted, and alkalosis is corrected.[36] In addition to volume expansion, provision of chloride was also a feature of studies used to substantiate this hypothesis. The classical hypothesis can be viewed from a different perspective in which changes in chloride are the cause of the alkalosis.[35] In rats, chloride ion depletion alone plays a role in the genesis and maintenance of metabolic alkalosis.[31–33,57] In rats with chronic hypochloremic alkalosis, chloride repletion (and correction of alkalosis) can be achieved without administration of sodium, without volume expansion, and without an increase in glomerular filtration rate (GFR).[83] The correction phase is associated with a decrease in plasma renin activity but with no change in plasma aldosterone concentration. It also has been shown that maintenance and correction of hypochloremic alkalosis primarily are dependent on total body chloride and its influence on renal function, and not on the demands of sodium and fluid homeostasis.[34] Ultimately, the correction of alkalosis is dependent on the kidney.[36] The principal mechanisms by which the kidneys correct metabolic alkalosis probably operate in the collecting ducts, especially in the cortical segment, where HCO_3^- can either be secreted or reabsorbed.[35]

Expanding the ECF without providing chloride does not correct hypochloremic alkalosis. Furosemide-induced hypochloremic alkalosis in humans eating an NaCl-free diet supplemented with 60 mEq potassium per day can be corrected with orally administered KCl without changes in weight or ECF volume.[75] In this study, five NaCl-depleted control subjects were given furosemide and a combination of KCl and NaCl intravenously to maintain their sodium deficit while correcting their chloride deficit. Subjects who were selectively sodium depleted did not become alkalotic.[75] It also has been shown that a 25% increase in ECF volume (created by intravenous infusion of 6% bovine albumin in 5% dextrose) has no effect on hypochloremic alkalosis in a rat model of hypochloremic alkalosis.[34]

These studies demonstrate that ECF volume, GFR, effective circulating volume, and sodium balance are not independent variables in the generation and maintenance of metabolic alkalosis.[65] However, it still could be concluded that chloride induces potassium conservation that in turn inhibits bicarbonate reabsorption because potassium balance was corrected even in studies during which choline-Cl instead of KCl was used to correct the alkalosis. When NaCl is supplied without potassium, however, alkalosis is corrected despite a persisting potassium deficit,[3,64] and administration of potassium without chloride does not correct alkalosis.[51] It has been speculated that hypokalemia in rats may cause hypochloremia by impairing recycling of potassium at the luminal membrane in the thick ascending limb of Henle's loop. This, in turn, impairs the effectiveness of the Na^+-K^+-$2Cl^-$ carrier, decreasing net chloride reabsorption.[36] It still is controversial whether hypokalemia induces metabolic alkalosis in humans.[30] Contrary to what occurs in rats, isolated potassium deficiency in dogs causes mild metabolic acidosis.[6,7] Chronic potassium depletion also is associated with metabolic acidosis in cats.[21]

Studies in rats with experimentally induced normovolemic and hypovolemic hypochloremic alkalosis showed no difference in the renal handling of chloride and bicarbonate between alkalotic and normal animals in the proximal convoluted tubule, loop of Henle, or distal convoluted tubule.[36] Key adjustments in anion excretion during the maintenance and correction of hypochloremic alkalosis were suspected to occur in the collecting tubule, especially in the cortical segment.[35] Sodium-independent chloride and bicarbonate transport, and secretion or reabsorption of HCO_3^- occur at this site.[35,36] Alterations in the delivery of HCO_3^- and Cl^- to the collecting tubules also may be important.[35]

The chloride depletion hypothesis for the genesis and maintenance of metabolic alkalosis was proposed as an extension of the classical hypothesis.[35,36] It states that chloride alone is essential for correction of the hypochloremic alkalosis and that it does so by a renal mechanism. Volume depletion is a common but not essential feature of the maintenance phase of alkalosis, and its persistence does not preclude correction of alkalosis. If adequate chloride is provided, restoration of depleted volume, however, may hasten correction of alkalosis by increasing GFR and decreasing proximal tubular reabsorption of fluid and bicarbonate.[35,36] The manner by which exogenous Cl^- repletion is detected and the kidney signaled to excrete HCO_3^-, and the cellular mechanisms by which these events occur in the various nephron segments remain to be determined.[35]

ROLE OF CHLORIDE IN ADAPTATION FOR ACID-BASE DISTURBANCES

Chloride excretion is an important mechanism in the kidney's adaptation to metabolic acidosis and chronic respiratory acid-base disturbances. In **metabolic acido-sis**, the kidneys increase net acid excretion (primarily by enhanced NH_4Cl excretion) beginning on day 1 and reaching a maximum after 5 to 6 days.[72] The increase in chloride ion excretion without an associated increase in sodium ion excretion increases plasma SID and returns $[HCO_3^-]$ and pH toward normal.

The increase in Pco_2 in **chronic respiratory acidosis** causes intracellular $[H^+]$ to increase in the renal tubular cells, resulting in stimulation of net acid excretion (primarily as NH_4Cl).[72] Chloruresis, negative chloride balance, enhanced fractional and absolute bicarbonate reabsorption, and enhanced net acid excretion typically are associated with the renal response to chronic respiratory acidosis.[36] The loss of chloride ions in the urine decreases urinary SID because Cl^- is accompanied by NH_4^+ (a weak cation) rather than Na^+. Thus plasma SID and consequently $[HCO_3^-]$ are increased. Hypochloremia is a common finding in dogs with chronic hypercapnia.[60,70,77,82] Conversely, renal H^+ ion excretion is decreased in **chronic respiratory alkalosis.** This effect probably is mediated by a decrease in intracellular $[H^+]$. In this setting, there is a decrease in NH_4Cl excretion in the urine and an increase in renal reabsorption of Cl^-. The increase in Cl^- reabsorption decreases plasma SID and consequently $[HCO_3^-]$ and is responsible for the hyperchloremia observed in dogs with chronic hypocapnia.[38]

CLINICAL APPROACH TO CHLORIDE DISORDERS

CORRECTED CHLORIDE

Changes in chloride concentration can result from changes in water balance or can be caused by a gain or loss of chloride. When changes in $[Cl^-]$ are caused by water balance alterations (i.e., increase or decrease in free water), $[Na^+]$ also changes. Changes in $[Cl^-]$ and $[Na^+]$ are proportional in this setting (e.g., a 10% gain in free water decreases $[Cl^-]$ and $[Na^+]$ by 10%). To account for changes in water balance, $[Cl^-]$ must be evaluated in conjunction with evaluation of changes in $[Na^+]$.[13] Therefore patient $[Cl^-]$ is "corrected" for changes in $[Na^+]$ concentration[13]:

$$Cl^- \text{ (corrected)} = Cl^- \text{ (measured)} \times \frac{Na^+ \text{ (normal)}}{Na^+ \text{ (measured)}}$$

where Cl^- (measured) and Na^+ (measured) are the patient's chloride and sodium concentrations, respectively, and Na^+ (normal) is the mean normal sodium concentration.

Assuming mean values for $[Na^+]$ of 146 mEq/L in dogs and 156 mEq/L in cats, and for $[Cl^-]$ of 110 mEq/L in dogs and 120 mEq/L in cats,[16] the Cl^- (corrected) can be estimated[13] in dogs as:

$$Cl^- \text{ (corrected)} = Cl^- \times 146/Na^+$$

and in cats as:

$$Cl^- \text{ (corrected)} = Cl^- \times 156/Na^+$$

Normal Cl^- (corrected) is approximately 107 to 113 mEq/L in dogs and approximately 117 to 123 mEq/L in cats.[13] These values may vary for different laboratories and different analyzers. Newer analyzers report higher chloride values unless the chloride calibration is deliberately changed.[89] Using the Cl^- (corrected) permits the division of chloride disorders into artifactual and corrected chloride changes (Table 4-1). In artifactual chloride changes, changes in free water are solely responsible for the chloride changes, whereas in corrected chloride changes, chloride itself is primarily changed. Algorithms for the evaluation of chloride abnormalities are presented in Figs. 4-1 through 4-3.

CHLORIDE MEASUREMENTS

Reference intervals for $[Cl^-]$ and $[Na^+]$ vary depending on the analytical method and performing laboratory, and these factors should be considered when interpreting and comparing clinical results. Chloride ions can be measured in plasma, serum, or blood; serum is preferred because serum chloride is stable for months. Chloride concentrations most commonly are measured by potentiometry, which is based on ion electrical potential. When the ion electrode is immersed in a solution containing chloride ions, an electrode potential proportional to the logarithm of the chloride ion activity is generated. Chloride ions then are measured by the chloride ion electrode based on this principle in combination with a reference electrode. Because of the much greater solubility of AgCl compared with AgI, the chloride electrode will be irreversibly damaged if immersed in solutions containing iodide ions, resulting in a falsely increased chloride concentration. A high interference also is observed when bromide and cyanide ions are measured, and the chloride electrode will only give reliable results if these ions are absent or in minimal amounts when compared with chloride ions. Some

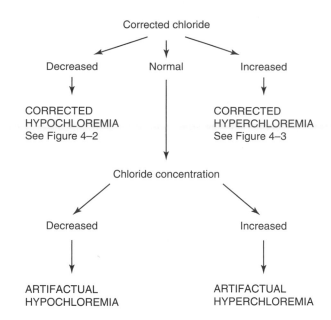

Fig. 4-1 Algorithm for evaluation of patients with chloride abnormalities.

laboratories still measure chloride concentration by flame photometry, which is based on ion concentration resulting from flame color change.

CLINICAL DISTURBANCES

DISORDERS ASSOCIATED WITH NORMAL Cl^- (CORRECTED)

Artifactual Hypochloremia and Artifactual Hyperchloremia

A change in the water content of plasma without an imbalance in the content of electrolytes dilutes or concentrates anions and cations. Consequently, $[Cl^-]$ and $[Na^+]$ will change in parallel. These changes usually are recognized by changes in sodium concentration (hypernatremia or hyponatremia), and this ion (and changes in osmolality) should receive primary attention (see Chapter 3).

TABLE 4-1   Classification of Chloride Disorders

Disorder	Cl^-	Na^+	Cl^- Corrected	Associated Acid-Base Disorder
Artifactual hyperchloremia	⇑	⇑	N	Concentration alkalosis
Artifactual hypochloremia	⇓	⇓	N	Dilution acidosis
Corrected hyperchloremia	⇑, N, ⇓	⇑, N, ⇓	⇑	Hyperchloremic acidosis
Corrected hypochloremia	⇑, N, ⇓	⇑, N, ⇓	⇓	Hypochloremic alkalosis

Source: de Morais HSA: Chloride ion in small animal practice: the forgotten ion, J Vet Emerg Crit Care 2:11-24, 1992.

Cl^-, *Chloride concentration;* Cl^- *corrected, corrected chloride concentration;* Na^+, *sodium concentration;* ⇑, *increased concentration;* N, *normal concentration;* ⇓, *decreased concentration.*

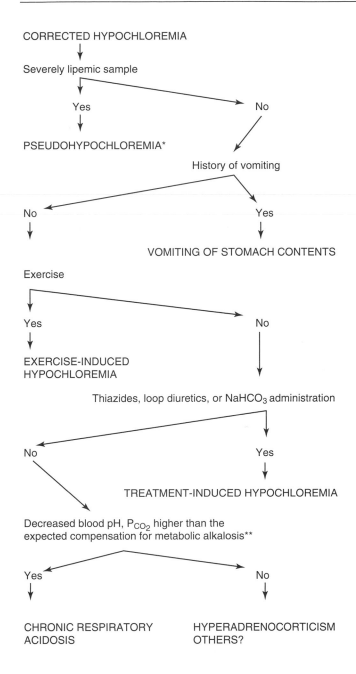

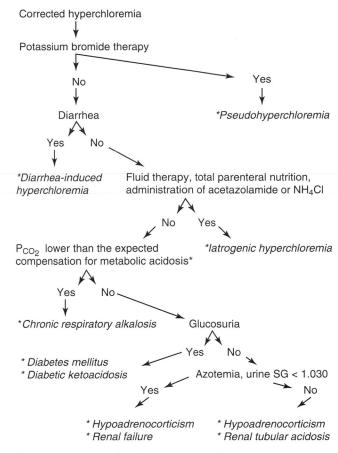

Fig. 4-3 Algorithm for evaluation of dogs with corrected hyperchloremia.

*Lipemia will underestimate chloride when chloride is measured by titrimetic methods.
**Expected compensation for metabolic alkalosis in dogs is a 0.35 mm Hg increase in P_{CO_2} for each 1 mEq/L increase in bicarbonate.

Fig. 4-2 Algorithm for evaluation of dogs with corrected hypochloremia.

High chloride concentration with normal Cl⁻ (corrected) (**artifactual hyperchloremia**) usually is associated with pure water loss (e.g., diabetes insipidus, essential hypernatremia) or hypotonic losses (e.g., osmotic diuresis). Patients with hypernatremia caused by sodium gain (e.g., hypertonic saline or $NaHCO_3$ administration,

hyperadrenocorticism) tend to have abnormal Cl⁻ (corrected). Low chloride concentration with normal Cl⁻ (corrected) (**artifactual hypochloremia**) has been associated with congestive heart failure, hypoadrenocorticism, and third-space loss of sodium and chloride. It also is associated with gastrointestinal loss, although in this setting one ion often is lost in excess of the other (e.g., chloride in patients with vomiting of stomach contents, sodium in patients with diarrhea), and the Cl⁻ (corrected) may be abnormal. Patients with hypoadrenocorticism may be presented with corrected hyperchloremia as a result of mineralocorticoid deficiency.

Patients with artifactual hypochloremia tend to have decreased SID and therefore a tendency toward acidosis (so-called dilutional acidosis), whereas patients with artifactual hyperchloremia tend to have increased SID and a tendency toward alkalosis (so-called concentration alkalosis).[14] These are the only situations in which $[HCO_3^-]$ changes in the same direction as $[Cl^-]$, and the change in $[Cl^-]$ is more pronounced.[12]

DISORDERS ASSOCIATED WITH ABNORMAL Cl⁻ (CORRECTED)

Corrected Hypochloremia

Decreased Cl⁻ (corrected) is associated with a tendency toward alkalosis (hypochloremic alkalosis) caused by the associated increase in SID.[14] Pseudohypochloremia may occur whenever chloride ion concentration is measured with a technique that is not ion-selective in lipemic or hyperproteinemic samples.[17,41] Chloride concentration in lipemic samples (triglyceride concentration >600 mg/dL) is underestimated by titrimetric methods but overestimated when colorimetric methods are used.[41] Clinical signs associated with pure hypochloremia in dogs and cats have not been reported but probably are related to the metabolic alkalosis that accompanies hypochloremia.[13] However, it has been shown that in euvolemic chloride depletion, GFR decreases acutely by as much as 15% to 20%, probably as a result of changes in tubuloglomerular feedback and internal shifts of fluid out of the ECF.[36,37] The clinical importance of these experimental observations is unknown, but hypochloremia itself may potentiate the decrease in GFR associated with hypovolemia in the most common causes of corrected hypochloremia (e.g., vomiting of stomach contents, therapy with loop diuretics). Chloride ion depletion also stimulates renin secretion in rats despite concurrent volume expansion and potassium infusion.[1] Renin release caused by hypochloremia probably is mediated by the macula densa. Any resultant increase in aldosterone secretion would increase potassium excretion in the urine and contribute to hypokalemia.

Corrected hypochloremia may be caused by excessive loss of chloride relative to sodium or by administration of substances containing proportionately more sodium than chloride as compared with the normal ECF composition. The former can occur with administration of diuretics that cause chloride ion wasting (e.g., loop diuretics, thiazides) or when the fluid lost has a high [Cl⁻], as in the case of vomiting of stomach contents or gastric conduit urinary diversions.[14,26,61] Loss of plasma during exercise in greyhounds also leads to corrected hypochloremia as a result of a greater loss of Cl⁻ than Na⁺.[81] The administration of substances containing proportionately more sodium than chloride (e.g., NaHCO₃) increases [Na⁺] without increasing [Cl⁻], therefore causing a decrease in Cl⁻ (corrected). Corrected hypochloremia in dogs with hyperadrenocorticism has been discussed previously. Unlike dogs with hypoadrenocorticism that have corrected hyperchloremia caused by the lack of mineralocorticoids, dogs with gastrointestinal diseases that mimic hypoadrenocorticism (i.e., presence of hyperkalemia and hyponatremia)[18] tend to develop corrected hypochloremia. In cats, acute tumor lysis syndrome,[8] primary hypoadrenocorticism,[68] anemia,[87] hemorrhagic pleural effusion,[87] and diabetic ketoacidosis[11] have been associated with corrected

hypochloremia. Vomiting may have been a contributory factor in the corrected hypochloremia observed in some of these cats.

An increase in renal chloride ion excretion and a decrease in plasma [Cl⁻] have been observed in dogs with experimentally induced chronic respiratory acidosis.[60,70,77,82] Consequently, patients with chronic hypercapnia may be presented with corrected hypochloremia.[45] Potential causes of corrected hypochloremia are listed in Box 4-2, and an algorithm for the differential diagnosis of corrected hypochloremia is presented in Fig. 4-2.

Treatment of patients with corrected hypochloremia should be directed at correcting the SID. Special attention also should be paid to the sodium concentration. Renal Cl⁻ conservation is enhanced in hypochloremic states, and renal chloride ion reabsorption does not return to normal until plasma [Cl⁻] is restored to normal or near normal.[36] Therefore patients with normal renal function should be expected to respond to therapy if the underlying disease process is corrected and chloride is provided. In cases in which expansion of extracellular volume is desired, intravenous infusion of 0.9% NaCl is the treatment of choice.[26] If hypokalemia also is present, KCl should be added to the fluid administered. In the rare situation in which volume expansion is not necessary, chloride can be administered using salts without sodium (e.g., KCl, NH₄Cl). Use of NaCl or KCl requires normal renal function to correct hypochloremia, whereas NH₄Cl requires intact hepatic and renal function.[52]

| **Box 4-2** | **Causes of Corrected Hypochloremia** |

Pseudohypochloremia
Lipemic samples (titrimetric methods)

Excessive Loss of Chloride Relative to Sodium
Vomiting of stomach contents*
Therapy with thiazides or loop diuretics*
Chronic respiratory acidosis
Hyperadrenocorticism
Exercise
Selected gastrointestinal diseases associated with hyperkalemia and hyponatremia in dogs without hypoadrenocorticism

Therapy with Solutions Containing High Sodium Concentration Relative to Chloride
Sodium bicarbonate
Sodium penicillin (extremely high doses)

Adapted from de Morais HSA: Chloride ion in small animal practice: the forgotten ion, *J Vet Emerg Crit Care* 2:11-24, 1992.
*More important causes in small animal practice.

Corrected Hyperchloremia

Increased Cl^- (corrected) is associated with a tendency toward acidosis (hyperchloremic acidosis) because of a decrease in SID. Pseudohyperchloremia may occur in patients receiving potassium bromide because bromide and other halides (e.g., iodides) are measured as chloride.[17,25] Bromide interferes with every chloride assay to some extent, but ion-selective electrodes are the most vulnerable to bromide interference.[23-25] If colorimetric methods are used to measure chloride concentration, other pigments such as hemoglobin and bilirubin may cause pseudohyperchloremia.[17] Lipemia also can cause pseudohyperchloremia when colorimetric methods are used.[41] Emulsified lipids in the photoelectric cell induce scattering of light resulting in overestimate of the true chloride content. This effect overcomes the decrease in chloride caused by increase in the plasma water fraction.[41]

Specific clinical signs associated with pure hyperchloremia in dogs and cats have not been reported but probably are related to the metabolic acidosis that accompanies hyperchloremia.[13] Potential causes of corrected hyperchloremia are listed in Box 4-3, and an algorithm for the differential diagnosis of corrected hyperchloremia is presented in Fig. 4-3.

Corrected hyperchloremia can be caused by chloride retention in renal failure[84,88] or by administration of

---

Box 4-3	**Causes of Corrected Hyperchloremia**

Pseudohyperchloremia
Lipemic samples (colorimetric methods)
Potassium bromide therapy

Excessive Loss of Sodium Relative to Chloride
Diarrhea

Excessive Gain of Chloride Relative to Sodium
Therapy with chloride salts (NH_4Cl, KCl)
Total parenteral nutrition
Fluid therapy (e.g., 0.9% NaCl, hypertonic saline, KCl-supplemented fluids)
Salt poisoning

Renal Chloride Retention
Renal failure
Renal tubular acidosis
Hypoadrenocorticism*
Diabetes mellitus*
Chronic respiratory alkalosis
Drug-induced: acetazolamide, spironolactone

Adapted from de Morais HSA: Chloride ion in small animal practice: the forgotten ion, *J Vet Emerg Crit Care* 2:11-24, 1992.
*May be associated with corrected hypochloremia in cats.

NH_4Cl to cats[10,27,55,79] and dogs.[43,44] Type I renal tubular acidosis also is associated with hyperchloremic acidosis in dogs[19,71] and cats.[5,22,86] The exact mechanism by which hyperchloremic acidosis occurs in distal renal tubular acidosis is not completely understood. However, there is a decrease in ammonium excretion,[72] and chloride replaces bicarbonate in the plasma, causing hyperchloremia.[52] Patients with diarrhea develop corrected hyperchloremia because of loss of a fluid with a high sodium and lower chloride ion concentration than those of plasma.

Patients with diabetes mellitus may have ketoacidosis with normal AG (hyperchloremia). The ketoacids are excreted in the urine at low serum concentrations; thus a patient with normal or near normal extracellular volume, renal perfusion, and GFR may excrete the ketoacids as fast as they are generated. The kidneys retain chloride in place of ketones in this situation, increasing chloride concentration while the AG remains unchanged.[29] Patients with diabetes also can develop corrected hyperchloremia during the resolving phase of the ketoacidotic crisis.[39,66] The hyperchloremia of the recovery phase has at least three causes. First, the administration of large volumes of isotonic saline can increase chloride concentration more than sodium concentration; second, KCl often is infused in large doses; and third, the ketones are lost in the urine, in exchange for NaCl.[2,63] In cats, however, ketoacidosis was associated with corrected hypochloremia in at least one report.[11] No information was provided about whether the cats in this report had vomited. In at least one ketoacidotic dog, corrected hypochloremia also was found.[87] Patients with hypoadrenocorticism and hypoaldosteronism have chloride retention and hyperchloremic metabolic acidosis because of the lack of mineralocorticoids. These patients typically are presented with decreased serum sodium and chloride concentrations caused by lack of aldosterone. The hyponatremia is more pronounced than the hypochloremia, and Cl^- (corrected) is increased.[13] Well-hydrated dogs with mineralocorticoid deficiency that are able to maintain serum sodium concentration usually have a mildly increased serum chloride concentration.

Drugs that cause chloride retention also can cause hyperchloremia. Potassium-sparing diuretics such as spironolactone act by decreasing the number of open aldosterone-sensitive sodium channels in the principal cells of the cortical collecting tubules.[72] Inhibition of sodium reabsorption at this site leads to hyperkalemia and hyperchloremic acidosis. Acetazolamide inhibits carbonic anhydrase in the proximal tubule, resulting in bicarbonaturia, urinary alkalinization, and in rats, but not in dogs, reduction in renal ammoniagenesis.[28,40] Chloride reabsorption proceeds normally in the ascending loop of Henle, resulting in chloride retention,[53] and use of acetazolamide is associated with hyperchloremia and metabolic acidosis.[46,72,74] Parenteral nutrition can cause hyperchloremia because some solutions have high concentrations of cationic amino acids (e.g., lysine-HCl, arginine-HCl) that release chloride and generate hydrogen ions.[47]

Fluid therapy is another important cause of hyperchloremia in hospitalized patients. Administration of isotonic saline, lactated Ringer's solution, or isotonic saline with 5% dextrose has been associated with corrected hyperchloremia in dogs.[9,73] Hyperchloremia can be exacerbated by intravenous infusion of 0.9% sodium chloride.[52] Isotonic sodium chloride solution supplemented with 20 mEq/L of KCl has a final sodium concentration of 154 mEq/L and a chloride concentration of 174 mEq/L. This solution has a much higher chloride concentration than plasma and is a common cause of corrected hyperchloremia in hospitalized patients.[13] Corrected hyperchloremia also has been associated with salt poisoning in dogs[16,48] and with administration of hypertonic saline in dogs and pigs.[13,62] Experimentally, chronic respiratory alkalosis causes renal chloride retention in dogs.[38] The observed hyperchloremia is part of the normal renal adaptation to chronic respiratory acid-base disorders. Therefore patients with chronic hypocapnia can be expected to have corrected hyperchloremia.

Treatment of corrected hyperchloremia should be directed at correction of the underlying disease process. The effects of fluid therapy on chloride concentration should be anticipated, especially in patients with diabetes mellitus or abnormal renal function. Special attention should be given to plasma pH because patients with corrected hyperchloremia tend to be acidotic. Bicarbonate therapy can be instituted whenever plasma pH is less than 7.2 or bicarbonate concentration is less than 12 mEq/L in patients with hyperchloremic metabolic acidosis.

CONCLUSION

Although it is the major anion in ECF, chloride has not received much attention in the clinical setting. It should be remembered that the chloride ion also is important in the metabolic regulation of acid-base balance. The kidneys regulate acid-base balance by changing the amount of chloride that is reabsorbed with sodium. Chloride is important in determining the patient's SID, and therefore changes in chloride concentration will reflect the patient's acid-base status. Corrected hypochloremia is associated with increased SID and metabolic alkalosis. Chloride is the only anion in ECF that can contribute to a substantial increase in SID. Administration of chloride is necessary for correction of hypochloremic metabolic alkalosis. Corrected hyperchloremia is associated with decreased SID and metabolic acidosis. Treatment with sodium bicarbonate should be carried out in hyperchloremic patients with pH less than 7.2.

REFERENCES

1. Abboud HE, Luke RG, Galla JH, et al: Stimulation of renin by acute selective chloride depletion in the rat, *Circ Res* 44:815-821, 1979.
2. Adrogué HJ, Eknoyan G, Suki WK: Diabetic ketoacidosis: role of the kidneys in the acid-base homeostasis re-evaluated, *Kidney Int* 25:591-598, 1984.
3. Atkins EL, Schwartz WB: Factors governing correction of the alkalosis associated with potassium deficiency: the critical role of chloride in the recovery process, *J Clin Invest* 41:218-229, 1962.
4. Bia M, Thier SO: Mixed acid-base disturbances: a clinical approach, *Med Clin North Am* 65:347-361, 1981.
5. Brown SA, Spyridakis LK, Crowell WA: Distal renal tubular acidosis and hepatic lipidosis in a cat, *J Am Vet Med Assoc* 189:1350-1352, 1986.
6. Burnell JM, Dawbron JK: Acid base parameters in potassium depletion in the dog, *Am J Physiol* 218:1583-1589, 1970.
7. Burnell JM, Teubner EJ, Simpson DP: Metabolic acidosis accompanying potassium deprivation, *Am J Physiol* 227:329-333, 1974.
8. Calia CM, Hohenhaus AE, Fox PR, et al: Acute tumor lysis syndrome in a cat with lymphoma, *J Vet Int Med* 10:409-411, 1996.
9. Chew DJ, Leonard M, Muir WW III: Effect of sodium bicarbonate infusion on serum osmolality, electrolyte concentration, and blood gas tensions in cats, *Am J Vet Res* 52:12-17, 1991.
10. Ching SV, Fettman MJ, Hamar DW, et al: The effect of chronic dietary acidification using ammonium chloride on acid-base and mineral metabolism in the adult cat, *J Nutr* 111:902-915, 1989.
11. Christopher MM, Broussard JD, Peterson ME: Heinz body formation associated with ketoacidosis in cats, *J Vet Int Med* 9:24-31, 1995.
12. de Morais HSA: A nontraditional approach to acid-base disorders. In DiBartola SP, editor: *Fluid therapy in small animal practice*, Philadelphia, 1992, WB Saunders, pp. 297-320.
13. de Morais HSA: Chloride ion in small animal practice: the forgotten ion, *J Vet Emerg Critic Care* 2:11-24, 1992.
14. de Morais HSA, Muir WW III: Strong ions and acid-base disorders. In Bonagura JD, Kirk RW, editors: *Current veterinary therapy XII*, ed 12, Philadelphia, 1995, WB Saunders, pp. 121-127.
15. de Rouffignac C, Elalouf JM: Hormonal regulation of chloride transport in the proximal and distal nephron, *Ann Rev Physiol* 50:123-140, 1988.
16. DiBartola SP, de Morais HSA: Case examples. In DiBartola SP, editor: *Fluid therapy in small animal practice*, Philadelphia, 1992, WB Saunders, pp. 599-688.
17. DiBartola SP, Green RA, de Morais HSA: Electrolyte and acid-base abnormalities. In Willard MD, Tvedten H, Turnwald GH, editors: *Small animal clinical diagnosis by laboratory methods*, ed 2, Philadelphia, 1994, WB Saunders, pp. 97-114.
18. DiBartola SP, Johnson SE, Davenport DJ, et al: Clinicopathologic findings resembling hypoadrenocorticism in dogs with primary gastrointestinal disease, *J Am Vet Med Assoc* 187:60, 1985.
19. DiBartola SP, Leonard PO: Renal tubular acidosis in a dog, *J Am Vet Med Assoc* 180:70-73, 1982.
20. Dobbins J: Gastrointestinal disorders. In Arieff AI, DeFronzo RA, editors: *Fluid, electrolyte, and acid-base disorders*, New York, 1985, Churchill Livingstone, pp. 827-849.

21. Dow SW, Fettman MJ, Smith KR, et al: Effects of dietary acidification and potassium depletion on acid-base balance, mineral metabolism and renal function in adult cats, *J Nutr* 120:569-578, 1990.

22. Drazner FH: Distal renal tubular acidosis associated with chronic pyelonephritis in a cat, *Calif Vet* 34:15-21, 1980.

23. Driscoll JL, Martin HF: Detection of bromism by an automated chloride method, *Clin Chem* 12:314-318, 1966.

24. Elin RJ, Robertson EA: Bromide interference with determination of chloride by each of four methods (letter), *Clin Chem* 27:778-779, 1981.

25. Emancipator K, Kroll MH: Bromide interference: is less really better? *Clin Chem* 8:1470-1473, 1990.

26. Fencl V, Rossing TH. Acid-base disorders in critical care medicine, *Ann Rev Med* 40:17-29, 1989.

27. Finco DR, Barsanti JA, Brown SA: Ammonium chloride as an urinary acidifier in cats: efficacy, safety and rationale for its use, *Mod Vet Pract* 67:537-541, 1986.

28. Fine A: Effects of carbonic anhydrase inhibition on renal ammoniagenesis in the dog, *Pharmacology* 33:217-220, 1986.

29. Gabow PA: Disorders associated with altered anion gap, *Kidney Int* 27:472-483, 1985.

30. Galla JH: Metabolic alkalosis, *J Am Soc Nephrol* 11:369-373, 2000.

31. Galla JH, Bonduris DN, Luke RG: Correction of chloride depletion metabolic alkalosis (CDA) without volume expansion (abstract), *Clin Res* 30:540A, 1982.

32. Galla JH, Bonduris DN, Luke RG: Effect of hypochloremia in glomerular filtration rate (GFR) on euvolemic rats (abstract), *Clin Res* 30:785A, 1982.

33. Galla JH, Bonduris DN, Luke RG: The correction of acute chloride-depletion alkalosis in the rat without volume expansion, *Am J Physiol* 244:F217-F221, 1983.

34. Galla JH, Bonduris DN, Luke RG, et al: Effects of chloride and extracellular fluid volume on bicarbonate reabsorption along the nephron in metabolic alkalosis in the rat: reassessment of the classical hypothesis of the pathogenesis of metabolic alkalosis, *J Clin Invest* 80:41-50, 1987.

35. Galla JH, Gifford JD, Luke RG, et al: Adaptations to chloride-depletion alkalosis, *Am J Physiol* 261:R771-R781, 1991.

36. Galla JH, Luke RG: Chloride transport and disorders of acid-base balance, *Ann Rev Physiol* 50:141-158, 1988.

37. Garella S, Cohen JJ, Northrup TE: Chloride-depletion metabolic alkalosis induces ECF volume depletion via internal fluid shifts in nephrectomized dogs, *Eur J Clin Invest* 21:273-279, 1991.

38. Gennari FJ, Goldstein MB, Schwartz W: The nature of the renal adaptation to chronic hypocapnia, *J Clin Invest* 51:1722-1730, 1972.

39. Goodkin DA, Krishna GG, Narins RG: The role of the anion gap in detecting and managing mixed metabolic acid-base disorders, *Clin Endocrinol Metab* 13:333-349, 1984.

40. Gougoux A, Vinay P, Zizian L, et al: Effect of acetazolamide on renal metabolism and ammoniagenesis in the dog, *Kidney Int* 31:1279-1290, 1987.

41. Graber ML, Quigg RJ, Slempsey WE, et al: Spurious hyperchloremia and decreased anion gap in hyperlipidemia, *Ann Int Med* 98:607-609, 1983.

42. Greger R: Chloride transport in thick ascending loop, distal convolution, and collecting duct, *Ann Rev Physiol* 50:111-122, 1988.

43. Halperin ML, Bun-Chen C: Influence of acute hyponatremia on renal ammoniagenesis in dogs with chronic metabolic acidosis, *Am J Physiol* 258:F328-F332, 1990.

44. Halperin ML, Vinay P, Gougoux A, et al: Regulation of the maximum rate of renal ammoniagenesis in the acidotic dog, *Am J Physiol* 248:F607-F615, 1985.

45. Hara Y, Nezu Y, Harada Y, et al: Secondary chronic respiratory acidosis in a dog following the cervical cord compression by an intradural glioma, *J Vet Med Sci* 64:863-866, 2002.

46. Haskins SC, Munger RJ, Helphrey MG, et al: Effects of acetazolamide on blood acid-base and electrolyte values in dogs, *J Am Vet Med Assoc* 179:792-796, 1981.

47. Heird WC, Dell B, Driscoll JM, et al: Metabolic acidosis resulting from intravenous alimentation with synthetic amino acids, *N Engl J Med* 287:943-945, 1972.

48. Hughes DE, Sokolowski J: Sodium chloride poisoning in the dog, *Canine Pract* 5:28-31, 1978.

49. Hulter HN, Licht JH, Sebastian A: K+ deprivation potentiates the renal acid excretory effect of mineralocorticoid: obliteration by amiloride, *Am J Physiol* 236:F48-F57, 1979.

50. Jones NL: *Blood gases and acid base physiology,* ed 2, New York, 1987, Thieme Medical Publishers.

51. Kassirer JP, Berkman PM, Lawrenz DR, et al: The critical role of chloride in the correction of hypokalemic alkalosis in man, *Am J Med* 38:172-189, 1965.

52. Koch SM, Taylor RW: Chloride ion in intensive care medicine, *Crit Care Med* 20:227-240, 1992.

53. Kreisberg RA, Wood BC: Drugs and chemical-induced metabolic acidosis, *Clin Endocrinol Metab* 12:391-411, 1983.

54. Lemieux G, Gervais M: Acute chloride depletion alkalosis: effect of anions on its maintenance and correction, *Am J Physiol* 207:1279-1286, 1964.

55. Lemieux G, Lemieux C, Duplessis S, et al: Metabolic characteristics of cat kidney: failure to adapt to metabolic acidosis, *Am J Physiol* 259:R277-R281, 1990.

56. Ling G, Stabenfeldt GH, Comer KM, et al: Canine hyperadrenocorticism: pretreatment clinical and laboratory evaluation of 117 cases, *J Am Vet Med Assoc* 174:1211-1215, 1979.

57. Luke RG, Galla JH: Chloride-depletion alkalosis with a normal extracellular fluid volume, *Am J Physiol* 254:F419-F424, 1983.

58. MacCallum WG, Lintz J, Vermilye HN, et al: The effect of pyloric obstruction relation to gastric tetany, *Bull John Hopkins Hosp* 31:1-7, 1920.

59. Madias NE, Bossed WH, Adrogué HJ: Ventilatory response to chronic metabolic acidosis and alkalosis in the dog, *J Appl Physiol* 56:1640-1646, 1984.

60. Madias NE, Wolf CJ, Cohen JJ: Regulation of acid-base equilibrium in chronic hypercapnia, *Kidney Int* 27:538-543, 1985.

61. McLoughlin MA, Walshaw R, Thomas MW, et al: Gastric conduit urinary diversion in normal dogs. Part II. Hypochloremic metabolic alkalosis, *Vet Surg* 21:33-39, 1992.

62. Moon PF, Kramer GC: Hypertonic saline-dextran resuscitation from hemorrhagic shock induces transient mixed acidosis, *Crit Care Med* 23:323-331, 1995.

63. Narins RG, Emmett M: Simple and mixed acid-base disorders: a practical approach, *Medicine* 59:161-187, 1980.

64. Needle MA, Kaloyanides GJ, Schwartz WB: The effects of selective depletion of hydrochloric acid on acid-base and electrolyte equilibrium, *J Clin Invest* 43:1836-1846, 1964.

65. Norris SH, Kurtzman NA: Does chloride play an independent role in the pathogenesis of metabolic alkalosis? *Semin Nephrol* 7:101-108, 1988.

66. Oh MS, Carrol HJ, Goldstein DA, et al: Hyperchloremic acidosis during the recovery phase of diabetic ketosis, *Ann Int Med* 89:925-927, 1978.

67. Penman RW, Luke RF, Jarboe TM: Respiratory effects of hypochloremic alkalosis and potassium depletion in the dog, *J Appl Physiol* 33:170-174, 1972.

68. Peterson ME, Greco DS, Orth DN: Primary hypoadrenocorticism in ten cats, *J Vet Int Med* 3:55-58, 1989.

69. Phillips SF: Small and large intestinal disorders: associated fluid and electrolyte complications. In Maxwell MH, Kleeman CR, Narins RG, editors: *Clinical disorders of fluid and electrolyte metabolism,* New York, 1987, McGraw-Hill, pp. 865-877.

70. Polak A, Haynie GD, Hays RM, et al: Effects of chronic hypercapnia on electrolyte and acid-base equilibrium. I. Adaptation, *J Clin Invest* 40:1223-1237, 1961.

71. Polzin DJ, Stevens JB, Osborne CA: Clinical application of the anion gap in evaluation of acid-base disorders in dogs, *Comp Cont Educ Pract Vet* 4:1021-1033, 1982.

72. Rose BD: *Clinical physiology of acid-base and electrolyte disorders,* ed 3, New York, 1989, McGraw-Hill.

73. Rose RJ: Some physiological and biochemical effects of the intravenous administration of five different electrolyte solutions in the dog, *J Vet Pharmacol Ther* 2:279-289, 1979.

74. Rose RJ, Caner J: Some physiological and biochemical effects of acetazolamide in the dog, *J Vet Pharmacol Ther* 2:215-221, 1979.

75. Rosen RA, Bruce JA, Dubovsky EV, et al: On the mechanism by which chloride corrects metabolic alkalosis in man, *Am J Med* 84:449-458, 1988.

76. Schild L, Giebisch G, Green R: Chloride transport in the proximal renal tubule, *Ann Rev Physiol* 50:97-110, 1988.

77. Schwartz WB, Brackelt NC, Cohen JJ: The response of extracellular hydrogen ion concentration to graded degrees of chronic hypercapnia: the physiologic limits of defense of pH, *J Clin Invest* 44:291-301, l965.

78. Schwartz WB, Hays RM, Polak A, et al: Effects of chronic hypercapnia on electrolyte and acid-base equilibrium. II.

Recovery, with special reference to the influence of chloride intake, *J Clin Invest* 40:1238-1249, 1961.

79. Senior DF, Sundstrom DA, Wolfson BB: Testing the effects of ammonium chloride and d-methionine on the urinary pH of cats, *Vet Med* 81:88-93, 1986.

80. Tietz NW, Pruden EL, Sigaard-Andersen O: Electrolytes, blood gases, and acid-base balance. Section one. Electrolytes. In Tietz NW, editor: *Textbook of clinical chemistry,* Philadelphia, 1986, WB Saunders, pp. 1172-1191.

81. Toll PW, Gaehtgens P, Neuhaus D, et al: Fluid, electrolyte, and packed cell volume shifts in racing greyhounds, *Am J Vet Res* 56:227-232, 1995.

82. van Ypersele de Strihou C, Gulyassy PF, Schwartz WB: Effects of chronic hypercapnia on electrolyte and acid-base equilibrium. III. Characteristics of the adaptive and recovery process as evaluated by provision of alkali, *J Clin Invest* 41:2246-2253, 1962.

83. Wall BM, Byrum GV, Galla JH, et al: Importance of chloride for the correction of chronic metabolic alkalosis in the rat, *Am J Physiol* 253:F1031-F1039, 1987.

84. Warnock DG: Uremic acidosis, *Kidney Int* 34:278-287, 1988.

85. Waters JH, Miller LR, Clack S, et al: Causes of metabolic acidosis in prolonged surgery, *Crit Care Med* 27:2142-2146, 1999.

86. Watson AD, Culvenor JA, Middleton DJ, et al: Distal renal tubular acidosis in a cat with pyelonephritis, *Vet Rec* 119:65-68, 1986.

87. Whitehair KJ, Haskins SC, Whitehair JG, et al: Clinical applications of quantitative acid-base chemistry, *J Vet Int Med* 9:1-12, 1995.

88. Widmer B, Gerhardt RE, Harrington JT, et al: Serum electrolyte and acid base composition: the influence of graded degrees of chronic renal failure, *Arch Intern Med* 139:1099-1102, 1979.

89. Winter SD, Pearson JR, Gabow PA, et al: The fall of serum anion gap, *Arch Intern Med* 150:311-313, 1990.

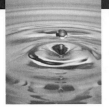

CHAPTER • 5

DISORDERS OF POTASSIUM: HYPOKALEMIA AND HYPERKALEMIA

Stephen P. DiBartola and Helio Autran de Morais

Potassium is the major intracellular cation in mammalian cells, whereas sodium is the major extracellular cation. Normally, the extracellular fluid (ECF) sodium concentration is approximately 140 mEq/L, and the ECF potassium concentration is approximately 4 mEq/L. This relationship is reversed in intracellular fluid (ICF), in which the sodium concentration is approximately 10 mEq/L and the potassium concentration is approximately 140 mEq/L. In experimental studies of dogs, control values for ICF sodium and potassium concentrations in skeletal muscle were 8.4 to 13.7 and 139 to 142 mEq/L, respectively.[16,96]

Total body potassium content in humans is approximately 50 to 55 mEq/kg body weight, and almost all of this potassium is readily exchangeable.[6,62] In one study of potassium depletion in dogs, the control value for total exchangeable potassium as determined by ^{42}K dilution was 47.1 mEq/kg body weight (range, 39.8 to 61.1 mEq/kg).[1] As much as 95% or more of total body potassium is located within cells, with muscle containing 60% to 75% of this potassium. Muscle potassium content in normal dogs and cats is approximately 400 mEq/kg.[16,96,132,171] As a solute, intracellular potassium is crucial for maintenance of normal cell volume. Intracellular potassium is also important for normal cell growth because it is required for the normal function of enzymes responsible for nucleic acid, glycogen, and protein synthesis.

The remaining 5% of the body's potassium is located in the ECF. Maintaining the ECF potassium concentration within narrow limits is critical to avoid the life-threatening effects of hyperkalemia on cardiac conduction. In humans, the serum potassium concentration is inversely correlated with the total body deficit of potassium (Fig. 5-1). Likewise, in dogs with potassium depletion induced by dietary restriction, the muscle potassium content was strongly correlated ($r = 0.87$) with the serum potassium concentration.[132] During translocation of potassium between ICF and ECF, however, the serum potassium concentration can change without any change in the total body potassium content. One of the most important func-

tions of potassium in the body is its role in generation of the normal resting cell membrane potential.

THE RESTING CELL MEMBRANE POTENTIAL

The normal relationship between ECF and ICF potassium concentrations is maintained by sodium, potassium-adenosinetriphosphatase (Na$^+$, K$^+$-ATPase) in cell membranes. This enzyme pumps sodium ions out of and potassium ions into the cell in a 3:2 Na/K ratio so that the intracellular concentration of potassium is much

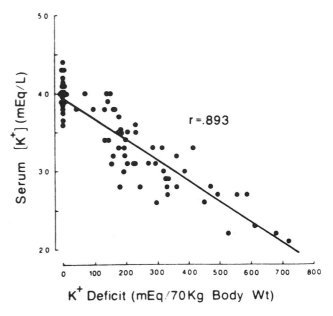

Fig. 5-1 Relationship of serum potassium concentration to bodily potassium deficit. The data are derived from seven metabolic balance studies carried out on 24 human subjects depleted of potassium. (From Raymond KH, Kunau RT: Hypokalemic states. In Maxwell MH, Kleeman CR, Narins RG, editors: *Clinical disorders of fluid and electrolyte metabolism,* ed 4, New York, 1987, McGraw-Hill, p. 519, with permission of the McGraw-Hill Companies.)

higher than its extracellular concentration. As a result, K^+ ions diffuse out of the cell down their concentration gradient. However, the cell membrane is impermeable to most intracellular anions (e.g., proteins and organic phosphates). Therefore a net negative charge develops within the cell as K^+ ions diffuse out, and a net positive charge accumulates outside the cell. Consequently, a potential difference is generated across the cell membrane.

The principal extracellular cation is sodium, and it enters the cell relatively slowly down its concentration and electrical gradients because the permeability of the cell membrane to potassium is 100-fold greater than its permeability to sodium. Diffusion of K^+ ions from the cell continues until the ECF acquires sufficient positive charge to prevent further diffusion of K^+ ions out of the cell. The ratio of the intracellular to extracellular concentrations of potassium ($[K^+]_I/[K^+]_O$) is the major determinant of the **resting cell membrane potential** as described by the Nernst equation:

$$E_m = -61 \log_{10} \frac{[K^+]_I}{[K^+]_O}$$

The Goldman-Hodgkin-Katz equation is a modification of the Nernst equation that allows prediction of E_m based on the ionic permeability characteristics of the cell membrane to sodium and potassium and the concentrations of these ions inside and outside the cell:

$$E_m = -61 \log_{10} \frac{rP_K[K^+]_I + P_{Na}[Na^+]_I}{rP_K[K^+]_O + P_{Na}[Na^+]_O}$$

where P_{Na} and P_K are the membrane permeabilities for sodium and potassium. The term r is included in the equation to account for the effect of the electrogenic Na^+,K^+-ATPase pump under steady-state conditions. This term is assigned the Na/K transport ratio of 3:2 so that $r = 1.5$. If the membrane permeability for potassium is assigned a value of 1.0 and the cell membrane is 100 times more permeable to potassium than sodium:

$$E_m = -61 \log_{10} \frac{1.5[K^+]_I + 0.01[Na^+]_I}{1.5[K^+]_O + 0.01[Na^+]_O}$$

For example, using the hypothetical ECF and ICF concentrations of sodium and potassium given at the beginning of this chapter:

$$E_m = -61 \log_{10} \frac{1.5[140] + 0.01[10]}{1.5[4] + 0.01[140]}$$

$$E_m = -61 \log_{10}(28.4) = -89 \text{ mV}$$

In one study of dogs with potassium deficiency, the predicted E_m was −86.6 mV and the measured E_m in skeletal muscle of control animals was −90.1 mV.[16] The resting cell membrane potential plays a vital role in the normal function of skeletal and cardiac muscle, nerve, and transporting epithelia.

THE THRESHOLD CELL MEMBRANE POTENTIAL

The **threshold cell membrane potential** is reached when sodium permeability increases to the point that sodium entry exceeds potassium exit, depolarization becomes self-perpetuating, and an action potential develops. The ability of specialized cells to develop an action potential is crucial to normal cardiac conduction, muscle contraction, and nerve impulse transmission. The excitability of a tissue is determined by the difference between the resting and threshold potentials (the smaller the difference, the greater the excitability).

Hypokalemia increases the resting potential (i.e., makes it more negative) and hyperpolarizes the cell, whereas hyperkalemia decreases the resting potential (i.e., makes it less negative) and initially makes the cell hyperexcitable (Fig. 5-2). If the resting potential decreases to less than the threshold potential, depolarization results, repolarization cannot occur, and the cell is no longer excitable. Translocation of potassium between body compartments results in a greater change in the ratio of intracellular to extracellular potassium concentrations ($[K^+]_I/[K^+]_O$) than does a change in total body potassium. In the former instance, the potassium concentrations of the two compartments change in opposite directions, whereas in the latter instance, they change in the same direction.

Membrane excitability also is affected by ionized calcium concentration and acid-base balance. Calcium affects the threshold potential rather than the resting potential. Ionized hypocalcemia increases membrane excitability by allowing self-perpetuating sodium permeability to be reached with a lesser degree of depolarization, whereas ionized hypercalcemia requires greater than normal depolarization for this threshold to be reached (see Fig. 5-2). Thus hypercalcemia counteracts hyperkalemia by normalizing the difference between the resting and threshold potentials, whereas hypocalcemia exacerbates the effect of hyperkalemia on membrane excitability. This principle is the basis for treating hyperkalemia with calcium salts (see Treatment of Hyperkalemia). Membrane excitability is increased by alkalemia and decreased by acidemia. As a result of these factors, clinical signs are not necessarily correlated with serum potassium concentrations. Electrocardiographic findings and muscle strength reflect the functional consequences of abnormalities in serum potassium concentration.

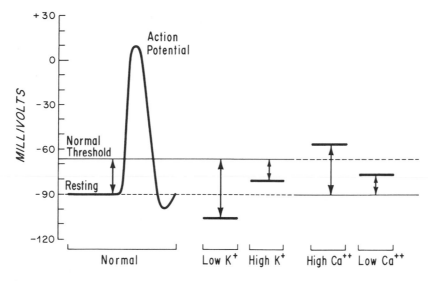

Fig. 5-2 Effects of serum calcium and potassium on membrane potentials of excitable tissues. The concentration of potassium in extracellular fluids affects the resting potential, whereas calcium concentrations alter the threshold potential. (From Leaf A, Cotran R: *Renal pathophysiology,* New York, 1976, Oxford University Press, p. 116.)

POTASSIUM BALANCE

EXTERNAL POTASSIUM BALANCE

External balance for potassium is maintained by matching output (primarily in the urine) to input (from the diet). In the normal animal, potassium enters the body only through the gastrointestinal tract, and virtually all ingested potassium is absorbed in the stomach and small intestine. Transport of potassium in the small intestine is passive, whereas active transport (responsive to aldosterone) occurs in the colon. Colonic secretion of potassium may play an important role in extrarenal potassium homeostasis in some disease states (e.g., chronic renal failure) (Fig. 5-3).

Potassium derived from the diet and endogenous cellular breakdown is removed from the body primarily by the kidneys and, to a much lesser extent, by the gastrointestinal tract. During zero balance, 90% to 95% of ingested potassium is excreted in the urine, and the remaining 5% to 10% is excreted in the stool. This pattern of output has been observed during control balance studies in normal dogs.[11,125,136,151,164] In a study of renal handling of potassium in dogs, 90% to 98% of potassium intake was eliminated from the body by the kidneys.[19]

Adaptation occurs during chronic potassium loading so that the animal is protected from hyperkalemia that could occur as a result of an acute potassium load. This effect results from enhanced renal and colonic excretion of potassium, as well as from enhanced uptake of potassium by liver and muscle, mediated by the effects of insulin and catecholamines. Potassium deprivation is associated with decreased aldosterone secretion, suppression of potassium secretion in the distal nephron, and increased reabsorption of potassium in the inner medullary collecting ducts. Skeletal muscle potassium concentration decreases, but brain and heart potassium concentrations are minimally affected during potassium depletion.[16,96,160] The colon adapts to potassium deprivation by decreasing its secretion of potassium.

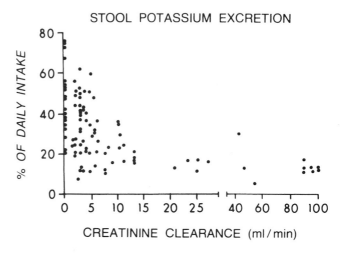

Fig. 5-3 Relationship between the degree of renal insufficiency and fecal potassium excretion. Data points are compiled from three studies comprising 98 balance periods in 40 human patients. Variation in dietary protein or sodium intake did not produce consistent changes in fecal potassium excretion; thus data points from these balance periods were included without special designation. (From Alexander EA, Perrone RD: Regulation of extrarenal potassium metabolism. In Maxwell MH, Kleeman CR, Narins RG, editors: *Clinical disorders of fluid and electrolyte metabolism,* ed 4, New York, 1987, McGraw-Hill, p. 112, with permission of the McGraw-Hill Companies.)

INTERNAL POTASSIUM BALANCE

Internal balance for potassium is maintained by translocation of potassium between ECF and ICF. One half to two thirds of an acute potassium load appears in the urine within the first 4 to 6 hours, and effective translocation of potassium from ECF to ICF is crucial in preventing life-threatening hyperkalemia until the kidneys have sufficient time to excrete the remainder of the potassium load. Endogenous insulin secretion and stimulation of β$_2$-adrenergic receptors by epinephrine promote cellular uptake of potassium in liver and muscle by increasing the activity of cell membrane Na$^+$, K$^+$-ATPase. The main effect of these hormones is to facilitate distribution of an acute potassium load and not to mediate minor adjustments in serum potassium concentration. The ECF concentration of potassium itself plays an important role in translocation because potassium movement into cells is facilitated by the change in chemical concentration gradient resulting from addition of potassium to ECF. The fraction of an acute potassium load taken up by the body is increased during chronic potassium depletion and decreased when total body potassium is excessive. In summary, any change in serum potassium concentration must arise from a change in intake, distribution, or excretion (Fig. 5-4).

EFFECT OF ACID-BASE BALANCE ON POTASSIUM DISTRIBUTION

The effect of acute pH changes on translocation of potassium between ICF and ECF is complex. In general, acidosis is associated with movement of potassium ions from ICF to ECF, and alkalosis is associated with movement of potassium ions from ECF to ICF. Early animal studies and observations in a small number of human patients led to the prediction that acute metabolic acidosis would be associated with a 0.6-mEq/L increment in serum potassium concentration for each 0.1-U decrement in pH. This rule of thumb has circulated widely among clinicians.[25,163,168]

However, a critical review of experimental studies in animals and humans demonstrated that changes in serum potassium concentration during acute acid-base disturbances were quite variable.[4] The change in serum potassium concentration was greatest during acute mineral acidosis. In dogs, the increase in serum potassium concentration after administration of a mineral acid (e.g., HCl or NH$_4$Cl) was very variable, ranging from a 0.17- to 1.67-mEq/L increment in serum potassium concentration per 0.1-U decrement in pH (mean, 0.75 mEq/L). The increment in serum potassium concentration during acute respiratory acidosis in dogs was much lower, averaging only 0.14 mEq/L per 0.1-U decrement in pH. The decrement in serum potassium concentration during metabolic alkalosis in dogs averaged 0.18 mEq/L per 0.1-U increment in pH, whereas it averaged 0.27 mEq/L per 0.1-U increment in pH during respiratory alkalosis. In another study, respiratory alkalosis induced by hyperventilation in anesthetized dogs caused a somewhat greater decrement in serum potassium concentration (0.4 mEq/L) for each 0.1-U increment in pH.[123] An increase in serum potassium concentration did not occur in acute metabolic acidosis caused by organic acids (e.g., lactic acid and ketoacids).[4,5,88,127,128,174] Acute infusion of β-hydroxybutyric acid in normal dogs caused an increase in insulin in portal venous blood and hypokalemia, presumably as a result of potassium uptake by cells. Conversely, acute infusion of HCl led to increased portal vein glucagon concentration and hyperkalemia, possibly caused by potassium release from cells.[5] In summary, only mineral acidosis is expected to cause any clinically relevant change in serum potassium concentration during acute acid-base disturbances.

Many factors probably contribute to the variable changes observed in serum potassium concentration during acute acid-base disturbances, including blood pH and HCO$_3$$^-$ concentration, nature of the acid anion (mineral versus organic), osmolality, hormonal activity (e.g., catecholamines, insulin, glucagon, and aldosterone), and the metabolic and excretory roles of the liver and kidney.[4] Hyperosmolality and lack of insulin are more likely to be responsible for hyperkalemia observed in patients with diabetic ketoacidosis than is the acidosis itself.

Hyperkalemia associated with acute metabolic acidosis induced by mineral acids is transient. In a study of acute and chronic metabolic acidosis induced in dogs by administration of HCl or NH$_4$Cl, hyperkalemia was observed after acute infusion of HCl, but hypokalemia

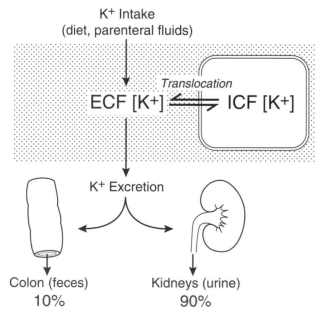

Fig. 5-4 Components of potassium homeostasis. *ECF,* Extracellular fluid; *ICF,* intracellular fluid. (Drawing by Tim Vojt.)

developed after 3 to 5 days of NH$_4$Cl administration.[110] The observed hypokalemia was associated with inappropriately high urinary excretion of potassium and increased plasma aldosterone concentration.[110] Similar findings have been reported in rats with chronic metabolic acidosis induced by NH$_4$Cl. Despite a total body deficit of potassium, rats with chronic metabolic acidosis did not conserve potassium appropriately.[152] This effect may be caused by a decreased filtered load of HCO$_3^-$, increased distal delivery of sodium, and increased distal tubular flow. Thus metabolic acidosis of at least 2 to 3 days' duration is associated with increased urinary potassium excretion and mild hypokalemia rather than hyperkalemia.[71]

RENAL HANDLING OF POTASSIUM

The kidney is the primary regulator of potassium balance. Potassium is filtered at the glomerulus, and approximately 70% of the filtered load is reabsorbed isosmotically with water and sodium in the proximal tubule. An additional 10% to 20% of filtered potassium is reabsorbed in the ascending limb of Henle's loop. Finally, 10% to 20% of the filtered load is delivered to the distal nephron, where final adjustments in potassium reabsorption and secretion are made. Potassium experiences either net reabsorption or secretion in the connecting tubule, cortical collecting duct, and first portion of the outer medullary collecting duct, depending on the body's needs. Net movement of potassium in these segments of the nephron determines urinary excretion of potassium. Potassium once again experiences reabsorption in the last portion of the outer medullary collecting duct and inner medullary collecting duct regardless of the body's needs.

MECHANISMS OF RENAL TUBULAR TRANSPORT OF POTASSIUM

The transepithelial electrical potential difference is lumen negative in the early proximal tubule, but no active transport mechanism for potassium has been discovered in this segment of the nephron. In the proximal tubule, potassium is reabsorbed along with water by solvent drag via the paracellular route. Apparently, water reabsorption increases the luminal concentration of potassium enough to overcome the unfavorable transepithelial potential difference. The transepithelial electrical potential difference becomes lumen positive in the late proximal tubule, and this facilitates reabsorption of potassium by the paracellular route. Transcellular transport of potassium in the proximal tubular cells occurs by means of potassium channels in both luminal and basolateral membranes and by a K$^+$-Cl$^-$ cotransporter in basolateral membranes (Fig. 5-5).

In the thick ascending limb of Henle's loop, the transepithelial electrical potential difference is strongly lumen positive, and most potassium reabsorption occurs by the paracellular route. Potassium channels in the luminal membranes allow potassium to exit the cell down its concentration gradient and facilitate the electrochemical gradient for potassium reabsorption via the paracellular route. Transcellular reabsorption of potassium is facilitated by the luminal Na$^+$-K$^+$-2Cl$^-$ cotransporter and by potassium channels and a K$^+$-Cl$^-$ cotransporter in the basolateral membranes (Fig. 5-6).

The mechanisms of renal potassium handling in the distal convoluted tubule are shown in Fig. 5-7. The thiazide-sensitive Na$^+$-Cl$^-$ cotransporter and the K$^+$-Cl$^-$ cotransporter in the luminal membranes of these tubular cells result in secretion of potassium and reabsorption of sodium while chloride is recycled across the luminal membrane. The basolateral Na$^+$, K$^+$-ATPase maintains a low intracellular concentration of sodium and a high intracellular concentration of potassium that facilitate sodium reabsorption and potassium secretion across the luminal membranes.

Principal cells are found in the connecting tubule and collecting duct and are responsible for potassium secretion. The basolateral membranes of principal cells are rich in Na$^+$, K$^+$-ATPase, which maintains a high intracellular potassium concentration. The luminal membranes of the principal cells contain an electrogenic sodium channel

Proximal Tubule

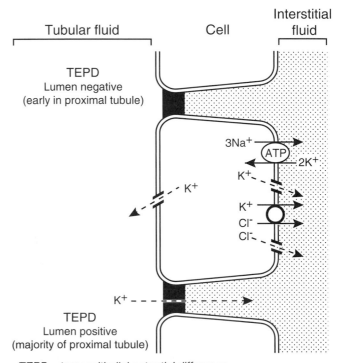

TEPD = transepithelial potential difference

Fig. 5-5 Renal tubular transport mechanisms for potassium in the proximal tubule. (Drawing by Tim Vojt.)

Thick Ascending Limb of Henle's Loop

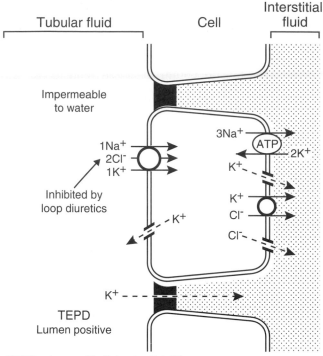

TEPD = transepithelial potential difference

Fig. 5-6 Renal tubular transport mechanisms for potassium in the thick ascending limb of Henle's loop. (Drawing by Tim Vojt.)

Distal Convoluted Tubule

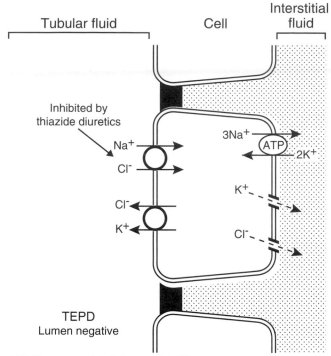

TEPD = transepithelial potential difference

Fig. 5-7 Renal tubular transport mechanisms for potassium in the distal convoluted tubule (early distal tubule). (Drawing by Tim Vojt.)

(ENaC). This sodium channel is directly blocked by the diuretics amiloride and triamterene, whereas spironolactone antagonizes the effect of aldosterone on the channel. Sodium movement through this channel renders the tubular lumen negative, and the resultant increase in lumen electronegativity facilitates secretion of K+ ions through luminal K+ channels (Fig. 5-8).

There are two types of intercalated cells in the distal nephron. Type A or α intercalated cells contain H+-ATPase and H+,K+-ATPase in their luminal membranes and Cl⁻-HCO₃⁻ countertransporters and Cl⁻ and K+ channels in their basolateral membranes. They also contain carbonic anhydrase. This arrangement allows the α intercalated cell to secrete H+ ions and reabsorb K+ and HCO₃⁻ ions. Potassium is actively transported across the luminal membranes of type α intercalated cells by H+, K+-ATPase and then diffuses down its concentration gradient through potassium channels in the basolateral membranes (Fig. 5-9). Type α intercalated cells are found in the connecting tubule, cortical collecting duct, and outer medullary collecting duct. Type B or β intercalated cells are found only in the cortical collecting ducts and secrete HCO₃⁻ ions. They are able to do so because their polarity is reversed as compared with type α intercalated cells (i.e., the H+-ATPase is in the baso-

lateral membrane, and the Cl⁻-HCO₃⁻ countertransporter is in the luminal membrane).

Potassium is reabsorbed from the last portion of the outer medullary collecting duct and throughout the inner medullary collecting duct. In these segments of the nephron, potassium is reabsorbed by the paracellular route despite a lumen-negative transepithelial potential difference because reabsorption of water increases the chemical concentration gradient sufficiently to overcome the unfavorable electrical gradient.

DETERMINANTS OF URINARY POTASSIUM EXCRETION

Three main factors affect potassium secretion in the distal nephron: the magnitude of the chemical concentration gradient for potassium between the tubular cells and tubular lumen, the tubular flow rate, and the transmembrane potential difference across the luminal membranes of the tubular cells. Gastrointestinal absorption of a potassium load increases the ECF concentration of potassium. This results in an increase in the number of K+ ions available for uptake at the basolateral membranes of the distal tubular cells by Na+, K+-ATPase, and the resulting increase in intracellular potassium concentration increases the chemical concentration gradient for

Collecting Duct

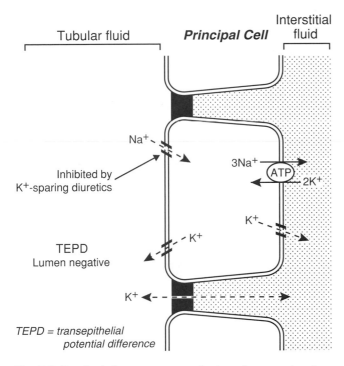

Fig. 5-8 Renal tubular transport mechanisms for potassium in the principal cells of the late distal tubule and collecting duct. (Drawing by Tim Vojt.)

Collecting Duct

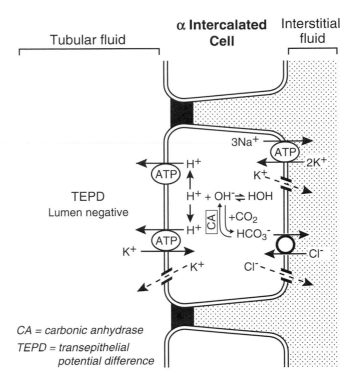

Fig. 5-9 Renal tubular transport mechanisms for potassium in the α intercalated cells of the late distal tubule and collecting duct. (Drawing by Tim Vojt.)

diffusion of K^+ ions out of the tubular cells across their luminal membranes.

Aldosterone is the most important hormone affecting urinary potassium excretion. Its secretion by the zona glomerulosa of the adrenal gland is stimulated directly by hyperkalemia and angiotensin II (produced in response to volume depletion), whereas adrenocorticotropic hormone (ACTH), hyponatremia, and decreased extracellular pH play permissive roles in promoting aldosterone secretion. Aldosterone release is inhibited by dopamine and atrial natriuretic factor, both of which are released in response to volume expansion.

Aldosterone increases reabsorption of Na^+ and secretion of K^+ and H^+ ions in the distal nephron. Its primary effect is to increase the number of open Na^+ channels in the luminal membranes of the principal cells. Sodium reabsorption via these luminal Na^+ channels is electrogenic (i.e., it generates electronegativity in the tubular lumen). This electronegativity can be dissipated either by K^+ or H^+ ion secretion or by Cl^- reabsorption in the distal nephron. Aldosterone increases the activity and number of Na^+, K^+-ATPase pumps in the basolateral membranes of the principal cells, and this effect may occur as a result of increased entry of Na^+ ions across the luminal membranes. Increased Na^+, K^+-ATPase activity in turn increases the intracellular K^+ concentration and facilitates K^+ secretion across the luminal membranes.

Aldosterone also increases the number of open K^+ channels in the luminal membrane, thus facilitating K^+ exit into tubular fluid.

Aldosterone can influence H^+ secretion in two ways. It directly promotes H^+ ion secretion in H^+-secreting type α intercalated cells by stimulation of the H^+-ATPase present in their luminal membranes. Aldosterone also promotes H^+ secretion in the distal tubule by stimulating electrogenic Na^+ reabsorption in principal cells and increasing lumen electronegativity, which favors enhanced H^+ secretion.

An increase in distal tubular flow enhances potassium secretion by rapidly moving secreted K^+ ions downstream and providing new tubular fluid from upstream in the nephron. This allows maintenance of a high chemical concentration gradient for potassium secretion and provides a "sink" for movement of K^+ ions into tubular fluid. A decrease in distal tubular flow has the opposite effect and promotes dissipation of the chemical gradient for diffusion of K^+ ions from principal cells into tubular fluid.

Lumen electronegativity is generated by sodium reabsorption through Na^+ channels in the luminal membranes of principal cells. Normally, some of this electronegativity is dissipated by passive Cl^- reabsorption. If a large concentration of a relatively nonresorbable anion (e.g., SO_4^{2-},

HCO_3^-, penicillin) is present in distal tubular fluid, less dissipation of the electronegativity occurs, and K^+ secretion is enhanced. This factor contributes to the pathophysiology of metabolic alkalosis. In this setting, there is less Cl^- and more HCO_3^- in the distal tubular fluid, and HCO_3^- is relatively nonresorbable in the cortical collecting duct. This is one reason metabolic alkalosis promotes urinary K^+ excretion. Amiloride is a diuretic that impairs luminal Na^+ entry into principal cells by decreasing the number of open Na^+ channels. This in turn reduces lumen electronegativity and impairs K^+ secretion. Thus the magnitude of distal tubular lumen electronegativity has an important effect on urinary K^+ excretion.

The Na^+ and Cl^- concentrations of distal tubular fluid usually have little effect on K^+ secretion. When the luminal Na^+ concentration is very low (<25 to 35 mEq/L), however, diffusion of Na^+ ions into distal tubular cells may be impaired sufficiently to produce an increase in the tubular cell transmembrane potential (making the cell interior more negative) and impeding diffusion of K^+ ions from the cell into the tubular lumen.[76,180,181] Extremely low luminal Cl^- concentrations (<10 mEq/L) may increase net potassium secretion, possibly because some fraction of K^+ reabsorption or secretion may be accomplished by K^+-Cl^- cotransport.[176] Such a mechanism may also play a role in the pathophysiology of enhanced urinary K^+ excretion during metabolic alkalosis. Antidiuretic hormone (ADH) helps minimize disruption of potassium balance during water deprivation by increasing the number of open luminal K^+ channels in principal cells and facilitating potassium excretion at a time when distal tubular flow is reduced.[30,61,165] Conversely, potassium excretion is not necessarily increased despite increased distal tubular flow during water diuresis because ADH is suppressed. Major factors affecting renal excretion of potassium are summarized in Fig. 5-10.

FACTORS INFLUENCING RENAL POTASSIUM EXCRETION

Sodium Intake

High sodium intake is associated with increased urinary potassium excretion as a result of increased potassium secretion in the connecting tubule and cortical collecting duct. Increased delivery of sodium to the distal nephron results in more sodium crossing the luminal membranes of the distal tubular cells down its concentration gradient. This increased entry of Na^+ ions into the tubular cells leads to increased activity of Na^+, K^+-ATPase in the basolateral membranes with removal of sodium to the peritubular interstitium and increased cellular uptake of potassium. This increased intracellular potassium then crosses the luminal membranes of the tubular cells and enters the tubular fluid down a favorable electrochemical gradient. Increased sodium delivery to the distal nephron

Distal Nephron

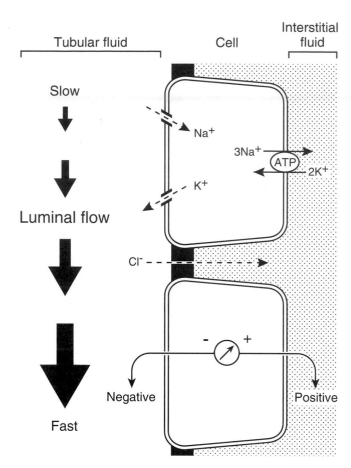

Fig. 5-10 Factors affecting urinary excretion of potassium. (Drawing by Tim Vojt.)

also increases the distal tubular fluid flow rate, which enhances the chemical concentration gradient for potassium between the tubular cell cytoplasm and tubular fluid.

Low sodium intake is associated with decreased renal potassium excretion as a result of mechanisms opposite to those described previously. In addition, increased potassium reabsorption by type α intercalated cells occurs in the medullary collecting duct. One reason for this increased reabsorption may be increased recycling of potassium into the medullary interstitium, which may play a role in the urinary concentrating mechanism when sodium intake is restricted.

Potassium Intake

High potassium intake is associated with increased urinary potassium excretion as a result of increased tubular secretion of potassium in the connecting tubule, cortical collecting duct, and outer medullary collecting duct. This occurs because of increased numbers and activity of Na^+, K^+-ATPase pumps and amplification of the basolateral membranes of principal cells, which results from an increased concentration of aldosterone. Therefore more potassium is actively pumped into the tubular cells from the peritubular interstitium, leaves the cells down a favorable electrochemical gradient, and enters the tubular fluid.

Low potassium intake results in decreased urinary excretion of potassium. In the presence of low potassium intake, there is decreased to absent tubular secretion by principal cells in the connecting tubule, cortical collecting duct, and outer medullary collecting duct and increased reabsorption by type α intercalated cells in the inner medullary collecting duct. The decrease in tubular secretion results from less potassium being available for peritubular uptake into the tubular cells by the Na^+, K^+-ATPase pump and a less favorable concentration gradient for potassium to leave the tubular cells and enter tubular fluid.

Dietary potassium intake also has a direct effect on the function of the luminal potassium channels in principal cells. A high potassium intake increases the activity of these channels by decreasing the phosphorylation of a specific tyrosine residue in the ROMK protein component of the channel, which in turn results in decreased removal of the channels from the luminal membranes. A low potassium diet has the opposite effect.[73,178]

Mineralocorticoids

An increased concentration of aldosterone results in increased urinary excretion of potassium as a result of increased secretion of potassium by tubular cells mainly in the cortical collecting duct. The actions of aldosterone on the principal cells result in increased uptake of potassium from the peritubular interstitium and increased movement of potassium into tubular fluid across the luminal membranes of the principal cells. A decreased transmembrane potential difference across the luminal membrane (as Na^+ ions enter from tubular fluid) allows potassium to exit more easily into the tubular fluid (i.e., the interior of the cell is now less negative compared with the tubular fluid). A decreased concentration of aldosterone results in decreased urinary excretion of potassium.

Hydrogen Ion Balance

Acute mineral metabolic acidosis decreases urinary excretion of potassium. Chronic metabolic acidosis actually may increase urinary excretion of potassium. If distal tubular flow remains constant, acute (<8 hours) mineral metabolic acidosis results in decreased urinary excretion of potassium because, during metabolic acidosis caused by administration of a mineral acid, H^+ ions enter cells to be buffered by intracellular proteins in exchange for K^+ ions that leave cells and enter the ECF.[163,168] When this ion exchange occurs across the basolateral membranes of the cells of the connecting tubule and cortical collecting ducts, the resulting decreased intracellular concentration of potassium is associated with less tubular secretion of potassium because of a less favorable chemical concentration gradient.

A critical factor determining whether acute metabolic acidosis causes this exchange of H^+ and K^+ ions across the cell membranes is the permeability of the anion associated with the acid. Chloride ions are relatively impermeable and cannot follow the H^+ ions into the cell, whereas lactate and ketoacid anions are more permeable and can follow H^+ ions into the cell so that K^+ ions do not need to be exchanged with H^+ ions for electroneutrality. As a result, acute mineral metabolic acidosis may be associated with H^+-K^+ exchange across cell membranes, but acute organic metabolic acidosis is not. Chronic (>3 days) metabolic acidosis caused by administration of a mineral acid leads to mild hypokalemia, possibly caused by stimulation of aldosterone secretion by the acidosis.[71,110,152] Even in acute acidosis, a decreased filtered load of bicarbonate can reduce sodium reabsorption in the proximal tubules and increase delivery of sodium and water to the distal nephron. This increases the distal tubular flow rate and enhances urinary potassium excretion.

During alkalosis, H^+ ions leave cells to titrate bicarbonate in the ECF in exchange for K^+ ions that enter the cells. The increased concentration of potassium in the distal tubular cells results in increased secretion of potassium because of a more favorable chemical concentration gradient. Alkalosis also appears to directly stimulate the basolateral Na^+, K^+-ATPase in the principal cells of the cortical collecting duct.

Diuretics

Many clinically important diuretics (furosemide, ethacrynic acid, thiazides, and mannitol) cause increased urinary excretion of potassium and may result in depletion of body potassium stores. These diuretics increase the distal tubular delivery of sodium and the distal tubular fluid flow rate and, as a result of these effects, cause increased urinary potassium excretion for the same reason as described earlier in the discussion of the effects of high sodium intake on potassium excretion.

NORMAL SERUM CONCENTRATIONS

Ion-selective potentiometry and flame photometry are methods used by clinical laboratories to measure sodium and potassium concentrations in body fluids. Electrolytes in plasma are excluded from the fraction of plasma (normally about 7%) that is occupied by solids (e.g., lipids and proteins) and are confined to the aqueous phase of plasma (about 93% of total plasma volume). Flame photometry and indirect potentiometry are affected by the exclusion of electrolytes from the fraction of plasma that is occupied by solids, whereas direct potentiometry is not.[173] The resulting error is usually small, but for serum sodium concentration it may be clinically relevant in patients with hyperlipemia (see Chapter 3). Potassium is present in ECF at a much lower concentration than sodium, and the effect of hyperlipemia on the measured serum potassium concentration is much less apparent.

Normal values for serum potassium concentration in dogs and cats vary slightly among laboratories but are expected to be 3.5 to 5.5 mEq/L, with an average value of approximately 4.5 mEq/L. Serum potassium concentrations exceed plasma concentrations because potassium is released from platelets during the clotting process. There is a positive correlation between platelet count and serum potassium concentration in dogs.[41,139] The difference between serum and plasma potassium concentrations is most pronounced in animals with thrombocytosis.[42,112,139] In one study, serum potassium concentration was greater than plasma potassium concentration by a mean of 0.63 mEq/L in dogs with normal platelet counts and by a mean of 1.55 mEq/L in dogs with thrombocytosis.[139]

The potassium content of erythrocytes varies in mammalian species, and hemolysis can result in hyperkalemia in species that have high red cell potassium concentrations (Table 5-1). Normal adult canine and feline red cells usually contain potassium in concentrations similar to those of plasma, and hemolysis is not associated with hyperkalemia.[35,40,57,83,137] In one study, storage of canine red cells in citrate-phosphate-dextrose-adenine for 40 days resulted in an increase in plasma potassium concentration from 5 to almost 9 mEq/L despite the fact that the original intracellular potassium concentration in the red cells was only 3.8 mEq/L.[137] Regardless of the underlying mechanism, this magnitude of increase in

plasma potassium concentration would be unlikely to result in detectable hyperkalemia in a recipient dog transfused with blood stored in this manner.

The potassium concentrations of red cells from neonatal dogs are higher than those of red cells from adult dogs.[35,119,130] Red cell concentrations of potassium decrease during the first weeks of life and reach normal adult concentrations by approximately 8 to 13 weeks of age. In one study, mean red cell potassium concentrations in puppies were 19.0 mEq/L at 1 day of age, 15.1 mEq/L at 5 weeks of age, and 8.7 mEq/L at 13 weeks of age.[35] Reticulocytes from adult dogs also contain higher potassium concentrations than do mature red cells.[108] In adult Akitas, red cell potassium concentrations may exceed 70 mEq/L, and hemolysis results in a progressive increase in plasma potassium concentration (up to 24 mEq/L) during storage of blood.[40,141]

Dogs may be divided genetically into two groups based on the presence or absence of Na+,K+-ATPase activity in the membranes of their mature red cells.[89,109] Dogs with red cell membrane Na+,K+-ATPase activity maintain high intracellular potassium concentrations, whereas those without red cell Na+,K+-ATPase activity maintain red cell potassium concentrations similar to those of plasma. Reticulocytes from low-potassium (LK) dogs possess Na+,K+-ATPase, but it is rapidly and completely degraded by a proteolytic process during cell maturation.[90,108] Reticulocytes from high-potassium (HK) dogs have twice as much Na+,K+-ATPase activity as reticulocytes from LK dogs, but in the HK dogs, degradation of the enzyme ceases early in maturation, and sufficient activity remains in the mature red cell to account for the observed high intracellular concentration of potassium.[108] The HK phenotype is inherited as an autosomal recessive trait and occurs with an incidence of 26% to 38% in the Shiba and Akita breeds in Japan and 42% in the Kindo breed in Korea.[68] Some dogs with the HK phenotype also accumulate large amounts of reduced glutathione in their erythrocytes (so-called HK/HG phenotype), which predisposes them to oxidative injury and hemolytic anemia associated with onion ingestion.[185]

Red cells of English springer spaniel dogs with phosphofructokinase deficiency had potassium concentrations of 19.2 to 28 mEq/L as compared with 5.1 to 7.7 mEq/L in control dogs, and hemolytic crises in affected dogs were associated with hyperkalemia.[74] The higher potassium concentration in the red cells of affected dogs was attributed in part to the large number of circulating reticulocytes (7% to 26%).

Hemolysis in Akitas (and presumably in other HK dogs) and thrombocytosis cause what has been called **pseudohyperkalemia** because these effects occur in vitro. Pseudohyperkalemia has also been reported in a dog with acute lymphoblastic leukemia before chemotherapy.[85] Leakage of potassium from the leukemic cells in vitro was thought to be responsible for pseudohyperkalemia in this

TABLE 5-1 Sodium and Potassium Concentrations of Mammalian Erythrocytes

Species	Sodium (mEq/L)	Potassium (mEq/L)
Human	10-21	104-155
Dog LK*	93-150	4-11
Dog HK*[109]	54	124
Cat	104-142	6-8
Horse	4-16	80-140
Cow LK*	72-102	7-37
Cow HK*	15	70
Sheep LK*	74-121	8-39
Sheep HK*	10-43	60-88
Swine	11-19	100-124

Sheep, cattle, and dogs demonstrate polymorphism with respect to their intracellular cation concentrations, depending on the level of Na+,K+-ATPase activity in the mature red cell membranes.
HK, High potassium; LK, low potassium.

case. Use of plasma from small blood samples collected in an excessive volume of tripotassium ethylenediaminetetraacetic acid may also result in measured hyperkalemia.

HYPOKALEMIA

CLINICAL AND LABORATORY FEATURES

Many dogs and cats with hypokalemia have no clinical signs. Muscular weakness, polyuria, polydipsia, and impaired urinary concentrating capacity are the clinical signs most likely to be recognized in dogs and cats with symptomatic hypokalemia. The pathophysiology of these clinical signs is discussed here.

The clinician should verify the abnormal serum potassium concentration with the laboratory, but measurement of potassium by flame photometry and ion-selective potentiometry is reliable, and errors are uncommon. The clinical history often provides information about the likely source of potassium loss (e.g., chronic vomiting and diuretic administration) or the possibility of translocation (e.g., insulin administration and alkalosis).

Determination of the fractional excretion of potassium (FE_K) may help differentiate renal and nonrenal sources of potassium loss. Fractional potassium excretion can be calculated and expressed as a percentage using:

$$\frac{(U_K/S_K)}{(U_{Cr}/S_{Cr})} \times 100$$

where U_K is the urine concentration of K (mEq/L), S_K is the serum concentration of K (mEq/L), U_{Cr} is the urine concentration of creatinine (mg/dL), and S_{Cr} is the serum concentration of creatinine (mg/dL).

The FE_K should be less than 4% for nonrenal sources of loss, and in the presence of hypokalemia, values above 4% may indicate inappropriate renal loss.[52] In one study, however, FE_K values for normal cats were $10.6 \pm 2.1\%$.[3] In another study of normal cats receiving a potassium-deficient diet, FE_K values decreased from 10% to 12% to 3% to 6%.[53] Thus FE_K values up to 6% should probably be considered normal in potassium-depleted animals with normal renal function. However, the clinical utility of FE_K calculations is limited by the fact that FE_K does not correlate well with 24-hour urinary excretion of potassium.[3,66] The occurrence of hypokalemia in patients with metabolic alkalosis suggests vomiting of stomach contents or diuretic administration as likely causes of potassium loss. In patients with hypokalemia and metabolic acidosis, diarrhea caused by small intestinal disease, chronic renal failure, and distal renal tubular acidosis are more likely causes of potassium loss (Fig. 5-11).

The effect of aldosterone on serum potassium excretion can also be evaluated by comparing urine and serum potassium concentrations after correcting the urine potassium concentration for reabsorption of solute-free water by the kidneys. This index has been called the transtubular potassium gradient (TTKG).[110,180,181] A value of 5.0 or higher has been said to indicate the presence of an aldosterone effect, whereas a value of 3.0 or less is expected in the absence of mineralocorticoid activity.[181] Use of the TTKG is valid only when the urine osmolality is greater than 300 mOsm/kg and the urine sodium concentration is greater than 25 mEq/L. The renal TTKG may be estimated according to the equation:

$$TTKG = [U_K/(U_{Osm}/S_{Osm})]/S_K$$

where U_K is the urine potassium concentration (mEq/L), S_K is the serum potassium concentration (mEq/L), U_{Osm} is the urine osmolality (mOsm/kg), and S_{Osm} is the serum osmolality (mOsm/kg).[180,181] Values for TTKG were estimated as 3.7 ± 0.9 in normal cats and 4.2 ± 1.3 in normal dogs.[44,48] Determination of TTKG was used in a dog with hypoadrenocorticism to assess the contribution of concurrent trimethoprim administration on the observed hyperkalemia.[148] The causes of hypokalemia are listed in Box 5-1, and the diagnostic approach to hypokalemia is presented in Fig. 5-11.

Effects of Potassium Depletion on Acid-Base Balance

Hypokalemia is often said to be associated with metabolic alkalosis, but early studies used diuretics or mineralocorticoids to induce potassium depletion. These methods probably caused disproportionate urinary loss of chloride relative to the chloride concentration of ECF, and chloride depletion presumably was the major factor responsible for development of metabolic alkalosis (see Chapter 10).

Pure potassium depletion apparently does cause metabolic alkalosis in rats, but in dogs it leads to metabolic acidosis.[16,26,69] When potassium depletion was produced during a 2- to 4-week period in dogs and care was taken to avoid chloride depletion, metabolic acidosis developed.[26,69] When potassium was restored to the diet, metabolic acidosis resolved within 5 days. The observed reduction in net acid excretion and metabolic acidosis that accompany dietary potassium depletion in the dog appear to be caused by a distal renal tubular acidification defect, which is promptly reversed by potassium repletion.[69] This acidification defect is at least partially related to decreased aldosterone secretion.[87]

Chronic potassium depletion also appears to lead to metabolic acidosis in cats. Adult cats were fed a potassium-restricted (0.2% potassium), 32% protein diet with or without 0.8% NH_4Cl.[53] Serum potassium concentrations decreased from 4.3 to 4.5 mEq/L to 3.1 to 3.5 mEq/L in the NH_4Cl-treated cats and to 3.6 to 3.8 mEq/L in the cats not receiving NH_4Cl. Urinary FE_K was appropriately reduced to 3% to 6% in both groups of cats. Potassium balance was decreased in both groups but

Hypokalemia

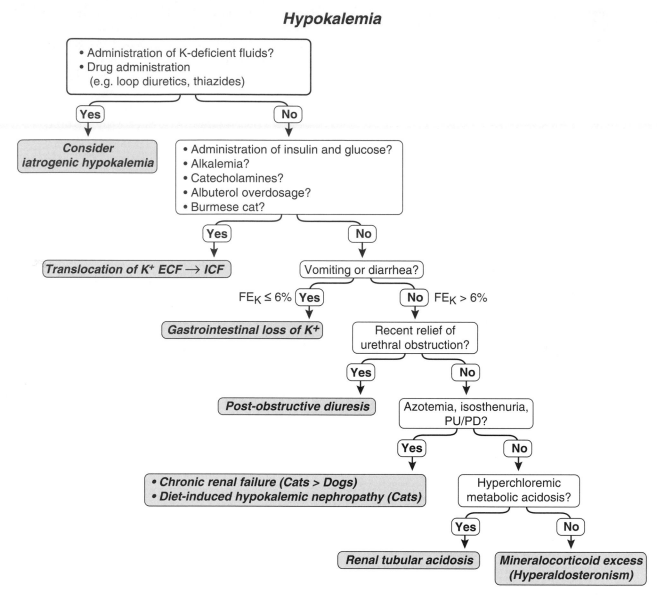

Fig. 5-11 Algorithm for the clinical approach to hypokalemia. (Drawing by Tim Vojt.)

became negative only in the NH_4Cl-treated cats. Metabolic acidosis developed in both groups but was more severe in cats treated with NH_4Cl. Metabolic acidosis resolved in both groups during potassium repletion.

Effects on Muscle

Muscle weakness develops when serum potassium concentration decreases to less than 3.0 mEq/L, increased creatine kinase concentration develops when serum potassium concentration decreases to less than 2.5 mEq/L, and frank rhabdomyolysis may occur when serum potassium concentration decreases to less than 2.0 mEq/L.[95] Rear limb weakness may be observed in dogs and cats with hypokalemia. In cats, weakness of the neck muscles with ventriflexion of the head is commonly

observed.[51,162] Forelimb hypermetria and a broad-based hind limb stance also may be observed in hypokalemic cats. Respiratory muscle paralysis required ventilatory support in two cats with potassium depletion and was thought to be the cause of death in an experimental study of potassium depletion in dogs.[51,132] Acute onset of hypokalemia and muscular weakness also have been reported in hyperthyroid cats.[126] Three of the four cats in this study received fluid therapy with lactated Ringer's solution and were treated by surgical thyroidectomy, but one cat developed hypokalemia before treatment.

The effects of progressive potassium depletion on skeletal muscle were studied in dogs and rats.[16] In both species, a progressive increase in ICF sodium concentration and a progressive decrease in ICF potassium con-

Box 5-1	Causes of Hypokalemia

Decreased intake
   Alone unlikely to cause hypokalemia unless diet is aberrant
   Administration of potassium-free (e.g., 0.9% NaCl, 5% dextrose in water) or deficient fluids (e.g., lactated Ringer's solution over several days)
   Bentonite clay ingestion (e.g., cat litter)
Translocation (ECF → ICF)
   Alkalemia
   Insulin/glucose-containing fluids
   Catecholamines
   Hypothermia?
   Hypokalemic periodic paralysis (Burmese cats)
   Albuterol overdosage
Increased loss
   Gastrointestinal (FE_K < 4-6%)
      Vomiting of stomach contents
      Diarrhea
   Urinary (FE_K > 4-6%)
      Chronic renal failure in cats
      Diet-induced hypokalemic nephropathy in cats
      Distal (type I) renal tubular acidosis (RTA)
      Proximal (type II) RTA after $NaHCO_3$ treatment
      Postobstructive diuresis
      Dialysis
      Mineralocorticoid excess
         Hyperadrenocorticism
         Primary hyperaldosteronism (adenoma, adenocarcinoma, hyperplasia)
      Drugs
         Loop diuretics (e.g., furosemide, ethacrynic acid)
         Thiazide diuretics (e.g., chlorothiazide, hydrochlorothiazide)
         Amphotericin B
         Penicillins
         Unknown mechanism
         Rattlesnake envenomation

centration were observed during potassium deficiency. In rats, hyperpolarization of the cell membrane (as predicted by the Goldman-Hodgkin-Katz equation) was detected by direct measurement at all stages of potassium depletion. In dogs, there was an initial hyperpolarization of the cell membrane (mean measured E_m, −92.4 mV) during moderate potassium deficiency because $[K^+]_O$ decreased proportionately more than $[K^+]_I$. There was a dramatic decrease in E_m (mean measured value, −54.8 mV) at the onset of muscle weakness and paralysis in dogs with severe potassium deficiency (serum potassium concentration, 1.6 mEq/L). In rats with potassium deficiency, predicted and measured E_m values were similar during both moderate and severe potassium deficiency, and paralysis was not observed. The inability to predict resting E_m in dogs with severe potassium depletion could be explained by an increase in the sodium permeability of the muscle cell membrane. This study also demonstrated the development of metabolic acidosis in dogs (pH, 7.29; HCO_3^-, 17.0 mEq/L) and metabolic alkalosis (pH, 7.54; HCO_3^-, 37.0 mEq/L) in rats with severe potassium deficiency.

Potassium is released from muscle cells during exercise, causing vasodilatation and increased blood flow.[95] This release of cellular potassium is impaired in states of potassium depletion, resulting in muscle ischemia. Muscle blood flow and potassium release increased markedly during exercise in normal but not in potassium-depleted dogs (serum potassium concentration, 2.3 mEq/L), and exercise caused rhabdomyolysis characterized by focal necrosis and inflammatory cell infiltration in potassium-depleted dogs.[96] Increased creatine kinase concentrations and electromyographic abnormalities have been observed in cats with hypokalemic polymyopathy, but histopathologic lesions are usually mild or absent.[51,162] In dogs with experimentally induced potassium depletion, electromyographic changes were not observed, and increased serum creatine kinase concentration and muscle histopathology were observed only in dogs that had experienced extremely rapid potassium depletion induced by administration of desoxycorticosterone acetate in addition to a potassium-deficient diet.[132] Intestinal ileus has been described in human patients with potassium depletion but usually is not recognized clinically in dogs and cats.

Effects on the Cardiovascular System

Electrocardiographic changes and cardiac arrhythmias may develop because hypokalemia delays ventricular repolarization, increases the duration of the action potential, and increases automaticity. The electrocardiographic changes associated with hypokalemia in human patients (e.g., decreased amplitude T waves, ST segment depression, and U waves) are not consistently observed in dogs and cats, but supraventricular and ventricular arrhythmias may occur. Prolongation of the QT interval and U waves have been reported in a dog with severe hypokalemia (2.0 mEq/L) caused by chronic vomiting and in dogs with experimentally induced potassium depletion (serum potassium concentration, 2.2 mEq/L).[13,77] In another study, development of hypokalemia in dogs over 5 days was associated with ST segment deviations, decreased amplitude T waves, and the appearance of U waves.[60] The appearance of T waves in normal dogs is variable (e.g., positive, negative, and biphasic), and interpretation of the effects of hypokalemia on ventricular repolarization is difficult unless a baseline electrocardiogram has been obtained previously. Hypokalemia potentiates the toxic effects of digitalis on cardiac conduction and may potentiate premature contractions. Hypokalemia also renders the myocardium refractory to the effects of class I antiarrhythmic agents (e.g., lidocaine, quinidine, procainamide). Therefore serum potassium concentration should be measured and hypokalemia should be corrected in dogs with ventricular arrhythmias unresponsive to antiarrhythmic therapy.

Effects on the Kidney

Potassium depletion produces functional and morphologic abnormalities in the kidneys, referred to as hypokalemic nephropathy. Renal vasoconstriction leads to decreases in renal blood flow and glomerular filtration rate (GFR). Polyuria and polydipsia are observed in potassium depletion and result from impaired responsiveness of the kidneys to ADH. Defective collecting duct responsiveness to ADH is associated with decreased medullary tonicity, increased medullary blood flow, and impaired cyclic adenosine monophosphate (cAMP) generation in response to ADH. The urinary concentrating defect in potassium depletion results from decreased expression of ADH-regulated aquaporin 2 water channels in the luminal membranes of the renal epithelial cells of the cortical and medullary collecting ducts.[10,113]

In one study, potassium depletion in dogs for an average of 51 days led to a decrease in total exchangeable potassium from 47.1 to 35.3 mEq/kg and a decrease in serum potassium concentration from more than 4.0 mEq/L to approximately 2.5 mEq/L.[1] These dogs experienced decreases in GFR, renal blood flow, and urinary concentrating capacity (U_{Osm} after 20 hours of water deprivation) of approximately 25%. In another study, potassium depletion (serum potassium concentration, 2.1 mEq/L) in dogs had little effect on GFR but caused a 45% reduction in maximal U_{Osm} (1902 to 1055 mOsm/kg).[15] In a clinical report, a dog with chronic vomiting and hypokalemia (2.0 mEq/L) developed polyuria, polydipsia, and a urinary concentrating defect that persisted after correction of hypokalemia.[77] These abnormalities were attributed to medullary washout of solute and were corrected by partial water restriction and dietary supplementation with NaCl and KCl. In yet another study, dogs subjected to potassium depletion (serum potassium concentration, 2.9 mEq/L) experienced a doubling of urine volume (596 to 1202 mL per 24 hours) and a 40% reduction in maximal urine osmolality (2006 to 1187 mOsm/kg).[149]

Potassium depletion increases renal ammoniagenesis and urinary net acid excretion, whereas potassium loading tends to have the opposite effect.[169] In the rat, increased ammoniagenesis during potassium depletion occurs primarily via enhanced phosphate-dependent glutaminase activity and increased mitochondrial ammoniagenesis in the proximal tubular cells of the renal cortex. The decrease in ammoniagenesis during potassium loading may occur in renal tubular cells from the outer medullary region. Many experimental studies on potassium depletion and renal regulation of acid-base balance have been performed in rats. The renal response of the dog to acute acidosis is known to differ somewhat from that of the rat, and care must be taken in extrapolating data about the renal response to potassium depletion in the rat to dogs.[170]

Proximal renal tubular sodium reabsorption is increased during potassium depletion, possibly as a result of an increase in the activity of the proximal Na^+-H^+ antiporter. However, distal sodium reabsorption is decreased during potassium depletion. This presumably occurs as a result of decreased aldosterone secretion and is a direct effect of decreased ECF potassium concentration on the zona glomerulosa of the adrenal glands. Decreased distal sodium reabsorption decreases K^+ and H^+ ion secretion by decreasing luminal electronegativity. This reduces potassium loss in the urine but also tends to impair renal acid excretion. Thus increased renal ammoniagenesis during potassium depletion may represent a mechanism for enhancing urinary excretion of fixed acid (as NH_4^+) at a time when distal H^+ ion secretion is impaired. Consequently, derangements in acid-base balance are minimized.

The cytoplasmic and mitochondrial enzyme activity profile of renal tubular cells during potassium depletion is strikingly similar to that observed during chronic metabolic acidosis.[169] This similarity suggests the possibility of a common effector mechanism for stimulation of renal ammoniagenesis. Intracellular pH would be a logical candidate for such an effector. As K^+ ions leave cells to maintain ECF potassium concentration during potassium depletion, H^+ ions enter cells and presumably lower intracellular pH. Reduced intracellular pH may in turn be the signal for increased renal ammoniagenesis from glutamine. Some studies have demonstrated reduced intracellular pH in renal tubular cells during potassium depletion, whereas others have found no change.[2,159]

Increased ammonia concentrations may activate the third component of complement (C3) and contribute to development of chronic tubulointerstitial disease by recruitment of immune cells.[124,175] Vacuolization of proximal tubular cells is observed in human patients, whereas similar lesions are observed in the distal nephron, mainly in the medullary collecting ducts, in potassium-depleted rats. Vacuolization of proximal tubular epithelial cells has also been reported in potassium-depleted dogs.[1]

SPECIFIC CAUSES OF HYPOKALEMIA IN DOGS AND CATS

Hypokalemia arises from decreased intake, translocation of potassium from ECF to ICF, and excessive loss of potassium by either the gastrointestinal or urinary route. Decreased intake of potassium alone is unlikely to cause hypokalemia, but it may be a contributing factor. In chronically ill animals, for example, prolonged anorexia, loss of muscle mass, and ongoing urinary potassium losses probably combine to cause hypokalemia. A specific cause for mild hypokalemia in hospitalized dogs and cats often cannot be identified. Such hypokalemia may resolve with successful treatment of the primary disease process. Iatrogenic hypokalemia may develop when potassium-deficient fluids are administered to anorexic patients in a hospital setting. For example, lactated Ringer's solution (potassium concentration, 4 mEq/L) is a replacement solution and does not provide sufficient potassium for maintenance needs in most animals. Solutions used for maintenance fluid therapy should contain 15 to 30 mEq/L potassium (see Chapter 14). Ingestion of certain types of clay has been associated with hypokalemia in humans because the clay can bind potassium in the gastrointestinal tract and impair its absorption, and hypokalemia has been reported in a cat after ingestion of clay cat litter containing bentonite.[75,86]

Translocation of potassium into cells may occur with alkalemia, insulin release, and catecholamine release. Alkalemia contributes to hypokalemia as K^+ ions enter cells in exchange for H^+ ions. Insulin promotes uptake of glucose and potassium by hepatic and skeletal muscle cells and may contribute to hypokalemia when glucose-containing fluids are administered. The stress of illness and the associated epinephrine release may also contribute to hypokalemia. Severe hypokalemia (1.9 mEq/L) was reported in a dog that had ingested the β_2-adrenergic agonist albuterol.[177] The mechanism of hypokalemia was presumably rapid uptake of extracellular potassium by liver and muscle cells. Hypokalemia has been associated with hypothermia, possibly as a result of potassium entry into cells.[146] Mild hypokalemia was reported in 78% of dogs suffering from rattlesnake envenomation.[22] Affected dogs also had transient echinocytosis that was not consistently associated with the observed hypokalemia.

A syndrome characterized by recurrent episodes of limb muscle weakness, neck ventriflexion, increased creatine kinase concentrations, and hypokalemia has been reported in related Burmese cats 4 to 12 months of age.[18,92,101,115,116] This syndrome may represent an animal model of hypokalemic periodic paralysis in humans, a familial disorder characterized by episodes of sudden translocation of potassium from ECF to ICF.

Gastrointestinal loss of potassium (e.g., vomiting of stomach contents) is an important cause of hypokalemia in small animals. Chloride depletion and sodium avidity related to volume depletion contribute to perpetuation of potassium depletion and metabolic alkalosis in this setting by enhancing urinary losses of K^+ and H^+ ions. The effects of metabolic alkalosis on potassium balance are discussed further in Chapter 10.

Urinary loss of potassium is another important cause of hypokalemia, and hypokalemia is common in cats with chronic renal failure. Approximately 20% to 30% of cats with chronic renal failure have hypokalemia at presentation, and in one study, chronic renal disease was the most common associated disorder observed in a survey of cats with hypokalemia.[46,52,56,105] Most dogs with chronic renal failure have normal serum potassium concentrations. For example, fewer than 10% of dogs with chronic renal failure caused by renal amyloidosis had hypokalemia at presentation.[47] Hypokalemia also commonly occurs during the postobstructive diuresis that follows relief of urethral obstruction in cats with idiopathic lower urinary tract disease.

Renal tubular acidosis may be associated with hypokalemia (see Chapter 10). In distal (type I) renal tubular acidosis, hypokalemia is usually present before treatment, and urinary potassium losses may result in part from increased aldosterone secretion. Hypokalemia has been reported in distal renal tubular acidosis in cats.[54,179] In proximal (type II) renal tubular acidosis, correction of acidosis requires large doses of $NaHCO_3$, and hypokalemia usually appears during therapy. This is a result of the increased delivery of Na^+ and HCO_3^- ions to the distal nephron. These factors enhance urinary potassium excretion by increasing distal tubular flow and lumen electronegativity (HCO_3^- is a relatively nonresorbable anion in the cortical collecting duct).

Finally, hypokalemic nephropathy characterized by chronic tubulointerstitial nephritis may develop in cats fed diets low in potassium and containing urinary acidifiers.[24,48,50,52] Stimulation of aldosterone secretion by chronic metabolic acidosis and decreased gastrointestinal absorption of potassium may contribute to potassium depletion in this syndrome.[53,152]

Mutations in genes that encode epithelial transport proteins and channels have been associated with rare disorders of renal tubular function that cause hypokalemia in humans. One of these familial disorders, Bartter's syndrome, is especially complex. It can be caused by mutations in the NKCC2 gene that codes for the luminal Na^+-K^+-$2Cl^-$ cotransporter found in the thick ascending limb of Henle's loop (type I), in the gene for the ROMK protein component of renal tubular potassium channels (type II), in the CLCNKB gene that codes for the ClC-Kb chloride channel in the basolateral membranes of tubular cells in the thick ascending limb (type III), or in the BSND gene that codes for barttin, a subunit protein of chloride channels that is required for proper insertion of the channels into the basolateral membrane (type IV).[84,158] Other rare diseases can arise from a loss of function mutation in the NCCT gene for the thiazide-sensitive Na^+-Cl^- cotransporter in the luminal membranes of the distal convoluted tubule (Gitelman's variant of Bartter's syndrome) or a gain of function mutation in the SCNN1 gene for the luminal sodium channel (ENaC) of the principal cells of the collecting duct (Liddle's syndrome). None of these rare tubular disorders have yet been recognized in veterinary medicine.

Mineralocorticoid excess is an uncommon cause of urinary potassium loss and hypokalemia in dogs and cats.

One report described hyperaldosteronism in a dog thought to be caused by adrenal hyperplasia of the adrenal zona glomerulosa.[21] Older dogs with hyperaldosteronism as a result of aldosterone-producing adenomas or adenocarcinomas are presented for evaluation of weakness and polyuria.[59,183] Mild to moderate hypertension may be detected, and hypokalemia, hypernatremia, mild metabolic alkalosis, dilute urine, and extremely high serum aldosterone concentrations (>3000 pmol/L; normal, 14 to 957 pmol/L) are present on laboratory evaluation. Dogs with adenomas respond well to surgical adrenalectomy, but those with adenocarcinomas experience recurrence of clinical signs if metastasis occurs. One affected dog had polyuria and hyperaldosteronism associated with a very small (2 mm) adrenal adenoma that initially was undetected by computed tomography, and the dog responded to treatment with spironolactone.[142] Ultimately, the tumor was identified and removed, and the dog recovered completely. Another dog with an adrenal adenocarcinoma had clinical and laboratory features of mineralocorticoid excess, but serum aldosterone concentration was undetectable.[140] Serum desoxycorticosterone concentration was measured and found to be abnormally high (288 ng/mL; normal, 16 to 46 ng/mL). After surgical removal of the tumor, serum potassium concentration normalized, but serum desoxycorticosterone concentration remained high, and the dog was treated with spironolactone. Hypokalemia also may be observed in dogs with hyperadrenocorticism because of the mineralocorticoid effects of endogenous steroids such as corticosterone and deoxycorticosterone, and it is more common in dogs with adrenal-dependent disease than in those with pituitary-dependent disease.[104,117]

Several cats (5 to 20 years of age) with hyperaldosteronism have been reported.[55,67,107,121,142] Affected cats are presented for evaluation of weakness (sometimes with ventriflexion of the neck), ataxia, weight loss, polyuria, polydipsia, and ocular abnormalities (e.g., mydriasis, blindness, and retinal detachments) associated with hypertension. Laboratory features consist of hypokalemia, hypernatremia, mild metabolic alkalosis, increased serum creatine kinase activity, dilute urine, extremely high serum aldosterone concentrations (>3000 pmol/L; normal, 194 to 388 pmol/L), and plasma renin activity that is low or at the low end of the normal reference range (0.2 to 0.5 ng/L/sec; normal, 0.2 to 1.4 ng/L/sec). In two affected cats, urinary FE_K was more than 50% and consistent with inappropriate kaliuresis.[67] In these two cats, chronic renal disease also was present and might have contributed to hypertension and increased FE_K. Hyperaldosteronism may be associated with hyperglycemia caused by insulin resistance, and one affected cat had diabetes mellitus that persisted despite removal of the adrenal tumor.[67] Aldosterone-producing adrenal tumors reported in cats have been 1 to 3 cm in diameter and were visualized on abdominal

ultrasonography. Cytological evaluation of fine needle aspirates is consistent with neuroendocrine neoplasia, and histologically these tumors are adenomas or adenocarcinomas. Surgical removal of the tumor is the treatment of choice, especially for adenomas. Spironolactone (2 to 4 mg/kg/day) and potassium supplementation (2 to 6 mEq/day) can be used to manage cats that are not surgical candidates.[67] In one cat, invasion of the caudal vena cava by an adenocarcinoma ultimately resulted in thromboembolism. See Chapter 10 for further discussion of states of mineralocorticoid excess.

Administration of loop or thiazide diuretics may cause hypokalemia as a result of increased flow rate in the distal tubules and increased secretion of aldosterone secondary to volume depletion. In one study, dogs with heart failure receiving furosemide had significantly lower mean serum potassium concentrations (mean serum potassium concentration, 3.9 mEq/L) than did normal dogs (mean serum potassium concentration, 4.4 mEq/L) or untreated dogs with arrhythmias (mean serum potassium concentration, 4.3 mEq/L).[33] Of the dogs treated with furosemide, 17% had serum potassium concentrations less than 3.0 mEq/L. In another study, 10 dogs with congestive heart failure treated with captopril, furosemide, and a sodium-restricted diet did not develop significant changes in serum electrolyte concentrations.[147] Penicillin derivatives may cause hypokalemia by acting as nonresorbable anions in the distal tubule and increasing secretion of potassium into tubular fluid. Amphotericin B may cause increased loss of potassium by binding to sterols in cell membranes and increasing permeability. Peritoneal dialysis can be complicated by hypokalemia if potassium-free dialysate is used for an extended time period.[38]

TREATMENT

Preparations available for parenteral use include KCl (2 mEq K$^+$/mL) and a potassium phosphate solution containing K_2HPO_4 and KH_2PO_4 (4.36 mEq K$^+$/mL). Potassium chloride is the additive of choice for parenteral therapy because chloride repletion is essential if vomiting or diuretic administration is the underlying cause of hypokalemia. Replacement of chloride is also essential for resolution of the metabolic alkalosis often present in such settings (see Chapter 10). When administered intravenously, KCl generally should not be infused at rates greater than 0.5 mEq/kg/hr to avoid potential adverse cardiac effects. A scale such as that shown in Table 5-2 may be used to estimate the amount of KCl to add to parenteral fluids based on serum potassium concentration.[79] Infusion rates greater than 0.5 mEq/kg/hr are required to normalize serum potassium concentration in hypokalemic patients with diabetic ketoacidosis treated with insulin. In hypokalemic human patients, potassium infusion rates up to 0.9 mEq/kg/hr were used safely in one study.[80] Careful mixing of

TABLE 5-2 Guidelines for Routine Intravenous Supplementation of Potassium in Dogs and Cats

Serum Potassium Concentration (mEq/L)	mEq KCl to Add to 250 mL Fluid	mEq KCl to Add to 1 L Fluid	Maximal Fluid Infusion Rate* (mL/kg/hr)
<2.0	20	80	6
2.1-2.5	15	60	8
2.6-3.0	10	40	12
3.1-3.5	7	28	18
3.6-5.0	5	20	25

From Greene RW, Scott RC: Lower urinary tract disease. In Ettinger SJ, editor: Textbook of veterinary internal medicine, Philadelphia, 1975, WB Saunders, p. 1572. *So as not to exceed 0.5 mEq/kg/hr.*

potassium chloride after addition to flexible bags of fluids is extremely important to prevent the patient from receiving a high concentration of potassium that could be life threatening. In one study, inadequate mixing of potassium chloride added to flexible bags of fluid was demonstrated to result in up to a fourfold increase in the concentration of potassium in the fluids.[43] For determination of serum potassium concentration, when submitting blood samples that have been drawn from intravenous catheters in patients receiving potassium-supplemented fluids, the initial volume of blood withdrawn should be discarded, and a second sample should be submitted to the laboratory to avoid results that may be spuriously high.

Infusion of potassium-containing fluids initially may be associated with a decrease in serum potassium concentration as a result of dilution, increased distal renal tubular flow, and cellular uptake of potassium, especially if the infused fluid also contains glucose.[52] This effect may be minimized by using a fluid that does not contain glucose, administering fluids at an appropriate rate, and beginning oral potassium supplementation as soon as possible. The concentration of potassium in the infused fluid generally should not exceed 60 mEq/L because higher concentrations of potassium may cause pain and sclerosis of peripheral veins.[145] Parenteral fluids containing up to 35 mEq/L have been used safely by the subcutaneous route.[64]

Careful potassium supplementation is important when using insulin to treat diabetic ketoacidosis. Chronic potassium depletion is usually present in affected patients as a result of loss of muscle mass, anorexia, vomiting, and polyuria. However, serum potassium concentrations are sometimes normal or even increased because of the effects of insulin deficiency and hyperosmolality on serum potassium concentration. Because blood glucose concentration decreases with insulin treatment, marked hypokalemia may develop if supplementation is not adequate.

Potassium gluconate (e.g., Kaon and Tumil-K) is recommended for oral supplementation. In one study,

orally administered KCl and $KHCO_3$ were not palatable to cats.[51] Dogs may require 2 to 44 mEq potassium per day, depending on body size.[82] In cats with hypokalemic nephropathy, the initial oral dosage of potassium gluconate is 5 to 8 mEq/day divided in two or three doses, whereas the maintenance dosage can usually be reduced to 2 to 4 mEq/day.[52] It is difficult to estimate the amount of potassium required to reestablish normal balance from the serum potassium concentration in a given patient because potassium is an intracellular solute. Thus the amount of potassium required for treatment must be determined by judicious supplementation and serial measurement of serum potassium concentration during treatment and recovery. Selected preparations available for oral potassium supplementation are listed in Table 5-3.

HYPERKALEMIA

Hyperkalemia is uncommon if renal function and urine output are normal. Soon after ingestion of a potassium load, cellular uptake of potassium is mediated by insulin, epinephrine, and the resulting increase in ECF potassium concentration itself. Renal excretion of the potassium load then follows. Sustained, chronic hyperkalemia is almost always associated with some impairment in urinary excretion of potassium.

CLINICAL AND LABORATORY FEATURES

The clinical manifestations of hyperkalemia reflect changes in cell membrane excitability and reflect the magnitude and the rapidity of onset of hyperkalemia. Muscle weakness develops with hyperkalemia, usually when serum potassium concentration exceeds 8.0 mEq/L. The electrocardiographic findings caused by hyperkalemia are often characteristic, and the electrocardiogram may be helpful in establishing a suspicion of hyperkalemia while awaiting results of the serum potassium concentration (Fig. 5-12).

The effects of hyperkalemia on the electrocardiogram have been studied in dogs and cats.[34,36,166,167] Increased

TABLE 5-3 Selected Preparations Available for Oral Potassium Supplementation

Chemical Name	Proprietary Name	Formulation	Unit	Total mg	mEqK+
Potassium chloride	Kaon-Cl[a]	Controlled release tablets	1 tablet	500	6.7
	Various	Controlled release tablets	1 tablet	600	8
	Klor-Con 8[b]	Controlled release tablets	1 tablet	600	8
	Slow-K[c]	Controlled release tablets	1 tablet	600	8
	K+10[d]	Controlled release tablets	1 tablet	750	10
	Kaon Cl-10[a]	Controlled release tablets	1 tablet	750	10
	Klor-Con 10[b]	Controlled release tablets	1 tablet	750	10
	Klotrix[e]	Controlled release tablets	1 tablet	750	10
	K-Tab[f]	Controlled release tablets	1 tablet	750	10
	K-Dur 10[g]	Controlled release tablets	1 tablet	750	10
	Ten-K[c]	Controlled release tablets	1 tablet	750	10
	K-Dur 20[g]	Controlled release tablets	1 tablet	1500	20
	K+8[d]	Extended release tablets	1 tablet	600	8
	Various	Extended release tablets	1 tablet	750	10
	Micro-K Extencaps[l]	Controlled release capsules	1 capsule	600	8
	Various	Controlled release capsules	1 capsule	750	10
	K-Lease[a]	Controlled release capsules	1 capsule	750	10
	K-Norm[m]	Controlled release capsules	1 capsule	750	10
	Micro-K 10 Extencaps[l]	Controlled release capsules	1 capsule	750	10
	Various	Liquid	15 ml (1 T)	1500	20
	Cena-K[n]	Liquid	15 ml (1 T)	1500	20
	Kaochlor 10%[a]	Liquid	15 ml (1 T)	1500	20
	Kaochlor S-F[a]	Liquid	15 ml (1 T)	1500	20
	Kay Ciel[o]	Liquid	15 ml (1 T)	1500	20
	Klorvess[i]	Liquid	15 ml (1 T)	1500	20
	Potasalan[p]	Liquid	15 ml (1 T)	1500	20
	Rum-K[q]	Liquid	15 ml (1 T)	2250	30
	Various	Liquid	15 ml (1 T)	3000	40
	Cena-K[n]	Liquid	15 ml (1 T)	3000	40
	Kaon-Cl 20%[a]	Liquid	15 ml (1 T)	3000	40
	K+Care[d]	Powder	1 packet	975	15
	Various	Powder	1 packet	1500	20
	Gen-K[s]	Powder	1 packet	1500	20
	Kay Ciel[o]	Powder	1 packet	1500	20
	K+Care[d]	Powder	1 packet	1500	20
	K-Lor[f]	Powder	1 packet	1500	20
	Klor-Con[b]	Powder	1 packet	1500	20
	Micro-K LS[l]	Powder	1 packet	1500	20
	K-vescent KCl[u]	Powder	1 packet	1500	20
	K+Care[d]	Powder	1 packet	1875	25
	Klor-Con/25[b]	Powder	1 packet	1875	25
	K-Lyte/Cl[t]	Powder	1 packet	1875	25
Potassium gluconate	Various	Tablets	1 tablet	500	2.13
	Mission[h]	Tablets	1 tablet	595	2.53
	Tumil-K[v]	Tablets	1 tablet	468	2
	Tumil-K[v]	Protein-based powder	0.65 g (1/4 t)	468	2
	Tumil-K[v]	Gel	2.34 g (1/2 t)	468	2
	Various	Liquid	15 ml (1 T)	4680	20
	Kaon[a]	Liquid	15 ml (1 T)	4680	20
	Kaylixir[p]	Liquid	15 ml (1 T)	4680	20
	K-G Elixir[r]	Liquid	15 ml (1 T)	4680	20
Potassium citrate	Urocit-K[h]	Tablets	1 tablet	540	5
		Tablets	1 tablet	1080	10
Potassium bicarbonate	K+Care ET[d]	Effervescent tablets	1 tablet	2002	20
	K+Care ET[d]	Effervescent tablets	1 tablet	2503	25

TABLE 5-3 Selected Preparations Available for Oral Potassium Supplementation—cont'd

Chemical Name	Proprietary Name	Formulation	Unit	Total mg	mEqK+
Potassium bicarbonate/ Potassium citrate	Effer-K[j]	Effervescent tablets	1 tablet		25
	Effervescent Potassium[k]	Effervescent tablets	1 tablet		25
	Klor-Con/EF[b]	Effervescent tablets	1 tablet		25
	K•Lyte[e]	Effervescent tablets	1 tablet		25
	K•Lyte DS[e]	Effervescent tablets	1 tablet		50
Potassium bicarbonate/ Potassium chloride	Klorvess[i]	Effervescent tablets	1 tablet		20
	K•Lyte/Cl[e]	Effervescent tablets	1 tablet		25
	K•Lyte/Cl 50[e]	Effervescent tablets	1 tablet		50
Potassium acetate/ Potassium bicarbonate/ Potassium citrate	Tri-K[n]	Liquid	15 ml (1 T)		45
Potassium gluconate/ Potassium citrate	Twin-K[r]	Liquid	15 ml (1 T)		20
Potassium gluconate/ Potassium chloride	Kolyum[m]	Liquid	15 ml (1 T)		20
Potassium chloride/ Potassium bicarbonate/ Potassium citrate	Klorvess Effervescent Granules[i]	Powder	1 packet		20

Chemical Name	Chemical Structure	Molecular Weight	mEqK+ per gram
Potassium chloride	KCl	74.6	13.4
Potassium bicarbonate	$KHCO_3$	100.1	10.0
Potassium citrate	$K_3C_6H_5O_7 \cdot H_2O$	324.3	9.25
Potassium gluconate	$KC_6H_{11}O_7$	234.1	4.3

NOTE: KCl is made for injection by various manufacturers; most preparations contain 2 mEq K+ per ml. A potassium phosphate preparation containing 4.36 mEq K+ per ml also is available (see Chapter 7).
[a] Adria Labs, Division of Pharmacia, Kalamazoo, MI 49001.
[b] Upsher-Smith, Minneapolis, MN 55447.
[c] Summit, Division of Novartis, East Hanover, NJ 04936.
[d] Alra, Gurnee, IL 60031.
[e] Bristol-Meyers Squib, Princeton, NJ 08540.
[f] Abbott Laboratories, Abbott Park, IL 60064.
[g] Key, Division of Schering-Plough, Kenilworth, NJ 07033.
[h] Mission Pharmacal, San Antonio, TX 78298.
[i] Sandoz, Division of Novartis, East Hanover, NJ 04936.
[j] Nomax, St. Louis, MO 63119.
[k] Rugby Labs, Duluth, GA 30097.
[l] Robins, Division of Wyeth Consumer Health, Madison, NJ 07940.
[m] Fison, Division of CellTech Pharmaceuticals, Rochester, NY 14623.
[n] Century, Indianapolis, IN 46256.
[o] Forest, New York, NY 10022.
[p] Lannett, Philadelphia, PA 19136.
[q] Fleming, Fenton, MO 63026.
[r] Boots, Division of Abbott Laboratories, Abbott Park, IL 60064.
[s] Goldline, Division of IVAX Pharmaceuticals, Miami, FL 33137.
[t] Mead Johnson Nutritionals, Evansville, IN 47721.
[u] Major, Livonia, MI 48150
[v] Virbac, Fort Worth, TX 76161.
T, Tablespoon; t, teaspoon.
Data from Facts and comparisons, St. Louis, MO 2003, Wolters Kluwer Health.

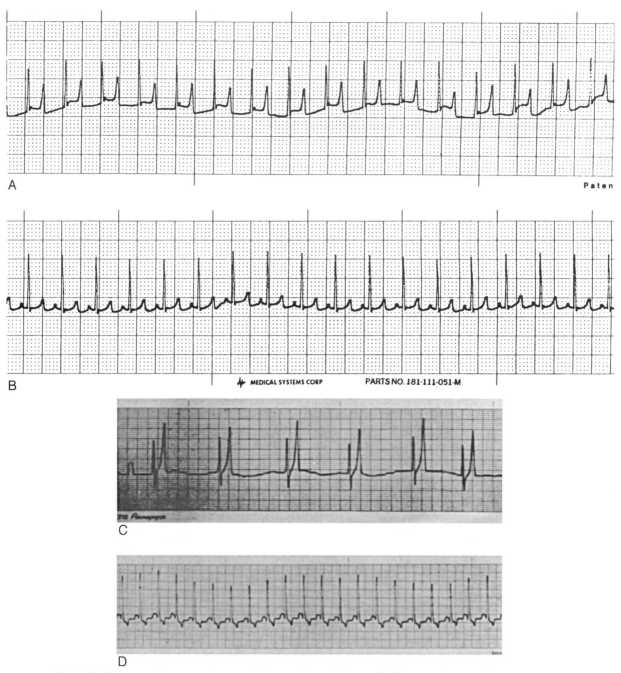

Fig. 5-12 Electrocardiograms of a cat and dog with hyperkalemia. **A,** Electrocardiogram from an 8-year-old female domestic shorthaired cat with oliguric acute renal failure and serum K^+ concentration of 7.8 mEq/L. **B,** Electrocardiogram of same cat after 2 mEq/kg $NaHCO_3$ administered intravenously over 30 minutes. **C,** Electrocardiogram of a dog with serum K^+ concentration of 9.6 mEq/L before treatment. Note tall, tented T waves and absence of P waves. **D,** Electrocardiogram of same dog 15 minutes after infusion of $NaHCO_3$. (Parts **C** and **D** from Chew DJ, DiBartola SP: *Manual of small animal nephrology and urology,* New York, 1986, Churchill Livingstone, p. 132.)

amplitude and narrowing or "tenting" of the T waves may occur with mild increases in serum potassium concentration, but these changes are inconsistent in dogs and cats. Shortening of the QT interval may also be observed. These changes reflect abnormally rapid repolarization. Moderate hyperkalemia may result in prolongation of the PR interval and widening of the QRS complex because of slowing of conduction through the atrioventricular system. With progression of hyperkalemia, conduction through the atrial muscle is impaired, and a decrease in the amplitude and widening of the P wave are observed. In severe hyperkalemia, atrial conduction ceases, the P waves disappear, and pronounced bradycardia with a sinoventricular rhythm may

Box 5-2	Causes of Hyperkalemia

Pseudohyperkalemia
Thrombocytosis
Hemolysis

Increased Intake
Unlikely to cause hyperkalemia in presence of normal
  renal function unless iatrogenic (e.g., continuous
  infusion of potassium-containing fluids at an excessively
  rapid rate)

Translocation (ICF → ECF)
Acute mineral acidosis (e.g., HCl, NH_4Cl)
Insulin deficiency (e.g., diabetic ketoacidosis)
Acute tumor lysis syndrome
Reperfusion of extremities after aortic thromboembolism
  in cats with cardiomyopathy
Hyperkalemic periodic paralysis (one case report in a
  pit bull)
Mild hyperkalemia after exercise in dogs with induced
  hypothyroidism
Infusion of lysine or arginine in total parenteral nutrition
  solutions
Drugs
  Nonspecific beta-blockers (e.g., propranolol)*
  Cardiac glycosides (e.g., digoxin)*

Decreased Urinary Excretion
Urethral obstruction
Ruptured bladder
Anuric or oliguric renal failure
Hypoadrenocorticism
Selected gastrointestinal disease (e.g., trichuriasis,
  salmonellosis, perforated duodenal ulcer)
Late pregnancy in greyhound dogs (mechanism unknown
  but affected dogs had gastrointestinal fluid loss)
Chylothorax with repeated pleural fluid drainage
Hyporeninemic hypoaldosteronism†
Drugs
  Angiotensin-converting enzyme inhibitors
    (e.g., enalapril)*
  Angiotensin receptor blockers (e.g., losartan)*
  Cyclosporin and tacrolimus*
  Potassium-sparing diuretics (e.g., spironolactone,
    amiloride, triamterene)*
  Nonsteroidal antiinflammatory drugs*
  Heparin*
  Trimethoprim*

*Likely to cause hyperkalemia only in conjunction with other
contributing factors (e.g., other drugs, decreased renal function,
concurrent administration of potassium supplements).
†Not well documented in veterinary medicine.

be observed. In extreme hyperkalemia, the QRS complex may merge with the T wave, creating a sine wave appearance, followed by ventricular fibrillation or ventricular asystole. During progressive hyperkalemia, atrial inexcitability, depressed conduction through the specialized tissues and ventricular muscle, and the potential for reentry lead to axis deviations, widening of the QRS complex, and ventricular asystole or ventricular fibrillation. Ventricular fibrillation in hyperkalemia is most likely the result of slow intraventricular conduction and decreased duration of the refractory period. These electrocardiographic changes have also been described in cats with hyperkalemia secondary to urethral obstruction, and they represent the most life-threatening functional consequences of hyperkalemia.[131] The causes of hyperkalemia are listed in Box 5-2, and the clinical approach to hyperkalemia is presented in Fig. 5-13.

SPECIFIC CAUSES OF HYPERKALEMIA IN DOGS AND CATS

Increased intake of potassium is unlikely to cause sustained hyperkalemia unless impaired renal excretion of potassium is present. Exceptions include iatrogenic hyperkalemia resulting from calculation errors during continuous infusion of potassium-containing fluids or administration of drugs known to predispose to hyperkalemia with concurrent potassium supplementation. Examples of the latter situation include concurrent use of nonspecific beta-blockers (e.g., propranolol) or angiotensin-converting enzyme inhibitors (e.g., enalapril) with potassium supplementation (KCl used as a salt substitute contains 13.4 mEq potassium/g) during treatment of heart failure (see Chapter 21).

Translocation of potassium from ICF to ECF can cause hyperkalemia. Acute metabolic acidosis caused by mineral acids (e.g., NH_4Cl and HCl) but not organic acids (e.g., lactic acid and ketoacids) causes potassium to shift out of cells in exchange for H^+ ions that enter cells to be buffered. The effect of acute inorganic metabolic acidosis on serum potassium concentration in dogs is variable and was characterized by a 0.16- to 1.67-mEq/L increment in serum potassium concentration per 0.1-U decrement in pH in a review of previously published studies.[4]

Induction of hypothyroidism in beagles led to a 41% decrease in the Na^+,K^+-ATPase content of skeletal muscle, which was associated with a decrease in the mean resting plasma sodium concentration (from 148 to 142 mEq/L) and an increase in the mean resting plasma potassium concentration (from 3.7 to 4.3 mEq/L).[153] Plasma potassium concentration also increased slightly after exercise in the hypothyroid dogs (up to a mean of approximately 5.0 mEq/L) but not in the euthyroid dogs presumably because decreased Na^+,K^+-ATPase in the hypothyroid dogs resulted in slower reuptake of potassium by muscle cells.

Insulin deficiency and hyperosmolality contribute to hyperkalemia in diabetic patients. Hyperosmolality may increase serum potassium concentration as water moves from ICF to ECF and potassium follows because of sol-

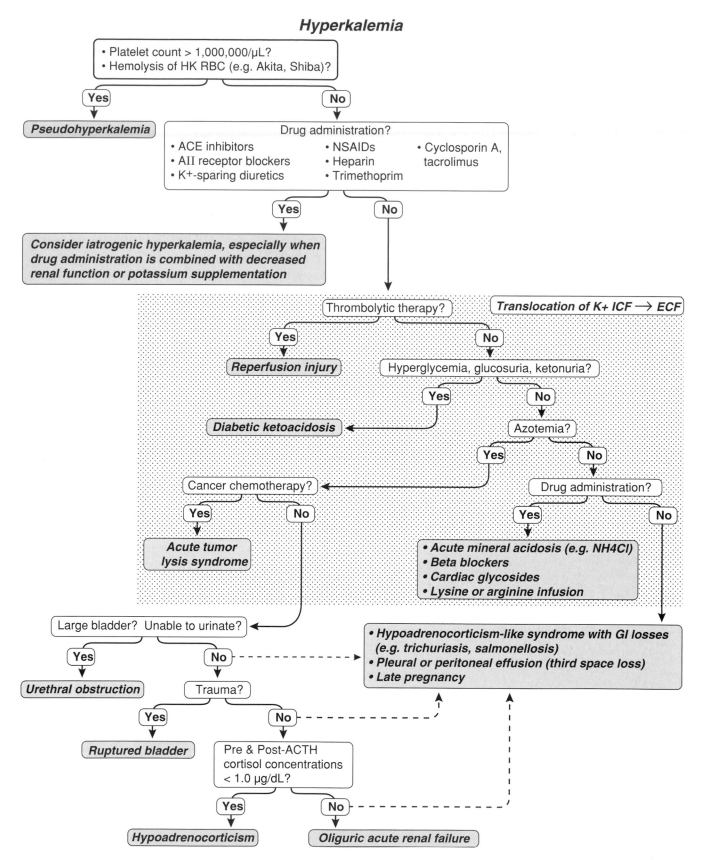

Fig. 5-13 Algorithm for the clinical approach to hyperkalemia. (Drawing by Tim Vojt.)

vent drag and as a result of the increased ICF potassium concentration resulting from cellular water loss. Most diabetic patients have total body depletion of potassium caused by urinary losses, muscle mass loss, anorexia, and vomiting. A normal or low serum potassium concentration in a patient with untreated diabetic ketoacidosis indicates serious total body depletion of potassium and the need for diligent potassium supplementation. Hypokalemia at presentation is more common than hyperkalemia in diabetic dogs and cats. In one study, 43% of dogs and 83% of cats with diabetes mellitus were hypokalemic at presentation as compared with 10% of affected dogs and 8% of affected cats that were hyperkalemic.[58] Other studies of cats with diabetes mellitus have confirmed that hyperkalemia is uncommon and that 44% to 70% of affected cats had hypokalemia at presentation.[23,37,120,155] Hypokalemia may also develop after treatment with insulin despite potassium supplementation of fluids.[106] Consequently, the clinician must pay close attention to potassium supplementation of patients with diabetic ketoacidosis.

Massive tissue breakdown may lead to transient hyperkalemia until the kidneys excrete the released potassium. Severe exercise may cause release of potassium from cells and transient hyperkalemia in humans, and this effect is less pronounced in conditioned subjects. In untrained dogs, exercise to the point of exhaustion resulted in an increase in mean serum potassium concentration from 4.4 to 6.0 mEq/L.[97] Exhaustive exercise was not associated with a significant increase in serum potassium concentration after the same dogs had been trained for 6 weeks. In racing greyhounds, no change in serum potassium concentration was observed immediately after racing, despite development of marked lactic acidosis.[88] Severe rhabdomyolysis and lethal hyperkalemia (serum potassium concentrations of 10.9 to 12.6 mEq/L) occurred in three cats with hypertrophic muscular dystrophy after restraint and anesthesia.[70] The sarcolemma of muscle cells in dystrophin-deficient animals is thought to be more sensitive to injury by anesthetic agents and intense activity resulting in release of intracellular contents. Life-threatening hyperkalemia developed in 16 of 46 (35%) cats with aortic thromboembolism treated with streptokinase because of reperfusion of ischemic muscle tissue and possibly decreased renal excretion associated with renal artery thrombosis.[121] Acute tumor lysis syndrome complicated by renal failure and hyperkalemia has been reported in dogs and cats with lymphoma treated by radiation and chemotherapy.[28,98,99] There is one case report of a young pit bull dog with episodic hind limb and neck weakness. Exercise or potassium challenge resulted in mild hyperkalemia.[91] This case may represent an example of hyperkalemic periodic paralysis. In quarter horses, hyperkalemic periodic paralysis is an autosomal dominant trait that causes recurrent episodes of muscle fasciculations and spasm.[118] It is caused by a mutation in the alpha subunit of the sodium channel of skeletal muscle that results in impaired channel inactivation.[29,81]

Decreased urinary excretion is the most important cause of hyperkalemia in small animal practice. The most common associated disorders are urethral obstruction, ruptured bladder, anuric or oliguric renal failure, and hypoadrenocorticism. The time required for development of hyperkalemia in cats after urethral obstruction is variable, but it may occur within 48 hours.[63,65] After relief of obstruction, hyperkalemia resolves within 24 hours, whereas azotemia and hyperphosphatemia require 48 to 72 hours to resolve.[65] After experimental bladder rupture in dogs, azotemia, hyperphosphatemia, and mild hyponatremia developed within 24 hours, whereas hyperkalemia did not develop until after 48 hours.[27] In a retrospective clinical study of uroperitoneum in cats, hyperkalemia was detected in 13 of 24 (54%) animals evaluated.[12]

In chronic renal failure, normal potassium balance is maintained, and hyperkalemia is uncommon and develops only if oliguria occurs. This renal adaptation is accomplished by increased FE_K in remnant nephrons (Fig. 5-14).[19,20,161] Fecal excretion of potassium also increases during chronic progressive renal disease and represents an extrarenal adaptation to maintain potassium balance (see Fig. 5-3). However, patients with chronic renal disease have reduced ability to tolerate an acute potassium load and may require 1 to 3 days to reestablish external potassium balance when intake of potassium is abruptly increased. Dogs with experimentally induced renal disease demonstrate decreased ability to excrete a potassium load. In the first 5 hours after a potassium load, dogs with experimentally induced renal disease excreted 30% to 37% of administered potassium, whereas control dogs excreted 56% to 67%.[19,20] Kaliuresis was blunted in the dogs with remnant kidneys despite exaggerated hyperkalemia and increased secretion of aldosterone, and approximately 24 hours were required for complete excretion of the potassium load.

Oliguria or anuria with hyperkalemia is more likely to occur in acute renal failure (e.g., ethylene glycol ingestion), but these findings may be observed terminally in chronic renal failure. Acute renal failure with oliguria or anuria is associated with hyperkalemia for several reasons. First, there has been insufficient time for renal adaptation to nephron loss, as occurs with chronic renal failure. Severe reductions in GFR and urine output result in inadequate distal tubular flow for effective urinary excretion of potassium. Finally, increased release of potassium from tissues during this catabolic state and acute metabolic acidosis may contribute to translocation of potassium from ICF to ECF.

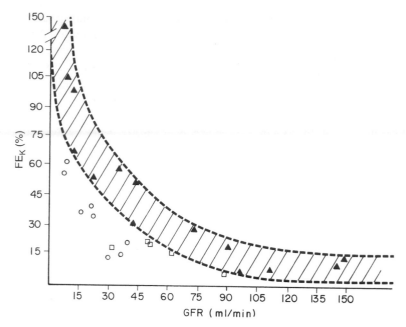

Fig. 5-14 Nomogram relating fractional potassium excretion (FE$_K$) to glomerular filtration rate (GFR). Values for patients with an intact hormonal and renal tubular secretory mechanism for potassium (closed triangles) are used to delineate the hatched area. The open squares and circles indicate patients with selective aldosterone deficiency and renal tubular secretory defects, respectively. (From Batlle DC, Arruda JA, Kurtzman NA: Hyperkalemic distal renal tubular acidosis associated with obstructive uropathy, *N Engl J Med* 304:373-380, 1981. Copyright ©1981 Massachusetts Medical Society. All rights reserved.)

Hyperkalemia, hyponatremia, and Na/K ratios less than 27:1 are usually, but not always, found in dogs and cats with hypoadrenocorticism.* In dogs with hypoadrenocorticism, hyperkalemia has been reported in 74% to 96%, hyponatremia in 56% to 100%, and Na/K ratios less than 27:1 in 85% to 100% of cases. Hyperkalemia was found in 9 of 10 cats with hypoadrenocorticism, whereas hyponatremia and Na/K ratios less than 27:1 were found in all 10 affected cats.[134] Treatment is begun immediately after a presumptive diagnosis of hypoadrenocorticism is made, but conclusive diagnosis requires results of an ACTH stimulation test.

If sodium intake is sufficient to maintain normal ECF volume and distal tubular flow rate, an animal with hypoadrenocorticism may be able to maintain potassium balance. Treatment of dogs with hypoadrenocorticism with fluids alone also often decreases serum potassium concentration into the normal range. However, usually these animals are presented with anorexia and vomiting that contribute to decreased ECF volume and urine output, and without adequate endogenous mineralocorticoids they are unable to excrete sufficient potassium to prevent frank hyperkalemia.

Electrolyte abnormalities similar to those found in dogs with hypoadrenocorticism (i.e., hyponatremia and hyperkalemia) can occur in dogs with gastrointestinal disease related to trichuriasis, salmonellosis, or perforated duodenal ulcer.[45,111] Hyperkalemia in affected dogs with trichuriasis is not caused by a deficiency of aldosterone because plasma aldosterone concentrations have been found to be normal or high.[78] Hyperkalemia and hyponatremia also have been observed in dogs and cats with chylous pleural and peritoneal effusions, in a dog with pleural effusion caused by a lung lobe torsion, in a dog with a neoplastic pleural effusion, in a dog with portal hypertension and peritoneal effusion associated with *Bartonella henselae* infection, and in cats with peritoneal effusion caused by neoplasia or feline infectious peritonitis.* The hyperkalemia observed in these situations is thought to arise from decreased renal excretion of potassium as a consequence of volume depletion (e.g., gastrointestinal fluid loss and third-space loss of fluid) and decreased distal renal tubular flow. Hyperkalemia and hyponatremia also have been reported in three female greyhounds late in pregnancy.[157] The underlying mechanism was unknown, but all of the dogs had a history of vomiting or diarrhea.

Hyporeninemic hypoaldosteronism is an important cause of unexplained asymptomatic hyperkalemia in human patients, but this disorder has rarely been recognized in veterinary medicine.[39] Many affected human patients have mild to moderate renal insufficiency caused by diabetic glomerulosclerosis or interstitial renal disease. Most of them have low plasma renin and aldosterone concentrations. Even in patients with normal plasma aldosterone concentrations, the concentration of this hormone must be considered abnormal in light of the hyperkalemia. Resting plasma cortisol concentrations and response to

---

*References 102,134,135,138,144,150,156,182.

*References 17,94,100,172,184,186.

ACTH are normal. Hyperchloremic metabolic acidosis and hypertension may be observed. It is unclear whether low aldosterone concentrations are a consequence of diminished renin secretion and lack of trophic effect of angiotensin II on the zona glomerulosa of the adrenal cortex or whether there is a primary adrenal defect in aldosterone secretion. To document this syndrome in veterinary patients would require demonstration of subnormal plasma renin and aldosterone concentrations or a subnormal increase in aldosterone after volume contraction or ACTH administration. Normally, aldosterone concentrations increase in response to ACTH in the dog.[183] In this study, one dog with diabetes mellitus was suspected to have hyporeninemic hypoaldosteronism based on a subnormal aldosterone response to ACTH.

Several drugs may contribute to hyperkalemia, especially when used in combination with one another, in conjunction with potassium supplementation, or in patients with renal sufficiency.[133] Nonspecific beta-blockers (e.g., propranolol) interfere with catecholamine-mediated uptake of potassium by liver and muscle by blocking β_2-adrenergic stimulation of cell membrane Na^+,K^+-ATPase. Similar to digoxin, cardiac glycoside toxins found in the plant oleander (e.g., oleandrin, digitoxigenin, and Nerium) inhibit Na^+,K^+-ATPase and can cause hyperkalemia and arrhythmias. The deleterious effects of oleandrin are blocked by infusion of fructose-1,6-diphosphate.[114] Angiotensin-converting enzyme inhibitors (e.g., enalapril) and angiotensin II receptor blockers (e.g., losartan) contribute to hyperkalemia by decreasing production of aldosterone by the adrenal glands and blunting glomerular efferent arteriolar constriction, which potentially can decrease delivery of sodium and water to the distal nephron and impair renal potassium excretion. Prostaglandins stimulate renin release, and use of nonsteroidal antiinflammatory drugs may contribute to development of hyperkalemia. These drugs also may impair the stimulatory effect of prostaglandins on potassium channels in the luminal membranes of renal tubular cells. Heparin impairs aldosterone production by decreasing the number and affinity of angiotensin II receptors in the zona glomerulosa of the adrenal glands and may contribute to hyperkalemia in the presence of other predisposing factors.[129] Potassium-sparing diuretics (e.g., spironolactone, amiloride, and triamterene) reduce urinary excretion of potassium and can cause hyperkalemia. Spironolactone competitively inhibits binding of aldosterone to its cytoplasmic receptor in the principal cells of the collecting duct. Amiloride and triamterene block sodium channels in the luminal membranes of the principal cells. Trimethoprim is similar in structure to amiloride and also inhibits sodium channels in the luminal membranes of the principal cells. Trimethoprim is most likely to cause hyperkalemia at high dosages, when urine pH is low (<6.0), and when used in patients with renal insufficiency.[133] The immunosuppressive drugs cyclosporin A and tacrolimus contribute to hyperkalemia in renal transplant patients by several mechanisms, including decreased aldosterone production, inhibition of Na^+,K^+-ATPase, and interference with luminal potassium channels in renal tubular cells. Infusions of total parenteral nutrition solutions containing lysine and arginine may contribute to hyperkalemia because these amino acids may enter cells in exchange for potassium. In many hospitalized animals, however, the cause of mild hyperkalemia cannot be determined. In these instances, hyperkalemia often resolves with appropriate fluid therapy and treatment of the primary disease.

TREATMENT

Appropriate treatment is dependent on the magnitude and rapidity of onset of the hyperkalemia, as well as the underlying cause. Abnormalities of serum ionized calcium concentration and acid-base balance may aggravate the functional consequences of hyperkalemia as reflected by muscular weakness and electrocardiographic changes. Thus if compatible electrocardiographic changes are observed, hyperkalemia should be treated regardless of its magnitude. An acute increase in serum potassium concentration to more than 6.5 mEq/L should be treated promptly. Asymptomatic animals with normal urine output and chronic hyperkalemia in the range of 5.5 to 6.5 mEq/L may not require immediate treatment, but a search for the underlying cause should be initiated.

Underlying diseases should be treated promptly (e.g., relief of urethral obstruction, establishment of urine output in patients with oliguria or anuria, and 0.9% NaCl and mineralocorticoids in patients with hypoadrenocorticism). Fluid therapy with lactated Ringer's solution (potassium concentration, 4 mEq/L) also ameliorates hyperkalemia by improving renal perfusion and enhancing urinary excretion of potassium. However, use of a potassium-free solution (e.g., 0.9% NaCl and 0.45% NaCl) has a greater dilutional effect on the ECF potassium concentration.

Hyperkalemia may be treated by antagonizing the effects of potassium on cell membranes using calcium gluconate, by driving potassium from ECF to ICF with sodium bicarbonate or glucose (with or without concurrent insulin administration), or by removing potassium from the body with a cation exchange resin or dialysis. First, any source of intake must be discontinued (e.g., potassium-containing fluids and potassium penicillin). The clinician also should review the history to verify that the patient is not currently being treated with any drug known to contribute to hyperkalemia (e.g., nonsteroidal antiinflammatory drugs, beta-blockers, angiotensin-converting enzyme inhibitors, and potassium-sparing diuretics).

Hyperkalemia decreases the resting potential of cells. By administering calcium gluconate, the ECF concentration of calcium is increased and the threshold potential is decreased, thus normalizing the difference between the resting and threshold potential and restoring normal membrane excitability (see Fig. 5-2). Administered calcium begins to work within minutes, but its effect lasts less than 1 hour. The dosage of calcium gluconate is 2 to 10 mL of a 10% solution to be administered slowly with electrocardiographic monitoring.

Glucose works by increasing endogenous insulin release and moving potassium into cells. Its effects begin within 1 hour and last a few hours. Glucose-containing fluids (5% or 10% dextrose) or 50% dextrose (1 to 2 mL/kg) can be used for this purpose. The combination of insulin with glucose may result in greater reduction in serum potassium concentration, but there is a risk of hypoglycemia.[8] Insulin (0.55 to 1.1 U/kg regular insulin added to parenteral fluids) and dextrose (2 g dextrose per unit of insulin added) have been recommended to treat hyperkalemia in cats with urethral obstruction.[154]

Sodium bicarbonate also works by moving K^+ ions into cells as H^+ ions leave cells to titrate administered HCO_3^- in the ECF. Bicarbonate begins to work within 1 hour, and its effects last a few hours. The usual dosage is 1 to 2 mEq/kg intravenously, and it can be repeated if necessary. In normal cats, 4 mEq/kg sodium bicarbonate given intravenously caused hypokalemia, hypernatremia, hyperosmolality, and decreased ionized calcium concentrations.[31,32] If a slow sinoventricular rhythm is present and caused by hyperkalemia, atropine (0.02 to 0.04 mg/kg) may increase the firing rate of the sinus node. An experimental study in dogs demonstrated no beneficial effect of alkalinization in treating hyperkalemia in anesthetized dogs. In this study, the effects of sodium bicarbonate were similar to those of hypertonic saline.[93] Sodium may have effects on cardiac muscle that account for reversal of hyperkalemic electrophysiologic changes.[14] In a study of hyperkalemic human patients with end-stage renal disease, sodium bicarbonate alone did not decrease plasma potassium concentration, and it did not potentiate the potassium-lowering effects of insulin or albuterol.[9]

The cation exchange resin polystyrene sulfonate (Kayexalate) can be used to bind potassium and release sodium in the gastrointestinal tract. Each gram binds 1 mEq of potassium and releases 1 to 3 mEq of sodium. It can be mixed with sorbitol (to prevent constipation) and given orally or diluted in tap water and given per rectum as a retention enema using a large Foley catheter. This approach takes a few hours to work and lasts several hours. Kayexalate must be used carefully in patients with impaired ability to excrete a sodium load (e.g., those with congestive heart failure or oliguric renal failure). Intestinal necrosis also is a reported complication of polystyrene sulfonate and sorbitol given postoperatively to human patients.[72,103]

Loop or thiazide diuretics increase the distal tubular flow rate and potassium secretion and may have adjunctive value in the treatment of hyperkalemia. The β_2 agonist albuterol increases cellular uptake of potassium by stimulating Na^+,K^+-ATPase activity and has been used to treat hyperkalemia in human patients with renal failure.[7] If all of these measures fail, the clinician must consider peritoneal dialysis (see Chapter 28).[38] Hemodialysis (see Chapter 29) is more efficient at removing potassium but is available only at selected referral institutions. The treatment of hyperkalemia is outlined in Box 5-3.

Box 5-3 **Therapeutic Considerations in Management of Hyperkalemia***

Establish venous access and administer potassium-deficient (lactated Ringer's) or potassium-free (0.9% NaCl, 0.45% NaCl) fluids.

Discontinue potassium intake (e.g., potassium-supplemented fluids, potassium-containing salt substitutes, potassium penicillin).

If possible, discontinue drugs that promote hyperkalemia (e.g., beta-blockers, angiotensin-converting enzyme inhibitors, potassium-sparing diuretics, prostaglandin inhibitors).

Administer 1-2 mEq/kg $NaHCO_3$ intravenously.[†]
  Or
Administer calcium gluconate 2-10 mL of a 10% solution slowly intravenously.
  Or
Administer 5-10% dextrose or 1-2 mL/kg 50% dextrose intravenously. Consider 0.55-1.1 U/kg regular insulin in parenteral fluids with 2 g dextrose per unit of insulin administered.

Consider administration of sodium polystyrene sulfonate (Kayexalate) orally (20 g with 100 mL 20% sorbitol) or by retention enema (50 g in 100-200 mL tap water).[‡]

Consider administration of loop (furosemide, 2-4 mg/kg) or thiazide (chlorothiazide, 10-40 mg/kg; hydrochlorothiazide, 2-4 mg/kg) diuretics.

If all other measures fail, institute peritoneal dialysis.

---

*The therapeutic measures to be used will vary with the clinical situation (see text for discussion).
†This is the treatment most commonly used at the Ohio State University Veterinary Teaching Hospital.
‡Oral administration of Kayexalate may cause nausea or vomiting. Sorbitol is added to the oral preparation to prevent constipation. Sorbitol should not be used when administering Kayexalate as a retention enema because of the possible risk of colonic necrosis.[103]

REFERENCES

1. Abbrecht PH: Effects of potassium deficiency on renal function in the dog, *J Clin Invest* 48:432, 1969.

2. Adam WR, Koretsky AP, Weiner MW: ^{32}P-NMR in vivo measurement of renal intracellular pH: effects of acidosis and K$^+$ depletion in rats, *Am J Physiol* 251:F904, 1986.

3. Adams LG, Polzin DG, Osborne CA, et al: Comparison of fractional excretion and 24-hour urinary excretion of sodium and potassium in clinically normal cats and cats with induced chronic renal failure, *Am J Vet Res* 52:718, 1991.

4. Adrogué HJ, Madias NE: Changes in plasma potassium concentration during acute acid base disturbances, *J Clin Invest* 71:456, 1981.

5. Adrogué HJ, Chap Z, Ishida T, et al: Role of the endocrine pancreas in the kalemic response to acute metabolic acidosis in conscious dogs, *J Clin Invest* 75:798, 1985.

6. Alexander EA, Perrone RD: Regulation of extrarenal potassium metabolism. In Maxwell MH, Kleeman CR, Narins RG, editors: *Clinical disorders of fluid and electrolyte metabolism*, New York, 1987, McGraw-Hill, pp. 105-117.

7. Allon M, Copkney C: Albuterol and insulin for treatment of hyperkalemia in hemodialysis patients, *Kidney Int* 38:869, 1990.

8. Allon M, Takeshian A, Shanklin N: Effect of insulin-plus-glucose infusion with or without epinephrine on fasting hyperkalemia, *Kidney Int* 43:212, 1993.

9. Allon M, Shanklin N: Effect of bicarbonate administration on plasma potassium in dialysis patients: interactions with insulin and albuterol, *Am J Kidney Dis* 28:508, 1996.

10. Amlal H, Krane CM, Chen Q, et al: Early polyuria and urinary concentrating defect in potassium deprivation, *Am J Physiol* 279:F655, 2000.

11. Atkins EL, Schwartz WB: Factors governing correction of the alkalosis associated with potassium deficiency: the critical role of chloride in the recovery process, *J Clin Invest* 41:218, 1962.

12. Aumann M, Worth LT, Drobatz KJ: Uroperitoneum in cats: 26 cases (1986-1995), *J Am Anim Hosp Assoc* 34:315, 1998.

13. Bahler RC, Rakita L: Cardiovascular function in potassium-depleted dogs, *Am Heart J* 81:650, 1971.

14. Ballantyne F, Davis LD, Reynolds EW: Cellular basis for reversal of hyperkalemic electrocardiographic changes by sodium, *Am J Physiol* 229:935, 1975.

15. Bennett CM: Urine concentration and dilution in hypokalemic and hypercalcemic dogs, *J Clin Invest* 49:1447, 1970.

16. Bilbrey GL, Herbin L, Carter NW: Skeletal muscle resting membrane potential in potassium deficiency, *J Clin Invest* 52:3011, 1973.

17. Bissett SA, Lamb M, Ward CR: Hyponatremia and hyperkalemia associated with peritoneal effusion in four cats, *J Am Vet Med Assoc* 218:1590, 2001.

18. Blaxter AC, Livesley P, Gruffydd-Jones T, et al: Periodic muscle weakness in Burmese kittens, *Vet Rec* 118:619, 1986.

19. Bourgoignie JJ, Kaplan M, Pincus J, et al: Renal handling of potassium in dogs with chronic renal insufficiency, *Kidney Int* 20:482, 1981.

20. Bourgoignie JJ, Gavellas G, van Putten V, et al: Potassium-aldosterone response in dogs with chronic renal insufficiency, *Miner Electrolyte Metab* 11:150, 1985.

21. Breitschwerdt EB, Meuten DJ, Greenfield CL, et al: Idiopathic hyperaldosteronism in a dog, *J Am Vet Med Assoc* 187:841, 1985.

22. Brown DE, Meyer DJ, Wingfield WE, et al: Echinocytosis associated with rattlesnake envenomation in dogs, *Vet Pathol* 31:654, 1994.

23. Bruskiewicz KA, Nelson RW, Feldman EC, et al: Diabetic ketosis and ketoacidosis in cats: 42 cases (1980-1995), *J Am Vet Med Assoc* 211:188, 1997.

24. Buffington CA, DiBartola SP, Chew DJ, et al: Effect of low potassium commercial nonpurified diet on renal function in adult cats, *J Nutr* 121:S91, 1991.

25. Burnell JM, Villamil MF, Uyeno BT, et al: The effect in humans of extracellular pH change on the relationship between serum potassium concentration and intracellular potassium, *J Clin Invest* 35:935, 1956.

26. Burnell JM, Teubner EJ, Simpson DP: Metabolic acidosis accompanying potassium deprivation, *Am J Physiol* 227:329, 1974.

27. Burrows CF, Bovee KC: Metabolic changes due to experimentally induced rupture of the canine urinary bladder, *Am J Vet Res* 35:1083, 1974.

28. Calia CM, Hohenhaus AE, Fox PR, et al: Acute tumor lysis syndrome in a cat with lymphoma, *J Vet Intern Med* 10:409, 1996.

29. Cannon SC, Hayward LJ, Beech J, et al: Sodium channel inactivation is impaired in equine hyperkalemic periodic paralysis, *J Neurophysiol* 73:1892, 1995.

30. Cassola AC, Giebisch G, Wang W: Vasopressin increases density of apical low-conductance K+ channels in rat CCD, *Am J Physiol* 264:F502, 1993.

31. Chew DJ, Leonard M, Muir WW: Effect of sodium bicarbonate infusions on ionized calcium and total calcium concentrations in serum of clinically normal cats, *Am J Vet Res* 50:145, 1989.

32. Chew DJ, Leonard M, Muir WW: Effect of sodium bicarbonate infusion on serum osmolality, electrolyte concentrations, and blood gas tensions in cats, *Am J Vet Res* 52:12, 1991.

33. Cobb M, Michell AR: Plasma electrolyte concentrations in dogs receiving diuretic therapy for cardiac failure, *J Small Anim Pract* 33:526, 1992.

34. Cohen HC, Gozo EG, Pick A: The nature and type of arrhythmias in acute experimental hyperkalemia in the intact dog, *Am Heart J* 82:777, 1971.

35. Coulter DB, Small LL: Sodium and potassium concentrations of erythrocytes from perinatal, immature, and adult dogs, *Cornell Vet* 63:462, 1972.

36. Coulter DB, Duncan RJ, Sander PD: Effects of asphyxia and potassium on canine and feline electrocardiograms, *Can J Comp Med* 39:442, 1975.

37. Crenshaw KL, Peterson ME: Pretreatment clinical and laboratory evaluation of cats with diabetes mellitus: 104 cases (1992-1994), *J Am Vet Med Assoc* 209:943, 1996.

38. Crisp MS, Chew DJ, DiBartola SP, et al: Peritoneal dialysis: 27 cases (1976-1987), *J Am Vet Med Assoc* 195:1262, 1989.

39. DeFronzo RA: Hyperkalemia and hyporeninemic hypoaldosteronism, *Kidney Int* 17:118, 1980.

40. Degen M: Pseudohyperkalemia in Akitas, *J Am Vet Med Assoc* 190:541, 1987.

41. Degen MA: Correlation of spurious potassium elevation and platelet count in dogs, *Vet Clin Pathol* 15:20, 1986.

42. Degen MA, Feldman BF, Turrel JM, et al: Thrombocytosis associated with a myeloproliferative disorder in a dog, *J Am Vet Med Assoc* 194:1457, 1989.

43. Dhein CR, Wardrop KJ: Hyperkalemia associated with potassium chloride administration in a cat, *J Am Vet Med Assoc* 206:1565, 1995.

44. DiBartola SP, Chew DJ, Jacobs G: Quantitative urinalysis including 24-hour protein excretion in the dog, *J Am Anim Hosp Assoc* 16:537, 1980.

45. DiBartola SP, Johnson SE, Davenport DJ, et al: Clinicopathologic findings resembling hypoadrenocorticism in dogs with primary gastrointestinal disease, *J Am Vet Med Assoc* 187:60, 1985.

46. DiBartola SP, Rutgers HC, Zack PM, et al: Clinicopathologic findings associated with chronic renal disease in cats: 74 cases (1973-1984), *J Am Vet Med Assoc* 190:1196, 1987.

47. DiBartola SP, Tarr MJ, Parker AT, et al: Clinicopathologic findings in dogs with renal amyloidosis: 59 cases (1976-1986), *J Am Vet Med Assoc* 195:358, 1989.

48. DiBartola SP, Buffington CA, Chew DJ, et al: Development of chronic renal disease in cats fed a commercial diet, *J Am Vet Med Assoc* 202:744, 1993.

49. Dow SW: Studies on potassium depletion in cats. *Proceedings of the 12th Annual Kal Kan Symposium for the Treatment of Small Animal Diseases,* 1989, p. 61.

50. Dow SW, Fettman MJ, LeCouteur RS, et al: Potassium depletion in cats: renal and dietary influences, *J Am Vet Med Assoc* 191:1569, 1987.

51. Dow SW, LeCouteur RA, Fettman MJ, et al: Potassium depletion in cats: hypokalemic polymyopathy, *J Am Vet Med Assoc* 191:1563, 1987.

52. Dow SW, Fettman MJ, Curtis CR, et al: Hypokalemia in cats: 186 cases (1984-1987), *J Am Vet Med Assoc* 194:1604, 1989.

53. Dow SW, Fettman MJ, Smith KR, et al: Effects of dietary acidification and potassium depletion on acid-base balance, mineral metabolism and renal function in adult cats, *J Nutr* 120:569, 1990.

54. Drazner FH: Distal renal tubular acidosis associated with chronic pyelonephritis in a cat, *Calif Vet* 34:15, 1980.

55. Eger CE, Robinson WF, Huxtable CRR: Primary aldosteronism (Conn's syndrome) in a cat: a case report and review of comparative aspects, *J Small Anim Pract* 24:293, 1983.

56. Elliott J, Barber PJ: Feline chronic renal failure: clinical findings in 80 cases diagnosed between 1992 and 1995, *J Small Anim Pract* 39:78, 1998.

57. Ellory JC, Tucker EM: Cation transport in red blood cells. In Agar NS, Board PG, (editors): *Red blood cells of domestic mammals,* Amsterdam, 1983, Elsevier Scientific Publishing, pp. 291-314.

58. Feldman EC, Nelson RW: Diabetes mellitus. In Feldman EC, Nelson RW, editors: *Canine and feline endocrinology,* ed 2, Philadelphia, 1996, WB Saunders, p. 401.

59. Feldman EC, Nelson RW: Canine hyperadrenocorticism (Cushing's syndrome). In Feldman EC, Nelson RW, editors): *Canine and feline endocrinology,* ed 3, Philadelphia, 2004, WB Saunders, pp. 359-360.

60. Felkai F: Electrocardiographic signs in ventricular repolarization of experimentally induced hypokalemia and appearance of the U wave in dogs, *Acta Vet Hung* 33:221, 1985.

61. Field MJ, Stanton BA, Giebisch G: Influence of ADH on renal potassium handling: a micropuncture and microperfusion study, *Kidney Int* 25:502, 1984.

62. Field MJ, Berliner RW, Giebisch GH: Regulation of renal potassium metabolism. In Maxwell MH, Kleeman GR, Narins RG, editors: *Clinical disorders of fluid and electrolyte metabolism,* New York, 1987, McGraw-Hill, pp. 119-146.

63. Finco DR: Induced feline urethral obstruction: response of hyperkalemia to relief of obstruction and administra-tion of parenteral fluids, *J Am Anim Hosp Assoc* 12:198, 1976.

64. Finco DR: Fluid therapy. In Kirk RW, editor: *Current veterinary therapy VI,* Philadelphia, 1977, WB Saunders, p. 8.

65. Finco DR, Cornelius LM: Characterization and treatment of water, electrolyte, and acid-base imbalances of induced urethral obstruction in the cat, *Am J Vet Res* 38:823, 1977.

66. Finco DR, Brown SA, Barsanti JA, et al: Reliability of using random urine samples for spot determination of fractional excretion of electrolytes in cats, *Am J Vet Res* 58:1184, 1997.

67. Flood SM, Randolph JF, Gelzer ARM, et al: Primary hyperaldosteronism in two cats, *J Am Anim Hosp Assoc* 35:411, 1999.

68. Fujise H, Higa K, Nakayama T, et al: Incidence of dogs possessing red blood cells with high K in Japan and East Asia, *J Vet Med Sci* 59:495, 1997.

69. Garella S, Chang B, Kahn SI: Alterations of hydrogen ion homeostasis in pure potassium depletion: studies in rats and dogs during the recovery phase, *J Lab Clin Med* 93:321, 1979.

70. Gaschen F, Gaschen L, Seiler G, et al: Lethal peracute rhabdomyolysis associated with stress and general anesthesia in three dystrophin-deficient cats, *Vet Pathol* 35:117, 1998.

71. Gennari FJ, Cohen JJ: Role of the kidney in potassium homeostasis: lessons from acid-base disturbances, *Kidney Int* 8:1, 1975.

72. Gerstman BB, Kirkman R, Platt R: Intestinal necrosis associated with postoperative orally administered sodium polystyrene sulfonate in sorbital, *Am J Kidney Dis* 20:159, 1992.

73. Giebisch G, Hebert SC, Wang WH: New aspects of renal potassium transport, *Eur J Physiol* 446:289, 2003.

74. Giger U, Harvey JW: Hemolysis caused by phosphofructokinase deficiency in English springer spaniels: seven cases (1983-1986), *J Am Vet Med Assoc* 191:453, 1987.

75. Gonzalez JJ, Owens W, Ungaro PC, et al: Clay ingestion: a rare cause of hypokalemia, *Ann Intern Med* 97:65, 1982.

76. Good DW, Velazquez H, Wright FS: Luminal influences on potassium secretion: low sodium concentration, *Am J Physiol* 246:F609, 1984.

77. Grauer GF, Kunze RS: Potassium depletion nephropathy and renal medullary washout: a case report, *Calif Vet* 33:8, 1979.

78. Graves T, Schall W, Refsal K, et al: Basal and ACTH-stimulated plasma aldosterone concentrations are normal or increased in dogs with trichuriasis-associated pseudohypoadrenocorticism, *J Am Vet Intern Med* 8:287, 1994.

79. Greene RW, Scott RC: Lower urinary tract disease. In Ettinger SJ, editor: *Textbook of veterinary internal medicine,* Philadelphia, 1975, WB Saunders, p. 1572.

80. Hamill RJ, Robinson LM, Wexler HR, et al: Efficacy and safety of potassium infusion therapy in hypokalemic critically ill patients, *Crit Care Med* 19:694, 1991.

81. Hanna WJ, Tsushima RG, Sah R, et al: The equine periodic paralysis Na+ channel mutation alters molecular transitions between the open and inactivated states, *J Physiol* 497:349, 1996.

82. Harrison JB, Sussman HH, Pickering DE: Fluid and electrolyte therapy in small animals, *J Am Vet Med Assoc* 137:637, 1960.

83. Harvey JW: Erythrocyte metabolism. In Kaneko JJ, editor: *Clinical biochemistry of domestic animals*, New York, 1989, Academic Press, p. 196.

84. Hebert SC: Bartter syndrome, *Curr Opin Nephrol Hypertens* 12:527, 2003.

85. Henry CJ, Lanevschi A, Marks SL, et al: Acute lymphoblastic leukemia, hypercalcemia, and pseudohyperkalemia in a dog, *J Am Vet Med Assoc* 208:237, 1996.

86. Hornfeldt CS, Westfall ML: Suspected bentonite toxicosis in a cat from ingestion of clay cat litter, *Vet Hum Toxicol* 38:365, 1996.

87. Hulter HN, Sebastian A, Sigala JF, et al: Pathogenesis of renal hyperchloremic acidosis resulting from dietary potassium restriction in the dog: role of aldosterone, *Am J Physiol* 238:F79, 1980.

88. Ilkiw JE, Davis PE, Church DB: Hematologic, biochemical, blood gas, and acid base values in greyhounds before and after exercise, *Am J Vet Res* 50:583, 1989.

89. Inaba M, Maede Y: Increase of Na^+ gradient-dependent L-glutamate and L-aspartate transport in high K^+ dog erythrocytes associated with high activity of (Na^+,K^+)-ATPase, *J Biol Chem* 259:312, 1984.

90. Inaba M, Maede Y: Na,K-ATPase in dog red cells: immunological identification and maturation-associated degradation by the proteolytic system, *J Biol Chem* 261: 16099, 1986.

91. Jezyk PF: Hyperkalemic periodic paralysis in a dog, *J Am Anim Hosp Assoc* 18:977, 1982.

92. Jones BR, Swinney GW, Alley MR: Hypokalemic myopathy in Burmese kittens, *N Z Vet J* 36:150, 1988.

93. Kaplan JL, Braitman LE, Dalsey WC, et al: Alkalinization is ineffective for severe hyperkalemia in nonnephrectomized dogs, *Acad Emerg Med* 4:93, 1997.

94. Kitchell BE, Fan TM, Kordick D, et al: Peliosis hepatitis in a dog infected with *Bartonella henselae*, *J Am Vet Med Assoc* 216:519, 2000.

95. Knochel JP: Neuromuscular manifestations of electrolyte disorders, *Am J Med* 72:521, 1982.

96. Knochel JP, Schlein EM: On the mechanism of rhabdomyolysis in potassium depletion, *J Clin Invest* 51: 1750, 1972.

97. Knochel JP, Blanchley JD, Johnson JH, et al: Muscle cell electrical hyperpolarization and reduced exercise hyperkalemia in physically conditioned dogs, *J Clin Invest* 75:740, 1985.

98. Laing EJ, Carter RF: Acute tumor lysis syndrome following treatment of canine lymphoma, *J Am Anim Hosp Assoc* 24:691, 1988.

99. Laing EJ, Fitzpatrick PJ, Binnington AG, et al: Half-body radiotherapy in the treatment of canine lymphoma, *J Vet Intern Med* 3:102, 1989.

100. Lamb WA, Muir P: Lymphangiosarcoma associated with hyponatremia and hyperkalemia in a dog, *J Small Anim Pract* 35:374, 1994.

101. Lieveley P, Gruffydd-Jones TJ: Episodic collapse and weakness in cats, *Vet Annu* 29:261, 1989.

102. Lifton SJ, King LG, Zerbe CA: Glucocorticoid deficient hypoadrenocorticism in dogs: 18 cases (1986-1995), *J Am Vet Med Assoc* 209:2076, 1996.

103. Lillemole KD, Romolo JL, Hamilton SR, et al: Intestinal necrosis due to sodium polystyrene (Kayexalate) in sorbitol enemas: clinical and experimental support for the hypothesis, *Surgery* 101:267-272, 1987.

104. Ling GV, Stabenfeldt GH, Comer KM, et al: Canine hyperadrenocorticism: pretreatment clinical and laboratory evaluation of 117 cases, *J Am Vet Med Assoc* 174: 1211, 1979.

105. Lulich JP, Osborne CA, O'Brien TD, et al: Feline renal failure: questions, answers, questions, *Compend Contin Educ Pract Vet* 14:127, 1992.

106. MacIntire DK: Treatment of diabetic ketoacidosis in dogs by continuous low-dose intravenous infusion of insulin, *J Am Vet Med Assoc* 202:1266, 1993.

107. MacKay AD, Holt PE, Sparkes AH: Successful surgical treatment of a cat with primary aldosteronism, *J Feline Med Surg* 1:117, 1999.

108. Maede Y, Inaba M: (Na^+,K^+)-ATPase and ouabain binding in reticulocytes from dogs with high K and low K erythrocytes and their changes during maturation, *J Biol Chem* 260:3337, 1985.

109. Maede Y, Inaba M, Taniguchi N: Increase of Na-K ATPase activity, glutamate, and aspartate update in dog erythrocytes associated with hereditary high accumulation of GSH, glutamate, glutamine, and aspartate, *Blood* 61:493, 1983.

110. Magner PO, Robinson L, Halperin RM, et al: The plasma potassium concentration in metabolic acidosis: a re-evaluation, *Am J Kidney Dis* 11:220, 1988.

111. Malik R, Hunt GB, Hinchliffe JM, et al: Severe whipworm infection in the dog, *J Small Anim Pract* 31:185, 1990.

112. Mandell CP, Goding B, Degen MA, et al: Spurious elevation of serum potassium in two cases of thrombocythemia, *Vet Clin Pathol* 17:32, 1988.

113. Marples D, Frokiaer J, Dorup J, et al: Hypokalemia-induced down regulation of aquaproin-2 water channel expression in rat kidney medulla and cortex, *J Clin Invest* 97:1960, 1996.

114. Markov AK, Payment MF, Hume AS, et al: Fructose-1,6-diphosphate in the treatment of oleander toxicity in dogs, *Vet Hum Toxicol* 41:9, 1999.

115. Mason KV: A hereditary disease in Burmese cats manifested as an episodic weakness with head nodding and neck ventroflexion, *J Am Anim Hosp Assoc* 24:147, 1988.

116. Mason KV: Hereditary potassium depletion in Burmese cats? *J Am Anim Hosp Assoc* 24:481, 1988.

117. Meijer JC: Canine hyperadrenocorticism. In Kirk RW, editor: *Current veterinary therapy VII*, Philadelphia, 1980, WB Saunders, p. 975.

118. Meyer TS, Fedde MR, Cox JH, et al: Hyperkalemic periodic paralysis in horses: a review, *Equine Vet J* 31:362, 1999.

119. Miles PR, Lee P: Sodium and potassium content and membrane transport properties in red blood cells from newborn puppies, *J Cell Physiol* 79:367, 1972.

120. Moise NS, Reimers TJ: Insulin therapy in cats with diabetes mellitus, *J Am Vet Med Assoc* 182:158, 1983.

121. Moore KE, Morris N, Dhupa N, et al: Retrospective study of streptokinase administration in 46 cats with arterial thromboembolism, *J Vet Emerg Crit Care* 10:245, 2000.

122. Moore LE, Biller DS, Smith TA: Use of abdominal ultrasonography in the diagnosis of primary hyperaldosteronism in a cat, *J Am Vet Med Assoc* 217:213, 2000.

123. Muir WW, Wagner AE, Buchanan C: Effects of acute hyperventilation on serum potassium in the dog, *Vet Surg* 19:83, 1990.

124. Nath KA, Hostetter MK, Hostetter TH: Pathophysiology of chronic tubulointerstitial disease in rats: interactions of

dietary acid load, ammonia, and complement component C3, *J Clin Invest* 76:667, 1985.

125. Needle MA, Kaloyanides GJ, Schwartz WB: The effects of selective depletion of hydrochloric acid on acid base and electrolyte equilibrium, *J Clin Invest* 43:1836, 1964.

126. Nemzek JA, Kruger JM, Walshaw R, et al: Acute onset of hypokalemia and muscular weakness in four hyperthyroid cats, *J Am Vet Med Assoc* 205:65, 1994.

127. Oster JR, Perez GO, Vaamonde CA: Relationship between blood pH and potassium and phosphorus during acute metabolic acidosis, *Am J Physiol* 235:F345, 1978.

128. Oster JR, Perez GO, Castro A, et al: Plasma potassium response to acute metabolic acidosis induced by mineral and nonmineral acids, *Miner Electrolyte Metab* 4:28, 1980.

129. Oster JR, Singer I, Fishman LM: Heparin-induced aldosterone suppression and hyperkalemia, *Am J Med* 98:575, 1995.

130. Parker JC: Dog red blood cells—adjustment in density in vivo, *J Gen Physiol* 61:146, 1973.

131. Parks J: Electrocardiographic abnormalities from serum electrolyte imbalance due to feline urethral obstruction, *J Am Anim Hosp Assoc* 11:102, 1975.

132. Patterson RE, Haut MJ, Montgomery CA, et al: Natural history of potassium-deficiency myopathy in the dog: role of adrenocorticosteroid in rhabdomyolysis, *J Lab Clin Med* 102:565, 1983.

133. Perazella MA: Drug-induced hyperkalemia: old culprits and new offenders, *Am J Med* 109:307, 2000.

134. Peterson ME, Greco DS, Orth DN: Primary hypoadrenocorticism in ten cats, *J Vet Intern Med* 3:55, 1989.

135. Peterson ME, Kintzer PP, Kass PH: Pretreatment clinical and laboratory findings in dogs with hypoadrenocorticism—225 cases (1979-1993), *J Am Vet Med Assoc* 208:85, 1996.

136. Polak A, Haynie GD, Hays RM, et al: Effects of chronic hypercapnia on electrolyte and acid base equilibrium, *J Clin Invest* 40:1223, 1961.

137. Price GS, Armstrong PJ, McLeod DA, et al: Evaluation of citrate-phosphate-dextrose-adenine as a storage medium for packed canine erythrocytes, *J Vet Intern Med* 2:126, 1988.

138. Rakich PM, Lorenz MD: Clinical signs and laboratory abnormalities in 23 dogs with spontaneous hypoadrenocorticism, *J Am Anim Hosp Assoc* 20:647, 1984.

139. Reimann KA, Knowlen GG, Tvedten HW: Factitious hyperkalemia in dogs with thrombocytosis: the effect of platelets on serum potassium concentration, *J Vet Intern Med* 3:47, 1989.

140. Reine NJ, Hohenhaus AE, Peterson ME, et al: Deoxycorticosterone-secreting adrenocortical carcinoma in a dog, *J Vet Intern Med* 13:386, 1999.

141. Rich LJ, Berneuter DC, Cowell RL: Elevated serum potassium associated with delayed separation of serum from clotted blood in dogs of the Akita breed, *Vet Clin Pathol* 15:12, 1986.

142. Rijnberk A, Kooistra HS, van Vonderen IK, et al: Aldosteronoma in a dog with polyuria as the leading symptom, *Domest Anim Endocrinol* 20:227, 2001.

143. Rijnberk A, Voorhout G, Kooistra HS, et al: Hyperaldosteronism in a cat with metastasized adrenocortical tumor, *Vet Q* 23:38, 2001.

144. Rogers W, Straus J, Chew D: Atypical hypoadrenocorticism in three dogs, *J Am Vet Med Assoc* 179:155, 1981.

145. Rose BD: Hypokalemia. In Rose BD, editor: *Clinical physiology of acid-base and electrolyte disorders*, New York, 1994, McGraw-Hill, p. 811.

146. Ross LA, Goldstein M: *Biochemical abnormalities associated with accidental hypothermia in a dog and cat*, St. Louis, 1981, American College of Veterinary Internal Medicine, p. 66.

147. Roudebush P, Allen TA, Kuehn NF, et al: The effect of combined therapy with captopril, furosemide, and a sodium-restricted diet on serum electrolyte concentrations and renal function in normal dogs and dogs with congestive heart failure, *J Vet Intern Med* 8:337, 1994.

148. Rubin SI, Toolan L, Halperin ML: Trimethoprim-induced exacerbation of hyperkalemia in a dog with hypoadrenocorticism, *J Vet Intern Med* 12:186, 1998.

149. Rutecki GW, Cox JW, Robertson GW, et al: Urinary concentrating ability and antidiuretic hormone responsiveness in the potassium-depleted dog, *J Lab Clin Med* 100:53, 1982.

150. Sadek D, Schaer M: Atypical Addison's disease in the dog: a retrospective survey of 14 cases, *J Am Anim Hosp Assoc* 32:159, 1996.

151. Sapir DG, Levine DZ, Schwartz WB: The effects of chronic hypoxemia on electrolyte and acid base equilibrium: an examination of normocapneic hypoxemia and of the influence of hypoxemia on the adaptation to chronic hypercapnia, *J Clin Invest* 46:369, 1967.

152. Scandling JD, Ornt DB: Mechanism of potassium depletion during chronic metabolic acidosis in the rat, *Am J Physiol* 252:F122, 1987.

153. Schaafsma IA, van Emst MG, Kooistra HS, et al: Exercise-induced hyperkalemia in hypothyroid dogs, *Domest Anim Endocrinol* 22:113, 2002.

154. Schaer M: The use of regular insulin in the treatment of hyperkalemia in cats with urethral obstruction, *J Am Anim Hosp Assoc* 11:106, 1975.

155. Schaer M: A clinical survey of thirty cats with diabetes mellitus, *J Am Anim Hosp Assoc* 13:23, 1977.

156. Schaer M, Chen CL: A clinical survey of 48 dogs with adrenocortical hypofunction, *J Am Anim Hosp Assoc* 19:443, 1983.

157. Schaer M, Halling KB, Collins KE, et al: Combined hyponatremia and hyperkalemia mimicking acute hypoadrenocorticism in three pregnant dogs, *J Am Vet Med Assoc* 218:897, 2001.

158. Schlingmann KP, Konrad M, Jeck N, et al: Salt wasting and deafness resulting from mutations in two chloride channels, *N Engl J Med* 350:1314, 2004.

159. Schoolwerth AC, Culpepper RM: Measurement of intracellular pH in suspensions of renal tubules from potassium-depleted rats, *Miner Electrolyte Metab* 16:191, 1990.

160. Schrock H, Kuschinsky W: Consequences of chronic potassium depletion for the ionic composition of brain, heart, skeletal muscle, and cerebrospinal fluid, *Miner Electrolyte Metab* 15:171, 1989.

161. Schultze RG, Taggart DD, Shapiro H, et al: On the adaptation in potassium excretion associated with nephron reduction in the dog, *J Clin Invest* 50:1061, 1971.

162. Schunk KL: Feline polymyopathy. *Proceedings of the American College of Veterinary Internal Medicine*, Washington DC, 1984, p. 197.

163. Schwartz WB, Orning KJ, Porter R: The internal distribution of hydrogen ions with varying degrees of metabolic acidosis, *J Clin Invest* 36:373, 1957.

164. Schwartz WB, Brackett NC, Cohen JJ: The response of extracellular hydrogen ion concentration to graded degrees of chronic hypercapnia: the physiologic limits of the defense of pH, *J Clin Invest* 44:291, 1965.

165. Sealey JE, Laragh JH: A proposed cybernetic system for sodium and potassium homeostasis: coordination of aldosterone and intrarenal physical factors, *Kidney Int* 6:281, 1974.

166. Surawicz B: Arrhythmias and electrolyte disturbances, *Bull N Y Acad Med* 43:1160, 1967.

167. Surawicz B: Relationship between electrocardiogram and electrolytes, *Am Heart J* 73:814, 1967.

168. Swan RC, Pitts RF: Neutralization of infused acid by nephrectomized dogs, *J Clin Invest* 34:205, 1955.

169. Tannen RL: Relationship of renal ammonia production and potassium homeostasis, *Kidney Int* 11:453, 1977.

170. Tannen RL, Sastrasinh S: Response of ammonia metabolism to acute acidosis, *Kidney Int* 11:453, 1984.

171. Theisen SK, DiBartola SP, Radin MJ, et al: Muscle potassium content and potassium gluconate supplementation in normokalemic cats with naturally occurring chronic renal failure, *J Vet Intern Med* 11:212, 1997.

172. Thompson MD, Carr AP: Hyponatremia and hyperkalemia associated with chylous pleural and peritoneal effusion in a cat, *Can Vet J* 43:610, 2002.

173. Tietz NW, Pruden EL, Siggaard-Andersen O: Electrolytes, blood gases, and acid-base balance. In Tietz NW, editor: *Textbook of clinical chemistry*, Philadelphia, 1986, WB Saunders, p. 1181.

174. Tobin RB: Varying role of extracellular electrolytes in metabolic acidosis and alkalosis, *Am J Physiol* 195:687, 1958.

175. Tolins JP, Hostetter MK, Hostetter TH: Hypokalemic nephropathy in the rat: role of ammonia in chronic tubular injury, *J Clin Invest* 79:1447, 1987.

176. Velazquez H, Wright FS, Good DW, et al: Luminal influences on potassium secretion: chloride replacement with sulfate, *Am J Physiol* 242:F46, 1982.

177. Vite CH, Gfeller RW: Suspected albuterol intoxication in a dog, *J Vet Emerg Crit Care* 4:7, 1994.

178. Wang WH: Regulation of renal potassium transport by dietary potassium intake, *Annu Rev Physiol* 66:547, 2004.

179. Watson ADJ, Culvenor JA, Middleton DJ, et al: Distal renal tubular acidosis in a cat with pyelonephritis, *Vet Rec* 119:65, 1986.

180. West ML, Bendz O, Chen CB, et al: Development of a test to evaluate the transtubular potassium concentration gradient in the cortical collecting duct in vivo, *Miner Electrolyte Metab* 12:226, 1986.

181. West ML, Marsden PA, Richardson RMA, et al: New clinical approach to evaluate disorders of potassium excretion, *Miner Electrolyte Metab* 12:234, 1986.

182. Willard MD, Schall WD, McCaw DE, et al: Canine hypoadrenocorticism: report of 37 cases and review of 39 previously reported cases, *J Am Vet Med Assoc* 180:59, 1982.

183. Willard MD, Refsal K, Thacker E: Evaluation of plasma aldosterone concentrations before and after ACTH administration in clinically normal dogs and in dogs with various diseases, *Am J Vet Res* 48:1713, 1987.

184. Willard MD, Fossum TW, Torrance A, et al: Hyponatremia and hyperkalemia associated with idiopathic or experimentally induced chylothorax in four dogs, *J Am Vet Med Assoc* 199:353, 1991.

185. Yamato O, Hayashi M, Kasai E, et al: Reduced glutathione accelerates the oxidative damage produced by sodium n-propylthiosulfate, one of the causative agents of onion-induced hemolytic anemia in dogs, *Biochim Biophys Acta* 1427:175, 1999.

186. Zenger E: Persistent hyperkalemia associated with nonchylous pleural effusion in a dog, *J Am Anim Hosp Assoc* 28:411, 1992.

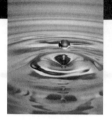

CHAPTER · 6

DISORDERS OF CALCIUM: HYPERCALCEMIA AND HYPOCALCEMIA

Patricia A. Schenck, Dennis J. Chew, Larry Allen Nagode, and Thomas J. Rosol

Calcium is required in the body for many vital intracellular and extracellular functions, as well as for skeletal support. Ionized calcium (iCa or Ca^{2+}) is required for enzymatic reactions, membrane transport and stability, blood coagulation, nerve conduction, neuromuscular transmission, muscle contraction, vascular smooth muscle tone, hormone secretion, bone formation and resorption, control of hepatic glycogen metabolism, and cell growth and division.[448] Intracellular calcium ion is one of the primary regulators of the cellular response to many agonists and serves as "an almost universal ionic messenger, conveying signals received at the cell surface to the inside of the cell."[421] In addition to serving as an intracellular messenger, the iCa concentration in the extracellular fluid (ECF) regulates cell function in many organs, including the parathyroid gland, kidney, and thyroid C cells by binding to a newly identified cell membrane–bound calcium-sensing receptor.[75] Normal homeostatic control mechanisms usually maintain the serum calcium concentration within a narrow range and guarantee an adequate supply of calcium for intracellular function. These mechanisms must be disrupted for hypercalcemia or hypocalcemia to develop. Abnormal serum calcium concentrations are of diagnostic value and contribute to the development of lesions and clinical signs. Technologic advances in the measurement of serum iCa concentration, parathyroid hormone (PTH), parathyroid hormone–related protein (PTHrP), and vitamin D metabolites have provided tools that allow greater diagnostic accuracy in the investigation of calcium disorders.

Veterinarians must frequently interpret abnormal serum calcium concentrations. Large deviations of serum calcium concentration from normal occur infrequently, but small deviations may be equally important because they also provide diagnostic clues to an underlying disease. The magnitude of altered serum calcium concentration often does not suggest a specific diagnosis or the extent of disease. Furthermore, a normal serum calcium concentration does not eliminate a disorder of calcium homeostasis.

NORMAL PHYSIOLOGY

OVERVIEW OF CALCIUM HOMEOSTASIS

Regulation of serum calcium concentration is complex and requires the integrated actions of PTH, vitamin D metabolites, and calcitonin (Fig. 6-1). PTH and calcitriol (1,25-dihydroxyvitamin D_3) are the main regulators of calcium homeostasis and have major regulatory effects on each other.[435] PTH is largely responsible for the minute-to-minute control of serum iCa concentration, whereas calcitriol maintains day-to-day control. In the fetus, the parathyroid glands and placenta produce PTHrP, which binds to PTH receptors and regulates calcium balance.[530] After birth, the parathyroid glands modify their pattern of hormone secretion and produce predominantly PTH. Other hormones, including adrenal corticosteroids, estrogens, thyroxine, growth hormone, glucagon, and prolactin, have less influence on calcium homeostasis but may play a role during growth, lactation, or certain disease states.

The intestine, kidney, and bone are the major target organs affected by calcium regulatory hormones. These interactions allow conservation of calcium in the ECF by renal tubular reabsorption, increased intestinal transport of calcium from the diet, and internal redistribution of calcium from bone (Fig. 6-2). The intestine and kidneys are the major regulators of calcium balance in health.[167] Normally, dietary calcium intake equals the amount of calcium lost in urine and feces. The enteric absorption of calcium depends on the physiologic status of the intestines (e.g., acidity, presence of other dietary components, integrity of the villi or presence of small intestinal disease, and degree of enterocyte stimulation by calcitriol). Non–protein-bound calcium is filtered by the glomerulus and undergoes extensive renal reabsorption. This process results in reclamation of more than 98% of the filtered calcium in health.[137,439]

The skeleton provides a major supply of calcium and phosphorus when intestinal absorption and renal

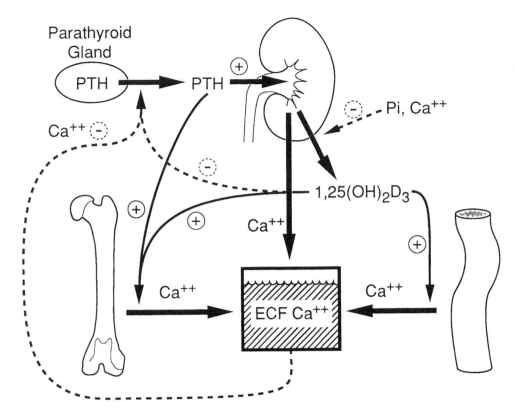

Fig. 6-1 Regulation of extracellular fluid (ECF) calcium concentration by the effects of parathyroid hormone (PTH) and calcitriol (1,25-dihydroxyvitamin D$_3$) on gut, kidney, bone, and parathyroid gland. The principal effect of PTH is to increase the ECF calcium concentration by mobilizing calcium from bone, increasing tubular calcium reabsorption, and, indirectly on the gut, by increasing calcitriol synthesis. The principal effect of calcitriol is to increase intestinal absorption of calcium, but it also exerts negative regulatory control of PTH synthesis and further calcitriol synthesis. (Modified from Habner JF, Rosenblatt M, Pott JT: Parathyroid hormone: biochemical aspects of biosynthesis, secretion, action, and metabolism, *Physiol Rev* 64:1000, 1984.)

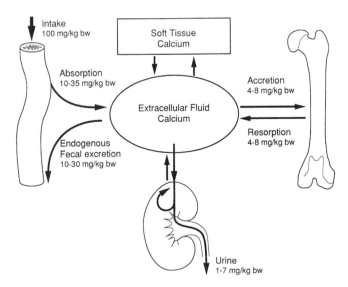

Fig. 6-2 Normal calcium balance showing the major organs that supply or remove calcium from extracellular fluid: bone, gut, and kidney. Total calcium input into extracellular fluid equals total calcium leaving the extracellular space. (Modified from Hazewinkel HAW: Dietary influences on calcium homeostasis and the skeleton. In *Purina international nutrition symposium*, Orlando, FL, Ralston Purina Company, Marriott World Center, January 15, 1991, p. 52.)

reabsorption inadequately maintain normal serum calcium concentrations. Bone calcium mobilization is important in the acute regulation of blood calcium.[395] Calcium and phosphorus can be mobilized from calcium phosphate in the bone ECF compartment, but these stores are rapidly depleted. The osteoblast is critical in limiting the distribution of calcium and phosphate between bone and ECF, and exchangeable bone water is separated from ECF water by the combined membranes of osteoblasts lining bone surfaces. For greater or prolonged release of calcium from bone, osteoclastic bone resorption must be activated. Osteoclasts secrete acid and proteases that result in dissolution of the mineralized matrix of bone and mobilize calcium and phosphorus.

Extracellular iCa concentration is the actively regulated fraction of total calcium (tCa).[76,111] When blood iCa concentration decreases, PTH secretion is stimulated. PTH exerts direct effects on bone and kidney and indirect effects on the intestine through calcitriol. PTH increases synthesis of calcitriol by activating renal mitochondrial 1α-hydroxylation of 25-hydroxycholecalciferol. Calcitriol increases calcium absorption from the intestine and acts with PTH to stimulate osteoclastic bone resorption.[99]

Calcitriol is necessary for differentiation of osteoclasts from precursor mononuclear cells. PTH increases osteoclast number and stimulates osteoclast function to increase bone resorption and the release of calcium from bone to blood. Calcitriol also induces renal transport mechanisms activated by PTH that increase tubular reabsorption of calcium from the glomerular filtrate, thus preventing calcium loss in urine.[366]

CALCIUM DISTRIBUTION WITHIN THE BODY

Approximately 99% of body calcium resides in the skeleton and is stored as hydroxyapatite, $Ca_{10}(PO_4)_6(OH)_2$. Most skeletal calcium is poorly exchangeable, and less than 1% is considered readily available. The small amount of rapidly exchangeable bone calcium arises from the ECF in bone that is present between osteoblasts and osteocytes and the bone matrix. Almost all of the nonskeletal calcium resides in the extracellular space, although small and biologically important quantities are found intracellularly.[448]

Extracellular Calcium

Calcium in plasma or serum exists in three fractions: ionized (iCa), complexed (bound to phosphate, bicarbonate, sulfate, citrate, and lactate), and protein bound (Fig. 6-3).

Extracellular Calcium

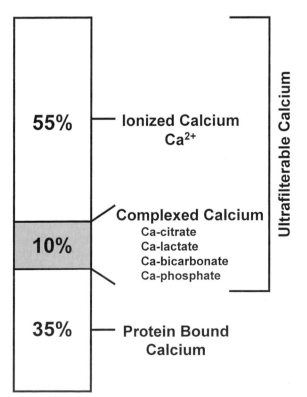

Fig. 6-3 Serum total calcium concentration consists of ionized (free), complexed, and protein-bound fractions.

In clinically normal dogs, protein-bound, complexed, and iCa account for approximately 34%, 10%, and 56% of serum tCa concentration, respectively.[472] Ionized calcium is the most important biologically active fraction in serum, although an active biologic role for complexed calcium has been suggested.[520] No biologic role for protein-bound calcium has been identified other than as a storage pool or buffering system for iCa.

Intracellular Calcium

Intracellular iCa is an important secondary messenger in the response to biochemical signals (such as hormones) transduced through the cell membrane.[420,448] Therefore intracellular iCa concentrations are maintained at a very low level (approximately 100 nM), 10,000-fold less than the serum concentration. This permits rapid diffusion into the cytoplasm from the ECF or endoplasmic reticulum. Intracellular calcium is rapidly buffered by cytosolic proteins and is transported into organelles or to the outside of the cell after an increase in intracellular iCa. If intracellular iCa is not maintained at a low concentration, it leads to toxicity and eventual cell death.

Most intracellular calcium is sequestered in organelles or bound to cellular membranes or proteins.[256] Sequestration of iCa in mitochondria blunts an increase in cytosolic iCa, whereas endoplasmic reticulum serves as a reservoir to increase cytosolic iCa when necessary. Binding of calcium to specific cytosolic or membrane proteins is an efficient method for regulation of intracellular iCa concentration. Protein binding provides intracellular iCa buffering and also may act as a messenger system when protein configuration and activity are altered. Calbindin, calmodulin, and troponin C are important intracellular calcium-binding proteins.[52]

Cell Membrane Calcium Ion Sensing Receptor. In 1993, a novel iCa-sensing receptor was cloned and sequenced.[73] The iCa receptor plays an integral role in iCa balance by regulating parathyroid chief cells, C cells, and renal epithelial cells.[72,235] In parathyroid chief cells and C cells, the iCa receptor directly regulates intracellular iCa concentration, which controls PTH and calcitonin secretion. Ionized magnesium (iMg) is also an agonist of the iCa receptor. Stimulation of the iCa receptor caused by increased extracellular iCa concentration in the kidney decreases NaCl, iCa, and iMg reabsorption in the proximal convoluted tubule and decreases water reabsorption in collecting ducts. This results in greater excretion of iCa and iMg in a more dilute urine.

Genetic diseases have been described related to both inactivating and activating mutations of the calcium receptor gene.[20] Inactivating mutations lead to severe neonatal hypercalcemia when homozygous and to familial hypocalciuric hypercalcemia when heterozygous.[512] Activating mutations of the calcium receptor produce hypoparathyroidism and hypocalcemia.[513] Autoantibodies produced against the calcium receptor may either disable it, producing hyperparathyroidism with hypercalcemia,[389,429] or activate it, producing hypoparathyroidism.[206,270] Drugs that bind the Ca^{2+}-sensing receptor may be useful to treat disorders of the parathyroid gland.

PARATHYROID HORMONE

STRUCTURE

PTH is an 84-amino acid single-chain polypeptide that is synthesized and secreted by chief cells of the parathyroid glands.[435] The amino acid sequence of PTH is known for the dog, cow, pig, rat, chicken, and human,[289,445] and most mammals appear to have very similar amino-terminal portions of the molecule.[366] Whereas the conserved amino end of PTH is vital for binding to cell membrane receptors, the role of the carboxyl terminus is to serve as a guide for PTH through the cellular secretory pathway.[303]

SYNTHESIS AND SECRETION

Synthesis, secretion, and degradation of PTH by chief cells are closely related. Little PTH is stored within the parathyroid glands,[216] and synthesis of new specific messenger RNA (mRNA) and translation to PTH are required to maintain secretion.[489] After secretion, PTH has a short half-life (3 to 5 minutes) in serum; thus a steady rate of secretion is necessary to maintain serum PTH concentrations. Circulating PTH has many forms, not all of which have bioactivity,[66,375] leading to potential confusion in assay interpretations.[464,510,569]

The amount of PTH available for secretion is a function of the balance of synthesis and degradation within chief cells (Fig. 6-4). Calcitriol, via the vitamin D receptor (VDR), and extracellular iCa concentration, via effects on the plasmalemmal calcium receptor,[103,104,427] control these parathyroid cell processes. Because calcitriol regulates expression of the calcium receptor gene,[94] calcitriol can be considered to exert overall control over PTH synthesis and secretion by the parathyroid cells. In general, the parathyroid gland has evolved most of its regulatory strategies to protect against hypocalcemia, with sensitive control of PTH synthesis and secretion being the dominant sites for regulation.[77,490] However, high serum iCa concentrations increase the rate of degradation of PTH within the gland to protect against hypercalcemia.[289]

Except for minor diurnal variation, PTH secretion is relatively constant but may have a mild pulsatile pattern in response to minor fluctuations in the concentration of serum iCa.[76] A relatively low rate of PTH secretion is needed normally to maintain serum iCa concentration. The basal secretory rate of PTH is approximately 25% of the maximal rate, and PTH is constantly secreted during normocalcemia. Complete inhibition of PTH secretion is not achieved even in the presence of severe hypercalcemia.[289]

Hypocalcemia is the principal stimulus for PTH secretion, but epinephrine, isoproterenol, dopamine, secretin, prostaglandin E_2, and stimulation of nerve endings within the parathyroid gland may have minor effects.[216] High concentrations of serum and intracellular iCa inhibit PTH secretion via increased arachidonic acid[57,96] and possibly subsequent eicosanoid production.[96] The control at PTH mRNA synthesis is also critically important.[489]

Calcitriol also plays an important role in the regulation of PTH synthesis and secretion.[492] Calcitriol inhibits PTH mRNA synthesis[491] and stimulates synthesis of the calcium receptor.[94] These relationships explain the requirement for adequate blood concentrations of calcitriol to maintain the ability of the parathyroid gland to respond to changes in extracellular calcium concentrations.[323,367] Increased intracellular iCa may also cooperate with calcitriol to reduce PTH synthesis in chief cells by inhibiting the expression of calreticulin (a blocker of VDR action).[481,548] Animals with uremia and reduced serum calcitriol concentrations have poorly regulated chief cell function that results in renal secondary hyperparathyroidism,[204,363] but a significant part of the hyperparathyroid response in uremic patients is the result of a glandular hyperplasia caused by the changes of both calcitriol and serum phosphorus.[8] Serum phosphorus concentrations are generally considered to regulate PTH secretion principally by indirect means. Renal calcitriol synthesis is reduced early in uremia by modest hyperphosphatemia, and the plasma iCa concentration may decrease because of reduced effects of calcitriol on the intestine, bone, and kidney. Markedly increased serum phosphorus concentrations (as seen in advanced renal failure) can lower the serum iCa concentration (mass law effect), resulting in an increase in PTH secretion because of the lowered calcium, but these effects do not occur early in renal failure when serum phosphorus is only moderately increased.[363]

Serum magnesium concentration has little role in the control of PTH secretion under normal conditions, but PTH secretion can be inhibited by very high concentrations of serum iMg.[435] Paradoxically, hypomagnesemia or magnesium depletion also results in inability to secrete PTH, but the cellular mechanism of this effect is unclear. This effect may be partially caused by reduced sensitivity of cell membrane receptors to iCa in the presence of low serum iMg concentrations.[216,347]

Set-point for PTH Secretion

The **set-point** for PTH secretion is defined as the ECF iCa concentration that occurs at the serum PTH concentration that is midway between maximal and minimal values of PTH obtained experimentally.[76] Normal serum iCa concentration is maintained slightly higher than the set-point; thus PTH release normally is less than half-maximal (Fig. 6-5).

Parathyroid Cell

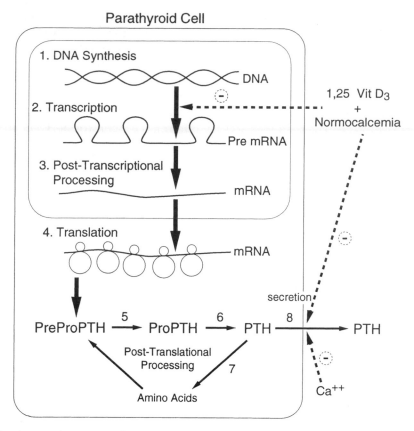

Fig. 6-4 Synthesis and secretion of parathyroid hormone. Note sites of regulation of PTH biosynthesis by extracellular ionized calcium or calcitriol (1,25-[OH]$_2$-vitamin D$_3$) interaction. (Modified from Habner JF, Rosenblatt M, Potts JT: Parathyroid hormone: biochemical aspects of biosynthesis, secretion, action, and metabolism, *Physiol Rev* 64:1004, 1984.)

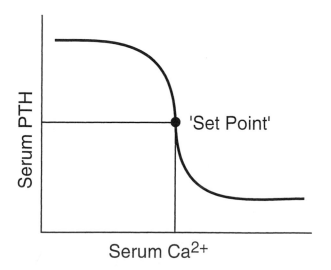

Fig. 6-5 Relationship between secretion rate of parathyroid hormone and plasma calcium concentration. Small changes in plasma calcium concentration cause large changes in parathyroid hormone secretion, but secretion is not completely suppressed by high plasma calcium concentrations.

The rate of PTH secretion is inversely proportional to the concentration of extracellular calcium, but this proportional secretion of PTH occurs only over a narrow range corresponding to a serum tCa concentration of 7.5 to 11.0 mg/dL.[216] An inverse sigmoidal curve with a steep slope results when the relationship between serum iCa concentration and PTH secretion is plotted over a larger range of calcium concentrations (see Fig. 6-5).[76] This ensures large changes in PTH secretion for relatively small changes in iCa concentration in the physiologic range and precise control of serum iCa concentration. An approximately 10% decrease in serum iCa concentration elicits a nearly maximal PTH secretory response. The rate of decrease of serum iCa concentration is also important, and rapid decreases in serum iCa result in larger increases in PTH secretion. A 2% to 3% decrease in iCa concentration, if rapid in onset, may result in a 400% increase in PTH secretion.[76]

The cell membrane calcium receptor is responsible for establishing the relationship of the set-point for PTH secretion and extracellular iCa concentration.[546]

The calcium receptor regulates PTH secretion indirectly by controlling the intracellular iCa concentration by means of (1) release of iCa from intracellular stores, and (2) cell membrane calcium channels. Calcium channels span the parathyroid chief cell membrane and are important in allowing extracellular iCa access to the interior of the cell.[176] The calcium channels are controlled by intracellular iCa concentration[77] and membrane regulatory G proteins, which interact with the cell membrane calcium receptor.[21]

Calcitriol plays an important role in controlling the parathyroid gland set-point by regulating (1) synthesis of the cell membrane calcium receptor,[71,94] (2) synthesis of cell membrane G proteins, and (3) function of cell membrane calcium channels.[366] Therefore adequate calcitriol is necessary to maintain the set-point for PTH secretion. The regulation of calcium receptor expression by calcitriol explains the observed "calcium set point" aberrations in control of PTH secretion in those with uremia.[329] These patients have deficits in calcitriol production,[112,563] as well as resistance in uremic parathyroids to calcitriol[151,396]; thus they are less able to induce synthesis of adequate numbers of calcium receptors.

Although regulations at each parathyroid cell may fail, thus producing abnormally increased PTH,[201,419] changes may also be seen in the maximal secretory capacity dependent mostly on parathyroid cell numbers.[462] It is likely that increased PTH secretion in patients with renal secondary hyperparathyroidism is primarily caused by parathyroid gland hyperplasia.[148] One important role of calcitriol therapy in these patients is to prevent or reverse the parathyroid cellular hyperplasia.[95,147,365]

Inhibition of PTH Synthesis and Secretion

This topic has become important with understanding of the toxicity of PTH in animals and humans with chronic renal failure (CRF) and accompanying secondary hyperparathyroidism.[10,330,363,398] Recently, increased awareness of PTH toxicity stems from established relations to cardiovascular disease[128] and mortality.[499] PTH secretion is inhibited by increased serum iCa concentration,[489,491] and the initial effect to decrease PTH secretion is rapid (occurring within 2 to 3 minutes), mediated by the calcium receptor with a cascade of resulting intracellular events[62,129,235] and involving mediation by arachidonate.[7] Slower effects are caused by inhibition of synthesis of PTH mRNA and its translation to hormone (Fig. 6-6).[489]

Calcitriol is an important inhibitor of PTH synthesis, and it completes a negative feedback loop from the kidney because PTH stimulates renal calcitriol synthesis. Short and long negative feedback loops complement each other to control normal secretion of PTH.[289] The long negative feedback loop is completed when an increased serum iCa concentration results from PTH stimulation of renal calcitriol production and subsequent enhanced gastrointestinal absorption of calcium. This effect takes hours to develop because calcium-binding proteins associated with calcium absorption must be induced in enterocytes.[67,549] The short negative feedback loop is mediated by the binding of calcitriol to VDRs in parathyroid cells, with inhibition of transcription of the PTH gene.[489] The calcitriol receptor (VDR) is expressed in parathyroid chief cells at concentrations equal to those in intestinal epithelial cells that regulate calcium absorption in the gastrointestinal tract. The VDR was found to be depleted in the parathyroid glands of dogs and humans with uremia because of lack of renal production of calcitriol.[70] After the VDR binds calcitriol, the VDR-calcitriol complex acts in the nucleus of the parathyroid chief cells by binding to specific regions of the PTH gene called vitamin D response elements (VDREs) and inhibiting transcription of the PTH gene (see Fig. 6-6).[289,363] For calcitriol to suppress synthesis of PTH, a normal concentration of iCa must be present because it would be inappropriate to suppress PTH synthesis in a hypocalcemic patient.

CLEARANCE AND METABOLISM OF PARATHYROID HORMONE

The intact PTH molecule (84 amino acids) circulates in the bloodstream with a half-life of 3 to 5 minutes and is removed by fixed macrophages.[289,435] A significant amount of cleavage is close to the amino terminus of the PTH molecule. Regardless of where the endopeptidase cleavage occurs, the amino-terminal portion of PTH is completely degraded within the phagocytes. Kidney and bone also participate in destruction of intact PTH.

Fragments of PTH are filtered by the glomeruli. This mechanism of excretion is most important for the excretion of the carboxyl-terminal PTH fragments because carboxyl-terminal PTH (released from either the parathyroid gland or Kupffer cells) is cleared only by glomerular filtration (Fig. 6-7). The carboxyl-terminal fragments of PTH are not important for calcium metabolism. The circulating half-life of carboxyl-terminal PTH is much longer than that of intact PTH, and serum concentrations of carboxyl-terminal PTH can be very high during primary or secondary hyperparathyroidism and can be nonspecifically increased during renal failure.

ACTIONS OF PARATHYROID HORMONE

PTH is the principal hormone involved in the minute-to-minute fine regulation of blood calcium concentration. It exerts its biologic actions directly by influencing the function of target cells primarily in bone and kidney and indirectly in the intestine to maintain plasma calcium at a concentration sufficient to ensure the optimal functioning of a wide variety of body cells.

In general, the most important biologic effects of PTH on calcium are to (1) increase the blood calcium

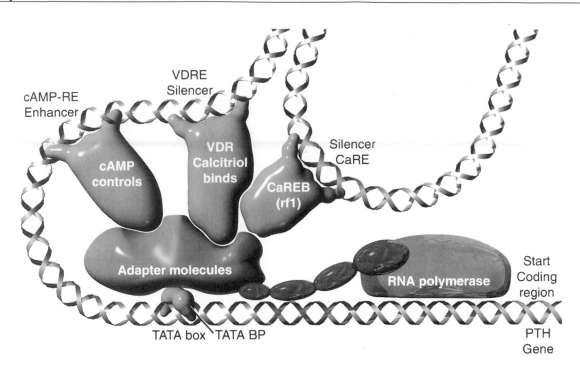

Fig. 6-6 Simplified depiction of events regulating transcription of the parathyroid hormone (PTH) gene by RNA polymerase. Only the three transcription factors best understood to interact in this regulation are shown. Cyclic AMP (cAMP) stimulates phosphorylation of a transcription factor that binds to a cAMP response element (cAMP-RE) on the gene and enhances transcription. In contrast, the vitamin D receptor (VDR)–calcitriol complex and calcium response element–binding protein (CaREB, rf1) bind to their respective vitamin D (VDRE) and calcium (CaRE) response elements of the PTH gene, which function as "silencers" or negative regulators of gene transcription. Note that for calcium to exert its negative effect by means of the CaREB transcription factor, calcitriol and the vitamin D receptor must also be present. The adapter molecules (shown as a single structure) diagrammatically represent about 30 proteins termed accessory transcription factors. The TATA box is part of the gene promoter to which the TATA box binding proteins (BPs) bind. (From Nagode LA, Chew DJ, Podell M: Benefits of calcitriol therapy and serum phosphorus control in dogs and cats with chronic renal failure, *Vet Clin North Am Small Anim Pract* 26:1293-1330, 1996.)

concentration; (2) increase tubular reabsorption of calcium, resulting in decreased calcium loss in the urine; (3) increase bone resorption and the numbers of osteoclasts on bone surfaces; and (4) accelerate the formation of the principal active vitamin D metabolite (1,25-dihydroxyvitamin D, or calcitriol) by the kidney through a trophic effect to both induce synthesis of and activate the 1α-hydroxylase in mitochondria of renal epithelial cells in the proximal convoluted tubules.

An important action of PTH on bone is to mobilize calcium from skeletal reserves into ECF.[97] The increase in blood calcium concentration results from an interaction of PTH with receptors on osteoblasts that stimulate increased calcium release from bone and direct an increase in osteoclastic bone resorption.[356]

The response of bone to PTH is biphasic. The immediate effects are the result of increasing the activity of existing bone cells. This rapid effect of PTH depends on the continuous presence of hormone and results in an increased flow of calcium from deep in bone to bone surfaces through the action of an osteocyte-osteoblast "pump" to make fine adjustments in the blood calcium concentration.[395] The later effects of PTH on bone are potentially of greater magnitude and are not dependent on the continuous presence of hormone. Osteoclasts are primarily responsible for the long-term action of PTH on increasing bone resorption and overall bone remodeling.[97,356]

PTH also has the potential to serve as an anabolic agent in bone and stimulate osteoblastic bone formation.[190,505] Intermittent administration of exogenous 1-34 PTH has been reported to increase bone mass in humans and animals.[507]

The ability of PTH to enhance the renal reabsorption of calcium is of considerable importance. This effect of PTH on tubular reabsorption of calcium is caused by, in part, a direct action on the distal convoluted tubule.[573] PTH may also increase calcium reabsorption in the ascending thick limb of Henle's loop indirectly by increasing the net positive charge in the nephron

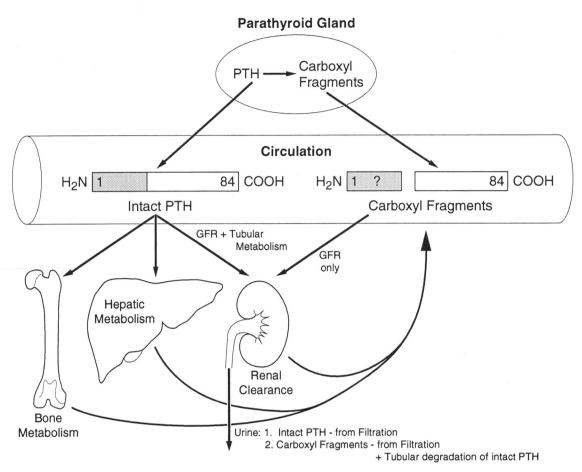

Fig. 6-7 Degradation and clearance of parathyroid hormone (PTH). PTH (1-84) is secreted intact from the parathyroid gland into the circulation. Biologically inactive carboxy-terminal (COOH) fragments of PTH are also secreted by the parathyroid gland, but amino-terminal PTH is not secreted and does not circulate in biologically relevant concentrations. Peripheral metabolism of intact PTH to carboxy-terminal PTH fragments occurs mostly in the liver but may also occur in the kidney and bone. Both intact PTH and carboxy-terminal PTH are cleared by glomerular filtration, but only intact PTH is metabolized in the liver, kidney, and bone. The half-life of intact PTH in vivo is short compared with that of the carboxy-terminal fragments of PTH. (Modified from Endres DB, Villaneuva R, Sharp CF, et al: Measurement of parathyroid hormone, *Endocrinol Metab Clin North Am* 18:614, 1989.)

lumen and creating a stimulus for diffusion out of the lumen. PTH also regulates the conversion of 25-hydroxycholecalciferol to calcitriol and other metabolites of vitamin D.

Parathyroid Hormone C-Terminal 7-84 as PTH Antagonist

It was originally thought that PTH 35-84 and other fragments cleaved between residues 24 and 43 dominated the carboxyl-terminal fragments of PTH secreted by chief cells. The C-terminal fragments can be measured using C-terminal-specific immunoassays. The function of PTH 35-84 and its receptor is unknown, but it may regulate bone cell function. The larger C-terminal fragment, PTH 7-84,[259] may be significantly increased in

renal secondary hyperparathyroidism[351] and can antagonize the effects of PTH 1-84 in vivo.[297] The antagonistic action of PTH 7-84 is likely attributable to binding to an alternate PTH receptor and not to the PTH1 receptor that is used by PTH 1-34 and PTH 1-84.[139,376]

Parathyroid Hormone Receptor

The receptor for N-terminal PTH (amino acids 1 to 34), the region important in calcium regulation, has been cloned and sequenced in humans, dogs, and other species.[1,378,496] It is a seven-transmembrane domain receptor that is expressed in renal epithelial cells, osteoblasts, and some other cells. The N-terminal regions of PTH and PTHrP bind this receptor with equal affinity. The PTH receptor is also located on many cell types, such as dermal fibroblasts, that are not associated with the action of PTH. It is assumed that the receptor functions as the binding protein for PTHrP in these tissues. The currently used terminology for this receptor is the PTH1 receptor, but it is often described as the PTH/PTHrP receptor. The PTH2 receptor is present in the brain and binds to both PTH and tuberoinfundibular peptide but not to PTHrP.[233]

PARATHYROID HORMONE–RELATED PROTEIN: A POLYHORMONE

PTHrP is not strictly a calcium-regulating hormone, but it was identified in 1982 as an important PTH-like factor that plays a central role in the pathogenesis of humoral hypercalcemia of malignancy (HHM).[437] PTHrP is produced widely in the body and has numerous actions in the developing fetus and adult animal independent of its role in cancer-associated hypercalcemia.[411] This is in contrast to PTH, which is produced by the parathyroid glands and functions principally in regulation of calcium balance. PTHrP has multiple actions that are specific to the N-terminal, midregion, and C-terminal regions of the protein, making PTHrP a true polyhormone.

Some of the actions of PTHrP involve normal regulation of calcium metabolism.[448] For example, PTHrP functions as a calcium-regulating hormone in the fetus and is produced by the fetal placenta.[317] In the adult, PTHrP circulates in the blood in low concentrations (<1 pM) but is produced by many different tissues and functions principally as an autocrine, paracrine, or intracrine cellular regulator. PTHrP is produced by the lactating mammary gland and is secreted into milk. Mammary gland production of PTHrP likely facilitates mobilization of calcium from maternal bones and may play a role in the transport of calcium into milk during lactation.[571,572] PTHrP acts as an abnormal systemic calcium-regulating hormone and mimics the actions of PTH in patients with HHM. PTHrP not only plays a major role in most forms of HHM but also has been demonstrated in many normal tissues, including epithelial cells of the skin and other organs; endocrine glands; smooth, skeletal, and cardiac muscle; lactating mammary gland; placenta; fetal parathyroid glands; bone; brain; and lymphocytes.[411,435] Therefore PTHrP functions as (1) a hormone in an endocrine manner in the fetus and lactating dams, (2) a paracrine factor in many fetal and adult tissues, and (3) an abnormal hormone in an endocrine manner in adults with HHM (Fig. 6-8). PTHrP is necessary for normal endochondral bone formation in the fetus and neonate. Knockout of the PTHrP gene results in short-limb dwarfism and death at birth as a result of a failure of car-

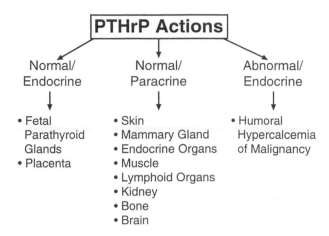

Fig. 6-8 Actions of parathyroid hormone–related protein (PTHrP).

tilage proliferation at the growth plates and premature ossification.[265]

PTHrP is a 139- to 173-amino acid peptide originally isolated from human and animal tumors associated with HHM.[437] PTHrP shares 70% sequence homology with PTH in its first 13 amino acids. The N-terminal region of PTHrP (amino acids 1 to 34) binds and stimulates PTH receptors in bone and kidney cells with affinity equal to that of PTH, so that PTHrP functions similarly to PTH in patients with HHM.[119,385] The midregion of PTHrP is responsible for stimulating iCa uptake by the fetal placenta,[317] and the C-terminal region can inhibit osteoclastic bone resorption.[171]

The complementary DNA (cDNA) for canine and feline PTHrP has been cloned and sequenced.[449,508] The sequence of canine PTHrP cDNA and gene indicated that the dog PTHrP gene is more closely related to the human PTHrP gene than are the PTHrP genes in rats, mice, and chickens.[212] The deduced amino acid sequence of the N-terminal region (amino acids 1 to 36) is identical in five mammalian species (dog, cat, human, rat, and mouse), and there is a high degree of homology of the midregion of PTHrP in these species.[324,449,504,508,575] The high degree of interspecies homology indicates the importance of the N terminus and midregion in the function of PTHrP.

There is less homology of the C-terminal region of canine PTHrP with that from other species. The function of the C-terminal region is unknown. PTHrP (107 to 111) and PTHrP (107 to 139) may inhibit osteoclastic bone resorption.[172,501] Increased urine concentrations of C-terminal PTHrP have been demonstrated in humans and mice with cancer-associated hypercalcemia[255,266] and in patients with renal failure.[84] Increased C-terminal PTH is also seen in the serum of patients with renal failure and indicates that the kidney is an important site of excretion of C-terminal PTHrP.

C-terminal PTHrP may have a longer serum half-life than N-terminal or midregion PTHrP.

PARATHYROID HORMONE–RELATED PROTEIN IN THE FETUS

Fetuses maintain higher concentrations of serum iCa than their dams. Fetal parathyroid glands produce low levels of PTH,[100] and PTHrP functions to maintain iCa balance in the fetus.[316,317] PTHrP is secreted by fetal parathyroid chief cells, and PTHrP is produced by the placenta, which is necessary for iCa uptake by the fetus.[571] The midregion of PTHrP is the most active portion that stimulates iCa and iMg transport by the placenta. The placenta expresses the iCa-sensing receptor, which may contribute to the regulation of placental calcium transport.[285] PTHrP is also produced by the uterus, where it is important in permitting relaxation of the smooth muscle of the muscularis as the fetuses grow.[514]

VITAMIN D

Vitamin D (calciferol) is classified as a secosteroid hormone.[243] In tetrapods, the role of vitamin D via the calcitriol-activated VDR has evolved into one dominated by calcium regulatory mechanisms, but the roles in primitive species, including regulation of detoxification enzymes, have commonly been retained in more evolved life forms.[544,559] These pleiotropic actions of vitamin D[304] include, among others, important roles as antiproliferative and prodifferentiative mediators[22] working in part via control of DNA replication[155] and roles as immunomodulators,[222] including effects on glomerulonephritis[393] and encephalitis.[193] A role of calcitriol to regulate expression of the insulin receptor has been described,[319] as has a role in muscle.[132] Of particular interest in uremic patients is the calcitriol increase of erythroid proliferation via burst-forming units.[18] These pleiotropic effects of calcitriol can be related to important clinical applications in patients with renal or other metabolic disease.[236] They may explain the clinical improvements noticed in dog and cat uremic patients treated preventatively with low doses of calcitriol[363] that were accomplished when calcitriol was used before any PTH elevation had occurred.

VITAMIN D METABOLISM

The cholecalciferol (parent vitamin D_3 of animal origin) metabolites 25-hydroxyvitamin D_3 (calcidiol), 1,25-dihydroxyvitamin D_3 (calcitriol), and 24,25-dihydroxyvitamin D_3 are the most important of at least 30 metabolites. In domestic mammals, the same three metabolites derived from vitamin D_2 (ergocalciferol of plant origin) are equally bioactive; thus generic use of the terms 1,25-dihydroxyvitamin D and calcitriol is assumed to include metabolites of vitamin D_3 or D_2 derived from animal or plant origin, respectively. The 25-hydroxyvitamin D that is produced in liver is the major circulating form of vitamin D[197] and serves as a pool for further activation by 1α-hydroxylation or catabolism by 24-hydroxylation.[227,383] Only 25-hydroxylation and 1α-hydroxylation are important in the function of vitamin D.[131]

Synthesis

In humans, the requirement for vitamin D can be met by consumption of vitamin D_2 or D_3 or by synthesis of vitamin D_3 (cholecalciferol) in the skin. Cholecalciferol is synthesized in the skin from 7-dehydrocholesterol after exposure to ultraviolet light. 7-Dehydrocholesterol forms previtamin D_3 in the presence of ultraviolet B light at 288 nm, followed by further thermal conversion from previtamin D_3 to vitamin D_3.[237] Dogs and cats inefficiently photosynthesize vitamin D in their skin and consequently are dependent on vitamin D in their diet.[245] Vitamin D ingested in the diet is absorbed intact from the intestine.

Vitamin D–binding protein transports vitamin D to the liver and other target sites (Fig. 6-9).[124] Hydroxylation of vitamin D occurs in the liver to produce 25-hydroxyvitamin D (calcidiol). The 25-hydroxylase activity is not influenced by calcium or phosphorus.[197] Calcidiol does not have any known action in normal animals,[131] but during vitamin D intoxication, high levels of calcidiol are produced by the liver and can induce hypercalcemia.

The most important step in bioactivation of vitamin D occurs as 25-hydroxyvitamin D is further hydroxylated to calcitriol in the proximal tubule of the kidney.[227] This reaction is tightly regulated by ionic and hormonal control mechanisms that modulate the activity of the hydroxylase enzyme systems (Fig. 6-10). The two principal enzyme systems involved are 25-hydroxyvitamin D-1α-hydroxylase (resulting in active calcitriol formation) and 25-hydroxyvitamin D-$24R$-hydroxylase (the first step of catabolism to inactive vitamin D metabolites). The activities of these enzymes are reciprocally regulated.[383]

The 1α-hydroxylase enzyme activity is localized within mitochondria of the convoluted tubules and portions of the straight proximal tubule of the kidney. Little extrarenal 1α-hydroxylation of 25-hydroxyvitamin D occurs in other tissues except in human and rat placenta and skin and in some lymphoproliferative disorders.[4,150] The 24-hydroxylation can also metabolize calcitriol, generating 1,24,25-trihydroxyvitamin D as the first step in the major catabolic pathway of calcitriol to biologically inactive calcitroic acid.[243] Inactive vitamin D catabolites are excreted through the bile into feces, which is the only important excretory route; less than 4% is excreted into urine.[131]

Stimulation of Calcitriol Synthesis. Serum PTH, calcitriol, phosphorus, and calcium concentrations are

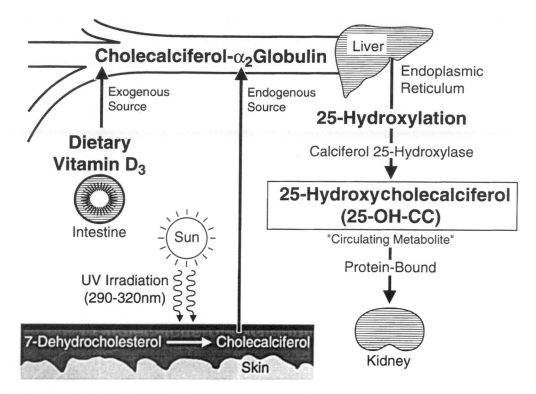

Fig. 6-9 Metabolism of vitamin D. The initial step of metabolic activation of vitamin D_3 from endogenous (photoactivation) and dietary sources is in the liver to form 25-hydroxycholecalciferol (25-hydroxyvitamin D_3). Photoactivation is poor in dogs and cats; consequently, they depend on dietary sources of vitamin D_3.

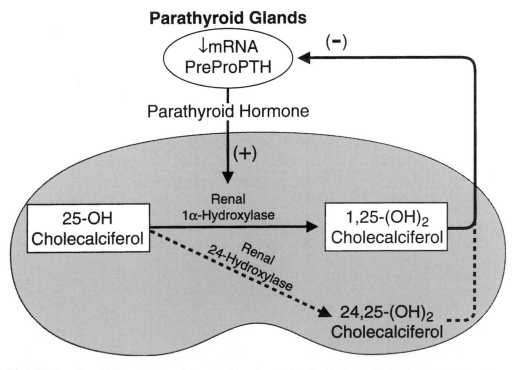

Fig. 6-10 Parathyroid hormone increases renal synthesis of 1,25-dihydroxycholecalciferol (calcitriol) by stimulating the 1α-hydroxylase activity in renal epithelial cells that converts 25-hydroxycholecalciferol to 1,25-dihydroxycholecalciferol. Negative feedback is exerted by 1,25-dihydroxycholecalciferol (calcitriol) on parathyroid chief cells to decrease the rate of PTH synthesis and secretion, which in turn decreases the rate of formation of 1,25-dihydroxycholecalciferol. Calcitriol also directly suppresses synthesis of the renal 1α-hydroxylase enzyme.

the principal regulators for renal calcitriol synthesis.[227] Chronic changes in serum calcium concentration regulate the synthesis of calcitriol, and these calcium changes can override signals from serum phosphorus and PTH concentrations.[248] Deficiencies of phosphorus, calcium, and calcitriol lead to increased calcitriol formation.[364] Low calcium or calcitriol concentrations lead to increased serum PTH concentrations. In the kidney, PTH mediates dephosphorylation of renal ferredoxin (renoredoxin) and results in increased synthesis of calcitriol.[199,487] Renoredoxin is the regulatory constituent of the 1α-hydroxylase enzyme system and is inhibited by phosphorylation in the presence of high concentrations of phosphorus or calcium in the renal tubule.[227] PTH not only activates the renal 1α-hydroxylase but also induces synthesis of the enzyme from the renal gene encoding it.[149,150]

Several drugs and hormones have effects on vitamin D metabolism, some of which are stimulatory.[60] Hypocalcemia and calcitonin directly stimulate 1α-hydroxylation independent of PTH.[65] Estrogens increase calcitriol synthesis after up-regulation of PTH receptors in the kidney,[65] and testosterone may also increase calcitriol synthesis.[582] Reduced dietary calcium intake can lead to stimulation of renal 1α-hydroxylase in the absence of detectable hypocalcemia.[582]

Inhibition of Calcitriol Synthesis. Calcitriol synthesis is inhibited by calcitriol, hypercalcemia, and phosphate loading.[65,227] Calcium directly and indirectly inhibits calcitriol synthesis.[166] The indirect action is caused by inhibition of PTH synthesis and secretion, thus removing the stimulus provided by PTH. The inhibitory effects of chronic hypercalcemia can override the stimulatory effects of increased PTH concentrations in calcitriol production, as may occur in primary hyperparathyroidism.[248] The inhibitory effects of high concentrations of phosphorus on calcitriol synthesis are important and affect the activity of existing enzyme molecules.[363,364]

Actions of Calcitriol

Calcitriol is the only natural form of vitamin D with significant biologic activity.[131,424] It is approximately 1000 times as effective as parent vitamin D and 500 times as effective as its precursor calcidiol (25-hydroxyvitamin D) in binding to the natural calcitriol receptor (VDR) in target cells.[366] Calcitriol increases serum calcium and phosphorus concentrations, and its major target organ for these effects is the intestine.[67] However, there is also an important contribution from bone,[502] and calcitriol stimulates the kidney to reabsorb both calcium and phosphorus from the glomerular filtrate. Calcitriol has multiple indirect effects on calcium balance, including up-regulation of calcitriol receptors in patients with uremia, regulation of PTH synthesis and secretion by the parathyroid

gland,[577] and prevention or reversal of parathyroid gland hyperplasia in the uremic patient.[191,363]

THE CALCITRIOL RECEPTOR

The VDR for calcitriol is present in many tissues in addition to bone, kidney, intestine, and parathyroid gland.[221] The importance of calcitriol in a tissue is proportional to the abundance of the VDR in the cells, and this is highly regulated.[287] Intestinal epithelial cells and parathyroid gland chief cells have equal and high concentrations of VDR. VDR genetic polymorphisms are thought to generate variation of efficiency of the VDR.[79,105] Calcitriol initially dissociates from its serum binding protein, diffuses across the cell membrane, and binds with its receptor.

Effects of Calcitriol on the Intestine

Calcitriol enhances the transport of calcium and phosphate from the intestinal lumen to plasma across the enterocyte.[68,549] Energy in the form of adenosine triphosphate (ATP) is required to transport calcium from the enterocytes into the blood and to absorb phosphate from the intestinal lumen. Calcitriol induces synthesis of the plasma membrane calcium pump (ATPase) that removes calcium from the enterocytes[394] and the Na^+-phosphate cotransport protein that transports phosphorus into the enterocyte. In addition, calcitriol increases the brush border permeability to calcium and induces the synthesis of calbindin-D 9k.[120,516] Calbindins serve as buffers to protect enterocytes from toxic concentrations of calcium ion while ferrying calcium across the cell.[549] Calcitriol also directly stimulates rapid calcium transport (transcaltachia) across the enterocyte.[380] Normal dogs have a progressive decrease in the number of calcitriol receptors and calbindin concentrations that regulate the efficiency of calcium absorption in enterocytes from the duodenum to the ileum.[283] Longer transit times in certain portions of the intestinal tract (e.g., ileum) can still lead to significant calcium absorption despite low transport efficiency.[549]

Effects of Calcitriol on Bone

Calcitriol is necessary for bone formation and mineralization because it ensures an adequate source of calcium and phosphorus from the intestinal tract. Deficiencies in vitamin D lead to impaired bone growth, such as rickets in growing animals and osteomalacia in adults.[435] Calcitriol is necessary for normal bone development and growth because it regulates the production of multiple bone proteins produced by osteoblasts, including alkaline phosphatase (ALP), collagen type I, osteocalcin, and osteopontin.[17,497] Calcitriol is also necessary for normal bone resorption because it promotes differentiation of monocytic hematopoietic precursors in the bone marrow into osteoclasts.[502] This relationship between calcitriol and osteoclasts explains the dependence of PTH on calcitriol for optimal bone resorption.[365]

Effects of Calcitriol on the Kidney

An important effect of calcitriol in the kidney is direct inhibition of 25-hydroxyvitamin D–1α-hydroxylase in the renal tubule, preventing overproduction of calcitriol.[424] In addition, calcitriol facilitates calcium and phosphorus reabsorption from the glomerular filtrate.[294] Calcitriol is necessary to work with PTH to reabsorb urinary calcium into blood. Glomerular podocytes contain the VDR for calcitriol and respond to low doses of calcitriol with decreased injury and loss of podocytes.[292] In glomerulonephritis, low doses of calcitriol decreased mesangial proliferative nephritis, which involved calcitriol abrogation of inflammatory mediators interleukin (IL)-1α, tumor necrosis factor-α (TNF-α), and IL-6 in the mesangium.[392] Although calcitriol has generally been thought to protect the kidneys during CRF by preventing the damage from excess PTH,[365,577] it is becoming clear that calcitriol has direct beneficial effects on the diseased kidney as well.

Effects of Calcitriol on the Parathyroid Gland

Calcitriol inhibits the production of PTH in the parathyroid gland by direct and indirect means.[486,491] Binding of calcitriol to its receptor in parathyroid chief cells directly inhibits PTH synthesis. Second, calcitriol stimulates intestinal calcium absorption, which indirectly reduces PTH secretion by increasing serum iCa concentration. Calcitriol suppression of PTH synthesis is dose dependent and occurs before serum iCa concentration is increased by the delayed effects of calcitriol on intestinal calcium transport.[494] Calcitriol may be considered the primary controlling factor for transcription of the PTH gene and subsequent synthesis of PTH because suppression of PTH synthesis cannot occur in the absence of calcitriol even in the presence of hypercalcemia (see Fig. 6-6).[364,491] PTH secretion decreases 12 to 24 hours after exposure to calcitriol. Whereas PTH stimulates renal calcitriol synthesis, calcitriol is a negative regulator of PTH. Long-standing calcitriol deficiency results in chief cell hypertrophy and hyperplasia, demonstrating that calcitriol is important in limiting cellular proliferation in the parathyroid gland.[491] Calcitriol treatment of uremia in dogs and humans has resulted in regression of parathyroid gland hyperplasia.[191,366] Calcitriol can be used in a preventative manner to avoid development of hyperparathyroidism in dogs and cats with early stages of CRF.[363] This has proven to be highly successful and is consistent with developing thinking in the human medical profession.[583]

Calcitriol in Therapy of Cancer

Many studies focus on the benefits of calcitriol therapy in cancer.[208,238] Part of the great interest stems from the antiproliferative role of calcitriol,[22] with specific effects on DNA replication genes[155] and with a potentially important effect on proliferation of blood vessel endothelial cells.[39] Studies are focused on human prostate cancer[288] and also on breast and colon cancers.[238] Although a discussion is beyond the scope of this chapter, its dynamic character indicates it will be important for many years to come.

CALCITONIN

Calcitonin is a 32-amino acid polypeptide hormone that is synthesized by C cells in the thyroid gland.[352,435] An important role of calcitonin is to limit the degree of postprandial hypercalcemia. This effect, in concert with PTH, acts to maintain serum iCa concentration within a narrow range. Calcitonin is secreted in response to hypercalcemia and also to a calcium-rich meal. Calcitonin secretion increases during hypercalcemia, but the effects of calcitonin on normal calcium homeostasis are considered to be minor. The major target site for calcitonin is bone, where it inhibits osteoclastic bone resorption. The effects of calcitonin in bone are transitory, which has limited the usefulness of calcitonin as a treatment for hypercalcemia. At high doses, calcitonin may promote urinary calcium excretion.[76]

NORMAL HOMEOSTATIC RESPONSE TO HYPOCALCEMIA

Hypocalcemia elicits corrective responses that are mediated by PTH and calcitriol.[435] Acute effects occur in seconds to minutes; subacute effects occur over several hours; and chronic effects occur over days to weeks. A marked increase in PTH secretion occurs in response to mild hypocalcemia, and this response occurs in seconds. Acute secretion of preformed PTH can maintain PTH concentrations for 1 to 1.5 hours during hypocalcemia. Hypocalcemia decreases the proportion of PTH that is degraded in the parathyroid chief cells, making more PTH available for secretion. This effect is relatively rapid (approximately 40 minutes). During increased PTH secretion, renal calcium reabsorption and phosphorus excretion are increased within minutes, whereas bone mobilization of calcium and phosphate occurs within 1 to 2 hours.

After several hours of hypocalcemia, increased PTH secretion stimulates the synthesis and secretion of calcitriol. Increased intestinal transport of calcium and phosphorus into blood follows, providing an external source of calcium in addition to the internal mobilization from bone. Hypocalcemia increases transcription of the PTH gene and synthesis of PTH mRNA, enhancing the ability of the chief cells to produce PTH. This effect also occurs within hours of hypocalcemia. Over days or weeks of hypocalcemia, further increases in PTH secretion are achieved largely by hypertrophy and hyperplasia of chief cells in the parathyroid gland.[454] In addition, the proportion of chief cells actively synthesizing PTH is increased.

NORMAL HOMEOSTATIC RESPONSE TO HYPERCALCEMIA

Most of the effects that occur during hypercalcemia are the opposite of those described earlier for hypocalcemia.[435] Hypercalcemia results in decreased PTH secretion, increased intracellular degradation of PTH in chief cells, and decreased PTH synthesis. Increased calcitonin secretion is stimulated in an attempt to minimize the magnitude of hypercalcemia. In addition, hyperplasia of C cells in the thyroid gland results if the hypercalcemic stimulus is sustained, but this mechanism is ineffective for controlling hypercalcemia because of the transitory effect of calcitonin on osteoclastic bone resorption.[382,441] Calcitriol synthesis is decreased both through direct inhibition by iCa and as a result of decreased stimulation because of decreased PTH concentration.

DIAGNOSTICS

Table 6-1 lists normal values for serum tCa,[111] iCa,[110] PTH,[366,526] PTHrP,[446] and vitamin D metabolites that are useful in the diagnostic workup of patients with calcium disorders.[435]

TOTAL CALCIUM

Despite the fact that only the iCa fraction is physiologically active, the calcium status of animals is usually initially based on evaluation of the serum tCa concentration. Measurement of tCa concentration is more readily available than iCa measurement, but it does not always accurately reflect the iCa concentration of the patient. The serum tCa concentration has been assumed to be directly proportional to iCa, but in many clinical conditions, this may lead to erroneous interpretation of laboratory data. In humans with disorders of calcium balance, measurement of serum tCa concentrations failed to predict serum iCa concentrations in 31% of all patients[515] and in 26% of patients with renal disease.[83] In 1633 canine samples, diagnostic disagreement between serum iCa and tCa was 27%, and in dogs with CRF, this disagreement was 36%.[475] In cats, serum iCa concentrations were only moderately correlated with serum tCa concentrations,[134] and a 40% diagnostic disagreement between serum iCa and tCa measurement was noted in 434 cats.[474] In dogs, tCa measurement overestimated normocalcemia and underestimated hypocalcemia,[475] and in cats, hypercalcemia and normocalcemia were underestimated, and hypocalcemia was overestimated when using serum tCa concentration to predict iCa status.[474]

Analytical Methods

Fasting serum or heparinized plasma samples should be submitted for analysis. Oxalate, citrate, and ethylenediaminetetraacetic acid (EDTA) anticoagulants should not be used because calcium is bound to these chemicals and becomes unavailable for analysis.[567]

Serum tCa concentrations vary with the method used. Isotope dilution with subsequent mass spectrometry constitutes the definitive method for calcium measurement but is not readily available.[189] For clinical determination of serum tCa concentration, simple colorimetric reactions and spectrophotometry are usually employed using automated or manual methods. *Ortho*-cresophthalein complexone is a metal dye that is commonly used to form a color complex with calcium. This method is accurate and reproducible.[189] Hemolysis can result in formation of an interfering hemoglobin-chromogen complex that falsely increases measured calcium concentration. High concentrations of bilirubin falsely decrease, and acetaminophen and hydralazine falsely increase serum tCa concentration. Lipemia can result in spuriously high calcium concentrations,[345] with values exceeding 20 mg/dL in some instances of severe lipemia.

Caution should be exercised in the interpretation of tCa measurements performed on small serum or plasma volumes. When submitted volume is inadequate, dilution

TABLE 6-1 Normal Serum Concentrations

	Dog	Cat
Total Calcium		
mg/dL	9.0-11.5	8.0-10.5
mmol/L	2.2-3.8	2.0-2.6
Ionized Calcium		
mg/dL	5.0-6.0	4.5-5.5
mmol/L	1.2-1.5	1.1-1.4
Parathyroid Hormone (PTH)		
Intact (pmol/L)	2-13*	0-4*
N-terminal (pg/mL)	15-55	8-28
Parathyroid Hormone Related protein (PTHrP) (pmol/L) (intact or N-terminal)	<1.0*	<1.0*
25-Hydroxyvitamin D (calcidiol) (nmol/L)	60-215*	65-170*
1,25-Dihyroxyvitamin D (calcitriol) (pg/mL)		
Adults	20-50	20-40
10-12-week-old	60-120	20-80

Data from Endocrine Diagnostic Section, Diagnostic Center for Population and Animal Health, Lansing, MI.

with water or saline is often performed. In an in-house commercial laboratory study, when samples were diluted 1:3, serum tCa concentrations were nearly 3 mg/dL lower than when analyzed in undiluted samples (Antech newsletter 05-1999).

Normal Values

The range for serum tCa concentration in normal dogs and cats is wide and varies among laboratories (see Table 6-1). Each laboratory should establish normal values. Variability may result from differences in age, diet, duration of fasting before sampling, and time of sampling, in addition to differences in analytical method.

Normal serum tCa concentrations in mature dogs and cats are approximately 10.0 and 9.0 mg/dL, respectively. No difference in serum tCa concentration has been ascribed to breed or sex in normal dogs and cats, but an effect of aging has been observed in the dog.[111,224] Dogs younger than 3 months of age have slightly higher mean serum calcium concentrations (approximately 11.0 mg/dL) than those for dogs older than 1 year (approximately 10.0 mg/dL), probably because of normal bone growth. In a small percentage of normal young dogs, serum tCa concentrations may be greater than 12.0 mg/dL and as high as 15.0 mg/dL.[379] Dietary calcium, phosphorus, and vitamin D supplementation should be evaluated in dogs with serum tCa concentrations greater than 12.0 mg/dL.

Adjusted Total Calcium

It has been reported that serum tCa concentrations should be "corrected" or "adjusted" relative to the total serum protein or albumin concentration to improve diagnostic interpretation.[174,341] Such correction seemed logical because binding of serum calcium to protein is substantial, and 80% to 90% of the calcium bound to proteins is bound to albumin. The correlation between serum tCa and serum albumin or total protein concentrations was moderate, and adjustment formulas were developed for use in dogs older than 1 year. These adjustment formulas were not recommended for use in cats because there was no linear relationship between serum tCa and serum albumin and total protein concentrations in this species.[179]

It has been assumed that serum tCa concentrations that correct into the normal range are associated with normal serum iCa concentration. Likewise, samples with values that fail to correct into the normal range are presumed to have abnormal serum iCa concentrations. However, these formulas were developed without verification by serum iCa measurements. Correction of serum tCa concentration for albumin did not improve the correlation between serum tCa and iCa concentrations.[350] In 1633 canine serum samples, the use of an adjustment formula to predict iCa status showed a higher diagnostic disagreement than did serum tCa measurement alone.[475] Diagnostic disagreement between tCa adjusted to total

protein and iCa measurement was 37% and was 38% between tCa adjusted to albumin and iCa measurement. In 490 dogs with CRF, diagnostic disagreement between adjusted tCa and iCa measurement increased to 53%, indicating the poor performance of the adjustment formulas in the prediction of iCa status. In all dogs, hypercalcemia and normocalcemia were overestimated, and hypocalcemia was underestimated when either adjustment formula was used. In dogs with CRF, however, hypercalcemia was overestimated, and normocalcemia and hypocalcemia were underestimated. Because of the high degree of diagnostic disagreement between adjusted tCa and iCa measurement, the use of adjustment formulas to predict iCa status cannot be recommended.

IONIZED CALCIUM

Ionized calcium is the biologically active form of calcium, and its homeostasis is important for many physiologic functions.[435] Calcium ion regulates its own homeostasis directly by binding to cell membrane receptors specific for iCa.[74] The cell membrane calcium receptors are present in parathyroid chief cells and C cells of the thyroid gland, in which iCa regulates PTH and calcitonin secretion, respectively. Calcium receptors are also present on renal tubular cells, and iCa directly regulates its own tubular reabsorption rate. Therefore serum iCa concentration is controlled by interacting feedback loops that involve iCa, phosphate, PTH, calcitriol, and calcitonin. These mechanisms help maintain serum iCa concentration in a narrow range.

For accurate assessment of calcium status, iCa must be measured directly. Ionized calcium measurement has been shown to be superior to serum tCa measurements in many conditions, especially in hyperparathyroidism, renal disease, hypoproteinemia and hyperproteinemia, acid-base disturbances, and critical illnesses.[205,475,580] Changes in the magnitude of serum protein concentration, individual protein binding capacity and affinity, serum pH, and complexed calcium all interact to determine the iCa concentration, independent of the tCa concentration. Fasting serum samples collected at the same time in the morning are advised.

Analytical Methods

Use of automated equipment with a calcium ion-selective electrode allows easy and accurate measurement of iCa in blood, plasma, or serum.[59] Newly developed electrodes minimize interference by other ions (e.g., magnesium, lithium, and potassium), protein, or hemolysis.[207] Nevertheless, differences among analyzers exist, and it is recommended that reference ranges be established for each analyzer.[246]

Recently, portable clinical analyzers have been developed for cage-side analysis of iCa concentration. These analyzers use a disposable cartridge containing an impregnated biosensor for iCa and other analytes. Heparinized whole blood is used for analysis, but caution should be exercised when interpreting these results. Ionized calcium concentrations in dogs are typically 0.05 to 0.26 mmol/L lower, and 0.05 to 0.14 mmol/L lower in cats, when heparinized whole blood is compared with serum iCa measurement.[213] The greatest underestimation of iCa concentration occurred when serum iCa concentrations were greater than 1.3 mmol/L. When iCa concentration in heparinized whole blood was measured using both ion-selective electrode methodology and portable clinical analyzer methods, correlation (r) was only 0.71.[361] The portable clinical analyzer method resulted in an iCa concentration that was approximately 2.6% lower than that measured with an ion-selective electrode.[308] However, in a study of dogs and horses, there were no differences in iCa concentrations using heparinized whole blood measured with an ion-selective electrode and portable clinical analyzer.[311] Because the quantity and type of heparin used and volume of blood collected also have an effect on iCa measurement, it is best to establish a rigid protocol for blood collection when using a portable clinical analyzer. Reference ranges should also be established for the analyzer using this standard protocol.

Sample Handling Techniques

Concentration of iCa can be determined in samples handled under both anaerobic and aerobic conditions. The most precise determination of iCa concentration and physiologic pH requires that samples be collected and processed anaerobically to ensure that no increase in pH occurs because of loss of CO_2. The pH of blood or serum has a significant effect on serum iCa concentration. Acidic pH favors dissociation of calcium from protein and increases the amount of iCa in the sample. Alkaline pH occurs with loss of CO_2 and favors calcium binding to protein, thus decreasing the amount of iCa. Mixing serum with air results in increased pH and decreased measured iCa concentration because of loss of CO_2 from the sample.[471] Exposure to air in partially filled serum tubes also can affect iCa concentration; tubes that were only 25% or 50% filled had 0.07 or 0.04 mmol/L lower concentrations of iCa when compared with measurement from tubes that were 100% filled.[535]

Ionized calcium can be measured in whole blood or heparinized plasma, but measurement is problematic. Heparinized canine blood provided stable iCa measurements when stored up to 9 hours at 4° C, but pH was significantly increased after 3 hours.[506] In practice, it may be impossible to analyze the sample within this period. The amount and type of heparin used for whole blood or plasma samples also affect the measurement of iCa. When zinc heparin is used as an anticoagulant, iCa concentration is overestimated most likely because of a decrease in pH, which displaces calcium from proteins.[312,314] Lithium heparin causes an underestimation in iCa concentration,[312] and an electrolyte-balanced heparin may underestimate or overestimate iCa concentration depending on whether hypocalcemia, normocalcemia, or hypercalcemia is present. The amount of heparin used is critical in the measurement of iCa in blood. Using syringes containing a premeasured quantity of lithium heparin or electrolyte-balanced heparin, iCa measurement was underestimated when a less than recommended quantity of blood was collected for analysis.[312,313] When using heparinized whole blood for measurement of iCa concentration, it is imperative to collect the same volume of blood for each sample to avoid the dilutional effects of heparin. Syringes containing a premeasured amount of dry heparin are preferable to coating a syringe manually with an unknown and variable quantity of liquid heparin.

Ionized calcium and pH are more stable in serum than in whole or heparinized blood. The analysis of serum eliminates the potential interference of heparin and allows a longer storage period before analysis. Silicone separator tubes should not be used; the iCa concentration was increased in serum separated by use of silicone separator tubes because of release of calcium from the silicone gel.[298] Measured iCa in canine and equine serum was stable after storage for 72 hours at 23° C or 4° C and for 7 days at 4° C.[470,471] Use of serum collected anaerobically and stored at 4° C allows sufficient time for shipment to a reference laboratory for anaerobic measurement of iCa and pH.

Ionized calcium may also be accurately measured in samples handled aerobically. Mathematical formulas have been developed to correct the iCa concentration in samples exposed to air (with increased pH) to the actual pH of the patient or to a pH of 7.4.[305,362] In a study of serum samples from 61 dogs and 21 cats, there was good correlation between iCa measured anaerobically and again aerobically after shipment to a diagnostic laboratory (Schenck and Chew, unpublished observations). These pH correction formulas are species specific, and formulas developed in humans should not be used. A mathematical correction formula should be derived for each species in each laboratory setting. Although not as precise as anaerobic measurement, aerobic measurement under proper laboratory conditions offers a diagnostically accurate methodology for iCa determination with simplified shipping and handling requirements.

Some iCa analyzers will automatically mathematically manipulate the iCa concentration and actual pH value of the sample and yield an adjusted value for iCa concentration that theoretically would occur at a pH of 7.4. These correction formulas were developed for use in humans and should not be used in animals. When using anaerobically collected samples, corrected iCa concentrations have not been advocated for use in humans because insight into the pathophysiology of the patient is gained by evaluation of the in vivo iCa concentration and pH.[188] This may be especially true for patients with renal disease.[455] If anaerobic sampling is possible (typically in an in-house setting), there is no necessity or benefit in correcting the iCa concentration to a pH of 7.4. Only when samples are handled aerobically is there a need for correction to a standard pH.

Normal Values

The range for serum iCa concentration in normal dogs and cats varies among laboratories but is approximately 5.0 to 5.8 mg/dL (1.25 to 1.45 mmol/L) in adult dogs[472] and 4.6 to 5.4 mg/dL (1.15 to 1.35 mmol/L) in adult cats.[134] An effect of aging has been observed in both the dog and cat. Young dogs and cats (up to 2 years of age) have serum iCa concentrations that are 0.1 to 0.4 mg/dL higher than those reported in older animals.[134,350] Normal values should be established for each laboratory based on age of animal, type of sample, and analyzer used.

Fractionation of Serum Calcium

In addition to measuring the ionized concentration in serum, the protein-bound and complexed fractions of calcium can be quantified using fractionation techniques. Ionized calcium and complexed calcium are diffusable, and together are referred to as ultrafilterable calcium. To separate protein-bound from ultrafilterable serum calcium, a micropartition system based on the filtration method has been used.[164,472] The micropartition system contains a filter through which ultrafilterable calcium (complexed and ionized) passes. It is important that serum be collected anaerobically before ultrafiltration to allow accurate measurement of the calcium fractions and to prevent changes in serum pH.

Protein-bound, ionized, and complexed calcium fractions in serum were 34%, 56%, and 10% in normal dogs[472] and 40%, 52%, and 8% in normal cats, respectively (Schenck, unpublished observations). Ultrafilterable calcium (ionized and complexed fractions) in dogs,[472] horses,[239] and cats (Schenck, unpublished observations) accounted for 66%, 63%, and 60% of serum tCa, respectively. The iCa fraction has the smallest variation, with larger variations occurring in the protein-bound and complexed fractions. This observation supports the concept that the iCa fraction is tightly regulated and represents the biologically active fraction of serum calcium.

Complexed and protein-bound calcium fractions have not been assessed in metabolic disorders associated with abnormal calcium concentrations. Measurement of the protein-bound and complexed calcium fractions in addition to the iCa fraction may facilitate detection of disease processes that affect calcium metabolism. In dogs with CRF, two subgroups have been identified based on calcium fractionation. Dogs with normal to elevated serum tCa concentrations had a significantly higher concentration of circulating complexed calcium as compared with those dogs with low concentrations of tCa, even though there was no difference in iCa or protein-bound calcium between groups.[473] Further studies are needed to determine whether prognosis or effectiveness of therapy differs between these groups.

PARATHYROID HORMONE

PTH circulates predominantly as intact PTH (1-84) and carboxyl-terminal fragments. Only intact PTH is biologically active, and it is best to measure this form in serum or plasma. Samples should be stored and shipped frozen to prevent degradation of intact PTH. Stability is best in plasma collected with EDTA, but serum is adequate if stored frozen after separation from blood. Because of sequence homology of human and animal PTH, commercial assays developed for humans have been used successfully for some veterinary species.[113] An amino-terminal–specific radioimmunoassay (RIA) was used for more than 50 mammalian species but is no longer commercially available.[364] A two-site immunoradiometric assay (IRMA) for intact human PTH has been validated in the dog and cat.[23,526] Normal values for serum PTH concentration are 2 to 13, 0 to 4, and 0 to 2 pmol/L in the dog, cat, and horse, respectively (Endocrine Diagnostic Section, Diagnostic Center for Population and Animal Health, Lansing, MI). The two-site assays have not proved useful for measurement of PTH in reptiles. Expected response of PTH in various conditions will be discussed later (see Hypercalcemia and Hypocalcemia).

The current two-site IRMA measures both the intact PTH-(1-84) and the PTH-(7-84) fragment because the amino-terminal antibodies react near the tenth amino acid.[69,126,375] A new third generation IRMA "whole" PTH assay has been developed for use in humans that measures only PTH-(1-84).[192] This new assay could offer a better measure of whole PTH especially in patients with secondary hyperparathyroidism because the PTH-(7-84) fragment is increased in these patients.[351] High concentrations of carboxyl-terminal PTH fragments, which occur in cats with CRF, may interfere with intact PTH immunoassays.[27] Using ratios of "whole" PTH versus "intact" PTH to clarify low bone turnover renal osteodystrophy[368] or dynamics of PTH secretion[463] have been attempted.[203,281] The "whole" PTH assay may also be of better diagnostic value in dogs than the "intact" PTH assay because PTH-(7-84) fragments may be increased in dogs as compared with humans.[159] Whole PTH (1-84) and intact PTH (1-84 and 7-84) have been measured in dogs, and it was observed that the whole PTH/intact PTH ratio in dogs (about 36%) was less than in humans, and the ratio did not change during acute hypocalcemia.[159] In preliminary studies in cats, a third generation PTH-(1-84) assay resulted in higher PTH values than a second generation assay that also measures the PTH-(7-84) fragment.[127] Although this is opposite of what is found in humans, it is not unexpected because cat and other mammalian PTH is more similar to human PTH in the first few amino acids than in the region of the tenth amino acid.

PARATHYROID HORMONE–RELATED PROTEIN

Two-site IRMA and N-terminal RIA are available for the measurement of human PTHrP.[44,286] These assays are useful for measuring biologically active PTHrP in the dog (see Cancer-Associated Hypercalcemia)[113,446] because of the high degree of sequence homology of PTHrP between species, especially in the N-terminal 111 amino acids.[86] An N-terminal RIA for human PTHrP did not prove useful for measuring circulating PTHrP in a small number of horses.[447] PTHrP is susceptible to degradation by serum proteases, and PTHrP concentrations must be measured in fresh or frozen plasma using EDTA as an anticoagulant. EDTA complexes with plasma calcium, which is required for function of many proteases. The addition of protease inhibitors such as aprotinin and leupeptin may provide further inhibition of proteolysis in plasma.[391]

The circulating forms of PTHrP are not completely understood because PTHrP rapidly undergoes proteolysis intracellularly and extracellularly after secretion into blood.[391] The forms of PTHrP that are present in vivo include intact PTHrP, an N-terminal peptide, a combined N-terminal and midregion peptide, a midregion peptide, and a C-terminal peptide.[85,574] Fragments that have PTH-like biologic activity in vivo include N-terminal PTHrP (1-36), PTHrP (1-86), and intact PTHrP (1-141). The two-site immunologic assays measure intact PTHrP (1-141) and PTHrP (1-86) because antibodies bind to the N terminus and midregion. The N-terminal RIAs measure intact PTHrP (1-141), PTHrP (1-86), and N-terminal PTHrP (1-36). The C-terminal PTHrP accumulates in the serum of human patients with renal failure, which suggests that C-terminal PTHrP peptides are excreted by the kidney, as occurs with PTH.[84]

VITAMIN D METABOLITES

Measurement of vitamin D metabolites is occasionally helpful in diagnosing disorders of calcium homeostasis (see Table 6-1). 25-Hydroxyvitamin D (calcidiol) and calcitriol are the metabolites of clinical interest for detection of hypovitaminosis D, hypervitaminosis D, and abnormalities of the renal hydroxylase system (e.g., renal failure). The metabolites are stable during refrigeration and freezing, but samples should not be exposed to light for long periods.

The metabolites of vitamin D are chemically identical in all species, thus receptor-binding assays or RIAs developed for use in humans are satisfactory for the measurement of the same metabolites in animals.[240,242] Young growing dogs have higher calcitriol concentrations than mature dogs, and most mammals appear to share this attribute during rapid growth.[339]

Concentrations of 25-hydroxyvitamin D are a good indicator of vitamin D ingestion or production in vivo and can be used to diagnose hypovitaminosis D or hypervitaminosis D.[102] Calcitriol assays can be used to detect genetic errors of vitamin D metabolism, low concentrations of calcitriol in patients with renal failure, or high concentrations of calcitriol in some patients with cancer-associated hypercalcemia.[435]

BONE BIOPSY AND BONE MARROW ASPIRATION

Bone marrow aspiration or core biopsy is frequently part of the diagnostic evaluation of animals without an obvious cause of hypercalcemia. Its greatest utility is in the discovery of lymphoma, myeloproliferative disease, or multiple myeloma. Biopsy of the iliac crest is recommended for standardization, particularly when histomorphometric analysis is available for the quantitative evaluation of bone formation and bone resorption. A procedure for iliac crest bone biopsy has been described.[117,443] Direct biopsy of focal bone lesions may be diagnostic, particularly when such lesions are caused by lymphoma, multiple myeloma, or a metastatic bone tumor.

HYPERCALCEMIA

Hypercalcemia is an uncommon but important electrolyte disturbance of dogs and cats. The frequency of finding hypercalcemia based on evaluation of serum tCa in more than 10,000 canine serum samples analyzed during a 6-month period at one private veterinary diagnostic laboratory was 1.5%.[89] Of these, 28% were found to be from young growing dogs, 62% were found to be transient, and 18% were persistent and associated with pathology.

Hypercalcemia can serve as a marker of disease or can create disease. Increases in serum iCa concentration above normal often have adverse pathophysiologic consequences. Hypercalcemia represents a clinically relevant increase above an individual animal's own normal serum calcium concentration, usually defined as a fasting serum tCa concentration greater than 12.0 mg/dL in dogs or greater than 11.0 mg/dL in cats. Ionized calcium measurements can provide greater sensitivity and specificity for the diagnosis of some hypercalcemic disorders. A serum iCa concentration greater than 6.0 mg/dL (1.5 mmol/L) in dogs and greater than 5.7 mg/dL (1.4 mmol/L) in cats constitutes ionized hypercalcemia.

TOXICITY OF HYPERCALCEMIA AND CLINICAL SIGNS

Excessive calcium ions are toxic to cells,[420] and increased serum iCa concentration decreases cellular function by causing alterations in cell membrane permeability and cell membrane calcium pump activity. Increased intracellular iCa content can ultimately result in cell death caused by deranged cellular function and reduced energy production. Although all tissues may be subject to the dangerous effects of hypercalcemia, effects on the central nervous system, gastrointestinal tract, heart, and kidneys are of most importance clinically.

Polydipsia, polyuria, anorexia, lethargy, and weakness are the most common clinical signs in dogs with hypercalcemia,[109,168] but individual animals often display remarkable differences in clinical signs despite similar magnitudes of hypercalcemia. The severity of clinical signs and development of lesions of hypercalcemia depend not only on the magnitude of hypercalcemia but also on its rate of development and duration. Simultaneous disturbances in other electrolyte concentrations and in acid-base balance, as well as organ dysfunction secondary to hypercalcemia, all contribute to clinical signs, laboratory abnormalities, and lesions. Box 6-1 lists the signs and conditions associated with hypercalcemia.

Clinical signs are most severe when hypercalcemia develops rapidly, as can occur with vitamin D intoxication or during rapid infusion of calcium-containing fluids. Dogs with similar magnitudes of hypercalcemia may display minimal clinical signs when hypercalcemia has developed gradually. Regardless of the rate of increase in serum calcium concentration, clinical signs become more severe as the magnitude of hypercalcemia increases. Serum tCa concentrations of 12.0 to 14.0 mg/dL may not be associated with severe clinical signs, but most animals with concentrations greater than 15.0 mg/dL show systemic signs. Dogs with serum calcium concentrations greater than 18 mg/dL are often severely ill, and concentrations greater than 20 mg/dL may constitute a life-threatening crisis. Exceptions do occur, however, and some dogs are severely affected by mild hypercalcemia, whereas others are relatively unaffected by severe hypercalcemia. Clinical signs and histopathologic changes are more likely to develop the longer hypercalcemia has been present, regardless of its magnitude. Progressive hypercalcemia may also contribute to the severity of clinical signs, as occurs in animals with malignant neoplasia or hypervitaminosis D related to rat bait ingestion.

Box 6-1	**Clinical Signs and Conditions Associated with Hypercalcemia**

Common	**Uncommon**
Polydipsia and polyuria	Constipation
Anorexia	Cardiac arrhythmia
Dehydration	Seizures or twitching
Lethargy	Death
Weakness	Acute intrinsic renal failure
Vomiting	Calcium urolithiasis
Prerenal azotemia	
Chronic renal failure	

Changes in serum sodium and potassium concentrations can magnify the clinical signs of hypercalcemia by their effects on cell membrane excitability, particularly in nerve and muscle (see Chapter 5). Acidosis increases the proportion of serum calcium that is ionized, worsening clinical signs, whereas alkalosis lessens toxicity and clinical signs by decreasing the proportion of calcium that is ionized.

Mineralization of soft tissues (especially the heart and kidneys) is an important complication of hypercalcemia. The serum phosphorus concentration at the time hypercalcemia develops is important in determining the extent of soft tissue mineralization. Soft tissue mineralization is most severe when the calcium (mg/dL) times phosphorus (mg/dL) product is greater than 60.[111] Soft tissue mineralization occurs regardless of the serum phosphorus concentration in severe hypercalcemia.

Renal Effects of Hypercalcemia

Abnormal renal function frequently accompanies hypercalcemia, and rapid deterioration in renal function occasionally occurs. The functional effects of hypercalcemia on the kidneys are readily reversible, but structural changes may not be reversible if renal lesions are advanced. Azotemia occurred commonly in 34 dogs with hypercalcemia related to malignancy, hypoadrenocorticism, CRF, and hypervitaminosis D.[290] The frequency of azotemia was higher in dogs with malignancy (71%) than in those with hypercalcemia related to primary hyperparathyroidism (11%). Azotemia caused by hypercalcemia can result from any combination of the following mechanisms: prerenal reduction in ECF volume (anorexia, hypodipsia, vomiting, and polyuria); renal vasoconstriction from ionized hypercalcemia; decreased permeability coefficient of the glomerulus (K_f); acute tubular necrosis from the ischemic and toxic effects of hypercalcemia; and CRF caused by nephron loss, nephrocalcinosis, tubulointerstitial inflammation, and interstitial fibrosis.

Decreased urinary concentrating ability and polyuria are early functional effects of hypercalcemia in dogs. The concentrating defect is often out of proportion to the observed reduction in glomerular filtration rate (GFR) and increase in serum creatinine or blood urea nitrogen (BUN) concentration. Urine specific gravity is consistently less than 1.030 in dogs and was less than 1.020 in more than 90% of hypercalcemic dogs in one study.[290] Urinary concentration may be well preserved in some cats with hypercalcemia that do not have CRF. Defective urinary concentrating ability results from a combination of reduced tubular reabsorption of sodium and impaired action of antidiuretic hormone on tubular cells of the collecting duct. This results in a form of nephrogenic diabetes insipidus characterized by hyposthenuria if the diluting segment of the nephron (medullary thick ascending limb of Henle's loop) is unaffected. These effects are caused by intrinsic responses of the kidney to hypercalcemia. Some of these effects are mediated by calcium-sensing receptors on the renal epithelial cells,[74] whereas others may be related to effects of hypercalcemia on aquaporin expression, cell trafficking, and delivery to apical membranes of the collecting tubules.[154,418,545] Additional direct effects of hypercalcemia on the kidney include reduced tubular calcium reabsorption and antagonism of the actions of PTH. These responses by the kidney facilitate calcium excretion and help to ameliorate the clinical effects of hypercalcemia. Renal medullary blood flow is increased in dogs with experimental hypercalcemia[81] and can result in medullary washout as another mechanism contributing to hyposthenuria. Isosthenuria develops if the diluting segments have been structurally altered by long-standing hypercalcemia. Polydipsia occurs as compensation for obligatory polyuria, but there is evidence that polydipsia can be caused by direct stimulation of the thirst center by hypercalcemia.[111] Mineralization of renal tubules, basement membranes, or the interstitium; tubular degeneration; and interstitial fibrosis are structural changes that may occur in the kidney secondary to hypercalcemia and can contribute to impaired urinary concentrating ability.

Dehydration is common owing to increased fluid losses from vomiting and polyuria. Substantial contraction of the ECF volume results in reduced GFR severe enough to increase BUN and serum creatinine concentrations and cause prerenal azotemia. The clinical axiom that dilute urine in association with azotemia is caused by intrinsic renal lesions may not be true in animals with hypercalcemia because the urinary concentrating defect can occur without structural renal lesions. This condition is commonly misdiagnosed as primary renal failure when it is actually prerenal failure caused by dehydration and a renal concentrating defect early in the course of hypercalcemia.

Intrarenal causes of azotemia during hypercalcemia can be functional or structural. Hypercalcemia can induce renal vasoconstriction, resulting in decreased renal blood flow (RBF) and GFR.[107] In an acute model of hypercalcemia, reduced RBF and GFR were observed consistently in conscious dogs when serum tCa concentration exceeded 20 mg/dL, but only one half of the dogs had significant reductions in GFR and RBF when serum calcium concentration was 15 to 20 mg/dL. Little effect on RBF and GFR was observed when serum calcium concentration was less than 15 mg/dL. These findings are in contrast to those in studies of anesthetized dogs, which demonstrated much more severe functional changes during hypercalcemia.[309] Impaired renal autoregulation related to the effects of hypercalcemia may result in azotemia at early stages of dehydration because GFR would otherwise be maintained by afferent arteriolar vasodilatation.

Acute intrinsic renal failure (AIRF) occasionally develops as a consequence of hypercalcemia, but chronic intrinsic renal failure is more common. Sustained renal vasoconstriction related to hypercalcemia may result in ischemic tubular injury, promoting development of both AIRF and chronic intrinsic renal failure and potentiating the direct toxic effects of calcium on tubular cells. The toxic effects of ionized hypercalcemia are enhanced by high concentrations of PTH in animals with CRF because excess PTH increases calcium entry into cells.[365] The ascending limb of Henle's loop and distal convoluted tubule show the earliest structural lesions, but lesions in the collecting system are ultimately the most pronounced. Thickening and mineralization of tubular basement membranes are most apparent in the proximal tubule. Tubular atrophy, mononuclear cell infiltration, and interstitial fibrosis occur in the chronic stages. Degenerative and necrotic tubules also are observed. Granular and tubular cell casts contribute to intrarenal obstruction and azotemia.[107,290]

Calcium-oxalate urolithiasis occasionally occurs in animals with long-standing hypercalcemia and has been described in dogs and cats with primary hyperparathyroidism. Nephrocalcinosis and linear mineralization along the renal diverticula are nonspecific findings discovered by radiography or ultrasonography in some dogs with long-standing hypercalcemia. Increased renal echogenicity and the medullary rim sign have been described during renal ultrasonography in dogs with hypercalcemia.[25,48] These changes can occur in other normocalcemic conditions and in forms of dystrophic mineralization.

Effects of Hypercalcemia on Other Organs

Anorexia, vomiting, and constipation can result from hypercalcemia by reduction of the excitability of gastrointestinal smooth muscle and from direct effects on the central nervous system. Gastric hyperacidity and subsequent gastric ulceration caused by increased secretion of gastrin and direct stimulation of hydrogen ion secretion from parietal cells by hypercalcemia may account for some of the vomiting. Gastrin concentration was increased in four of six dogs with hypercalcemia in one preliminary report.[61] Increased gastrin concentration occurs secondary to reduced renal clearance as a consequence of the hypercalcemia. Decreased excitability of skeletal muscle contributes to generalized weakness. Lethargy is commonly observed in severe hypercalcemia because of direct effects on the central nervous system and rarely can progress to stupor and coma. Seizures and muscle twitching are unusual neuromuscular manifestations of hypercalcemia.[251]

Clinically important cardiac effects of hypercalcemia are not commonly detected in dogs and cats, but PR interval prolongation and QT interval shortening can be observed on the electrocardiogram. Serious arrhythmias (including ventricular fibrillation) can be caused by the direct effects of severe hypercalcemia or may be a consequence of mineralization of cardiac tissue. Hypertension has been demonstrated in humans and rats during both acute and chronic hypercalcemia. The increase in blood pressure is proportional to the increase in serum calcium concentration in acute studies.[92] In a study of acute hypercalcemia, hypertension was attributed to a direct effect of calcium on vascular smooth muscle and to an indirect effect of calcium to increase secretion of catecholamine with activation of adrenergic receptors.[156] Whether hypertension is a clinically relevant complication in dogs and cats with hypercalcemia is unknown.

MECHANISMS AND DIFFERENTIAL DIAGNOSIS OF HYPERCALCEMIA

Increased entry of calcium into ECF, decreased egress of calcium from ECF, reduced plasma volume, or a combination of these factors must occur for hypercalcemia to develop (Fig. 6-11). Increased calcium input can arise from increased intestinal absorption, increased bone resorption, or increased renal tubular reabsorption of calcium. Decreased glomerular filtration and decreased bone accretion result in decreased egress of calcium from ECF. Volume contraction is common in the presence of hypercalcemia because of the effects of anorexia, vomiting, and obligatory polyuria. The mechanisms of hypercalcemia vary with the specific causes, but much attention has been focused on the importance of increased bone resorption.

Box 6-2 provides a list of possibilities in the differential diagnosis for hypercalcemia. Characterization of the hypercalcemia as transient or persistent, pathologic or nonpathologic, mild or severe, progressive or static, and acute or chronic is helpful in determining its cause. Persistent, pathologic hypercalcemia occurs most often in association with malignancy. Most studies in dogs attribute hypercalcemia to malignancy in more than 50% of the cases,[41,157,534] although in one series malignancy accounted for only one third of the cases.[290] Hypoadrenocorticism, renal failure, primary hyperparathyroidism, hypervitaminosis D, and inflammatory disorders sporadically account for hypercalcemia in dogs. It is often difficult to determine the cause of hypercalcemia in animals with mild or transient hypercalcemia. No definitive diagnosis could be made for 2% to 9% of hypercalcemic dogs in two reports.[157,534] No definitive diagnosis was reported in 13% of cats with hypercalcemia in one report, but the actual percentage is much higher based on sample submissions to veterinary endocrinology laboratories.[467]

In serum samples from 332 hypercalcemic cats, 80% had parathyroid-independent hypercalcemia, 10% had parathyroid-dependent hypercalcemia, and 10% were equivocal.[56] Approximately 10% of these hypercalcemic cats had PTHrP levels above the reference range, suggesting malignancy as the cause. Hypercalcemic cats have parathyroid-independent hypercalcemia more commonly than do dogs. Samples from 5722 hypercalcemic

dogs from the same laboratory categorized the hypercalcemia as parathyroid dependent in about 40%, parathyroid independent in 50%, and equivocal in 10%.[423]

GENERAL APPROACH TO DIAGNOSTIC WORKUP OF PATIENTS WITH HYPERCALCEMIA

It is important to ensure that the hypercalcemia initially detected is repeatable, especially if the magnitude of hypercalcemia is modest. The likely cause of the hypercalcemia will be obvious in some patients from findings in the history (hypervitaminosis D) or from physical examination (masses and effusions). When the cause is not immediately apparent, body cavity imaging with chest radiographs, abdominal radiographs, and abdominal ultrasound is recommended to determine whether organomegaly or infiltrative processes are present that could account for the hypercalcemia. Fine needle aspiration, needle biopsy, or wedge biopsy of abnormal tissues will often yield the cause of the hypercalcemia. Patients with cytopenias (neutropenia, anemia, and thrombocytopenia) should undergo bone marrow evaluation if the diagnosis has not already been established by other means. Bone marrow evaluation in the absence of cytopenias does not often result in a diagnosis. Radiographs of painful bones may reveal lesions associated with hypercalcemia. Aspiration of focal bone lesions may reveal the cause of the hypercalcemia. Bone survey of all bones is sometimes useful in finding lesions even in those without demonstrable bone pain (multiple myeloma). Bone scintigraphy may be considered in those in which a diagnosis is lacking despite exhaustive diagnostics.

High frequency ultrasonography of the cervical region can be performed to help determine whether the hypercalcemia is parathyroid dependent (large parathyroid glands) or parathyroid independent. In parathyroid-independent hypercalcemia, parathyroid glands are not enlarged or may not be identified; some may be atrophic if ionized hypercalcemia of malignancy or hypervitaminosis D has been long standing.

If the increase in serum tCa is minimal, measurement of serum iCa is important to determine whether the increase is clinically significant. Measurement of iCa in patients with renal failure is essential because renal failure can be associated with nonionized or ionized hypercalcemia. Serum iCa should be measured in association with PTH determination to assess the appropriateness of PTH response to serum iCa concentration.

If the cause of hypercalcemia is not apparent following history, physical examination, hematology, routine serum biochemistry, and body cavity imaging, then measurement of calcium-regulating hormones is needed to establish or suggest a definitive cause. The first step is to determine whether the hypercalcemia is parathyroid dependent (disease of the parathyroid glands is causing the hypercalcemia) or parathyroid independent (normal parathyroid glands suppress PTH secretion in response

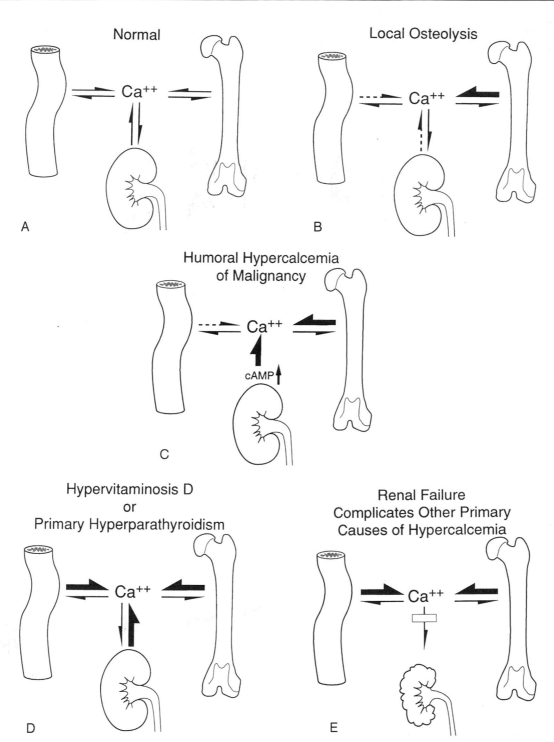

Fig. 6-11 Patterns of calcium transport between extracellular fluid and gut, kidney, and bone in various states of hypercalcemia. **A,** Normal. **B,** Osteolysis. **C,** Humoral hypercalcemia of malignancy. **D,** Hypervitaminosis D or primary hyperparathyroidism. **E,** Hypercalcemia complicated by renal failure. Size of arrows is proportional to the degree of calcium influx or efflux. Dashed arrows indicate possible response of decreased PTH secretion to hypercalcemia of nonparathyroid origin. (Modified from Mundy GR: Malignancy and hypercalcemia—humoral hypercalcemia of malignancy, hypercalcemia associated with osteolytic metastases. In Mundy GR, editor: *Calcium homeostasis: hypercalcemia and hypocalcemia,* London, 1989, Martin Dunitz, p. 65.)

Box 6-2 — Conditions Associated with Hypercalcemia

Nonpathologic
Nonfasting (minimal increase)
Physiologic growth of young
Laboratory error
Spurious
  Lipemia
  Detergent contamination of sample or tube

Transient or Inconsequential
Hemoconcentration
Hyperproteinemia
Hypoadrenocorticism
Severe environmental hypothermia (very rare)

Pathologic or Consequential—Persistent
Parathyroid dependent
  Primary hyperparathyroidism
    Adenoma (common)
    Adenocarcinoma (rare)
    Hyperplasia (uncommon)
Parathyroid independent
  Malignancy-associated (most common cause in dogs)
    Humoral hypercalcemia of malignancy
      Lymphoma (common)
      Anal sac apocrine gland adenocarcinoma (common)
      Carcinoma (sporadic): lung, pancreas, skin, nasal cavity, thyroid, mammary gland, adrenal medulla
      Thymoma (rare)
    Hematologic malignancies (bone marrow osteolysis, local osteolytic hypercalcemia)
      Lymphoma
      Multiple myeloma
      Myeloproliferative disease (rare)
      Leukemia (rare)
    Metastatic or primary bone neoplasia (very uncommon)
  Idiopathic hypercalcemia (most common association in cats)
  Chronic renal failure (with and without ionized hypercalcemia)
  Hypervitaminosis D
    Iatrogenic
    Plants (calcitriol glycosides)
    Rodenticide (cholecalciferol)
    Antipsoriasis creams (calcipotriol or calcipotriene)
  Granulomatous disease
    Blastomycosis
    Dermatitis
    Panniculitis
    Injection reaction
  Acute renal failure (diuretic phase)
  Skeletal lesions (nonmalignant) (uncommon)
    Osteomyelitis (bacterial or mycotic)
    Hypertrophic osteodystrophy
    Disuse osteoporosis (immobilization)
  Excessive calcium-containing intestinal phosphate binders
  Excessive calcium supplementation (calcium carbonate)
  Hypervitaminosis A
  Raisin/grape toxicity
  Hypercalcemic conditions in human medicine
    Milk-alkali syndrome (rare in dogs)
    Thiazide diuretics
    Acromegaly
    Thyrotoxicosis (rare in cats)
    Postrenal transplantation
    Aluminum exposure (intestinal phosphate binders in dogs and cats?)

to hypercalcemia). Measurement of PTHrP is helpful if malignancy is suspected, but PTHrP concentrations are not always increased in malignancy. If extensive imaging methodologies are not available, measurement of serum iCa, PTH, and PTHrP may be performed before extensive body cavity imaging or bone marrow evaluation. Measurement of 25-hydroxyvitamin D is useful in cases of potential cholecalciferol or ergocalciferol ingestion. Measurement of 1,25-dihydroxyvitamin D (calcitriol) is occasionally useful if excess calcitriol is the cause of hypercalcemia. The anticipated changes in calcium hormones and serum biochemistry in disorders causing hypercalcemia are noted in Table 6-2.

NONPATHOLOGIC HYPERCALCEMIA

Serum calcium concentrations in animals may be mildly increased after feeding; consequently, a 12-hour fast is recommended before blood sampling. Laboratory error or detergent contamination of the serum or sample tube may result in artifactual hypercalcemia.[345] Lipemia frequently causes erroneously high serum tCa concentrations because of colorimetric interference. Normal young growing dogs may have mildly higher serum calcium concentrations than older dogs.[350]

Transient or Inconsequential Hypercalcemia

Inconsequential hypercalcemia does not cause injury, resolves rapidly, or is only mild. Dehydration can result in mild hypercalcemia attributed to hemoconcentration. Furthermore, dehydration and volume contraction stimulate increased sodium and calcium reabsorption in the kidney. An increased serum concentration of protein, especially albumin, can result in an increased serum tCa concentration as more calcium binds to protein. Dehydration in dogs is occasionally associated with serum tCa concentrations of 12.0 to 13.5 mg/dL that rapidly return to normal after dehydration is corrected. Increased serum tCa and decreased iCa concentrations can occur transiently after plasma transfusion because of excess citrate–calcium ion complexes.[350]

TABLE 6-2 Anticipated Changes in Calcemic Hormones and Serum Biochemistry Associated with Disorders of Hypercalcemia

	tCa	iCa	alb	Corr tCa	Pi	PTH	PTHrP	25(OH)-D	1,25 (OH)₂-D	PTG ULS, Surgery
Primary hyperparathyroidism	↑	↑	N	N	↓N	↑N	N	N	N↑	Single ↑
Nutritional secondary hyperparathyroidism	N↓	N↓	N	N↓	N↑	↑	N	↓N	N↓	Multiple ↑
Renal secondary hyperparathyroidism	N↓↑	N↓	N	N	↑N	↑	N	N↓	N↓	Multiple ↑
Tertiary hyperparathyroidism	↑	↑	N	↑	↑	↑	N	N↓	↓N	Multiple ↑
Malignancy Associated										
Humoral hypercalcemia	↑	↑	N→	↑N	↓N	→N	↑N	N	↓N↑	→
Local osteolytic	↑	↑	N→	↑N	N↑	→N	N↑	N	N	→
Hypervitaminosis D										
Cholecalciferol	↑	↑	N	↑	↑N	→	N	↑	N↑	N→
Calcitriol	↑	↑	N	↑	N↑	→	N	N	↑→	→N
Calcipotriene	↑	↑	N	↑	↑N	→	N	N	N	N→
Hypoadrenocorticism	↑	↑	N→	↑	↑N	↓N	N	N	↓N	N→
Hypervitaminosis A	↑	↑	N	↑	N	→N	N	N	N↓	→N
Idiopathic (cat)	↑	N↑	N↓	N	N↑	N→	N	N	N↓→	→N
Dehydration	↑	N↑	↑N	N	N↑	N→	N	N	N	N↑→
Aluminum exposure (renal failure)	↑	↑	N	↑	↑N	N→	N	N	N	N↑↓
Hyperthyroidism (cat)	↑	↑	N	↑	N↑	N↑↓	N	N	N↓	N↑
Raisin/grape toxicity (dog)	↑	—	N	↑	N↑	—	—	—	—	—

↓, Decreased concentration; ↑, increased concentration; N, normal; tCa, serum total calcium; iCa, serum ionized calcium; alb, albumin; Corr tCa, corrected total calcium; Pi, inorganic phosphorus; PTH, parathyroid hormone; PTHrP, parathyroid hormone–related protein; 25(OH)-D, 25-hydroxyvitamin D; 1,25(OH)2-D, 1,25-dihydroxyvitamin D; PTG, parathyroid gland; ULS, ultrasound.

Hypoadrenocorticism

Hypoadrenocorticism is the second most common cause of hypercalcemia in dogs (after malignancy), accounting for 11% to 45% of cases in five studies,[111,157,290,534,560] but no cases were reported in one study.[41] Hypercalcemia was reported in 28% to 31% of dogs with glucocorticoid- and mineralocorticoid-deficient hypoadrenocorticism,[402,405] in some dogs with glucocorticoid-deficient hypoadrenocorticism,[302] and in 1 of 10 cats.[403] Hypoadrenocorticism is rarely recognized in cats, and hypercalcemia is present in only 8% of cases.[32] Hypercalcemia was present in one cat with iatrogenic secondary hypoadrenocorticism and diabetes mellitus.[495] Magnitude of hypercalcemia was greatest in the most severely affected dogs, but the mechanism is unknown. A correlation between the degree of hyperkalemia and hypercalcemia was detected when the serum potassium concentration was greater than 6.0 to 6.5 mEq/L, and serum tCa concentration was often 11.4 to 13.5 mg/dL.[168] Increases in serum iCa may or may not develop in hypoadrenocorticism.[543] Serum tCa concentration rapidly returns to normal after 1 to 2 days of corticosteroid replacement therapy in dogs,[402] and IV volume expansion can return serum calcium concentration to normal within a few hours. Hypoadrenocorticism should always be included in the differential diagnosis of hypercalcemia because clinical signs of hypoadrenocorticism and hypercalcemia are similar.

Chronic Renal Failure

The finding of hypercalcemia and primary renal azotemia poses a special diagnostic problem because hypercalcemia can cause renal failure or develop as a consequence of CRF. Serum PTH concentration is often increased in patients with hypercalcemia related to renal failure, and these animals must be differentiated from those with primary hyperparathyroidism. Serum iCa concentration is increased in primary hyperparathyroidism but is usually normal or low in patients with CRF.[114,290]

Deleterious effects of hypercalcemia occur in patients with renal failure only if it is associated with increases in serum iCa concentration. Consequently, clinical signs of hypercalcemia are uncommon in CRF patients, and measurement of serum iCa concentration to assess calcium status in CRF patients is critical. In CRF patients, the serum tCa measurement incorrectly assessed iCa status in 36% of dogs and 32% of cats.[474,475] The use of the "adjusted tCa" value incorrectly assessed iCa status in approximately 53% of dogs with CRF. In dogs, serum tCa measurement or adjusted tCa measurement overestimated hypercalcemia and underestimated hypocalcemia. In cats with CRF, serum tCa measurement overestimated normocalcemia and underestimated hypercalcemia. Thus to accurately assess calcium status in patients with CRF, iCa concentration must be directly measured.

Fewer than 10% of all dogs with CRF have increased serum iCa concentrations. In one study, approximately 6% exhibited ionized hypercalcemia.[114] In a recent study of 490 dogs with CRF, 9% exhibited hypercalcemia, 55% were normocalcemic, and 36% were hypocalcemic based on serum iCa concentrations.[475] Cats with CRF appear to have a higher incidence of ionized hypercalcemia as compared with dogs. In 102 cats with CRF, 29% were hypercalcemic, 61% were normocalcemic, and 10% were hypocalcemic based on iCa concentration.[474]

Many dogs and cats with CRF have normal serum tCa concentrations.[138,173,345] Hypercalcemia based on measurement of serum tCa concentration occurs sporadically in dogs and cats with CRF and is usually listed as second or third in frequency of causes of hypercalcemia in dogs. Elevated tCa occurs in up to 14% of dogs with CRF, with a range of 12.1 to 15.2 mg/dL.[114,173,290,367] In 71 hypercalcemic cats, CRF was noted in 38%.[467] In cats with CRF, the reported incidence of serum total hypercalcemia ranged from 11.5%[138] to 58%.[24]

The incidence of elevated tCa increases with severity of azotemia. In 73 cats with CRF, serum tCa was increased in 8%, 18%, and 32% of those with mild, moderate, or severe azotemia, respectively.[24] However, increases in serum iCa do not show a strong association with the degree of azotemia.[127] In 47 of the previous 73 cats with CRF, iCa was increased in 0%, 9%, and 6% of those with mild, moderate, or severe azotemia, respectively.[24] Hypercalcemia was also not correlated with serum phosphorus concentration in dogs with experimental renal failure.[381,531]

The parathyroid glands must be present for hypercalcemia to develop,[531] and partial parathyroidectomy ameliorates hypercalcemia in some dogs with CRF.[173] Treatment of dogs with CRF and hypercalcemia with low-dose calcitriol to reduce PTH synthesis and secretion can result in decreased iCa concentration. Low-dose calcitriol therapy does not appreciably increase intestinal calcium absorption.[363,364] In patients with CRF, increased serum PTH concentration (renal secondary hyperparathyroidism) contributes to the progression of renal disease.[364] Oral administration of low doses of calcitriol reduces toxic concentrations of PTH, improves quality of life, reduces progression of renal disease, and leads to prolongation of life.[365,479]

Some cases of ionized hypercalcemia and CRF may be associated with the use of calcium carbonate intestinal phosphate binders. In these cases, serum iCa concentration rapidly returns to normal after discontinuation of treatment. In humans with CRF, therapeutic use of calcitriol is limited by development of hypercalcemia in patients also being treated with calcium-based dietary phosphorus binders.[121,365] In veterinary medicine, use of aluminum-based phosphorus binders or sevelamer (Renagel, Genzyme Corporation, Cambridge, MA) largely precludes this problem.[9] "Noncalcemic analogues" of calcitriol have been developed for use in humans,[493] such as paricalcitol (Zemplar, Abbott Laboratories, Abbott Park, IL), 22-oxacalcitriol (OCT), and doxercalciferol (Hectorol, Bone Care International, Middleton, WI).[146] These analogues have a very short half-life (several minutes), and this short half-life is responsible for their weak stimulation of intestinal calcium absorption. Doses of noncalcemic analogues needed to suppress PTH synthesis are approximately eightfold higher than that of calcitriol[493] and are up to 12 times the cost. If hypercalcemia develops with calcitriol therapy, a twice-weekly dosing strategy of calcitriol is used. This dosing regimen will suppress PTH but be much less effective at stimulating intestinal calcium absorption. Noncalcemic analogues are not needed and are financially impractical in veterinary medicine.

Ionized hypercalcemia occurs in patients with CRF who receive excessive doses of calcitriol. Hypercalcemia is very uncommon in animals treated with the lower dosages of calcitriol (2.5 to 4.0 ng/kg daily). If hypercalcemia is caused by excessive calcitriol, the serum tCa concentration decreases during the week after its discontinuation. Most CRF patients who develop an elevated tCa during low-dose calcitriol treatment have normal or low serum iCa concentrations. Serum tCa concentration may not decrease when calcitriol is discontinued if the increased serum tCa concentration is caused by increased complexed calcium.

The mechanisms of increased serum tCa concentration in CRF have not been well characterized.[173,290,435,531] In dogs with CRF, serum total hypercalcemia, and normal iCa concentrations, the increase in serum tCa is caused by an increase in the complexed calcium fraction.[473] In CRF, organic anions such as citrates, phosphates, lactates, bicarbonates, and oxalates are capable of complexing with calcium. Complexed calcium accounted for 24% of serum tCa in those dogs with CRF and elevated serum tCa as compared with 11% in those dogs with CRF and low serum tCa. Increased PTH-mediated bone resorption as a consequence of CRF could increase serum tCa concentration. If elevated iCa is also present, then reduced GFR caused by loss of renal mass could cause increased iCa concentration as the filtered load of calcium declines. Hyperplasia of parathyroid gland chief cells could account for increased PTH secretion and serum calcium concentration because chief cells secrete small amounts of PTH that are nonsuppressible regardless of serum iCa concentration.[201]

Tertiary hyperparathyroidism refers to the condition of a subset of patients with CRF who develop ionized hypercalcemia and excessive PTH secretion that is not inhibited by high serum iCa concentration. It is likely that such patients had high PTH concentrations in association with normal or low serum iCa concentration (renal secondary hyperparathyroidism) earlier in the clinical course of CRF. Autonomous secretion of PTH from the parathyroid gland is unlikely, but the set-point for PTH secretion may be altered in CRF such that higher concentrations of iCa are necessary to inhibit PTH secretion.[202] Decreased serum calcitriol concentrations, decreased numbers of calcitriol receptors in the parathyroid gland, and decreased calcitriol–VDR interactions with chief cell DNA caused by uremic toxins may contribute to this increase in set-point,[70,247,396] as may decreased levels of the calcium receptor, which both establishes the set-point and depends on calcitriol functionality for synthesis of its mRNA from the parathyroid cells' DNA.[94] Ten dogs with CRF and increased serum tCa concentration were compared with those with normal serum tCa concentration (Fig. 6-12). Serum aminoterminal PTH concentration was markedly increased in both groups of uremic dogs, but those with increased tCa had higher PTH concentrations. Calcitriol concentration was decreased to a similar extent in both groups. It was proposed that the hypercalcemic and more markedly hyperparathyroid uremic dogs might have had greater calcitriol receptor (VDR) deficits in their parathyroid cells, which would lead to poorly controlled PTH synthesis and chief cell hyperplasia.[367] Deficient calcitriol functionality caused by VDR deficits would also lead to calcium receptor deficits and the "set-point" elevations involved in the observed hypercalcemia.[94]

Aluminum accumulation in the development of hypercalcemia in dogs or cats with renal disease being treated with aluminum-containing intestinal phosphate binders has not been investigated despite the fact that such treatment is common. Experimental dogs exposed to aluminum developed mild hypercalcemia within minutes of a single intravenous injection. During chronic daily exposure to aluminum during a period of weeks, serum calcium concentration progressively increased, and azotemia developed.[226]

Two of 15 cats with CRF developed hypercalcemia while eating a phosphate-restricted veterinary diet designed for treatment of renal failure. Hypercalcemia in these cats was associated with a decrease in serum phosphorus and low or undetectable PTH concentrations. Serum calcium returned to normal, and PTH and phosphorus increased with the feeding of a maintenance diet.[26]

PATHOLOGIC OR CONSEQUENTIAL HYPERCALCEMIA

Cancer-Associated Hypercalcemia

The most common cause of hypercalcemia in dogs is cancer-associated hypercalcemia. Cancer is third in frequency of association with hypercalcemia in cats. There are three mechanisms (Fig. 6-13) of increased serum calcium concentration induced by neoplasms: (1) HHM, (2) hypercalcemia induced by metastases of solid tumors

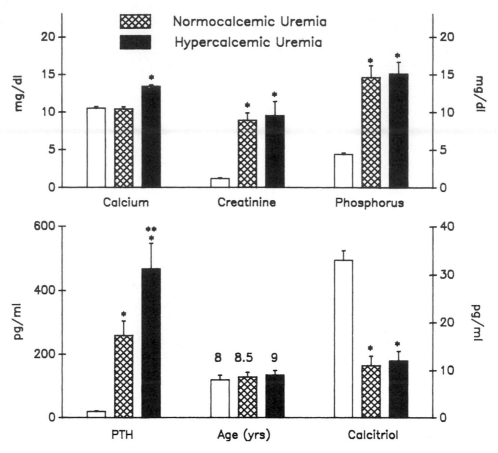

Fig. 6-12 Comparison of biochemical data for dogs with renal failure and hypercalcemia or normocalcemia. Dogs with renal failure were normalized for age and had similar concentrations of serum creatinine, phosphorus, and calcitriol. Serum concentrations of PTH were greater in the hypercalcemic dogs than in the normocalcemic dogs. Data are mean ± SEM. For normal and hypercalcemic uremic dogs, n = 10; for normocalcemic uremic dogs, n = 20. Significant differences were *P < 0.0001 (from normal) and **P < 0.02 (from normocalcemic uremia PTH) by Student's *t* test. (From Nagode LA, Steinmeyer CL, Chew DJ, et al.: Hyper- and normo-calcemic dogs with chronic renal failure: relations of serum PTH and calcitriol to parathyroid gland Ca++ set-point. In Norman AW, Schaefer K, Grigoleit HG, et al, editors: *Vitamin D 1988. Chemical, biochemical and clinical endocrinology,* Berlin, 1988, Walter de Gruyter & Co., pp. 799-800.)

to bone (local osteolytic hypercalcemia [LOH]), and (3) hematologic malignancies growing in the bone marrow (LOH).[436,437]

Humoral Hypercalcemia of Malignancy. HHM is a syndrome associated with many tumors in people and animals.[437] Characteristic clinical findings in patients with HHM include hypercalcemia, hypophosphatemia, hypercalciuria (often with decreased fractional calcium excretion), increased fractional excretion of phosphorus, increased nephrogenous cyclic adenosine monophosphate (cAMP), and increased osteoclastic bone resorption. Hypercalcemia is induced by humoral effects on bone, kidney, and possibly the intestine (Fig. 6-14).[438] Increased osteoclastic bone resorption is a consistent finding in HHM and increases calcium release from bone. The kidney plays a critical role in the pathogenesis

of hypercalcemia because PTHrP stimulates calcium reabsorption, which binds and activates renal PTH-PTHrP receptors. The level of renal function in the patient may also contribute to the development of hypercalcemia. Animals with dehydration or impaired renal function are more susceptible to developing hypercalcemia or may have more severe hypercalcemia because of decreased renal excretion of calcium. In some forms of HHM, increased serum 1,25-dihydroxyvitamin D concentrations may increase calcium absorption from the intestine.[446]

Malignancies that are commonly associated with HHM in dogs include T-cell lymphoma and adenocarcinomas derived from the apocrine glands of the anal sac.[33,436,553,561] Dogs with cancer and HHM are expected to have shorter survival. In addition, sporadic cases of HHM occur in dogs with thymoma, myeloma,

Cancer-Associated Hypercalcemia

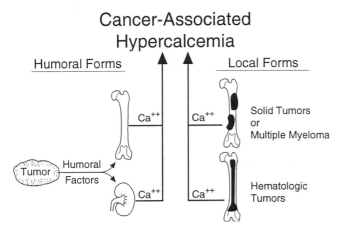

Fig. 6-13 Pathogenesis of cancer-associated hypercalcemia. Humoral and local forms of cancer-associated hypercalcemia increase circulating concentrations of calcium by stimulation of osteoclastic bone resorption and increased renal tubular reabsorption of calcium.

Humoral Factors and HHM

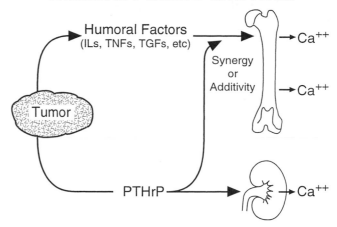

Fig. 6-14 Humoral factors such as parathyroid hormone–related protein (PTHrP), interleukin-1 (IL-1), tumor necrosis factors (TNFs), or transforming growth factors (TGFs) produced by tumors induce humoral hypercalcemia of malignancy (HHM) by acting as systemic hormones and stimulating osteoclastic bone resorption or increasing tubular reabsorption of calcium.

melanoma, or carcinomas originating in the lungs, pancreas, thyroid gland, skin, mammary gland, nasal cavity, and adrenal medulla.[56,417,436-438] Tumors associated with hypercalcemia in cats include lymphosarcoma, multiple myeloma, squamous cell carcinoma, bronchogenic carcinoma/adenocarcinoma, osteosarcoma, fibrosarcoma, undifferentiated sarcoma, undifferentiated renal carcinoma, anaplastic carcinoma of the lung and diaphragm, and thyroid carcinoma.* Lymphosarcoma and squamous cell carcinoma are the two most common causes of hypercalcemia in cats.[467] Of 11 hypercalcemic cats with lymphosarcoma, two each had renal, generalized, gastrointestinal, or mediastinal involvement, and one each had laryngeal, nasal, or cutaneous disease.[56,115,152,158,467] Squamous cell carcinoma has been found in mandibular, maxillary, pulmonary, and ear canal locations.[56,250,276,467]

Excessive secretion of biologically active PTHrP plays a central role in the pathogenesis of hypercalcemia in most forms of HHM, but cytokines such as IL-1, TNF-α, and transforming growth factor (TGF)-α and -β or calcitriol may have synergistic or cooperative actions with PTHrP (see Fig. 6-14). Before PTHrP was identified, it was recognized that tumors associated with HHM induced a syndrome that mimicked primary hyperparathyroidism with secretion of a PTH-like factor that was antigenically unrelated to PTH.[359,552]

PTHrP binds to the N-terminal PTH-PTHrP receptor in bone and kidney but does not cross-react immunologically with native PTH (Fig. 6-15). PTHrP stimulates adenylyl cyclase and increases intracellular calcium in bone and kidney cells by binding to and activating the cell membrane PTH-PTHrP receptors. This binding results in

stimulation of osteoclastic bone resorption, increased renal tubular calcium reabsorption, and decreased renal tubular phosphate reabsorption. IL-1 stimulates bone resorption in vivo and in vitro and is synergistic with PTHrP.[335,437] TGF-α and -β can stimulate bone resorption in vitro and have been identified in tumors associated with HHM, including adenocarcinomas derived from apocrine glands of the anal sac in dogs.[340]

Lymphoma. Hypercalcemia is found in 20% to 40% of dogs with lymphoma (Fig. 6-16).[297,316] Most dogs with lymphoma and hypercalcemia have HHM because increased osteoclastic resorption is present in bones without evidence of tumor metastasis. Lymphoma is an uncommon cause of mild HHM in ferrets.[268] Lymphomas associated with HHM are usually of the T-cell type.[553] T-cell lymphoma occurred in 22% of dogs with lymphoma, and hypercalcemia only occurred in dogs with CD4+ lymphoma in one study.[459] The pathogenesis of hypercalcemia in dogs with lymphoma and HHM resembles that occurring in humans with lymphoma or leukemia induced by human T-cell lymphotropic virus type I (HTLV-I). Neoplastic cells from humans with HTLV-I–induced lymphoma have increased PTHrP production.[428]

Most dogs with lymphoma and hypercalcemia have T-cell lymphoma.[511,553] Dogs with T-cell lymphoma were significantly more likely to have early relapse and death compared with those with B-cell lymphoma. Shorter remissions and survival times have been noted by others for T-cell lymphoma compared with B-cell lymphoma in dogs.[211] In another study, 46 (32.8%) of 140

References 11,42,56,115,152,158,229,250,276,467,484.

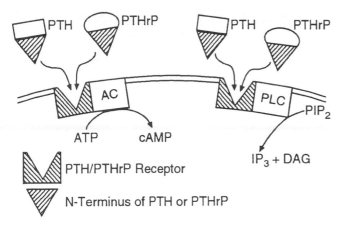

Fig. 6-15 Parathyroid hormone–related protein (PTHrP) induces many of the effects of parathyroid hormone (PTH) by interacting with the PTH receptor in bone and kidney and activating adenylyl cyclase (AC) to form cyclic AMP (cAMP) and phospholipase C (PLC) to form inositol triphosphate (IP$_3$) and diacylglycerol (DAG) from phosphatidylinositol (PIP$_2$). Stimulation of the PTH receptor results in increased osteoclastic bone resorption and renal tubular reabsorption of calcium, inhibition of renal tubular reabsorption of phosphorus, and stimulation of renal production of 1,25-dihydroxyvitamin D$_3$ (calcitriol).

lymphomas were classified as T cell in origin, and 16 of these dogs (35%) were hypercalcemic.[185] In 37 dogs with lymphoma and hypercalcemia, calcium concentration was not related to prognosis; mean remission was 10.4 months, and median remission was 6 months.[434] The presence of a mediastinal mass had an adverse effect on remission in these hypercalcemic dogs. Serum tCa concentration may return to normal despite minimal reduction in tumor mass following chemotherapy, as happened in 5 of 12 dogs with lymphoma and initial hypercalcemia.[556] The finding of hypercalcemia in dogs with lymphoma was not prognostic for survival or time to remission, but T-cell origin lymphoma did adversely affect prognosis.[275,511,538]

Most dogs with lymphoma and HHM have increased circulating PTHrP concentrations, but concentrations are lower than in dogs with carcinomas and HHM, and PTHrP concentrations are not correlated with serum calcium concentration (Fig. 6-17).[446] These findings indicate that PTHrP is an important marker of HHM in dogs with lymphoma but is not the sole humoral factor responsible for stimulation of osteoclasts and development of hypercalcemia. It is likely that cytokines such as IL-1 or TNF function synergistically with PTHrP to induce HHM in dogs with lymphoma (see Fig. 6-14).[436,437]

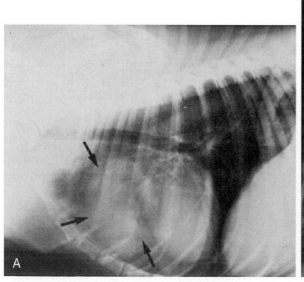

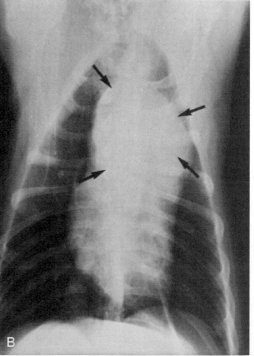

Fig. 6-16 Lateral **(A)** and ventrodorsal **(B)** thoracic radiographs of a 5-year-old boxer dog with hypercalcemia of malignancy caused by mediastinal lymphoma (arrows). Severe hypercalcemia (serum total calcium concentration, 20.6 mg/dL) was detected on initial presentation. (From Chew DJ, Carothers M: Hypercalcemia, *Vet Clin North Am* 19:272, 1989.)

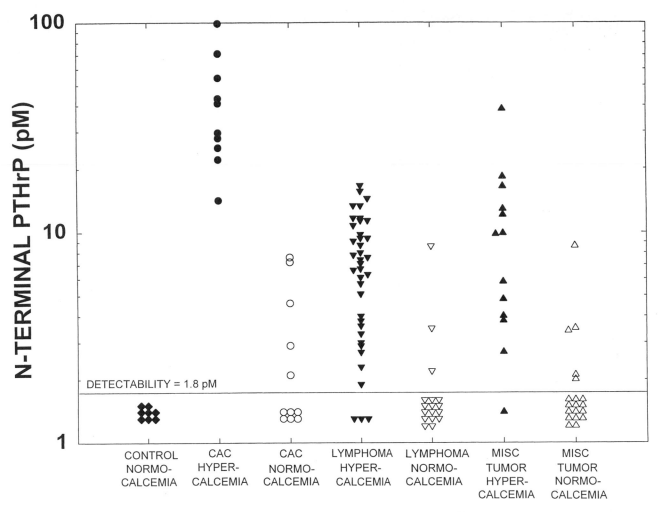

Fig. 6-17 Circulating N-terminal parathyroid hormone–related protein (PTHrP) concentrations in normal dogs (CONTROL); dogs with hypercalcemia (>12 mg/dL) and anal sac adenocarcinomas (CAC), lymphoma, or miscellaneous tumors (MISC TUMOR); and dogs with normocalcemia (<12 mg/dL) and anal sac adenocarcinomas, lymphoma, or miscellaneous tumors. (From Rosol TJ, Nagode LA, Couto CG, et al: Parathyroid hormone–related protein, parathyroid hormone, and 1,25-dihydroxyvitamin D in dogs with cancer-associated hypercalcemia, *Endocrinology* 131:1157, 1992. ©The Endocrine Society.)

Some dogs and human patients with lymphoma and hypercalcemia have increased serum calcitriol concentrations, which may contribute to the induction of hypercalcemia.[446,482] Some lymphocytes contain the 1α-hydroxylase (similar to that found in renal tubules) that converts 25-hydroxyvitamin D to the active metabolite 1,25-dihydroxyvitamin D (calcitriol). Therefore lymphomas that retain this capability may synthesize excessive calcitriol, which could increase calcium absorption from the intestinal tract and facilitate development of hypercalcemia.

An early report indicated that a mediastinal mass was detected in most dogs with lymphoma and hypercalcemia.[343] However, a recent report indicates that the presence of a cranial mediastinal mass was not required for development of hypercalcemia in dogs, and mediastinal masses were not disproportionately more common in those dogs with hypercalcemia.[49]

Canine Adenocarcinoma Derived from Apocrine Glands of the Anal Sac. The adenocarcinoma derived from apocrine glands of the anal sac of dogs consistently fulfills the criteria for HHM.[342,344,430] This tumor appears primarily in middle-aged (mean, 10 years) dogs and rarely metastasizes to bone. Clinical signs are referable to hypercalcemia (polyuria, polydipsia, anorexia, and weakness), a mass in the perineum (tenesmus, ribbonlike stools, increased odor, and protruding mass), a mass in the sublumbar region, or more distant metastases. Apocrine adenocarcinomas often require rectal and anal sac palpation to confirm their presence because their size ranges from 7 mm to 6 × 8 cm (Fig. 6-18). Dogs

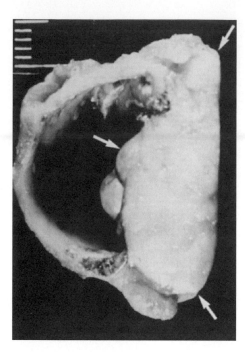

Fig. 6-18 Hypercalcemia of malignancy associated with apocrine gland adenocarcinoma of the anal sac in an elderly female dog. Transverse section of the anal sac and associated malignancy (arrows). (From Chew DJ, Meuten DJ: Disorders of calcium and phosphorus metabolism, *Vet Clin North Am* 12:417, 1982.)

with this tumor and HHM have hypercalcemia (tCa, 12 to 24 mg/dL); hypophosphatemia; decreased immunoreactive PTH concentration; increased urinary excretion of calcium, phosphorus, and cAMP; and increased osteoclastic bone resorption.[33,344,561] This tumor should not be confused with the common perianal adenomas or the uncommon perianal adenocarcinomas that arise from the circumanal glands and have entirely different biologic behavior. Perianal adenomas and adenocarcinomas affect primarily male dogs and are not associated with hypercalcemia.[539]

Hypercalcemia was present at the time of diagnosis in 80% to 100% of affected dogs in early studies.[330,331] Recent reports in dogs with earlier detection note the incidence of hypercalcemia to be lower, at 33%,[453] 27%,[561] and 53% of cases.[33] Early reports also noted a strong bias toward the occurrence of this tumor in female dogs, but equal sex distribution has been more recently noted.[561] In some instances, the finding of hypercalcemia during routine serum biochemistry testing prompts rectal palpation and subsequent discovery of an apocrine gland adenocarcinoma. Surgical removal or radiation therapy of the adenocarcinoma results in rapid return to normal of serum calcium and phosphorus concentrations, increased serum PTH concentration, and decreased calcitriol concentration.[446] Postsurgical survival of dogs with apocrine gland adenocarcinoma and hypercalcemia

ranged from 2 to 21 months, with a mean of 8.8 months. Sublumbar metastases occur in a high percentage (72%) of affected dogs and are associated with recrudescence of the biochemical alterations in serum and urine.[33] In one study, dogs with hypercalcemia and anal sac adenocarcinoma had shorter survival times compared with normocalcemic dogs with this tumor (356 versus 584 days)[561]; in another study, survival was not influenced by the presence of hypercalcemia.[33]

Most dogs with HHM have increased concentrations of circulating PTHrP (see Fig. 6-17). Plasma concentrations of PTHrP are highest (10 to 100 pmol/L) in dogs with apocrine adenocarcinomas of the anal sac and sporadic carcinomas associated with HHM.[446] Serum calcium concentrations in affected dogs correlate well with circulating PTHrP concentrations, which is consistent with the concept that PTHrP plays a primary role in the pathogenesis of HHM in these dogs. Dogs with apocrine adenocarcinomas and normocalcemia may have increased plasma PTHrP concentrations (2 to 15 pmol/L), but the concentrations are lower than in dogs with hypercalcemia.

Some dogs with apocrine adenocarcinomas have inappropriate concentrations (normal or increased) of calcitriol for the degree of hypercalcemia.[446] This finding suggests that the humoral factors produced by the neoplastic cells are capable of stimulating renal 1α-hydroxylase and increasing the formation of calcitriol even in the presence of increased serum calcium concentration. PTH concentrations were not increased in hypercalcemic dogs and were significantly lower than those observed in dogs with primary hyperparathyroidism. Parathyroid glands from dogs with apocrine adenocarcinoma were atrophic or inactive, and there was nodular hyperplasia of C cells in the thyroid glands because of prolonged hypercalcemia.[344]

Hematologic Malignancies. Some types of hematologic malignancies present in the bone marrow produce hypercalcemia by inducing bone resorption locally.[436,437] This effect occurs most commonly in multiple myeloma and lymphoma. Hypercalcemia has been reported in 17% of dogs with multiple myeloma.[331] A number of paracrine factors or cytokines may be responsible for the stimulation of bone resorption in this setting. The cytokines most often implicated in the pathogenesis of local bone resorption are IL-1, TNF-α, and TNF-β (lymphotoxin).[328,360] Other cytokines or factors that may play a role include IL-6, TGF-α and -β, and PTHrP.[48] Production of small amounts of PTHrP by a tumor in bone may stimulate local bone resorption without inducing a systemic response. Prostaglandins (especially prostaglandin E$_2$) may also be responsible for local stimulation of bone resorption.

Some dogs with lymphoma and hypercalcemia have localized bone resorption associated with metastases to medullary cavities without evidence of increased bone resorption at sites distant from the tumor metastases.[343] Hypercalcemic dogs with lymphoma and bone metastases had decreased PTH and calcitriol concentrations, increased excretion of hydroxyproline, calcium, phosphorus, and increased concentrations of the prostaglandin E$_2$ metabolite 13,14-dihydro-15-ketoprostaglandin E$_2$. Prostaglandin E$_2$ may be an important local mediator of bone resorption in these dogs. Other potential mediators include IL-1 and TNFs.

Tumors Metastatic to Bone. Solid tumors that metastasize widely to bone can produce hypercalcemia by the induction of local bone resorption associated with tumor growth. This is not common in animals but is an important cause of cancer-associated hypercalcemia in humans.[436,450,451] Tumors that often metastasize to bone and induce hypercalcemia in human patients include breast and lung carcinomas. Carcinomas of the mammary gland, prostate, liver, and lung were most frequently reported to metastasize to bone in dogs, and the humerus, femur, and vertebrae were the most common sites of metastasis.[345,452] Primary bone tumors are not often associated with hypercalcemia in dogs or cats.

The pathogenesis of enhanced bone resorption is not well understood, but two primary mechanisms are secretion of cytokines or factors that stimulate local bone resorption and indirect stimulation of bone resorption by tumor-induced cytokine secretion from local immune or bone cells.[195] Cytokines or factors that may be secreted by tumor cells and stimulate local bone resorption include PTHrP,[416] TGF-α and -β, and prostaglandins (especially prostaglandin E$_2$). In some cases, bone-resorbing activity can be inhibited by indomethacin, which suggests that prostaglandins are either directly or indirectly associated with stimulation of bone resorption. The cytokines most often implicated in indirect stimulation of bone resorption by local immune cells include IL-1 and TNFs.

Malignant neoplasms with osseous metastases may cause moderate to severe hypercalcemia and hypercalciuria, but serum ALP activity and phosphorus concentrations are usually normal or only moderately increased. It is believed these changes are caused by release of calcium and phosphorus into the blood from areas of bone destruction at rates greater than can be cleared by the kidney and intestine. Bone involvement can be multifocal but is usually sharply demarcated and localized to the area of metastasis.

Primary Hyperparathyroidism

Primary hyperparathyroidism is an uncommon cause of hypercalcemia in dogs[37,82] and is even less common in cats.[133,263] In hypercalcemic cats, primary hyperparathyroidism was found in 4 of 71 cases.[467] Excessive and inappropriate secretion of PTH by the parathyroid glands relative to the serum iCa concentration characterizes this condition. Primary hyperparathyroidism was caused by a solitary parathyroid gland adenoma in approximately 90% of dogs, whereas parathyroid gland carcinoma and parathyroid gland hyperplasia each accounted for 5% of cases in one large series.[168] Adenomas occurred with nearly equal frequency in the external and internal parathyroid glands in one study,[37] but external gland adenomas predominated in another report in dogs.[565] Idiopathic parathyroid gland hyperplasia may affect one or more glands and has been reported in six older dogs.[135] Although remnant parathyroid tissue may be found in the cranial mediastinum near the base of the heart, neoplastic transformation has not been reported at this site in dogs or cats. An ectopic parathyroid gland adenoma cranial to the thoracic inlet has been described in one dog.[564] In cats, the underlying lesion is typically benign, owing to an adenoma, bilateral cystadenomas, or hyperplasia,[133,163,467,503] but unilateral or bilateral carcinomas have also been diagnosed.[168,263,326,412]

Primary parathyroid gland hyperplasia has been reported in two German shepherd dog puppies.[517] Diffuse hyperplasia was present in all four parathyroid glands. In retrospect, this family of German shepherd dogs probably had an inactivating mutation in the gene for the calcium-sensing receptor. Mutations in one or both of the calcium-sensing receptor genes in humans result in familial hypocalciuric hypercalcemia or neonatal severe hypercalcemia, respectively, because of inadequate ability to sense extracellular calcium concentration and coordinate the appropriate cellular response.[414] The affected puppies had a disease syndrome that mimicked neonatal severe hypercalcemia in humans. Neonatal severe hypercalcemia is lethal unless total parathyroidectomy is performed early in life to markedly reduce increased PTH concentrations.

Dogs with primary hyperparathyroidism are older, with a mean age of 10.5 years (range, 5 to 15 years).[168] The mean age in affected cats was 12.9 years (range, 8 to 15 years).[263] No sex predisposition has been noted, but keeshonds constituted 36% of affected dogs, and five of eight cats were Siamese.[345] Parathyroid gland masses usually cannot be palpated in dogs, but 50% of cats with primary hyperparathyroidism had a palpable cervical mass.[133,263] Clinical signs related to hypercalcemia are either mild (e.g., lethargy, polydipsia, polyuria, and weakness) or absent in many affected dogs.[37,168] In one study, most owners of affected dogs were not convinced that their dogs had a serious illness,[37] but some owners retrospectively recognized subtle signs after hypercalcemia resolved.[168] More prominent clinical signs and serious consequences can occur when hyperparathyroidism and severe hypercalcemia are long standing and associated with renal failure.[111,112] Clinical signs referable to the lower urinary tract have been reported to occur in

27% of dogs as a result of urolithiasis or bacterial urinary tract infection.[168] Calcium-containing uroliths (calcium phosphate, calcium oxalate, or mixtures) occurred in approximately 30% of dogs and in a cat with primary hyperparathyroidism.[168,277,326] Urolithiasis is attributed to hypercalcemia and subsequent hypercalciuria. Interestingly, hypercalcemia arising from other causes has not been associated with urolithiasis except in cats with idiopathic hypercalcemia (IHC).[476]

The diagnostic workup to confirm primary hyperparathyroidism often begins with the fortuitous finding of increased serum calcium concentration on routine clinical chemistry testing.[168] The diagnosis of primary hyperparathyroidism is easy in dogs and cats that have increased serum tCa concentration, normal renal function, and increased concentration of immunoreactive PTH. The appropriateness of the PTH concentration must be interpreted in relation to the serum iCa concentration. Additional support for the diagnosis of primary hyperparathyroidism is provided by the finding of increased serum iCa concentration, increased serum ALP, low serum phosphorus concentration, increased or normal calcitriol concentration, undetectable PTHrP, and calcium-containing uroliths. The most consistent laboratory abnormality in dogs with primary hyperparathyroidism is increased serum calcium concentration.[168]

Hypercalcemia results from a combination of effects following PTH binding to receptors in kidney and bone. PTH also acts indirectly to increase serum iCa concentration by enhancing renal conversion of 25-hydroxyvitamin D to calcitriol. Hypophosphatemia secondary to PTH-enhanced urinary excretion of phosphorus was observed in 5 of 21 dogs.[37] Serum phosphorus concentration is typically low,[168] and calcitriol concentrations were mildly increased or in the high-normal range in three of four dogs with primary hyperparathyroidism.[446]

The diagnosis of primary hyperparathyroidism is more challenging when PTH is within the reference range. A PTH concentration in the upper part of the reference range in association with hypercalcemia is inappropriate. Confirmed primary hyperparathyroidism has been noted in dogs and cats with hypercalcemia and reference range PTH concentrations.[168,263] In a cat with persistent hypercalcemia related to primary hyperparathyroidism, PTH concentration was increased on two occasions but within the reference range on five other occasions.[133] PTH concentrations measured in blood collected from either the left or right jugular vein did not differ, and sampling from a specific side was not valuable for localizing the site of an enlarged parathyroid gland.[170] Circulating PTHrP concentrations were undetectable in six dogs with primary hyperparathyroidism.[446]

Ultrasonography of the neck is helpful in the diagnosis of primary hyperparathyroidism in dogs and cats, but it requires an ultrasound unit with a high-frequency (7.5- to 10-MHz) transducer to achieve the necessary level of resolution rather than the widely available 5- or 7.5-MHz units used for abdominal studies.[168,564] With a 10-MHz linear transducer, the parathyroid glands of normal dogs can routinely be identified especially in larger dogs.[426] Parathyroid gland masses greater than 5 mm can usually be identified, and some masses as small as 2 mm may be detected. Enlarged parathyroid glands are expected to be hypoechoic or anechoic, well marginated, and easily contrasted with thyroid tissue. False-positive results are rare, but false-negative findings may occur. Ultrasonography correctly identified the presence and location of a solitary parathyroid gland mass in 10 of 11 dogs in a prospective study in which the mass was confirmed at surgery.[170] Sonography identifies the location of the parathyroid gland tumor and allows presurgical planning.

Double-phase scintigraphy of the parathyroid glands using ^{99m}Tc sestamibi was useful in the diagnosis of parathyroid gland adenoma in initial reports from two dogs.[333,570] In a study of 15 dogs with hypercalcemia, scintigraphy correctly identified 3 of 3 dogs with hypercalcemia of malignancy as negative for hyperfunctioning parathyroid glands.[332] Scintigraphy identified only one of six dogs with parathyroid gland adenoma and only one of six dogs with parathyroid hyperplasia. Based on these results, parathyroid gland scintigraphy is not recommended to identify abnormal parathyroid glands because of very poor sensitivity and specificity.

Surgical exploration of the cervical region in patients with parathyroid gland adenoma or carcinoma usually reveals enlargement of one parathyroid gland, and the remaining three are small or impossible to identify because hypercalcemia results in atrophy of normal parathyroid tissue. Primary parathyroid gland hyperplasia may affect more than one gland, and clinical signs can recur if only the largest gland is removed surgically. Parathyroid gland tumors may be difficult to identify if the tumor is embedded in fat or if it arises from the internal parathyroid gland. Failure to visualize a parathyroid gland tumor is rarely attributed to the occurrence of a tumor in ectopic parathyroid tissue. Methylene blue infusion to enhance visualization of parathyroid glands should be reserved for patients in whom a tumor is strongly suspected but not readily identified during surgery because clinically relevant side effects of methylene blue administration include hemolytic anemia and acute renal failure.[175]

Ultrasound-guided chemical ablation was used safely and effectively as an alternative treatment to surgery in eight dogs with a solitary parathyroid gland mass and hypercalcemia.[310] Serum tCa and iCa concentrations were within reference ranges 24 hours after treatment in seven dogs and within 5 days in one dog. Transient hypocalcemia developed in four dogs during the first 5 days after treatment; one dog required treatment for hypocalcemic tetany. Dysphonia was noted in two of eight dogs in this study, but Horner's syndrome, laryngeal paralysis, and death were not encountered as has been described with ethanol injection of thyroid glands of hyperthyroid cats.[200,540,558] It is likely that the low volume of ethanol injected into a single parathyroid mass provides less potential for leakage beyond the parathyroid mass.

Ultrasonographically guided radiofrequency heat ablation of parathyroid masses in dogs has become the preferred treatment at some referral hospitals. In one study, 11 dogs with either one or two masses on ultrasonography were treated by radiofrequency heat following anesthesia and insertion of a 20-gauge over-the-needle catheter into the mass.[415] Hypocalcemia developed in five of the eight successfully treated dogs, all of which required treatment. The only other adverse effect was a transient voice change in one dog.

Hypervitaminosis D

Hypervitaminosis D refers to toxicity resulting from excess cholecalciferol (vitamin D_3) or ergocalciferol (vitamin D_2). Metabolites of vitamin D can also exert toxicity, and the term hypervitaminosis D has been extended clinically to include toxicity from 25-hydroxyvitamin D, dihydrotachysterol, and 1,25-dihydroxyvitamin D (calcitriol), as well as newer analogues of calcitriol. Vitamin D toxicity is better referred to as 25-hydroxyvitamin D toxicity because vitamin D is rapidly transformed into this metabolite in vivo.[188] Vitamin D and its immediate metabolite, 25-hydroxyvitamin D, have little biologic activity at physiologic concentrations because they have low binding affinity for the VDR. Pharmacologic concentrations of 25-hydroxyvitamin D that occur during hypervitaminosis D exert hypercalcemic effects because 25-hydroxyvitamin D competes with calcitriol for binding to the VDR in target tissues.[153,366] Hypercalcemia results from increased intestinal absorption of calcium, but increased osteoclastic bone resorption and calcium reabsorption from renal distal tubules may also contribute.

Vitamin D intoxication and hypercalcemia may result from excessive dietary supplementation or may be caused iatrogenically during the treatment of hypoparathyroidism. Accurate dosing with cholecalciferol and ergocalciferol is difficult because they have a slow onset and prolonged duration of action.[37,485] Hypercalcemia developed in 7 of 16 hypoparathyroid dogs during treatment with vitamin D and calcium salt supplementation.[37] Ingestion of toxic plants that contain glycosides of calcitriol (e.g., *Cestrum diurnum*, *Solanum malacoxylon*, and *Trisetum flavescens*) is a potential cause of hypercalcemia in small animals.[390] Vitamin D toxicity associated with ingestion of *C. diurnum* has been reported in a cat.[142] *C. diurnum*, day-blooming jessamine, has achieved increasing popularity as a house plant and should not be confused with jasmine, which is an indoor climbing plant without active vitamin D metabolites.[80]

A diagnosis of hypervitaminosis D in dogs and cats increased with the introduction of cholecalciferol-containing rodenticides in 1985, but this source of intoxication is less common today. Cholecalciferol bait is delivered as pellets that are palatable to some animals and are very toxic when ingested. One manufacturer claimed a low hazard to dogs (oral median lethal dose, 88 mg/kg), but toxicity at a lower dosage (10 mg/kg) was demonstrated.[153,214] High-risk groups include dogs weighing 12 kg or less and those younger than 9 months. Recovery from previous cholecalciferol toxicity can be a risk factor for subsequent occurrence because removal of the source from the premises may not be possible.[108] Toxicity in four cats has also been reported.[353,401] One reason for the few reports of vitamin D toxicity in cats is that they appear to be resistant to cholecalciferol toxicity when the diet is otherwise complete and balanced.[488]

Clinical signs are usually vague and include anorexia, lethargy, vomiting, tremors, constipation, and polyuria. These signs are usually attributed to the effects of hypercalcemia. Hypercalcemia is reversible with early and aggressive therapy by providing enough time for 25-hydroxyvitamin D to be eliminated from the body.[102,140,153] Death occurred in approximately 45% of dogs after developing hypercalcemia from hypervitaminosis D in early reports,[153,214,318,457] but the survival rate was higher in dogs of a later series.[102]

Hypercalcemia usually develops within 24 hours after ingestion,[214] and hypercalcemia is often severe unless serum samples were obtained within 24 hours of ingestion. Mild hyperphosphatemia is often noted. Azotemia is initially absent but can develop subsequently. Serum creatinine concentration usually is less than 3 mg/dL unless treatment has been delayed, in which case azotemia may be marked. It may take as long as 72 hours for azotemia to develop as a result of renal lesions caused by hypercalcemia. Measurement of serum 25-hydroxyvitamin D concentration can provide conclusive evidence for hypervitaminosis D after exposure to cholecalciferol or ergocalciferol. Serum concentrations of 25-hydroxyvitamin D were increased to at least twice the upper limit of normal, with a mean concentration approximately 10 times normal in dogs with hypervitaminosis D,[102] and were increased for weeks to months in some instances.[140] In 10 episodes of cholecalciferol intoxication, concentrations of cholecalciferol were increased above the normal range for 10 to 61 days.[108] The half-life for cholecalciferol was 29 days in experimental dogs.[457] Serum calcitriol concentrations were also increased early in the syndrome,[102] but suppression of calcitriol synthesis occurs later. Hypervitaminosis D with hypercalcemia, azotemia, high concentrations of 25-hydroxyvitamin D, and/or renal calcification has been described in cats from Japan fed fish-based commercial cat food.[220,354,465] Cholecalciferol content of these diets exceeded the dietary requirements of vitamin D by more than 100 times.

Renal disease and failure occurred within 4 to 14 months in a large number of cats fed a commercial cat food containing 30 times the vitamin D requirement.[355] All commercial cat foods provide vitamin D in excess of the minimal requirements, and there is no regulated upper limit on the quantity of vitamin D that can be included. Other factors may modulate the toxicity of hypervitaminosis D, such as increased dietary calcium and phosphorus or dietary reduction in magnesium.[488]

Hypercalcemia attributed to the effects of increased calcitriol occasionally occurs during calcitriol treatment in animals with hypoparathyroidism and rarely during treatment of renal secondary hyperparathyroidism. When hypercalcemia is observed, it is usually in patients given doses more than 3.5 ng/kg daily. Discontinuation of calcitriol should result in normocalcemia within 1 week. Dosing with calcitriol at twice the daily dosage every other day up-regulates fewer intestinal epithelial cells for calcium absorption and decreases the chance for further development of hypercalcemia. Formulation errors have also been encountered in which the concentration of calcitriol in a compounded product was too high. There are no veterinary preparations of calcitriol; thus the available preparations of calcitriol must be diluted in pharmaceutical oils for appropriate dosing. Hypercalcemia has also been encountered when dosing errors have been made (mg/kg amounts given as opposed to ng/kg amounts). High serum concentrations of calcitriol have been observed in some dogs with lymphoma and hypercalcemia,[446] but it is not clear whether the excess calcitriol was synthesized by the tumor or by the kidneys under stimulation of PTHrP.

Topical ointments containing potent vitamin D analogues (calcipotriene) for treatment of human psoriasis can result in hypercalcemia when toxic quantities are ingested by dogs.* Minimal toxic dose is 10 µg/kg; minimal lethal dose is 65 µg/kg; and the oral LD50 is between 100 and 150 µg/kg in dogs.[218] In 25 dogs with calcipotriene ingestion, 28% died, and 50% experienced AIRF. Phosphorus, tCa, and iCa are elevated with calcipotriene toxicity.[215,218] The affinity of calcipotriene for vitamin D–binding protein is much lower than that of calcitriol; thus free calcipotriene is readily available for binding to VDRs. The rapid binding to VDRs accounts for the rapid onset of hypercalcemia and hyperphosphatemia and also for the rapid catabolism of calcipotriene. Hypercalcemia decreases after several days rather than being prolonged for weeks to months as seen in cholecalciferol toxicity. Exposure to calcipotriene has not yet been reported in cats, although there are two anecdotal reports (one in Ireland and one in Australia; Boyd Jones, personal communication) of cats that developed hypercalcemia after licking calcipotriene from their owner's skin. Telephone calls to animal poison control centers indicate that exposure to this ointment has been increasing in dogs.[327] Whether calcipotriene cross-reacts with calcitriol in the measurement of vitamin D metabolites has not yet been determined, but it is not detected by methods to measure 25-hydroxyvitamin D.

Granulomatous Disease

Hypercalcemia can result from calcitriol synthesis by activated macrophages during granulomatous inflammation. Normal macrophages express 1α-hydroxylase activity (which converts 25-hydroxyvitamin D to calcitriol) when stimulated by interferon or lipopolysaccharide. Macrophages in granulomatous inflammation express such activity without stimulation.[150] Blastomycosis is a granulomatous disease in dogs that is occasionally (6% to 14% of cases) associated with hypercalcemia. Hypercalcemia is usually mild but can be severe.[13,141] Reports of granulomatous diseases associated with hypercalcemia include two cats with disseminated histoplasmosis[234] and dogs with coccidioidomycosis or schistosomiasis.[168,529] In one dog with schistosomiasis, PTHrP levels were undetectable,[433] but in two other dogs with schistosomiasis, PTHrP levels were increased with no malignancy found at necropsy.[186] In cats, elevated calcitriol concentrations were documented in cases of *Nocardia* and atypical mycobacteria infection.[338] Cats with blastomycosis, cryptococcosis, actinomyces, and injection site granulomas (Chew and Peterson, unpublished observations on injection site granuloma)[338,467,500] have been noted with hypercalcemia possibly because of enhanced synthesis of calcitriol.[141] Severe hypercalcemia was observed in association with noninfectious granulomatous dermatitis in two dogs in which excess synthesis of calcitriol was suspected (Kwochka and Chew, unpublished observations). PTH, PTHrP, and 25-hydroxyvitamin D concentrations were not increased. Hypercalcemia resolved as the inflammation subsided. Nodular panniculitis with hypercalcemia has been reported in dogs, and calcitriol concentrations were two to three times normal in one instance.[157,408]

Idiopathic Hypercalcemia of Cats

Hypercalcemia may be less common in cats than in dogs, although the incidence of hypercalcemia from primary care practices is not reported. Within the past 10 years, IHC has been recognized in cats[336,346] and is now the most common cause of ionized hypercalcemia in cats in the United States. Even though some suggest that IHC is a local geographic phenomenon,[168] it is widespread across the United States and is being recognized in other parts of the world.

In IHC, serum calcium concentration may be increased for months to more than 1 year. In 427 cases of feline IHC, 46% had no clinical signs, 18% had mild weight loss with no other clinical signs, 6% had inflam-

---

References 91,163,218,231,252-254,525.

matory bowel disease, 5% had chronic constipation, 4% were vomiting, and 1% were anorectic.[476] Uroliths or renoliths were observed in 15%, and calcium oxalate stones were noted in 10% of cases. Cats ranged in age from 0.5 to 20 years, and longhaired cats accounted for 27% of the cases (compared with an overall submission rate of 14% from longhaired cats). There was no sex predilection. Serum iCa concentration was increased; PTH concentration was in the lower half of the reference range; and PTHrP was negative in all samples. Concentration of iMg was normal, and mean concentration of 25-hydroxyvitamin D was within the reference range. Calcitriol was measured in a small number of these cats and was suppressed. In another study, 1 of 7 cats exhibited an increased concentration of calcitriol, and 2 of 11 cats had increased PTHrP in the absence of underlying neoplasia following extensive diagnostic evaluation, survival for many months, and necropsy.[346] It appears that excessive PTH, 25-hydroxyvitamin D, or calcitriol concentration is not the cause of IHC in most cats. However, normal concentrations of calcitriol could result in hypercalcemia if there are mutations of the VDR or an increase in number of calcitriol receptors. Normal concentrations of iMg indicate that PTH secretion is not inhibited by decreased or excess iMg.[476] Renal function, based on BUN and serum creatinine concentration, is usually normal initially, but some cats develop CRF secondary to long-standing IHC.[346] Results of serology testing for feline leukemia virus and feline immunodeficiency virus have been negative, and serum thyroxine concentrations have been normal. Chronic acidosis could explain chronic elevations of iCa,[116] but venous blood gas analysis has not revealed significant acid-base disturbances. Exploration of the cervical region has not identified primary hyperparathyroidism, and subtotal parathyroidectomy has not resolved hypercalcemia in cats in which this procedure was performed.[346]

As many as 35% of cats with calcium oxalate urinary stones have hypercalcemia. Even though the specifics of the underlying diagnoses were not detailed,[386] it is likely that most had IHC. The occurrence of ureterolithiasis in cats was very uncommon before 1993. Eleven cases of calcium oxalate ureterolithiasis were recently described in cats, and four had mild to moderate hypercalcemia.[295] It appears that the frequency of hypercalcemia in calcium oxalate stone-forming cats has decreased substantially (Lulich, personal communications, 2003).

Specific treatment for IHC is impossible because the pathogenesis remains unknown. Increased bone resorption, increased intestinal absorption, or decreased renal excretion of calcium or combinations of these mechanisms could be responsible for hypercalcemia. The feeding of increased dietary fiber decreased serum calcium in some cats[336] but not in others.[346] The beneficial effect of a higher fiber diet may be because of decreased intestinal absorption of dietary calcium. The effects of fiber on intestinal absorption are complex and depend on the types and amounts of fiber in the diet and other nutrients present.

The feeding of veterinary renal diets may result in normocalcemia in some cats with IHC. These diets are generally low in calcium and phosphorus and are considered alkalinizing or at least less acidifying than maintenance diets. Some cats that show an initial decrease in serum calcium concentration following any type of dietary change will have a return to hypercalcemia over time.

In those cats that do not respond to a change in diet, prednisone therapy may result in a long-term decrease in iCa. The effects of glucocorticosteroid treatment may last for months to years in some cats with doses of 5 to 20 mg prednisone/cat/day. There is an escape from the effects of glucocorticosteroid treatment in some cats and a return to hypercalcemia despite maximal doses of prednisone. When dietary modification and treatment with prednisolone have been unsuccessful in resolving IHC, intravenous pamidronate treatment can be considered.

Beneficial effects from the chronic administration of subcutaneous fluids or oral furosemide to cats with IHC have not been evaluated. Treatment with calcimimetics could be of benefit. Calcimimetics interact with the calcium receptor and are effective in decreasing calcium, phosphorus, and PTH in human patients.[50]

Uncommon Causes of Hypercalcemia

AIRF in dogs is occasionally associated with mild hypercalcemia. Hypercalcemia may occur more commonly after conversion of oliguria to polyuria, possibly as calcium salts that were deposited during oliguria are mobilized from soft tissues. Sudden improvement in renal function also may result in rapid decrease of serum phosphorus concentration, changing mass law interactions between phosphorus and calcium and resulting in transient hypercalcemia. Mild hypercalcemia (11.5 to 12.5 mg/dL) is observed uncommonly in some dogs with severe oliguria and decreased GFR during intrinsic renal failure. Animals with severe hyperphosphatemia during AIRF usually have normal or low serum calcium concentrations.

Nonmalignant skeletal lesions are occasionally associated with hypercalcemia in dogs. Bacterial and fungal osteomyelitis can potentially result in hypercalcemia if the rate of osteolysis is sufficient.[106] Neonatal septicemia has been associated with hypercalcemia on rare occasion in puppies after septic embolization of bone and subsequent osteolysis.[106] Mild hypercalcemia occurs in some dogs with hypertrophic osteodystrophy, and the hypercalcemia may be aggravated by ascorbic acid supplementation.[509] Hypothermia has caused hypercalcemia in one cat.[391] One cat with pancreatitis and hypercalcemia has been described, even though hypocalcemia is more common in cases of pancreatitis.[231] In one report, a dog receiving intermittent calcium therapy for hypocalcemia developed hypercalcemia and acute pancreatic hemorrhage that may have been related to excessive calcium therapy.[371] Dehydration may cause mild and reversible hypercalcemia, especially with normal kidney function. Disuse osteoporosis after prolonged immobilization can rarely contribute to the development of mild hypercalcemia because weight bearing is necessary to maintain the balance between new bone formation and resorption of old bone. Serum total hypercalcemia has been noted in a small percentage of hyperthyroid cats,[25,467] but iCa concentration is normal. In cats with untreated hyperthyroidism, mild ionized hypercalcemia that resolved following conversion to euthyroidism with treatment has been uncommonly noted (Chew, unpublished observations). Overuse of calcium-containing intestinal phosphate binders can occasionally cause hypercalcemia.[106] An unusual case of hypercalcemia was attributed to the chronic ingestion of calcium carbonate in the form of limestone rocks.[273] Malignant histiocytosis in dogs was reported in association with hypercalcemia in one dog.[534]

The ingestion of large amounts of grapes or raisins may result in hypercalcemia. Seven of 10 dogs with renal failure associated with grape or raisin ingestion had increased serum tCa concentrations (12.3 to 26 mg/dL) and increased serum phosphorus (6.4 to 22 mg/dL) 24 hours to several days following ingestion.[215] In four dogs, ingestion was estimated to be from 0.41 to 1.1 ounces of grapes or raisins per kilogram of body weight. Oliguria or anuria was noted in 5 of 10 dogs, and 5 of 10 dogs survived. These cases were clustered from 1999 to 2001, and raisin/grape toxicity has not been previously reported.

Vomiting following ingestion of what appears to be a trivial quantity of raisins or grapes in some dogs leads to the development of AIRF usually within 48 hours. Not all dogs that consume grapes or raisins develop clinical signs or acute renal failure. Of 132 dogs reported with raisin or grape ingestion, 33 developed no clinical signs or azotemia, and 14 of 133 dogs developed clinical signs but no azotemia.[160] Of 132 cases, 43 dogs developed clinical signs and AIRF. The pathogenesis of nephrotoxicity associated with raisins and grapes remains unknown, but it is speculated that ochratoxin may be a toxic component.[409] Tubular degeneration and necrosis of varying severity are consistently described and most pronounced in proximal tubules.[160,357]

In some cases of grape/raisin ingestion with AIRF, mild to severe hypercalcemia develops, and in some dogs, serum tCa concentration can change dramatically from day to day during various treatments.[334] With acute renal failure following ingestion of raisins or grapes, hypercalcemia was detected in 93% of affected dogs, and tCa ranged from 8 to 26 mg/dL.[160,215] Of 40 dogs, 23 (57.5%) survived, and 17 (42.5%) failed to survive; 15 of 23 underwent complete resolution of azotemia. Initial

and peak serum tCa concentration and initial and peak calcium x phosphorus product were significantly higher in those that did not survive as compared with those that did survive. Hypercalcemia was documented in 1 of 3 dogs evaluated within 24 hours of ingestion, in 2 of 8 dogs within 24 to 48 hours, and in 12 of 13 dogs evaluated for the first time 48 to 72 hours after ingestion. Total calcium concentration returned to the normal range in a median of 11 days (range, 2 to 51 days). Unfortunately, iCa measurements have yet to be reported for any dogs with raisin toxicity, AIRF, and hypercalcemia based on serum tCa. Because many dogs with severe AIRF have hyperphosphatemia, some of the increased serum tCa may be because of complex formation with phosphate. The observation that serum tCa concentration can dramatically increase or decrease daily during treatment suggests that its origin is related to extracellular or intravascular fluid volume dynamics.

A favorable outcome is possible in about 50% of cases, but several weeks of hospitalization with intensive fluid treatment is often needed in those with AIRF, especially if oliguric. About 50% of affected dogs can be expected to develop oliguria or anuria.[160,215,334] A case of AIRF with a fatal outcome occurred after ingestion of 450 g of raisins in a vizsla dog despite intensive treatment including peritoneal dialysis.[397] Aggressive treatment has been recommended for any dogs suspected of having ingested large, or even small, quantities of grapes or raisins, including induction of emesis, gastric lavage, and administration of activated charcoal, followed by intravenous fluid therapy for a minimum of 48 hours.[215] However, some dogs may consume relatively large quantities of grapes or raisins without development of ill effects.

Hypercalcemia was reported in a dog with a retained fetus and endometritis.[232] Serum PTH was suppressed, and 25-hydroxyvitamin D concentration was within the normal range. Biopsy of the removed uterus documented neutrophilic inflammation but no granulomatous inflammation as a possible cause of the hypercalcemia. Serum iCa was normal 4 days after surgical removal of the uterus, and serum tCa was normal 6 weeks later.

Humoral hypercalcemia of benignancy is a phrase used to describe the association of humoral factors such as PTHrP and hypercalcemia in the absence of malignancy.[186,279] One dog with massive mammary gland hyperplasia, severe ionized hypercalcemia, and increased PTHrP in the absence of malignancy at necropsy has been observed (Chew, unpublished observations). This phenomenon has rarely been described in humans.[258,269]

TREATMENT OF HYPERCALCEMIA
Philosophy of Treatment

There is no absolute serum calcium concentration that can be used as a guideline for the decision to treat hypercalcemia aggressively.[109,174] The magnitude of hypercalcemia, its rate of development, whether the serum calcium concentration is stable or progressively increasing, and the modifying effects of other electrolyte and acid-base disturbances must all be considered when deciding on a treatment plan. The clinical condition of the animal ultimately dictates how aggressive treatment should be, but a serum calcium concentration of 16 mg/dL or greater has been recommended as a basis for aggressive therapy.[174] Animals with serum calcium concentrations approaching 20 mg/dL should be considered candidates for crisis management. Animals with serum calcium concentrations less than 16 mg/dL may also require aggressive treatment, depending on the degree of neurologic, cardiac, and renal dysfunction induced by the hypercalcemia and concurrent deleterious factors. Acidosis can magnify the effects of hypercalcemia at all serum calcium concentrations by shifting more calcium to the ionized fraction. The serum phosphorus concentration at the time of hypercalcemia is also an important modulating factor in clinical decision making because soft tissue mineralization is potentiated by hyperphosphatemia. Animals with rapid and progressive development of hypercalcemia usually display serious clinical signs that require aggressive therapy.

Definitive Therapy

Removal of the underlying cause is the definitive treatment for hypercalcemia. Most animals with pathologic hypercalcemia have an associated malignancy that is quickly diagnosed but often not readily treated. Complete excision of isolated neoplasms (e.g., apocrine gland adenocarcinoma of the anal sac and parathyroid gland adenoma) abolishes hypercalcemia. In animals with disseminated metastases, multicentric neoplasia, or nonresectable primary malignancy, the tumor burden and hypercalcemia may be decreased by appropriate chemotherapy, radiation therapy, and immunotherapy. Chemotherapy may disrupt neoplastic cellular metabolism to such an extent that the tumor may no longer be able to synthesize enough humoral factors to sustain hypercalcemia. Decreased serum calcium concentrations can occur despite lack of obvious reduction in tumor size in these instances.

Antifungal treatment with amphotericin B, ketoconazole, or itraconazole effectively lowers increased serum calcium concentrations in dogs with systemic mycoses as the infectious agent is eradicated and inflammation resolves. For animals with hypercalcemia associated with hypoadrenocorticism, replacement therapy with mineralocorticoids and glucocorticoids after fluid volume replacement definitively manages the condition. Discontinuing all vitamin D supplementation in animals with hypervitaminosis D and hypercalcemia removes the external cause of intoxication, but excessive body stores of vitamin D may continue to contribute to hypercalcemia for several weeks.

Supportive Therapy

Supportive therapy is often necessary to decrease serum calcium concentration to a less toxic level while waiting for a definitive diagnosis to be established, for definitive treatment to reduce serum calcium concentration permanently, or for chronic management of hypercalcemia when the underlying cause cannot be removed. Box 6-3 and Table 6-3 list general and specific treatments for the management of hypercalcemia. Unfortunately, no single treatment protocol is consistently effective for all causes of hypercalcemia. Consequently, regimens must be tailored for the individual patient. Supportive treatments reduce the magnitude of hypercalcemia by increasing renal calcium excretion, inhibiting bone resorption, promoting soft tissue deposition of calcium, causing a shift of intravascular calcium to other body compartments, promoting extrarenal calcium loss, reducing calcium transport across the gut, or some combination of these effects.[109,291,327]

Initial Considerations for Treatment

Parenteral fluids, furosemide, sodium bicarbonate, glucocorticoids, or combinations of these treatments effectively reduce serum calcium concentrations in most animals. Repeatable serum hypercalcemia should be confirmed before prescribing aggressive treatments. It is not necessary to reduce serum calcium concentration to within normal limits, but substantial resolution of serious clinical signs may occur when serum tCa concentration decreases by as little as 1 to 3 mg/dL.

Box 6-3	**General Treatment of Hypercalcemia**

Definitive
    Remove underlying cause

Supportive
    Initial considerations
        Fluids (0.9% sodium chloride)
        Furosemide
        Calcitonin
    Secondary considerations
        Glucocorticosteroids
        Bisphosphonates
    Tertiary considerations
        Sodium bicarbonate
        Mithramycin (severe toxicity)
        Ethylenediamine tetraacetic acid (EDTA) (severe toxicity)
        Dialysis
    Future considerations
        Calcium channel blockers
        Somatostatin congeners
        Calcium receptor agonists
        Nonhypercalcemic calcitriol analogues

TABLE 6-3 Specific Treatment of Hypercalcemia

Treatment	Dose	Indications	Comments
Volume Expansion			
Subcutaneous saline (0.9%)*	75-100 mL/kg/day	Mild hypercalcemia	Contraindicated if peripheral edema is present.
Intravenous saline (0.9%)*	100-125 mL/kg/day	Moderate to severe hypercalcemia	Contraindicated in congestive heart failure and hypertension. Minimal decreases of calcium as single therapy when cause is severe pathologic hypercalcemia.
Diuretics			
Furosemide	2-4 mg/kg BID to TID IV, SQ, PO	Moderate to severe hypercalcemia	Volume expansion is necessary before use of this drug. Rapid onset of action.
Alkalinizing Agent			
Sodium bicarbonate	1 mEq/kg IV slow bolus; may give up to 4 mEq/kg total dose	Severe hypercalcemia	Requires close monitoring. Rapid onset of action.
Glucocorticoids			
Prednisone	1-2.2 mg/kg BID PO, SQ, IV	Moderate to severe hypercalcemia	Use of these drugs before identification of etiology may make definitive diagnosis difficult or impossible.
Dexamethasone	0.1-0.22 mg/kg BID IV, SQ		
Bone Resorption Inhibitors			
Calcitonin	4-6 IU/kg SQ BID to TID	Hypervitaminosis D	Response may be short-lived. Vomiting may occur. Rapid onset of action.
Bisphosphonates			
EHDP–didronel	15 mg/kg SID to BID	Moderate to severe hypercalcemia	Delayed onset of action.
Clodronate	20-25 mg/kg in a 4-hr IV infusion		Clodronate is approved for use in humans in Europe; availability in U.S. may be limited.
Pamidronate	1.3 mg/kg in 150 mL 0.9% saline a 2-hr IV infusion; can repeat in 1 week		Very expensive
Mithramycin	25 µg/kg IV in 5% dextrose over 2 to 4 hr every 2 to 4 weeks	Severe hypercalcemia, refractory HHM	Limited use in dogs and cats. Nephrotoxicity, hepatoxicity, thrombocytopenia.
Miscellaneous			
Sodium EDTA	25-75 mg/kg/hr	Severe hypercalcemia	Nephrotoxicity
Peritoneal dialysis	Low calcium dialysate	Severe hypercalcemia	Short duration of response. Use in hypercalcemia not reported.

Potassium supplementation is necessary. Add 5 to 40 mEq KCl/L depending on serum potassium concentration.
BID, Twice daily; TID, thrice daily; PO, oral; IV, intravenous; SQ, subcutanous; SID, once daily; HHM, humoral hypercalcemia of malignancy.

Fluid Therapy. Parenteral fluid therapy is an important first treatment for all animals with hypercalcemia. The first goal of fluid therapy is to correct dehydration because hemoconcentration contributes to increased serum calcium concentration. In addition, the kidney responds during ECF volume contraction with more avid reabsorption of sodium and calcium from the glomerular ultrafiltrate. Correction of dehydration abrogates this effect and allows calciuresis and natriuresis to occur.

Dehydration should be corrected with intravenous fluids within 4 to 6 hours of presentation in animals with severe clinical signs attributable to hypercalcemia. Additional expansion of ECF volume with parenteral fluids is then indicated, but sufficient fluid for rehydration and volume expansion is often provided simultaneously. Fluid therapy alone may be sufficient in some animals to reduce the magnitude of hypercalcemia adequately when the initial serum calcium concentration is less than 14 mg/dL, but often other treatments must be added. Normocalcemia may be restored by fluid therapy alone if hypercalcemia was initially mild (12 to 13 mg/dL).

Physiologic saline (0.9% NaCl) is the solution of choice for correction of the intravascular volume deficit and for further slight volume expansion. Slight volume expansion with 0.9% NaCl promotes calcium loss in urine secondary to increased GFR and increased filtered load of calcium, and competition from the additional sodium ions results in reduced renal tubular calcium reabsorption and enhanced calciuresis.

ECF volume expansion with lactated Ringer's solution (6 mg/dL calcium) in dogs results in decreased total protein, tCa, and iCa concentrations. Decreases in tCa concentration were greater (12.4%) than those observed for iCa concentration (3.5%).[425] Thus volume expansion with solutions that contain some calcium can be beneficial because the dilutional effect supersedes the effect of the additional calcium that is administered. However, physiologic saline (0.9% NaCl) is preferred because it is devoid of additional calcium and contains more sodium than that in lactated Ringer's solution (154 versus 130 mEq/L). Consequently, 0.9% NaCl results in a more rapid reduction in serum calcium concentration. An initial fluid volume of two to three times maintenance needs (120 to 180 mL/kg/day) usually corrects dehydration, provides maintenance needs, and results in mild volume expansion. The use of sodium phosphate is not recommended because of the potential detrimental effects of soft tissue mineralization.[174]

Diuretics (Calciuretics). Administration of furosemide follows rehydration and fluid volume expansion as second in importance for treatment of persistent hypercalcemia. Furosemide promotes enhanced urinary calcium loss, but calciuresis does not follow the use of all diuretics. In particular, thiazides should not be used because they may result in hypocalciuria and potentially may aggravate hypercalcemia. Furosemide (5 mg/kg intravenously, followed by 5 mg/kg/hr as an infusion) acutely decreases serum tCa by a maximum of approximately 3 mg/dL.[384] It is important to match the increased volume of urine lost with an increased volume of parenteral fluids to prevent dehydration and to gain maximal calciuresis. Less aggressive regimens of furosemide administration may be effective in combination with other treatments or for chronic management of hypercalcemia. Adequate hydration before and during furosemide administration is essential; otherwise, diuresis may increase serum calcium concentration through hemoconcentration. Diuresis, natriuresis, and calciuresis were greater in greyhounds given a continuous rate infusion of furosemide (0.66 mg/kg bolus, followed by 0.66 mg/kg/hr for 8 hours) compared with intermittent furosemide (3 mg/kg at 0 and 4 hours).[5]

Sodium Bicarbonate. Infusion of sodium bicarbonate has been advocated for acute or crisis management of hypercalcemia, but most often it is mentioned for use in the presence of metabolic acidosis.[5,109,290] Serum iCa concentration is reduced as acidosis is corrected or mild alkalosis is created because more calcium becomes bound to serum proteins, and there is increased binding of calcium to bicarbonate.[425] Decreases in ionized and tCa concentrations after bicarbonate infusions have been observed in dogs[345] and cats.[110] A dosage of 1 to 4 mEq/kg sodium bicarbonate has been recommended to obtain the desired reduction in calcium concentration,[110,290] but it may not be necessary to provide continuous bicarbonate infusion because the effect can last for as long as 3 hours after a single dose of bicarbonate in normal cats.[110] Reduction in serum calcium concentration is slight after administration of sodium bicarbonate alone, but the effect increases with larger doses. Sodium bicarbonate infusion is most likely to be helpful in combination with other treatments.

Steroids. Glucocorticosteroids can contribute to a significant reduction in serum iCa concentration in hypercalcemic animals with lymphoma, apocrine gland adenocarcinoma of the anal sac, multiple myeloma, thymoma, hypoadrenocorticism, hypervitaminosis D, hypervitaminosis A, or granulomatous disease, but they have little effect on serum iCa concentration in animals with other causes of hypercalcemia (Box 6-4). Some cats with IHC also have a substantial decrease in serum iCa concentration after glucocorticoid treatment. Steroids exert their effect mainly by reducing bone resorption, decreasing intestinal calcium absorption, and increasing renal calcium excretion.[107,302]

Cytotoxicity against neoplastic lymphocytes after glucocorticoids can result in a dramatic and rapid reduction in serum calcium concentration in dogs with lymphoma. Whenever possible, however, glucocorticoids should be withheld from animals for which a diagnosis has not yet been established because lymphocytolysis can make a definitive histopathologic diagnosis of lymphoma much more difficult or impossible. A challenge test for the diagnosis of occult lymphoma has been proposed using L-asparaginase at 20,000 IU/m^2 intravenously in an effort to disturb tumor cell metabolism but not cause cytolysis. Calcium concentrations are measured at baseline and then every 12 to 24 hours for 72 hours. A complete return of serum calcium concentration to normal suggests occult lymphoma.[168] Once a diagnosis of lymphoma has been made, prednisone is usually administered at 1 to 2 mg/kg twice daily concomitant with chemotherapy.

Decreased bone resorption after administration of glucocorticoids may be the result of impaired osteoclast maturation and decreased numbers of calcitriol receptors in bone.[498] Cortisol antagonizes the effects of vitamin D on the intestine in rats.[219] In dogs, chronic oral administration of prednisone (1.2 to 1.5 mg/kg/day) resulted in decreased serum calcitriol concentrations but caused no change in the number of calcitriol receptors or calcium-binding proteins in enterocytes.[283] Granulomatous diseases associated with increased calcitriol synthesis and hypercalcemia are often sensitive to the effects of glucocorticoids in reducing the serum calcium concentration.[424,483] However, caution is advised because the underlying disease (e.g., systemic mycosis) may be worsened. Hypercalcemia associated with hypervitaminosis A can also be steroid responsive.[38]

Calcitonin. Calcitonin treatment may be useful in animals with severe hypercalcemia. Calcitonin should be considered instead of prednisone for treatment of animals without a definitive diagnosis. Calcitonin rapidly decreases the magnitude of hypercalcemia primarily by reducing the activity and formation of osteoclasts. A maximal decrement in serum tCa concentration of approximately 3 mg/dL can be expected.[111] The only known adverse effects of calcitonin are anorexia and vomiting, but relatively few treated dogs and cats have been evaluated. Calcitonin treatment is expensive; the magnitude

of its effect is unpredictable; its effects may be short-lived (hours); and resistance often develops in a few days. Receptor down-regulation is thought to be responsible for development of resistance, a phenomenon that may be delayed by concurrent glucocorticoid treatment. The effectiveness of calcitonin may be restored after discontinuing treatment for 24 to 48 hours.[327] Despite these limitations, calcitonin in combination with pamidronate is considered the best therapy for severe malignancy-associated hypercalcemia in humans.[118,480]

The dosage of calcitonin in animals has been extrapolated from that used in humans (4 IU/kg intravenously, followed by 4 to 8 IU/kg subcutaneously once or twice daily).[291] Calcitonin is listed as an antidote on packages of cholecalciferol-containing (vitamin D) rat poison, and treatment with calcitonin has been reported in dogs with hypercalcemia resulting from cholecalciferol toxicity. The dosage of calcitonin used in these dogs was 8 IU/kg subcutaneously every 24 hours,[183] 5 IU/kg subcutaneously every 6 hours,[194] and 4 to 7 IU/kg subcutaneously every 6 to 8 hours.[140] Short-term calcitonin treatment (6 U/kg subcutaneously every 8 hours for 2 days) was not effective in controlling hypercalcemia in dogs when measured 4 days after ingestion of cholecalciferol.[457] Vomiting was common within 2 hours of calcitonin administration. Calcitonin (4 U/kg every 4 hours for the first day and then 8 mg/kg twice daily for the next 3 days) decreased serum tCa from nearly 18 mg/dL to 13 to 15 mg/dL, but the effect only lasted 4 to 8 hours.[232] Calcitonin has also been used as part of combination therapy for treatment of hypercalcemia in a cat with granulomatous disease.[338]

Bisphosphonates. Bisphosphonates (formerly misnamed diphosphonates) are drugs (pyrophosphate analogues) that have been developed to inhibit bone resorption.[53,431] The hypocalcemic effects of bisphosphonates during malignancy are bone related because there is no effect on tumor mass. Bisphosphonates decrease osteoclast activity and function, despite increased numbers of osteoclasts present as a result of local or humoral mechanisms of osteolysis. Inhibition of resorption requires 1 to 2 days. Long-term bisphosphonate administration can lead to decreased osteoclast numbers through lethal injury of osteoclasts and decreased recruitment of new osteoclasts. Etidronate was the first bisphosphonate to be used clinically, and the activity of newer bisphosphonates is often compared with that of etidronate. Etidronate and clodronate are non-amino bisphosphonates. The addition of an amine group to one of the side chains increases the antiresorptive action in bone (alendronate, residronate, ibandronate, and zoledronate). The greatest potency to date has been obtained in those compounds containing a tertiary amine (zoledronate).[349] Clodronate, pamidronate, alendronate, and residronate have potencies 10, 100,

1000, and 5000 times as great as that of etidronate, respectively.[181] Ibandronate is approximately 5000 times and zoledronate is more than 10,000 times the potency of etidronate.[372,374] Zoledronate is 100 to 850 times more active than pamidronate.[54]

Inhibition of bone resorption by pamidronate occurs earlier and is maintained longer than that induced by etidronate. Intravenous infusion of pamidronate has been the treatment of choice for severe hypercalcemia associated with malignancy in humans,[55,118,125] controlling cancer-induced hypercalcemia in more than 70%[466] to 90% of human patients.[55] The use of intravenous zoledronate is the new treatment of choice because of its increased potency over pamidronate, as well as the more convenient infusion protocol of only 15 minutes.* Serum tCa decreases more rapidly, and maintenance of normocalcemia is nearly twice as long when treated with zoledronate compared with pamidronate.[557]

Bisphosphonate treatment occasionally has been associated with the development of renal impairment in humans and AIRF in experimental animals.[315] This effect was seen after multiple doses and in some with preexisting renal disease.[22,315,325,399] Renal toxicity in dogs may be more likely when doses of 10 mg/kg or more of pamidronate are given.[456] The rate of infusion and the particular bisphosphonate chosen influence the possibilities for nephrotoxicity.[3,349] Dehydration should be corrected before bisphosphonates are administered to lessen chances of renal injury. Depending on the bisphosphonate used, several hours of 0.9% saline infusion may be required to attenuate potential adverse effects. Pamidronate infusion in humans with hypercalcemia and underlying renal failure was shown to be safe in some studies.[36,315,533]

In a model of cholecalciferol-induced hypercalcemia, dogs treated with pamidronate (1.3 mg/kg in 150 mL saline administered intravenously over 2 hours) starting 1 day following ingestion lost less weight and had significantly lower serum concentrations of phosphorus, tCa, and iCa than those treated with saline or calcitonin. Mean serum tCa decreased to within the reference range, and values for iCa decreased but not to the same degree as that for tCa following pamidronate treatment.[457] In a subsequent study, three different doses of pamidronate were given to dogs after a single dose of cholecalciferol.[456] Clinical signs were fewest in dogs given the two higher doses of pamidronate. All dogs given any dosage of pamidronate were alert and lost less weight compared with saline treatment. The decreases in serum tCa were dose dependent. Pamidronate lessened the reduction in GFR in a dose-dependent manner, but GFR was still reduced by 20% to 25% on day 14 (end of study). Minimal histopathologic lesions were seen in dogs treated with the low and intermediate doses of pamidronate; no lesions were detected in dogs treated with the high dose of pamidronate. It appears that doses of pamidronate at 2.0 mg/kg are most effective in dogs with cholecalciferol toxicity.

Clodronate was used clinically to treat hypercalcemia of malignancy in one dog and hypervitaminosis D in another dog.[408] Serum iCa and tCa concentrations were normal at 36 and 48 hours after a 4-hour infusion of clodronate (20 to 25 mg/kg), but long-term results were not reported. In a dog with severe hypercalcemia associated with adenocarcinoma of the anal sac, a single 2-hour infusion of pamidronate rapidly reduced serum tCa and iCa that had not previously responded to intravenous fluids, calcitonin, and furosemide.[262] In seven dogs with clinical calcipotriene toxicity, pamidronate (1.3 to 2.0 mg/kg intravenously) resulted in a decrease in tCa, phosphorus, and creatinine.[215] In another clinical report, seven dogs and two cats were given pamidronate (1.05 to 2.0 mg/kg intravenously) for a variety of disease processes, and treatment rapidly decreased serum calcium without evidence of toxicosis.[244] In dogs with bone tumors, intravenous pamidronate (1 mg/kg given over 2 hours as a constant rate infusion) was administered every 28 days depending on progression of the bone tumor.[162] One hundred thirty-three doses of intravenous pamidronate were given to this group of 33 dogs. Only one dog developed renal toxicity 16 days following the second pamidronate treatment; this dog also had paraneoplastic hypercalcemia. Based on these findings, pamidronate at multiple doses may safely and effectively lower both serum total and iCa concentrations in patients with hypercalcemia resulting from various disease processes.

Oral bisphosphonate therapy is generally designed for maintenance treatment after a course of intravenous bisphosphonates has been effective in the control of hypercalcemia. Less than 5% of orally administered bisphosphonate is absorbed from the gastrointestinal tract,[182] which limits the usefulness of oral forms of etidronate, clodronate, and alendronate.[210] Food in the stomach markedly reduces the oral absorption of some bisphosphonates.[198] Increasing the dose can slightly increase the oral absorption of bisphosphonates.[349] Etidronate is generally administered orally to dogs at 10 to 40 mg/kg/day in divided doses, and it has had some effectiveness in reduction of hypercalcemia associated with lymphoma, myeloma, primary hyperparathyroidism, and hypervitaminosis D in dogs (Chew and Couto, unpublished observations). A puppy with hypercalcemia and primary hyperparathyroidism was also successfully treated using etidronate.[517] There is concern about the oral administration of some bisphosphonates to humans because nausea, vomiting, abdominal pain, dyspepsia, esophagitis, and esophageal reflux can be adverse effects.[47] Both clodronate and alendronate have been used orally in humans,[34,249] but

---

*References 35,78,321,322,373,399,557.

there are no clinical studies in dogs or cats using these drugs orally.

Both clodronate and pamidronate have safely and effectively been given subcutaneously for the control of hypercalcemia in people.[149,432] Use of subcutaneous clodronate was better tolerated than subcutaneous pamidronate.[541,542] The subcutaneous route has not yet been investigated for use in dogs or cats with hypercalcemia.

Other Miscellaneous Treatments. Mithramycin is a potent inhibitor of osteoclastic bone resorption.[440,443] Significant toxicity, including thrombocytopenia, hepatic necrosis, renal necrosis, and hypocalcemia, unfortunately has been reported with the use of this drug.[111,174,290] Mithramycin was safe when two doses of 0.1 mg/kg were administered intravenously 1 week apart to eight normal beagle dogs. Mithramycin decreased serum iCa concentration in these normal dogs without adverse side effects such as hepatotoxicity, nephrotoxicity, or bone marrow hypoplasia, but some shivering occurred during the infusion. Osteoclastic bone resorption was significantly reduced.[443] Mithramycin was used to treat cancer-associated hypercalcemia in client-owned dogs.[444] A single infusion of 0.1 mg/kg to two dogs resulted in normal serum tCa concentration within 24 hours, but severe hepatocellular necrosis associated with marked vomiting, diarrhea, and fever resulted in death shortly thereafter. To decrease additional episodes of toxicity, the dosage of mithramycin was decreased to 25 µg/kg for the remaining dogs in this study. Serum calcium concentration returned to the normal range in six of nine dogs within 24 to 48 hours of treatment. Toxicity at this dosage was minimal, but the calcium-lowering effect lasted only 24 to 72 hours in three dogs. PTHrP concentrations and tumor size remained unchanged after treatment, and the lowering of serum calcium concentration was attributed to decreased osteoclastic bone resorption. Mithramycin is seldom prescribed because of its toxicity in hypercalcemic dogs at higher dosages and the short-lived effect at lower dosages.

During a hypercalcemic crisis, EDTA can be infused at a dosage of 25 to 75 mg/kg/hr. Administered EDTA combines with circulating calcium to form a soluble complex that then is excreted by the kidneys.[111] This treatment is considered a rescue method designed to allow other modalities time to take effect. Use of EDTA should be reserved for crisis situations because EDTA is nephrotoxic at higher dosages. A 2-hour infusion of EDTA in normal dogs at 25 mg/kg/hr did not have detrimental effects on the kidneys.[527]

Hemodialysis or peritoneal dialysis with calcium-free dialysate may be used to lower serum calcium concentration when other methods fail.[93,282] Dialysis may be particularly helpful in animals with severe intrinsic renal failure caused by hypercalcemia. Clinical experience with this method of treatment in animals is limited.

Future Considerations

Calcimimetics are a new class of compounds that are able to activate the calcium receptor, stopping PTH secretion.[161,536] Cinacalcet (Sensipar, Amgen Inc., Thousand Oaks, CA) has been marketed for use in human renal secondary hyperparathyroidism.[50,187,369] This drug is expensive, and it is available only as a solid tablet, making its use in small animals problematic because creating smaller doses is very difficult. Despite their action on calcium receptors throughout the body rather than exclusively on the calcium receptors of the parathyroid glands, calcimimetics may have promise in treating hypercalcemias of any type, including idiopathic hypercalcemia of cats. In the future, calcimimetics for veterinary use may be developed.

The calcium channel blocker diltiazem reduces the magnitude of hypercalcemia and soft tissue mineralization in vitamin D toxicosis in chicks[153] and may be effective in hypercalcemia of other causes. The toxic effects of hypercalcemia on the cardiovascular system of dogs can be blunted by verapamil,[30,579,581] and this drug may prove useful for stabilizing dogs and cats with severe hypercalcemia until other measures to decrease serum calcium concentration become effective.

Most treatments for HHM have focused on counteracting the effects of excess PTHrP rather than inhibiting PTHrP secretion. Somatostatin congeners inhibit secretion of certain hormones, and one congener, lanreotide, successfully reduced serum calcium and PTHrP concentrations in a human patient with HHM.[12] Similar results were observed in other tumors in humans treated with octreotide.[348,358,410,532]

Nonhypercalcemic analogues of calcitriol have been reported to inhibit cell proliferation and PTHrP production by neoplastic tissue in vitro.[337,576] These new modalities for treating hypercalcemia in conditions associated with increased PTHrP appear to be safe, are easy to use, and are effective.[290]

Gallium nitrate is an antineoplastic, radioprotectant drug that has hypocalcemic properties related to its ability to reduce the solubility of hydroxyapatite in bone and inhibit osteoclast function. Gallium nitrate has been considered for treatment of refractory hypercalcemia, but it requires constant infusion.[43,291,382,547] Gallium nitrate was more effective in control of hypercalcemia for longer periods than etidronate or pamidronate in a recent study of humans. Treatment with gallium nitrate may be more effective than bisphosphonates in cancer-related hypercalcemia in those with the highest concentrations of PTHrP.[301] The cytoprotectant amifostine (investigational drug WR-2721) inhibits PTH secretion and may have effectiveness in animals with hyperparathyroidism.[551] Use of amifostine has been limited to humans, and its adverse effects include nausea, vomiting, somnolence, and hypotension.[43]

Additional Specific Treatments for Hypervitaminosis D

In hypervitaminosis D associated with cholecalciferol intoxication, treatment may be necessary for several weeks because of the long half-lives of cholecalciferol and vitamin D metabolites. Consequently, aggressive fluid therapy for 1 week or more may be required to correct the severe hypercalcemia that is often encountered. Prednisone and furosemide therapy should be continued as maintenance therapy for 1 month. In addition, a low-calcium diet is important to reduce intestinal absorption of calcium. The diet provided can be a commercially available veterinary food or a homemade diet consisting mostly of macaroni and lean ground beef. Dairy products should be strictly avoided. Non–calcium-containing intestinal phosphorus binders may also be beneficial to counteract the effects of hyperphosphatemia. This treatment may be particularly important because the magnitude of soft tissue mineralization is most severe in animals with hypercalcemia induced by vitamin D toxicosis. Aluminum hydroxide at 30 to 90 mg/kg/day in divided doses is recommended during the first 2 weeks, with dosage and duration of treatment adjusted based on serial measurements of serum phosphorus concentration. Other unproven methods for treatment include anticonvulsants to increase hepatic metabolism of cholecalciferol, intestinal calcium binders to reduce intestinal calcium absorption, and calcium channel blockers to decrease the toxic intracellular effects of persistent hypercalcemia.[153]

When hypervitaminosis D is caused by excess calcitriol in patients with granulomatous disease, chloroquine, hydroxychloroquine, and ketoconazole may be used as supplemental therapeutic agents or as substitutes for glucocorticoids because they impair conversion of 25-hydroxyvitamin D to 1,25-dihydroxyvitamin D by macrophages.[155,435]

HYPOCALCEMIA

INTRODUCTION

Hypocalcemia based on serum tCa is a relatively common laboratory abnormality and was observed in 13.5% of serum biochemical profiles of dogs in one clinical study.[111] Based on serum iCa measurement in 1633 sick dogs, the prevalence of hypocalcemia was 31%,[475] and in 434 sick cats, the prevalence was 27%.[192] On the basis of serum tCa concentration, hypocalcemia is usually defined as a concentration less than 8.0 mg/dL in dogs and less than 7.0 mg/dL in cats. When serum iCa concentration is used, hypocalcemia is generally defined as a concentration less than 5.0 mg/dL (1.25 mmol/L) in dogs and less than 4.5 mg/dL (1.1 mmol/L) in cats. The most likely reason for submission of samples to measure calcium regulatory hormones in animals with hypocalcemia is for those with persistent hypocalcemia that is moderate to severe in magnitude and for which a known cause cannot be identified; most will be submitted with suspicion for a diagnosis of primary hypoparathyroidism.

In human patients, large and unexplained differences between ionized and tCa concentrations have been found in hypocalcemic conditions.[296] This discordance is also seen in dogs and cats and is not predictable. Based on serum tCa measurement in 1633 sick dogs, 27% were classified hypocalcemic, but when iCa was measured, 31% were hypocalcemic.[475] Using serum tCa measurement in 434 sick cats, 49% were classified hypocalcemic, but when iCa was measured, only 27% were actually hypocalcemic. Thus in dogs, tCa measurement underestimated ionized hypocalcemia, and in cats, hypocalcemia was overestimated when using serum tCa concentration to predict iCa status.

CONSEQUENCES OF HYPOCALCEMIA AND CLINICAL SIGNS

Clinical signs related to hypocalcemia are identical regardless of the underlying cause (Box 6-5). Low serum iCa increases excitability of neuromuscular tissue, which accounts for many of the clinical signs of hypocalcemia.

Box 6-5	**Clinical Signs Associated with Hypocalcemia**

Common
  None
  Muscle tremors or fasciculations
  Facial rubbing (paresthesia?)
  Muscle cramping
  Stiff gait
  Behavioral change
    Restlessness or excitation
    Aggression
    Hypersensitivity to stimuli
    Disorientation

Occasional
  Panting
  Pyrexia
  Lethargy
  Anorexia
  Prolapse of third eyelid (cats)
  Posterior lenticular cataracts
  Tachycardia or electrocardiographic alterations
    (prolonged QT interval)

Uncommon
  Polyuria or polydipsia
  Hypotension
  Respiratory arrest or death

Animals with mild decreases in iCa concentration may display no obvious clinical signs. The duration and magnitude of ionized hypocalcemia and the rate of decline in iCa concentration interact to determine the severity of clinical signs. Clinical signs in dogs often are not obvious until serum tCa concentration is less than 6.5 mg/dL, and some dogs show surprisingly few signs despite severe hypocalcemia (serum tCa concentration, <5.0 mg/dL), especially if the underlying disease has been chronic and there has been sufficient time for physiologic adaptation. Acute development of hypocalcemia is usually associated with severe clinical signs. In its most severe forms, hypocalcemia can cause death as a result of circulatory effects (e.g., hypotension and decreased myocardial contractility) and respiratory arrest from paralysis of respiratory muscles. Serum tCa concentration less than 4.0 mg/dL can cause left-sided myocardial failure[145] and death,[169] especially if the decline in serum calcium concentration was rapid.

Other electrolyte and acid-base abnormalities can either magnify or diminish the signs of hypocalcemia. Correction of hypokalemia in cats with concurrent hypocalcemia may precipitate the onset of clinical signs of hypocalcemia.[136,370] Patients with chronic hypocalcemia often display intermittent clinical signs despite seemingly stable serum tCa concentrations. Although unpredictable, clinical signs often follow periods of exercise or excitement that may be associated with respiratory alkalosis and subsequent decreases in iCa concentration. Rapid infusion of alkali to correct metabolic acidosis can cause seizures in animals with marginal or previously compensated hypocalcemia through further reduction in iCa concentration.

Clinical signs in dogs with chronic hypocalcemia (primary hypoparathyroidism) include seizures, muscle tremors or fasciculations, muscle cramping, stiff gait, and behavioral changes (e.g., restlessness, excitation, aggression, hypersensitivity to stimuli, and disorientation).[82,111,136,485] Seizures often begin as focal muscle tremors that become more widespread. Most dogs in one series had a seizure during the initial 24 to 48 hours of hospitalization, a much higher frequency than encountered with idiopathic epilepsy.[169] Seizure activity associated with hypocalcemia may not be similar to that in idiopathic epilepsy because affected dogs may remain partially conscious and retain urinary continence during the seizure.[169,406] Seizures are often preceded by apprehension or nervousness. The seizures may be as short as 60 seconds or as long as 30 minutes in some dogs. Most seizures resolve without treatment but often recur despite treatment with anticonvulsants. Growling attributable to pain or behavior change occurred in approximately 40% of dogs, and intense rubbing of the face with the paws or on the ground was observed in more than 50% of dogs. These signs were attributed to either paresthesias or pain from facial muscle spasms.[82,169]

Pyrexia may be caused by increased muscular activity with or without seizures. Lethargy and weakness are seen in approximately 33%, and polyuria and polydipsia occur in about 25% of cases, as a result of psychogenic mechanisms or renal injury (nephrocalcinosis) from hypercalciuria associated with PTH deficiency in animals with hypoparathyroidism.[460,485] Anterior and posterior lenticular cataracts occurred in more than 33% of affected dogs[82,284] and also in cats.[169,404] Tachycardia and electrocardiographic abnormalities (increased QT interval) may also be encountered. Both hypertension and hypotension have been reported during hypocalcemia in humans.[92,145]

Neuromuscular signs in cats with chronic hypocalcemia associated with primary hypoparathyroidism are similar to those in dogs (e.g., muscle tremors, weakness, and generalized seizures).[404] Anorexia and lethargy appear to be more common in cats than in dogs with primary hypoparathyroidism, but seizures have not been reported to be induced by excitement, as occurs in dogs. Prolapse of the third eyelid is occasionally observed in cats with acute hypocalcemia but is not a prominent finding during chronic hypocalcemia.

Clinical signs associated with acute postoperative hypocalcemia are similar in dogs and cats and are related to neuromuscular excitability. Focal twitching of facial muscles and vibrissae may be noticed before more generalized muscle tremors or seizures develop. Tetany or facial twitching has not been observed in cats after thyroidectomy until serum tCa concentration is less than 6.9 mg/dL.[169,404,406] Severe hypocalcemia (<6.5 mg/dL) is often associated with muscular twitching, tetany, or seizures. Anorexia and lethargy are not often considered primary signs of hypocalcemia, but both signs decrease in cats during calcium infusion after thyroidectomy, suggesting a relationship between hypocalcemia and these signs.

APPROACH TO HYPOCALCEMIA

Hypocalcemia develops when bone mobilization of calcium is reduced, skeletal calcium accretion is enhanced, urinary losses of calcium are increased, gastrointestinal absorption of calcium is reduced, calcium is translocated intracellularly, or as a result of a combination of these mechanisms. Much like the initial approach to hypercalcemia, it is helpful to make the initial distinction as to whether hypocalcemia is parathyroid dependent or parathyroid independent. Ionized calcium concentration must be evaluated in conjunction with PTH concentration to determine whether PTH production is appropriate. Patients with low iCa and low PTH concentrations have absolute hypoparathyroidism (parathyroid dependent). A normal reference range PTH when iCa is low is inappropriate because normal parathyroid glands should respond with increased PTH. Hypocalcemic patients with increased PTH are classified as having parathyroid-independent hypocalcemia. Normograms to determine the adequacy of the increased response of PTH to low iCa have not been established for dogs or cats. In cases of parathyroid-independent hypocalcemia, hypocalcemia exists from redistribution of calcium into other body spaces, excess phosphorus effects, or from deficiencies of vitamin D or dietary calcium. Patients with persistent moderate to severe hypocalcemia based on serum tCa should be evaluated for iCa and PTH concentrations; measurement of 25-hydroxyvitamin D and serum phosphorus is also helpful, and in rare circumstances, measurement of calcitriol may help provide a definitive diagnosis. The conditions associated with hypocalcemia in dogs and cats are listed in Box 6-6 according to their relative frequency regardless of clinical signs or severity of decreased serum calcium concentration. The anticipated changes in calcium hormones and serum biochemistry in disorders causing hypocalcemia are noted in Table 6-4.

DIFFERENTIAL DIAGNOSIS AND MECHANISMS OF HYPOCALCEMIA

Hypoalbuminemia

Hypoalbuminemia is the most common associated condition but perhaps the least important for clinical consequences, and it occurs in nearly one half of the dogs with hypocalcemia.[111] Hypocalcemia associated with hypoalbuminemia is usually mild (serum tCa concentration, 7.5 to 9.0 mg/dL in dogs), and no signs referable to the functional effects of low serum calcium concentration are observed. Application of calcium correction formulas to serum tCa concentrations in dogs or cats with hypoproteinemia or hypoalbuminemia has been advocated in the past. However, these correction formulas do not improve the prediction of actual iCa concentration and in many cases increase the level of diagnostic discordance.[475] Use of correction formulas to adjust serum tCa concentration to serum total protein or albumin concentration is not recommended.

Renal Failure

Renal failure is the second most common disorder associated with hypocalcemia in dogs.[111] Decreased calcitriol synthesis by diseased kidneys and, to a lesser extent, mass law interactions of calcium with markedly increased serum phosphorus concentration are probable causes of the hypocalcemia observed in dogs and cats with CRF. To decrease iCa concentration by 0.1 mg/dL, serum phosphorus concentration must increase by 3.7 mg/dL.[6] Calcitriol deficits are more important because hypocalcemia results from reduced intestinal calcium absorption and increased skeletal resistance to PTH.[366] Animals with CRF and decreased serum tCa concentration are most often asymptomatic, possibly because of an increase in iCa concentration that accompanies metabolic acidosis.

Box 6-6 **Conditions Associated with Hypocalcemia**

Common
Hypoalbuminemia
Chronic renal failure
Puerperal tetany (eclampsia)
Acute renal failure
Acute pancreatitis
Undefined cause (mild hypocalcemia)

Occasional
Soft tissue trauma or rhabdomyolysis
Hypoparathyroidism
  Primary
    Idiopathic or spontaneous
    Postoperative bilateral thyroidectomy
  After sudden reversal of chronic hypercalcemia
  Secondary to magnesium depletion or excess
Ethylene glycol intoxication
Phosphate enema
After $NaHCO_3$ administration

Uncommon
Laboratory error
Improper sample anticoagulant (EDTA)
Infarction of parathyroid gland adenoma
Rapid intravenous infusion of phosphates
Acute calcium-free intravenous infusion (dilutional)
Intestinal malabsorption or severe starvation
Hypovitaminosis D
Blood transfusion (citrated anticoagulant)
Hypomagnesemia
Nutritional secondary hyperparathyroidism
Tumor lysis syndrome

Human
Pseudohypoparathyroidism
Drug-induced
Hypercalcitonism
Osteoblastic bone neoplasia (prostate cancer)

Serum tCa concentration was 8.0 mg/dL or less in 10% of 268 dogs with clinical CRF, whereas low serum iCa concentrations were detected in 40% of affected dogs.[114] In 23 dogs with CRF, iCa represented 40% of tCa as compared with 51% of tCa in normal dogs.[280] Serum iCa was low in 56%, normal in 26%, and high in 17% of the dogs with CRF. Thus iCa concentration was low in the majority of dogs despite the presence of metabolic acidosis in 83% of dogs, which would be expected to increase iCa.[280] Hypocalcemia was diagnosed more frequently in a study of 489 dogs with CRF when determined by iCa measurement. Based on serum tCa measurement, hypocalcemia was noted in only 19% of dogs with CRF; when iCa concentration was measured, hypocalcemia was observed in 29% of dogs with CRF.[475]

TABLE 6-4 Anticipated Changes in Calcemic Hormones and Serum Biochemistry Associated with Disorders of Hypocalcemia

	tCa	iCa	alb	Corr tCa	Pi	PTH	PTHrP	25(OH)-D	1,25 (OH)₂-D	PTG ULS, Surgery
Primary hypoparathyroidism	↓	↓	N	↓	↑N	↓N	N	N	N↓	Multiple ↓
Pseudohypoparathyroidism	↓	N↓	N	↓	↑N	↑	N	N	N↑	N↑
Sepsis/critical care	N	↓	N	N	N↑	↑N	N	N	N	N
Ethylene glycol toxicity	↓	↓	N	↓	↑N	↑	N	N	↓N	N
Paraneoplastic	↓	↓	N	↓	↓↑	↑N	N	N	N	N↑
Phosphate enema	↓	↓	N	↓	↑	↑	N	N	N↓↑	N
Eclampsia	↓	↓N	N	↓	↓	Mild ↑, N	N	N	N↓↑	N
Hypoalbuminemia	↓	N	↓	N	N	N↑	N	N	N↑	N↑

↓, Decreased concentration; ↑, increased concentration; N, normal; tCa, serum total calcium; iCa, serum ionized calcium; alb, albumin; Corr tCa, corrected total calcium; Pi, inorganic phosphorus; PTH, parathyroid hormone; PTHrP, parathyroid hormone related protein; 25(OH)-D, 25-hydroxyvitamin D; 1,25(OH)2-D, 1,25-dihydroxyvitamin D; PTG, parathyroid gland; ULS, ultrasound.

In 74 cats with clinical CRF, 15% were hypocalcemic based on serum tCa.[138] In cats with CRF, hypocalcemia was found more commonly with higher magnitudes of azotemia.[24] In 73 cats with CRF, none had hypocalcemia based on tCa, but 3% of cats with moderate CRF and 23% of cats with advanced CRF did have hypocalcemia. In 47 cats with CRF, 14% with moderate CRF and 56% with advanced CRF had ionized hypocalcemia. Mean iCa for cats with advanced CRF was significantly lower than values from normal cats or cats with mild and moderate CRF. Hypocalcemia was underappreciated when based on results of tCa measurement, especially with advancing azotemia.

AIRF and postrenal failure can result in hypocalcemia that is more likely to be symptomatic because the degree of hyperphosphatemia is often greater than that observed in CRF. Dogs with AIRF had a mean serum tCa concentration of 9.8 ± 1.7 mg/dL, but iCa was not reported.[537]

Emergency and Critical Care

Ionized hypocalcemia is common in critically ill humans in the intensive care setting and is more common in septic patients.[101,307,584] The magnitude of hypocalcemia is correlated to severity of illness. Hypocalcemia with critical illness probably also occurs in veterinary patients.[136] The causes of hypocalcemia in critical illness appear to be multifactorial because sepsis, systemic inflammatory response syndrome, hypomagnesemia, blood transfusions, and AIRF have been associated with hypocalcemia.[136,306,578,584] In humans, hypocalcemia associated with critical illness involves decreased PTH secretion, hypercalcitonism, and altered calcium binding to proteins.[422] The cause of the hypocalcemia is not related to enhanced urinary calcium excretion, decreased bone mobilization, or blunted secretion of PTH in septic patients.[307] The presence of proinflammatory cytokines during sepsis is related to the development of hypocalcemia in septic patients.[307] PTH is commonly elevated in this population even when normocalcemia exists.[101,307]

Up to 88% of hospitalized human patients had decreased iCa that correlated to severity of illness but not any specific diagnosis.[584] The impact of hypocalcemia on patient survival has not yet been determined, although in one study, hypocalcemia and higher levels of PTH were more frequently associated with fatality.[101]

Ionized calcium concentration decreased in experimental dogs with hemorrhage-caused hypotension and continued to decline during replacement of blood volume with citrated whole blood.[51] Hemorrhage also decreases iCa concentration in clinical dogs. Massive transfusions in 10 dogs resulted in significant ionized hypocalcemia.[261]

Cardiopulmonary resuscitation (CPR) may result in hypocalcemia. Dogs developed ionized hypocalcemia within 5 minutes of starting CPR in dogs with prolonged cardiac arrest and continued to decrease after 20 minutes.[88,377] Serum tCa was not concordant with changes in iCa because mean serum tCa did not change, and iCa concentrations were negatively associated with lactate concentrations. Decreased iCa was most likely related to formation of complexes with lactate.

In horses with enterocolitis, decreased iCa was identified in nearly 80% of patients.[524] Ionized hypocalcemia was associated with decreased iMg, increased serum phosphorus, decreased fractional urinary excretion of calcium, and increased PTH in 71% of cases. Hypocalcemia in 29% of these horses was a result of inadequate secretion of PTH, although impaired mobilization of calcium from bone and loss or sequestration of calcium within the gastrointestinal tract could not be excluded.

Acute pancreatitis may be associated with hypocalcemia. In 46 cats with acute pancreatitis, iCa concentration was low in 61% of cats.[272] Suggested mechanisms to account for low iCa in acute pancreatitis include sequestration of calcium into peripancreatic fat (saponification), increased free fatty acids, increased calcitonin secondary to increased glucagonemia, and PTH resistance or deficit resulting from the effects of hypomagnesemia.[40,136,257,461]

In dogs with diabetes mellitus, 47% had ionized hypocalcemia.[228] Normal iCa concentrations were noted in 49.4% of dogs from this study, and 3.5% had ionized hypercalcemia. Acute pancreatitis was diagnosed in 13% of these dogs, which could be the mechanism in some but not all of those with hypocalcemia.

Puerperal tetany (eclampsia) typically occurs between 1 and 3 weeks postpartum in females of small dog breeds and is attributed to loss of calcium into milk during lactation, although parathyroid gland dysfunction has not been conclusively excluded.[19,169] Proposed mechanisms for hypocalcemia include a poor dietary source of calcium, major loss of calcium during lactation, fetal skeletal ossification, and abnormal parathyroid gland function, including parathyroid gland atrophy. Hypophosphatemia may accompany the hypocalcemia, and clinical signs rarely occur before whelping.[98] In 31 dogs with periparturient hypocalcemia, iCa was less than the reference range, and small breed dogs with large litters were typical.[143] Median time from whelping to detection of clinical signs was 14 days, but variation was wide. Clinical signs most often included seizures, trembling, twitching, shaking, and stiffness. Nontypical signs included panting, behavioral changes, collapse, and whining; vomiting, diarrhea, and choking were rare. Rectal temperature was elevated, attributable to increased muscle activity. After treatment with intravenous calcium gluconate (mean dose, 115 mg/kg), iCa concentration normalized within 25 minutes in 90% of dogs. Most dogs received more than one injection of calcium gluconate, but the total calcium dose given did not correlate to initial iCa concentration. In one lactating bitch, severe hypocalcemia and hypomagnesemia occurred in association with acute onset of gastric and bladder atony, congestive heart failure, weakness, and paresis without muscle fasciculation or seizures.[14]

Puerperal tetany is rare in cats.[550] Eclampsia was described in four cats in which hypocalcemia developed 3 to 17 days before parturition.[165] Signs of depression, weakness, tachypnea, and mild muscle tremors were most common; vomiting and anorexia were less common, and prolapse of the third eyelid occurred in some cats. Hypothermia, instead of hyperthermia as seen in dogs, was observed. All cats responded to parenteral calcium gluconate initially and to oral calcium supplementation throughout gestation and lactation.

Ionized hypocalcemia is common in cats with urethral obstruction and is likely to develop in cats that also have hyperkalemia and metabolic acidosis. Cats with severe ionized hypocalcemia can exhibit compromised vital functions, although most survive with relief of urethral obstruction. In 199 cats with urethral obstruction, iCa was below the reference range in 34%, normal in 47%, and above the reference range in 19%.[299] Of those with low iCa, 14% had moderate and 6% had severe hypocalcemia. In an earlier study, 75% of cats with urethral obstruction exhibited low iCa.[144] Most of these cats had elevated tMg probably from reduced renal function at the time of obstruction. Hypomagnesemia is not likely to account for the development of hypocalcemia in these cats, but iMg was not measured. Calcium regulatory hormones were not evaluated in either of these studies. Alkalinizing infusions designed to correct metabolic acidosis or for translocation of potassium into cells are often considered for treatment of cats with urethral obstruction, but these can decrease tCa and iCa concentrations.[110]

Rhabdomyolysis is sometimes associated with hypocalcemia, but clinical signs of hypocalcemia are rare. Mild hypocalcemia in dogs and cats with severe vehicular muscle trauma is occasionally observed (Chew, personal observations). Hypocalcemia likely occurs as a consequence of translocation of calcium into the damaged muscles. Symptomatic hypocalcemia resulting in death of three dystrophin-deficient cats occurred following anesthesia or mild exertion during restraint and subsequent acute rhabdomyolysis.[196] Hypocalcemia was documented along with hyperphosphatemia, increased liver transaminases, and massive increases in creatine kinase. Hypocalcemia has been described in some dogs with fatal *Vipera xanthina palestinae* envenomation.[15] The origin of the hypocalcemia may be multifactorial, including muscle necrosis. Renal transplantation in 14 cats resulted in decreased iCa in the 5-day postoperative period.[568] All cats also had decreased serum iMg but normal tMg.

Small Intestinal Diseases

Hypocalcemia may occur in association with gastrointestinal disease. Ionized calcium concentration was below the reference range (mean, 0.99 ± 0.19 mmol/L; reference range, 1.13 to 1.33 mmol/L) in 12 dogs with intestinal lymphangiectasia.[293] Ten of 13 dogs had hypoalbuminemia with a mean of 2.12 ± 0.70 g/dL, and "corrected" serum tCa was discordant with iCa measurement. Mechanisms for hypocalcemia could include calcium/fatty acid complexes in the intestinal lumen that could decrease intestinal calcium absorption. Hypovitaminosis D from malabsorption or hypomagnesemia may have contributed to hypocalcemia but was not evaluated. No dogs had clinical signs associated with hypocalcemia.

In five Yorkshire terriers and a shih tzu with protein-losing enteropathy, iCa and tMg concentrations were moderately to severely low.[87,271] Concentration of PTH was increased (secondary hyperparathyroidism), and 25-hydroxyvitamin D concentration was below the reference range. It is not clear whether the apparent elevation in PTH was increased to an appropriate level in the face of low iCa, or whether maximum production was suppressed because of the effects of hypomagnesemia. Intravenous supplementation with fluids containing magnesium salts resulted in increases in PTH and iCa; 25-hydroxyvitamin D remained below the reference range.[87] Following 8 weeks of treatment for inflammatory bowel disease, calcium homeostasis was normal based on normal iCa, PTH, tMg, and 25-hydroxyvitamin D concentrations. Magnesium repletion apparently resulted in resolution of hypocalcemia largely because of increased PTH secretion, whereas 25-hydroxyvitamin D concentration was still low. Resolution of weakness may have been the result of correction of hypocalcemia, hypomagnesemia, or both.

Alkali Administration

The administration of alkaline agents may result in the development of hypocalcemia. Symptomatic hypocalcemia was documented in a cat treated for salicylate intoxication with sodium bicarbonate.[2] Muscle fasciculation increased during treatment with sodium bicarbonate, and serum tCa was low. A single dose of intravenous sodium bicarbonate at 4 mEq/L to cats resulted in a maximal decrease of iCa 10 minutes following infusion; iCa remained below baseline for 3 hours.[110] Part of the decrease in iCa was attributed to dilution and part to increased pH of serum, but most of the decrease was the result of unidentified factors. Similar findings were noted in dogs receiving sodium bicarbonate infusion.[345] Twitching has been observed on rare occasion during or shortly after infusion of sodium bicarbonate solutions to cats with urethral obstruction and to dogs or cats with renal failure (Chew, personal observations) presumably because of decreases in serum iCa.

Acute Reversal of Chronic Hypercalcemia

The sudden correction of chronic hypercalcemia can result in hypocalcemia as a result of parathyroid gland atrophy and inadequate ability to synthesize and secrete PTH. This happens frequently in dogs with primary hyperparathyroidism caused by parathyroid gland adenoma following surgical excision of the affected parathyroid gland(s). The degree of parathyroid gland atrophy depends on the magnitude of hypercalcemia and its duration before correction. Two dogs with spontaneous infarction of a parathyroid gland adenoma have been reported with the development of hypocalcemia and clinical signs.[442] Rapid correction of hypercalcemia following chemotherapy for lymphosarcoma or surgical excision of anal sac adenocarcinoma often results in mild hypocalcemia that is usually not associated with clinical signs, but clinical signs of hypocalcemia may occur.[241] Persistent hypocalcemia has been observed in dogs following parathyroidectomy in association with hypomagnesemia. In three dogs, hypocalcemia resolved following supplementation with magnesium salts, but calcium regulatory hormones were not measured (Chew, unpublished observations).

Tumor Lysis Syndrome

Tumor lysis syndrome occurs when there is rapid destruction of sensitive tumor cells (usually lymphoid or bone marrow tumors) following chemotherapy.[400] Release of intracellular products can result in hyperkalemia, hyperphosphatemia, and hyperuricemia. Hypocalcemia can develop as calcium-phosphate salts are deposited into soft tissues by mass-law effects from markedly increased serum phosphorus[90,388,413] and may be associated with the development of AIRF. Tumor lysis syndrome is a rarely reported cause of symptomatic hypocalcemia in dogs,[388,413] although it may be more common than previously reported because The Ohio State University oncology service has documented seven cases (Couto, personal communication, 2004).

Nutritional Secondary Hyperparathyroidism

Vitamin D deficiency and nutritional secondary hyperparathyroidism associated with low calcium and/or high phosphorus concentrations in the diet results in low serum iCa and phosphorus concentrations, with an increase in PTH secretion. Nutritional secondary hyperparathyroidism may also occur when severe gastrointestinal disease is present, limiting the absorption of calcium and vitamin D. Increased PTH secretion tends to return serum iCa concentration to normal, but decreases serum phosphorus concentration.[567] The occurrence of nutritional secondary hyperparathyroidism has decreased dramatically since the advent of feeding commercially available, nutritionally complete and balanced pet food.[264] Nutritional secondary hyperparathyroidism was induced in adult beagles by feeding a diet high in phosphorus and low in calcium, with a calcium to phosphorus ratio of 1:10.[123] A significant increase in PTH production was seen at 10 weeks of feeding, and cancellous bone volume was reduced by 20% to 30%. Under experimental conditions, puppies fed a low-calcium, normal phosphorus content diet exhibited increased concentrations of PTH and calcitriol, with a decrease in 24,25-dihydroxyvitamin D concentration.[223] In five German shepherd dog puppies fed a diet consisting of 80% steamed rice and 20% raw meat, nutritional secondary hyperparathyroidism was observed.[267] This diet apparently had an adequate calcium concentration but contained an excess of phosphorus. All puppies showed moderate to marked fibrous osteodystrophy.

Serum iCa and phosphorus concentrations were below the reference range in six young cats with nutritional secondary hyperparathyroidism.[522] Clinical signs referable to hypocalcemia (excitation, muscle twitching, seizures) and spontaneous fractures of bones were present in most cats. Renal secondary hyperparathyroidism preferentially affects the bones of the face (fibrous osteodystrophy), whereas nutritional secondary hyperparathyroidism tends to cause osteopenia of the long bones and vertebrae. Calcitriol concentration was mildly increased in three of four cats in which it was measured, whereas 25-hydroxyvitamin D was mildly decreased in three of three cats. PTH concentrations were increased in all cats and ranged from a minimal increase in one cat to a marked increase of 4 to 9.7 times the upper range in the remaining five cats. Cats had been fed meat only (three cats), meat combined with vegetables (two cats), or vegetables only (one cat). Dietary calcium intake was less than one tenth of the minimal nutritional requirement; dietary intake of phosphorus was mildly below the minimal requirements in five of six cats. An unfavorable calcium to phosphorus ratio existed for all diets. A case of type 2 vitamin D–dependent rickets was described in a 4-month-old cat examined because of vomiting, diarrhea, muscle tremors, and mydriasis of acute onset.[478] Serum tCa and tMg concentrations were decreased, and serum phosphorus, calcitriol, and PTH concentrations were increased, excluding hypoparathyroidism as the cause of hypocalcemia. Calcitriol and calcium salt supplementation resulted in the return to normocalcemia.

Exotic animals may be at increased risk for the development of nutritional secondary hyperparathyroidism because nutritional requirements are not always known. Nutritional secondary hyperparathyroidism was documented in a 3-month-old tiger cub that was fed only beef with no calcium or vitamin supplementation.[566] This tiger cub was reluctant to walk, exhibited osteodystrophy of the lumbosacral vertebrae, and had an elevated serum PTH concentration. Clinical signs improved after administration of vitamin D and calcium.

With the feeding of BARF (biologically appropriate raw food, or bones and raw food) and other homemade diets, the occurrence of nutritional secondary hyperparathyroidism is more likely. In a recent report, 6-week-old, large-breed puppies from two litters were fed a BARF diet on weaning.[130] Puppies were weak, exhibited pain, and had abnormal-appearing joints, and some were unable to stand. In puppies that were radiographed, osteopenia was noted, with pathologic fractures apparent in multiple long bones. In euthanized puppies, the long bones were pliable, and cortices were thin. Parathyroid glands were prominent, and histologically, fibrous osteodystrophy was present in bones. Nutritional secondary hyperparathyroidism was attributable to a diet low in calcium and an inappropriate calcium to phosphorus ratio.

EFFECTS OF DRUGS

Drug administration may cause a decrease in iCa. A significant decrease in iCa was observed in dogs administered enrofloxacin at 5 mg/kg intramuscularly once daily for 14 days.[130] Mean iCa decreased to its nadir on day 3, remained below normal at day 10, and normalized by day 14 despite continued administration of enrofloxacin.

The administration of mithramycin or bisphosphonates can cause mild hypocalcemia as a side effect in humans, but symptomatic hypocalcemia is rare.[125,519] The potential for development of hypocalcemia exists in dogs following mithramycin administration because normal dogs and those with malignancy-associated hypercalcemia undergo significant decreases in serum iCa and tCa.[443,444] Use of mithramycin is reserved for emergency management of hypercalcemia refractory to other treatments because of severe toxicity in some dogs.

Phosphate enema administration can result in hypocalcemia after rapid absorption of phosphate, hyperphosphatemia, and subsequent mass law interaction with serum calcium. This is particularly a problem in cats and small dogs in which death can occur.[16,260,468,523] Serum tCa decreased within 45 minutes of administration of a hypertonic phosphate enema to cats and persisted for 4 hours.[16] Mean serum phosphorus was more than 14 mg/dL within 15 minutes, and increases persisted for 4 hours. Serum tCa concentrations were negatively correlated to serum phosphorus. Mild hypernatremia, severe hyperphosphatemia (mean, 37.6 mg/dL), and hypocalcemia were noted in five cats. Phosphate enemas should not be used in small dogs, cats, or in debilitated patients of any size.

Hypoparathyroidism

Hypoparathyroidism is an absolute or relative deficiency of PTH secretion that can be permanent or transient. Hypocalcemia and clinical signs referable to low iCa concentration are the hallmarks of advanced hypoparathyroidism. Hypoparathyroidism in dogs is most commonly idiopathic, whereas surgical removal of or injury to the parathyroid gland during thyroidectomy to correct hyperthyroidism is the most common cause in cats.

Idiopathic chronic inflammation of parathyroid tissue occurs sporadically in both dogs and cats but more commonly in dogs. It is presumed that parathyroiditis has an immune-mediated mechanism. Histopathologic study of affected parathyroid glands reveals inflammatory cell infiltration (lymphocytes, plasma cells, and neutrophils), fibrosis, and loss of secretory cells.[82,169,404,406,485] Clinical signs occurred 1 to 26 weeks (mean, 7 weeks) before diagnosis of primary hypoparathyroidism in cats[404] and 1 day to 25 weeks (mean, 3 weeks) before diagnosis in dogs.[82] Primary hypoparathyroidism and parathyroiditis occur in dogs and cats of any age but more frequently in female dogs and male cats. In 735 dogs with primary hypoparathyroidism, 62% were female and 38% were male.[423] Mean age was 7.0 ± 3.9 years, with 71% of diagnoses occurring in purebred dogs. The highest odds ratios for hypoparathyroidism correcting for breed popularity occurred in the standard schnauzer, Scottish terrier, miniature schnauzer, West Highland white terrier, and dachshund. Reduced risk was identified for the German shepherd dog, shih tzu, and Labrador retriever. In another study, 357 dogs were diagnosed with primary hypoparathyroidism over a 2-year period.[477] Mixed-breed dogs accounted for 25% of the cases, with 13% schnauzers, 7% Labrador retrievers, 5% dachshunds, 4% Yorkshire terriers, 4% poodles, 3% golden retrievers, and 3% Scottish terriers without correction for breed popularity. There were 59 other dog breeds represented with an incidence of less than 3% each.

Serum tCa concentration is usually less than 6.5 mg/dL (often 4.0 to 4.9 mg/dL) in dogs with primary hypoparathyroidism. Dogs that have episodes of tetany or seizures often have serum tCa concentration less than 6.0 mg/dL. Serum phosphorus concentration is greater than serum calcium concentration in nearly all affected dogs and cats, and most have hyperphosphatemia. Parathyroid gland biopsy may confirm the diagnosis of lymphocytic parathyroiditis as the cause of primary hypoparathyroidism, but the parathyroid glands can be difficult or impossible to locate during surgical exploration because of atrophy and fibrosis. Parathyroid gland biopsy is not recommended to confirm hypoparathyroidism since the advent of validated PTH assays for use in the dog and cat.

Diagnosis of Hypoparathyroidism. Inappropriately low concentrations of PTH result in hypocalcemia, hyperphosphatemia, and decreased concentrations of 1,25-dihydroxyvitamin D (calcitriol). Hypocalcemia results from increased urinary loss of calcium (hypercalciuria), reduced bone resorption, and decreased intestinal absorption of calcium. Hyperphosphatemia results from decreased urinary loss of phosphorus (hypophosphaturia) that overrides the effects of decreased bone resorption and decreased intestinal absorption of phosphorus (secondary to calcitriol deficit) on serum phosphorus concentration. PTH is a potent stimulator and phosphorus is a potent inhibitor of the 25-hydroxyvitamin D–1α-hydroxylase enzyme system in renal tubules. Consequently, the absence of PTH and the presence of hyperphosphatemia act together to decrease renal synthesis of calcitriol. Decreased concentrations of calcitriol contribute to hypocalcemia via decreased intestinal calcium absorption. Hypocalcemia unrelated to low PTH concentrations may arise from increased uptake of calcium by bone after rapid correction of long-standing hyperparathyroidism or hyperthyroidism, both of which are associated with loss of bone calcium before treatment ("hungry bone" syndrome).[501,516,563]

Definitive diagnosis of primary hypoparathyroidism is based on the combination of clinical signs (see Box 6-5), low iCa concentration, and PTH concentration inappropriately low to the magnitude of ionized hypocalcemia. Hypoparathyroidism is the only possible diagnosis when low serum calcium concentration, high serum phosphorus concentration, normal renal function, and low PTH concentration are present in combination. Low serum calcium and high serum phosphorus concentrations can be encountered during nutritional and renal secondary hyperparathyroidism, after phosphate-containing enemas, and during tumor lysis syndrome, but PTH is increased in all of these conditions.

PTH should be measured in patients with chronic hypocalcemia of undetermined etiology. Primary hypoparathyroidism requires lifelong treatment, and confirmation of the diagnosis with PTH measurement is recommended. It is not necessary to measure PTH routinely in patients with postsurgical hypocalcemia because this effect is usually transient and the cause obvious. PTH concentrations should be determined for patients in which hypocalcemia does not resolve. Absolute hypoparathyroidism is present if a PTH concentration below the reference range is detected simultaneously with hypocalcemia. Relative hypoparathyroidism is present if PTH concentration is inappropriately low but remains within the normal reference range. Increased serum phosphorus and decreased calcitriol concentrations provide further support for a diagnosis of hypoparathyroidism.[217]

Causes of Hypoparathyroidism. The causes of hypoparathyroidism can be divided into three categories: (1) suppressed secretion of PTH without parathyroid gland destruction,[111,136] (2) sudden correction of chronic hypercalcemia, and (3) absence or destruction of the parathyroid glands. The most common category of hypoparathyroidism in dogs and cats is absence or destruction of the parathyroid glands.

Postoperative hypocalcemia develops 1 to 3 days after thyroidectomy in approximately 20% to 30% of cats.[46,177,180,209,555] Some cats developed hypocalcemia as late as 1 to 2 weeks after surgery. The surgical technique

used for thyroidectomy influences the chances that hypocalcemia will develop, and hypocalcemia occurred in more than 80% of cats when original extracapsular technique was used.[177] Bilateral thyroidectomy results in loss of the two internal parathyroid glands, and hypoparathyroidism is permanent in patients in which the external parathyroid glands are completely removed during bilateral thyroidectomy. Hypocalcemia and hypoparathyroidism do not develop if the two external parathyroid glands are not excised or damaged during thyroidectomy. Normocalcemia can be maintained with one completely functional parathyroid gland.

Hypoparathyroidism is usually transient when the external parathyroid glands are retained but have their blood supply disrupted (parathyroid gland ischemia after physical trauma, vessel stretching, suture, cautery, or transection) during surgery. Permanent hypoparathyroidism is rare, but it may take as long as 3 months to be certain whether remaining parathyroid tissue can recover by hyperplasia.[46,406,460] Similar injury to parathyroid glands can occur during any extensive surgery of the neck in dogs[225,278] or cats or after exploration of the neck for unilateral parathyroid gland removal. Restored vascular supply to damaged parathyroid tissue seems unlikely as the mechanism for recovery from hypocalcemia. It is more likely that hyperplasia and hypertrophy of parathyroid gland remnants left behind during surgery or ectopic parathyroid tissue achieve sufficient mass to synthesize adequate amounts of PTH. Experimental cats subjected to parathyroidectomy predictably developed hypocalcemia and low serum PTH concentration, but, interestingly, the hypocalcemia resolved, although the PTH concentrations remained low.[178] Autotransplantation of parathyroid tissue after bilateral thyroparathyroidectomy was associated with reduced morbidity and rapid return of serum calcium concentrations to normal in experimental cats.[387]

Long-standing ionized hypercalcemia causes normal parathyroid tissue to atrophy. If hypercalcemia is nonparathyroid in origin, PTH concentrations will already be low. Rapid correction of hypercalcemia results in hypocalcemia because the atrophic parathyroid glands cannot respond immediately to the need for increased PTH secretion. Surgical removal of a single parathyroid gland tumor (usually an adenoma) commonly causes postoperative hypocalcemia in this manner. Hypocalcemia severe enough to require treatment is likely to develop within 24 to 48 hours. Nearly 50% of dogs with primary hyperparathyroidism can be expected to develop clinical signs of hypocalcemia 3 to 6 days after surgical removal of a parathyroid gland tumor. Hypocalcemia is more likely to develop in dogs with higher presurgical iCa concentrations. More than one half of hyperparathyroid dogs exhibit a rapid decrease in serum iCa concentration that normalizes within 24 hours of surgery. Serum iCa concentrations in the remaining dogs usually normalize by

2 or 3 days after surgery, but some require as long as 5 days. Hypoparathyroidism resolves for most affected dogs in 8 to 12 weeks. Cats develop hypocalcemia less frequently than dogs after surgical correction of primary hyperparathyroidism.[133,263]

Hypoparathyroidism following spontaneous infarction of a parathyroid gland tumor previously causing hypercalcemia is a rare condition that can result in acute hypocalcemia in dogs.[442] The rapid correction of cancer-associated hypercalcemia (e.g., with tumor excision and chemotherapy) can be associated with hypocalcemia and low PTH concentration, but hypocalcemia is usually minor and transient.

Both acute hypermagnesemia and severe magnesium depletion may suppress PTH secretion.[58,422,521] As with hypocalcemia, mild acute hypomagnesemia stimulates PTH secretion, but severe magnesium depletion decreases PTH secretion, increases end-organ resistance to PTH, and may impair calcitriol synthesis. The end-organ resistance to PTH that develops during magnesium depletion may persist for days after magnesium repletion and resumption of normal PTH concentrations in humans. Until recently, hypomagnesemia has been reported rarely in dogs and cats with hypoparathyroidism. Normal serum tMg does not guarantee a normal iMg concentration because there is substantial discordance between these two measurements.

Magnesium depletion can cause functional hypoparathyroidism, and measurement of serum iMg concentration is recommended to exclude or identify this form of hypoparathyroidism. Serum tMg concentrations in dogs and cats with primary hypoparathyroidism usually have been normal when measured.[82,169] In 357 dogs with primary hypoparathyroidism, mean iCa and mean PTH concentrations were below the reference range.[477] The iMg concentration was below the reference range in 39%, within the reference range in 55%, and above the reference range in 6% of dogs with hypoparathyroidism. Of the 55% of dogs with iMg within the reference range, 69% had an iMg concentration within the lower half of the reference range, and only 31% had an iMg concentration within the upper half of the reference range.

Despite the relative paucity of published reports from cats, hypoparathyroidism was diagnosed in 27 cats during a 2-year period.[477] Of cats with hypoparathyroidism, 59% were domestic shorthairs, 22% were an unspecified breed, and 15% were Siamese. Mean serum iCa concentration was below the reference range, and mean PTH concentration was in the lower half of the reference range. The iMg concentration was below the reference range in 37%, within the reference range in 59%, and above the reference range in 4%. Of the 59% of cats with iMg within the reference range, 88% had an iMg concentration within the lower half of the reference range,

and only 12% had an iMg concentration within the upper half of the reference range. These results suggest that a large number of dogs and cats with hypoparathyroidism also exhibit subnormal or marginal iMg concentrations. The impact of magnesium supplementation in the treatment of hypoparathyroidism should be investigated. Although primary hypoparathyroidism is usually diagnosed in older cats, it has been reported in a 6-month-old kitten initially evaluated for lethargy, inappetence, muscle tremors, and seizures.[31]

Most causes of primary hypoparathyroidism have been attributed to immune destruction of parathyroid tissue. Early reports of hypoparathyroidism in dogs and cats did not consistently evaluate magnesium status and used tMg when it was reported. Based on discordance of magnesium status using iMg versus tMg, hypomagnesemia based on tMg assessments may have underestimated a role for hypomagnesemia in the genesis of hypoparathyroidism in animals. Hypomagnesemia may decrease cell membrane receptor sensitivity to iCa and PTH, as well as decrease PTH synthesis.[300] Serum iMg concentration should be measured when iCa and PTH concentrations are determined.

The potential role of magnesium depletion in the development of postthyroidectomy hypocalcemia in cats has not been explored. Magnesium depletion could play a role in the development of postoperative hypocalcemia in cats with hyperthyroidism because hyperthyroidism can be associated with magnesium depletion.[169]

Canine distemper virus (CDV)-induced parathyroid hypofunction may contribute to development of hypocalcemia. Dogs infected with CDV had reduced serum tCa concentrations associated with ultrastructural evidence of parathyroid gland inactivity, degeneration, and viral inclusions.[554]

Miscellaneous Causes of Hypocalcemia

Metabolites of ethylene glycol can chelate calcium and become deposited in soft tissues, resulting in hypocalcemia. Both dogs and cats exhibit hypocalcemia after ethylene glycol ingestion.[518] Seizures have been observed in dogs within hours of ingestion; renal function was normal at this time (Chew, personal observations). Hypocalcemia often develops later when renal function is severely reduced from acute renal failure and when hyperphosphatemia is severe.

Acute decreases in iCa concentrations are most commonly caused by acute respiratory alkalosis in humans.[422] It is likely that this phenomenon also occurs in dogs and cats subjected to the stresses of hypocalcemia and a visit to a veterinary clinic. This could explain the phenomenon of mild stress-induced seizures or tetany in dogs that have hypocalcemia, as the alkalosis shifts some calcium to the protein-bound state, causing more severe ionized hypocalcemia.

TREATMENT OF HYPOCALCEMIA

Puerperal tetany is the condition most likely to require correction of hypocalcemia acutely, but chronic treatment is not needed. Hypoparathyroidism is the only condition requiring acute and chronic treatment to alleviate clinical signs of hypocalcemia. Other conditions associated with hypocalcemia are transient or result in minimal decreases in serum calcium concentration, do not cause obvious clinical signs, and only occasionally necessitate calcium replacement therapy. No treatment is indicated for hypocalcemia attributable entirely to hypoalbuminemia or hypoproteinemia, assuming that the iCa fraction is normal.

Treatment is individualized based on severity of clinical signs, magnitude of hypocalcemia, rapidity of decline in serum calcium concentration, and trend of serial serum calcium measurements (i.e., further decrease or stability). Aggressive treatment is prescribed for patients with severe clinical signs of hypocalcemia, patients with severe ionized hypocalcemia with or without signs, and patients in which serum calcium concentration is steadily or rapidly declining. Acute, subacute, and chronic rescue treatment regimens are available using supplementation with calcium salts and vitamin D metabolites. The goal of therapy is to increase serum calcium concentration to a level that alleviates the signs of hypocalcemia, minimizes the likelihood of the development of hypercalcemia, and reduces the magnitude of hypercalciuria (especially in patients with hypoparathyroidism). It is usually not necessary or desirable to return serum calcium concentration completely to normal because many clinical signs improve dramatically with slight increases in serum calcium concentration, and the consequences of overcorrection can be serious. For suspected temporary postsurgical hypoparathyroidism, it is desirable to keep the serum calcium concentration relatively low to maximize compensatory hypertrophy of remaining parathyroid glands.

In patients with hypoparathyroidism, no treatment regimen completely compensates for the full range of physiologic actions of the absent PTH. Vitamin D metabolite treatment corrects the low intestinal absorption of calcium but does not completely protect the kidneys from hypercalciuria as would occur in the presence of PTH. Similarly, vitamin D metabolites do not exert as powerful an effect on bone in the absence of PTH. Replacement therapy with once-daily subcutaneous injections of human PTH (1-34) in human subjects was highly effective in providing good 24-hour control of serum calcium concentration.[562] Use of synthetic human amino-terminal PTH for treatment of veterinary patients is possible because the amino-terminal portions of PTH are highly conserved, function *in vivo* in animals, and would be unlikely to elicit an immune response.

Hypocalcemia severe enough to cause clinical signs should be anticipated in dogs undergoing parathyroidectomy as treatment for hypercalcemia related to a parathyroid gland adenoma. Animals with very high concentrations of serum calcium, PTH, and serum ALP may be at greater risk of developing postoperative hypocalcemia. Postoperative hypocalcemia in this instance is the consequence of acute hypoparathyroidism resulting from chronic suppression of remaining parathyroid glands and calcium uptake into "hungry" bones. Hypocalcemia should be anticipated in cats that undergo bilateral thyroidectomy because up to 30% of cats can be expected to have transiently lowered serum calcium concentrations.

Therapy should be instituted before the development of tetany. Preemptive therapy to increase serum calcium concentration may be a good choice for animals with marked hypocalcemia with no apparent clinical signs or for those in which serum calcium concentration is steadily or rapidly declining. Prophylactic therapy to prevent hypocalcemia in dogs undergoing surgery for hyperparathyroidism should be considered, especially in dogs with severe hypercalcemia. Active vitamin D metabolites should be started before surgery in these instances because there is a lag time until maximal effect is achieved. Vitamin D metabolites given at the time of surgery or just after surgery fail to prevent development of hypocalcemia.

Autotransplantation of normal parathyroid glands is a treatment option to minimize postoperative hypocalcemia when it is obvious that damage has been done to the parathyroid glands during surgery (bilateral extracapsular thyroidectomy). Autotransplantation of normal parathyroid glands was studied in experimental cats following bilateral extracapsular thyroparathyroidectomy.[387] External parathyroid glands were harvested and dissected from thyroid tissue, and small pieces of parathyroid tissue were embedded into the sternohyoideus muscle. Cats showed an average decrease of 44% in serum tCa with the nadir occurring 1.9 days following surgery. Hypocalcemia was present a median of 14 days in cats having parathyroidectomy and autotransplantation in this study compared with a median of 71 days in cats of a previous report involving parathyroidectomy without autotransplantation.[178] Seven of eight cats with autotransplantation of parathyroid glands regained normocalcemia within 20 days without oral calcium salt supplementation.[387]

Acute Management of Hypocalcemia Causing Tetany or Seizures

Tetany or seizures caused by hypocalcemia require treatment with intravenously administered calcium salts. Calcium is administered to effect, at a dosage of 5 to 15 mg/kg of elemental calcium (0.5 to 1.5 mL/kg of 10% calcium gluconate) over a 10- to 20-minute period.[111,169,406,407] The calcium content of different calcium salts varies considerably (Table 6-5). There is no difference in effectiveness of calcium salts administered intravenously to correct hypocalcemia when the dose is based on elemental calcium content. Calcium gluconate is often the calcium salt of choice because it is nonirritating if the solution is inadvertently injected perivascularly. In contrast, calcium chloride is extremely irritating to tissues but provides more elemental calcium in each milliliter of solution (see Table 6-5).

The heart rate and electrocardiogram should be monitored during acute infusions of calcium salts. Bradycardia may signal the onset of cardiotoxicity arising from excessively rapid infusion of calcium. Sudden elevation of the ST segment or shortening of the QT interval also may indicate cardiotoxicity resulting from the calcium infusion. Not all clinical signs abate immediately after acute correction of hypocalcemia; some may persist for 30 to 60 minutes. Nervousness, panting, and behavioral changes may persist despite return of normocalcemia during this period, perhaps reflecting a lag in equilibration between cerebrospinal fluid and ECF calcium concentrations.[169,274,460] Hyperthermia that resulted from increased muscle activity or seizures may also take time to dissipate.

Subacute Management of Hypocalcemia

The initial bolus injection of elemental calcium can be expected to decrease signs of hypocalcemia for as little as 1 hour to as long as 12 hours if the underlying cause of hypocalcemia has not been corrected. Vitamin D metabolites should be administered as soon as possible because some of them require a few days before intestinal calcium transport is maximized. Calcitriol exerts initial effects on the intestine within 3 to 4 hours.[549] Additional parenteral calcium salt administration is necessary until therapy with vitamin D metabolites is effective at maintaining serum calcium concentration at an acceptable level.

Multiple intermittent intravenous injections of calcium salts can be administered to control clinical signs, but this method is not recommended because wide fluctuations in serum calcium concentration are observed. Instead, continuous intravenous infusion of calcium is recommended at 60 to 90 mg/kg/day elemental calcium (2.5 to 3.75 mg/kg/hr) until oral medications provide control of serum calcium concentration.[82,169,406,407] Initial doses in the higher range are administered to patients with more severe hypocalcemia, and the dose decreased according to the serum calcium concentration achieved. The intravenous dose of calcium is further reduced as oral calcium salts and vitamin D metabolites become more effective.

Ten milliliters of 10% calcium gluconate provides 93 mg of elemental calcium. A convenient method for infusing calcium is available when intravenous fluids are given at a maintenance volume of 60 mL/kg/day (2.5 mL/kg/hr). Approximately 1, 2, or 3 mg/kg/hr elemental calcium is provided by adding 10, 20, or 30 mL of 10% calcium gluconate, respectively, to each 250-mL bag of fluids. Calcium salts should not be added to fluids that contain lactate, acetate, bicarbonate, or phosphates because calcium salt precipitates can occur. Alkalinizing fluids that contain or generate bicarbonate should be avoided because they can decrease iCa and may unmask clinical signs of hypocalcemia in animals with borderline hypocalcemia.

Subcutaneous administration of calcium gluconate has been regarded as safe for use in dogs with hypocalcemia when diluted to at least 1:1 by volume. The use of calcium chloride is too caustic to ever be given subcutaneously. However, a recent report raises concerns about the safety of calcium gluconate administration subcutaneously. A 6-month-old border collie with hypoparathyroidism was initially treated with intravenous calcium gluconate, followed by oral calcitriol and calcium carbonate.[469] This dog then received subcutaneous calcium gluconate three times daily for 2 days, and calcium gluconate was diluted as previously recommended. Fever and pain, swelling, and erythema of the ventral abdomen were obvious after 2 days of subcutaneous calcium gluconate treatments. Initial skin biopsy revealed calcinosis cutis with pyogranulomatous dermatitis and dermoepidermal separation. The dog's condition worsened; ulceration involving about 80% of the skin developed over the trunk; and the dog was euthanized. A second skin biopsy revealed severe pyogranulomatous panniculitis with mineralization of adipocytes.

Reports of this reaction to the subcutaneous administration of calcium gluconate had not previously been reported in dogs despite its extensive use by some institutions (Feldman, personal communication, 2005). Unfortunately, we are aware of at least three other dogs with similar severe reactions to the subcutaneous administration of properly diluted calcium gluconate as treatment for primary hypoparathyroidism, resulting in euthanasia for most (Chew, personal communications, 2003, 2004). Differences in an individual animal's susceptibility to the effects of calcium salts on subcutaneous tissues could account for severe reactions in some dogs. All dogs with this severe tissue reaction were also receiving calcitriol, which may potentiate more local dramatic effects in the subcutaneous tissues as compared with less active vitamin D metabolites (cholecalciferol, ergocalciferol, and dihydrotachysterol) commonly used in the past.

There are only two reports of cats with primary hypoparathyroidism that were treated with subcutaneous administration of calcium gluconate. No adverse effects were noted in one report.[184] Iatrogenic calcinosis cutis, skin necrosis, and scarring occurred at sites of diluted calcium gluconate injection and sites where injected

TABLE 6-5 Treatment of Hypocalcemia

Drug	Preparation	Calcium Content	Dose	Comment
Parenteral Calcium*				
Calcium gluconate	10% solution	9.3 mg of Ca/mL	a. Slow IV to effect (0.5-1.5 mL/kg IV)	Stop if bradycardia or shortened QT interval occurs
			b. 5-15 mg/kg/hr IV	Infusion to maintain normal Ca
			c. SQ diluted calcium salts	SQ calcium salts can cause severe skin necrosis/mineralization; no longer recommended as safe
Calcium chloride	10% solution	27.2 mg of Ca/mL	5-15 mg/kg/hr IV	Only given IV because extremely caustic perivascularly
Oral Calcium†				
Calcium carbonate	Many sizes	40% tablet	25-50 mg/kg/day	Most common calcium supplement
Calcium lactate	325- and 650-mg tablets	13% tablet	25-50 mg/kg/day	
Calcium chloride	Powder	27.2%	25-50 mg/kg/day	May cause gastric irritation
Calcium gluconate	Many sizes	10%	25-50 mg/kg/day	

				Time for maximal effect to occur:	Time for toxicity effect to resolve:
Vitamin D					
Vitamin D$_2$ (ergocalciferol)			Initial: 4000-6000 U/kg/day; Maintenance: 1000-2000 U/kg once daily to once weekly	5-21 days	1-18 weeks
Dihydrotachysterol			Initial: 0.02-0.03 mg/kg/day Maintenance: 0.01-0.02 mg/kg every 24-48 hours	1-7 days	1-3 weeks
1,25-(OH)$_2$D$_3$ (calcitriol)			Initial: 20-30 ng/kg/day for 3-4 days Maintenance: 5-15 ng/kg/day	1-4 days	2-14 days

*Do not mix calcium solutions with bicarbonate-containing fluids as precipitation may occur.
†Calculate dose on elemental calcium content. IV, Intravenous; SQ, subcutaneous.

fluids pooled in one cat.[458] This cat survived. Because of the severity of adverse reactions that have recently been observed in dogs and a cat, the administration of subcutaneous fluids containing calcium gluconate is no longer recommended as a safe and predictable treatment.

Subacute and Chronic Maintenance

Supplemental elemental calcium is administered orally (see Table 6-5) to guarantee adequate calcium for intestinal absorption after treatment with vitamin D metabolites. Oral calcium administered by pill or slurry is most important during initial treatment, especially if the animal is not eating. Active intestinal transport of calcium is under the control of calcitriol when calcium intake is low, but vitamin D–independent (passive) intestinal absorption of calcium occurs when calcium intake is high. The passive mechanisms for intestinal calcium transport can be used therapeutically before the actions of vitamin D take effect in the intestine. In most patients, normal dietary intake of calcium is sufficient to maintain adequate serum calcium concentrations in the presence of vitamin D metabolite treatment. Consequently, oral calcium salt supplementation can be tapered and discontinued in many instances as vitamin D compounds reach maximal effect.

Calcium carbonate is the most widely used oral preparation of the calcium salts because it contains the greatest percentage of elemental calcium. This approach allows fewer pills to be administered. The degree of calcium ionization from its salt and its bioavailability for absorption vary for each calcium salt and with conditions in the intestine. Consequently, it is not a simple matter to determine the bioavailable elemental calcium content of a specific oral calcium salt. Oral calcium is usually administered at 25 to 50 mg/kg/day elemental calcium in divided doses. Oral calcium carbonate serves as an intestinal phosphate binder in addition to providing calcium for intestinal absorption. It is advisable to continue oral calcium carbonate therapy for its intestinal phosphate-binding effects if serum phosphorus concentration remains increased. Lower serum phosphorus concentrations may allow increased endogenous synthesis of calcitriol because phosphate inhibits renal synthesis of calcitriol.

Vitamin D preparations (see Table 6-5) include ergocalciferol, cholecalciferol, dihydrotachysterol (DHT), 25-hydroxycholecalciferol (calcidiol), 1α-hydroxycholecalciferol, and calcitriol. Ergocalciferol, DHT, and calcitriol are the preparations most commonly used in veterinary medicine. Lifelong treatment with some form of vitamin D metabolite is necessary for patients with primary hypoparathyroidism or postoperative hypocalcemia that fails to resolve spontaneously.

Ergocalciferol is favored by some because of its low cost,[422] but it has several features that make it the least attractive agent for treatment of hypocalcemia. Ergocalciferol and its immediate metabolite, 25-hydroxyergocalciferol, have low VDR avidity; thus high doses are necessary. Ergocalciferol is highly lipid soluble, and several weeks are required to saturate body stores and achieve a maximal effect. It also has a long half-life. Consequently, prolonged periods of hypercalcemia occur after overdose with ergocalciferol. In addition, there is extreme individual variation in the dose of ergocalciferol required to achieve a target serum calcium concentration. Use of loading doses reduces the time required to achieve a maximal effect (see Table 6-5).

DHT is a synthetic vitamin D analogue with onset of maximal effect and biologic half-life between those of ergocalciferol and calcitriol. The polarity and lower dose requirements of DHT limit its storage in fat compared with ergocalciferol. Toxicity resulting from hypercalcemia still can be prolonged (up to 30 days), and there is wide variation in the dose required to achieve a target serum calcium concentration. Use of loading doses reduces the time to maximal effect.

Calcitriol is the vitamin D metabolite of choice to provide calcemic actions because it has the most rapid onset of maximal action and the shortest biologic half-life. Calcitriol is approximately 1000 times as effective as parent vitamin D and 500 times as effective as its precursor, calcidiol (25-hydroxyvitamin D), in binding to the VDR. The dose of calcitriol can be adjusted frequently because of its short half-life and rapid effects on serum calcium concentration. If hypercalcemia occurs, it abates quickly after dose reduction. The half-life of calcitriol in blood is 4 to 6 hours, whereas its biologic half-life is 2 to 4 days. Loading protocols for use of calcitriol in animals have not been reported, but it is logical to use a loading protocol when more rapid correction of serum calcium concentration is desirable. A calcitriol dosage of 30 to 60 ng/kg/day has been recommended.[82,169] This dosage may be satisfactory as a loading dose, but in our experience it is too high for chronic maintenance therapy. Calcitriol dosages for chronic maintenance therapy in humans range from 10 to 40 ng/kg/day, and doses are divided and given twice daily.[217,422,562] We have used loading dosages of 20 to 30 ng/kg/day for 3 to 4 days and maintenance dosages of 10 to 20 ng/kg/day in most patients. The dose of calcitriol is divided and given twice daily to ensure sustained priming effects on intestinal epithelium for calcium transport. Calcitriol is commercially available in 0.25- and 0.50-μg capsules (250 and 500 ng per capsule, respectively; Rocaltrol, Hoffman-LaRoche, Basel, Switzerland). It is likely that reformulation of calcitriol in doses suitable for a variety of animal sizes will be necessary. It may be useful to prescribe calcitriol in liquid formulation so that small adjustments in dosage can be made accurately. A number of specialty pharmacies reformulate human drugs for veterinary use and can create any calcitriol dose needed.

CLINICAL FOLLOW-UP AND POTENTIAL COMPLICATIONS

Periods of hypocalcemia and hypercalcemia occur sporadically in patients during initial efforts to manage serum calcium concentration. Daily measurement of serum tCa concentration during stabilization is necessary. Weekly serum calcium measurements should suffice during maintenance therapy until target serum calcium concentration has been achieved and maintained. Measurement of serum tCa concentration is recommended every 3 months thereafter in animals with permanent hypoparathyroidism. Serum calcium concentration should be adjusted to just below the reference range. This not only lessens the likelihood that hypercalcemia will develop but also reduces the magnitude of hypercalciuria that occurs in patients with PTH deficiency. Maintaining a mildly decreased serum calcium concentration also ensures a continued stimulus for hypertrophy of the remaining parathyroid tissue in patients with postoperative hypoparathyroidism.

A change in dosage of vitamin D metabolites should only occur after maximal effect has occurred and should be altered gradually. The time lag for maximal effect varies with the different vitamin D metabolites (see Table 6-5). Dosage increases of 10% to 25% are recommended when serum calcium concentration is still below the target level.[406,407] Vitamin D metabolite and calcium salt supplementation should be discontinued temporarily in patients that develop hypercalcemia.

Hypercalcemia is a serious adverse effect of treatment that can result in death or renal damage causing acute or CRF.[106,111,290] Early signs of hypercalcemia should be explained to owners, who should be instructed to seek veterinary attention immediately if clinical signs suggest hypercalcemia. Clinical signs of hypercalcemia that clients are likely to recognize include polydipsia, polyuria, anorexia, vomiting, and lethargy. Animals with severe hypercalcemia require hospitalization. Fluids, furosemide, corticosteroids, bisphosphonates, calcitonin, or some combination may be required. All patients with symptomatic, vitamin D metabolite-induced hypercalcemia should be given a calcium-restricted diet because increased intestinal absorption of calcium contributes substantially to the development of hypercalcemia in hypervitaminosis D.

Patients that maintain serum iCa concentrations in the target zone are often managed successfully for years. Twenty-four of 25 dogs with primary hypoparathyroidism were managed successfully for more than 5 years,[169] and long-term management was successful in a small number of cats.[404] Patients that develop episodic or prolonged hypercalcemia during treatment have a poor prognosis. Management with calcitriol is easier and more successful in inducing and maintaining serum iCa concentrations in the target zone than are older therapeutic approaches.

Hypercalciuria, nephrocalcinosis, urolithiasis, and reduced renal function have occurred in humans treated for chronic hypoparathyroidism.[217,521,562] As many as 80% of human patients treated for 2 years or longer have decreased creatinine clearance.[562] These abnormalities can be attributed to episodes of hypercalcemia and hyperphosphatemia and to hypercalciuria that occurs in the absence of the actions of PTH on the renal tubules.

In the absence of PTH, hypercalciuria occurs more readily at all serum iCa concentrations and is especially severe as iCa concentrations approach the normal range, which increases the filtered load of calcium. Nephrocalcinosis, reduced renal function, and CRF have also been suspected in veterinary patients receiving long-term treatment for hypoparathyroidism, but the risk for these disorders has not been critically evaluated.[406]

Vitamin D metabolite treatment is gradually tapered and then discontinued in patients with postsurgical hypoparathyroidism because hypocalcemia is usually transient. Most cats are able to maintain normal serum iCa concentrations 2 weeks after thyroidectomy, although some may take as long as 3 months. Dogs with hypocalcemia usually require 6 to 12 weeks of treatment after removal of a parathyroid gland adenoma. A reduction in dose of vitamin D metabolites is usually begun 1 month after initiation of therapy. If serum iCa concentration declines substantially, the previous dose is resumed, and reduction is attempted again 1 or 2 months later. Permanent hypoparathyroidism is likely if failure to maintain acceptable serum iCa concentration occurs after reduction of the vitamin D metabolite dose at 3 months.

REFERENCES

1. Abou-Samra AB, Juppner H, Force T, et al: Expression cloning of a common receptor for parathyroid hormone and parathyroid hormone-related peptide from rat osteoblast-like cells: a single receptor stimulates intracellular accumulation of both cAMP and inositol trisphosphates and increases intracellular free calcium, *Proc Natl Acad Sci U S A* 89:2732-2736, 1992.
2. Abrams KL: Hypocalcemia associated with administration of sodium bicarbonate for salicylate intoxication in a cat, *J Am Vet Med Assoc* 191:235-236, 1987.
3. Adami S, Zamberlan N: Adverse effects of bisphosphonates. A comparative review, *Drug Saf* 14:158-170, 1996.
4. Adams JS, Sharma OP, Diz MM, et al: Ketoconazole decreases the serum 1,25-dihydroxyvitamin D and calcium concentration in sarcoidosis-associated hypercalcemia, *J Clin Endocrinol Metab* 70:1090-1095, 1990.
5. Adin DB, Taylor AW, Hill RC, et al: Intermittent bolus injection versus continuous infusion of furosemide in normal adult greyhound dogs, *J Vet Intern Med* 17:632-636, 2003.
6. Adler AJ, Ferran N, Berlyne GM: Effect of inorganic phosphate on serum ionized calcium concentration in vitro: a reassessment of the "trade-off hypothesis," *Kidney Int* 28:932-935, 1985.
7. Almaden Y, Canalejo A, Ballesteros E, et al: Regulation of arachidonic acid production by intracellular calcium in parathyroid cells: effect of extracellular phosphate, *J Am Soc Nephrol* 13:693-698, 2002.
8. Almaden Y, Felsenfeld AJ, Rodriguez M, et al: Proliferation in hyperplastic human and normal rat parathyroid glands: role of phosphate, calcitriol, and gender, *Kidney Int* 64:2311-2317, 2003.
9. Almirall J, Lopez T, Vallve M, et al: Safety and efficacy of sevelamer in the treatment of uncontrolled hyperphosphataemia of haemodialysis patients, *Nephron Clin Pract* 97:c17-22, 2004.

10. Amin M, Fawzy A, Hamid MA, et al: Pulmonary hypertension in patients with chronic renal failure: role of parathyroid hormone and pulmonary artery calcifications, *Chest* 124:2093-2097, 2003.

11. Anderson TE, Legendre AM, McEntee MM: Probable hypercalcemia of malignancy in a cat with bronchogenic adenocarcinoma, *J Am Anim Hosp Assoc* 36:52-55, 2000.

12. Anthony LB, May ME, Oates JA: Case report: lanreotide in the management of hypercalcemia of malignancy. *Am J Med Sci* 309:312-314, 1995.

13. Arceneaux KA, Taboada J, Hosgood G: Blastomycosis in dogs: 115 cases (1980-1995), *J Am Vet Med Assoc* 213:658-664, 1998.

14. Aroch I, Ohad DG, Baneth G: Paresis and unusual electrocardiographic signs in a severely hypomagnesaemic, hypocalcaemic lactating bitch, *J Small Anim Pract* 39:299-302, 1998.

15. Aroch I, Segev G, Klement E, et al: Fatal Vipera xanthina palestinae envenomation in 16 dogs, *Vet Hum Toxicol* 46:268-272, 2004.

16. Atkins CE, Tyler R, Greenlee P: Clinical, biochemical, acid-base, and electrolyte abnormalities in cats after hypertonic sodium phosphate enema administration, *Am J Vet Res* 46:980-988, 1985.

17. Aubin JE, Heersche JN: Vitamin D and osteoblasts. In Feldman D, editor: *Vitamin D*, New York, 1997, Academic Press, pp. 313-328.

18. Aucella F, Scalzulli RP, Gatta G, et al: Calcitriol increases burst-forming unit-erythroid proliferation in chronic renal failure. A synergistic effect with r-HuEpo, *Nephron Clin Pract* 95:c121-127, 2003.

19. Austad R, Bjerkas E: Eclampsia in the bitch, *J Small Anim Pract* 17:793-798, 1976.

20. Bai M, Quinn S, Trivedi S, et al: Expression and characterization of inactivating and activating mutations in the human Ca2+o-sensing receptor, *J Biol Chem* 271:19537-19545, 1996.

21. Bai M: Structure-function relationship of the extracellular calcium-sensing receptor, *Cell Calcium* 35:197-207, 2004.

22. Banerjee D, Asif A, Striker L, et al: Short-term, high-dose pamidronate-induced acute tubular necrosis: the postulated mechanisms of bisphosphonate nephrotoxicity, *Am J Kidney Dis* 41:E18, 2003.

23. Barber PJ, Elliott J, Torrance AG: Measurement of feline intact parathyroid hormone: assay validation and sample handling studies, *J Small Anim Pract* 34:614-620, 1993.

24. Barber PJ, Elliott J: Feline chronic renal failure: calcium homeostasis in 80 cases diagnosed between 1992 and 1995, *J Small Anim Pract* 39:108-116, 1998.

25. Barber PJ, Elliott J: Study of calcium homeostasis in feline hyperthyroidism, *J Small Anim Pract* 37:575-582, 1996.

26. Barber PJ, Rawlings JM, Markwell PJ, et al: Effect of dietary phosphate restriction on renal secondary hyperparathyroidism in the cat, *J Small Anim Pract* 40:62-70, 1999.

27. Barber PJ, Torrance AG, Elliott J: Carboxyl fragment interference in assay of feline parathyroid hormone, *J Vet Intern Med* 8:168, 1994.

28. Barr FJ, Patterson MW, Lucke VM, et al: Hypercalcemic nephropathy in three dogs: sonographic appearance, *Vet Radiol* 30:169-173, 1989.

29. Barrett S, Sheafor SE, Hillier A, et al: Challenging cases in internal medicine "What's your diagnosis?" *Vet Med* 93:35-44, 1998.

30. Basoglu A, Sevinc M, Sen I, et al: The blocking effect of verapamil in hypercalcemic dogs, *Turkish J Vet Anim Sci* 21:331-333, 1997.

31. Bassett JR: Hypocalcemia and hyperphosphatemia due to primary hypoparathyroidism in a six-month-old kitten, *J Am Anim Hosp Assoc* 34:503-507, 1998.

32. Behrend EN, Kemppainen R: Adrenocortical disease. In August J, editor: *Consultations in feline internal medicine 4*, Philadelphia, 1980, WB Saunders, pp. 159-168.

33. Bennett PF, DeNicola DB, Bonney P, et al: Canine anal sac adenocarcinomas: clinical presentation and response to therapy, *J Vet Intern Med* 16:100-104, 2002.

34. Bereket A, Erdogan T: Oral bisphosphonate therapy for vitamin D intoxication of the infant, *Pediatrics* 111:899-901, 2003.

35. Berenson J, Hirschberg R: Safety and convenience of a 15-minute infusion of zoledronic acid, *Oncologist* 9:319-329, 2004.

36. Berenson JR, Rosen L, Vescio R, et al: Pharmacokinetics of pamidronate disodium in patients with cancer with normal or impaired renal function, *J Clin Pharmacol* 37:285-290, 1997.

37. Berger B, Feldman EC: Primary hyperparathyroidism in dogs: 21 cases (1976-1986), *J Am Vet Med Assoc* 191:350-356, 1987.

38. Bergman SM, O'Mailia J, Krane NK, et al: Vitamin-A-induced hypercalcemia: response to corticosteroids. *Nephron* 50:362-364, 1988.

39. Bernardi RJ, Johnson CS, Modzelewski RA, et al: Antiproliferative effects of 1alpha,25-dihydroxyvitamin D(3) and vitamin D analogs on tumor-derived endothelial cells, *Endocrinology* 143:2508-2514, 2002.

40. Bhattacharya SK, Luther RW, Pate JW, et al: Soft tissue calcium and magnesium content in acute pancreatitis in the dog: calcium accumulation, a mechanism for hypocalcemia in acute pancreatitis, *J Lab Clin Med* 105:422-427, 1985.

41. Bienzle D, Jacobs RM, Lumsden JH: Relationship of serum total calcium to serum albumin in dogs, cats, horses and cattle, *Can Vet J* 34:360-364, 1993.

42. Bienzle D, Silverstein DC, Chaffin K: Multiple myeloma in cats: variable presentation with different immunoglobulin isotypes in two cats, *Vet Pathol* 37:364-369, 2000.

43. Bilezikian JP, Singer FR: Acute management of hypercalcemia due to parathyroid hormone and parathyroid hormone-related protein. In Bilezikian JP, Levine MA, Marcus R, editors: *The parathyroids*, New York, 1994, Raven Press, pp. 359-372.

44. Bilezikian JP: Clinical utility of assays for parathyroid hormone-related protein, *Clin Chem* 38:179-181, 1992.

45. Biller DS, Bradley GA, Partington BP: Renal medullary rim sign: ultrasonographic evidence of renal disease, *Vet Radiol Ultrasound* 33:286-290, 1992.

46. Birchard SJ, Peterson ME, Jacobson A: Surgical treatment of feline hyperthyroidism: results of 85 cases, *J Am Anim Hosp Assoc* 20:705-709, 1984.

47. Biswas PN, Wilton LV, Shakir SA: Pharmacovigilance study of alendronate in England, *Osteoporos Int* 14:507-514, 2003.

48. Black KS, Mundy GR: Other causes of hypercalcemia: local and ectopic secretion syndromes. In Bilezikian JP, Marcus R, Levine MA, editors: *The parathyroids*, New York, 1994, Raven Press, pp. 341-358.

49. Blackwood L, Sullivan M, Lawson H: Radiographic abnormalities in canine multicentric lymphoma: a review of 84 cases, *J Small Anim Pract* 38:62-69, 1997.

50. Block GA, Martin KJ, de Francisco AL, et al: Cinacalcet for secondary hyperparathyroidism in patients receiving hemodialysis, *N Engl J Med* 350:1516-1525, 2004.

51. Blumenthal SR, Williams TC, Barbee RW, et al: Effects of citrated whole blood transfusion in response to hemorrhage, *Lab Anim Sci* 49:411-417, 1999.

52. Boden SD, Kaplan FS: Calcium homeostasis, *Orthop Clin North Am* 21:31-42, 1990.

53. Body JJ, Coleman RE, Piccart M: Use of bisphosphonates in cancer patients, *Cancer Treat Rev* 22:265-287, 1996.

54. Body JJ: Clinical research update: zoledronate, *Cancer* 80(suppl):1699-1701, 1997.

55. Body JJ: Hypercalcemia of malignancy, *Semin Nephrol* 24:48-54, 2004.

56. Bolliger AP, Graham PA, Richard V, et al: Detection of parathyroid hormone-related protein in cats with humoral hypercalcemia of malignancy, *Vet Clin Pathol* 31:3-8, 2002.

57. Bourdeau A, Souberbielle JC, Bonnet P, et al: Phospholipase-A2 action and arachidonic acid metabolism in calcium-mediated parathyroid hormone secretion, *Endocrinology* 130:1339-1344, 1992.

58. Bourke E, Delaney V: Assessment of hypocalcemia and hypercalcemia, *Clin Lab Med* 13:157-181, 1993.

59. Bowers GN Jr, Brassard C, Sena SF: Measurement of ionized calcium in serum with ion-selective electrodes: a mature technology that can meet the daily service needs, *Clin Chem* 32:1437-1447, 1986.

60. Bowman AR, Epstein S: Drug and hormone effects on vitamin D metabolism. In Feldman D, editor: *Vitamin D*, New York, 1997, Academic Press, pp. 797-829.

61. Bregazzi VS, Fettman MJ, Twedt DC: Hypergastrinemia associated with hypercalcemia in the dog, *J Vet Intern Med* 14:389, 2000.

62. Breitwieser GE, Miedlich SU, Zhang M: Calcium sensing receptors as integrators of multiple metabolic signals, *Cell Calcium* 35:209-216, 2004.

63. Brenza HL, DeLuca HF: Regulation of 25-hydroxyvitamin D3 1alpha-hydroxylase gene expression by parathyroid hormone and 1,25-dihydroxyvitamin D3, *Arch Biochem Biophys* 381:143-152, 2000.

64. Brenza HL, Kimmel-Jehan C, Jehan F, et al: Parathyroid hormone activation of the 25-hydroxyvitamin D3-1alpha-hydroxylase gene promoter, *Proc Natl Acad Sci U S A* 95:1387-1391, 1998.

65. Breslau NA: Normal and abnormal regulation of 1,25-(OH)2D synthesis, *Am J Med Sci* 296:417-425, 1988.

66. Bringhurst FR: Circulating forms of parathyroid hormone: peeling back the onion, *Clin Chem* 49:1973-1975, 2003.

67. Bronner F: Mechanisms and functional aspects of intestinal calcium absorption, *J Exp Zoolog A Comp Exp Biol* 300:47-52, 2003.

68. Bronner F: Mechanisms of intestinal calcium absorption, *J Cell Biochem* 88:387-393, 2003.

69. Brossard JH, Cloutier M, Roy L, et al: Accumulation of a non-(1-84) molecular form of parathyroid hormone (PTH) detected by intact PTH assay in renal failure: importance in the interpretation of PTH values, *J Clin Endocrinol Metab* 81:3923-3929, 1996.

70. Brown AJ, Dusso A, Lopez-Hilker S, et al: 1,25-(OH)2D receptors are decreased in parathyroid glands from chronically uremic dogs, *Kidney Int* 35:19-23, 1989.

71. Brown AJ, Zhong M, Finch J, et al: Rat calcium-sensing receptor is regulated by vitamin D but not by calcium, *Am J Physiol* 270:F454-460, 1996.

72. Brown EM, Conigrave A, Chattopadhyay N: Receptors and signaling for calcium ions, In Bilezikian JP, Marcus R, Levine MA, editors: *The parathyroids,* San Diego, 2001, Academic Press, pp. 127-142.

73. Brown EM, Gamba G, Riccardi D, et al: Cloning and characterization of an extracellular Ca(2+)-sensing receptor from bovine parathyroid, *Nature* 366:575-580, 1993.

74. Brown EM, Hebert SC: Calcium-receptor-regulated parathyroid and renal function, *Bone* 20:303-309, 1997.

75. Brown EM, Pollak M, Seidman CE, et al: Calcium-ion-sensing cell-surface receptors, *N Engl J Med* 333:234-240, 1995.

76. Brown EM: Extracellular Ca2+ sensing, regulation of parathyroid cell function, and role of Ca2+ and other ions as extracellular (first) messengers, *Physiol Rev* 71:371-411, 1991.

77. Brown EM: Homeostatic mechanisms regulating extracellular and intracellular calcium metabolism. In Bilezikian JP, Marcus R, Levine MA, editors: *The parathyroids,* New York, 1994, Academic Press, pp. 15-54.

78. Brown JE, Neville-Webbe H, Coleman RE: The role of bisphosphonates in breast and prostate cancers, *Endocr Relat Cancer* 11:207-224, 2004.

79. Brown MA, Haughton MA, Grant SF, et al: Genetic control of bone density and turnover: role of the collagen 1alpha1, estrogen receptor, and vitamin D receptor genes, *J Bone Miner Res* 16:758-764, 2001.

80. Brownie CF: Confusion over jasmine and jessamine, *J Am Vet Med Assoc* 191:613-614, 1987.

81. Brunette MG, Vary J, Carriere S: Hyposthenuria in hypercalcemia. A possible role of intrarenal blood-flow (IRBF) redistribution, *Pflugers Arch* 350:9-23, 1974.

82. Bruyette DS, Feldman EC: Primary hypoparathyroidism in the dog. Report of 15 cases and review of 13 previously reported cases, *J Vet Intern Med* 2:7-14, 1988.

83. Burritt MF, Pierides AM, Offord KP: Comparative studies of total and ionized serum calcium values in normal subjects and patients with renal disorders, *Mayo Clin Proc* 55:606-613, 1980.

84. Burtis WJ, Brady TG, Orloff JJ, et al: Immunochemical characterization of circulating parathyroid hormone-related protein in patients with humoral hypercalcemia of cancer, *N Engl J Med* 322:1106-1112, 1990.

85. Burtis WJ, Dann P, Gaich GA, et al: A high abundance midregion species of parathyroid hormone-related protein: immunological and chromatographic characterization in plasma, *J Clin Endocrinol Metab* 78:317-322, 1994.

86. Burtis WJ: Parathyroid hormone-related protein: structure, function, and measurement, *Clin Chem* 38:2171-2183, 1992.

87. Bush WW, Kimmel SE, Wosar MA, et al: Secondary hypoparathyroidism attributed to hypomagnesemia in a dog with protein-losing enteropathy, *J Am Vet Med Assoc* 219:1732-1734, 1708, 2001.

88. Cairns CB, Niemann JT, Pelikan PC, et al: Ionized hypocalcemia during prolonged cardiac arrest and closed-chest CPR in a canine model, *Ann Emerg Med* 20:1178-1182, 1991.

89. Caldin M, Tommaso F, Lubas G, et al: Incidence of persistent hypercalcemia in dogs and its diagnostic approach. In *European Society of Veterinary Internal Medicine Congress,* Dublin, Ireland, 2001.

90. Calia CM, Hohenhaus AE, Fox PR, et al: Acute tumor lysis syndrome in a cat with lymphoma, *J Vet Intern Med* 10:409-411, 1996.

91. Campbell A: Calcipotriol poisoning in dogs, *Vet Rec* 141:27-28, 1997.

92. Campese VM: Calcium, parathyroid hormone, and blood pressure, *Am J Hypertens* 2:34S-44S, 1989.

93. Camus C, Charasse C, Jouannic-Montier I, et al: Calcium free hemodialysis: experience in the treatment of 33 patients with severe hypercalcemia, *Intensive Care Med* 22:116-121, 1996.

94. Canaff L, Hendy GN: Human calcium-sensing receptor gene. Vitamin D response elements in promoters P1 and P2 confer transcriptional responsiveness to 1,25-dihydroxyvitamin D, *J Biol Chem* 277:30337-30350, 2002.

95. Canalejo A, Almaden Y, Torregrosa V, et al: The in vitro effect of calcitriol on parathyroid cell proliferation and apoptosis, *J Am Soc Nephrol* 11:1865-1872, 2000.

96. Canalejo A, Canadillas S, Ballesteros E, et al: Importance of arachidonic acid as a mediator of parathyroid gland response, *Kidney Int Suppl* June:S10-13, 2003.

97. Canalis E, Hock JM, Raisz LG: Anabolic and catabolic effects of parathyroid hormone on bone and interactions with growth factors. In Bilezikian JP, Marcus R, Levine MA, editors: *The parathyroids,* New York, 1994, Raven Press, pp. 65-82.

98. Capen CC, Martin SL: Calcium metabolism and disorders of parathyroid glands, *Vet Clin North Am* 7:513-548, 1977.

99. Capen CC, Rosol TJ: Hormonal control of mineral metabolism. In Bojrab MJ, editors: *Disease mechanisms in small animal surgery,* Philadelphia, 1993, Lea & Febiger, pp. 841-857.

100. Care AD: The placental transfer of calcium, *J Dev Physiol* 15:253-257, 1991.

101. Carlstedt F, Lind L, Rastad J, et al: Parathyroid hormone and ionized calcium levels are related to the severity of illness and survival in critically ill patients, *Eur J Clin Invest* 28:898-903, 1998.

102. Carothers M, Chew DJ, Nagode LA: 25-OH-cholecalciferol intoxication in dogs. In *Proceedings Am Coll Vet Intern Med Forum,* 1994.

103. Chang W, Shoback D: Extracellular Ca2+-sensing receptors—an overview, *Cell Calcium* 35:183-196, 2004.

104. Chen RA, Goodman WG: Role of the calcium-sensing receptor in parathyroid gland physiology, *Am J Physiol Renal Physiol* 286:F1005-1011, 2004.

105. Cheteri MB, Stanford JL, Friedrichsen DM, et al: Vitamin D receptor gene polymorphisms and prostate cancer risk, *Prostate* 59:409-418, 2004.

106. Chew DJ, Capen CC: Hypercalcemic nephropathy and associated disorders. In Kirk RW, editor: *Current veterinary therapy VII,* Philadelphia, 1980, WB Saunders, pp. 1067-1072.

107. Reference deleted in pages.

108. Chew DJ, Carothers M, Nagode LA, et al: 25-OH-cholecalciferol intoxication in 12 dogs (14 episodes). In *Proceedings of the 39th Annual Congress of World Small Animal Veterinary Association,* Berlin, Germany, 1993.

109. Chew DJ, Carothers M: Hypercalcemia, *Vet Clin North Am Small Anim Pract* 19:265-87, 1989.

110. Chew DJ, Leonard M, Muir W 3rd: Effect of sodium bicarbonate infusions on ionized calcium and total calcium concentrations in serum of clinically normal cats, *Am J Vet Res* 50:145-150, 1989.

111. Chew DJ, Meuten DJ: Disorders of calcium and phosphorus metabolism, *Vet Clin North Am Small Anim Pract* 12:411-438, 1982.

112. Chew DJ, Meuten DJ: Primary hyperparathyroidism. In Kirk RW, editor: *Current veterinary therapy VIII,* Philadelphia, 1983, WB Saunders, pp. 880-884.

113. Chew DJ, Nagode L, Rosol TJ, et al: Utility of diagnostic assays in the evaluation of hypercalcemia and hypocalcemia: parathyroid hormone, vitamin D metabolites, parathyroid hormone-related protein, and ionized calcium. In Bonagura JD, editor: *Kirk's current veterinary therapy XII: small animal practice,* Philadelphia, 1995, WB Saunders, pp. 378-383.

114. Chew DJ, Nagode LA: Renal secondary hyperparathyroidism. In *Proc Soc Comp Endocrinol,* 1990.

115. Chew DJ, Schaer M, Liu S-K, et al: Pseudohyperparathyroidism in a cat, *J Natl Cancer Inst* 11:46-52, 1975.

116. Ching SV, Fettman MJ, Hamar DW, et al: The effect of chronic dietary acidification using ammonium chloride on acid-base and mineral metabolism in the adult cat, *J Nutr* 119:902-915, 1989.

117. Ching SV, Norrdin RW: Histomorphometric comparison of measurements of trabecular bone remodeling in iliac crest biopsy sites and lumbar vertebrae in cats, *Am J Vet Res* 51:447-450, 1990.

118. Chisholm MA, Mulloy AL, Taylor AT: Acute management of cancer-related hypercalcemia, *Ann Pharmacother* 30:507-513, 1996.

119. Chorev M, Alexander JM, Rosenblatt M: Interactions of parathyroid hormone and parathyroid hormone-related protein with their receptors. In Bilezikian JP, Marcus R, Levine MA, editors: *The parathyroids,* San Diego, 2001, Academic Press, pp. 53-92.

120. Christakos S, Beck JD, Hyliner SJ: Calbindin-D 28K. In Feldman D, editor: *Vitamin D,* New York, 1997, Academic Press, pp. 209-221.

121. Coburn JW, Maung HM: Use of active vitamin D sterols in patients with chronic kidney disease, stages 3 and 4, *Kidney Int Suppl* June:S49-53, 2003.

122. Coburn JW: An update on vitamin D as related to nephrology practice: 2003, *Kidney Int Suppl* November: S125-130, 2003.

123. Cook SD, Skinner HB, Haddad RJ: A quantitative histologic study of osteoporosis produced by nutritional secondary hyperparathyroidism in dogs, *Clin Orthop Relat Res* May:105-120, 1983.

124. Cooke NE, Haddad JG: Vitamin D binding protein. In Feldman D, editor: *Vitamin D,* New York, 1997, Academic Press, pp. 87-101.

125. Coukell AJ, Markham A: Pamidronate. A review of its use in the management of osteolytic bone metastases, tumour-induced hypercalcaemia and Paget's disease of bone, *Drugs Aging* 12:149-168, 1998.

126. D'Amour P, Brossard JH, Rousseau L, et al: Amino-terminal form of parathyroid hormone (PTH) with immunologic similarities to hPTH(1-84) is overproduced in primary and secondary hyperparathyroidism, *Clin Chem* 49:2037-2044, 2003.

127. Davainis GM, Chew DJ, Nagode LA, et al: Calcium regulation in the cat with chronic renal failure. In *European Society of Veterinary Internal Medicine/European Society of Veterinary Endocrinology Annual Meeting,* Dublin, Ireland, 2001.

128. De Boer IH, Gorodetskaya I, Young B, et al: The severity of secondary hyperparathyroidism in chronic renal insufficiency is GFR-dependent, race-dependent, and associated with cardiovascular disease, *J Am Soc Nephrol* 13:2762-2769, 2002.

129. De Luisi A, Hofer AM: Evidence that Ca(2+) cycling by the plasma membrane Ca(2+)-ATPase increases the "excitability" of the extracellular Ca(2+)-sensing receptor, *J Cell Sci* 116:1527-1538, 2003.

130. DeLay J, Laing J: Nutritional osteodystophy in puppies fed a BARF diet, *AHL Newsletter* 6:23, 2002.

131. DeLuca HF, Krisinger J, Darwish H: The vitamin D system: 1990, *Kidney Int Suppl* 29:S2-8, 1990.

132. Demay M: Muscle: a nontraditional 1,25-dihydroxyvitamin D target tissue exhibiting classic hormone-dependent vitamin D receptor actions, *Endocrinology* 144:5135-5137, 2003.

133. den Hertog E, Goossens MM, van der Linde-Sipman JS, et al: Primary hyperparathyroidism in two cats, *Vet Q* 19:81-84, 1997.

134. Deniz A, Mischke R: [Ionized calcium and total calcium in the cat], *Berl Munch Tierarztl Wochenschr* 108:105-108, 1995.

135. DeVries SE, Feldman EC, Nelson RW, et al: Primary parathyroid gland hyperplasia in dogs: six cases (1982-1991), *J Am Vet Med Assoc* 202:1132-1136, 1993.

136. Dhupa N, Proulx J: Hypocalcemia and hypomagnesemia, *Vet Clin North Am Small Anim Pract* 28:587-608, 1998.

137. DiBartola SP, Chew DJ, Jacobs G: Quantitative urinalysis including 24-hour protein excretion in the dog, *J Am Anim Hosp Assoc* 16:537-546, 1980.

138. DiBartola SP, Rutgers HC, Zack PM, et al: Clinicopathologic findings associated with chronic renal disease in cats: 74 cases (1973-1984), *J Am Vet Med Assoc* 190:1196-1202, 1987.

139. Divieti P, John MR, Juppner H, et al: Human PTH-(7-84) inhibits bone resorption in vitro via actions independent of the type 1 PTH/PTHrP receptor, *Endocrinology* 143:171-176, 2002.

140. Dougherty SA, Center SA, Dzanis DA: Salmon calcitonin as adjunct treatment for vitamin D toxicosis in a dog, *J Am Vet Med Assoc* 196:1269-1272, 1990.

141. Dow SW, Legendre AM, Stiff M, et al: Hypercalcemia associated with blastomycosis in dogs, *J Am Vet Med Assoc* 188:706-709, 1986.

142. Drazner FH: Hypercalcemia in the dog and cat, *J Am Vet Med Assoc* 178:1252-1256, 1981.

143. Drobatz KJ, Casey KK: Eclampsia in dogs: 31 cases (1995-1998), *J Am Vet Med Assoc* 217:216-219, 2000.

144. Drobatz KJ, Hughes D: Concentration of ionized calcium in plasma from cats with urethral obstruction, *J Am Vet Med Assoc* 211:1392-1395, 1997.

145. Drop LJ: Ionized calcium, the heart, and hemodynamic function, *Anesth Analg* 64:432-451, 1985.

146. Drueke TB, McCarron DA: Paricalcitol as compared with calcitriol in patients undergoing hemodialysis, *N Engl J Med* 349:496-499, 2003.

147. Drueke TB: Cell biology of parathyroid gland hyperplasia in chronic renal failure, *J Am Soc Nephrol* 11:1141-1152, 2000.

148. Drueke TB: Parathyroid gland hyperplasia in uremia, *Kidney Int* 59:1182-1183, 2001.

149. Duncan AR: The use of subcutaneous pamidronate, *J Pain Symptom Manage* 26:592-593, 2003.

150. Dusso AS, Finch J, Brown A, et al: Extrarenal production of calcitriol in normal and uremic humans, *J Clin Endocrinol Metab* 72:157-164, 1991.

151. Dusso AS: Vitamin D receptor: mechanisms for vitamin D resistance in renal failure, *Kidney Int Suppl* June:S6-9, 2003.

152. Dust A, Norris AM, Valli VEO: Cutaneous lymphosarcoma with IgG monoclonal gammopathy, serum hyperviscosity and hypercalcemia in a cat, *Can Vet J* 23:235-239, 1982.

153. Dzanis DA, Kallfelz FA: Recent knowledge of vitamin D toxicity in dogs. In *Proceedings Am Coll Vet Intern Med Forum*, vol 6, 1988.

154. Earm JH, Christensen BM, Frokiaer J, et al: Decreased aquaporin-2 expression and apical plasma membrane delivery in kidney collecting ducts of polyuric hypercalcemic rats, *J Am Soc Nephrol* 9:2181-2193, 1998.

155. Eelen G, Verlinden L, van Camp M, et al: The effects of 1alpha,25-dihydroxyvitamin D3 on the expression of DNA replication genes, *J Bone Miner Res* 19:133-146, 2004.

156. Eiam-Ong S, Punsin P, Sitprija V, et al: Acute hypercalcemia-induced hypertension: the roles of calcium channel and alpha-1 adrenergic receptor, *J Med Assoc Thai* 87:410-418, 2004.

157. Elliott J, Dobson J, Dunn J, et al: Hypercalcemia in the dog: a study of 40 cases, *J Small Anim Pract* 32:564-571, 1991.

158. Engelman RW, Tyler RD, Good RA, et al: Hypercalcemia in cats with feline-leukemia-virus-associated leukemia-lymphoma, *Cancer* 56:777-781, 1985.

159. Estepa JC, Lopez I, Felsenfeld AJ, et al: Dynamics of secretion and metabolism of PTH during hypo- and hypercalcaemia in the dog as determined by the "intact" and "whole" PTH assays, *Nephrol Dial Transplant* 18:1101-1107, 2003.

160. Eubig PA: Acute renal failure in dogs subsequent to the ingestion of grapes or raisins: a retrospective evaluation of 43 dogs (1992-2002), *J Vet Intern Med* in press, 2005.

161. Falchetti A: Calcium agonists in hyperparathyroidism, *Expert Opin Investig Drugs* 13:229-244, 2004.

162. Fan TM, de Lorimier LP, Charney SC, et al: Evaluation of intravenous pamidronate administration in 33 cancer-bearing dogs with primary or secondary bone involvement, *J Vet Intern Med* 19:74-80, 2005.

163. Fan TM, Simpson KW, Trasti S, et al: Calcipotriol toxicity in a dog, *J Small Anim Pract* 39:581-586, 1998.

164. Farese G, Mager M, Blatt WF: A membrane ultrafiltration procedure for determining diffusible calcium in serum, *Clin Chem* 16:226-228, 1970.

165. Fascetti AJ, Hickman MA: Preparturient hypocalcemia in four cats, *J Am Vet Med Assoc* 215:1127-1129, 1999.

166. Favus MJ, Langman CB: Evidence for calcium-dependent control of 1,25-dihydroxyvitamin D3 production by rat kidney proximal tubules, *J Biol Chem* 261:11224-11229, 1986.

167. Favus MJ: Intestinal absorption of calcium, magnesium, and phosphorus. In Coe FL, Favus MJ: *Disorders of bone and mineral metabolism*, New York, 1992, Raven Press, pp. 57-81.

168. Feldman EC, Nelson RW: Hypercalcemia and primary hyperparathyroidism. In Feldman EC, editor: *Canine and feline endocrinology and reproduction*, Philadelphia, 2004, WB Saunders, pp. 660-715.

169. Feldman EC, Nelson RW: Hypocalcemia and primary hypoparathyroidism. In Feldman EC, editor: *Canine and feline endocrinology and reproduction*, Philadelphia, 2004, WB Saunders.

170. Feldman EC, Wisner ER, Nelson RW, et al: Comparison of results of hormonal analysis of samples obtained from selected venous sites versus cervical ultrasonography for localizing parathyroid masses in dogs, *J Am Vet Med Assoc* 211:54-56, 1997.

171. Fenton AJ, Kemp BE, Hammonds RG Jr, et al: A potent inhibitor of osteoclastic bone resorption within a highly conserved pentapeptide region of parathyroid hormone-related protein; PTHrP[107-111], *Endocrinology* 129:3424-3426, 1991.

172. Fenton AJ, Kemp BE, Kent GN, et al: A carboxyl-terminal peptide from the parathyroid hormone-related

protein inhibits bone resorption by osteoclasts, *Endocrinology* 129:1762-1768, 1991.

173. Finco DR, Rowland GN: Hypercalcemia secondary to chronic renal failure in the dog: a report of four cases, *J Am Vet Med Assoc* 173:990-994, 1978.

174. Finco DR: Interpretations of serum calcium concentration in the dog, *Comp Contin Educ* 5:778-787, 1983.

175. Fingeroth JM, Smeak DD: Intravenous methylene blue infusion for intraoperative identification of parathyroid gland tumors in dogs. Part III: Clinical trials and results in three dogs, *J Am Anim Hosp Assoc* 24:673-678, 1988.

176. Fitzpatrick LA, Brandi ML, Aurbach GD: Control of PTH secretion is mediated through calcium channels and is blocked by pertussis toxin treatment of parathyroid cells, *Biochem Biophys Res Commun* 138:960-965, 1986.

177. Flanders JA, Harvey HJ, Erb HN: Feline thyroidectomy. A comparison of postoperative hypocalcemia associated with three different surgical techniques, *Vet Surg* 16:362-366, 1987.

178. Flanders JA, Neth S, Erb HN, et al: Functional analysis of ectopic parathyroid activity in cats, *Am J Vet Res* 52:1336-1340, 1991.

179. Flanders JA, Scarlett JM, Blue JT, et al: Adjustment of total serum calcium concentration for binding to albumin and protein in cats: 291 cases (1986-1987), *J Am Vet Med Assoc* 194:1609-1611, 1989.

180. Flanders JA: Surgical therapy of the thyroid, *Vet Clin North Am Small Anim Pract* 24:607-621, 1994.

181. Fleisch H: Bisphosphonates. Pharmacology and use in the treatment of tumour-induced hypercalcaemic and metastatic bone disease, *Drugs* 42:919-944, 1991.

182. Fleisch H: Mechanisms of action of the bisphosphonates, *Medicina (B Aires)* 57(suppl 1):65-75, 1997.

183. Fooshee SK, Forrester SD: Hypercalcemia secondary to cholecalciferol rodenticide toxicosis in two dogs, *J Am Vet Med Assoc* 196:1265-1268, 1990.

184. Forbes S, Nelson RW, Guptill L: Primary hypoparathyroidism in a cat, *J Am Vet Med Assoc* 196:1285-1287, 1990.

185. Fournel-Fleury C, Ponce F, Felman P, et al: Canine T-cell lymphomas: a morphological, immunological, and clinical study of 46 new cases, *Vet Pathol* 39:92-109, 2002.

186. Fradkin JM, Braniecki AM, Craig TM, et al: Elevated parathyroid hormone-related protein and hypercalcemia in two dogs with schistosomiasis, *J Am Anim Hosp Assoc* 37:349-355, 2001.

187. Franceschini N, Joy MS, Kshirsagar A: Cinacalcet HCl: a calcimimetic agent for the management of primary and secondary hyperparathyroidism, *Expert Opin Investig Drugs* 12:1413-1421, 2003.

188. Fraser D, Jones G, Kooh SW, et al: *Calcium and phosphate metabolism*, Philadelphia, 1986, WB Saunders, pp. 1317-1372.

189. Fraser D, Jones G, Kooh SW: Calcium and phosphate metabolism. In Tietz NW, editor: *Fundamentals of clinical chemistry*, Philadelphia, 1987, WB Saunders, pp. 705-728.

190. Frolik CA, Black EC, Cain RL, et al: Anabolic and catabolic bone effects of human parathyroid hormone (1-34) are predicted by duration of hormone exposure, *Bone* 33:372-379, 2003.

191. Fukagawa M, Kitaoka M, Kurokawa K: Renal failure and hyperparathyroidism. In Feldman D, editor: *Vitamin D*, New York, 1997, Academic Press, pp. 1227-1239.

192. Gao P, Scheibel S, D'Amour P, et al: Development of a novel immunoradiometric assay exclusively for biologically active whole parathyroid hormone 1-84: implica-

tions for improvement of accurate assessment of parathyroid function, *J Bone Miner Res* 16:605-614, 2001.

193. Garcion E, Sindji L, Nataf S, et al: Treatment of experimental autoimmune encephalomyelitis in rat by 1,25-dihydroxyvitamin D3 leads to early effects within the central nervous system, *Acta Neuropathol (Berl)* 105:438-448, 2003.

194. Garlock SM, Matz ME, Shell LG: Vitamin D3 rodenticide toxicity in a dog, *J Am Anim Hosp Assoc* 27:356-360, 1991.

195. Garrett IR: Bone destruction in cancer, *Semin Oncol* 20(suppl 2):4-9, 1993.

196. Gaschen F, Gaschen L, Seiler G, et al: Lethal peracute rhabdomyolysis associated with stress and general anesthesia in three dystrophin-deficient cats, *Vet Pathol* 35:117-123, 1998.

197. Gascon-Barre M: The vitamin D 25-hydroxylase. In Feldman D, editor: *Vitamin D*, New York, 1997, Academic Press, pp. 41-56.

198. Gertz BJ, Holland SD, Kline WF, et al: Studies of the oral bioavailability of alendronate, *Clin Pharmacol Ther* 58:288-298, 1995.

199. Ghazarian JG: The renal mitochondrial hydroxylases of the vitamin D3 endocrine complex: how are they regulated at the molecular level? *J Bone Miner Res* 5:897-903, 1990.

200. Goldstein RE, Long C, Swift NC, et al: Percutaneous ethanol injection for treatment of unilateral hyperplastic thyroid nodules in cats, *J Am Vet Med Assoc* 218:1298-1302, 2001.

201. Goodman WG, Belin T, Gales B, et al: Calcium-regulated parathyroid hormone release in patients with mild or advanced secondary hyperparathyroidism, *Kidney Int* 48:1553-1558, 1995.

202. Goodman WG, Veldhuis JD, Belin TR, et al: Calcium-sensing by parathyroid glands in secondary hyperparathyroidism, *J Clin Endocrinol Metab* 83:2765-2772, 1998.

203. Goodman WG: New assays for parathyroid hormone (PTH) and the relevance of PTH fragments in renal failure, *Kidney Int Suppl* November:S120-124, 2003.

204. Goodman WG: Recent developments in the management of secondary hyperparathyroidism, *Kidney Int* 59:1187-1201, 2001.

205. Gosling P: Analytical reviews in clinical biochemistry: calcium measurement, *Ann Clin Biochem* 23:t146-156, 1986.

206. Goswami R, Brown EM, Kochupillai N, et al: Prevalence of calcium sensing receptor autoantibodies in patients with sporadic idiopathic hypoparathyroidism, *Eur J Endocrinol* 150:9-18, 2004.

207. Gouget B, Gourmelin Y, Blanchet F, et al: Ca2+ measurement with ion selective electrodes. The French coordinated evaluation of seven analyzers, for a better clinical relevance and acceptance, *Ann Biol Clin (Paris)* 46:419-434, 1988.

208. Grant WB, Garland CF: Evidence supporting the role of vitamin D in reducing the risk of cancer, *J Intern Med* 252:178-179; author reply 179-180, 2002.

209. Graves TK: Complications of treatment and concurrent illness associated with hyperthyroidism in cats. In Bonagura JD: *Kirk's current veterinary therapy XII: small animal practice*, Philadelphia, 1995, WB Saunders, pp. 369-372.

210. Green MD: Oral bisphosphonates and malignancy, *Med J Aust* 167:211-212, 1997.

211. Greenlee PG, Filippa DA, Quimby FW, et al: Lymphomas in dogs. A morphologic, immunologic, and clinical study, *Cancer* 66:480-490, 1990.

212. Grone A, McCauley LK, Capen CC, et al: Cloning and sequencing of the 3′-region of the canine parathyroid hormone-related protein gene and analysis of alternate mRNA splicing in two canine carcinomas, *Domest Anim Endocrinol* 22:169-177, 2002.

213. Grosenbaugh DA, Gadawski JE, Muir WW: Evaluation of a portable clinical analyzer in a veterinary hospital setting, *J Am Vet Med Assoc* 213:691-694, 1998.

214. Gunther R, Felice LJ, Nelson RK, et al: Toxicity of a vitamin D3 rodenticide to dogs, *J Am Vet Med Assoc* 193:211-214, 1988.

215. Gwaltney-Brant S, Holding JK, Donaldson CW, et al: Renal failure associated with ingestion of grapes or raisins in dogs, *J Am Vet Med Assoc* 218:1555-1556, 2001.

216. Habener JF, Rosenblatt M, Potts JT Jr: Parathyroid hormone: biochemical aspects of biosynthesis, secretion, action, and metabolism, *Physiol Rev* 64:985-1053, 1984.

217. Halabe A, Arie R, Mimran D, et al: Hypoparathyroidism—a long-term follow-up experience with 1 alpha-vitamin D3 therapy, *Clin Endocrinol (Oxf)* 40:303-307, 1994.

218. Hare WR, Dobbs CE, Slayman KA, et al: Calcipotriene poisoning in dogs, *Vet Med* 95:770-778, 2000.

219. Harrison HE, Harrison HC: Transfer of Ca45 across intestinal wall in vitro in relation to action of vitamin D and cortisol, *Am J Physiol* 199:265-271, 1960.

220. Haruna A, Kawai K, Takab T, et al: Dietary calcinosis in the cat, *J Anim Clin Res Round* 1:9-16, 1992.

221. Haussler MR, Haussler CA, Jurutka PW, et al: The nuclear vitamin D receptor: from clinical radioreceptor assay of the vitamin D hormone to genomics, proteomics and a novel ligand, *J Clin Ligand Assay* 25:221-228, 2002.

222. Hayes CE, Nashold FE, Spach KM, et al: The immunological functions of the vitamin D endocrine system, *Cell Mol Biol (Noisy-le-grand)* 49:277-300, 2003.

223. Hazewinkel HA, Tryfonidou MA: Vitamin D3 metabolism in dogs, *Mol Cell Endocrinol* 197:23-33, 2002.

224. Hazewinkel HA: Dietary influences on calcium homeostasis and the skeleton. In *Proceedings of the 1st Purina Int Nutr Symp*, 1991.

225. Henderson RA, Powers RD, Perry L: Development of hypoparathyroidism after excision of laryngeal rhabdomyosarcoma in a dog, *J Am Vet Med Assoc* 198:639-643, 1991.

226. Henry DA, Goodman WG, Nudelman RK, et al: Parenteral aluminum administration in the dog: I. Plasma kinetics, tissue levels, calcium metabolism, and parathyroid hormone, *Kidney Int* 25:362-369, 1984.

227. Henry H: The 25-hydroxyvitamin D 1-alpha-hydroxylase. In Feldman D, editor: *Vitamin D,* New York, 1997, Academic Press, pp. 57-68.

228. Hess RS, Saunders HM, Van Winkle TJ, et al: Concurrent disorders in dogs with diabetes mellitus: 221 cases (1993-1998), *J Am Vet Med Assoc* 217:1166-1173, 2000.

229. Hickford FH, Stokol T, vanGessel YA, et al: Monoclonal immunoglobulin G cryoglobulinemia and multiple myeloma in a domestic shorthair cat, *J Am Vet Med Assoc* 217:1029-1033, 1007-1008, 2000.

230. Hilbe M, Sydler T, Fischer L, et al: Metastatic calcification in a dog attributable to ingestion of a tacalcitol ointment, *Vet Pathol* 37:490-492, 2000.

231. Hill RC, Van Winkle TJ: Acute necrotizing pancreatitis and acute suppurative pancreatitis in the cat. A retrospective study of 40 cases (1976-1989), *J Vet Intern Med* 7:25-33, 1993.

232. Hirt RA, Kneissl S, Teinfalt M: Severe hypercalcemia in a dog with a retained fetus and endometritis, *J Am Vet Med Assoc* 216:1423-1425, 1412, 2000.

233. Hoare SR, Usdin TB: Molecular mechanisms of ligand recognition by parathyroid hormone 1 (PTH1) and PTH2 receptors, *Curr Pharm Des* 7:689-713, 2001.

234. Hodges RD, Legendre AM, Adams LG, et al: Itraconazole for the treatment of histoplasmosis in cats, *J Vet Intern Med* 8:409-413, 1994.

235. Hofer AM, Brown EM: Extracellular calcium sensing and signalling, *Nat Rev Mol Cell Biol* 4:530-538, 2003.

236. Holick MF: Noncalcemic actions of 1,25-dihydroxyvitamin D3 and clinical applications, *Bone* 17(suppl):107S-111S, 1995.

237. Holick MF: Photobiology of vitamin D. In Feldman D, editor: *Vitamin D,* New York, 1997, Academic Press, pp. 33-40.

238. Holick MF: Vitamin D: importance in the prevention of cancers, type 1 diabetes, heart disease, and osteoporosis, *Am J Clin Nutr* 79:362-371, 2004.

239. Holley DC, Evans JW: Determination of total and ultrafilterable calcium and magnesium in normal equine serum, *Am J Vet Res* 38:259-262, 1977.

240. Hollis BW, Kamerud JQ, Kurkowski A, et al: Quantification of circulating 1,25-dihydroxyvitamin D by radioimmunoassay with 125I-labeled tracer, *Clin Chem* 42:586-592, 1996.

241. Horn B, Irwin PJ: Transient hypoparathyroidism following successful treatment of hypercalcaemia of malignancy in a dog, *Aust Vet J* 78:690-692, 2000.

242. Horst RL, Reinhardt TA, Hollis BW: Improved methodology for the analysis of plasma vitamin D metabolites, *Kidney Int Suppl* 29:S28-35, 1990.

243. Horst RL, Reinhardt TA: Vitamin D metabolism. In Feldman D, editor: *Vitamin D,* New York, 1997, Academic Press, pp. 13-31.

244. Hostutler RA, Chew DJ, Jaeger JQ, et al: Uses and effectiveness of pamidronate disodium for treatment of dogs and cats with hypercalcemia, *J Vet Intern Med* 19:29-33, 2005.

245. How KL, Hazewinkel HA, Mol JA: Dietary vitamin D dependence of cat and dog due to inadequate cutaneous synthesis of vitamin D, *Gen Comp Endocrinol* 96:12-18, 1994.

246. Hristova EN, Cecco S, Niemela JE, et al: Analyzer-dependent differences in results for ionized calcium, ionized magnesium, sodium, and pH, *Clin Chem* 41:1649-1653, 1995.

247. Hsu CH, Patel SR: Altered vitamin D metabolism and receptor interaction with the target genes in renal failure: calcitriol receptor interaction with its target gene in renal failure, *Curr Opin Nephrol Hypertens* 4:302-306, 1995.

248. Hulter HN, Halloran BP, Toto RD, et al: Long-term control of plasma calcitriol concentration in dogs and humans. Dominant role of plasma calcium concentration in experimental hyperparathyroidism, *J Clin Invest* 76:695-702, 1985.

249. Hung SH, Tsai WY, Tsao PN, et al: Oral clodronate therapy for hypercalcemia related to extensive subcutaneous fat necrosis in a newborn, *J Formos Med Assoc* 102:801-804, 2003.

250. Hutson CA, Willauer CC, Walder EJ, et al: Treatment of mandibular squamous cell carcinoma in cats by use of mandibulectomy and radiotherapy: seven cases (1987-1989), *J Am Vet Med Assoc* 201:777-781, 1992.

251. Ihle SL, Nelson RW, Cook JR Jr: Seizures as a manifestation of primary hyperparathyroidism in a dog, *J Am Vet Med Assoc* 192:71-72, 1988.

252. Imaizumi T, Tsuruta M, Kitagaki T, et al: [Single dose toxicity studies of calcipotriol (MC903) in rats and dogs], *J Toxicol Sci* 21(suppl 2):277-285, 1996.

253. Imaizumi T, Tsuruta M, Koike Y, et al: [A 26-week repeated percutaneous dose toxicity study of calcipotriol (MC903) in dogs], *J Toxicol Sci* 21(suppl 2):365-387, 1996.

254. Imaizumi T, Tsuruta M, Koike Y, et al: A 4-week repeated percutaneous dose toxicity study of calcipotriol (MC903) followed by a 4-week recovery test in dogs, *J Toxicol Sci* 21(suppl 2):309-323, 1996.

255. Imamura H, Sato K, Shizume K, et al: Urinary excretion of parathyroid hormone-related protein fragments in patients with humoral hypercalcemia of malignancy and hypercalcemic tumor-bearing nude mice, *J Bone Miner Res* 6:77-84, 1991.

256. Irvine RF: Calcium transients: mobilization of intracellular Ca2+, *Br Med Bull* 42:369-374, 1986.

257. Izquierdo R, Bermes E Jr, Sandberg L, et al: Serum calcium metabolism in acute experimental pancreatitis, *Surgery* 98:1031-1037, 1985.

258. Jackson IT, Saleh J, van Heerden JA: Gigantic mammary hyperplasia in pregnancy associated with pseudohyperparathyroidism, *Plast Reconstr Surg* 84:806-810, 1989.

259. John MR, Goodman WG, Gao P, et al: A novel immunoradiometric assay detects full-length human PTH but not amino-terminally truncated fragments: implications for PTH measurements in renal failure, *J Clin Endocrinol Metab* 84:4287-4290, 1999.

260. Jorgensen LS, Center SA, Randolph JF, et al: Electrolyte abnormalities induced by hypertonic phosphate enemas in two cats, *J Am Vet Med Assoc* 187:1367-1368, 1985.

261. Jutkowitz LA, Rozanski EA, Moreau JA, et al: Massive transfusion in dogs: 15 cases (1997-2001), *J Am Vet Med Assoc* 220:1664-1669, 2002.

262. Kadar E, Rush JE, Wetmore L, et al: Electrolyte disturbances and cardiac arrhythmias in a dog following pamidronate, calcitonin, and furosemide administration for hypercalcemia of malignancy, *J Am Anim Hosp Assoc* 40:75-81, 2004.

263. Kallet AJ, Richter KP, Feldman EC, et al: Primary hyperparathyroidism in cats: seven cases (1984-1989), *J Am Vet Med Assoc* 199:1767-1771, 1991.

264. Kallfelz FA: Nutritional supplements in small animal practice: boon or bane? In *Proceedings of the 8th Am Coll Vet Intern Med Forum*, Washington, DC, 1990.

265. Karaplis AC, Luz A, Glowacki J, et al: Lethal skeletal dysplasia from targeted disruption of the parathyroid hormone-related peptide gene, *Genes Dev* 8:277-289, 1994.

266. Kasahara H, Tsuchiya M, Adachi R, et al: Development of a C-terminal-region-specific radioimmunoassay of parathyroid hormone-related protein, *Biomed Res* 13:155-161, 1992.

267. Kawaguchi K, Braga IS 3rd, Takahashi A, et al: Nutritional secondary hyperparathyroidism occurring in a strain of German shepherd puppies, *Jpn J Vet Res* 41:89-96, 1993.

268. Kawasaki T: Creatinine unreliable indicator of renal failure in ferrets, *J Small Anim Exotic Med* 1:28-29, 1991.

269. Khosla S, van Heerden JA, Gharib H, et al: Parathyroid hormone-related protein and hypercalcemia secondary to massive mammary hyperplasia, *N Engl J Med* 322:1157, 1990.

270. Kifor O, McElduff A, LeBoff MS, et al: Activating antibodies to the calcium-sensing receptor in two patients with autoimmune hypoparathyroidism, *J Clin Endocrinol Metab* 89:548-556, 2004.

271. Kimmel SE, Waddell LS, Michel KE: Hypomagnesemia and hypocalcemia associated with protein-losing enteropathy in Yorkshire terriers: five cases (1992-1998), *J Am Vet Med Assoc* 217:703-706, 2000.

272. Kimmel SE, Washabau RJ, Drobatz KJ: Incidence and prognostic value of low plasma ionized calcium concentration in cats with acute pancreatitis: 46 cases (1996-1998), *J Am Vet Med Assoc* 219:1105-1109, 2001.

273. Kirby R, Iverson W, Schaer M: Hypercalcemic nephropathy in a young dog resembling human milk alkali syndrome, *J Am Anim Hosp Assoc* 28:119-123, 1992.

274. Kirk GR, Breazile JE, Kenny AD: Pathogenesis of hypocalcemic tetany in the thyroparathyroidectomized dog, *Am J Vet Res* 35:407-408, 1974.

275. Kiupel M, Teske E, Bostock D: Prognostic factors for treated canine malignant lymphoma, *Vet Pathol* 36:292-300, 1999.

276. Klausner JS, Bell FW, Hayden DW, et al: Hypercalcemia in two cats with squamous cell carcinomas, *J Am Vet Med Assoc* 196:103-105, 1990.

277. Klausner JS, Fernandez FR, O'Leary TP, et al: Canine primary hyperparathyroidism and its association with urolithiasis, *Vet Clin North Am Small Anim Pract* 16:227-239, 1986.

278. Klein MK, Powers BE, Withrow SJ, et al: Treatment of thyroid carcinoma in dogs by surgical resection alone: 20 cases (1981-1989), *J Am Vet Med Assoc* 206:1007-1009, 1995.

279. Knecht TP, Behling CA, Burton DW, et al: The humoral hypercalcemia of benignancy. A newly appreciated syndrome, *Am J Clin Pathol* 105:487-492, 1996.

280. Kogika MM, Lustoza MD, Notomi MK, et al: Serum ionized calcium evaluation in healthy dogs and in dogs with chronic renal failure. In *Proceedings of the World Small Anim Vet Assoc*, 2002.

281. Koller H, Zitt E, Staudacher G, et al: Variable parathyroid hormone(1-84)/carboxylterminal PTH ratios detected by 4 novel parathyroid hormone assays, *Clin Nephrol* 61:337-343, 2004.

282. Koo WS, Jeon DS, Ahn SJ, et al: Calcium-free hemodialysis for the management of hypercalcemia, *Nephron* 72:424-428, 1996.

283. Korkor AB, Kuchibotla J, Arrieh M, et al: The effects of chronic prednisone administration on intestinal receptors for 1,25-dihydroxyvitamin D3 in the dog, *Endocrinology* 117:2267-2273, 1985.

284. Kornegay JN: Hypocalcemia in dogs, *Compend Contin Educ* 4:1785-1792, 1982.

285. Kovacs CS, Ho-Pao CL, Hunzelman JL, et al: Regulation of murine fetal-placental calcium metabolism by the calcium-sensing receptor, *J Clin Invest* 101:2812-2820, 1998.

286. Kremer R, Goltzman D: Assays for parathyroid hormone-related protein. In Bilezikian JP, Marcus R, Levine MA, editors: *The parathyroids*, New York, 1994, Raven Press, pp. 321-340.

287. Krishnan AV, Feldman D: Regulation of vitamin D receptor abundance. In Feldman D, editor: *Vitamin D*, New York, 1997, Academic Press, pp. 179-200.

288. Krishnan AV, Shinghal R, Raghavachari N, et al: Analysis of vitamin D-regulated gene expression in LNCaP human prostate cancer cells using cDNA microarrays, *Prostate* 59:243-251, 2004.

289. Kronenberg HM, Bringhurst FR, Segre GV, et al: Parathyroid hormone biosynthesis and metabolism. In Bilezikian JP, Marcus R, Levine MA, editors: *The parathyroids*, San Diego, 2001, Academic Press, pp. 17-30.

290. Kruger JM, Osborne CA, Nachreiner RF, et al: Hypercalcemia and renal failure. Etiology, pathophysiology, diagnosis, and treatment, *Vet Clin North Am Small Anim Pract* 26:1417-1445, 1996.

291. Kruger JM, Osborne CA, Polzin DJ: Treatment of hypercalcemia. In Kirk RW, editor: *Current veterinary therapy IX*, Philadelphia, 1986, WB Saunders, pp. 75-90.

292. Kuhlmann A, Haas CS, Gross ML, et al: 1,25-Dihydroxyvitamin D3 decreases podocyte loss and podocyte hypertrophy in the subtotally nephrectomized rat, *Am J Physiol Renal Physiol* 286:F526-533, 2004.

293. Kull PA, Hess RS, Craig LE, et al: Clinical, clinicopathologic, radiographic, and ultrasonographic characteristics of intestinal lymphangiectasia in dogs: 17 cases (1996-1998), *J Am Vet Med Assoc* 219:197-202, 2001.

294. Kumar R: Vitamin D and the kidney. In Feldman D, editor: *Vitamin D*, New York, 1997, Academic Press, pp. 275-292.

295. Kyles AE, Stone EA, Gookin J, et al: Diagnosis and surgical management of obstructive ureteral calculi in cats: 11 cases (1993-1996), *J Am Vet Med Assoc* 213:1150-1156, 1998.

296. Ladenson JH, Lewis JW, McDonald JM, et al: Relationship of free and total calcium in hypercalcemic conditions, *J Clin Endocrinol Metab* 48:393-397, 1979.

297. Langub MC, Monier-Faugere MC, Wang G, et al: Administration of PTH-(7-84) antagonizes the effects of PTH-(1-84) on bone in rats with moderate renal failure, *Endocrinology* 144:1135-1138, 2003.

298. Larsson L, Ohman S: Effect of silicone-separator tubes and storage time on ionized calcium in serum, *Clin Chem* 31:169-170, 1985.

299. Lee JA, Drobatz KJ: Characterization of the clinical characteristics, electrolytes, acid-base, and renal parameters in male cats with urethral obstruction, *J Vet Emerg Crit Care* 13:227-233, 2003.

300. Levi J, Massry SG, Coburn JW, et al: Hypocalcemia in magnesium-depleted dogs: evidence for reduced responsiveness to parathyroid hormone and relative failure of parathyroid gland function, *Metabolism* 23:323-335, 1974.

301. Leyland-Jones B: Treating cancer-related hypercalcemia with gallium nitrate, *J Support Oncol* 2:509-516; discussion 516-520, 2004.

302. Lifton SJ, King LG, Zerbe CA: Glucocorticoid deficient hypoadrenocorticism in dogs: 18 cases (1986-1995), *J Am Vet Med Assoc* 209:2076-2081, 1996.

303. Lim SK, Gardella TJ, Baba H, et al: The carboxy-terminus of parathyroid hormone is essential for hormone processing and secretion, *Endocrinology* 131:2325-2330, 1992.

304. Lin R, White JH: The pleiotropic actions of vitamin D, *Bioessays* 26:21-28, 2004.

305. Lincoln SD, Lane VM: Serum ionized calcium concentration in clinically normal dairy cattle, and changes associated with calcium abnormalities, *J Am Vet Med Assoc* 197:1471-1474, 1990.

306. Lind L, Bucht E, Ljunghall S: Pronounced elevation in circulating calcitonin in critical care patients is related to the severity of illness and survival, *Intensive Care Med* 21:63-66, 1995.

307. Lind L, Carlstedt F, Rastad J, et al: Hypocalcemia and parathyroid hormone secretion in critically ill patients, *Crit Care Med* 28:93-99, 2000.

308. Lindemans J, Hoefkens P, van Kessel AL, et al: Portable blood gas and electrolyte analyzer evaluated in a multiinstitutional study, *Clin Chem* 45:111-117, 1999.

309. Lins LE: Renal function in hypercalcemic dogs during hydropenia and during saline infusion, *Acta Physiol Scand* 106:177-186, 1979.

310. Long CD, Goldstein RE, Hornof WJ, et al: Percutaneous ultrasound-guided chemical parathyroid ablation for treatment of primary hyperparathyroidism in dogs, *J Am Vet Med Assoc* 215:217-221, 1999.

311. Looney AL, Ludders J, Erb HN, et al: Use of a handheld device for analysis of blood electrolyte concentrations and blood gas partial pressures in dogs and horses, *J Am Vet Med Assoc* 213:526-530, 1998.

312. Lyon ME, Bremner D, Laha T, et al: Specific heparin preparations interfere with the simultaneous measurement of ionized magnesium and ionized calcium, *Clin Biochem* 28:79-84, 1995.

313. Lyon ME, Guajardo M, Laha T, et al: Electrolyte balanced heparin may produce a bias in the measurement of ionized calcium concentration in specimens with abnormally low protein concentration, *Clin Chim Acta* 233:105-113, 1995.

314. Lyon ME, Guajardo M, Laha T, et al: Zinc heparin introduces a preanalytical error in the measurement of ionized calcium concentration, *Scand J Clin Lab Invest* 55:61-65, 1995.

315. Machado CE, Flombaum CD: Safety of pamidronate in patients with renal failure and hypercalcemia, *Clin Nephrol* 45:175-179, 1996.

316. MacIsaac RJ, Caple IW, Danks JA, et al: Ontogeny of parathyroid hormone-related protein in the ovine parathyroid gland, *Endocrinology* 129:757-764, 1991.

317. MacIsaac RJ, Heath JA, Rodda CP, et al: Role of the fetal parathyroid glands and parathyroid hormone-related protein in the regulation of placental transport of calcium, magnesium and inorganic phosphate, *Reprod Fertil Dev* 3:447-457, 1991.

318. MacKenzie CP: Poisoning in four dogs by a compound containing warfarin and calciferol, *J Small Anim Pract* 28:433-445, 1987.

319. Maestro B, Davila N, Carranza MC, et al: Identification of a vitamin D response element in the human insulin receptor gene promoter, *J Steroid Biochem Mol Biol* 84:223-230, 2003.

320. Mahgoub A, Hirsch PF, Munson PL: Calcium-lowering action of glucocorticoids in adrenalectomized-parathyroidectomized rats. Specificity and relative potency of natural and synthetic glucocorticoids, *Endocrine* 6:279-283, 1997.

321. Major P, Lortholary A, Hon J, et al: Zoledronic acid is superior to pamidronate in the treatment of hypercalcemia of malignancy: a pooled analysis of two randomized, controlled clinical trials, *J Clin Oncol* 19:558-567, 2001.

322. Major P: The use of zoledronic acid, a novel, highly potent bisphosphonate, for the treatment of hypercalcemia of malignancy, *Oncologist* 7:481-491, 2002.

323. Malberti F, Surian M, Cosci P: Improvement of secondary hyperparathyroidism and reduction of the set point of calcium after intravenous calcitriol, *Kidney Int Suppl* 41:S125-130, 1993.

324. Mangin M, Ikeda K, Broadus AE: Structure of the mouse gene encoding parathyroid hormone-related peptide, *Gene* 95:195-202, 1990.

325. Markowitz GS, Fine PL, Stack JI, et al: Toxic acute tubular necrosis following treatment with zoledronate (Zometa), *Kidney Int* 64:281-289, 2003.

326. Marquez GA, Klausner JS, Osborne CA: Calcium oxalate urolithiasis in a cat with a functional parathyroid adenocarcinoma, *J Am Vet Med Assoc* 206:817-819, 1995.

327. Martin LG: Hypercalcemia and hypermagnesemia, *Vet Clin North Am Small Anim Pract* 28:565-585, 1998.

328. Martin TJ, Grill V: Hypercalcemia in cancer, *J Steroid Biochem Mol Biol* 43:123-129, 1992.

329. Martin-Salvago M, Villar-Rodriguez JL, Palma-Alvarez A, et al: Decreased expression of calcium receptor in parathyroid tissue in patients with hyperparathyroidism secondary to chronic renal failure, *Endocr Pathol* 14:61-70, 2003.

330. Massry SG: Pathogenesis of uremic toxicity, Part 1. Parathryoid hormone as a uremic toxin. In Massry SG, Glassock RJ, editors: *Textbook of nephrology*, Baltimore, 1989, Williams & Wilkins, pp. 1126-1144.

331. Matus RE, Leifer CE, MacEwen EG, et al: Prognostic factors for multiple myeloma in the dog, *J Am Vet Med Assoc* 188:1288-1292, 1986.

332. Matwichuk CL, Taylor SM, Daniel GB, et al: Double-phase parathyroid scintigraphy in dogs using technetium-99M-sestamibi, *Vet Radiol Ultrasound* 41:461-469, 2000.

333. Matwichuk CL, Taylor SM, Wilkinson AA, et al: Use of technetium Tc 99m sestamibi for detection of a parathyroid adenoma in a dog with primary hyperparathyroidism, *J Am Vet Med Assoc* 209:1733-1736, 1996.

334. Mazzaferro S, Barberi S, Scarda A, et al: Ionised and total serum magnesium in renal transplant patients, *J Nephrol* 15:275-280, 2002.

335. McCauley LK, Rosol TJ, Stromberg PC, et al: Effects of interleukin-1 alpha and cyclosporin A in vivo and in vitro on bone and lymphoid tissues in mice, *Toxicol Pathol* 19:1-10, 1991.

336. McClain HM, Barsanti JA, Bartges JW: Hypercalcemia and calcium oxalate urolithiasis in cats: a report of five cases, *J Am Anim Hosp Assoc* 35:297-301, 1999.

337. McElwain MC, Modzelewski RA, Yu WD, et al: Vitamin D: an antiproliferative agent with potential for therapy of squamous cell carcinoma, *Am J Otolaryngol* 18:293-298, 1997.

338. Mealey KL, Willard MD, Nagode LA, et al: Hypercalcemia associated with granulomatous disease in a cat, *J Am Vet Med Assoc* 215:959-962, 946, 1999.

339. Meller Y, Kestenbaum RS, Yagil R, et al: The influence of age and sex on blood levels of calcium-regulating hormones in dogs, *Clin Orthop Relat Res* Jul-Aug:296-299, 1984.

340. Merryman JI, Rosol TJ, Brooks CL, et al: Separation of parathyroid hormone-like activity from transforming growth factor-alpha and -beta in the canine adenocarcinoma (CAC-8) model of humoral hypercalcemia of malignancy, *Endocrinology* 124:2456-2463, 1989.

341. Meuten DJ, Chew DJ, Capen CC, et al: Relationship of serum total calcium to albumin and total protein in dogs, *J Am Vet Med Assoc* 180:63-67, 1982.

342. Meuten DJ, Cooper BJ, Capen CC, et al: Hypercalcemia associated with an adenocarcinoma derived from the apocrine glands of the anal sac, *Vet Pathol* 18:454-471, 1981.

343. Meuten DJ, Kociba GJ, Capen CC, et al: Hypercalcemia in dogs with lymphosarcoma. Biochemical, ultrastructural, and histomorphometric investigations, *Lab Invest* 49:553-562, 1983.

344. Meuten DJ, Segre GV, Capen CC, et al: Hypercalcemia in dogs with adenocarcinoma derived from apocrine glands of the anal sac. Biochemical and histomorphometric investigations, *Lab Invest* 48:428-435, 1983.

345. Meuten DJ: Hypercalcemia, *Vet Clin North Am* 14:891-910, 1984.

346. Midkiff AM, Chew DJ, Randolph JF, et al: Idiopathic hypercalcemia in cats, *J Vet Intern Med* 14:619-626, 2000.

347. Miki H, Maercklein PB, Fitzpatrick LA: Effect of magnesium on parathyroid cells: evidence for two sensing receptors or two intracellular pathways? *Am J Physiol* 272:E1-6, 1997.

348. Miller D, Edmonds MW: Hypercalcemia due to hyperparathyroidism treated with a somatostatin analogue, *CMAJ* 145:227-228, 1991.

349. Milner RJ, Farese J, Henry CJ, et al: Bisphosphonates and cancer, *J Vet Intern Med* 18:597-604, 2004.

350. Mischke R, Hanies R, Lange K, et al: [The effect of the albumin concentration on the relation between the concentration of ionized calcium and total calcium in the blood of dogs], *Dtsch Tierarztl Wochenschr* 103:199-204, 1996.

351. Miwa N, Nitta K, Kimata N, et al: An evaluation of 1-84 PTH measurement in relation to bone alkaline phosphatase and bone Gla protein in hemodialysis patients, *Nephron Clin Pract* 94:c29-32, 2003.

352. Mol JA, Kwant MM, Arnold IC, et al: Elucidation of the sequence of canine (pro)-calcitonin. A molecular biological and protein chemical approach, *Regul Pept* 35:189-195, 1991.

353. Moore FM, Kudisch M, Richter K, et al: Hypercalcemia associated with rodenticide poisoning in three cats, *J Am Vet Med Assoc* 193:1099-1100, 1988.

354. Morita T, Awakura T, Shimada A, et al: Vitamin D toxicosis in cats: natural outbreak and experimental study, *J Vet Med Sci* 57:831-837, 1995.

355. Morris JG: Vitamin D synthesis by kittens, *Vet Clin Nutr* 3:88-92, 1996.

356. Morris SA, Bilezikian JP: Signal transduction in bone physiology: messenger systems for parathyroid hormone. In Bilezikian JP, Raisz LG, Rodan GA, editors: *Principles of bone biology*, New York, 1996, Academic Press, pp. 1203-1215.

357. Morrow CMK, Valli VE, Volmer PA, et al: Canine renal pathology associated with grape or raisin ingestion: 10 cases, *J Vet Diagn Invest* 17:223-231, 2005.

358. Mosdell KW, Visconti JA: Emerging indications for octreotide therapy, part 1, *Am J Hosp Pharm* 51:1184-1192, 1994.

359. Moseley JM, Kubota M, Diefenbach-Jagger H, et al: Parathyroid hormone-related protein purified from a human lung cancer cell line, *Proc Natl Acad Sci U S A* 84:5048-5052, 1987.

360. Mundy GR, Oyajobi B: Other local and ectopic hormone syndromes associated with hypercalcemia. In Bilezikian JP, Marcus R, Levine MA, editors: *The parathyroids*, San Diego, 2001, Academic Press, pp. 691-706.

361. Murthy JN, Hicks JM, Soldin SJ: Evaluation of i-STAT portable clinical analyzer in a neonatal and pediatric intensive care unit, *Clin Biochem* 30:385-389, 1997.

362. Nachreiner RF, Refsal KR: The use of parathormone, ionized calcium and 25-hydroxyvitamin D assays to diagnose calcium disorders in dogs. In *Proc Am Coll Vet Intern Med Forum*, vol 8, 1990.

363. Nagode LA, Chew DJ, Podell M: Benefits of calcitriol therapy and serum phosphorus control in dogs and cats with chronic renal failure. Both are essential to prevent of suppress toxic hyperparathyroidism, *Vet Clin North Am Small Anim Pract* 26:1293-1330, 1996.

364. Nagode LA, Chew DJ, Steinmeyer CL: The use of low doses of calcitriol in the treatment of renal secondary hyperparathyroidism. In *Proc 15th Waltham Symposium (Endocrinology)*, Columbus, OH, 1992.

365. Nagode LA, Chew DJ: Nephrocalcinosis caused by hyperparathyroidism in progression of renal failure: treat-

ment with calcitriol, *Semin Vet Med Surg (Small Anim)* 7:202-220, 1992.

366. Nagode LA, Chew DJ: The use of calcitriol in treatment of renal disease of the dog and cat. In *Proc 1st Purina Int Nutr Symp*, 1991.

367. Nagode LA, Steinmeyer CL, Chew DJ, et al: Hyper- and normo-calcemic dogs with chronic renal failure: relations of serum PTH and calcitriol to PTG Ca++ set-point. In Norman AW, Schaefer K, Grigoleit HG, et al, editors: *Vitamin D. Molecular, cellular and clinical endocrinology,* Berlin, 1988, Walter de Gruyter, pp. 799-800.

368. Negri AL, Alvarez Quiroga M, Bravo M, et al: [Whole PTH and 1-84/84 PTH ratio for the non invasive determination of low bone turnover in renal osteodysthrophy], *Nefrologia* 23:327-332, 2003.

369. Nemeth EF, Heaton WH, Miller M, et al: Pharmacodynamics of the type II calcimimetic compound cinacalcet HCl, *J Pharmacol Exp Ther* 308:627-635, 2004.

370. Nemzek JA, Kruger JM, Walshaw R, et al: Acute onset of hypokalemia and muscular weakness in four hyperthyroid cats, *J Am Vet Med Assoc* 205:65-68, 1994.

371. Neuman NB: Acute pancreatic hemorrhage associated with iatrogenic hypercalcemia in a dog, *J Am Vet Med Assoc* 166:381-383, 1975.

372. Neves M, Gano L, Pereira N, et al: Synthesis, characterization and biodistribution of bisphosphonates Sm-153 complexes: correlation with molecular modeling interaction studies, *Nucl Med Biol* 29:329-338, 2002.

373. Neville-Webbe H, Coleman RE: The use of zoledronic acid in the management of metastatic bone disease and hypercalcaemia, *Palliat Med* 17:539-553, 2003.

374. Neville Webbe HL, Holen I, Coleman RE: The anti-tumour activity of bisphosphonates, *Cancer Treat Rev* 28:305-319, 2002.

375. Nguyen-Yamamoto L, Rousseau L, Brossard JH, et al: Origin of parathyroid hormone (PTH) fragments detected by intact-PTH assays, *Eur J Endocrinol* 147:123-131, 2002.

376. Nguyen-Yamamoto L, Rousseau L, Brossard JH, et al: Synthetic carboxyl-terminal fragments of parathyroid hormone (PTH) decrease ionized calcium concentration in rats by acting on a receptor different from the PTH/PTH-related peptide receptor, *Endocrinology* 142:1386-1392, 2001.

377. Niemann JT, Cairns CB: Hyperkalemia and ionized hypocalcemia during cardiac arrest and resuscitation: possible culprits for postcountershock arrhythmias? *Ann Emerg Med* 34:1-7, 1999.

378. Nissenson RA: Receptors for parathyroid hormone and parathyroid hormone-related protein: signaling and regulation. In Bilezikian JP, Marcus R, Levine MA, editors: *The parathyroids,* San Diego, 2001, Academic Press, pp. 93-104.

379. *Normal blood values for cats and normal blood values for dogs,* St. Louis, 1975, Ralston-Purina Co.

380. Norman AW: Rapid biological responses mediated by 1,25-dihydroxyvitamin D3: a case study of transcaltachia (rapid hormonal stimulation of intestinal calcium transport). In Feldman D, editor: *Vitamin D,* New York, 1997, Academic Press, pp. 233-256.

381. Norrdin RW, Miller CW, LoPresti CA, et al: Observations on calcium metabolism, 47Ca absorption, and duodenal calcium-binding activity in chronic renal failure: studies in Beagles with radiation-induced nephropathy, *Am J Vet Res* 41:510-515, 1980.

382. Okada H, Merryman JI, Rosol TJ, et al: Effects of humoral hypercalcemia of malignancy and gallium nitrate on thyroid C cells in nude mice: immunohistochemical and ultrastructural investigations, *Vet Pathol* 31:349-357, 1994.

383. Omdahl JL, May B: The 25-hydroxyvitamin D 24-hydroxylase. In Feldman D, editor: *Vitamin D,* New York, 1997, Academic Press, pp. 69-86.

384. Ong SC, Shalhoub RJ, Gallagher P, et al: Effect of furosemide on experimental hypercalcemia in dogs, *Proc Soc Exp Biol Med* 145:227-233, 1974.

385. Orloff JJ, Reddy D, de Papp AE, et al: Parathyroid hormone-related protein as a prohormone: posttranslational processing and receptor interactions, *Endocr Rev* 15:40-60, 1994.

386. Osborne CA, Lulich JP, Thumchai R, et al: Feline urolithiasis. Etiology and pathophysiology, *Vet Clin North Am Small Anim Pract* 26:217-232, 1996.

387. Padgett SL, Tobias KM, Leathers CW, et al: Efficacy of parathyroid gland autotransplantation in maintaining serum calcium concentrations after bilateral thyroparathyroidectomy in cats, *J Am Anim Hosp Assoc* 34:219-224, 1998.

388. Page RL: Acute tumor lysis syndrome, *Semin Vet Med Surg (Small Anim)* 1:58-60, 1986.

389. Pallais JC, Kifor O, Chen YB, et al: Acquired hypocalciuric hypercalcemia due to autoantibodies against the calcium-sensing receptor, *N Engl J Med* 351:362-369, 2004.

390. Panciera DL: Diagnostic approach to disorders of calcium homeostasis. In August J, editor: *Consultations in feline internal medicine 2,* Philadelphia, 1994, WB Saunders.

391. Pandian MR, Morgan CH, Carlton E, et al: Modified immunoradiometric assay of parathyroid hormone-related protein: clinical application in the differential diagnosis of hypercalcemia, *Clin Chem* 38:282-288, 1992.

392. Panichi V, Migliori M, Taccola D, et al: Effects of 1,25(OH)2D3 in experimental mesangial proliferative nephritis in rats, *Kidney Int* 60:87-95, 2001.

393. Panichi V, Migliori M, Taccola D, et al: Effects of calcitriol on the immune system: new possibilities in the treatment of glomerulonephritis, *Clin Exp Pharmacol Physiol* 30:807-811, 2003.

394. Pannabecker TL, Chandler JS, Wasserman RH: Vitamin-D-dependent transcriptional regulation of the intestinal plasma membrane calcium pump, *Biochem Biophys Res Commun* 213:499-505, 1995.

395. Parfitt AM: Bone and plasma calcium homeostasis, *Bone* 8(suppl 1):S1-8, 1987.

396. Patel SR, Ke HQ, Vanholder R, et al: Inhibition of calcitriol receptor binding to vitamin D response elements by uremic toxins, *J Clin Invest* 96:50-59, 1995.

397. Penny D, Henderson SM, Brown PJ: Raisin poisoning in a dog, *Vet Rec* 152:308, 2003.

398. Perkovic V, Hewitson TD, Kelynack KJ, et al: Parathyroid hormone has a prosclerotic effect on vascular smooth muscle cells, *Kidney Blood Press Res* 26:27-33, 2003.

399. Perry CM, Figgitt DP: Zoledronic acid: a review of its use in patients with advanced cancer, *Drugs* 64:1197-1211, 2004.

400. Persons DA, Garst J, Vollmer R, et al: Tumor lysis syndrome and acute renal failure after treatment of non-small-cell lung carcinoma with combination irinotecan and cisplatin, *Am J Clin Oncol* 21:426-429, 1998.

401. Peterson EN, Kirby R, Sommer M, et al: Cholecalciferol rodenticide intoxication in a cat, *J Am Vet Med Assoc* 199:904-906, 1991.

402. Peterson ME, Feinman JM: Hypercalcemia associated with hypoadrenocorticism in sixteen dogs, *J Am Vet Med Assoc* 181:802-804, 1982.

403. Peterson ME, Greco DS, Orth DN: Primary hypoadrenocorticism in ten cats, *J Vet Intern Med* 3:55-58, 1989.

404. Peterson ME, James KM, Wallace M, et al: Idiopathic hypoparathyroidism in five cats, *J Vet Intern Med* 5:47-51, 1991.

405. Peterson ME, Kintzer PP, Kass PH: Pretreatment clinical and laboratory findings in dogs with hypoadrenocorticism: 225 cases (1979-1993), *J Am Vet Med Assoc* 208:85-91, 1996.

406. Peterson ME: Hypoparathyroidism. In Kirk RW, editor: *Current veterinary therapy IX: small animal practice,* Philadelphia, 1986, WB Saunders, pp. 1039-1045.

407. Peterson ME: Treatment of canine and feline hypoparathyroidism, *J Am Vet Med Assoc* 181:1434-1436, 1982.

408. Petrie G: Management of hypercalcemia using dichloromethylene bisphosphonate (clodronate). In *Proc Cong Eur Soc Vet Intern Med,* vol 6, 1996.

409. Petzinger E, Ziegler K: Ochratoxin A from a toxicological perspective, *J Vet Pharmacol Ther* 23:91-98, 2000.

410. Pezzilli R, Billi P, Barakat B, et al: Octreotide for the treatment of hypercalcemia related to B cell lymphoma, *Oncology* 54:517-518, 1997.

411. Philbrick WM, Wysolmerski JJ, Galbraith S, et al: Defining the roles of parathyroid hormone-related protein in normal physiology, *Physiol Rev* 76:127-173, 1996.

412. Phillips DE, Radlinsky MG, Fischer JR, et al: Cystic thyroid and parathyroid lesions in cats, *J Am Anim Hosp Assoc* 39:349-354, 2003.

413. Piek CJ, Teske E: [Tumor lysis syndrome in a dog], *Tijdschr Diergeneeskd* 121:64-66, 1996.

414. Pollak MR, Brown EM, Chou YH, et al: Mutations in the human Ca(2+)-sensing receptor gene cause familial hypocalciuric hypercalcemia and neonatal severe hyperparathyroidism, *Cell* 75:1297-1303, 1993.

415. Pollard RE, Long CD, Nelson RW, et al: Percutaneous ultrasonographically guided radiofrequency heat ablation for treatment of primary hyperparathyroidism in dogs, *J Am Vet Med Assoc* 218:1106-1110, 2001.

416. Powell GJ, Southby J, Danks JA, et al: Localization of parathyroid hormone-related protein in breast cancer metastases: increased incidence in bone compared with other sites, *Cancer Res* 51:3059-3061, 1991.

417. Pressler BM, Rotstein DS, Law JM, et al: Hypercalcemia and high parathyroid hormone-related protein concentration associated with malignant melanoma in a dog, *J Am Vet Med Assoc* 221:263-265, 240, 2002.

418. Procino G, Carmosino M, Tamma G, et al: Extracellular calcium antagonizes forskolin-induced aquaporin 2 trafficking in collecting duct cells, *Kidney Int* 66:2245-2255, 2004.

419. Ramirez JA, Goodman WG, Belin TR, et al: Calcitriol therapy and calcium-regulated PTH secretion in patients with secondary hyperparathyroidism, *Am J Physiol* 267:E961-967, 1994.

420. Rasmussen H, Barrett P, Smallwood J, et al: Calcium ion as intracellular messenger and cellular toxin, *Environ Health Perspect* 84:17-25, 1990.

421. Rasmussen H: The cycling of calcium as an intracellular messenger, *Sci Am* 261:66-73, 1989.

422. Reber PM, Heath H 3rd: Hypocalcemic emergencies, *Med Clin North Am* 79:93-106, 1995.

423. Refsal KR, Provencher-Bolliger AL, Graham PA, et al: Update on the diagnosis and treatment of disorders of calcium regulation, *Vet Clin North Am Small Anim Pract* 31:1043-1062, 2001.

424. Reichel H, Koeffler HP, Norman AW: The role of the vitamin D endocrine system in health and disease, *N Engl J Med* 320:980-991, 1989.

425. Renoe BW, McDonald JM, Ladenson JH: Influence of posture on free calcium and related variables, *Clin Chem* 25:1766-1769, 1979.

426. Reusch C: [Ultrasonography of the parathyroid glands in dogs—a review], *Schweiz Arch Tierheilkd* 143:55-62, 2001.

427. Riccardi D: The role of extracellular calcium in the regulation of intracellular calcium and cell function (II). Some answers and more questions, *Cell Calcium* 35:179-181, 2004.

428. Richard V, Lairmore MD, Green PL, et al: Humoral hypercalcemia of malignancy: severe combined immunodeficient/beige mouse model of adult T-cell lymphoma independent of human T-cell lymphotropic virus type-1 tax expression, *Am J Pathol* 158:2219-2228, 2001.

429. Rickels MR, Mandel SJ: Hypocalciuric hypercalcemia and autoantibodies against the calcium-sensing receptor, *N Engl J Med* 351:2237-2238; author reply 2237-2238, 2004.

430. Rijnberk A, Elsinghorst TA, Koeman JP, et al: Pseudohyperparathyroidism associated with perirectal adenocarcinomas in elderly female dogs, *Tijdschr Diergeneeskd* 103:1069-1075, 1978.

431. Rodan GA, Balena R: Bisphosphonates in the treatment of metabolic bone diseases, *Ann Med* 25:373-378, 1993.

432. Roemer-Becuwe C, Vigano A, Romano F, et al: Safety of subcutaneous clodronate and efficacy in hypercalcemia of malignancy: a novel route of administration, *J Pain Symptom Manage* 26:843-848, 2003.

433. Rohrer CR, Phillips LA, Ford SL, et al: Hypercalcemia in a dog: a challenging case, *J Am Anim Hosp Assoc* 36:20-25, 2000.

434. Rosenberg MP, Matus RE, Patnaik AK: Prognostic factors in dogs with lymphoma and associated hypercalcemia, *J Vet Intern Med* 5:268-271, 1991.

435. Rosol TJ, Capen CC: Calcium-regulating hormones and diseases of abnormal mineral (calcium, phosphorus, magnesium) metabolism. In Kaneko JJ, Harvey JW, Bruss ML, editors: *Clinical biochemistry of domestic animals,* San Diego, 1997, Academic Press, pp. 619-702.

436. Rosol TJ, Capen CC: Cancer-associated hypercalcemia. In Feldman BF, Zinkl JG, Jain NC, editors: *Schalm's veterinary hematology,* Philadelphia, 2000, Lippincott Williams & Wilkins, pp. 660-666.

437. Rosol TJ, Capen CC: Mechanisms of cancer-induced hypercalcemia, *Lab Invest* 67:680-702, 1992.

438. Rosol TJ, Capen CC: Pathogenesis of humoral hypercalcemia of malignancy, *Domest Anim Endocrinol* 5:1-21, 1988.

439. Rosol TJ, Capen CC: Pathophysiology of calcium, phosphorus, and magnesium metabolism in animals, *Vet Clin North Am Small Anim Pract* 26:1155-1184, 1996.

440. Rosol TJ, Capen CC: The effect of low calcium diet, mithramycin, and dichlorodimethylene bisphosphonate on humoral hypercalcemia of malignancy in nude mice transplanted with the canine adenocarcinoma tumor line (CAC-8), *J Bone Miner Res* 2:395-405, 1987.

441. Rosol TJ, Capen CC: Tumors of the parathyroid gland and circulating parathyroid hormone-related protein associated with persistent hypercalcemia, *Toxicol Pathol* 17:346-356, 1989.

442. Rosol TJ, Chew DJ, Capen CC, et al: Acute hypocalcemia associated with infarction of parathyroid gland

adenomas in two dogs, *J Am Vet Med Assoc* 192:212-214, 1988.

443. Rosol TJ, Chew DJ, Couto CG, et al: Effects of mithramycin on calcium metabolism and bone in dogs, *Vet Pathol* 29:223-229, 1992.

444. Rosol TJ, Chew DJ, Hammer AS, et al: Effect of mithramycin on hypercalcemia in dogs, *J Am Anim Hosp Assoc* 30:244-250, 1994.

445. Rosol TJ, McCauley LK, Steinmeyer CL, et al: Nucleotide sequence of canine preproparathyroid hormone. In Dacke C, Danks J, Caple I, et al, editors: *The comparative endocrinology of calcium regulation*, Bristol, UK, 1996, Journal of Endocrinology Ltd., pp. 201-203.

446. Rosol TJ, Nagode LA, Couto CG, et al: Parathyroid hormone (PTH)-related protein, PTH, and 1,25-dihydroxyvitamin D in dogs with cancer-associated hypercalcemia, *Endocrinology* 131:1157-1164, 1992.

447. Rosol TJ, Nagode LA, Robertson JT, et al: Humoral hypercalcemia of malignancy associated with ameloblastoma in a horse, *J Am Vet Med Assoc* 204:1930-1933, 1994.

448. Rosol TJ, Chew DJ, Nagode LA, et al: Pathophysiology of calcium metabolism, *Vet Clin Pathol* 24:49-63, 1995.

449. Rosol TJ, Steinmeyer CL, McCauley LK, et al: Sequences of the cDNAs encoding canine parathyroid hormone-related protein and parathyroid hormone, *Gene* 160:241-243, 1995.

450. Rosol TJ, Tannehill-Gregg SH, Corn S, et al: Animal models of bone metastasis, *Cancer Treat Res* 118:47-81, 2004.

451. Rosol TJ, Tannehill-Gregg SH, LeRoy BE, et al: Animal models of bone metastasis, *Cancer* 97(suppl):748-757, 2003.

452. Rosol TJ: Pathogenesis of bone metastases: role of tumor-related proteins, *J Bone Miner Res* 15:844-850, 2000.

453. Ross JT, Scavelli TD, Matthiesen DT, et al: Adenocarcinoma of the apocrine glands of the anal sac in dogs: a review of 32 cases, *J Am Anim Hosp Assoc* 27:349-355, 1991.

454. Roth SI, Capen CC: Ultrastructural and functional correlations of the parathyroid gland, *Int Rev Exp Pathol* 13:161-221, 1974.

455. Rudnicki M, Frolich A, Haaber A, et al: Actual ionized calcium (at actual pH) vs adjusted ionized calcium (at pH 7.4) in hemodialyzed patients, *Clin Chem* 38:1384, 1992.

456. Rumbeiha WK, Fitzgerald SD, Kruger JM, et al: Use of pamidronate disodium to reduce cholecalciferol-induced toxicosis in dogs, *Am J Vet Res* 61:9-13, 2000.

457. Rumbeiha WK, Kruger JM, Fitzgerald SF, et al: Use of pamidronate to reverse vitamin D3-induced toxicosis in dogs, *Am J Vet Res* 60:1092-1097, 1999.

458. Ruopp JL: Primary hypoparathyroidism in a cat complicated by suspect iatrogenic calcinosis cutis, *J Am Anim Hosp Assoc* 37:370-373, 2001.

459. Ruslander DA, Gebhard DH, Tompkins MB, et al: Immunophenotypic characterization of canine lymphoproliferative disorders. *In Vivo* 11:169-172, 1997.

460. Russo EA, Lees GE: Treatment of hypocalcemia. In Kirk RW, editor: *Current veterinary therapy IX: small animal practice,* Philadelphia, 1986, WB Saunders, pp. 91-94.

461. Ryzen E, Rude RK: Low intracellular magnesium in patients with acute pancreatitis and hypocalcemia, *West J Med* 152:145-148, 1990.

462. Salusky IB, Goodman WG: Parathyroid gland function in secondary hyperparathyroidism, *Pediatr Nephrol* 10:359-363, 1996.

463. Santamaria R, Almaden Y, Felsenfeld A, et al: Dynamics of PTH secretion in hemodialysis patients as determined by the intact and whole PTH assays, *Kidney Int* 64:1867-1873, 2003.

464. Santini SA, Carrozza C, Vulpio C, et al: Assessment of parathyroid function in clinical practice: which parathyroid hormone assay is better? *Clin Chem* 50:1247-1250, 2004.

465. Sato R, Yamagishi H, Naito Y, et al: Feline vitamin D toxicosis caused by commercially available cat food, *J Jpn Vet Med Assoc* 46:577-581, 1993.

466. Saunders Y, Ross JR, Broadley KE, et al: Systematic review of bisphosphonates for hypercalcaemia of malignancy, *Palliat Med* 18:418-431, 2004.

467. Savary KC, Price GS, Vaden SL: Hypercalcemia in cats: a retrospective study of 71 cases (1991-1997), *J Vet Intern Med* 14:184-189, 2000.

468. Schaer M, Cavanaugh P, Hause W, et al: Iatrogenic hyperphosphatemia, hypocalcemia, and hypernatremia in a cat, *J Am Anim Hosp Assoc* 13:39, 1977.

469. Schaer M, Ginn PE, Fox LE, et al: Severe calcinosis cutis associated with treatment of hypoparathyroidism in a dog, *J Am Anim Hosp Assoc* 37:364-369, 2001.

470. Schenck PA, Chew DJ, Brooks CL: Effects of storage on serum ionized calcium and pH from horses with normal and abnormal ionized calcium concentrations, *Vet Clin Pathol* 25:118-120, 1996.

471. Schenck PA, Chew DJ, Brooks CL: Effects of storage on serum ionized calcium and pH values in clinically normal dogs, *Am J Vet Res* 56:304-307, 1995.

472. Schenck PA, Chew DJ, Brooks CL: Fractionation of canine serum calcium, using a micropartition system, *Am J Vet Res* 57:268-271, 1996.

473. Schenck PA, Chew DJ: Determination of calcium fractionation in dogs with chronic renal failure, *Am J Vet Res* 64:1181-1184, 2003.

474. Schenck PA, Chew DJ: Diagnostic discordance of total calcium and adjusted total calcium in predicting ionized calcium concentration in cats with chronic renal failure and other diseases. In *Proceedings of the 10th Congress of the International Society of Animal Clinical Biochemistry*, Gainesville, FL, 2002.

475. Schenck PA, Chew DJ: Prediction of serum ionized calcium concentration by serum total calcium measurement in dogs, *Am J Vet Res* 66:1330-1336, 2005.

476. Schenck PA, Chew DJ, Refsal K, et al: Calcium metabolic hormones in feline idiopathic hypercalcemia, *J Vet Intern Med* 18:442, 2004.

477. Schenck PA: Serum ionized magnesium concentrations in dogs and cats with hypoparathyroidism. In *Proceedings of the Am Coll Vet Intern Med Meeting*, Baltimore, MD, 2005.

478. Schreiner CA, Nagode LA: Vitamin D-dependent rickets type 2 in a four-month-old cat, *J Am Vet Med Assoc* 222:337-339, 315-316, 2003.

479. Schwarz U, Amann K, Orth SR, et al: Effect of 1,25 (OH)2 vitamin D3 on glomerulosclerosis in subtotally nephrectomized rats. *Kidney Int* 53:1696-1705, 1998.

480. Sekine M, Takami H: Combination of calcitonin and pamidronate for emergency treatment of malignant hypercalcemia, *Oncol Rep* 5:197-199, 1998.

481. Sela-Brown A, Russell J, Koszewski NJ, et al: Calreticulin inhibits vitamin D's action on the PTH gene in vitro and may prevent vitamin D's effect in vivo in hypocalcemic rats, *Mol Endocrinol* 12:1193-1200, 1998.

482. Seymour JF, Gagel RF: Calcitriol: the major humoral mediator of hypercalcemia in Hodgkin's disease and non-Hodgkin's lymphomas, *Blood* 82:1383-1394, 1993.

483. Sharma OP: Vitamin D, calcium, and sarcoidosis, *Chest* 109:535-539, 1996.

484. Sheafor SE, Gamblin RM, Couto CG: Hypercalcemia in two cats with multiple myeloma, *J Am Anim Hosp Assoc* 32:503-508, 1996.

485. Sherding RG, Meuten DJ, Chew DJ, et al: Primary hypoparathyroidism in the dog, *J Am Vet Med Assoc* 176:439-444, 1980.

486. Sherwood LM, Cantley L, Russell J: Effects of calcium and 1,25-(OH)2D3 on the synthesis and secretion of parathyroid hormone. In Cohn DV, Martin TJ, Meunier PJ, editors: *Calcium regulation and bone metabolism: basic and clinical aspects,* Amsterdam, 1987, Elsevier Science Publishers, pp. 778-781.

487. Siegel N, Wongsurawat N, Armbrecht HJ: Parathyroid hormone stimulates dephosphorylation of the renoredoxin component of the 25-hydroxyvitamin D3-1 alpha-hydroxylase from rat renal cortex, *J Biol Chem* 261:16998-17003, 1986.

488. Sih TR, Morris JG, Hickman MA: Chronic ingestion of high concentrations of cholecalciferol in cats, *Am J Vet Res* 62:1500-1506, 2001.

489. Silver J, Kilav R, Naveh-Many T: Mechanisms of secondary hyperparathyroidism, *Am J Physiol Renal Physiol* 283:F367-F376, 2002.

490. Silver J, Kronenberg HM: Parathyroid hormone—molecular biology and regulation. In Bilezikian JP, Raisz LG, Rodan GA, editors: *Principles of bone biology,* San Diego, 1996, Academic Press, pp. 325-337.

491. Silver J, Naveh-Many T: Vitamin D and the parathyroid glands. In Feldman D, editor: *Vitamin D,* San Diego, 1997, Academic Press, pp. 353-367.

492. Silver J, Yalcindag C, Sela-Brown A, et al: Regulation of the parathyroid hormone gene by vitamin D, calcium and phosphate, *Kidney Int Suppl* 73:S2-7, 1999.

493. Slatopolsky E, Finch J, Brown A: New vitamin D analogs, *Kidney Int Suppl* June:S83-87, 2003.

494. Slatopolsky E, Lopez-Hilker S, Delmez J, et al: The parathyroid-calcitriol axis in health and chronic renal failure, *Kidney Int Suppl* 29:S41-47, 1990.

495. Smith SA, Freeman LC, Bagladi-Swanson M: Hypercalcemia due to iatrogenic secondary hypoadrenocorticism and diabetes mellitus in a cat, *J Am Anim Hosp Assoc* 38:41-44, 2002.

496. Smock SL, Vogt GA, Castleberry TA, et al: Molecular cloning and functional characterization of the canine parathyroid hormone/parathyroid hormone related peptide receptor (PTH1), *Mol Biol Rep* 28:235-243, 2001.

497. St. Arnaud R, Glorieux FH: Vitamin D and bone development. In Feldman D, editor: *Vitamin D,* San Diego, 1997, Academic Press, pp. 293-303.

498. Stern PH: Vitamin D and bone, *Kidney Int Suppl* 29:S17-21, 1990.

499. Stevens LA, Djurdjev O, Cardew S, et al: Calcium, phosphate, and parathyroid hormone levels in combination and as a function of dialysis duration predict mortality: evidence for the complexity of the association between mineral metabolism and outcomes, *J Am Soc Nephrol* 15:770-779, 2004.

500. Storms TN, Clyde VL, Munson L, et al: Blastomycosis in nondomestic felids, *J Zoo Wildl Med* 34:231-238, 2003.

501. Strewler GJ: Physiological actions of PTH and PTHrP: Skeletal actions. In Bilezikian JP, Marcus R, Levine MA, editors: *The parathyroids,* San Diego, 2001, Academic Press, pp. 213-226.

502. Suda T, Takahashi N: Vitamin D and osteoclastogenesis. In Feldman D, editor: *Vitamin D,* San Diego, 1997, Academic Press, pp. 329-340.

503. Sueda MT, Stefanacci, JD: Ultrasound evaluation of the parathyroid glands in two hypercalcemic cats, *Vet Radiol Ultrasound* 41:448-451, 2000.

504. Suva LJ, Winslow GA, Wettenhall RE, et al: A parathyroid hormone-related protein implicated in malignant hypercalcemia: cloning and expression, *Science* 237:893-896, 1987.

505. Swarthout JT, D'Alonzo RC, Selvamurugan N, et al: Parathyroid hormone-dependent signaling pathways regulating genes in bone cells, *Gene* 282:1-17, 2002.

506. Szenci O, Brydl E, Bajcsy CA: Effect of storage on measurement of ionized calcium and acid-base variables in equine, bovine, ovine, and canine venous blood, *J Am Vet Med Assoc* 199:1167-1169, 1991.

507. Takahashi HE, Tanizawa T, Hori M, et al: Effect of intermittent administration of human parathyroid hormone (1-34) on experimental osteopenia of rats induced by ovariectomy, *Cell Mater* 113-117, 1991.

508. Tannehill-Gregg S, Kergosien E, Rosol TJ: Feline head and neck squamous cell carcinoma cell line: characterization, production of parathyroid hormone-related protein, and regulation by transforming growth factor-beta, *In Vitro Cell Dev Biol Anim* 37:676-683, 2001.

509. Teare JA, Krook L, Kallfelz FA, et al: Ascorbic acid deficiency and hypertrophic osteodystrophy in the dog: a rebuttal, *Cornell Vet* 69:384-401, 1979.

510. Terry AH, Orrock J, Meikle AW: Comparison of two third-generation parathyroid hormone assays, *Clin Chem* 49:336-337, 2003.

511. Teske E, van Heerde P, Rutteman GR, et al: Prognostic factors for treatment of malignant lymphoma in dogs, *J Am Vet Med Assoc* 205:1722-1728, 1994.

512. Tfelt-Hansen J, Chattopadhyay N, Yano S, et al: Calcium-sensing receptor induces proliferation through p38 mitogen-activated protein kinase and phosphatidylinositol 3-kinase but not extracellularly regulated kinase in a model of humoral hypercalcemia of malignancy, *Endocrinology* 145:1211-1217, 2004.

513. Thakker RV: Diseases associated with the extracellular calcium-sensing receptor, *Cell Calcium* 35:275-282, 2004.

514. Thiede MA, Daifotis AG, Weir EC, et al: Intrauterine occupancy controls expression of the parathyroid hormone-related peptide gene in preterm rat myometrium, *Proc Natl Acad Sci U S A* 87:6969-6973, 1990.

515. Thode J, Juul-Jorgensen B, Bhatia HM, et al: Comparison of serum total calcium, albumin-corrected total calcium, and ionized calcium in 1213 patients with suspected calcium disorders, *Scand J Clin Lab Invest* 49:217-223, 1989.

516. Thomasset M: Calbindin-D 9K. In Feldman D, editor: *Vitamin D,* New York, 1997, Academic Press, pp. 223-232.

517. Thompson KG, Jones LP, Smylie WA, et al: Primary hyperparathyroidism in German shepherd dogs: a disorder of probable genetic origin, *Vet Pathol* 21:370-376, 1984.

518. Thrall MA, Grauer GF, Mero KN: Clinicopathologic findings in dogs and cats with ethylene glycol intoxication, *J Am Vet Med Assoc* 184:37-41, 1984.

519. Thurlimann B, Waldburger R, Senn HJ, et al: Plicamycin and pamidronate in symptomatic tumor-related hypercalcemia: a prospective randomized crossover trial, *Ann Oncol* 3:619-623, 1992.

520. Toffaletti J: Ionized calcium measurement: analytical and clinical aspects, *Lab Management* July:31-35, 1983.
521. Tohme JF, Bilezikian JP: Hypocalcemic emergencies, *Endocrinol Metab Clin North Am* 22:363-375, 1993.
522. Tomsa K, Glaus T, Hauser B, et al: Nutritional secondary hyperparathyroidism in six cats, *J Small Anim Pract* 40:533-539, 1999.
523. Tomsa K, Steffen F, Glaus T: [Life threatening metabolic disorders after application of a sodium phosphate containing enema in the dog and cat.], *Schweiz Arch Tierheilkd* 143:257-261, 2001.
524. Toribio RE, Kohn CW, Chew DJ, et al: Comparison of serum parathyroid hormone and ionized calcium and magnesium concentrations and fractional urinary clearance of calcium and phosphorus in healthy horses and horses with enterocolitis, *Am J Vet Res* 62:938-947, 2001.
525. Torley D, Drummond A, Bilsland DJ: Calcipotriol toxicity in dogs, *Br J Dermatol* 147:1270, 2002.
526. Torrance AG, Nachreiner R: Human-parathormone assay for use in dogs: validation, sample handling studies, and parathyroid function testing, *Am J Vet Res* 50:1123-1127, 1989.
527. Torrance AG, Nachreiner R: Intact parathyroid hormone assay and total calcium concentration in the diagnosis of disorders of calcium metabolism in dogs, *J Vet Intern Med* 3:86-89, 1989.
528. Tras B, Maden M, Bas AL, et al: Investigation of biochemical and haematological side-effects of enrofloxacin in dogs, *J Vet Med A Physiol Pathol Clin Med* 48:59-63, 2001.
529. Troy GC, Forrester D, Cockburn C, et al: Heterobilharzia americana infection and hypercalcemia in a dog: a case report, *J Am Anim Hosp Assoc* 23:35-40, 1987.
530. Tucci J, Hammond V, Senior PV, et al: The role of fetal parathyroid hormone-related protein in transplacental calcium transport, *J Mol Endocrinol* 17:159-164, 1996.
531. Tuma SN, Mallette LE: Hypercalcemia after nephrectomy in the dog: role of the kidneys and parathyroid glands, *J Lab Clin Med* 102:213-219, 1983.
532. Tweedy CR, Rees GM: Octreotide acetate in the treatment of hypercalcemia accompanying small cell carcinoma, *South Med J* 85:561, 1992.
533. Tyrrell CJ, Collinson M, Madsen EL, et al: Intravenous pamidronate: infusion rate and safety, *Ann Oncol* 5(suppl 7):S27-29, 1994.
534. Uehlinger P, Glaus T, Hauser B, et al: [Differential diagnosis of hypercalcemia—a retrospective study of 46 dogs], *Schweiz Arch Tierheilkd* 140:188-197, 1998.
535. Unterer S, Lutz H, Gerber B, et al: Evaluation of an electrolyte analyzer for measurement of ionized calcium and magnesium concentrations in blood, plasma, and serum of dogs, *Am J Vet Res* 65:183-187, 2004.
536. Urena P, Frazao JM: Calcimimetic agents: review and perspectives, *Kidney Int Suppl* June:S91-96, 2003.
537. Vaden SL, Levine J, Breitschwerdt EB: A retrospective case-control of acute renal failure in 99 dogs, *J Vet Intern Med* 11:58-64, 1997.
538. Vail DM, Kisseberth WC, Obradovich JE, et al: Assessment of potential doubling time (Tpot), argyrophilic nucleolar organizer regions (AgNOR), and proliferating cell nuclear antigen (PCNA) as predictors of therapy response in canine non-Hodgkin's lymphoma, *Exp Hematol* 24:807-815, 1996.
539. Vail DM, Withrow SJ, Schwarz PD, et al: Perianal adenocarcinoma in the canine male: a retrospective study of 41 cases, *J Am Anim Hosp Assoc* 26:329-334, 1990.
540. Walker MC, Schaer M: Percutaneous ethanol treatment of hyperthyroidism in a cat, *Feline Practice* 28:10-12, 1998.
541. Walker P, Watanabe S, Lawlor P, et al: Subcutaneous clodronate, *Lancet* 348:345-346, 1996.
542. Walker P, Watanabe S, Lawlor P, et al: Subcutaneous clodronate: a study evaluating efficacy in hypercalcemia of malignancy and local toxicity, *Ann Oncol* 8:915-916, 1997.
543. Walser M, Robinson BHB, Duckett JW Jr: The hypercalcemia of adrenal insufficiency, *J Clin Invest* 42:456-465, 1963.
544. Walters MR: Newly identified effects of the vitamin D endocrine system: update 1995. In Bikle DD, Negrovilar A, editors: *Hormonal regulation of bone mineral metabolism*, Bethesda, 1995, Endocrine Society, pp. 47-56.
545. Wang W, Li C, Kwon TH, et al: AQP3, p-AQP2, and AQP2 expression is reduced in polyuric rats with hypercalcemia: prevention by cAMP-PDE inhibitors, *Am J Physiol Renal Physiol* 283:F1313-1325, 2002.
546. Ward DT: Calcium receptor-mediated intracellular signalling, *Cell Calcium* 35:217-228, 2004.
547. Warrell RP Jr, Murphy WK, Schulman P, et al: A randomized double-blind study of gallium nitrate compared with etidronate for acute control of cancer-related hypercalcemia, *J Clin Oncol* 9:1467-1475, 1991.
548. Waser M, Mesaeli N, Spencer C, et al: Regulation of calreticulin gene expression by calcium, *J Cell Biol* 138:547-557, 1997.
549. Wasserman RH: Vitamin D and the intestinal absorption of calcium and phosphorus. In Feldman BF, editor: *Vitamin D*, New York, 1997, Academic Press, pp. 259-273.
550. Waters CB, Scott-Moncrieff JC: Hypocalcemia in cats, *Compend Contin Educ* 14:497-506, 1992.
551. Weaver ME, Morrissey J, McConkey C Jr, et al: WR-2721 inhibits parathyroid adenylate cyclase, *Am J Physiol* 252:E197-201, 1987.
552. Weir EC, Burtis WJ, Morris CA, et al: Isolation of 16,000-dalton parathyroid hormone-like proteins from two animal tumors causing humoral hypercalcemia of malignancy, *Endocrinology* 123:2744-2751, 1988.
553. Weir EC, Norrdin RW, Matus RE, et al: Humoral hypercalcemia of malignancy in canine lymphosarcoma, *Endocrinology* 122:602-608, 1988.
554. Weisbrode SE, Krakowka S: Canine distemper virus-associated hypocalcemia, *Am J Vet Res* 40:147-149, 1979.
555. Welches CD, Scavelli TD, Matthiesen DT, et al: Occurrence of problems after three techniques of bilateral thyroidectomy in cats, *Vet Surg* 18:392-396, 1989.
556. Weller RE, Theilen GH, Madewell BR: Chemotherapeutic responses in dogs with lymphosarcoma and hypercalcemia, *J Am Vet Med Assoc* 181:891-893, 1982.
557. Wellington K, Goa KL: Zoledronic acid: a review of its use in the management of bone metastases and hypercalcaemia of malignancy, *Drugs* 63:417-437, 2003.
558. Wells AL, Long CD, Hornof WJ, et al: Use of percutaneous ethanol injection for treatment of bilateral hyperplastic thyroid nodules in cats, *J Am Vet Med Assoc* 218:1293-1297, 2001.
559. Whitfield GK, Dang HT, Schluter SF, et al: Cloning of a functional vitamin D receptor from the lamprey (Petromyzon marinus), an ancient vertebrate lacking a calcified skeleton and teeth, *Endocrinology* 144:2704-2716, 2003.
560. Willard MD, Schall WD, McCaw DE, et al: Canine hypoadrenocorticism: report of 37 cases and review of 39 previously reported cases, *J Am Vet Med Assoc* 180:59-62, 1982.

561. Williams LE, Gliatto JM, Dodge RK, et al: Carcinoma of the apocrine glands of the anal sac in dogs: 113 cases (1985-1995), *J Am Vet Med Assoc* 223:825-831, 2003.

562. Winer KK, Yanovski JA, Cutler GB Jr: Synthetic human parathyroid hormone 1-34 vs calcitriol and calcium in the treatment of hypoparathyroidism, *JAMA* 276:631-636, 1996.

563. Winkelmayer WC, Levin R, Avorn J: The nephrologist's role in the management of calcium-phosphorus metabolism in patients with chronic kidney disease, *Kidney Int* 63:1836-1842, 2003.

564. Wisner ER, Nyland TG: Ultrasonography of the thyroid and parathyroid glands, *Vet Clin North Am Small Anim Pract* 28:973-991, 1998.

565. Wisner ER, Penninck D, Biller DS, et al: High-resolution parathyroid sonography, *Vet Radiol Ultrasound* 38:462-466, 1997.

566. Won DS, Park C, In YJ, et al: A case of nutritional secondary hyperparathyroidism in a Siberian tiger cub, *J Vet Med Sci* 66:551-553, 2004.

567. Woo J, Cannon DC: *Metabolic intermediates and inorganic ions*, ed 17, Philadelphia, 1984, WB Saunders, pp. 133-179.

568. Wooldridge JD, Gregory CR: Ionized and total serum magnesium concentrations in feline renal transplant recipients, *Vet Surg* 28:31-37, 1999.

569. Worth GK, Vasikaran SD, Retallack RW, et al: Major method-specific differences in the measurement of intact parathyroid hormone: studies in patients with and without chronic renal failure, *Ann Clin Biochem* 41:149-154, 2004.

570. Wright KN, Breitschwerdt EB, Feldman JM, et al: Diagnostic and therapeutic considerations in a hypercalcemic dog with multiple endocrine neoplasia, *J Am Anim Hosp Assoc* 31:156-162, 1995.

571. Wysolmerski JJ, Stewart AF, Martin JT: Physiological actions of PTH and PTHrP: epidermal, mammary, reproductive, and pancreatic tissues. In Bilezikian JP, Marcus R, Levine MA, editors: *The parathyroids*, San Diego, 2001, Academic Press, pp. 275-292.

572. Wysolmerski JJ: The evolutionary origins of maternal calcium and bone metabolism during lactation, *J Mammary Gland Biol Neoplasia* 7:267-276, 2002.

573. Yanagawa N, Lee DBN: Renal handling of calcium and phosphorus. In Coe FL, Favus MJ, editors: *Disorders of bone and mineral metabolism*, New York, 1992, Raven Press, pp. 3-40.

574. Yang KH, dePapp AE, Soifer NE, et al: Parathyroid hormone-related protein: evidence for isoform- and tissue-specific posttranslational processing, *Biochemistry* 33:7460-7469, 1994.

575. Yasuda T, Banville D, Rabbani SA, et al: Rat parathyroid hormone-like peptide: comparison with the human homologue and expression in malignant and normal tissue, *Mol Endocrinol* 3:518-525, 1989.

576. Yu J, Papavasiliou V, Rhim J, et al: Vitamin D analogs: new therapeutic agents for the treatment of squamous cancer and its associated hypercalcemia, *Anticancer Drugs* 6:101-108, 1995.

577. Yudd M, Llach F: Current medical management of secondary hyperparathyroidism, *Am J Med Sci* 320:100-106, 2000.

578. Zaloga GP, Chernow B: The multifactorial basis for hypocalcemia during sepsis. Studies of the parathyroid hormone-vitamin D axis, *Ann Intern Med* 107:36-41, 1987.

579. Zaloga GP, Malcolm D, Holaday J, et al: Verapamil reverses calcium cardiotoxicity, *Ann Emerg Med* 16:637-639, 1987.

580. Zaloga GP, Willey S, Tomasic P, et al: Free fatty acids alter calcium binding: a cause for misinterpretation of serum calcium values and hypocalcemia in critical illness, *J Clin Endocrinol Metab* 64:1010-1014, 1987.

581. Zawada ET Jr, Saelens DA, Lembke JM: Influence of calcium infusion on plasma atrial natriuretic peptide in conscious dogs: intervention with calcium antagonist, verapamil, *Miner Electrolyte Metab* 16:369-377, 1990.

582. Zelikovic I, Chesney RW: Vitamin D and mineral metabolism: the role of the kidney in health and disease, *World Rev Nutr Diet* 59:156-216, 1989.

583. Zitterman A: Vitamin D in preventive medicine: are we ignoring the evidence? *Br J Nutr* 89:552-572, 2003.

584. Zivin JR, Gooley T, Zager RA, et al: Hypocalcemia: a pervasive metabolic abnormality in the critically ill, *Am J Kidney Dis* 37:689-698, 2001.

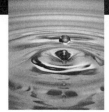

CHAPTER · 7

DISORDERS OF PHOSPHORUS: HYPOPHOSPHATEMIA AND HYPERPHOSPHATEMIA

Stephen P. DiBartola and Michael D. Willard

Phosphorus plays an essential role in cellular structure and function.[86] A constituent of structural phospholipids in cell membranes and of hydroxyapatite in bone, phosphorus also is an integral component of nucleic acids and of phosphoproteins involved in mitochondrial oxidative phosphorylation. Energy for essential metabolic processes (e.g., muscle contraction, neuronal impulse conduction, epithelial transport) is stored in high-energy phosphate bonds of adenosine triphosphate (ATP). The compound 2,3-diphosphoglyccrate (2,3-DPG) dccrcascs the affinity of hemoglobin for oxygen and facilitates the delivery of oxygen to tissues. Cyclic adenosine monophosphate (cAMP) is an intracellular second messenger for many polypeptide hormones. Phosphate is also an important urinary buffer, and urinary phosphate constitutes the majority of titratable acidity (see Chapter 9).

Phosphorus is important in the intermediary metabolism of protein, fat, and carbohydrate and as a component of glycogen. It stimulates glycolytic enzymes (e.g., hexokinase, phosphofructokinase) and participates in the phosphorylation of many glycolytic intermediates. Nicotinamide adenine dinucleotide phosphate ($NADP^+$) is a coenzyme for important biochemical reactions. Phosphate regulates the activity of enzymes such as the glutaminase essential for ammoniagenesis (stimulated by increased phosphate concentrations) and the 1α-hydroxylase required for vitamin D activation (stimulated by decreased phosphate concentrations).

PHYSICAL CHEMISTRY

Phosphorus exists in organic (phospholipids and phosphate esters) and inorganic (orthophosphoric and pyrophosphoric acids) forms in the body. Almost all serum phosphorus is in the form of orthophosphate. Orthophosphoric acid is governed by the following set of equilibria:

$$H_3PO_4 \rightleftharpoons H_2PO_4^{1-} + H^+ \rightleftharpoons HPO_4^{2-} + H^+ \rightleftharpoons PO_4^{3-} + H^+$$
$$\text{pKa 2.0} \qquad \text{pKa 6.8} \qquad \text{pKa 12.4}$$

The pKa for the reaction between $H_2PO_4^{1-}$ and HPO_4^{2-} is 6.8 at the ionic strength and temperature of extracellular fluid (ECF), and these are the two prevailing ionic species at the normal ECF pH of 7.4. At this pH, H_3PO_4 and PO_4^{3-} are present in negligible amounts, and plasma inorganic phosphorus principally consists of $H_2PO_4^{1-}$ and HPO_4^{2-}. At a pH of 7.4, the $HPO_4^{2-}:H_2PO_4^{1-}$ ratio is 4.0, and the average valence of phosphate in serum reflects this ratio. There is four times as much HPO_4^{2-} as $H_2PO_4^{1-}$ at a pH of 7.4, and therefore the average valence of phosphate at this pH is $(4/5)(-2) + (1/5)(-1) = -1.8$. Because the valence and number of milliequivalents (mEq) of phosphate in ECF are influenced by pH, it is easier to measure phosphate in millimoles (mmol) or milligrams (mg) of elemental phosphorus. Serum phosphorus concentrations typically are reported as elemental phosphorus and expressed as milligrams of elemental phosphorus per deciliter of serum. One millimole of phosphate contains 31 mg of elemental phosphorus. To convert mg/dL to mmol/L, divide mg/dL by 3.1. At a pH of 7.4, 1 mmol of phosphate equals 1.8 mEq, and conversion from mmol/L to mEq/L requires multiplication by 1.8.

Even though phosphorus circulates in organic and inorganic forms, clinical laboratories typically measure inorganic phosphate. Approximately 10% to 20% of the inorganic phosphate in serum is protein bound, and the remainder circulates as free anion or is complexed to sodium, magnesium, or calcium. The free and complexed fractions are available for ultrafiltration by the renal glomeruli.

BODY STORES AND DISTRIBUTION

Phosphate is the body's major intracellular anion, and translocation in and out of the intracellular compartment can rapidly change serum phosphorus concentration. Gradual changes in total body phosphate can be accommodated without noticeable changes in serum phosphorus concentration, resembling the situation with potassium (the major intracellular cation). Approximately 80% to 85% of total body phosphate is inorganic hydroxyapatite in bone, whereas 15% is in soft tissues such as muscle.[55,83] Most soft tissue phosphorus is organic and can be readily converted to the inorganic form as needed. The ECF compartment contains less than 1% of total body phosphorus stores.

NORMAL SERUM CONCENTRATIONS

Normal serum phosphorus concentrations in adult dogs range from 2.5 to 6.0 mg/dL, but they are higher in dogs younger than 1 year.[15,72,119,154] Serum phosphorus concentrations are highest in puppies less than 8 weeks of age (up to 10.8 mg/dL may be considered normal) and gradually decrease into the adult range after 1 year of age.[68] Sex-related changes are not reported.[121] The effect of age is less pronounced in cats, but immature cats have a tendency for higher serum concentrations.[30] Bone growth and an increase in renal tubular reabsorption of phosphorus mediated by growth hormone presumably contribute to this age effect. Feeding also affects serum phosphorus concentration. A carbohydrate meal or infusion (e.g., 5% dextrose) decreases serum phosphorus concentration because phosphate shifts into intracellular fluid as a result of stimulation of glycolysis and formation of phosphorylated glycolytic intermediates in muscle, liver, and adipose cells. In contrast, protein intake increases serum phosphorus concentration because of the relatively high phosphorus content of protein-rich diets.

Time of sampling affects the observed serum phosphorus concentration. People have substantial variation in serum phosphorus concentrations throughout the day.[92] Acid-base balance also influences serum phosphorus concentration. Respiratory alkalosis stimulates glycolysis (by activating phosphofructokinase) and decreases serum phosphorus concentration. Thus the measured serum phosphorus concentration is affected by several variables and does not accurately indicate total body phosphorus stores. Measuring serum phosphorus concentration after a 12-hour fast minimizes confounding factors, but the clinician must understand that the magnitude of hypophosphatemia or hyperphosphatemia may be incorrectly assessed if only one serum or plasma sample is analyzed.

Hemolysis may affect laboratory results because phosphate is present in erythrocytes. Human erythrocytes contain 8 μmol/dL red cells, whereas canine erythrocytes contain 35 μmol/dL and feline erythrocytes contain 26 μmol/dL.[28] Hyperlipidemia and hyperproteinemia sometimes cause overestimation of serum phosphorus concentration, depending on the methodology used.[63,90]

Thrombocytosis and monoclonal gammopathy also may cause spurious increases in serum phosphorus concentration.[87,95,100] Mannitol and other drugs may interfere with some assay systems, leading to erroneous measured values.[57,157] Icterus and hemolysis were reported to result in artifactual hypophosphatemia in dogs with immune-mediated hemolytic anemia.[67] Artifactual hypophosphatemia can occur in some automated systems but not in others. Thus occurrence of hypophosphatemia in patients without known predisposing factors should prompt consideration of laboratory error.

DIETARY INTAKE

The average phosphorus content of commercial pet foods is approximately 1% on a dry matter basis. Dogs and cats ingest 0.5 to 3.0 g of phosphorus per day, depending on their body size and energy requirements. The source of dietary phosphorus markedly affects absorption and excretion of phosphorus in cats.[53] The amount of phosphorus absorbed by the gastrointestinal tract, the amount excreted in the urine, and the extent of postprandial hyperphosphatemia were increased when monobasic and dibasic salts of phosphorus were fed but decreased when phosphorus originated from poultry, meat, and fish meal.

INTESTINAL ABSORPTION

Ingested organic phosphate is hydrolyzed in the gastrointestinal tract, liberating inorganic phosphate for absorption. Net intestinal phosphate absorption (i.e., the difference between dietary and fecal phosphate) is approximately 60% to 70% of the ingested load, and absorption is a linear function of phosphorus intake. In an animal in zero phosphorus balance, urinary phosphate excretion equals net intestinal phosphate absorption.

Intestinal phosphate absorption occurs via two mechanisms. Passive diffusion is the principal route and occurs primarily through the paracellular pathway. Active mucosal phosphate transport is a sodium-dependent, saturable carrier-mediated process. Calcitriol (1,25-dihydroxycholecalciferol) increases active intestinal mucosal phosphate transport, but this mechanism is probably important only during dietary phosphate deficiency. Both transport mechanisms function in the duodenum, whereas diffusion is the primary mechanism in the jejunum and ileum. Intestinal alkaline phosphatases may facilitate absorption by freeing inorganic phosphate for transport. Optimal phosphate transport occurs in an alkaline environment, and HPO_4^{-2} is the main ionic species transported. Decreased intestinal phosphate absorption may occur with vitamin D deficiency and in malabsorptive states.

There is no evidence of a direct effect of parathyroid hormone (PTH) on intestinal phosphate absorption, and observed effects are probably mediated by the role of PTH in conversion of 25-hydroxycholecalciferol to calcitriol. High dietary ratios of calcium to phosphorus (>3 to 4) may suppress intestinal phosphate absorption, presumably through binding of phosphate by calcium and formation of poorly absorbed calcium phosphate complexes. During phosphate deprivation, the kidney dramatically reduces phosphate excretion to negligible amounts in fewer than 3 days. Obligatory gastrointestinal loss continues for at least 3 weeks, but there is a diminution in the amount lost.[92] This gastrointestinal loss may cause a cumulative negative phosphorus balance during phosphate deprivation.

RENAL HANDLING

The kidney adjusts tubular reabsorption of filtered phosphate to maintain zero balance. Normally, 80% to 90% of the filtered phosphate load is reabsorbed by the renal tubules, and renal dysfunction is the most common cause of hyperphosphatemia.[29,141]

Phosphate crosses the luminal membranes of the proximal renal tubular cells by brush border sodium-phosphate cotransporters. The main transport protein in the proximal tubules (type IIa sodium-phosphate cotransporter) translocates three sodium ions and one divalent phosphate ion across the luminal membrane and thus promotes luminal electronegativity.[148] Luminal entry is the rate-limiting step and the target for physiologic and pathophysiologic mechanisms that alter phosphate reabsorption.[106] High dietary intake of phosphorus decreases proximal tubular reabsorption, whereas low dietary intake can result in nearly 100% proximal tubular reabsorption of phosphate. These dietary effects occur independently of changes in the plasma concentrations of phosphaturic hormones. PTH is the most important regulator of renal phosphate transport, and it decreases the tubular transport maximum for phosphate reabsorption (T_{maxPi}) in the proximal tubule where most phosphate reabsorption occurs. Apparently, no reabsorption occurs in the thin ascending limb or thick ascending limb of Henle's loop, and the presence of a reabsorptive mechanism in the distal convoluted tubule is uncertain. Phosphate reabsorption is inhibited in the early proximal tubule by volume expansion with saline, but there may be a more distal reabsorptive site (at some point beyond the last portion of the proximal tubule accessible by micropuncture) that is sensitive to PTH and unaffected by saline volume expansion.

The effects of calcitriol on renal phosphate transport are difficult to separate from the effects of calcitriol on PTH secretion and on phosphate transport in other organs (e.g., intestine, bone). Growth hormone increases proximal renal tubular phosphate reabsorption, which partially accounts for the increased serum phosphorus concentrations found in immature animals. Insulin and thyroxine also increase proximal tubular reabsorption of phosphate, whereas calcitonin and atrial natriuretic peptide inhibit proximal tubular phosphate reabsorption. High doses of adrenocorticotropic hormone (ACTH) or glucocorticoids increase renal phosphate excretion and may decrease serum phosphorus concentration.

The effects of acid-base balance on proximal tubular transport of phosphate are complex.[106] Acute metabolic acidosis does not affect renal tubular reabsorption of phosphate, but chronic metabolic acidosis results in decreased proximal tubular transport, an effect possibly mediated by glucocorticoids. Respiratory acidosis decreases and respiratory alkalosis increases proximal tubular reabsorption of phosphate. Volume expansion increases urinary phosphate excretion and causes natriuresis because phosphate is cotransported with sodium in the proximal tubule.

HYPOPHOSPHATEMIA

CLINICAL EFFECTS OF HYPOPHOSPHATEMIA

Hypophosphatemia can have many detrimental effects. The most severe cellular damage seems to occur when there is concurrent phosphate depletion.[92] Hypophosphatemia decreases erythrocyte concentrations of ATP, which increases erythrocyte fragility, leading to hemolysis. Hemolysis usually is not observed until serum phosphorus concentration decreases to 1.0 mg/dL or less. Hypophosphatemia also reduces erythrocyte 2,3-DPG concentrations, which impairs oxygen delivery to tissues. Leukocytes in hypophosphatemic patients have impaired chemotaxis, phagocytosis, and bacterial killing.[35] This altered function may promote sepsis in hypophosphatemic patients receiving total parenteral nutrition. Platelet-associated abnormalities include shortened survival time, impaired clot retraction, megakaryocytosis in the bone marrow, and thrombocytopenia. In starved dogs made hypophosphatemic by infusion of amino acids, hemolytic anemia, thrombocytopenia, and impaired clot retraction resulted, ostensibly because of depletion of cellular ATP stores.[156] Clinically, hemolysis has been reported in hypophosphatemic dogs and cats with diabetic ketoacidosis, hepatic lipidosis, and other disorders.[2,75,152] Hemolysis was reported in four other hypophosphatemic diabetic cats, but cause and effect were obscured by the possibility of Heinz body anemia.[21]

Neuromuscular effects of hypophosphatemia include weakness and pain associated with rhabdomyolysis, as well as anorexia, vomiting, and nausea secondary to intestinal ileus.[83,84] Decreased phosphate may impair central nervous system glucose utilization and ATP production, leading to metabolic encephalopathy, which has a wide range of manifestations in people (e.g., coma, seizure, confusion, irritability).[92,155] Reversible impairment of cardiac contractility occurs in dogs with experimentally induced hypophosphatemia and in people with naturally occurring hypophosphatemia.[59,60,158] Hypophosphatemia also causes proximal tubular bicarbonate wasting, reduction in titratable acidity, and impaired renal ammoniagenesis. However, serious acid-base disturbances do not arise in phosphate-deprived dogs.[134] Phosphate deficiency produces bone demineralization via effects of PTH and calcitriol, and release of carbonate from bone may prevent serious metabolic acidosis. Hypomagnesemia frequently is found in hypophosphatemic people, but the reasons for this association are not clear.[30]

CAUSES OF HYPOPHOSPHATEMIA

Hypophosphatemia may be caused by translocation of phosphate from extracellular to intracellular fluid (maldistribution), increased loss (decreased renal reabsorption of phosphate), or decreased intake (decreased intestinal absorption of phosphate).[92,122] Clinical conditions associated with hypophosphatemia are presented in Box 7-1.

Translocation related to administration of a carbohydrate load (e.g., 5% dextrose infusion) is a common cause of hypophosphatemia in hospitalized people.[13,74] Insulin facilitates entry of glucose and phosphate into cells, where glucose is phosphorylated to glycolytic intermediates. Interestingly, infusion of a higher concentration (e.g., 10% dextrose) for a shorter time seems to be less detrimental than infusing 4% glucose continuously.[92] Malnourished patients receiving total parenteral nutrition are particularly susceptible to hypophosphatemia because of the accelerated rate of tissue repair as phosphate is incorporated into new cells and phosphate utilization during glycolysis.[83,122] Respiratory alkalosis likewise causes translocation because it stimulates glycolysis by activating phosphofructokinase.[83] This effect has been demonstrated in experimental dogs but was marked only when hyperventilation was combined with glucose administration.[17] Increased intracellular pH may be more important than increased extracellular pH for causing hypophosphatemia in respiratory alkalosis, which could explain why severe hypophosphatemia may occur in people with severe respiratory failure who are mechanically ventilated.[92]

Diabetic patients are especially at risk for hypophosphatemia. They often have total body phosphate deficits because of loss of muscle mass, urinary phosphate losses, and impaired tissue use of phosphate related to insulin deficiency. Most diabetic cats in one study had mild hypophosphatemia at presentation, whereas 20 of 48 ketotic cats in another study were hypophosphatemic.[21,130] Another study found only 7 of 104 diabetic cats to be hypophosphatemic. However, stratification of the cats into ketoacidotic and nonketoacidotic groups revealed that 5 of 38 ketoacidotic cats were hypophosphatemic and only 2 of 66 nonketotic cats were hypophosphatemic.[36] Interestingly, serum phosphorus concentrations are often normal to increased at presentation in diabetic people, perhaps because of metabolic acidosis by organic acids (e.g., β-hydroxybutyrate), insulin deficiency, osmotic effects of hyperglycemia, or renal insufficiency.[81,108]

Administration of large doses of insulin makes hypophosphatemia even more likely in diabetic ketoacidotic patients. Severe hypophosphatemia has been reported in dogs and cats treated for diabetic ketoacidosis.[2,21,152] Hypophosphatemia developed or worsened after insulin administration, and clinical signs (e.g., hemolysis, seizures) thought related to hypophosphatemia developed in 11 animals. Interestingly, four of these cats developed hemolytic anemia despite intravenous supplementation of potassium phosphate, and it is not clear whether the anemia was caused by inadequate phosphate supplementation or Heinz body formation.[21]

Although it is not documented in dogs and cats, hypophosphatemia may occur in people with certain rapidly growing tumors. Ostensibly, the rapidly dividing cells use phosphorus, removing it from the blood.[92]

Increased urinary loss of phosphorus often produces moderate hypophosphatemia in primary hyperparathyroidism, but clinical signs are caused by hypercalcemia.*

Box 7-1	**Causes of Hypophosphatemia**

Maldistribution (Translocation)
- Treatment of diabetic ketoacidosis
- Carbohydrate load or insulin administration
- Respiratory alkalosis or hyperventilation
- Total parenteral nutrition or nutritional recovery
- Hypothermia

Increased Loss (Reduced Renal Reabsorption)
- Primary hyperparathyroidism
- Renal tubular disorders (e.g., Fanconi's syndrome)
- Proximally acting diuretics (e.g., carbonic anhydrase inhibitors) (?)*
- Eclampsia
- Hyperadrenocorticism (?)

Decreased Intake (Reduced Intestinal Absorption)
- Dietary deficiency (?)
- Vomiting (?)
- Malabsorption (?)
- Phosphate binders
- Vitamin D deficiency

Laboratory Error

*(?) Importance in veterinary medicine uncertain.

---

*References 11,27,82,91,151,153.

If 2.5 mg/dL is considered the lower limit of normal, serum phosphorus concentration was decreased in approximately one third of reported cases associated with parathyroid adenoma, but in six of six cases associated with parathyroid hyperplasia.[40] Hypophosphatemia is seen inconsistently in cats with primary hyperparathyroidism.[39,77] The fractional excretion of phosphorus (FE_{Pi}) was increased in a few affected dogs.[151] The normal FE_{Pi} was found to be 7.5% ± 4.6% in 10 normal dogs but 10% to 23% in a dog with primary hyperparathyroidism.[27]

Fanconi's syndrome in basenjis is associated with decreased renal fractional reabsorption of phosphate, but serum phosphorus concentrations are normal.[16] The renal tubular transport abnormality may be caused by metabolic or membrane defects affecting sodium transport, and the observed phosphaturia may be secondary to natriuresis.[101] Loop diuretics (e.g., furosemide) and distally acting diuretics (e.g., thiazides) have little effect on renal phosphate excretion, but proximally acting diuretics (e.g., carbonic anhydrase inhibitors) may increase renal excretion of phosphate secondary to their effects on proximal tubular sodium reabsorption. In one study, acetazolamide (10 mg/kg intravenously three times daily) did not cause hypophosphatemia when administered to dogs over a 7-day period.[123] Eclampsia in the bitch may be associated with hypophosphatemia and hypocalcemia.[7,9] Presumably, increased PTH secretion in response to hypocalcemia leads to decreased renal reabsorption of phosphate.

Hypophosphatemia caused by dietary deficiency is unlikely in animals eating commercial diets with adequate protein content. A low-protein, low-phosphorus diet designed to dissolve struvite calculi (Prescription Diet S/D, Hill's Pet Nutrition, Inc., Topeka, KS) did not cause significant hypophosphatemia when fed to dogs over a 6-month period.[1] Urinary phosphorus excretion decreased and calcium excretion increased in this study. Although vomiting and malabsorptive diseases potentially can cause phosphate loss, these disorders rarely cause hypophosphatemia in dogs or cats.[29] Canine malabsorptive intestinal disorders often are characterized by hypocalcemia related to hypoalbuminemia, but serum phosphorus concentrations typically are normal.[18,52]

People have become hypophosphatemic after administration of magnesium and aluminum-containing antacids.[94] Whether phosphate depletion occurs depends on the patient's phosphorus intake, dosage of the phosphate binding agent, duration of administration, and the preexisting phosphate balance of the patient. Vitamin D deficiency may cause hypophosphatemia because hypocalcemia increases PTH secretion, which increases renal phosphate excretion. Decreased intestinal phosphate absorption presumably also plays a role in this setting.

It has been stated that 38% of hyperadrenocortical dogs have hypophosphatemia, but actual serum phosphorus concentrations were not reported.[113] In one study, an identifiable cause of hypophosphatemia could not be found in the majority of dogs with this serum biochemical abnormality.[29] Hypophosphatemia, hypercalcemia, hyperglycemia, azotemia, hypokalemia, and acidosis have been reported in a dog and cat with hypothermia caused by exposure to low environmental temperature.[124] The mechanisms responsible for these electrolyte and acid-base disturbances are uncertain, but translocation seems likely.

Disorders of renal tubular phosphate transport associated with hypophosphatemia in humans include X-linked hypophosphatemia, autosomal dominant hypophosphatemic rickets, oncogenic hypophosphatemic osteomalacia, and hereditary hypophosphatemic rickets with hypercalciuria.[148] Naturally occurring mutations in the npt2 gene encoding the type IIa sodium-phosphate cotransporter have not been identified in these disorders, but rather mutations have been found in other phosphate-regulating genes. X-linked hypophosphatemia is caused by a mutation in the PHEX gene (i.e., phosphate-regulating gene with homology to endopeptidases on the X chromosome), which is expressed in bone, whereas autosomal dominant hypophosphatemic rickets is caused by a mutation in the FGF-23 gene, a member of the fibroblast growth factor family. Oncogenic hypophosphatemic osteomalacia occurs as a result of secretion of a humoral phosphaturic factor secreted by neoplastic cells. Hereditary hypophosphatemic rickets with hypercalciuria is similar to X-linked hypophosphatemia and autosomal dominant hypophosphatemic rickets except that it is associated with appropriately increased serum concentrations of calcitriol, whereas the other hereditary disorders are not. Renal tubular disorders of phosphate transport have not been conclusively identified in dogs and cats, but hypophosphatemia, increased urinary FE_{Pi}, low serum 25-hydroxycholecalciferol concentration, osteopenia, and pathologic fractures were reported in a young cat thought to have abnormal renal tubular phosphate transport and defective hepatic 25-hydroxylation of vitamin D.[69]

TREATMENT OF HYPOPHOSPHATEMIA

Prevention, when possible, is preferred to therapy. The clinician should anticipate potential hypophosphatemia and either administer supplemental phosphorus (e.g., patients receiving total parenteral nutrition or insulin treatment for diabetic ketoacidosis) or carefully monitor the patient for hypophosphatemia (e.g., patients receiving phosphate binders).

If hypophosphatemia occurs, one should seek to correct the underlying condition responsible for it. Whether phosphorus is administered depends on the magnitude of the hypophosphatemia and whether clinical signs are present. Asymptomatic animals with low serum phosphorus concentrations but without phosphorus depletion and those with serum phosphorus concentrations greater than 1.8 mg/dL and unlikely to decrease any lower (e.g., primary hyperparathyroidism) often do not require phosphate administration.

Phosphate supplementation is appropriate for asymptomatic patients deemed at risk for developing symptomatic hypophosphatemia (e.g., diabetic ketoacidotic cat with serum phosphorus concentration of 1.6 mg/dL) and for patients with clinical signs believed to result from hypophosphatemia. Interestingly, treatment of asymptomatic hypophosphatemia in diabetic people is controversial and is recommended only when severe (<2.0 mg/dL).[80] However, clinical experience in veterinary medicine suggests that anticipatory phosphorus supplementation is reasonable in some ketoacidotic cats.

Oral phosphate administration is safe but slow and unacceptable in vomiting patients and perhaps in patients with diarrhea. If the enteral route is chosen, feeding skim or low-fat milk or a buffered laxative (e.g., Phospho-Soda, Fleet Pharmaceuticals, Lynchburg, VA) usually is effective. Patients symptomatic because of hypophosphatemia generally need parenteral replacement therapy. Administering phosphate intravenously is potentially dangerous because it may cause hypocalcemia, tetany, soft tissue mineralization, renal failure, or hyperphosphatemia.[83] Therefore phosphorus administration typically has consisted of injecting small amounts slowly over hours to days and monitoring the patient repeatedly (e.g., 0.01 to 0.06 mmol/kg/hr in dogs and cats with measurement of serum phosphorus concentration every 6 to 8 hours).[75,152] Although such caution is wise, it is noteworthy that more aggressive phosphorus administration has been used in people (i.e., 0.16 to 0.64 mmol/kg over 4 to 12 hours in patients receiving total parenteral nutrition).[30] Other groups have used similarly large doses over even shorter times (e.g., 0.4 to 0.8 mmol/kg depending on the degree of hypophosphatemia over 30 minutes in patients with cardiac disease), also without problems.[158] Sodium phosphate and potassium phosphate are commonly used, but administration of glucose phosphate has been reported.[158] Selection of the particular form of phosphorus to administer is based on the patient's serum electrolyte concentrations.

Currently, it seems safest to administer phosphate by constant-rate infusion at rates that have been used successfully in dogs and cats and to monitor the serum phosphorus concentration every 6 to 8 hours. Theoretically, adding phosphorus to fluids containing calcium may cause precipitation of calcium phosphate, but this appears to depend on relative concentrations of calcium and phosphorus. Phosphorus usually is administered after diluting it in physiologic saline solution. The volume of distribution for administered phosphate varies tremendously among hypophosphatemic people, and redistribution of phosphate can occur rapidly. Therefore the dose necessary to replete a patient and the patient's response to therapy cannot be predicted. In two studies of hypophosphatemic cats, total amounts of phosphorus infused intravenously ranged from 0.138 to 1.26 mmol/kg, indicating a wide range of total body phosphate deficits.[2,75]

A conservative approach is to assume that intravenously administered phosphate remains in the ECF compartment (actually much of it enters the intracellular fluid). Development of hyperphosphatemia is unlikely with this approach. Prophylactic parenteral phosphate therapy (such as may be used for patients with diabetic ketoacidosis) may be reasonably estimated by giving one fourth to one half of the supplemented potassium as potassium phosphate and the rest as potassium chloride. However, decreased urinary phosphate excretion that develops during hypophosphatemia may persist during treatment and predispose to hyperphosphatemia. The products available for oral and parenteral use are summarized in Tables 7-1 through 7-3.

HYPERPHOSPHATEMIA

CLINICAL EFFECTS OF HYPERPHOSPHATEMIA

Increased serum phosphorus concentration decreases serum calcium concentration so that the calcium phosphate solubility product ($[Ca] \times [Pi]$) remains constant. Hypocalcemia (which may cause tetany) and soft tissue mineralization are the major clinical consequences of hyperphosphatemia.[149] After phosphate administration,

TABLE 7-1 Oral Preparations of Compounds Used as Phosphate Binders

Name of Product	Chemical Name	Company	Preparations
Basaljel*	Aluminum carbonate gel	Wyeth-Ayerst	Capsules, suspension, tablets
Aluminum hydroxide	Aluminum hydroxide gel	Various manufacturers	Tablets, capsules, suspension
Calcium carbonate	Calcium carbonate	Various manufacturers	Tablets, suspension
PhosLo	Calcium acetate	Braintree	Tablets, capsules
Calcium citrate	Calcium citrate	Various manufacturers	Tablets
Renagel	Sevelamer HCl	Genzyme	Tablets, capsules

Product discontinued.

TABLE 7-2 Preparations for Phosphate Supplementation (Preparations for Parenteral Use)

Compound	Composition (per mL)	pH	Osmolality (mOsm/kg)	Phosphate (mmol/mL)	Sodium (mEq/mL)	Potassium (mEq/mL)
Sodium phosphate	142 mg Na_2HPO_4, 276 mg $NaH_2PO_4 \bullet H_2O$	5.70	5580	3.000	4.0	0
Potassium phosphate	236 mg K_2HPO_4 224 mg KH_2PO_4	6.60	5840	3.003	0	4.36

TABLE 7-3 Preparations for Phosphate Supplementation (Preparations for Oral Use)

Product	Composition	Phosphorus mg	Phosphorus mEq	Phosphate mg	Phosphate mEq	Potassium mg	Potassium mEq	Company	Prep
K-Phos Neutral	Dibasic sodium phosphate, monobasic potassium phosphate, monobasic sodium phosphate	250	14.1	45	1.1	298	13	Beach	Tablets
Uro-KP Neutral	Dibasic sodium phosphate, monobasic potassium phosphate, monobasic sodium phosphate	250	14.1	49	1.3	250	11	Star	Tablets
Neutro-Phos	Dibasic sodium phosphate, monobasic potassium phosphate, monobasic sodium phosphate	250	14.1	278	7.1	164	7.1	Ortho-McNeill	Powder
Neutra-Phos-K	Dibasic potassium phosphate, monobasic potassium phosphate	250	14.1	556	14.2	0	0	Ortho-McNeill	Powder
K-Phos Original	Monobasic potassium phosphate	114	3.7	144	3.7	0	0	Beach	Tablet
K-Phos M.F.	Monobasic potassium phosphate, monobasic sodium phosphate	126	4.0	45	1.1	67	2.9	Beach	Tablet
K-Phos No. 2	Monobasic potassium phosphate, monobasic sodium phosphate	250	8.0	88	2.2	134	5.8	Beach	Tablet

Amounts given per tablet or per 75 mL of reconstituted liquid.
Prep, *Preparation.*

deposition of calcium and phosphate in bone and soft tissue may contribute to hypocalcemia. The magnitude of hypocalcemia is related to the rate at which serum phosphorus concentration increases, but the exact relationship is unpredictable. The risk of soft tissue mineralization increases when the $[Ca] \times [Pi]$ solubility product exceeds 60 to 70.

CAUSES OF HYPERPHOSPHATEMIA

Hyperphosphatemia in dogs and cats is primarily caused by decreased renal excretion, but increased intake and translocation also may be responsible (Box 7-2).[149]

Translocation occurring during treatment of hemolymphatic malignancies may cause tumor lysis syndrome (i.e., hyperphosphatemia, hypocalcemia, hyperkalemia, hyperuricemia, and oliguric acute renal failure). Myeloblasts and lymphoblasts may contain up to four times as much phosphate as normal cells, and destruction of these cells causes release of phosphate. This syndrome is uncommon in small animal practice. In one study of dogs with multicentric lymphosarcoma, serum phosphorus concentrations were normal before therapy and did not change after treatment.[109] Urinary phosphorus excretion increased but probably because urine volume increased. There was no

Box 7-2   Causes of Hyperphosphatemia

Maldistribution (Translocation)
- Tumor cell lysis
- Tissue trauma or rhabdomyolysis
- Hemolysis
- Metabolic acidosis

Increased Intake
- Gastrointestinal
  - Phosphate enemas
  - Vitamin D intoxication (e.g., cholecalciferol-containing rodenticides, calcipotriene)
- Parenteral
  - Intravenous phosphate

Decreased Excretion
- Acute or chronic renal failure
- Uroabdomen or urethral obstruction
- Hypoparathyroidism
- Acromegaly (?)*
- Hyperthyroidism

Physiologic: Young Growing Animal

Laboratory Error (e.g., Lipemia, Hyperproteinemia) Depending on Methodology

*(?) Importance in veterinary medicine uncertain.

change in FE_{Pi} or renal function (as assessed by endogenous creatinine clearance). Chemotherapy in these dogs consisted of prednisone, vincristine, and L-asparaginase. However, acute tumor lysis syndrome has been reported in some animals with lymphosarcoma treated with chemotherapy with or without radiation therapy.[26,88,89] Severe hyperphosphatemia (23.6 and 13.7 mg/dL) occurred in a dog and a cat (respectively), and mild hyperphosphatemia (7.4 and 7.7 mg/dL) occurred in two other affected dogs.[26,88] Thus it may be prudent to promote diuresis by intravenous administration of fluids before beginning chemotherapy in patients with lymphosarcoma suspected of having large tumor burdens (e.g., hepatosplenomegaly).

Massive tissue injury with rhabdomyolysis may cause hyperphosphatemia. Subsequent development of acute renal failure related to myoglobinuria further contributes to hyperphosphatemia.[145] Hyperphosphatemia may occur after aortic thromboembolism in cats and was more common in nonsurvivors in one study.[144] Hemolysis can produce hyperphosphatemia because of the phosphorus content of erythrocytes. Lactic acidosis and diabetic ketoacidosis can be associated with hyperphosphatemia because acidosis caused by organic acids apparently results in breakdown of ATP to AMP and inorganic phosphate by an unknown mechanism.[108]

Increased intake of phosphorus may occur with intravenous administration of phosphate-containing fluids. Such therapy is uncommon in veterinary practice, except in treatment of diabetic ketoacidosis and total parenteral nutrition.[21,152] Increased absorption of phosphorus from the alimentary tract may occur with colonic infusion of hypertonic enema solutions or oral administration of sodium phosphate.[43] Such enemas have caused severe hyperphosphatemia in small dogs and cats.[8,73,131] Clinical signs in cats receiving phosphate enemas include lethargy, ataxia, vomiting, bloody diarrhea, mucous membrane pallor, and stupor. Laboratory abnormalities included marked hyperglycemia and hyperphosphatemia, mild hypernatremia, and lactic acidosis.[8] Severe hyperphosphatemia, azotemia, and metabolic acidosis were reported in a cat treated with a phosphate-containing urinary acidifier (pHos-pHaid) at twice the recommended dosage.[62]

Vitamin D increases intestinal absorption of calcium and phosphorus and may produce hyperphosphatemia in addition to hypercalcemia. In one study, administration of vitamin D_2 to dogs for 3 weeks caused hypercalcemia and azotemia, but serum phosphorus concentrations remained normal.[146] However, intoxication with cholecalciferol-containing rodenticides causes azotemia, hypercalcemia, and hyperphosphatemia in dogs and cats.[44,56,64,97,105] Topical medications containing calcipotriene, an analogue of calcitriol, also can cause hypercalcemia, hyperphosphatemia, metastatic soft tissue mineralization, and acute renal failure if ingested by dogs.[48,66,112]

Decreased urinary excretion is the main cause of hyperphosphatemia, and chronic renal failure is the most common cause of hyperphosphatemia in adult dogs and cats.[29] Chronic renal disease causes a progressive decrease in glomerular filtration rate (GFR), and the filtered load of phosphate (GFR × serum phosphorus concentration) decreases as GFR decreases. If phosphorus intake remains constant, phosphorus retention and transient hyperphosphatemia result. However, sustained hyperphosphatemia does not usually develop in early chronic renal failure because there is a compensatory increase in phosphate excretion by remnant nephrons. The effects of PTH on the kidney mediate this increase in the FE_{Pi}. When GFR decreases to 20% of normal or less (i.e., late chronic renal failure), this compensatory mechanism is exhausted, and hyperphosphatemia develops.

Renal secondary hyperparathyroidism is a consistent finding in progressive renal disease.[139,141] Hyperphosphatemia inhibits renal 1α-hydroxylase, which is present in the renal tubules (this inhibition impairs conversion of 25-hydroxycholecalciferol to calcitriol and thus reduces intestinal calcium absorption), and decreases serum ionized calcium concentration by the mass law effect ([Ca] × [Pi] = constant). The resultant hypocalcemia and the decreased serum calcitriol concentration stimulate PTH secretion. This increased PTH secretion increases renal excretion of phosphate and release of calcium and phosphate from bone. It also stimulates production of calcitriol. These actions normalize serum phosphorus and ionized calcium concentrations. Thus calcium and phosphorus balance is maintained by a progressive increase in serum PTH concentration (in early chronic renal failure). However, as renal tubular destruction progresses, there are fewer proximal renal tubules and a decrease in the amount of 1α-hydroxylase enzyme present. This reduction in 1α-hydroxylase means that it is harder for increased concentrations of PTH to increase serum calcium concentration. It also means that calcitriol is not available to inhibit PTH secretion.[107] As serum phosphate concentrations persistently remain increased, other changes also occur. Persistent hyperphosphatemia in rats increases the number and size of parathyroid cells. This is important because some percentage of each cell's secretion is autonomous, and parathyroid hyperplasia means that there is a greater amount of nonsuppressible PTH secretion. Chronically increased PTH concentration leads to bone demineralization and other toxic effects of uremia (e.g., bone marrow suppression, uremic encephalopathy). In addition, uremia decreases the number of parathyroid gland calcitriol receptors, which subsequently decreases the responsiveness of parathyroid glands to the inhibitory effect of calcitriol on PTH release.[19,85,102,143] Thus both decreased calcitriol production and decreased numbers of parathyroid gland calcitriol receptors promote development of renal secondary hyperparathyroidism.

Renal secondary hyperparathyroidism can be prevented or reversed in dogs with experimentally induced chronic renal disease by reducing dietary phosphorus intake in proportion to the decrease in GFR.[78,138,140] Early in the course of chronic renal disease, decreased phosphorus intake stimulates renal 1α-hydroxylase activity, which increases calcitriol production. Increased calcitriol enhances intestinal calcium absorption, increases serum ionized calcium concentration, and decreases PTH secretion. Late in the course of chronic renal disease, the kidneys are unable to produce sufficient calcitriol to promote normal intestinal absorption of calcium. Phosphorus restriction in advanced renal disease still decreases PTH secretion by unknown mechanisms independent of serum ionized calcium or calcitriol concentrations.[143] These observations form the basis for restricting phosphorus in the medical management of chronic renal failure.

Phosphorus restriction also may prevent renal disease progression by minimizing renal interstitial mineralization.[3] In rats with experimentally induced chronic renal failure, detrimental histologic changes (e.g., interstitial mineralization, inflammation, fibrosis) could be prevented and residual renal function maintained by dietary phosphorus restriction.[71,79] In cats with experimentally induced renal disease, histologic changes were prevented by phosphorus restriction.[125] In a study in rats with 80%

nephrectomy, diet was carefully controlled so that only phosphorus intake differed between groups, and a beneficial effect of phosphorus restriction was clearly demonstrated with regard to mortality, proteinuria, histologic changes, creatinine clearance, and serum lipid concentrations over a period of 14 weeks.[95] Similar beneficial effects were observed in dogs with 90% nephrectomy fed diets differing only in phosphorus content and followed for 12 months.[20] A similar experiment using 48 dogs with experimentally induced renal failure found that the amount of dietary phosphorus was more important in clinical management than the amount of dietary protein.[54] In studies of cats with naturally occurring chronic renal failure, renal secondary hyperparathyroidism was successfully managed using a combination of dietary restriction of phosphorus and administration of phosphate binders.[10,45]

In contrast to findings in early chronic renal failure, hyperphosphatemia is typical in acute renal failure because of insufficient time for compensatory mechanisms to develop. Hyperphosphatemia also occurs in uroabdomen or urethral obstruction because of urine reabsorption from the peritoneal cavity or decreased GFR caused by increased intratubular pressure resulting from urinary tract obstruction.[24,51]

Hypoparathyroidism in people causes mild hyperphosphatemia because renal reabsorption of phosphate is increased in the absence of PTH. Mild hyperphosphatemia also occurs in dogs with hypoparathyroidism but is overshadowed by the effects of hypocalcemia (e.g., muscle tremors, tetany, seizures, ataxia, behavioral aberrations).[22,23,103,136] Hyperphosphatemia has also been reported in cats with hypoparathyroidism.[118]

Acromegalic people may develop hyperphosphatemia because of growth hormone's effects on renal tubular phosphate reabsorption. Mild hyperphosphatemia has been reported in some acromegalic dogs and cats.[49,114,116] Thyroxine increases renal tubular phosphate reabsorption, which contributes to the increased serum phosphorus concentrations observed in hyperthyroid cats.[113,147,150] Hyperphosphatemia was reported in 21% of hyperthyroid cats in one study.[115]

TREATMENT OF HYPERPHOSPHATEMIA

Volume expansion with saline dilutes ECF phosphate and enhances renal phosphate excretion in dehydrated patients. Increasing GFR by volume expansion increases the filtered load of phosphate, and natriuresis impairs proximal tubular phosphate reabsorption. Administration of glucose (and insulin if necessary) may temporarily decrease serum phosphorus concentration by promoting phosphorus entry into cells, although such therapy is rarely, if ever, necessary. All sources of phosphorus intake should be curtailed. In the diet, phosphorus restriction is accomplished primarily by protein restriction. As a rule, low-protein diets are also low in phosphorus. Calcium salts should not be administered to hyperphosphatemic patients because of the risk of metastatic soft tissue calcification. Iatrogenic calcinosis cutis recently has been reported in a dog and cat with hypoparathyroidism given calcium gluconate subcutaneously.[126,132]

In patients with severe, chronic renal failure, low-phosphorus diets are helpful but often insufficient. Dialysis is unpredictable because phosphate is a poorly diffusible ion. Therefore the most practical and effective way to treat hyperphosphatemia in patients with stable chronic renal failure is to decrease intestinal phosphate absorption by orally administered phosphate binders. Such administration helps prevent ingested and endogenously secreted phosphate from being absorbed. Phosphate binders work because the cation in the binder combines with dietary phosphate, producing insoluble, nonabsorbable phosphate compounds. Adsorption of phosphate ions on the surface of binder particles may also contribute to their effect. The rate at which a binder dissolves depends on its water solubility, the pH of the environment, and the dosage.[135]

The most widely used oral phosphate-binding agents contain aluminum or calcium and hydroxide, carbonate, or acetate (see Table 7-1).[33,70,141] The appropriate dosage must be determined empirically, but 90 to 100 mg/kg/day divided two or three times daily is a reasonable starting point. Lower dosages of calcium acetate (50 to 60 mg/kg/day) may be sufficient because it has a greater capacity to bind phosphate than does calcium carbonate.[98] Magnesium-containing compounds are not useful as phosphate binders because they cause diarrhea, and limited ability to excrete magnesium in renal failure patients increases the risk of hypermagnesemia.

Aluminum hydroxide and aluminum carbonate are commonly used phosphate binders. Aluminum hydroxide reduces intestinal phosphorus absorption in normal and uremic people.[32] Aluminum is a better binding agent for phosphate than calcium or magnesium in the acidic gastric environment.[135] This effect is less important at the higher intestinal pH. Aluminum-containing gels are better tolerated by many dogs and cats when given as tablets or capsules, but the desiccated form has a lower phosphate binding capacity than the liquid gel.[128] Aluminum oxide gel prepared to maximize phosphate binding has been studied in dogs.[128,129] Constipation is a common side effect of aluminum-containing phosphate binders.

In people undergoing hemodialysis, osteomalacia and dialysis encephalopathy have been correlated with the aluminum content of dialysis water.[110] In one study, encephalopathy occurred in dialysis patients receiving aluminum hydroxide despite a negligible aluminum content of dialysis water.[4] Aluminum can be absorbed from the intestinal tract in normal people[76] and uremic people,[12,32] and aluminum-induced bone disease can occur in nondialyzed patients after oral administration of aluminum hydroxide.[5] The toxicity of aluminum-containing

phosphate binders in human patients with renal failure is now well established, and they have been replaced by calcium-containing phosphate binders.[46] It still is unclear whether aluminum-containing phosphate binders represent a hazard to dogs with chronic renal failure.

Calcium salts such as calcium carbonate and calcium acetate also have been used as phosphate binders. Calcium carbonate decreases intestinal phosphate absorption in normal and uremic people.* Calcium citrate also has been advocated as a phosphate binder but should not be given with aluminum-containing compounds because citrate enhances aluminum absorption.[37,59,104,111,137] Nausea, constipation, and hypercalcemia are potential side effects of calcium-containing phosphate binders. Simultaneous use of calcitriol and calcium-containing phosphate binders to manage renal secondary hyperparathyroidism increases the risk of hypercalcemia. Calcium acetate binds more phosphate than either calcium citrate or calcium carbonate, and less calcium is absorbed from the intestine during its use.[135] Calcium acetate binds phosphate better than aluminum carbonate at the neutral pH found in the small intestine, but aluminum carbonate is better at the lower gastric pH.[135] In vivo, both were about equally effective.

Phosphate binders are most effective when given with meals. In one study, calcium acetate reduced intestinal absorption of phosphate best when ingested just before or after a meal but was much less effective if given 2 hours after eating.[133] Approximately one third as much phosphate was removed from the body when calcium acetate was given during fasting versus as when it was given with a meal. The endogenous phosphate removed probably originated from basal intestinal secretions or passive diffusion into the intestine. Ingestion of a meal also decreased the absorption of calcium from the calcium acetate. Thus calcium-containing phosphate binders should be given with meals to reduce the risk of hypercalcemia.

The search for new phosphorus binders has continued because of the bone toxicity and encephalopathy associated with use of aluminum-containing compounds and the hypercalcemia and soft tissue (including cardiovascular) calcification associated with use of calcium-containing compounds.[46] Sevelamer hydrochloride is a cross-linked polymeric resin that binds phosphorus and releases chloride. It does not contain aluminum or calcium. Sevelamer reduces the risk of vascular and renal calcification that occurs in human patients with chronic renal failure treated with calcium-containing compounds.[34] It is very expensive, causes some adverse gastrointestinal effects, and has the potential to bind other substances (e.g., bile acids, cholesterol, vitamins) in addition to phosphorus. Initial reports suggested that sevelamer was similar in effective-

---

*References 6,31,57,93,99,142.

ness to calcium acetate in binding phosphorus but with less risk of hypercalcemia.[14] However, a recent study found calcium acetate superior to sevelamer in control of hyperphosphatemia and calcium-phosphorus product.[120] Sevelamer decreased serum bicarbonate concentrations in this study, presumably as a result of the release and absorption of the hydrochloride moiety.

Lanthanum carbonate also contains no aluminum and no calcium, is not absorbed from the gastrointestinal tract, and acts as an efficient phosphorus binder.[46] Its effects are similar to those of calcium carbonate but without risk of bone toxicity or hypercalcemia.[41] Lanthanum is excreted primarily in bile and should not accumulate in patients with renal failure, but its long-term safety is unknown.

Phosphate binder effectiveness is monitored by measuring fasting serum phosphorus concentration. The goal is to maintain the serum phosphorus concentration in the normal range. In normophosphatemic patients with early renal insufficiency, one may monitor fasting FE_{Pi} to determine the efficacy of phosphate restriction. Dogs with spontaneous chronic renal failure (mean serum creatinine concentration, 2.3 mg/dL) had significantly higher FE_{Pi} values than control dogs (23% versus 5%), respectively, and FE_{Pi} decreased in both groups after feeding of Prescription Diet K/D.[65] In one dog with chronic renal failure, FE_{Pi} was below the mean value for the chronic renal failure group despite increased serum PTH concentration. It has been suggested that FE_{Pi} values less than 30% are indicative of adequate phosphate restriction.[50] This method is limited by the wide range of normal values for FE_{Pi}.[42,127] The response to phosphate binders may be relatively slow because the pool of accumulated phosphate is large and the persistent osteolytic effects of PTH provide a large endogenous phosphate load. Thus the clinician should not be discouraged if the patient responds slowly to phosphate binder therapy.

REFERENCES

1. Abdullahi SU, Osborne CA, Leininger JR, et al: Evaluation of a calculolytic diet in female dogs with induced struvite urolithiasis, Am J Vet Res 45:1508-1519, 1984.
2. Adams LG, Hardy RM, Weiss DJ, et al: Hypophosphatemia and hemolytic anemia associated with diabetes mellitus and hepatic lipidosis in cats, J Vet Intern Med 7:266-271, 1993.
3. Alfrey AC: Effect of dietary phosphate restriction on renal function and deterioration, Am J Clin Nutr 47:153-156, 1988.
4. Alfrey AC, LeGendre GR, Kaehny WD: The dialysis encephalopathy syndrome: possible aluminum intoxication, N Engl J Med 294:184-188, 1976.
5. Andreoli SP, Bergstein JM, Sherrard DJ: Aluminum intoxication from aluminum-containing phosphate binders in children with azotemia not undergoing dialysis, N Engl J Med 310:1079-1084, 1984.
6. Andreoli SP, Dunson J, Bergstein JM: Calcium carbonate is an effective phosphorus binder in children with chronic renal failure, Am J Kidney Dis 9:206-210, 1987.
7. Aroch I, Srebro H, Shpigel NY: Serum electrolyte concentrations in bitches with eclampsia, Vet Rec 145:318-320, 1999.
8. Atkins CE, Tyler R, Greenlee P: Clinical, biochemical, acid-base, and electrolyte abnormalities in cats after hypertonic sodium phosphate enema administration, Am J Vet Res 46:980-988, 1985.
9. Austad R, Bjerkas E: Eclampsia in the bitch, J Small Anim Pract 17:795-798, 1976.
10. Barber PJ, Rawlings JM, Markwell PJ, et al: Effect of dietary restriction on renal secondary hyperparathyroidism in the cat, J Small Anim Pract 40:62-70, 1999.
11. Berger B, Feldman EC: Primary hyperparathyroidism in dogs: 21 cases (1976-1986), J Am Vet Med Assoc 191:350-356, 1987.
12. Berlyne GM, Ben-Ari J, Pest D, et al: Hyperaluminaemia from aluminum resins in renal failure, Lancet 2:494-496, 1970.
13. Betro MG, Pain RW: Hypophosphatemia and hyperphosphatemia in a hospital population, Lancet 1:273-276, 1972.
14. Bleyer AJ, Burke SK, Dillon M, et al: A comparison of the calcium-free phosphate binder sevelamer hydrochloride with calcium acetate in the treatment of hyperphosphatemia in hemodialysis patients, Am J Kidney Dis 33:694-701, 1999.
15. Bloom F: The blood chemistry of the dog and cat, New York, 1960, Gamma Publications.
16. Bovee KC, Joyce T, Blazer-Yost B, et al: Characterization of renal defects in dogs with a syndrome similar to Fanconi syndrome in man, J Am Vet Med Assoc 174:1094-1099, 1979.
17. Brautbar N, Leibovici H, Massry SG: On the mechanism of hypophosphatemia during acute hyperventilation: evidence for increased muscle glycolysis, Miner Electrolyte Metab 9:45-50, 1983.
18. Breitschwerdt EB, Halliwell WH, Foley CW, et al: A hereditary diarrhetic syndrome in the basenji characterized by malabsorption, protein losing enteropathy, and hypergammaglobulinemia, J Am Anim Hosp Assoc 16:551-560, 1980.
19. Brown AJ, Dusso A, Lopez-Hilker S, et al: 1,25-$(OH)_2$D receptors are decreased in parathyroid glands from chronically uremic dogs, Kidney Int 35:19-23, 1989.
20. Brown S, Finco D, Crowell WA, et al: Beneficial effect of moderate phosphate restriction in partially nephrectomized dogs on a low protein diet (abstract), Kidney Int 31:380, 1987.
21. Bruskiewicz KA, Nelson RW, Feldman EC, et al: Diabetic ketosis and ketoacidosis in cats: 42 cases (1980-1995), J Am Vet Med Assoc 211:188-192, 1997.
22. Bruyette DS, Feldman EC: Primary hypoparathyroidism in the dog, J Vet Intern Med 2:7-14, 1988.
23. Burk RL, Schaubhut CW: Spontaneous primary hypoparathyroidism in a dog, J Am Anim Hosp Assoc 11:784-785, 1975.
24. Burrows CF, Bovee KC: Metabolic changes due to experimentally-induced rupture of the canine urinary bladder, Am J Vet Res 35:1083-1088, 1974.
25. Busse JC, Gelbard MA, Byrnes JJ, et al: Pseudohyperphosphatemia and dysproteinemia, Arch Intern Med 147:2045-2046, 1987.
26. Calia CM, Hohenhaus AE, Fox PR, et al: Acute tumor lysis syndrome in a cat with lymphoma, J Vet Intern Med 10:409-411, 1996.

27. Carillo JM, Burk RL, Bode C: Primary hyperparathyroidism in a dog, *J Am Vet Med Assoc* 174:67-71, 1979.

28. Carlson GP: Fluid, electrolyte, and acid base balance. In Kaneko JJ, editor: *Clinical biochemistry of domestic animals*, ed 4, New York, 1989, Academic Press, pp. 543-575.

29. Chew DJ, Meuten DJ: Disorders of calcium and phosphorus metabolism, *Vet Clin North Am* 12:411-438, 1982.

30. Clark CL, Sacks GS, Dickerson RN, et al: Treatment of hypophosphatemia in patients receiving specialized nutrition support using a graduated dosing scheme. Results from a prospective clinical trial, *Crit Care Med* 23:1504-1511, 1995.

31. Clarkson EM, McDonald SJ, deWardener HE: The effect of a high intake of calcium carbonate in normal subjects and patients with chronic renal failure, *Clin Sci* 30:425-438, 1966.

32. Clarkson EM, Luck VA, Hynson WV, et al: The effect of aluminum hydroxide on calcium, phosphorus, and aluminum balances, the serum parathyroid hormone concentration and the aluminum content of bone in patients with chronic renal failure, *Clin Sci* 43:519-531, 1972.

33. Coburn JW, Salusky IB: Control of serum phosphorus in uremia, *N Engl J Med* 320:1140-1142, 1989.

34. Cozzolino M, Staniforth ME, Liapis H, et al: Sevelamer hydrochloride attenuates kidney and cardiovascular calcifications in long-term experimental uremia, *Kidney Int* 64:1653-1661, 2003.

35. Craddock PR, Yawata Y, VanSanten L, et al: Acquired phagocyte dysfunction, *N Engl J Med* 290:1403-1407, 1974.

36. Crenshaw KL, Peterson ME: Pretreatment of clinical and laboratory evaluation of cats with diabetes mellitus: 104 cases (1992-1994), *J Am Vet Med Assoc* 209:943-949, 1996.

37. Cushner HM, Copley JB, Lindberg JS, et al: Calcium citrate, a non–aluminum-containing phosphate-binding agent for treatment of CRF, *Kidney Int* 33:95-99, 1988.

38. Delmez JA, Kelber J, Norword KY, et al: Magnesium carbonate as a phosphorus binder: a prospective controlled crossover study, *Kidney Int* 49:163-167, 1996.

39. den Hertog E, Goossens MM, van der Linde-Sipman JS, et al: Primary hyperparathyroidism in two cats, *Vet Q* 19:81-84, 1997.

40. DeVries SE, Feldman EC, Nelson RW, et al: Primary parathyroid gland hyperplasia in dogs: six cases (1982-1991), *J Am Vet Med Assoc* 202:1132-1136, 1993.

41. D'Haese PC, Spasovski GB, Sikole A, et al: A multicenter study on the effects of lanthanum carbonate (Fosrenol™) and calcium carbonate on renal bone disease in dialysis patients, *Kidney Int* 63:S73-S78, 2003.

42. DiBartola SP, Chew DJ, Jacobs G: Quantitative urinalysis including 24-hour urinary protein excretion in the dog, *J Am Anim Hosp Assoc* 16:537-546, 1980.

43. DiPalma JA, Buckley SE, Warner BA, et al: Biochemical effects of oral sodium phosphate, *Dig Dis Sci* 41:749-753, 1996.

44. Dougherty SA, Center SA, Dzanis DA: Salmon calcitonin as adjunct treatment for vitamin D toxicosis in a dog, *J Am Vet Med Assoc* 196:1269-1272, 1990.

45. Elliott J, Rawlings JM, Markwell PJ, et al: Survival of cats with naturally-occurring chronic renal failure: effect of dietary management, *J Small Anim Pract* 41:235-242, 2000.

46. Emmett M: A comparison of clinically useful phosphorus binders for patients with chronic renal failure, *Kidney Int* 66:S25-S32, 2004.

47. Reference deleted in Pages.

48. Fan TM, Simpson KW, Trasti S, et al: Calcipotriol toxicity in a dog, *J Small Anim Pract* 39:581-586, 1998.

49. Feldman EC, Nelson RW: Disorders of growth hormone. In *Canine and feline endocrinology and reproduction*, ed 2, Philadelphia, 1996, WB Saunders, p. 60.

50. Finco DR: The role of phosphorus restriction in the management of chronic renal failure in the dog and cat, *Proc 7th Kal Kan Symposium*, 1983, pp. 131-134.

51. Finco DR, Cornelius LM: Characterization and treatment of water, electrolyte, and acid-base imbalances of induced urethral obstruction in the cat, *Am J Vet Res* 38:823-830, 1977.

52. Finco DR, Duncan JR, Schall WD, et al: Chronic enteric disease and hypoproteinemia in 9 dogs, *J Am Vet Med Assoc* 163:262-271, 1973.

53. Finco DR, Barsanti JA, Brown SA: Influence of dietary source of phosphorus on fecal and urinary excretion of phosphorus and other minerals by male cats, *Am J Vet Res* 50:263-266, 1989.

54. Finco DR, Brown SA, Crowell WA, et al: Effects of dietary phosphorus and protein in dogs with chronic renal failure, *Am J Vet Res* 53:2264-2271, 1992.

55. Fitzgerald F: Clinical hypophosphatemia, *Annu Rev Med* 29:177-189, 1978.

56. Fooshee SK, Forrester SD: Hypercalcemia secondary to cholecalciferol rodenticide toxicosis in two dogs, *J Am Vet Med Assoc* 196:1265-1268, 1990.

57. Fournier A, Moriniere P, Sebert JL, et al: Calcium carbonate, an aluminum-free agent for control of hyperphosphatemia, hypocalcemia, and hyperparathyroidism in uremia, *Kidney Int* 29:S114-S119, 1986.

58. Fraser D, Hones G, Kooh SW, et al: Calcium and phosphate metabolism. In Tietz NW, editor: *Fundamentals of clinical chemistry*, Philadelphia, 1987, WB Saunders, pp. 705-728.

59. Froment DH, Molitoris BA, Buddington B, et al: Site and mechanism of enhanced gastrointestinal absorption of aluminum by citrate, *Kidney Int* 36:978-984, 1989.

60. Fuller TJ, Carter NW, Barcenas C, et al: Reversible changes of the muscle cell in experimental phosphorus deficiency, *J Clin Invest* 57:1019-1024, 1976.

61. Fuller TJ, Nichols WW, Brenner BJ, et al: Reversible depression in myocardial performance in dogs with experimental phosphorus deficiency, *J Clin Invest* 62:1194-1200, 1978.

62. Fulton RB, Fruechte LK: Poisoning induced by administration of a phosphate-containing urinary acidifier in a cat, *J Am Vet Med Assoc* 198:883-885, 1991.

63. Glick MR, Ryder KW, Glick SJ: *Interferographs*, Indianapolis, 1991, Science Enterprises Inc.

64. Gunther R, Felice LJ, Nelson RK: Toxicity of a vitamin D_3 rodenticide to dogs, *J Am Vet Med Assoc* 193:211-214, 1988.

65. Hansen B, DiBartola SP, Chew DJ, et al: Clinical and metabolic findings in dogs with spontaneous chronic renal failure fed two different diets, *Am J Vet Res* 53:326-334, 1992.

66. Hare R, Dobbs C, Sayman K, et al: Calcipotriene poisoning in dogs, *Vet Med* 95:770-778, 2000.

67. Harkin KR, Braselton WE, Tvedten H: Pseudohypophosphatemia in two dogs with immune-mediated hemolytic anemia, *J Vet Intern Med* 12:178-181, 1998.

68. Harper EJ, Hackett RM, Wilkinson J, et al: Age-related variations in hematologic and plasma biochemical test results in Beagles and Labrador Retrievers, *J Am Vet Med Assoc* 223:1436-1442, 2003.

69. Henik RA, Forrest LJ, Friedman AL: Rickets caused by excessive renal phosphate loss and apparent abnormal vitamin D metabolism in a cat, *J Am Vet Med Assoc* 215:1644-1649, 1999.

70. Hercz G, Coburn JW: Prevention of phosphate retention and hyperphosphatemia in uremia, *Kidney Int* 32:S215-S220, 1987.

71. Ibels LS, Alfrey AC, Haut L, et al: Preservation of function in experimental renal disease by dietary restriction of phosphate, *N Engl J Med* 298:122, 1978.

72. Ikeuchi J, Yoshizaki T, Hirata M: Plasma biochemistry values of young Beagle dogs, *J Toxicol Sci* 16:49-59, 1991.

73. Jorgensen LS, Center SA, Randolph JF, et al: Electrolyte abnormalities induced by hypertonic phosphate enemas in two cats, *J Am Vet Med Assoc* 187:1367-1368, 1985.

74. Juan D, Elrazak MA: Hypophosphatemia in hospitalized patients, *JAMA* 242:163-164, 1979.

75. Justin RB, Hohenhaus AE: Hypophosphatemia associated with enteral alimentation in cats, *J Vet Intern Med* 9:228-233, 1995.

76. Kaehny WD, Hegg AP, Alfrey AC: Gastrointestinal absorption of aluminum from aluminum-containing antacids, *N Engl J Med* 296:1389-1390, 1977.

77. Kallet AJ, Richter KP, Feldman EC, et al: Primary hyperparathyroidism in cats: seven cases (1984-1989), *J Am Vet Med Assoc* 199:1767-1771, 1991.

78. Kaplan MA, Canterbury JM, Bourgoignie JJ, et al: Reversal of hyperparathyroidism in response to dietary phosphorus restriction in the uremic dog, *Kidney Int* 15:43, 1979.

79. Karlinsky ML, Haut L, Buddington B, et al: Preservation of renal function in experimental glomerulonephritis, *Kidney Int* 17:293, 1980.

80. Kassirer JP, Hricik DE, Cohen JJ: Phosphate. In *Repairing body fluids: principles and practice*, Philadelphia, 1989, WB Saunders, pp. 110-117.

81. Kebler R, McDonald FD, Cadnapaphornchai P: Dynamic changes in serum phosphorus level in diabetic ketoacidosis, *Am J Med* 79:571-576, 1985.

82. Klausner JS, O'Leary TP, Osborne CA: Calcium urolithiasis in two dogs with parathyroid adenomas, *J Am Vet Med Assoc* 191:1423-1426, 1987.

83. Knochel JP: The pathophysiology and clinical characteristics of severe hypophosphatemia, *Arch Intern Med* 137:203-220, 1977.

84. Knochel JP: Skeletal muscle in hypophosphatemia and phosphorus deficiency, *Adv Exp Med Biol* 103:357-366, 1978.

85. Korkor AB: Reduced binding of [^{3}H]1,25-dihydroxyvitamin D$_3$ in the parathyroid glands of patients with renal failure, *N Engl J Med* 316:1573, 1987.

86. Kreisberg RA: Phosphorus deficiency and hypophosphatemia, *Hosp Pract* 12:121-128, 1977.

87. Kristensen AT, Klausner JS, Weiss DJ, et al: Spurious hyperphosphatemia in a dog with chronic lymphocytic leukemia and an IgM monoclonal gammopathy, *Vet Clin Pathol* 20:45-48, 1991.

88. Laing EJ, Carter RF: Acute tumor lysis syndrome following treatment of canine lymphoma, *J Am Anim Hosp Assoc* 24:691-696, 1988.

89. Laing EJ, Fitzpatrick PJ, Norris AM, et al: Half-body radiotherapy in the treatment of canine lymphoma, *J Vet Intern Med* 3:102-108, 1989.

90. Leehey DJ, Daugirdas JT, Ing TS, et al: Spurious hyperphosphatemia due to hyperlipidemia, *Arch Intern Med* 145:743-744, 1985.

91. Legendre AM, Merkley DF, Carrig CB, et al: Primary hyperparathyroidism in a dog, *J Am Vet Med Assoc* 168:694-696, 1976.

92. Levine BS, Kleeman CR: Hypophosphatemia and hyperphosphatemia: clinical and pathophysiologic aspects. In Narins RG, editor: *Clinical disorders of fluid and electrolyte metabolism*, ed 5, New York, 1994, McGraw-Hill, pp. 1045-1090.

93. Lopez S, Galceran T, Slatopolsky E: Evaluation of calcium carbonate as an effective phosphorus-binding agent in the dog, *Clin Res* 32:452A, 1984.

94. Lotz M, Zisman E, Bartter FC: Evidence for a phosphorus depletion syndrome in man, *N Engl J Med* 278:409-415, 1968.

95. Lumlertgul D, Burke TJ, Gillum DM, et al: Phosphate depletion arrests progression of chronic renal failure independent of protein intake, *Kidney Int* 29:658, 1986.

96. Lutomski DM, Bower RH: The effect of thrombocytosis on serum potassium and phosphorus concentrations, *Am J Med Sci* 307:255-258, 1994.

97. MacKenzie CP, Burnie AG, Head KW: Poisoning in four dogs by a compound containing warfarin and calciferol, *J Small Anim Pract* 28:433-445, 1987.

98. Mai ML, Emmett ME, Sheikh MS, et al: Calcium acetate, an effective phosphorus binder in patients with renal failure, *Kidney Int* 36:690-695, 1989.

99. Malberti F, Surian M, Colussi G, et al: Calcium carbonate: a suitable alternative to aluminum hydroxide as phosphate binder, *Kidney Int* 33:S184-S185, 1988.

100. Mavrikakis M, Vaiopoulos G, Athanassiades P, et al: Pseudohyperphosphatemia in multiple myeloma, *Am J Hematol* 51:178-179, 1996.

101. McNamara PD, Rea CT, Bovee KC, et al: Cystinuria in dogs: comparison of the cystinuric component of the Fanconi syndrome in basenji dogs to isolated cystinuria, *Metabolism* 38:8-15, 1989.

102. Merke J, Hugel U, Zlotkowski A, et al: Diminished parathyroid 1,25-dihydroxycholecalciferol receptors in experimental uremia, *Kidney Int* 32:350-353, 1987.

103. Meyer DJ, Terrell TG: Idiopathic hypoparathyroidism in a dog, *J Am Vet Med Assoc* 168:858-860, 1976.

104. Molitoris BA, Froment DH, MacKenzie TA, et al: Citrate: a major factor in the toxicity of orally administered aluminum compounds, *Kidney Int* 36:949-953, 1989.

105. Moore FM, Kudisch M, Richter K, et al: Hypercalcemia associated with rodenticide poisoning in three cats, *J Am Vet Med Assoc* 193:1099-1100, 1988.

106. Murer H, Hernando N, Forster I, et al: Proximal tubular phosphate reabsorption: molecular mechanisms, *Physiol Rev* 80:1373-1409, 2000.

107. Nagode LA, Chew DJ, Podell M: Benefits of calcitriol therapy and serum phosphorus control in dogs and cats with renal failure, *Vet Clin North Am* 26:1293-1330, 1996.

108. Oster JR, Perez GO, Vaamonde CA: Relationship between blood pH and potassium and phosphorus during acute metabolic acidosis, *Am J Physiol* 235:F345-F351, 1978.

109. Page RL, Leifer CE, Matus RE: Uric acid and phosphorus excretion in dogs with lymphosarcoma, *Am J Vet Res* 47:910-912, 1986.

110. Parkinson IS, Ward MK, Kerr DNS: Dialysis encephalopathy, bone disease, and anemia: the aluminum intoxication syndrome during regular hemodialysis, *J Clin Pathol* 34:1285-1294, 1981.

111. Partridge NA, Regnier FE, White JL, et al: Influence of dietary constituents on intestinal absorption of aluminum, *Kidney Int* 35:1413-1417, 1989.

112. Pesillo SA, Khan SA, Rozanski EA, et al: Calcipotriene toxicosis in a dog successfully treated with pamidronate disodium, *J Vet Emerg Crit Care* 12:177-181, 2002.

113. Peterson ME: Hyperadrenocorticism, *Vet Clin North Am* 14:731-749, 1984.

114. Peterson ME: Endocrine disorders in cats: four emerging diseases, *Comp Contin Educ Pract Vet* 10:1353-1362, 1988.

115. Peterson ME, Kintzer PP, Cavanagh PG, et al: Feline hyperthyroidism: pretreatment clinical and laboratory evaluation of 131 cases, *J Am Vet Med Assoc* 183:103-110, 1983.

116. Peterson ME, Taylor RS, Greco DS, et al: Spontaneous acromegaly in the cat. *Proc Am Coll Vet Intern Med*, Washington, DC, 1986, pp. 14-43.

117. Peterson ME, Taylor RS, Greco DS, et al: Acromegaly in 14 cats, *J Vet Intern Med* 4:192-201, 1990.

118. Peterson ME, James KM, Wallace M, et al: Idiopathic hypoparathyroidism in five cats, *J Vet Intern Med* 5:47-51, 1991.

119. Pickrell JA, Schluter SJ, Belasich JJ, et al: Relationship of age of normal dogs to blood serum constituents and reliability of measured single values, *Am J Vet Res* 35:897-903, 1974.

120. Qunibi WY, Hootkins RE, McDowell LL, et al: Treatment of hyperphosphatemia in hemodialysis patients: the Calcium Acetate Renagel Evaluation (CARE Study), *Kidney Int* 65:1914-1926, 2004.

121. Ralston Purina Company: *Normal blood values for cats and normal blood values for dogs,* St. Louis, 1975, Ralston Purina Company.

122. Ritz E: Acute hypophosphatemia, *Kidney Int* 22:84-94, 1982.

123. Rose RJ, Carter J: Some physiological and biochemical effects of acetazolamide in the dog, *J Vet Pharmacol Ther* 2:215-221, 1979.

124. Ross LA, Goldstein M: Biochemical abnormalities associated with accidental hypothermia in a dog and cat. Abstract. *Proc Am Coll Vet Intern Med,* St. Louis, 1981, p. 66.

125. Ross LA, Finco DR, Crowell WA, et al: Effect of dietary phosphorus restriction on the kidneys of cats with reduced renal mass, *Am J Vet Res* 43:1023, 1982.

126. Ruopp JL: Primary hypoparathyroidism in a cat complicated by suspect iatrogenic calcinosis cutis, *J Am Anim Hosp Assoc* 37:370-373, 2001.

127. Russo EA, Lees GE, Hightower D: Evaluation of renal function in cats, using quantitative urinalysis, *Am J Vet Res* 47:1308-1312, 1986.

128. Rutherford E, Mercado A, Hruska K, et al: An evaluation of a new and effective phosphorus binding agent, *Trans Am Soc Artif Intern Organs* 19:446-449, 1973.

129. Rutherford E, King S, Perry B, et al: Use of a new phosphate binder in chronic renal insufficiency, *Kidney Int* 17:528-534, 1980.

130. Schaer M: A clinical survey of 30 cats with diabetes mellitus, *J Am Anim Hosp Assoc* 13:23-27, 1977.

131. Schaer M, Cavanaugh P, Hause W, et al: Iatrogenic hyperphosphatemia, hypocalcemia and hypernatremia in a cat, *J Am Anim Hosp Assoc* 13:39-41, 1977.

132. Schaer M, Gin PE, Fox LE, et al: Severe calcinosis cutis associated with treatment of hypoparathyroidism in a dog, *J Am Anim Hosp Assoc* 37:364-369, 2001.

133. Schiller LR, Santa Ana CA, Sheikh MS, et al: Effect of the time of administration of calcium acetate on phosphorus binding, *N Engl J Med* 320:1110-1113, 1989.

134. Schmidt RW: Effects of phosphate depletion on acid-base status in dogs, *Metabolism* 27:943-952, 1978.

135. Sheikh MS, Maguire JA, Emmett M, et al: Reduction of dietary phosphorus absorption by phosphorus binders: a theoretical, in vitro, and in vivo study, *J Clin Invest* 83:66-73, 1989.

136. Sherding RF, Meuten DJ, Chew DJ, et al: Primary hypoparathyroidism in the dog, *J Am Vet Med Assoc* 176:439-444, 1980.

137. Slanina P, Falkeborn Y, Frech W, et al: Aluminum concentration in the brain and bone of rats fed citric acid, aluminum citrate or aluminum hydroxide, *Food Chem Toxicol* 27:391-397, 1984.

138. Slatopolsky E, Bricker NS: The role of phosphorus restriction in the prevention of secondary hyperparathyroidism in chronic renal disease, *Kidney Int* 4:141, 1973.

139. Slatopolsky E, Caglar S, Pennell JP, et al: On the pathogenesis of hyperparathyroidism in chronic renal insufficiency in the dog, *J Clin Invest* 50:492, 1971.

140. Slatopolsky E, Caglar S, Gradowska L, et al: On the prevention of secondary hyperparathyroidism in experimental chronic renal disease using "proportional reduction" of dietary phosphorus intake, *Kidney Int* 2:147, 1972.

141. Slatopolsky E, Rutherford WE, Rosenbaum R, et al: Hyperphosphatemia, *Clin Nephrol* 7:138-146, 1977.

142. Slatopolsky E, Weerts C, Lopez-Hilker S, et al: Calcium carbonate as a phosphate binder in patients with chronic renal failure undergoing dialysis, *N Engl J Med* 315:157-161, 1986.

143. Slatopolsky E, Lopez-Hilker S, Delmez J, et al: The parathyroid-calcitriol axis in health and chronic renal failure, *Kidney Int* 38:S41-S47, 1990.

144. Smith SA, Tobias AH, Jacob KA, et al: Arterial thromboembolism in cats: acute crisis in 127 cases (1992-2001) and long-term management with low-dose aspirin in 24 cases, *J Vet Int Med* 17:73-83, 2003.

145. Spangler WL, Muggli FM: Seizure-induced rhabdomyolysis accompanied by renal failure in a dog, *J Am Vet Med Assoc* 172:1190-1194, 1978.

146. Spangler WL, Gribble DH, Lee TC: Vitamin D intoxication and the pathogenesis of vitamin D nephropathy in the dog, *Am J Vet Res* 40:73-83, 1979.

147. Taylor JA, Jacobs RM, Lumsden JH, et al: Perspectives on the diagnosis of feline hyperthyroidism, *Can Vet J* 30:477-481, 1989.

148. Tenenhouse HS, Murer H: Disorders of renal tubular phosphate transport, *J Am Soc Nephrol* 14:240-247, 2003.

149. Thatte L, Oster JR, Singer I, et al: Review of the literature: severe hyperphosphatemia, *Am J Med Sci* 310:167-174, 1995.

150. Turrel JM, Feldman EC, Nelson RW, et al: Thyroid carcinoma causing hyperthyroidism in cats: 14 cases (1981-1986), *J Am Vet Med Assoc* 193:359-364, 1988.

151. Weir EC, Morrdin RW, Barthold SW, et al: Primary hyperparathyroidism in a dog: biochemical, bone, histomorphometric, and pathologic findings, *J Am Vet Med Assoc* 189:1471-1474, 1986.

152. Willard MD, Zerbe CA, Schall WD, et al: Severe hypophosphatemia associated with diabetes mellitus in six dogs and one cat, *J Am Vet Med Assoc* 190:1007-1010, 1987.

153. Wilson JW, Harris SG, Moor WD, et al: Primary hyperparathyroidism in a dog, *J Am Vet Med Assoc* 164:942-946, 1974.

154. Wolford ST, Schroer RA, Gohs FX, et al: Effect of age on serum chemistry profile, electrophoresis and thyroid hormones in Beagle dogs two weeks to one year of age, *Vet Clin Pathol* 17:35-42, 1988.

155. Yawata Y, Craddock P, Hebbel R, et al: Hyperalimentation hypophosphatemia: hematologic and neurologic

dysfunction due to ATP depletion, *Clin Res* 31:729A, 1973.

156. Yawata Y, Hebbel RP, Silvis S, et al: Blood cell abnormalities complicating the hypophosphatemia of hyperalimentation: erythrocyte and platelet ATP deficiency associated with hemolytic anemia and bleeding in hyperalimented dogs, *J Lab Clin Med* 84:643-653, 1974.

157. Young DS: *Effects of drugs on clinical laboratory tests,* Washington, DC, 1995, AACC Press.

158. Zazzo JF, Troche G, Ruel P, et al: High incidence of hypophosphatemia in surgical intensive care patients. Efficacy of phosphorus therapy on myocardial function, *Intensive Care Med* 21:826-831, 1995.

APPENDIX TO CHAPTER 7

Calculation of Amount of PO_4^{3-} and H_3PO_4 Present in Extracellular Fluid at a pH of 7.4

The Henderson-Hasselbalch equation is derived from the formula for the dissociation constant of an acid. For the ionic species of phosphate of interest:

$$pH = pKa + \log([PO_4^{3-}]/[HPO_4^{2-}])$$
$$7.4 = 12.4 + \log(x)$$
$$\log(x) = -5.0$$
$$x = 0.00001$$
$$[PO_4^{3-}]/[HPO_4^{2-}] = 0.00001$$
$$[HPO_4^{2-}]/[PO_4^{3-}] = 100,000$$

Thus at a pH of 7.4, there are 100,000 molecules of HPO_4^{2-} for every molecule of PO_4^{3-}.

$$pH = pKa + \log([H_2PO_4^{1-}]/[H_3PO_4])$$
$$7.4 = 2.0 + \log(x)$$
$$\log(x) = 5.4$$
$$x = 251,189$$
$$[H_2PO_4^{1-}]/[H_3PO_4] = 251,189$$

Thus at a pH of 7.4, there are 251,189 molecules of $H_2PO_4^{1-}$ for every molecule of H_3PO_4.

$$pH = pKa + \log([HPO_4^{2-}]/[H_2PO_4^{1-}])$$
$$7.4 = 6.8 + \log(x)$$
$$\log(x) = 0.6$$
$$x = 4.0$$
$$[HPO_4^{2-}]/[H_2PO_4^{1-}] = 4.0$$

From these calculations, it can be determined that, at a pH of 7.4, there will be 1,004,756 molecules of HPO_4^{2-}, 251,189 molecules of $H_2PO_4^{1-}$, and 10 molecules of PO_4^{3-} for every molecule of H_3PO_4. Therefore it can be seen that the amounts of H_3PO_4 and PO_4^{3-} present in ECF at a pH of 7.4 can be safely ignored.

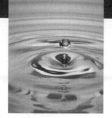

CHAPTER · 8

DISORDERS OF MAGNESIUM: MAGNESIUM DEFICIT AND EXCESS

Shane Bateman

Historically, magnesium has received very little attention in veterinary medicine as an electrolyte worthy of consideration. Studies conducted in animal models in the early twentieth century documented the devastating effects of dietary magnesium deficit in dogs.[22,23,111,157] For the ensuing decades, magnesium did not receive any significant attention. Dietary magnesium became a topic of interest in the 1970s and 1980s as a potential risk factor for cats with struvite urolithiasis and urethral obstruction.[28,87,120] Today, following significant study of the syndrome in cats and identification of numerous other risk factors, magnesium in the diet is no longer considered a risk factor for the formation of feline urolithiasis.[20,21,52,85] Since then, magnesium research in veterinary medicine has begun to document some of the clinical issues related to magnesium, but more work is needed.

Veterinary critical care has made significant developmental strides during the past 20 years as it follows in the footsteps of its human counterpart discipline. Magnesium has gained considerable importance within the discipline of critical care because of the prevalence of magnesium-related metabolic dysfunction documented in human and veterinary patient populations. Study of magnesium-related disease has proven to be difficult, most likely because approximately 99% of the body's magnesium is stored inside the cell, where it participates in vital behind-the-scenes metabolic activities of the cell. As technology has advanced, however, our understanding of the important role magnesium plays in maintaining normal homeostasis of body systems, such as the cardiovascular and neuromuscular systems, has increased significantly. At the beginning of the twenty-first century, the field of magnesium study is rich and ripe with opportunities. Our efforts have only just begun to scratch the surface of understanding the importance of magnesium.

MAGNESIUM REGULATION AND BALANCE

DISTRIBUTION OF MAGNESIUM

The precise distribution of magnesium in the bodies of dogs and cats under differing conditions has not been well studied. The distribution of magnesium within the bodies of humans has been documented more effectively. In humans, current estimates suggest that only about 1% of the total body magnesium is located outside the cell in the extracellular fluids (ECFs) and that the remaining 99% is located in intracellular stores.[119] Approximately two thirds (67%) of body magnesium is stored in the bone with calcium and phosphorus, 20% is found in muscle tissue, and 11% is found in other soft tissues not including muscle.[117] Bone and muscle account for the major intracellular stores of magnesium in humans. Exchange between intracellular magnesium and the ECF is difficult to study, but current estimates suggest that only 15% of these stores are considered to be exchangeable with the ECF. It appears that bone, muscle, and red blood cell stores of magnesium are very slow to liberate magnesium to the extracellular pool, and that soft tissues are much more able to liberate magnesium to the extracellular space in humans.[119] In dogs, however, similar radioisotope studies suggest that bone magnesium is the most labile pool and will be scavenged during a magnesium deficit.[13] Regulatory control of magnesium shifts between intracellular and extracellular spaces is poorly understood and is likely to be complex and multifactorial. Extracellular magnesium is present in three forms (like calcium): an ionized or free form (55%) that is thought to constitute the biologically active fraction, a protein-bound form (20% to 30%) and a complexed form (15% to 25%). Unlike calcium, which is approximately 40% protein bound, magnesium is only 20% to 30% bound to protein and so is less affected by changes

210

in albumin concentration.[84,117] Inside the cell, magnesium is complexed to many organic compounds where it plays a pivotal role. Current estimates indicate that only about 1% to 2% of the intracellular magnesium is present in the ionized or free form. Presumably, magnesium also shifts between the free and complexed intracellular forms as well, but the precise regulatory mechanisms governing those shifts are not understood at this time.

GASTROINTESTINAL HANDLING OF MAGNESIUM

The primary site of magnesium absorption appears to be the ileum, but the jejunum and colon also contribute substantially to net absorption.[63,65] The mechanisms of magnesium absorption from the ileum are the most well studied at this time. Much research remains to completely understand the complexities of gastrointestinal magnesium absorption. Several key mechanisms are currently well understood. Two pathways for intestinal magnesium absorption exist: an unsaturable passive paracellular route and a saturable active transcellular route (Fig. 8-1).[63,65,74] The paracellular movement of magnesium occurs through the tight junctions between epithelial cells. The driving forces for paracellular magnesium movement are the transepithelial magnesium concentration gradient, the transepithelial voltage gradient formed

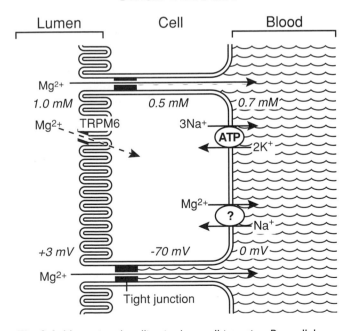

Small Intestine

Fig. 8-1 Magnesium handling in the small intestine. Paracellular transport of magnesium occurs via tight junctions down a favorable electrochemical gradient. Transcellular transport of magnesium occurs down favorable electrochemical gradients into the cell and is postulated to occur through TRPM6 channels. The net movement of sodium and water favors the net reabsorption of magnesium.

by salt and water absorption, and the permeability of the tight junctions to magnesium.[75] The transepithelial concentration gradient generally favors absorption of magnesium from the gut and is influenced by the gut intraluminal ionized magnesium concentration (chelated or complexed magnesium species do not contribute). Thus total dietary intake of magnesium and intake of dietary constituents that influence the amount of magnesium that is complexed or chelated may influence the net absorption of magnesium. Net movement of salt and water creates the transepithelial voltage gradient. A small positive intraluminal voltage results in a small force favoring transepithelial cation movement. Solvent drag created by sodium and water reabsorption will also result in transepithelial movement of magnesium and other ions. Therefore water and salt reabsorption from the gut have a significant influence on magnesium absorption.

The permeability of the paracellular tight junctions is currently an area of intense study and interest. Numerous proteins exist in the tight junction that serve as ion channels and influence permeability of many ions. Specific magnesium ion channels in the gut epithelial tight junctions have not been conclusively identified. Proteins regulating magnesium movement through the renal epithelial tight junctions have been identified (paracellin-1 [PCLN-1]), leading to speculation that a similar protein may exist in the gut as well. Once identified conclusively, further study will be required to determine whether this tight junction protein is selectively permeable and under what influences such selectivity is expressed.

Active transcellular magnesium movement from the gut is an area of very recent and exciting discovery. Study of numerous inherited conditions of impaired magnesium handling in humans led to an improved understanding of magnesium transport across the gut epithelium and a hypothesis that several magnesium transport proteins exist in both the luminal and basolateral cell membranes of gut epithelial cells.[31] Identification of two very unique ion channels has only recently occurred. A unique family of genes called the transient receptor potential (TRP) family codes for both proteins. Both proteins are in the M subfamily and are labeled TRPM6 and TRPM7, respectively. TRPM6 and TRPM7 are found extensively in membrane surfaces of the small intestine, colon, and distal collecting tubule of the kidney, all sites that are involved in magnesium regulation.[80,99,139] These two proteins are unique because they are the only known ion channels that combine a protein channel with an intracellular protein kinase or enzyme. As a result, much speculation has occurred about the role of the attached enzyme in magnesium homeostasis.[80,99,139] One study suggests that magnesium–adenosine triphosphate (Mg-ATP) is the substrate for the enzyme portion of these channels, resulting in inhibition of magnesium entry through the channel into the cell.[100] This finding has led to speculation that increasing intracellular levels of magnesium are able to thus inhibit intracellular entry of magnesium through this mechanism and that this constitutes the energy requiring active transport mechanism of transepithelial magnesium transport. Alternatively, others speculate that magnesium movement into the cell through TRPM6 and TRPM7 occurs via a favorable voltage gradient and that the active phase of magnesium transport across the cell occurs at the basolateral membrane, possibly connected to active sodium-magnesium exchange.[75]

In the kidney, calcium and several additional hormones influence transcellular and paracellular magnesium transport mechanisms. It is likely that similar control mechanisms influence magnesium reabsorption in the gut. The specific actions of each of these influences and the precise mechanisms of action have yet to be established. The influence of calcium and hormones on the renal handling of magnesium is much better studied and understood. However, some evidence does exist to support the positive influence of parathyroid hormone (PTH) and 1,25-dihydroxycholecalciferol (1,25[OH]$_2$D$_3$) levels on reabsorption of magnesium from the gut.[64,82]

The percentage of magnesium absorbed by transcellular and paracellular mechanisms depends primarily on the dietary concentration of magnesium. When magnesium intake is high, then a large concentration gradient exists, and most absorption likely occurs through the paracellular route with small quantities absorbed across the cell. Conversely, when magnesium intake is poor and a low concentration gradient exists, paracellular magnesium transport is less efficient, and active transcellular magnesium transport plays a much larger role in maintaining adequate magnesium balance.

RENAL HANDLING OF MAGNESIUM

Although the gut plays a crucial role in magnesium balance, the kidney is the site of control and regulation of magnesium balance. Various segments of the nephron play an important role in magnesium homeostasis. Numerous hormonal and other influences also play a role in the maintenance of magnesium balance. The complex interactions of many factors that may influence each other are the focus of intense research. Two factors have greatly assisted in elucidating the cellular physiologic principles guiding magnesium handling by the kidney. Genetic mapping and the accompanying molecular biological technology combined with investigation of several rare inherited renal magnesium handling disorders have contributed to new breakthroughs in the understanding of renal magnesium handling.

Proximal Tubule

Approximately 80% of total serum magnesium is filtered by the glomerulus and enters the proximal tubule. Studies in numerous mammalian species have documented that approximately 10% to 15% of magnesium is reabsorbed within the proximal tubule.[116] This is in sharp contrast to most other major cations, for which at least 60% of reabsorption occurs in the proximal tubule. The reabsorption process in this segment of the nephron appears to occur via passive and unsaturable mechanisms and is unchanged by numerous other factors that play a role in other nephron segments. Based on available data, absorption of magnesium in this tubular segment appears to occur through paracellular transport, but the precise mechanism is not known.

Loop of Henle

The loop of Henle is the site of the majority of magnesium absorption from the kidney. Approximately 60% to 70% of filtered magnesium is reabsorbed in the cortical thick ascending limb of the loop of Henle.[116,137] The medullary thick ascending limb does not appear to participate in magnesium balance.[143] Evidence gathered to date indicates that magnesium absorption in this segment occurs via the paracellular pathway through tight junctions between renal epithelial cells. Numerous factors may influence the transport of magnesium (Fig. 8-2). The principal force allowing magnesium transport in the loop, as in the gut, appears to be the electropositive luminal environment created by the movement of sodium and chloride from the lumen to the interstitial space.[116] In addition, magnesium movement through the tight junctions occurs as a result of "solvent drag" created by the salt and water movement. The positive intraluminal charge facilitates movement of magnesium (and calcium) from the lumen to the interstitium through a paracellular "pore" or channel. Recently, a tight junction protein called PCLN-1 or claudin-16 was discovered that is now thought to be the primary divalent cation channel permitting paracellular movement of magnesium and calcium in the thick ascending limb.[17,31,137,146] A study in humans with inherited defects in this protein has demonstrated significant impairment of magnesium and calcium reabsorption in the thick ascending limb with no change in sodium and chloride reabsorption.[17] A similar genetic anomaly has been documented in Japanese Black cattle that develop early renal failure.[66,105,135] When compared with each other, renal handling of magnesium and calcium appears to be similar in both the bovine and human conditions.[106]

Changes in the transepithelial voltage and paracellular permeability to magnesium strongly influence magnesium absorption from the thick ascending limb.[31] Increases in salt movement from the lumen will concurrently elevate the transepithelial electrical potential and facilitate magnesium absorption. Numerous factors can influence both of these properties, resulting in an increase or decrease in magnesium absorption. Hormones such as PTH, calcitonin, glucagon, antidiuretic hormone, aldosterone, and insulin all act to increase magnesium absorption from the lumen.[31] Conversely,

Thick Ascending Limb Loop of Henle

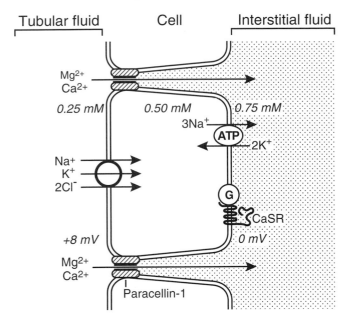

Fig. 8-2 Magnesium transport in the cortical thick ascending limb of the loop of Henle. Magnesium transport occurs exclusively through paracellular tight junction cation pore paracellin-1. Transport of magnesium through paracellin-1 down a favorable electrical gradient is enhanced by net reabsorption of sodium and water and the influence of cation-sensing receptor (CaSR).

prostaglandin E_2, hypokalemia, hypophosphatemia, and acidosis can all act to decrease magnesium absorption.[31]

In addition to the above influences on paracellular absorption of magnesium, a basolateral extracellular receptor, termed the calcium/magnesium sensing receptor or cation-sensing receptor (CaSR), also appears to play a crucial role.[31,143] The CaSR senses extracellular calcium and magnesium concentrations at the basolateral membrane and is coupled to intracellular inhibitory G proteins, which will inhibit and neutralize the effect of other hormonal influences mentioned above.[31,33,143] Activation of the CaSR in the loop appears to decrease salt absorption (sodium, magnesium, and calcium).[33] To what effect, if any, the CaSR may play a role in altering the permeability of PCLN-1 to magnesium transport is not known. Some researchers have suspected that there is a selective effect on paracellular permeability to magnesium that cannot adequately be explained by changes in voltage and hormonal influences, leading to speculation that the CaSR may influence PCLN-1 permeability.[34] The CaSR is also found throughout the gut, and although its function there, related to magnesium balance, is not completely understood, it likely plays a very similar role in both organs.[75]

Distal Convoluted Tubule

The distal convoluted tubule (DCT) does not appear to act as a mass transporter of magnesium as the ascending loop does, but instead it is the site for many complex influences to determine the final magnesium excretion (Fig. 8-3). The DCT normally reabsorbs approximately 10% to 15% of the filtered magnesium.[33,143] When necessary it can be very efficient at reabsorbing magnesium, reabsorbing as much as 70% to 80% of the magnesium that is delivered from the thick ascending limb.[33,143] There does not appear to be any ability to further reabsorb or secrete magnesium in nephron segments distal to the DCT; thus the final concentration of magnesium in the urine is principally determined by the DCT.

Reabsorption of magnesium in the DCT appears to occur only through active transcellular routes. Passive paracellular transport does not appear to occur to any sig-

Distal Convoluted Tubule

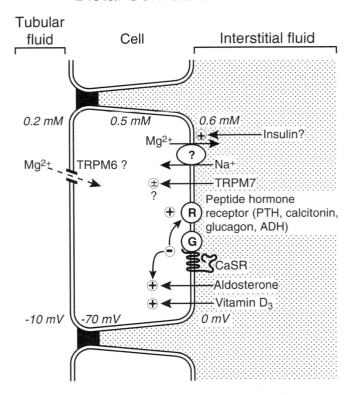

Fig. 8-3 Magnesium transport in the distal convoluted tubule. Magnesium transport occurs exclusively via transcellular mechanisms down a favorable electrical gradient and is postulated to occur through TRPM6 ion channels. Basolateral movement of magnesium is postulated to occur via a sodium-magnesium transporter. Several peptide hormones exert a positive influence on magnesium reabsorption by binding to a peptide hormone receptor *(PTH, parathyroid hormone; ADH, antidiuretic hormone)* or via non–receptor-mediated mechanisms. The cation-sensing receptor (CaSR) has a net negative influence on magnesium reabsorption by inhibiting the positive effects of other hormones. TRPM7 ion channels may be involved in basolateral magnesium sensing by the cell.

nificant degree. As a result, the absorption of magnesium via this route is an energy-requiring saturable process. The transcellular transport of magnesium is dependent on favorable transepithelial concentration and voltage gradients, similar to the gut.[33] Mounting evidence suggests that the principal entry for magnesium into the cell is through the unique transient receptor proteins, TRPM6 and TRPM7.[31,33,80,99] One research group has further speculated that TRPM6 is the principal apical or luminal receptor protein facilitating transport of magnesium from the environment to the ECF, and that TRPM7's role is less well defined, perhaps functioning more as an extracellular sensing mechanism that provides feedback to the cell.[139] The unique protein kinase activity that these ion channels possess suggests that their role in the cell is complex and serves some regulatory process.

Although evidence that influx of magnesium into the cell via TRPM6 (and possibly TRPM7) is mounting, there is not yet a documented mechanism of magnesium efflux from the basolateral cell membrane. Based on available evidence, several authors speculate that a sodium/magnesium countertransporter is likely to exist.[33,143] The presence of a sodium/magnesium countertransporter appears to exist in human red blood cells, and insulin appears to be at least one of the regulating influences on its function.[51]

Although the precise mechanisms for magnesium entry and exit from the DCT cells remain to be completely identified and described, the influence of other factors on magnesium transport in DCT cells has been more completely studied. Through complex intracellular signaling pathways, numerous hormones play a role in regulating magnesium transport. PTH, glucagon, antidiuretic hormone, insulin, aldosterone, 1,25-dihydroxycholecalciferol, prostaglandin E$_2$, β-adrenergic agonists, and increased sympathetic stimulation via the renal nerve have all been shown to play a role in increasing magnesium conservation.[33] The intracellular signaling pathways that occur following activation of the receptor by any of these hormones/factors are complex and interrelated. As a result, the role of each individual factor, particularly amid the "noise" of multiple simultaneous influences, is difficult to predict. Regardless, however, the sheer number of regulatory signals being sent to this portion of the nephron underscores the importance of magnesium balance within the organism.

Like the gut and the thick ascending limb, the DCT also possesses significant concentrations of the CaSR. Further study of this receptor suggests that there may be the potential for separate binding sites for both calcium and magnesium.[33] Thus the receptor may be able to sense the extracellular concentrations of both ions and send independent signals to intracellular regulators, allowing for completely separate control of magnesium and calcium balance. Once activated with magnesium, however, the CaSR sends a strong inhibitory signal via G

proteins, which negate the positive influence of peptide and steroid hormones and vitamin D$_3$ on magnesium transport.[33] How it accomplishes this is not yet clear. Possible sites of action include the purported basolateral sodium/magnesium countertransporter or gating of the TRPM6 or TRPM7 ion channels.[33]

The influence of other electrolyte and acid-base abnormalities also can exert a powerful negative effect on magnesium transport in the DCT. As in the loop of Henle, hypokalemia, hypophosphatemia, and acidosis all decrease magnesium reabsorption.[33] The precise mechanism of how these factors influence magnesium transport is not known, and it is likely that each has a different mechanism. Therefore their combined effect can be additive because they influence magnesium transport in different ways.

EFFECTS OF LACTATION

The nutrient composition of both dog and cat milk has been recently studied.[1,2] Magnesium content of both cat and dog milk appears to be modestly higher during the first 2 to 3 days of lactation, or in the colostrum of both of these species, and then tends to remain at a constant level throughout the remainder of the lactation period.[1,2] This is in sharp contrast to calcium levels that increase consistently throughout the lactation.[1,2]

The contrasting presentation of postparturient hypocalcemia among species is an area that has not been completely explained and is thus an area in which further study is needed. The classic tetanic presentation of postparturient hypocalcemia in dogs is markedly different from the paretic presentation of cattle. In addition, the tetanic presentation of hypomagnesemia or "grass tetany" in cattle adds further evidence to suggest that neuromuscular transmission is affected by complex interactions between calcium and magnesium. A case report of a lactating bitch with significant hypocalcemia and hypomagnesemia that presented with paresis rather than tetany adds to the speculation that the type of presentation is dependent on numerous electrolyte factors and interactions among them.[8] A follow-up retrospective study of serum electrolyte concentrations in 27 bitches with eclampsia or postparturient hypocalcemia revealed that 12 (44%) were concurrently hypomagnesemic, further suggesting that magnesium concentrations may play a role in the pathophysiology of eclampsia in the dog and that magnesium concentrations should be assessed in bitches with eclampsia.[9]

Undoubtedly, lactation does play a role in gut and renal handling of magnesium. Elevation of PTH, in addition to calcium concentration, most likely plays a role in magnesium conservation during lactation to supply the mammary glands with sufficient magnesium. The pathophysiology of calcium and magnesium handling during lactation and the exact triggers that result in eclampsia will require further study.

MANIFESTATIONS OF MAGNESIUM DEFICIT

A large body of research is present in the scientific literature evaluating the effects of magnesium deficit induced in animal models. Rodent models have been most commonly used, but early literature also evaluated the effects of magnesium-deficient diets in young growing dogs. Several of these early canine studies showed dramatic changes that occurred within 2 weeks of introduction of the diet with increasing severity until 5 to 7 weeks when the animals were euthanized.[13,22,23,111,157] Poor growth rates and numerous dermatological and soft tissue problems, such as dry brittle hair and nails, peripheral vasodilation, and swelling and splaying of the paws, were identified in the early weeks of these trials. After 5 to 7 weeks, however, neuromuscular signs including seizure activity were noted and were postulated to contribute to the death of these animals.[111,157] In two studies, significant myocardial necrosis with associated fibrosis and calcification was also noted after euthanasia.[149,164] Results of these trials assisted researchers in understanding magnesium's physiologic role in the organism. As technology has improved, so too has our understanding of the central role magnesium plays in the maintenance of healthy organisms.

Magnesium's importance to living organisms can be traced through early development of life.[3] Primeval oceans contained large quantities of magnesium, and the earth's crust at the time was predominantly composed of iron-magnesium silicate. As early plants perfected photosynthesis, magnesium played a core role in energy production as a component of chlorophyll. As animal life developed, magnesium played another core role in the production of ATP. In fact, as life has developed on earth, magnesium and calcium appear to have played complementary roles to each other, with magnesium being involved in energy production and cell metabolism, and calcium's role defined more by the essential role it plays in structural stability (bone) and movement (neuromuscular activity). Magnesium's evolution as a "behind-the-scenes" ion that keeps the inner machinery of the cell running smoothly and supplied with ample amounts of energy has perhaps contributed to the long period in which it received little clinical attention. However, this electrolyte recently has been placed under greater scrutiny, and it has been the focus of clinical research activity.

Magnesium plays a pivotal role in many cellular metabolic processes. Although magnesium is the second most abundant intracellular cation, most of the intracellular magnesium is bound to numerous molecules that regulate energy production, storage, and utilization.[4] Magnesium plays a vital role in the mitochondria during oxidative phosphorylation and anaerobic metabolism of glucose.[4] In addition, magnesium participates in a number of other important intracellular events, such as the synthesis and degradation of DNA, the binding of ribosomes to RNA, adenine nucleotide synthesis, and the production of important intracellular second messengers like cyclic adenosine monophosphate (cAMP).[4,112] Perhaps most well known is magnesium's function as a cofactor with ATP as the driving force behind intracellular ion pumping activity. Significant ion pumps such as the membrane-bound Na^+,K^+-ATPase, HCO_3^--ATPase, and Ca^{2+}-ATPase all require Mg^{2+}-ATP to maintain effective ionic gradients within and outside the cell.[4,94] As a result, magnesium has an important function in maintaining appropriate intracellular potassium concentrations and serves to regulate cytoplasmic calcium concentrations by stimulating the sequestration of calcium into the endoplasmic and sarcoplasmic reticula. The importance of magnesium's intracellular role becomes apparent clinically in several conditions.

CARDIOVASCULAR SYSTEM

Contraction of both cardiac and smooth muscle is a complex sequence of events that is orchestrated by many factors and requires rapid shifting of intracellular ions to maintain appropriate concentration gradients. Intracellular calcium, released from the sarcoplasmic reticulum or entering the cell from the extracellular space, is the initiating factor in muscle contraction. Magnesium (both intracellular ionized magnesium level and extracellular level) plays an important regulatory role in the intracellular cycling of calcium in muscle cells. It is a cofactor for the Ca^{2+}-ATPase that rapidly shunts intracellular calcium back into the sarcoplasmic reticulum after the contraction cycle is complete. In addition, there is some evidence to suggest that extracellular magnesium may act as a calcium channel blocker for some cell membrane-bound calcium channels, limiting the influx of extracellular calcium into the cytosol.[71,94] Intracellular and extracellular magnesium levels thus play an important role in cardiac excitability, contraction, and conduction through their regulatory effects on calcium movement.

Cardiac conduction electrophysiology is complex and involves finely orchestrated movement of sodium and calcium ions into and of potassium out of the myocytes to propagate an action potential and depolarize the cell. Rapid restoration of those electrolytes against their normal electrochemical gradients occurs to allow the cell to repolarize itself and prepare for the next action potential to occur. Magnesium has several roles in this process. First, magnesium is a cofactor for the ionic pumps that rapidly pump sodium out of the cell, potassium back into the cell, and calcium out of the cell or back into the sarcoplasmic reticulum. In addition, magnesium serves as an important gating mechanism to control the movement of intracellular calcium as described above, and it also acts to prevent leaking of potassium from inside the cell. Intracellular calcium overload triggered during myocardial ischemia by mediators such as lysophosphatidyl choline (LPC) has been implicated as an important cause of ventricular arrhythmias that result from ischemic conditions.[115] Magnesium may act as an antiarrhythmic agent by limiting intracellular calcium overload in such conditions.[115]

Cardiac arrhythmias are clinical manifestations that can arise from derangements of intracellular or extracellular electrolyte concentrations of magnesium, potassium, and calcium.[70,122] Common arrhythmias documented in humans in which magnesium deficit has been implicated as a cause of, or contributing to the severity of, include atrial fibrillation, supraventricular tachycardia, torsade de pointes, ventricular ectopy, ventricular tachycardias, and toxic digitalis arrhythmias.[119,130,166] Some but not all of these arrhythmias may have an association with hypomagnesemia in veterinary patients, but no definitive studies have documented the prevalence of various pathophysiologic causes of arrhythmias in veterinary patients.

Magnesium's effect on the peripheral vasculature is also significant. Magnesium appears to control or exert a powerful role in calcium cycling in the smooth muscle of the peripheral vasculature, with higher intracellular concentrations of magnesium producing a relaxing or vasodilating effect.[84,94,140] Low concentrations of intracellular magnesium appear to have the opposite or vasoconstricting effect. As a result, magnesium deficit has been implicated as a potential contributing cause in the constellation of causes of systemic hypertension.[84,140] The recent discovery of TRPM6 and TRPM7 channels in vascular smooth muscle cells further implicates the important role magnesium has to play in the complex control of vascular smooth muscle.[153] Research has also shown that magnesium plays an interesting role in the production of inflammatory cytokines and reactive oxygen species that have been postulated to play an important role in many common diseases of the cardiovascular system of humans.[84,140,160-163] The origin of this research interest was the cardiac necrosis and lesions in the myocytes of animal models fed magnesium-deficient diets.[161] The cause of these lesions and cardiac dysfunction appears to be reactive oxygen species that originate from neuropeptide substance P–induced activation of macrophages, neutrophils, and mast cells and an increase in important up-regulating inflammatory cytokines such as tumor necrosis factor α and interleukin-1.[160-163] A study investigating a potential link between feline cardiomyopathy and magnesium status has been reported.[55] It was not successful in showing any link between magnesium and feline hypertrophic cardiomyopathy but included only a small number of cats and did not robustly evaluate magnesium status. Animal models evaluating cardiac effects of magnesium deficit have also shown an increased susceptibility to ischemic and reperfusion injury, indicating that magnesium also has a protective antioxidant effect.[94,163]

The effect of magnesium on the electrocardiogram of dogs fed magnesium-deficient diets has been reported several times with very conflicting results.[109,149,164] One study reported a concurrently developing hypokalemia with an increase in peaked T waves and slight depression of the ST segment in addition to various arrhythmias.[109] A second study reported a decrease in the PQ and QRS distances and an increased incidence of negative T waves but did not evaluate concurrent electrolyte disturbances.[149] A third study reported yet another set of findings that included an increased incidence of mild hypocalcemia but normokalemia and transient RST segment and T wave changes that were not consistent or frequent enough to allow the authors to make any definitive conclusions about electrocardiographic changes associated with hypomagnesemia.[164]

NEUROMUSCULAR SYSTEM

The role of magnesium in neuromuscular transmission is important as evidenced by the severe clinical signs that may manifest in deficient states. Currently, our understanding of the precise role of magnesium in neuromuscular transmission is limited. In general, magnesium depletion leads to an increased neuronal excitability and enhanced neuromuscular transmission, with the opposite effects predominating in states of magnesium excess.

In small animal patients, neuromuscular signs of hypomagnesemia are rare. Perhaps the most instructive example of acute central nervous system magnesium deficit is "grass tetany" or "grass staggers" of cattle. In this condition, increased neuronal hyperexcitability and neuromuscular transmission occur, causing severe muscle tetany and seizure activity that frequently results in death. Chronic forms of magnesium deficit in humans have also been implicated in any number of neurological and neuromuscular conditions, including migraine headache, sudden infant death syndrome, age-related dementias, chronic fatigue syndrome, and many other psychiatric and sleep-related disorders.[42-44,46,47,49] An acute neurological condition similar to grass tetany and suspected to have been caused by magnesium deficit has also been described in a high school football team.[83] The pathophysiology of the acute and chronic clinical forms of magnesium deficit is likely to be multifactorial, but several contributing causes have been postulated. A decrease in neuronal magnesium concentration is thought to increase the likelihood of calcium binding to prejunctional acetylcholine vesicles, increasing release of acetylcholine into the neuromuscular cleft and increasing the likelihood of muscle contractions.[58]

In addition, magnesium has been shown to block N-methyl-D-aspartate (NMDA) receptors within the central nervous system. NMDA receptors are involved in numerous central nervous system functions, including pain sensation and excitatory neurotransmitter activities.[40] Some researchers have also speculated that NMDA receptor blockade by magnesium may play a role in bronchial smooth muscle relaxation.[136] Other causes that have been identified as potential contributing factors to neuromuscular effects of magnesium deficit include increased excitatory neurotransmitter release, decreased inhibitory neurotransmitter release, production of inflammatory neuropeptides (substance P), loss of antioxidant reserves, and the important influence of magnesium on numerous intracellular second messenger systems.[42,44]

ELECTROLYTE DISTURBANCES

Numerous concurrent electrolyte disturbances have been reported in association with magnesium deficit. Most commonly reported, in several species, and best studied is the depletion of potassium. During a magnesium-deficient state, the simultaneous occurrence of intracellular potassium loss and decreased ability for potassium to reenter the cell leads to a significant intracellular depletion of potassium. In some cases, a refractory state of hypokalemia occurs despite aggressive supplementation with potassium and resolves only when the magnesium deficit has also been corrected.[62,168] Several mechanisms may contribute to hypokalemia. Magnesium's function as a cofactor for most ATPase pumps likely plays a dominant role. Reduced Na,K-ATPase function will lead to a net loss of potassium outside the cell and a net gain of sodium in the cell.[168] In addition, a magnesium deficit also decreases the function of the Na-K-Cl cotransport system, thus decreasing potassium reentry into the cell.[53,168] Evidence also suggests that the concentration of Na-K pumps decreases in the cell membrane in response to intracellular potassium depletion that further compounds potassium reentry into the cell.[39] Finally, magnesium appears to act from both within and outside the cell to prevent potassium leak from the cell through potassium channels and other mechanisms that are less well understood.[168] Overall, magnesium acts to maintain appropriate intracellular potassium stores. In the kidney, where significant potassium reabsorption occurs through Na,K-ATPase activity and Na-K-Cl cotransport, magnesium stimulates and permits normal reabsorption to occur. Therefore depletion of magnesium has a permissive effect on intracellular loss, leading to extracellular accumulation of potassium, which is subsequently lost from the body because of ineffective potassium reabsorption mechanisms in the kidney. Frequently, this potassium deficiency is refractory to normal supplementation efforts until the magnesium deficit has also been corrected.[62,168]

Further complicating the relationship between potassium and magnesium is the influence of potassium on magnesium reabsorption in the kidney. In the distal collecting tubule, hypokalemia has been shown to decrease magnesium reabsorption concurrently.[33] Although the amount of magnesium reabsorbed in this segment of the nephron is not large, it may play a significant role. Thus it appears that potassium and magnesium have a complex interaction in which each assists in the regulation and control of the other. Therefore deficits of one ion often lead to deficits in the other, and an inciting causal factor may be difficult to find in many situations.

Hypocalcemia is also frequently reported as a concurrent electrolyte abnormality in humans with a magnesium deficit. The role of magnesium in regulating intracellular calcium flux is complex. It is not yet known whether a magnesium deficit contributes to net loss of calcium from the intracellular environment. The most likely origin of the concurrent deficiency of calcium and magnesium is loss through the kidney combined with decreased liberation from bone stores. Because magnesium and calcium are the most important divalent cations in the body, reabsorption of these ions, not surprisingly, occurs via similar pathways in the kidney. The influence of multiple hormones, the CaSR and a shared PCLN-1 passive transport pore, is likely to result in similar overall net patterns of loss or gain of divalent cations. In addition, there is some evidence in a canine model to suggest that chronic magnesium deficit impairs the skeletal response to PTH and may decrease the parathyroid gland function.[56,86] In humans, a severe magnesium deficit is thought to result in impaired release and impaired activity of PTH. Magnesium's role as a cofactor in the production of the intracellular signaling molecule cAMP is thought to be a contributing cause to this state of functional hypoparathyroidism.[6,59,130] Although unrelated to the presence of hypocalcemia, a recent study in a mouse model of bone and mineral metabolism has revealed that dietary magnesium deficit is related to significant impairment of bone growth, decreased osteoblast and increased osteoclast numbers, and significant stimulation of important cytokines of inflammation, suggesting that magnesium has a significant but as yet undocumented role in bone metabolism.[129]

PATHOGENESIS OF MAGNESIUM DEFICIT

Numerous causes for magnesium deficit have been documented. Most commonly, magnesium deficit occurs in hospitalized ill patients as a result of the combined causes of lack of dietary intake in conjunction with excessive loss through the gastrointestinal tract because of diarrhea or through the kidney because of excessive diuresis. Numerous specific causes have been reported to contribute in human patients as shown in Box 8-1.[37,94,119,166] Causes of magnesium deficit in veterinary patients have not been as well documented or reported, although the general mechanisms of magnesium loss are likely to be common among many species.

Box 8-1	**Causes of Magnesium Deficit**[37,94,119,166]

Gastrointestinal
Reduced intake/starvation/malnutrition
Chronic diarrhea
Gastric suction
Malabsorption syndromes
Short bowel syndrome
Gastric bypass surgery
Colonic neoplasia
Familial or inherited

Renal
Diabetes mellitus/diabetic ketoacidosis
Diuretics (except potassium sparing agents)
Osmotic agents (including hyperglycemia)
Intrinsic renal causes of diuresis
   Postobstructive
   Polyuric acute failure
   Hyperaldosteronism
   Hyperthyroidism
Renal tubular acidosis
Concurrent electrolyte disorders
   Hypokalemia
   Hypercalcemia/hyperparathyroidism
   Hypophosphatemia
Drugs
   Gentamicin
   Carbenicillin
   Ticarcillin
   Cyclosporin
   Cisplatin
Postrenal transplantation
Familial or inherited

Miscellaneous
Excessive loss from:
   Lactation
Redistribution
   Acute myocardial infarction
   Acute pancreatitis
   Insulin
   Catecholamine excess
Idiopathic

PREVALENCE OF MAGNESIUM DEFICIT

Serum hypomagnesemia is one of the most commonly reported electrolyte disturbances in a human critical care population. Numerous studies have been conducted on several differing critical care populations (pediatric, adult, and elderly), and all have revealed serum hypomagnesemia in 4% to 65% of patients tested.* Increased

*References 27,92,126,132,156,166.

mortality has also been reported in human patients with measurable hypomagnesemia when compared with normomagnesemic control subjects.[126,147] Although debate continues to swirl as to whether a magnesium deficit is a contributing cause to the mortality rate or simply an epiphenomenon of more severely ill patients, it would appear that magnesium deficit is an independent risk factor for mortality in critically ill humans.

Very few studies of the prevalence of hypomagnesemia in small animal veterinary patients have been published. Only three studies of the prevalence of magnesium abnormalities in hospitalized ill dogs and cats have been published. Two prospective studies have reported on dogs and cats that were admitted to a critical care unit.[93,151] In these studies, the point prevalence of hypomagnesemia at admission in dogs was reported to be 54% of 48 dogs, and the period prevalence of hypomagnesemia during hospitalization for 57 cats was reported to be 28%.[93,151] A third retrospective study reported a point prevalence of hypomagnesemia in a group of hospitalized dogs that were not necessarily confined to a critical care unit as 6.1% of 3102 dogs.[76] Abstracts for three additional studies in critically ill dogs and cats report a period prevalence of 33.6% of 70 animals (50 dogs and 20 cats), a point prevalence of 50% of 101 dogs, and a point prevalence of 39% of 65 animals (42 dogs and 23 cats) (Chew, unpublished data).[35,174] Based on these reports, it appears that hypomagnesemia is a very common finding of hospitalized dogs and cats that are admitted to a critical care unit.

However, the reported incidence of concurrent electrolyte abnormalities in these patients does not mirror that found in humans. In dogs, it was common to see concurrent hypokalemia.[35,76,174] However, only one study reported concurrent hypocalcemia in dogs (Chew, unpublished data). Unexpectedly, two studies in dogs reported concurrent abnormalities in sodium.[93,174] In two of the feline studies, hypokalemia and hypocalcemia were reported, but there was not sufficient information available to determine the significance (Chew, unpublished data).[35] In the published feline study, no concurrent association with other electrolyte disturbances was reported.[151] Although several studies reported mortality statistics, it is extremely difficult to interpret these findings without benefit of illness scoring systems (e.g., APACHE II).

Numerous veterinary researchers have also reported their findings of the prevalence of serum hypomagnesemia in specific disease conditions. Prospective studies of gastric dilatation-volvulus syndrome and parvoviral enteritis in dogs reported no significant abnormalities of serum magnesium.[14,90] A prospective study of Cavalier King Charles spaniels with myxomatous mitral valve disease reported significant serum hypomagnesemia in affected dogs.[108] A prospective study of cats with diabetes mellitus or diabetic ketoacidosis (DKA) reported a point prevalence of ionized hypomagnesemia of 62% of diabetic cats and 57% of DKA cats.[104] A prospective study of 14 feline renal transplant patients documented a period prevalence of ionized hypomagnesemia of 94%.[175] Interestingly, concurrent hypocalcemia and hypokalemia were documented in the majority of cats with magnesium deficit in this study. A prospective study of cats with chronic renal failure documented ionized hypomagnesemia, hypercalcemia, and elevated parathyroid levels (Chew, unpublished data). One case report and one case series of five dogs have reported hypomagnesemia and hypocalcemia in dogs with protein-losing enteropathy.[24,77] The significance of these studies cannot be overlooked, and they lend strong support to the central concept that magnesium deficit is common in ill and hospitalized dogs and cats. Currently, there is insufficient evidence to know whether a magnesium deficit contributes to mortality in this population of patients. As a result, we cannot also answer the question of whether treatment with magnesium contributes a significant benefit to survival or outcome.

DIAGNOSIS OF MAGNESIUM DEFICIT

The diagnosis of a magnesium deficit continues to be controversial. The fact that 99% of the body's magnesium stores are located within cells presents a diagnostic challenge for clinicians hoping to identify depletion of the body's magnesium. Given our currently limited ability to peer inside of cells on a routine basis clinically, it should not be surprising that diagnosis of magnesium deficit is difficult and controversial. Despite the challenges, however, numerous diagnostic methods have emerged in concert with the renewed clinical interest in magnesium during the past 20 years. These efforts can be broadly divided into two separate categories: methods that assess magnesium (ionized and total) in various tissues (including blood), and methods that assess magnesium-handling physiology.

The challenge of choosing a tissue to sample from to detect a magnesium deficit is to choose one that is most often reflective of a true total body deficit of magnesium. Total serum magnesium is the most commonly used method of assessing magnesium status because of the ease of obtaining serum samples from patients and the relative simplicity of and the ability to automate the assay. More recently, the development of technology that allowed measurement of ionized serum magnesium has emerged and is becoming widely available. There is no question that blood forms the main method of magnesium transport from dietary ingestion, urinary retention, and movement of magnesium between intracellular stores. Cellular intake of magnesium occurs when ionized magnesium crosses from the blood through the cell membrane and then is complexed and harnessed into the intracellular magnesium-dependent activities. Ionized magnesium appears to equilibrate rapidly across the cell membrane; thus extracellular ionized magnesium may be reflective of intracellular stores. However, the larger question is how reflective of a total body magnesium deficit is a blood sample? Total serum magnesium represents 1% of the body's magnesium stores, and ionized serum magnesium represents 0.2% to 0.3% of the total body magnesium stores. The lack of a gold standard test to compare both total serum magnesium and ionized serum magnesium assays contributes to the confusion regarding diagnosis of a magnesium deficit. Although it is attractive because of its simplicity, serum magnesium does not correlate with the diagnosis of a suspected magnesium deficit based on clinical signs, nor does it appear to correlate well with serum ionized magnesium.*

There may be several factors to consider when interpreting the results of a blood magnesium sample, such as adequate dietary intake of magnesium and the rapidity of loss of magnesium from the patient. Patients who lose magnesium rapidly will tend to draw heavily from the serum magnesium to replace an acute intracellular need and may be more likely to have low total serum or ionized serum magnesium levels. Chronic mild inadequate dietary intake of magnesium may allow sufficient time for compensatory mechanisms to increase gastrointestinal absorption, renal reabsorption, and possibly skeletal liberation of sufficient magnesium to maintain normal serum and total body magnesium.[48,50] When these compensatory mechanisms are active, they may be much more effective in coping with an additional acute loss and allowing normal serum levels to be maintained. Based on these alterations between serum and ionized fractions, one study suggested the use of a ratio between total serum and ionized magnesium as being more helpful.[48] Concurrent hormone activity, albumin concentration, sample handling, and acid-base status of the patient may all play a role in serum magnesium concentration (Chew, unpublished data).† In addition, redistribution of magnesium from the serum compartment has been reported to occur in acute pancreatitis and myocardial infarction of humans and thus could also affect the serum magnesium status and add further difficulty in interpretation of serum magnesium levels. Several studies have also called into question the ion-selective probe technology that has been used to measure ionized serum magnesium.[25,32] In combination, these factors add a large degree of uncertainty to the interpretation of blood magnesium levels.

Measurement of magnesium in red blood cells, white blood cells, and muscle tissue has also been investigated

---

*References 50,69,78,104,119,175.
†References 48,69,78,89,155,170.

as potential assays that are more reflective of intracellular magnesium stores.[14,50,133,141] Because of the complexity of the assays, none have found common clinical usage. In addition, results have not consistently correlated with the clinical assessment of magnesium deficit.[133,141] Newer technologies that may be able to assess intracellular ionized magnesium concentrations, such as nuclear magnetic resonance spectroscopy and fluorescent intracellular probes, hold much promise because they are noninvasive, can assess magnesium in several different tissues, and they assess intracellular magnesium stores.[88,159] Such technology has not yet found widespread clinical usage but is an important research technology.

Assessment of physiologic magnesium handling has been evaluated in one of two ways: assessment of renal magnesium handling and testing magnesium retention. Both are based on the concept that active renal retention of magnesium during total magnesium deficit should occur. In addition, they assume that renal function and renal magnesium handling are adequate and appropriate to the patient's current status. These assays cannot be used in patients with inadequate renal function or in which some defect of renal magnesium handling may be present. Urinary magnesium excretion (24-hour), urinary magnesium clearance, and urinary fractional excretion of magnesium have all been used as methods of evaluating renal magnesium handling. Patients with a magnesium deficit or who have inadequate dietary intake of magnesium would be expected to retain magnesium to a much more significant degree than normal patients. Although these assays have not been widely tested in clinical patients, they have been used as a helpful tool in assessing patients with inadequate dietary magnesium intake and thus increased renal reabsorptive compensatory mechanisms.[103,148] Many human physicians favor the use of a magnesium retention test when assessing magnesium status of their patients. Several studies have evaluated the use of this test in human patients and found it to correlate well with clinical suspicion of magnesium deficit.[68,131] However, one study suggests that the magnesium retention test assesses loss of magnesium from the exchangeable bone stores, which may not be reflective of total body magnesium deficit.[30] The magnesium loading test has not been standardized in human medicine, and several variations of the test are reported.[121] Although a study of a magnesium loading test has been completed in dogs, the results have not been published.[96]

The diagnosis of magnesium deficit is challenging. Currently, there is no consensus regarding the best assay for diagnosis; there are several new technologies that are very promising but have not reached widespread clinical use; and more questions than answers still exist. From the available veterinary literature, it would appear that both ionized serum magnesium and total serum magnesium may be useful when results are low and are consistent with clinical suspicion of a magnesium deficit. It must be emphasized that a normal result does not rule out a magnesium deficit. Clinical suspicion must still play an important role. The magnesium retention test holds promise, but no reference interval has been established for veterinary patients, and thus it needs to be evaluated more completely in veterinary species.

PHARMACOLOGIC USES OF MAGNESIUM

In addition to their use as therapy in patients with magnesium deficit, magnesium salts have been used to treat a number of disparate disease processes in humans. Although their use as a therapeutic agent in many of these conditions remains unproven, rigorous clinical trials have not been performed to validate the use of magnesium. The use of magnesium as prophylaxis for migrainous headache in children, as protection from endotoxin challenge, as management for cardiovascular signs of pheochromocytoma, as an adjunctive analgesic agent, and as an adjunctive means of controlling muscular spasms of tetanus are examples of magnesium use in this category.* Therapeutic use of magnesium has been more completely studied in several other diseases, but its therapeutic efficacy is still controversial. Diseases such as myocardial infarction, acute severe asthma, hypertension, and diabetes mellitus are examples that fit this category.† Finally, several conditions have been well studied, and the efficacy of magnesium in conditions such as eclampsia/preeclampsia and several types of cardiac arrhythmias, such as digitalis toxicity, torsade de pointes, and ventricular ectopy, has been shown.‡

In small animal veterinary medicine, there are several conditions that warrant consideration of magnesium as a therapeutic agent. For most dogs and cats being fed a commercial food, a dietary magnesium deficit is not a concern. Most commercial dog and cat foods have abundant magnesium supplementation. Therefore the at-risk population for magnesium deficit is predominantly hospitalized dogs and cats, particularly those who have been anorexic for several days and in whom excessive gastrointestinal or renal loss of magnesium could be occurring (see Box 8-1). Patients meeting such criteria should be evaluated for a magnesium deficit. Documented hypomagnesemia or a magnesium retention test suspected of being abnormal (normal values have not been established in small animal patients) should prompt the clinician to consider magnesium therapy to correct the deficit. Although increased mortality has been reported to occur in humans with a magnesium deficit, therapy with magnesium salts has not been studied to determine whether therapeutic

---

*References 10-12,26,40,72,73,79,97,114,134,150,154,158,171-173.
†References 5,7,15,16,38,60,61,91,110,123-125,127,128,136,138,142, 145,152,165,167,169,177.
‡References 19,29,40,54,57,70,81,98,107,113,115,118,122,144.

intervention with magnesium in such patients changes the clinical outcome. Patients with refractory hypokalemia or hypocalcemia despite seemingly appropriate supplementation should also be evaluated for a magnesium deficit and treated accordingly if one is detected. Bitches presenting with eclampsia should have their magnesium status evaluated in addition to their calcium status. In addition, there are two kinds of patient populations that are routinely encountered in small animal emergency and critical care medicine that are frequently identified with a magnesium deficit. Patients in heart failure with concurrent ventricular arrhythmias and who are being medicated with loop diuretics and/or digitalis constitute one high-risk group. Significantly better control of arrhythmias such as torsade de pointes, ventricular ectopy, and digitalis toxicity is frequently gained in humans from supplementation with magnesium and potassium and correction of underlying electrolyte disturbances and normalization of the myocyte's electrophysiological state.[70,122] Ventricular arrhythmias resulting from an overload of intracellular calcium induced by ischemia and LPC production may also benefit from magnesium administration.[115] The other high-risk population is patients diagnosed with diabetes mellitus and in particular DKA. In diabetic patients, more rapid correction of electrolyte disturbances should be expected when magnesium is used as an adjunctive therapeutic agent. Improved speed of correction of metabolic and electrolyte disturbances in this condition should result in a decreased length and cost of hospitalization. There is also some evidence from human medicine to suggest that magnesium may improve insulin sensitivity and thus glycemic control in diabetic patients.[18,60,110,124]

Magnesium therapy could also be considered experimental or unproven therapy for conditions such as bronchial asthma, pain, tetanus infections, and neuroprotection and cardioprotection following ischemia, hyperkalemia, sepsis, and hypertension (especially related to pheochromocytoma). Very little research has been conducted in veterinary patients related to magnesium's effect on any of these conditions. Limited research has been conducted in a dog model showing magnesium to have a positive effect on bronchoconstriction and pulmonary hypertension.[67,176] An in vitro study of the effects of magnesium on hyperkalemia has also been performed on canine myocardial cells revealing a significant attenuation of the detrimental electrophysiological effects of hyperkalemia.[81] Although none of these results are substantial enough to justify the routine clinical use of magnesium for these conditions at this time, they are significant enough to stimulate further study in these areas. In fact, further research related to the therapeutic use of magnesium in any of the conditions mentioned above could easily be conducted in veterinary patients and could serve as a valuable model for human diseases.

Administration of magnesium in dogs and cats has not been studied sufficiently to determine appropriate dosages for administration. However, the safety of administration of magnesium salts is great. Doses severalfold outside the normal therapeutic range were required to produce significant adverse effects in an anesthetized healthy dog model of magnesium administration.[102] As a result of its relative safety in patients with normal renal function, clinical use of magnesium should not be discouraged because of the lack of study evaluating appropriate dosing. Patients most likely to present with hypermagnesemia are patients that have an impaired renal ability to excrete or clear magnesium; therefore magnesium should be used with extreme caution in such patients and only after assessing magnesium levels. The published dose range for magnesium in dogs has been extrapolated from human medicine and tested empirically.[36] Parenteral magnesium generally is administered intravenously using either the chloride or sulfate salt, both of which are available commercially in several concentrations. Doses for magnesium supplementation can be found in Table 8-1. A rapid loading dose can be administered over minutes in severe cases or when required in emergency situations. Alternatively, in patients who do not require emergent therapy, the same emergency loading dose can be administered during the first 24 hours, followed by a slower administration on subsequent days. A continuous intravenous infusion is usually given following the loading dose until the patient's dietary intake is sufficient to maintain adequate magnesium levels. Severely depleted animals can be maintained on a fast replacement dose for multiple days. Mildly affected animals can be maintained on a slow replacement dose. Magnesium salt solution concentrations greater than 20% should not be administered. Magnesium salt solutions are not compatible with calcium- or bicarbonate-containing solutions. One human magnesium research group has strongly recommended the use of the chloride versus the sulfate salt, citing a greater risk of toxicity from magnesium sulfate.[41,45] However, widespread clinical use of the magnesium sulfate salt has continued, perhaps because of the lack of evidence in human studies to support the allegation of toxicity.

MAGNESIUM EXCESS

Hypermagnesemia is much less clinically significant than magnesium deficit in veterinary medicine. In the two prospective prevalence studies of magnesium abnormalities performed on hospitalized veterinary patients, the period prevalence documented for hypermagnesemia in 57 cats was 18%, and the point prevalence documented for hypermagnesemia in 48 dogs was 13%.[93,151] In these patients, renal insufficiency or postrenal azotemia was frequently documented. Because magnesium is predominantly excreted in the urine, it is not surprising that decreased ability to excrete magnesium from the kidney may result in hypermagnesemia. Iatrogenic overdose, either through parenteral administration or through oral supplementation, is another common cause of

TABLE 8-1 Dose Ranges for Magnesium Salts

		mEq Mg/g of salt	mEq/kg/day	mEq/kg/hr	mg/kg/hr
Rapid replacement					
	$MgSO_4$	8.12	0.75-1.00	0.03-0.04	3.7-4.9
	$MgCl_2$	9.25	0.75-1.00	0.03-0.04	3.2-4.3
		mEq Mg/g of salt	**mEq/kg/day**	**mEq/kg/hr**	**mg/kg/hr**
Slow replacement					
	$MgSO_4$	8.12	0.3-0.5	0.013-0.02	1.6-2.5
	$MgCl_2$	9.25	0.3-0.5	0.013-0.02	1.4-2.2
		mEq/kg	**mg/kg**	**Duration**	
Emergency/loading					
	$MgSO_4$	0.15-0.3	19-37	5 min-1 h (emerg)	
	$MgCl_2$	0.15-0.3	16-32	24 h (load)	
		mEq/kg/day			
Oral	Several	1-2			

hypermagnesemia in humans but has not been reported in small animal veterinary patients. It appears, based on these very limited data and the lack of clinical case reports of syndromes of hypermagnesemia in the veterinary literature, that elevation of magnesium rarely occurs to such an extent that it produces clinical symptoms in small animal patients. Symptoms reported in human patients include loss of deep tendon reflexes, impaired respiration caused by weak respiratory musculature, mild to moderate hypotension, and electrophysiological derangements of cardiac conduction and cutaneous flushing.[101]

A study of magnesium administration to anesthetized normal dogs at a rate of 0.12 mEq/kg/min revealed that significant adverse cardiovascular effects were not detected until plasma levels exceeded 12.2 mEq/L, which was achieved after a cumulative infusion of 1 to 2 mEq/kg of magnesium.[102] In this model, dangerous arrhythmias and significant hypotension were detected at cumulative doses of 3.9 mEq/kg.[102] Death occurred when cumulative infusions reached 5.9 to 10.9 mEq/kg.[102] Given currently recommended dosage infusions of magnesium, it would be very unlikely to reach these toxic levels; however, the effect of underlying pathologic states could contribute significantly to signs of toxicity at lower doses. Therefore magnesium administration should be used cautiously with careful attention to blood pressure and electrocardiographic monitoring. In the rare circumstance that significant clinical signs attributable to hypermagnesemia are detected, therapy should first consist of immediate discontinuation of any parenteral magnesium supplementation and initiating saline diuresis and administering loop diuretics. If renal function is impaired, peritoneal dialysis or hemodialysis

may be required. Administration of calcium can be considered to antagonize some of the cardiac effects in patients in whom cardiac arrest has occurred.[95]

REFERENCES

1. Adkins Y, Lepine AJ, Lonnerdal B: Changes in protein and nutrient composition of milk throughout lactation in dogs, *Am J Vet Res* 62:1266, 2001.
2. Adkins Y, Zicker SC, Lepine A, et al: Changes in nutrient and protein composition of cat milk during lactation, *Am J Vet Res* 58:370, 1997.
3. Aikawa JK: *Magnesium: It's biological significance*, Boca Raton, FL, 1981, CRC Press, Inc.
4. Alghamdi SMG, Cameron EC, Sutton RAL: Magnesium deficiency—pathophysiologic and clinical overview, *Am J Kidney Dis* 24:737, 1994.
5. Alter HJ, Koepsell TD, Hilty WM: Intravenous magnesium as an adjuvant in acute bronchospasm: a meta-analysis, *Ann Emerg Med* 36:191, 2000.
6. Anast CS, Winnacker JL, Forte LR: Impaired release of parathyroid hormone in magnesium deficiency, *J Clin Endocrinol Metab* 42:707, 1976.
7. Antman EM: Magnesium in acute myocardial infarction: overview of available evidence, *Am Heart J* 132:487, 1996.
8. Aroch I, Ohad DG, Baneth G: Paresis and unusual electrocardiographic signs in a severely hypomagnesaemic, hypocalcaemic lactating bitch, *J Small Anim Pract* 39:299, 1998.
9. Aroch I, Srebro H, Shpigel NY: Serum electrolyte concentrations in bitches with eclampsia, *Vet Rec* 145:318, 1999.
10. Attygalle D, Rodrigo N: Magnesium sulphate for control of spasms in severe tetanus. Can we avoid sedation and artificial ventilation? *Anaesthesia* 52:956, 1997.
11. Attygalle D, Rodrigo N: Magnesium sulphate for the control of spasms in severe tetanus, *Anaesthesia* 54:302, 1999.
12. Attygalle D, Rodrigo N: Magnesium as first line therapy in the management of tetanus: a prospective study of 40 patients, *Anaesthesia* 57:811, 2002.

13. Barnes BA, Mendelson J: The measurement of exchangeable magnesium in dogs, *Metabolism* 12:184, 1963.

14. Bebchuk TN, Hauptman JG, Braselton WE, et al: Intracellular magnesium concentrations in dogs with gastric dilatation-volvulus, *Am J Vet Res* 61:1415, 2000.

15. Bernstein WK, Khastgir T, Khastgir A, et al: Lack of effectiveness of magnesium in chronic stable asthma—a prospective, randomized, double-blind, placebo-controlled, crossover trial in normal subjects and in patients with chronic stable asthma, *Arch Intern Med* 155:271, 1995.

16. Bessmertny O, DiGregorio RV, Cohen H, et al: A randomized clinical trial of nebulized magnesium sulfate in addition to albuterol in the treatment of acute mild-to-moderate asthma exacerbations in adults, *Ann Emerg Med* 39:585, 2002.

17. Blanchard A, Jeunemaitre X, Coudol P, et al: Paracellin-1 is critical for magnesium and calcium reabsorption in the human thick ascending limb of henle, *Kidney Int* 59:2206, 2001.

18. Brown IR, McBain AM, Chalmers J, et al: Sex difference in the relationship of calcium and magnesium excretion to glycaemic control in type 1 diabetes mellitus, *Int J Clin Chem* 283:119, 1999.

19. Brugada P: Magnesium: an antiarrhythmic drug, but only against very specific arrhythmias, *Eur Heart J* 21:1116, 2000.

20. Buffington CA, Chew DJ, Dibartola SP: Lower urinary-tract disease in cats—is diet still a cause? *J Am Vet Med Assoc* 205:1524, 1994.

21. Buffington CA, Rogers QR, Morris JG: Effect of diet on struvite activity product in feline urine, *Am J Vet Res* 51:2025, 1990.

22. Bunce GE, Chiemchaisri Y, Phillips PH: The mineral requirements of the dog IV. Effect of certain dietary and physiologic factors upon the magnesium deficiency syndrome, *J Nutr* 76:23, 1962.

23. Bunce GE, Jenkins KJ, Phillips PH: The mineral requirements of the dog III. The magnesium requirement, *J Nutr* 76:17, 1962.

24. Bush WW, Kimmel SE, Wosar MA, et al: Secondary hypoparathyroidism attributed to hypomagnesemia in a dog with protein-losing enteropathy, *J Am Vet Med Assoc* 219:1732, 2001.

25. Cecco SA, Hristova EN, Rehak NN, et al: Clinically important intermethod differences for physiologically abnormal ionized magnesium results, *Am J Clin Pathol* 108:564, 1997.

26. Ceneviva GD, Thomas NJ, Kees-Folts D: Magnesium sulfate for control of muscle rigidity and spasms and avoidance of mechanical ventilation in pediatric tetanus, *Pediatr Crit Care Med* 4:480, 2003.

27. Chernow B, Bamberger S, Stoiko M, et al: Hypomagnesemia in patients in postoperative intensive care, *Chest* 95:391, 1989.

28. Chow FhC, Dysart I, Hamar DW, et al: Effect of dietary additives on experimentally produced feline urolithiasis, *Feline Pract* 6:51, 1976.

29. Cohen L, Kitzes R: Magnesium-sulfate and digitalis-toxic arrhythmias, *JAMA* 249:2808, 1983.

30. Cohen L, Laor A: Correlation between bone magnesium concentration and magnesium retention in the intravenous magnesium load test, *Magnes Res* 3:271, 1990.

31. Cole DEC, Quamme GA: Inherited disorders of renal magnesium handling, *J Am Soc Nephrol* 11:1937, 2000.

32. Csako G, Rehak NN, Elin RJ: Falsely high ionized magnesium results by an ion-selective electrode method in severe hypomagnesemia, *Eur J Clin Chem Clin Biochem* 35:701, 1997.

33. Dai LJ, Ritchie G, Kerstan D, et al: Magnesium transport in the renal distal convoluted tubule, *Physiol Rev* 81:51, 2001.

34. Desfleurs E, Wittner M, Simeone S, et al: Calcium-sensing receptor: regulation of electrolyte transport in the thick ascending limb of henle's loop, *Kidney Blood Pressure Res* 21:401, 1998.

35. Dhupa N: Serum magnesium abnormalities in a small animal intensive care unit population (abstract), *J Vet Intern Med* 8:157, 1994.

36. Dhupa N: Magnesium therapy. In Bonagura J, editor: *Kirk's current veterinary therapy XII,* Philadelphia, 1995, WB Saunders.

37. Dhupa N, Proulx J: Hypocalcemia and hypomagnesemia, *Vet Clin North Am Small Anim Pract* 28:587, 1998.

38. Dominguez LJ, Barbagallo M, Di Lorenzo G, et al: Bronchial reactivity and intracellular magnesium: a possible mechanism for the bronchodilating effects of magnesium in asthma, *Clin Sci* 95:137, 1998.

39. Dorup I: Effects of K+, Mg2+ deficiency and adrenal steroids on Na+, K+-pump concentration in skeletal muscle, *Acta Physiol Scand* 156:305, 1996.

40. Dube L, Granry JC: The therapeutic use of magnesium in anesthesiology, intensive care and emergency medicine: a review, *Can J Anaesth* 50:732, 2003.

41. Durlach J, Bac P, Bara M, et al: Is the pharmacological use of intravenous magnesium before preterm cerebroprotective or deleterious for premature infants? Possible importance of the use of magnesium sulphate, *Magnes Res* 11:323, 1998.

42. Durlach J, Bac P, Bara M, et al: Physiopathology of symptomatic and latent forms of central nervous hyperexcitability due to magnesium deficiency: a current general scheme, *Magnes Res* 13:293, 2000.

43. Durlach J, Bac P, Durlach V, et al: Are age-related neurodegenerative diseases linked with various types of magnesium depletion? *Magnes Res* 10:339, 1997.

44. Durlach J, Bac P, Durlach V, et al: Neurotic, neuromuscular and autonomic nervous form of magnesium imbalance, *Magnes Res* 10:169, 1997.

45. Durlach J, Bara M, Theophanides T: A hint on pharmacological and toxicological differences between magnesium chloride and magnesium sulphate, or of scallops and men, *Magnes Res* 9:217, 1996.

46. Durlach J, Pages N, Bac P, et al: Biorhythms and possible central regulation of Mg status, phototherapy, darkness therapy and chronopathological forms of Mg depletion, *Magnes Res* 15:49, 2002.

47. Durlach J, Pages N, Bac P, et al: Chronopathological forms of magnesium depletion with hypofunction or with hyperfunction of the biological clock, *Magnes Res* 15:263, 2002.

48. Durlach J, Pages N, Bac P, et al: Importance of the ratio between ionized and total Mg in serum or plasma: new data on the regulation of Mg status and practical importance of total Mg concentration in the investigation of Mg imbalance, *Magnes Res* 15:203, 2002.

49. Durlach J, Pages N, Bac P, et al: Magnesium deficit and sudden infant death syndrome (SIDS): SIDS due to magnesium deficiency and SIDS due to various forms of magnesium depletion: possible importance of the chronopathological form, *Magnes Res* 15:269, 2002.

50. Elin RJ: Magnesium—the 5th but forgotten electrolyte, *Am J Clin Pathol* 102:616, 1994.

51. Ferreira A, Rivera A, Romero JR: Na+/Mg2+ exchange is functionally coupled to the insulin receptor, *J Cell Physiol* 199:434, 2004.

52. Finco DR, Barsanti JA, Crowell WA: Characterization of magnesium-induced urinary disease in the cat and comparison with feline urologic syndrome, *Am J Vet Res* 46:391, 1985.

53. Flatman PW, Creanor J: Regulation of Na+-K+-2Cl(−) cotransport by protein phosphorylation in ferret erythrocytes, *J Physiol* 517:699, 1999.

54. Frakes MA, Richardson LE: Magnesium sulfate therapy in certain emergency conditions, *Am J Emerg Med* 15:182, 1997.

55. Freeman L, Brown D, Smith F: Magnesium status and the effect of magnesium supplementation in feline hypertrophic cardiomyopathy, *Can J Vet Res* 61:227, 1997.

56. Freitag JJ, Martin KJ, Conrades MB, et al: Evidence for skeletal resistance to parathyroid hormone in magnesium deficiency. Studies in isolated perfused bone, *J Clin Invest* 64:1238, 1979.

57. Frick M, Darpo B, Ostergren J, et al: The effect of oral magnesium, alone or as an adjuvant to sotalol, after cardioversion in patients with persistent atrial fibrillation, *Eur Heart J* 21:1177, 2000.

58. Ghoneim MM, Long JP: The interaction between magnesium and other neuromuscular blocking agents, *Anesthesiology* 32:23, 1970.

59. Glendinning P, Need AG, Nordin BEC: Hypocalcemia. In Morri H, Nishizawa Y, Massry S, editors: *Calcium in internal medicine,* London, 2002, Springer-Verlag.

60. Guerrero-Romero F, Tamez-Perez HE, Gonzalez-Gonzalez G, et al: Oral magnesium supplementation improves insulin sensitivity in non-diabetic subjects with insulin resistance. A double-blind placebo-controlled randomized trial, *Diabetes Metab* 30:253, 2004.

61. Hagg E, Carlberg BC, Hillorn VS, et al: Magnesium therapy in type 1 diabetes. A double blind study concerning the effects on kidney function and serum lipid levels, *Magnes Res* 12:123, 1999.

62. Hamill-Ruth RJ, McGory R: Magnesium repletion and its effect on potassium homeostasis in critically ill adults: results of a double-blind, randomized, controlled trial, *Crit Care Med* 24:38, 1996.

63. Hardwick LL, Jones MR, Brautbar N, et al: Site and mechanism of intestinal magnesium absorption, *Miner Electr Metab* 16:174, 1990.

64. Hardwick LL, Jones MR, Brautbar N, et al: Magnesium absorption—mechanisms and the influence of vitamin-D, calcium and phosphate, *J Nutr* 121:13, 1991.

65. Hayashi H, Hoshi T: Properties of active magnesium flux across the small-intestine of the guinea-pig, *Jpn J Physiol* 42:561, 1992.

66. Hirano T, Hirotsune S, Sasaki S, et al: A new deletion mutation in bovine claudin-16 (cl-16) deficiency and diagnosis, *Anim Genet* 33:118, 2002.

67. Hirota K, Sato T, Hashimoto Y, et al: Relaxant effect of magnesium and zinc on histamine-induced bronchoconstriction in dogs, *Crit Care Med* 27:1159, 1999.

68. Holm CN, Jepsen JM, Sjogaard G, et al: A magnesium load test in the diagnosis of magnesium deficiency, *Hum Nutr* 41:301, 1987.

69. Huijgen HJ, Sanders R, Cecco SA, et al: Comparison of three commercially available ion-selective electrodes for ionized magnesium determination in serum: a two-center study, *Clin Chem* 44:480, 1998.

70. Iseri LT, Allen BJ, Ginkel ML, et al: Ionic biology and ionic medicine in cardiac-arrhythmias with particular reference to magnesium, *Am Heart J* 123:1404, 1992.

71. Iseri LT, French JH: Magnesium—nature's physiologic calcium blocker, *Am Heart J* 108:188, 1984.

72. James MF: Magnesium sulphate for the control of spasms in severe tetanus, *Anaesthesia* 53:605, 1998.

73. James MF, Cronje L: Pheochromocytoma crisis: the use of magnesium sulfate, *Anesth Analg* 99:680, 2004.

74. Karbach U, Rummel W: Cellular and paracellular magnesium transport across the terminal ileum of the rat and its interaction with the calcium transport, *Gastroenterology* 98:985, 1990.

75. Kerstan D, Quamme GA: Intestinal absorption of magnesium. In Morri H, Nishizawa Y, Massry S, editors: *Calcium in internal medicine,* London, 2002, Springer-Verlag.

76. Khanna C, Lund EM, Raffe M, et al: Hypomagnesemia in 188 dogs: a hospital population-based prevalence study, *J Vet Intern Med* 12:304, 1998.

77. Kimmel SE, Waddell LS, Michel KE: Hypomagnesemia and hypocalcemia associated with protein-losing enteropathy in Yorkshire terriers: five cases (1992-1998), *J Am Vet Med Assoc* 217:703, 2000.

78. Koch SM, Warters RD, Mehlhorn U: The simultaneous measurement of ionized and total calcium and ionized and total magnesium in intensive care unit patients, *J Crit Care* 17:203, 2002.

79. Koinig H, Wallner T, Marhofer P, et al: Magnesium sulfate reduces intra- and postoperative analgesic requirements, *Anesth Analg* 87:206, 1998.

80. Konrad M, Schlingmann KP, Gudermann T: Insights into the molecular nature of magnesium homeostasis, *Am J Physiol-Renal Physiol* 286:F599, 2004.

81. Kraft LF, Katholi RE, Woods WT, et al: Attenuation by magnesium of the electrophysiologic effects of hyperkalemia on human and canine heart-cells, *Am J Cardiol* 45:1189, 1980.

82. Krejs GJ, Nicar MJ, Zerwekh JE, et al: Effect of 1,25-dihydroxyvitamin-D3 on calcium and magnesium absorption in the healthy-human jejunum and ileum, *Am J Med* 75:973, 1983.

83. Langley WF, Mann D: Central-nervous-system magnesium-deficiency, *Arch Intern Med* 151:593, 1991.

84. Laurant P, Touyz RM: Physiological and pathophysiological role of magnesium in the cardiovascular system: implications in hypertension, *J Hypertens* 18:1177, 2000.

85. Lekcharoensuk C, Osborne CA, Lulich JP, et al: Association between dietary factors and calcium oxalate and magnesium ammonium phosphate urolithiasis in cats, *J Am Vet Med Assoc* 219:1228, 2001.

86. Levi J, Massry SG, Coburn JW, et al: Hypocalcemia in magnesium-depleted dogs: evidence for reduced responsiveness to parathyroid hormone and relative failure of parathyroid gland function, *Metabolism* 23:323, 1974.

87. Lewis LD, Chow FHC, Taton GF, et al: Effect of various dietary mineral concentrations on the occurrence of feline urolithiasis, *J Am Vet Med Assoc* 172:559, 1978.

88. London RE: Methods for measurement of intracellular magnesium: NMR and fluorescence, *Ann Rev Physiol* 53:241, 1991.

89. Lum G: Clinical utility of magnesium measurement, *Lab Med* 35:106, 2004.

90. Mann FA, Boon GD, Wagner-Mann CC, et al: Ionized and total magnesium concentrations in blood from dogs with naturally acquired parvoviral enteritis, *J Am Vet Med Assoc* 212:1398, 1998.

91. Marik PE, Varon J, Fromm R: The management of acute severe asthma, *J Emerg Med* 23:257, 2002.

92. Martin BJ, Black J, McLelland AS: Hypomagnesemia in elderly hospital admissions—a study of clinical significance, *Q J Med* 78:177, 1991.

93. Martin L, Matteson V, Wingfield W, et al: Abnormalities of serum magnesium in critically ill dogs: incidence and implications, *J Vet Emerg Crit Care* 4:15, 1994.

94. Martin L, Wingfield W, Van Pelt D, et al: Magnesium in the 1990's: implications for veterinary critical care, *J Vet Emerg Crit Care* 3:105, 1993.

95. Martin LG: Hypercalcemia and hypermagnesemia, *Vet Clin North Am Small Anim Pract* 28:565, 1998.

96. Martin LG: Intravenous magnesium loading test as a method of evaluating magnesium status in the dog. In Proceedings of the Fourth International Veterinary Emergency Critical Care Symposium, San Antonio, TX, 1994.

97. McCartney CJL, Sinha A, Katz J: A qualitative systematic review of the role of N-methyl-D-aspartate receptor antagonists in preventive analgesia, *Anesth Analg* 98:1385, 2004.

98. McLean RM: Magnesium and its therapeutic uses—a review, *Am J Med* 96:63, 1994.

99. Montell C: Mg2+ homeostasis: the Mg(2+)nificent TRMP chanzymes, *Curr Biol* 13:R799, 2003.

100. Nadler MJS, Hermosura MC, Inabe K, et al: LTRPC7 is a mg-atp-regulated divalent cation channel required for cell viability, *Nature* 411:590, 2001.

101. Nakatsuka K, Inaba M, Ishimura I: Hyper- and hypo-magnesemia. In Morri H, Nishizawa Y, Massry S, editors: *Calcium in internal medicine,* London, 2002, Springer-Verlag.

102. Nakayama T, Nakayama H, Miyamoto M, et al: Hemodynamic and electrocardiographic effects of magnesium sulfate in healthy dogs, *J Vet Intern Med* 13:485, 1999.

103. Norris CR, Christopher MM, Howard KA, et al: Effect of a magnesium-deficient diet on serum and urine magnesium concentrations in healthy cats, *Am J Vet Res* 60:1159, 1999.

104. Norris CR, Nelson RW, Christopher MM: Serum total and ionized magnesium concentrations and urinary fractional excretion of magnesium in cats with diabetes mellitus and diabetic ketoacidosis, *J Am Vet Med Assoc* 215:1455, 1999.

105. Ohba Y, Kitagawa H, Kitoh K, et al: A deletion of the paracellin-1 gene is responsible for renal tubular dysplasia in cattle, *Genomics* 68:229, 2000.

106. Ohba Y, Kitoh K, Nakamura H, et al: Renal reabsorption of magnesium and calcium by cattle with renal tubular dysplasia, *Vet Rec* 151:384, 2002.

107. Olerich M, Rude R: Should we supplement magnesium in critically ill patients? *New Horiz* 2:186, 1994.

108. Olsen LH, Kristensen AT, Haggstrom J, et al: Increased platelet aggregation response in Cavalier King Charles Spaniels with mitral valve prolapse, *J Vet Intern Med* 15:209, 2001.

109. Ono I: The effect of varying dietary magnesium on the electrocardiogram and blood electrolytes of dogs, *Jpn Circ J* 26:677, 1962.

110. Orchard TJ: Magnesium and type 2 diabetes mellitus, *Arch Intern Med* 159:2119, 1999.

111. Orent ER, Kruse HD, McCollum EV: Studies on magnesium deficiency in animals II. Species variation in symptomology of magnesium deprivation, *Am J Physiol* 101:454, 1932.

112. Page S, Salem M, Laughlin MR: Intracellular Mg2+ regulates ADP phosphorylation and adenine nucleotide synthesis in human erythrocytes, *Am J Physiol-Endocrinol Metab* 37:E920, 1998.

113. Perticone F, Adinolfi L, Bonaduce D: Efficacy of magnesium-sulfate in the treatment of torsade-de-pointes, *Am Heart J* 112:847, 1986.

114. Poopalalingam R, Chin EY: Rapid preparation of a patient with pheochromocytoma with labetolol and magnesium sulfate, *Can J Anaesth* 48:876, 2001.

115. Prielipp RC, Butterworth JF 4th, Roberts PR, et al: Magnesium antagonizes the actions of lysophosphatidyl

choline (LPC) in myocardial cells: a possible mechanism for its antiarrhythmic effects, *Anesth Analg* 80:1083, 1995.

116. Quamme GA, de Rouffignac C: Epithelial magnesium transport and regulation by the kidney, *Front Biosci* 5:D694, 2000.

117. Quamme GA, Dirks JH: Magnesium metabolism. In Narins RG, editor: *Clinical disorders of fluid and electrolyte metabolism,* New York, 1994, McGraw-Hill, Inc.

118. Rasmussen HS, Thomsen PEB: The electrophysiological effects of intravenous magnesium on human sinus node, atrioventricular node, atrium, and ventricle, *Clin Cardiol* 12:85, 1989.

119. Reinhart RA: Magnesium-metabolism—a review with special reference to the relationship between intracellular content and serum levels, *Arch Intern Med* 148:2415, 1988.

120. Rich LJ, Dysart I, Chow FH, et al: Urethral obstruction in male cats: experimental production by addition of magnesium and phosphate to diet, Feline Pract 4:44, 1974.

121. Rob PM, Dick K, Bley N, et al: Can one really measure magnesium deficiency using the short-term magnesium loading test? *J Intern Med* 246:373, 1999.

122. Roden DM: Magnesium treatment of ventricular arrhythmias, *Am J Cardiol* 63:G43, 1989.

123. Rodrigo G, Rodrigo C, Burschtin O: Efficacy of magnesium sulfate in acute adult asthma: a meta-analysis of randomized trials, *Am J Emerg Med* 18:216, 2000.

124. Rodriguez-Moran M, Guerrero-Romero F: Oral magnesium supplementation improves insulin sensitivity and metabolic control in type 2 diabetic subjects—a randomized double-blind controlled trial, *Diabetes Care* 26:1147, 2003.

125. Rowe BH, Bretzlaff JA, Bourdon C, et al: Intravenous magnesium sulfate treatment for acute asthma in the emergency department: a systematic review of the literature, *Ann Emerg Med* 36:181, 2000.

126. Rubeiz GJ, Thillbaharozian M, Hardie D, et al: Association of hypomagnesemia and mortality in acutely ill medical patients, *Crit Care Med* 21:203, 1993.

127. Rubenowitz E, Axelsson G, Rylander R: Magnesium in drinking water and death from acute myocardial infarction, *Am J Epidemiol* 143:456, 1996.

128. Rubenowitz E, Motin I, Axelsson G, et al: Magnesium in drinking water in relation to morbidity and mortality from acute myocardial infarction, *Epidemiology* 11:416, 2000.

129. Rude RK, Gruber HE, Wei LY, et al: Magnesium deficiency: effect on bone and mineral metabolism in the mouse, *Calcif Tissue Int* 72:32, 2003.

130. Rude RK, Singer FR: Magnesium deficiency and excess, *Annu Rev Med* 32:245, 1981.

131. Ryzen E, Elbaum N, Singer FR, et al: Parenteral magnesium tolerance testing in the evaluation of magnesium deficiency, *Magnesium* 4:137, 1985.

132. Ryzen E, Wagers PW, Singer FR, et al: Magnesium-deficiency in a medical ICU population, *Crit Care Med* 13:19, 1985.

133. Sacks GS, Brown RC, Dickerson RN, et al: Mononuclear blood cell magnesium content and serum magnesium concentration in critically ill hypomagnesemic patients after replacement therapy, *Nutrition* 13:303, 1997.

134. Salem M, Kasinski N, Munoz R, et al: Progressive magnesium deficiency increases mortality from endotoxin challenge—protective effects of acute magnesium replacement therapy, *Crit Care Med* 23:108, 1995.

135. Sasaki Y, Kitagawa H, Kitoh K, et al: Pathological changes of renal tubular dysplasia in Japanese black cattle, *Vet Rec* 150:628, 2002.

136. Sato T, Hirota K, Matsuki A, et al: The role of the N-methyl-D-aspartic acid receptor in the relaxant effect of

ketamine on tracheal smooth muscle, *Anesth Analg* 87:1383, 1998.

137. Satoh J, Romero MF: Mg2+ transport in the kidney, *Biometals* 15:285, 2002.

138. Schenk P, Vonbank K, Schnack B, et al: Intravenous magnesium sulfate for bronchial hyperreactivity: a randomized, controlled, double-blind study, *Clin Pharmacol Ther* 69:365, 2001.

139. Schmitz C, Perraud AL, Fleig A, et al: Dual-function ion channel/protein kinases: novel components of vertebrate magnesium regulatory mechanisms, *Pediatr Res* 55:734, 2004.

140. Seelig MS: Consequences of magnesium deficiency on the enhancement of stress reactions—preventive and therapeutic implications (a review), *J Am Coll Nutr* 13:429, 1994.

141. Seelig MS, Altura BM: How best to determine magnesium status: a new laboratory test worth trying, *Nutrition* 13:376, 1997.

142. Seelig MS, Elin RJ, Antman EM: Magnesium in acute myocardial infarction: still an open question, *Can J Cardiol* 14:745, 1998.

143. Shah GM: Renal handling of magnesium. In Morri H, Nishizawa Y, Massry S, editors: *Calcium in internal medicine*, London, 2002, Springer-Verlag.

144. Shattock MJ, Hearse DJ, Fry CH: The ionic basis of the antiischemic and antiarrhythmic properties of magnesium in the heart, *J Am Coll Nutr* 6:27, 1987.

145. Silverman RA, Osborn H, Runge J, et al: IV magnesium sulfate in the treatment of acute severe asthma—a multicenter randomized controlled trial, *Chest* 122:489, 2002.

146. Simon DB, Lu Y, Choate KA, et al: Paracellin-1, a renal tight junction protein required for paracellular Mg2+ resorption, Science 285:103, 1999.

147. Soliman HM, Mercan D, Lobo SSM, et al: Development of ionized hypomagnesemia is associated with higher mortality rates, *Crit Care Med* 31:1082, 2003.

148. Stewart AJ, Hardy J, Kohn CW, et al: Validation of diagnostic tests for determination of magnesium status in horses with reduced magnesium intake, *Am J Vet Res* 65:422, 2004.

149. Syllm-Rapoport I: Electrocardiographic studies in dogs with experimental magnesium deficiency, *J Pediatr* 60:801, 1962.

150. Thwaites CL, Farrar JJ: Magnesium sulphate as a first line therapy in the management of tetanus, *Anaesthesia* 58:286, 2003.

151. Toll J, Erb H, Birnbaum N, et al: Prevalence and incidence of serum magnesium abnormalities in hospitalized cats, *J Vet Intern Med* 16:217-221, 2001.

152. Tosiello L: Hypomagnesemia and diabetes mellitus—a review of clinical implications, *Arch Intern Med* 156:1143, 1996.

153. Touyz RM, He Y, Yao G: Presence of functionally active Mg2+ uptake channels, TRPM6 and TRPM7, in vascular smooth muscle cells from wky and shr-differential regulation by aldosterone and angiotensin, *Am J Hypertens* 17:P389, 2004.

154. Tramer MR, Schneider J, Marti RA, et al: Role of magnesium sulfate in postoperative analgesia, *Anesthesiology* 84:340, 1996.

155. Unterer S, Lutz H, Gerber B, et al: Evaluation of an electrolyte analyzer for measurement of ionized calcium and magnesium concentrations in blood, plasma, and serum of dogs, *Am J Vet Res* 65:183, 2004.

156. Verive MJ, Irazuzta J, Steinhart CM, et al: Evaluating the frequency rate of hypomagnesemia in critically ill pediatric patients hy using multiple regression analysis and a computer-based neural network, *Crit Care Med* 28:3534, 2000.

157. Vitale JJ, Hellerstein EE, Nakamura M: Effects of magnesium-deficient diet upon puppies, *Circ Res* 9:387, 1961.

158. Wang F, Van den Eeden SK, Ackerson LM, et al: Oral magnesium oxide prophylaxis of frequent migrainous headache in children: a randomized, double-blind, placebo-controlled trial, *Headache* 43:601, 2003.

159. Wary C, Brillault-Salvat C, Bloch G, et al: Effect of chronic magnesium supplementation on magnesium distribution in healthy volunteers evaluated by P[31]-NMRS and ion selective electrodes, *Br J Clin Pharmacol* 48:655, 1999.

160. Weglicki WB, Mak IT: Commentary on magnesium deficiency, substance P receptor up-regulation and NO overproduction, *Magnes Res* 9:331, 1996.

161. Weglicki WB, Mak IT, Kramer JH, et al: Role of free radicals and substance P in magnesium deficiency, *Cardiovasc Res* 31:677, 1996.

162. Weglicki WB, Phillips TM: Pathobiology of magnesium deficiency—a cytokine neurogenic inflammation hypothesis, *Am J Physiol* 263:R734, 1992.

163. Weglicki WB, Phillips TM, Mak IT, et al: Cytokines, neuropeptides, and reperfusion injury during magnesium deficiency, *Ann N Y Acad Sci* 723:246, 1994.

164. Wener J, Pintar K, Simon MA: The effects of prolonged hypomagnesemia on the cardiovascular system in young dogs, *Am Heart J* 67:221, 1964.

165. Werner HA: Status asthmaticus in children—a review, *Chest* 119:1913, 2001.

166. Whang R: Magnesium deficiency—pathogenesis, prevalence, and clinical implications, *Am J Med* 82:24, 1987.

167. Whang R, Sims G: Magnesium and potassium supplementation in the prevention of diabetic vascular disease, *Med Hypotheses* 55:263, 2000.

168. Whang R, Whang DD, Ryan MP: Refractory potassium repletion—a consequence of magnesium deficiency, *Arch Intern Med* 152:40, 1992.

169. White J, Campbell R: Magnesium and diabetes: a review, *Ann Pharmacother* 27:775, 1993.

170. Whyte K, Addis GJ, Whitesmith R, et al: Adrenergic control of plasma magnesium in man, *Clin Sci* 72:135, 1987.

171. Wilder-Smith CH, Knopfli R, Wilder-Smith OH: Perioperative magnesium infusion and postoperative pain, *Acta Anaesthesiol Scand* 41:1023, 1997.

172. Wilder-Smith OH, Arendt-Nielsen L, Gaumann D, et al: Sensory changes and pain after abdominal hysterectomy: a comparison of anesthetic supplementation with fentanyl versus magnesium or ketamine, *Anesth Analg* 86:95, 1998.

173. Williams S: Use of magnesium to treat tetanus, *Br J Anaesth* 88:152, 2002.

174. Wingfield WE, Matteson VL: Ionized and serum magnesium in normal and critically ill dogs. In Proceedings of the Fifth International Veterinary Emergency Critical Care Symposium, 1996, San Antonio, TX.

175. Wooldridge JD, Gregory CR: Ionized and total serum magnesium concentrations in feline renal transplant recipients, *Vet Surg* 28:31, 1999.

176. Yoshioka H, Hirota K, Sato T, et al: Spasmolytic effect of magnesium sulfate on serotonin-induced pulmonary hypertension and bronchoconstriction in dogs, *Acta Anaesthesiol Scand* 45:435, 2001.

177. Ziegelstein RC, Hilbe JM, French WJ, et al: Magnesium use in the treatment of acute myocardial infarction in the United States (observations from the second national registry of myocardial infarction), *Am J Cardiol* 87:7, 2001.

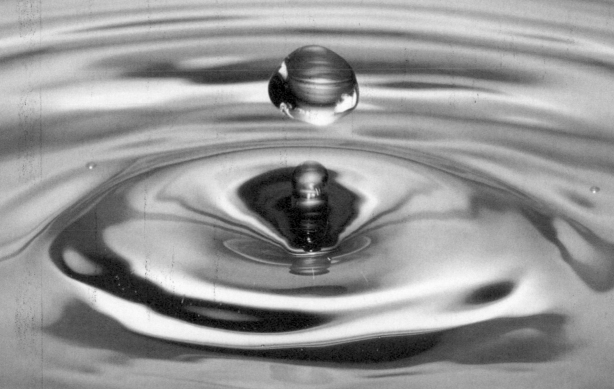

ACID-BASE DISORDERS

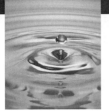

CHAPTER · 9

INTRODUCTION TO ACID-BASE DISORDERS

Stephen P. DiBartola

To Faraday we are indebted for naming the products of dissociation, ions—and thus we came by "hydrogen ions," a term now synonymous with proton. Tiny though it is, I suppose no constituent of living matter has so much power to influence biological behavior. . . .

A. Baird Hastings, Ann N Y Acad Sci 133:16, 1966.

Metabolic processes each day yield 50 to 100 mEq of H^+ ions (**fixed** or **nonvolatile acid**) from the metabolism of proteins and phospholipids and 10,000 to 15,000 mmol of CO_2 (**volatile acid**) from the metabolism of carbohydrate and fat. Carbon dioxide is potentially an acid by virtue of its ability to combine with H_2O in the presence of carbonic anhydrase to form carbonic acid (H_2CO_3). Carbon dioxide is continuously removed by alveolar ventilation so that the partial pressure of CO_2 (PCO_2) is kept constant at approximately 40 mm Hg.

CONCEPT OF ACIDITY

The most commonly used concept of acids and bases is that of Brönsted and Lowry, who stated that an **acid** is a proton donor and a **base** a proton acceptor. In the following equation, HA is an acid and A^- is a base:

$$HA \rightleftharpoons H^+ + A^-$$

In aqueous solutions, protons or H^+ ions are normally bound by electrostatic interaction to H_2O, resulting in the formation of hydronium ions, designated H_3O^+. Conventionally, however, the term **hydrogen ion** and the symbol H^+ are used to refer to protons in aqueous solutions.

The acidity of a solution refers to the chemical **activity** of its constituent H^+ ions. Chemical activity is related to chemical **concentration** by the **activity coefficient,** a factor that varies directly with temperature and inversely with the ionic strength of the solution. Physiologic control of body temperature and osmolality and the dilute nature of body fluids result in this factor being near unity, and the difference between activity and concentration is negligible in body fluids.

The concentrations of most important electrolytes in body fluids (e.g., Na^+, K^+, Cl^-, HCO_3^-) are in the range of milliequivalents per liter, whereas the concentration of H^+ is in the range of nanoequivalents per liter. That is, hydrogen ions are present at one-millionth the concentration of other electrolytes. What, then, accounts for the emphasis on hydrogen ions in biology and medicine? The answer lies in the fact that hydrogen ions are highly reactive. The proteins of the body have many dissociable groups. These may gain or lose protons as [H^+] changes, resulting in alterations in charge and molecular configuration that may adversely affect protein structure and function. The [H^+] of body fluids must be kept constant so that detrimental changes in enzyme function and cellular structure do not occur. The range of [H^+] compatible with life is 16 to 160 nEq/L.

CONCEPT OF pH

The concept of pH was introduced by Sørensen to allow easier notation for the wide range of [H^+] found in chemical systems. The term pH is defined as the negative base 10 logarithm of the hydrogen ion concentration expressed in equivalents per liter or the base 10 logarithm of the reciprocal of the hydrogen ion concentration:

$$pH = -\log_{10}[H^+] = \log_{10}\left(\frac{1}{[H^+]}\right)$$

Thus at the normal extracellular fluid (ECF) [H^+] of 40 nEq/L (4×10^{-8} Eq/L):

$$
\begin{aligned}
[H^+] &= 4 \times 10^{-8} \text{ Eq/L} \\
pH &= -\log_{10}(4 \times 10^{-8}) \\
&= -\log_{10}4 - \log_{10}10^{-8} \\
&= -(0.602) - (-8) \\
&= 8 - 0.602 \\
&= 7.398
\end{aligned}
$$

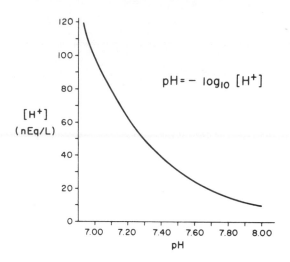

Fig. 9-1 Exponential relationship between [H⁺] and pH. (From Madias NE, Cohen JJ: Acid-base chemistry and buffering. In Cohen JJ, Kassirer JP, editors: *Acid-base,* Boston, 1982, Little, Brown & Co., p. 5.)

There is an inverse relationship between pH and $[H^+]$: the greater the $[H^+]$, the lower the pH. Furthermore, pH and $[H^+]$ vary not linearly with one another but exponentially as shown in Fig. 9-1. The $[H^+]$ for a given pH within the physiologic range is given in Table 9-1.

LAW OF MASS ACTION

The **law of mass action** states that the velocity of a reaction is proportional to the product of the concentrations of the reactants. For the acid just described, there are two opposing reactions:

$$HA \rightarrow H^+ + A^-$$
$$H^+ + A^- \rightarrow HA$$

The velocity of the first reaction can be written:

$$v_1 = k_1[HA]$$

and the velocity of the second reaction:

$$v_2 = k_2[H^+][A^-]$$

At equilibrium, the rates of the two opposing reactions exactly counterbalance one another and the two velocities are equal:

$$k_1[HA] = k_2[H^+][A^-]$$

Rearranging and substituting a new constant, K_a, the ionization, or dissociation, constant for the acid HA:

$$k_1/k_2 = K_a = \frac{[H^+][A^-]}{[HA]}$$

The ionization, or dissociation, constant for an acid is an indication of the strength of that acid. A large value for K_a means that $[H^+]$ and $[A^-]$ are much greater than $[HA]$; that is, the acid is a strong one and is largely dissociated. A small value for K_a means that $[H^+]$ and $[A^-]$ are much smaller than $[HA]$; that is, the acid is a weak one and little of it is dissociated. Hydrochloric acid (HCl) and sulfuric acid (H_2SO_4) are strong acids and dissociate almost completely in aqueous solutions, whereas NH_4^+ is a weak acid (i.e., it is a strong base) and dissociates to a small extent.

Taking the base 10 logarithm of both sides of the dissociation equilibrium equation yields:

$$\log K_a = \log \frac{[H^+][A^-]}{[HA]}$$
$$\log K_a = \log([H^+]) + \log \frac{[A^-]}{[HA]}$$

Multiplying by -1 yields:

$$-\log K_a = -\log([H^+]) - \log \frac{[A^-]}{[HA]}$$

Applying the concept of pH to both the hydrogen ion concentration and dissociation constant, K_a:

$$pK_a = pH - \log \left(\frac{[A^-]}{[HA]}\right)$$
$$pH = pK_a + \log \left(\frac{[A^-]}{[HA]}\right)$$

This is the commonly used Henderson-Hasselbalch form of the dissociation equilibrium equation. Occasionally, the term **salt** or **base** is substituted for A^- and the term **acid** for HA:

$$pH = pK_a + \log \frac{[salt]}{[acid]}$$

CONCEPT OF BUFFERING

A **buffer** is a compound that can accept or donate protons (hydrogen ions) and minimize a change in pH. A buffer solution consists of a weak acid and its conjugate salt. When a strong acid is added to a buffer solution containing a weaker acid and its salt, the dissociated protons from the strong acid are donated to the salt of the weak acid and the change in pH is minimized.

Consider an aqueous solution with equal amounts of Na_2HPO_4 and NaH_2PO_4. The pK_a for this buffer pair is 6.8:

$$pH = pK_a + \log \frac{[salt]}{[acid]}$$

TABLE 9-1 Conversions Between pH and [H⁺]

pH Units	[H⁺]* (nEq/L)	pH Units	[H⁺] (nEq/L)	pH Units	[H⁺] (nEq/L)	pH Units	[H⁺] (nEq/L)
8.00	10	7.64	23	7.29	51	6.94	115
7.99	10	7.63	23	7.28	52	6.93	117
7.98	10	7.62	24	7.27	54	6.92	120
7.97	11	7.61	25	7.26	55	6.91	123
7.96	11	7.60	25	7.25	56	6.90	126
7.95	11	7.59	26	7.24	58	6.89	129
7.94	11	7.58	26	7.23	59	6.88	132
7.93	12	7.57	27	7.22	60	6.87	135
7.92	12	7.56	28	7.21	62	6.86	138
7.91	12	7.55	28	7.20	63	6.85	141
7.90	13	7.54	29	7.19	65	6.84	145
7.89	13	7.53	30	7.18	66	6.83	148
7.88	13	7.52	30	7.17	68	6.82	151
7.87	13	7.51	31	7.16	69	6.81	155
7.86	14	7.50	32	7.15	71	6.80	159
7.85	14	7.49	32	7.14	72	6.79	162
7.84	14	7.48	33	7.13	74	6.78	166
7.83	15	7.47	34	7.12	76	6.77	170
7.82	15	7.46	35	7.11	78	6.76	174
7.81	15	7.45	35	7.10	79	6.75	178
7.80	16	7.44	36	7.09	81	6.74	182
7.79	16	7.43	37	7.08	83	6.73	186
7.78	17	7.42	38	7.07	85	6.72	191
7.77	17	7.41	39	7.06	87	6.71	196
7.76	17	7.40	40	7.05	89	6.70	200
7.75	18	7.39	41	7.04	91	6.69	204
7.74	18	7.38	42	7.03	93	6.68	209
7.73	19	7.37	43	7.02	95	6.67	214
7.72	19	7.36	44	7.01	98	6.66	219
7.71	19	7.35	45	7.00	100	6.65	224
7.70	20	7.34	46	6.99	102	6.64	229
7.69	20	7.33	47	6.98	105	6.63	234
7.68	21	7.32	48	6.97	107	6.62	240
7.67	21	7.31	49	6.96	110	6.61	245
7.66	22	7.30	50	6.95	112	6.60	251
7.65	22						

From Cohen JJ, Kassirer JP: Clinical evaluation of acid-base disorders. In Cohen JJ, Kassirer JP, editors: Acid-base, Boston, 1982, Little, Brown & Co., p. 409.

*Values for [H⁺] are given to the nearest nEq/L.

$$pH = 6.8 + \log \frac{[Na_2HPO_4]}{[NaH_2PO_4]}$$

If the amounts of Na_2HPO_4 and NaH_2PO_4 are equal, their ratio is 1.0:

$$pH = 6.8 + \log(1.0)$$
$$= 6.8$$

Consider adding 1 mmol of HCl to this solution. The protons from the HCl are donated to the salt of the buffer pair (Na_2HPO_4), converting it to its conjugate acid (NaH_2PO_4). If 10 mmol of each phosphate salt was present initially, the new ratio of Na_2HPO_4/NaH_2PO_4 would be 9/11 or 0.82 and:

$$pH = 6.8 + \log(0.82)$$
$$= 6.8 + (-0.086)$$
$$= 6.71$$

By contrast, an aqueous solution containing 1 mmol/L HCl (10^{-3} Eq/L) would have a pH of 3.0.

By solving the dissociation equilibrium equation for $[H^+]$, the same can be shown:

$$[H^+] = K_a \frac{[HA]}{[A^-]}$$

For the previously described solution of sodium phosphate:

$$[H^+] = K_a \frac{[NaH_2PO_4]}{[Na_2HPO_4]}$$

The K_a for this reaction is 1.6×10^{-7} Eq/L, and if there are equal amounts of the two phosphate salts present ($[NaH_2PO_4] = [Na_2HPO_4]$):

$$[H^+] = 1.6 \times 10^{-7} \text{ Eq/L}$$
$$= 160 \text{ nEq/L (pH 6.80)}$$

After addition of 1 mmol of HCl:

$$[H^+] = (1.6 \times 10^{-7})(11 \times 10^{-3})/(9 \times 10^{-3})$$
$$= 1.95 \times 10^{-7} \text{ Eq/L}$$
$$= 195 \text{ nEq/L (pH 6.71)}$$

By contrast, an aqueous solution containing 1 mmol/L HCl would have $[H^+] = 0.001$ mol/L or 1 million nmol/L. Thus 99.98% of the added hydrogen ions have been buffered by the sodium phosphate solution.

If the amount of strong acid (e.g., HCl) or base (e.g., NaOH) added to a solution of a weak acid and its salt (i.e., a buffer solution) is plotted against pH, the resulting relationship is called a **titration** or **buffer** curve (Fig. 9-2). The curve is sigmoidal, and its slope is greatest in the midregion, over which the curve is approximately linear. In the pH range associated with the midregion of the curve, the change in pH is smallest for a given amount of added acid or base and buffer capacity is greatest at the midpoint of the curve. At this point, there are equal amounts of the weak acid and its conjugate salt, and as shown by the Henderson-Hasselbalch equation, pH = pK_a. The region of best buffer capacity extends approximately 1.0 pH unit on either side of the pK_a. Thus a buffer is most effective within one pH unit of its pK_a. The pK_a values for some important biologic compounds are listed in Table 9-2.

ISOHYDRIC PRINCIPLE

Regardless of the number of buffers present, a solution can have only one $[H^+]$ and one pH. Using the law of mass action or the Henderson-Hasselbalch equation, the ratio of acid to salt forms of any buffer in the solution can be calculated. This has been called the **isohydric principle.** The implication of the isohydric principle is that the

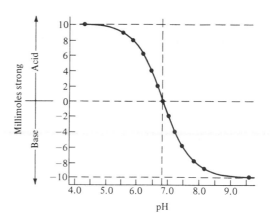

Fig. 9-2 Titration curve for an aqueous solution containing a phosphate buffer. (From Rose BD: *Clinical physiology of Acid-base and electrolyte disorders*, ed 3, New York, 1989, McGraw-Hill, p. 269, with permission of the McGraw-Hill Companies.)

behavior of any buffer pair in a complex solution can be predicted by knowledge of the dissociation constant and concentrations of any one buffer pair. In clinical practice, the bicarbonate–carbonic acid buffer pair is the one used to monitor acid-base balance in body fluids.

TABLE 9-2 pK_a Values of Biologically Important Compounds*

Compound	pK_a
Phosphoric acid	2.0
Citric acid	2.9
Carbonic acid (pK_a)	3.6
Acetoacetic acid	3.6
Lactic acid	3.9
Citrate^{1-}	4.3
Acetic acid	4.6
3-Hydroxybutyric acid	4.7
Creatinine	5.0
Citrate^{2-}	5.6
Uric acid	5.8
Organic phosphates	6.0-7.5
Carbonic acid (pK_a')	6.1
Imidazole group of histidine	6.4-7.0
Oxygenated hemoglobin	6.7
Phosphate^{1-}	6.8
α-Amino (amino-terminal)	7.4-7.9
Deoxygenated hemoglobin	7.9
Ammonium	9.2
Bicarbonate	9.8
Phosphate^{2-}	12.4

*Compounds with pK_a values in the range of 6.4-8.4 are most useful as buffers in biologic systems. The pK_a values for the imidazole group of histidine and for α-amino (amino-terminal) amino groups are for those side groups in proteins. The pK_a range for organ phosphates refers to such intracellular compounds as adenosine triphosphate, adenosine diphosphate, and 2,3-diphosphoglycerate.

The relative importance of a given buffer in the body is based on its concentration in the relevant body fluid, its pK_a, and the prevailing $[H^+]$ (40 nmol/L in ECF). The bicarbonate–carbonic acid system is unique among buffers in that carbonic acid is in equilibrium with dissolved CO_2, the concentration of which normally is kept constant by alveolar ventilation.

THE BICARBONATE–CARBONIC ACID SYSTEM: PHYSICAL CHEMISTRY

Gaseous CO_2 produced in the tissues is soluble in water, and the concentration of dissolved CO_2 in body fluids is proportional to the partial pressure of CO_2 in the gas phase (P_{CO_2}):

$$[CO_{2diss}] = \alpha(P_{CO_2})$$

where α is a factor called the **solubility coefficient of CO_2**. The solubility coefficient of CO_2 has a value of 0.0301 mmol/L/mm in arterial plasma at 37° C. Thus:

$$[CO_{2diss}] = 0.0301\ P_{CO_2}$$

Dissolved CO_2 combines with water to form carbonic acid:

$$CO_{2diss} + H_2O \rightarrow H_2CO_3$$

The uncatalyzed reaction proceeds slowly, but its rate is dramatically increased by the enzyme carbonic anhydrase, which is present in abundance in the body (e.g., red cells, renal tubular cells). In the body, therefore, the hydration of CO_2 to form H_2CO_3 reaches equilibrium almost instantaneously. Normally, the equilibrium is so far to the left that there are approximately 340 molecules of dissolved CO_2 for each molecule of carbonic acid.[42]

The dissociation of carbonic acid can be expressed using the law of mass action:

$$K_a = \frac{[H^+][HCO_3^-]}{[H_2CO_3]}$$

K_a for this reaction is 2.72×10^{-4} mol/L (pK_a=3.57). The ratio of bicarbonate to carbonic acid at the normal $[H^+]$ of body fluids can be calculated by rearranging this equation:

$$\frac{[HCO_3^-]}{[H_2CO_3]} = \frac{K_a}{[H^+]}$$
$$= 2.72 \times 10^{-4}/4 \times 10^{-8}$$
$$= 6.8 \times 10^3$$

Thus at $[H^+]$ = 40 nmol/L (pH 7.40), there are 6800 bicarbonate ions and 340 molecules of dissolved CO_2 for each molecule of carbonic acid.

The reaction of dissolved CO_2 in aqueous body fluids can be summarized as:

$$CO_{2diss} + H_2O \rightleftarrows H_2CO_3 \rightleftarrows H^+ + HCO_3^-$$

However, the number of carbonic acid molecules is negligible compared with the numbers of dissolved CO_2 molecules and HCO_3^- ions. Therefore this equation can be simplified:

$$CO_{2diss} + H_2O \rightleftarrows H^+ + HCO_3^-$$

The law of mass action for this equilibrium can be expressed as:

$$K_a = \frac{[H^+][HCO_3^-]}{[CO_{2diss}][H_2O]}$$

The concentration of water in dilute body fluids remains virtually unchanged by this reaction and can be incorporated into K_a to yield another constant, K'_a:

$$K'_a = \frac{[H^+][HCO_3^-]}{[CO_{2diss}]}$$

Solving for $[H^+]$ yields:

$$[H^+] = \frac{K'_a[CO_{2diss}]}{[HCO_3^-]}$$

In body fluids at 37° C, K'_a is approximately equal to 8×10^{-7} mol/L and pK'_a equals 6.1. An approximate value of 6.1 for this pK'_a is valid at temperatures ranging from 30 to 40° C (86 to 104° F) and pH values ranging from 7.0 to 7.6.[37]

A formula for $[H^+]$ in nanomoles per liter or nanoequivalents per liter is obtained by expressing K'_a in nanomoles per liter or nanoequivalents per liter:

$$[H^+] = \frac{800[CO_{2diss}]}{[HCO_3^-]}$$

Using the solubility coefficient for carbon dioxide yields:

$$[H^+] = \frac{800\ (0.0301)\ P_{CO_2}}{[HCO_3^-]} = \frac{24\ P_{CO_2}}{[HCO_3^-]}$$

This is the Henderson equation and has been used extensively in the clinical evaluation of acid-base disturbances. It shows clearly that the $[H^+]$ (and thus pH) of body fluids is determined by the **ratio** of P_{CO_2} to HCO_3^- concentration. The Henderson-Hasselbalch equation is derived by expressing $[H^+]$ and K'_a in moles per liter or equivalents per liter and converting the equation to logarithmic form:

$$[H^+] = \frac{K'_a\,[CO_{2diss}]}{[HCO_3^-]}$$

$$\log[H^+] = \log K'_a + \log \frac{[CO_{2diss}]}{[HCO_3^-]}$$

Multiplying by −1, we obtain:

$$-\log[H^+] = -\log K'_a - \log \frac{[CO_{2diss}]}{[HCO_3^-]}$$

$$pH = pK'_a + \log \frac{[HCO_3^-]}{[CO_{2diss}]}$$

Substituting 6.1 for the value of pK'_a and applying the solubility coefficient for CO_2, we obtain:

$$pH = 6.1 + \log \frac{[HCO_3^-]}{0.03 \times P{CO_2}}$$

This is the clinically relevant form of the equation and shows that in body fluids, pH is a function of the **ratio** between HCO_3^- concentration and $P{CO_2}$.

BODY BUFFERS

Body buffers can be divided into **bicarbonate,** which is the primary buffer system of **ECF,** and **nonbicarbonate** buffers (e.g., proteins and inorganic and organic phosphates), which constitute the primary **intracellular** buffer system. Bone is a prominent source of buffer and can contribute calcium carbonate and, to a lesser extent, calcium phosphate during chronic metabolic acidosis. Bone may even account for up to 40% of the buffering of an acute acid load in the dog.[9] After administration of $NaHCO_3$, carbonate can be deposited in bone.

BICARBONATE AS A BUFFER IN EXTRACELLULAR FLUID

If a buffer is most effective within 1 pH unit of its pK_a, what accounts for the importance of the bicarbonate system (pK'_a 6.1 versus ECF pH 7.4)? One factor is the high concentration of HCO_3^- (approximately 24 mEq/L versus 2 mEq/L for phosphate). However, the most important factor is that the bicarbonate–carbonic acid buffer pair functions as an open system. In a **closed** system, the bicarbonate and carbonic acid or dissolved CO_2 concentrations must change in a reciprocal manner as the following reaction is driven to the left or right:

$$CO_{2diss} + H_2O \rightleftharpoons H_2CO_3 \rightleftharpoons H^+ + HCO_3^-$$

In the body, the system is **open**, and carbonic acid, in the presence of carbonic anhydrase, forms CO_2, which is eliminated entirely from the system by alveolar ventilation. Thus the "acid" member of the buffer pair is free to change directly with the "salt" member as compensation for metabolic acidosis occurs. If $P{CO_2}$ is kept constant at 40 mm Hg, the effectiveness of the bicarbonate–carbonic acid system is increased dramatically. In response to metabolic acidosis, however, the body goes even further, and $P{CO_2}$ is reduced below the normal value of 40 mm Hg, thus increasing the effectiveness of this buffer pair even more.

Consider a closed system in which the bicarbonate–carbonic acid system is the only buffer pair. We will assume the following conditions at the start: $[H^+] = 40$ nmol/L, $[HCO_3^-] = 24$ mmol/L, $P{CO_2} = 40$ mm Hg (dissolved $CO_2 = 1.2$ mmol/L), and pH = 7.40. If 5 mmol of HCl is added to this closed system, $[HCO_3^-]$ is titrated and decreases to 19 mmol/L, $P{CO_2}$ increases to 206 mm Hg (dissolved $CO_2 = 1.2 + 5 = 6.2$ mmol/L), $[H^+]$ increases to 260 nmol/L, and pH decreases to 6.58, a value incompatible with life.

Consider now what would happen if the system were open and the $P{CO_2}$ kept constant at 40 mm Hg by a factor external to the system (i.e., alveolar ventilation). What would happen now if 5 mmol of HCl were added, assuming the same starting conditions? The $[HCO_3^-]$ again decreases to 19 mmol/L, but $P{CO_2}$ is fixed at 40 mm Hg (dissolved $CO_2 = 1.2$ mmol/L). The $[H^+]$ can be calculated from the Henderson equation: $[H^+] = 24(40)/19 = 50$ nmol/L. The pH is 7.30.

Consider now what would happen if, rather than being kept constant, the $P{CO_2}$ actually decreased to 36.5 mm Hg. This is what would be expected in a patient with metabolic acidosis if we use the rule of thumb that $P{CO_2}$ decreases by 0.7 mm Hg per 1.0 mEq/L decrement in plasma HCO_3^- concentration. In this setting, $[HCO_3^-]$ still decreases to 19 mmol/L, but $P{CO_2}$ is 36.5 mm Hg, and dissolved $CO_2 = 0.0301(36.5) = 1.1$ mmol/L. Again, the $[H^+]$ can be calculated from the Henderson relationship: $[H^+] = 24(36.5)/19 = 46$ nmol/L. The pH in this setting is 7.34, just slightly below the starting pH of 7.40. This, in essence, is what happens in the body in response to metabolic acidosis and illustrates the dramatic effect achieved because the bicarbonate–carbonic acid system is an open system with $P{CO_2}$ closely regulated by alveolar ventilation.

PROTEINS AS BUFFERS

Plasma proteins play a limited role in extracellular buffering, whereas intracellular proteins play an important role in the total buffer response of the body. The buffer effect of proteins is the result of their dissociable side groups. For most proteins, including hemoglobin, the most important of these dissociable groups is the imidazole ring of histidine residues (pK_a, 6.4 to 7.0).

Amino-terminal amino groups (pK_a, 7.4 to 7.9) also contribute somewhat to the buffer effect of proteins. Other side groups are relatively unimportant because their pK_a values are either too high or too low to be useful in the normal physiologic range of pH. The pK_a values for the dissociable groups of proteins are listed in Table 9-3.

Hemoglobin is responsible for more than 80% of the nonbicarbonate buffering capacity of whole blood, whereas plasma proteins contribute 20%. Of the plasma proteins, albumin is much more important than are the globulins. The buffer value of albumin is 0.12 to 0.14 mmol/g/pH unit, whereas that of globulins is 0 to 0.08 mmol/g/pH unit.[38,69,71] The difference results from a larger number of histidine (Fig. 9-3) residues in albumin.

The **isoelectric point** (pI) is the pH at which a substance has no tendency to move in an electric field and thus has no net charge. For proteins, this means that the sum of the charges on the negative side groups (e.g., R–COO$^-$) equals the sum of the charges on the positive side groups (e.g., R–NH$_3^+$). At physiologic pH (7.4), plasma proteins are polyanions because their pIs range from 5.1 to 5.7. The net negative charge on plasma proteins in mEq/L can be calculated as[38]:

$$[Pr] \times \beta \times (pH - pI)$$

where [Pr] is the concentration of plasma proteins in grams per liter, β is the buffer value of plasma proteins in millimoles per gram per pH unit, pH is the ECF pH, and pI is the isoelectric point of plasma proteins. Using this formula, it can be calculated that, at a normal plasma protein concentration of 7 g/dL, average buffer value of 0.1 mmol/g/pH unit, and pI range of 5.1 to 5.7, plasma proteins contribute 12 to 16 mEq/L of negative charge. In dogs, the mean contribution of charge by plasma proteins is approximately 16 mEq/L.[16,74]

TABLE 9-3 pK'_a Values for Dissociable Groups Found in Proteins

Dissociable Group (Amino Acid)	pK'_a
α-Carboxyl	3.6-3.8
β-Carboxyl (aspartic acid)	≈4.0
γ-Carboxyl (glutamic acid)	≈4.0
Imidazole (histidine)	6.4-7.0
α-Amino	7.4-7.9
Sulfhydryl (cysteine)	≈9.0
ε-Amino (lysine)	9.8-10.6
Phenolic (tyrosine)	8.5-10.9
Guanidino (arginine)	11.9-13.3

From Madias NE, Cohen JJ: Acid-base chemistry and buffering. In Cohen JJ, Kassirer JF, editors: Acid-base, Boston, 1982, Little, Brown & Co., p. 16.

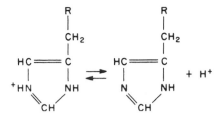

Fig. 9-3 The imidazole group of histidine. (From Madias NE, Cohen JJ: Acid-base chemistry and buffering. In Cohen JJ, Kassirer JP, editors: *Acid-base,* Boston, 1982, Little, Brown & Co., p. 16.)

PHOSPHATES AS BUFFERS

The most important intracellular buffers are proteins and inorganic and organic (e.g., adenosine triphosphate [ATP], adenosine diphosphate [ADP], 2,3-diphosphoglycerate) phosphates. The pK_a value for $H_2PO_4^-$ is 6.8, and pK_a values for organic phosphates range from 6.0 to 7.5. Inorganic phosphate is a more important buffer intracellularly, where its concentration is high (approximately 40 mEq/L in skeletal muscle cells), and less important in ECF, where its concentration is much lower (approximately 2 mEq/L). Inorganic phosphate is an important buffer in urine because the range of pH in tubular fluid (6.0 to 7.0) includes the pK_a of the Na_2HPO_4/NaH_2PO_4 system (6.8). This buffer pair functions in the excretion of **titratable acidity** in urine (see section on Titratable Acidity later in this chapter).

PHYSIOLOGIC LINES OF DEFENSE IN ACID-BASE DISTURBANCES

An overview of the body buffer response is provided by contrasting the body's response to a nonvolatile, or fixed, acid (e.g., HCl) and its response to the volatile acid CO_2. The hydrogen ions from a fixed acid load immediately titrate bicarbonate ions in ECF and then titrate intracellular buffers (e.g., proteins, phosphates). This physicochemical response occurs within minutes and protects ECF pH. Alveolar ventilation is stimulated, and P_{CO_2} is decreased to below normal. This response, which begins immediately and is complete within hours, minimizes the change in pH because the ratio of HCO_3^- to P_{CO_2} is normalized. Finally, the kidneys regenerate titrated HCO_3^-, pH increases, alveolar ventilation decreases, and P_{CO_2} returns to normal. The renal response begins within hours but requires 2 to 5 days to reach maximal effectiveness.

The volatile acid CO_2 cannot be buffered by HCO_3^-, and the hydrogen ions resulting from the dissociation of carbonic acid must titrate intracellular buffers, such as proteins (especially hemoglobin in red cells) and phosphates. Renal adaptation is characterized by increased

HCO_3^- reabsorption and net acid excretion, mechanisms that require 2 to 5 days to achieve maximal effectiveness. The buffer response of the body to the primary acid-base disorders is considered in more depth in the chapters on those disorders (see Chapters 10 and 11).

TERMINOLOGY

The terms **acidosis** and **alkalosis** refer to the pathophysiologic processes that cause net accumulation of acid or alkali in the body. The terms **acidemia** and **alkalemia** refer specifically to the pH of ECF. In **acidemia** the ECF pH is lower than normal, and the $[H^+]$ is higher than normal. In **alkalemia** the ECF pH is higher than normal, and the $[H^+]$ is lower than normal. The distinction between these terms is important. For example, a patient with chronic respiratory alkalosis may have a blood pH within the normal range because of effective renal compensation in this setting. Such a patient has **alkalosis** but does not have **alkalemia**. Patients with **mixed** acid-base disturbances can have blood pH values within the normal range as a result of the presence of two counterbalancing acid-base disturbances (see the following section on simple and mixed acid-base disorders).

PRIMARY ACID-BASE DISTURBANCES

Acidosis and alkalosis can each be of metabolic or respiratory origin, and as a result, there are four primary acid-base disturbances: metabolic acidosis, respiratory acidosis, metabolic alkalosis, and respiratory alkalosis. The metabolic disturbances refer to a net excess or deficit of nonvolatile, or fixed, acid, whereas the respiratory disturbances refer to the net excess or deficit of volatile acid (dissolved CO_2).

Metabolic acidosis is characterized by a decreased plasma HCO_3^- concentration and decreased pH (increased $[H^+]$) caused by either HCO_3^- loss or buffering of a noncarbonic (nonvolatile or fixed) acid. **Metabolic alkalosis** is characterized by an increased plasma HCO_3^- concentration and increased pH (decreased $[H^+]$), usually caused by a disproportionate loss of chloride ions from the body (i.e., loss of fluid with

a chloride concentration greater than that of ECF) or hypoalbuminemia (because albumin is a weak acid). In the absence of volume depletion or renal dysfunction, it is extremely difficult to produce metabolic alkalosis by administration of alkali. **Respiratory acidosis** is characterized by increased PCO_2 (hypercapnia) caused by alveolar hypoventilation. **Respiratory alkalosis** is characterized by decreased PCO_2 caused by alveolar hyperventilation (hypocapnia). In one study, metabolic acidosis was the most common acid-base disturbance encountered in dogs.[17]

Each **primary** metabolic or respiratory acid-base disturbance is accompanied by a **secondary**, or **adaptive**, change in the opposing component of the system (Table 9-4). The adaptive response involves the component opposite the one disturbed and returns the pH of the system toward but not completely to normal. Overcompensation does not occur. For example, metabolic acidosis is accompanied by a secondary or adaptive respiratory alkalosis. Respiratory acidosis is accompanied by a secondary or adaptive metabolic alkalosis.

SIMPLE AND MIXED ACID-BASE DISORDERS

An acid-base disorder is said to be **simple** if it is limited to the **primary** disorder and the **expected** secondary, or adaptive, response. The magnitude of the **expected** responses is considered in detail in the chapters devoted to the **primary** acid-base disorders (see Chapters 10 and 11). A **mixed** acid-base disorder is one that is characterized by the presence of at least two separate primary acid-base abnormalities occurring in the same patient. A **mixed** acid-base disorder should be suspected whenever the secondary, or adaptive, response exceeds or falls short of that expected. In dogs, for example, the expected response to metabolic acidosis is a 0.7-mm Hg decrease in PCO_2 for each 1.0-mEq/L decrement in plasma HCO_3^- concentration caused by metabolic acidosis (see Chapter 10 for more details).

Consider a dog with these normal blood gas values: pH 7.39, $[H^+]$ = 41 nEq/L, $[HCO_3^-]$ = 21 mEq/L, and PCO_2 = 36 mm Hg. This dog becomes ill and is observed to have the following blood gas values: pH 7.22, $[H^+]$ =

TABLE 9-4 Characteristics of Primary Acid-Base Disturbances

Disorder	pH	$[H^+]$	Primary Disturbance	Compensatory Response
Metabolic acidosis	↓	↑	↓ $[HCO_3^-]$	↓ PCO_2
Metabolic alkalosis	↑	↓	↑ $[HCO_3^-]$	↑ PCO_2
Respiratory acidosis	↓	↑	↑ PCO_2	↑ $[HCO_3^-]$
Respiratory alkalosis	↑	↓	↓ PCO_2	↓ $[HCO_3^-]$

From Rose BD: Clinical physiology of acid-base and electrolyte disorders, ed 3, New York, 1989, McGraw-Hill, p. 470, with permission of the McGraw-Hill Companies.

60 nEq/L, [HCO_3^-] = 14 mEq/L, and PCO_2 = 35 mm Hg. If the dog had a **simple** metabolic acidosis, using the rule of thumb described before, we would have expected the following results: pH 7.27, [H^+] = 53 nEq/L, [HCO_3^-] = 14 mEq/L, and PCO_2 = 31 mm Hg. Thus the dog has a **mixed** acid-base disorder characterized by both metabolic and respiratory acidoses.

Consider a patient with the following blood gas values: pH 7.40, [H^+] = 40 nEq/L, [HCO_3^-] = 31 mEq/L, and PCO_2 = 51 mm Hg. This patient is neither **alkalemic** nor **acidemic** because blood pH is 7.40; however, based on the PCO_2 and [HCO_3^-], the patient is not normal. This patient has a **mixed** disorder characterized by metabolic alkalosis and respiratory acidosis. The two disorders have counterbalancing effects, resulting in a normal pH. Mixed acid-base disorders are considered in detail in Chapter 12.

COMPENSATORY RESPONSES FOR PRIMARY ACID-BASE DISTURBANCES

The guidelines for secondary or adaptive responses are listed in Table 9-5 for reference. Note that there are single rules of thumb for each of the **metabolic** acid-base disorders but two rules of thumb (one each for acute and chronic disorders) for the **respiratory** acid-base disorders. This is a consequence of the fact that the adaptive respiratory response to metabolic disorders begins immediately and is complete within hours. Conversely, the response to respiratory disorders occurs in two phases. In the first phase, there is immediate titration of predominantly intracellular nonbicarbonate buffers, resulting in an initial change in plasma HCO_3^- concentration. The second phase is carried out by the kidneys and is characterized by alterations in net acid excretion and bicarbonate reabsorption. This response begins within hours but takes 2 to 5 days to achieve maximal effectiveness. Thus there are two expected compensatory responses: acute (<24 hours) and chronic (>48 hours). One caution about rules of thumb is that they define the

average response and not 95% confidence intervals. Acid-base maps depict 95% confidence intervals and, although more awkward to use, allow the clinician to consider normal variation in response (Fig. 9-4). Thus a patient should be considered to have a mixed disorder only when the blood gas value in question deviates considerably from the calculated expected value. Guidelines for establishing a diagnosis of mixed acid-base disorder are discussed in Chapter 12.

MEASUREMENT OF BLOOD GASES

Most blood gas analyzers measure pH and PCO_2. The HCO_3^- concentration is calculated. **Total CO_2 content** is determined by adding a strong acid to plasma or serum and measuring the amount of CO_2 produced according to the following reaction:

$$H^+ + HCO_3^- \rightleftharpoons H_2CO_3 \rightleftharpoons CO_2 + H_2O$$

The term **total CO_2 content** refers to the fact that this method includes both dissolved CO_2 and HCO_3^- present in the sample. As a result, total CO_2 content is greater than HCO_3^- concentration in normal individuals by approximately 1 to 2 mEq/L:

$$\begin{aligned} CO_{2diss} + HCO_3^- &= 0.0301 \times PCO_2 + HCO_3^- \\ &= 0.0301(40) + 24 \\ &= 25.2 \text{ mEq/L} \end{aligned}$$

If a sample to be analyzed for total CO_2 content is handled aerobically, the dissolved CO_2 is released to the atmosphere, and the value obtained is approximately equal to the HCO_3^- concentration.

Total CO_2 concentrations determined by automated chemistry analysis may differ substantially from those obtained by standard blood gas analysis. In one study of normal dogs and cats, factors implicated in this discrepancy included underfilling of blood collection tubes, delays between sampling and analysis, and freshness of laboratory reagents.[31] According to the results of this

TABLE 9-5 Expected Renal and Respiratory Compensations to Primary Acid-Base Disorders in Dogs

Disorder	Primary Change	Compensatory Response
Metabolic acidosis	↓ [HCO_3^-]	0.7-mm Hg decrement in PCO_2 for each 1-mEq/L decrement in [HCO_3^-]
Metabolic alkalosis	↑ [HCO_3^-]	0.7-mm Hg increment in PCO_2 for each 1-mEq/L increment in [HCO_3^-]
Acute respiratory acidosis	↑ PCO_2	1.5-mEq/L increment in [HCO_3^-] for each 10-mm Hg increment in PCO_2
Chronic respiratory acidosis	↑ PCO_2	3.5-mEq/L increment in [HCO_3^-] for each 10-mm Hg increment in PCO_2
Acute respiratory alkalosis	↓ PCO_2	2.5-mEq/L decrement in [HCO_3^-] for each 10-mm Hg decrement in PCO_2
Chronic respiratory alkalosis	↓ PCO_2	5.5-mEq/L decrement in [HCO_3^-] for each 10-mm Hg decrement in PCO_2

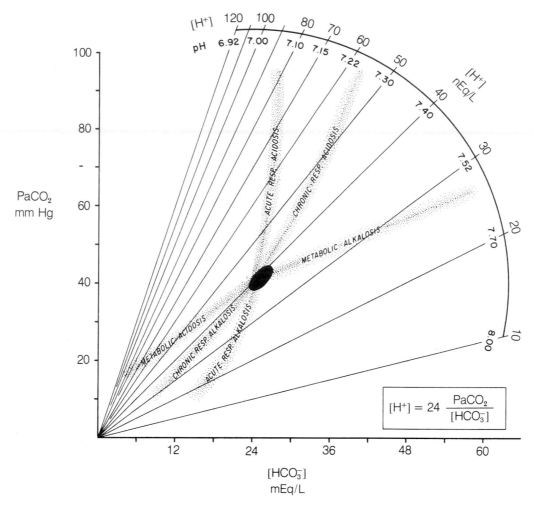

Fig. 9-4 Acid-base map or template. The shaded areas exemplify the ranges of $PaCO_2$-bicarbonate relationships characteristic of graded degrees of simple acid-base disorders. (From Harrington JT, Cohen JJ, Kassirer JP: Introduction to the clinical acid-base disturbances. In Cohen JJ, Kassirer JP, editors: *Acid-base,* Boston, 1982, Little, Brown & Co., p. 379.)

study, values for total CO_2 obtained by routine blood gas analysis may be up to 5 mmol/L higher than those obtained by automated analysis. Another study comparing total CO_2 measurement by three different methods (radiometer blood gas analyzer, Coulter DACOS analyzer [Beckman Coulter, Fullerton, CA], and Kodak Ektachem DTE analyzer [Eastman Kodak, Rochester, NY]) found lower than expected agreement among the different methods of analysis.[32] In this study, sample storage for 7 hours resulted in a decrease of approximately 2 mmol/L in total CO_2 concentration.

CO_2 combining power is the total CO_2 content of a plasma sample that has been equilibrated in vitro at 37° C with CO_2 at a partial pressure of 40 mm Hg. This method overestimates total CO_2 content when the patient's PCO_2 is less than 40 mm Hg and underestimates total CO_2 content when the patient's PCO_2 is more than 40 mm Hg. It is no longer commonly used in clinical medicine.

Standard bicarbonate is the concentration of bicarbonate in the plasma of fully oxygenated whole blood after equilibration with CO_2 at a partial pressure of 40 mm Hg at 37° C. The **base excess** (BE) is the amount of strong acid or base required to titrate 1 L of blood to pH 7.40 at 37° C while PCO_2 is held constant at 40 mm Hg.[5,6,59] It usually is derived from the Siggaard-Andersen alignment nomogram using measurements of pH, PCO_2, and hematocrit. BE is changed only by nonvolatile, or fixed, acids and thus is considered to reflect metabolic acid-base disturbances. In general, a negative value for BE (i.e., a **base deficit**) indicates metabolic acidosis, whereas a positive value indicates metabolic alkalosis.

One problem with the concept of standard bicarbonate is the assumption that the CO_2 titration curve of a whole blood sample is similar to that of the intact organism. This is not true because in the isolated blood sample, all of the buffering of the CO_2 equilibrated with the sample is done by the hemoglobin and other nonbicarbonate buffers in

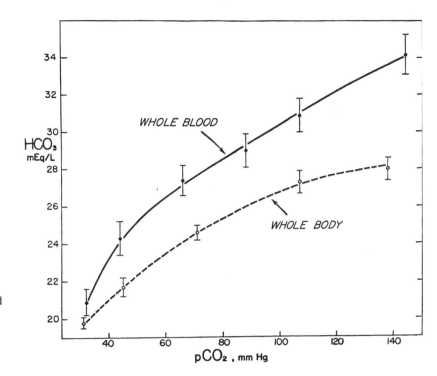

Fig. 9-5 Comparison of the CO_2 titration curves for whole blood and whole body using data derived from the dog. (Reproduced from the *Journal of Clinical Investigation* 43:783, 1964, by copyright permission of the American Society for Clinical Investigation.)

the sample, and the HCO_3^- generated can be distributed only within that sample. In vivo, however, other intracellular buffers are involved, the HCO_3^- produced has a larger volume of distribution, and the observed increase in HCO_3^- concentration would be less (Fig. 9-5).[14] Another problem with standard bicarbonate and BE determinations is that abnormalities of these values do not necessarily imply the presence of a primary metabolic acid-base disturbance. Rather, the change in HCO_3^- concentration may represent the normal adaptive change resulting from renal compensation for a respiratory acid-base disturbance. Debate continues about whether standard bicarbonate and BE are any more useful than bicarbonate in the evaluation of acid-base disturbances.[56,57] Regardless of the approach used, all of the aids devised to facilitate interpretation of blood gas data are merely graphic representations of the classic Henderson-Hasselbalch equation, and there is no substitute for a thorough understanding of the underlying principles of acid-base physiology.[67]

Whole-blood buffer base is the sum of the concentrations of all buffer anions contained in whole blood and includes HCO_3^-, hemoglobin, plasma proteins, phosphates, and any other potential buffer anions.[60] Its normal value is 40 to 50 mEq/L and is similar to Stewart's **strong ion difference** (see Chapter 13).[63,73] Changes in the Pco_2 of the whole blood sample do not change the value of the **whole blood buffer base** because a change in the nonbicarbonate buffers results in a reciprocal change in HCO_3^- concentration. The **whole body buffer base** decreases with metabolic acidosis and increases with metabolic alkalosis, regardless of changes in Pco_2 in the sample.

The calculations of **standard bicarbonate** and **whole blood buffer base** were introduced before the concept of whole body titration was developed[23] and represented an attempt to use in vitro titration of whole blood samples to separate the respiratory and metabolic components of acid-base disturbances. These methods do not account for other buffering effects in the body (e.g., intracellular proteins other than hemoglobin, intracellular organic phosphates, bone carbonate).

SAMPLE COLLECTION AND HANDLING

Proper collection and handling of samples for blood gas analysis are as important as accurate measurement of pH and Pco_2 by the blood gas analyzer.[24] In small animals, arterial samples usually are taken from the femoral artery. This procedure can be performed in unanesthetized dogs with minimal discomfort and restraint but is difficult in unanesthetized cats. Samples for venous blood gas analysis usually are taken from the jugular vein. However, venous stasis and muscular activity can result in accumulation of acid metabolites. Thus an attempt should be made to obtain a free-flowing venous sample by releasing digital pressure on the vein after venipuncture has been achieved.

For femoral artery samples, the hair over the medial thigh is clipped, and the puncture site is disinfected. A 3-mL syringe with a 25-gauge needle is coated with a small amount of heparin (1000 U/mL). Enough heparin is drawn into the syringe to coat the interior of the entire barrel, and air is expelled, leaving the dead space of the syringe filled with heparin. The dead space of 1- to 5-mL syringes is 0.1 to 0.2 mL, and this volume provides more than enough heparin for anticoagulation.[51] Dilution of the sample with heparin should be avoided because it can cause erroneously low values for pH, P_{CO_2}, and HCO_3^-.[25,28,51]

An assistant restrains the dog in lateral recumbency, and the rear limb closest to the table is extended. The artery is located by palpating the femoral pulse and is immobilized beneath the first and second fingers of the operator's free hand. The artery is punctured with the needle directed at an angle approximately perpendicular to the course of the vessel. At least 1.5 mL of blood is withdrawn, and the site of puncture is manually compressed for 3 to 5 minutes after needle withdrawal to prevent hematoma formation. If necessary, air bubbles are dislodged by flicking the barrel of the syringe with the index finger and expelling any air from the hub of the syringe. Usually, the needle is inserted into a rubber stopper to prevent exposure of the sample to room air. A tightly fitting cap placed over the hub of the syringe may be superior.[51] The syringe is rolled between the palms of the hands to mix the sample.

The P_{CO_2} of dry room air is extremely low, and the P_{CO_2} of the blood sample decreases, and its pH increases if it is exposed to air.[51] The P_{O_2} of room air is higher than that of arterial or venous blood, and the P_{O_2} of the sample increases if it is exposed to air. The increase is much greater for venous than arterial blood samples. Air bubbles may also cause an increase in P_{O_2} and a decrease in P_{CO_2} if they occupy 10% or more of the sample volume.

Analysis of the sample within 15 to 30 minutes of collection is desirable. The P_{CO_2} of a blood sample increases and the pH decreases as the sample is allowed to stand before analysis. The rate of change is much greater at 25° C than at 4° C. These changes in P_{CO_2} and pH are accompanied by decreased glucose and increased lactate concentrations and are attributed to glycolysis by white cells, red cells, and platelets. Aerobic metabolism by white cells also decreases P_{O_2}. By cooling the blood sample, these changes are minimized. Therefore if the sample cannot be analyzed soon after collection, the syringe should be immersed in a mixture of ice and water. Samples are stable for up to 2 hours at 4° C, but P_{CO_2} begins to increase and pH to decrease after 20 to 30 minutes at 25° C.[40]

Arterial samples are preferred to venous ones because oxygenation of blood can be evaluated, and the sample is not affected by stasis of blood flow and local tissue metabolism. The most conspicuous difference between arterial and venous samples is the difference in P_{O_2}, which reflects oxygenation of blood in the lungs and utilization in the tissues. Conversely, arterial samples may not reflect the acid-base status in peripheral tissues. This may present a problem during cardiopulmonary resuscitation (see Chapter 10). The P_{CO_2} is slightly higher and the pH is slightly lower in venous samples because of local tissue metabolism. Free-flowing capillary blood that has been "arterialized" by warming the skin punc-

ture site is used as an alternative to arterial samples in human medicine.

Capillary blood obtained from the caudal medial ear margin of unanesthetized dogs had blood gas values similar to those of arterial samples and did not require induction of arteriolar vasodilatation by warming ("arterialization").[52] In a study of cats, arterialized capillary blood was obtained from the cut claw after previously warming the paw.[62] In this study, mean P_{O_2} and P_{CO_2} did not differ from those of arterial blood, but mean pH was significantly higher (7.432 versus 7.419). Capillary blood is collected directly into a heparinized capillary tube; a small metal "flea" is added for mixing; and the ends of the tube are sealed with clay. During states of peripheral vascular collapse (e.g., hypovolemic shock), capillary blood does not provide meaningful blood gas values for comparison with those of arterial samples.[52,70]

NORMAL VALUES

Normal blood gas values for dogs and cats should be established with the laboratory performing the analysis. Extreme care must be taken in obtaining blood samples to establish a normal range because hyperventilation related to fear or pain, increased muscular activity related to struggling, and delays during sample transport and analysis may have effects on the resulting normal range. A review of previously published data provided the following guidelines for normal arterial blood gas values in dogs and cats[26]:

	Dog	**Cat**
pH	7.407 (7.351-7.463)	7.386 (7.310-7.462)
P_{CO_2} (mm Hg)	36.8 (30.8-42.8)	31.0 (25.2-36.8)
HCO_3^- (mEq/L)	22.2 (18.8-25.6)	18.0 (14.4-21.6)
P_{O_2} (mm Hg)	92.1 (80.9-103.3)	106.8 (95.4-118.2)

Studies of normal unanesthetized dogs yielded venous blood gas results as follows: pH 7.397 (7.351 to 7.443), P_{CO_2} 37.4 (33.6 to 41.2) mm Hg, and HCO_3^- 22.5 (20.8 to 24.2) mEq/L.[52,74] In one of these studies, venous P_{O_2} values were reported to be 52.1 (47.9 to 56.3) mm Hg.[52] Studies of normal unanesthetized cats indicated venous blood gas values as follows: pH 7.343 (7.277 to 7.409), P_{CO_2} 38.7 (32.7 to 44.7) mm Hg, and HCO_3^- 20.6 (18.0 to 23.2) mEq/L.[11,27,46]

When sampling sites were compared using unanesthetized normal dogs, blood gas data from three different venous sites (jugular vein, pulmonary artery, and cephalic vein) were similar, but P_{CO_2} was higher and pH was lower when venous data were compared with results obtained for the carotid artery.[30] The respiratory compensation for metabolic acidosis in these dogs ranged from a 1.1- to 1.3-mm Hg decrement in P_{CO_2} for each 1-mEq/L decrement in HCO_3^-, whereas the respiratory compensation for metabolic alkalosis ranged from a 0.4- to 0.6-mm Hg increment in P_{CO_2} for each 1-mEq/L increment in HCO_3^- for arterial, mixed venous, and jugular venous samples. The increment was 1.3 mm Hg per 1-mEq/L increment in HCO_3^- for the cephalic samples, which had the highest PCO_2 values, presumably because they were the only samples not collected under free-flowing conditions. Data for the normal dogs in this study are reproduced in Table 9-6.

Aging in humans has been associated with a decrease in PaO_2 and an increase in the alveolar-to-arterial PO_2 gradient, $P(A - a)O_2$. Mild or no changes in these values were observed in geriatric dogs, and no significant changes in acid-base balance were found in geriatric dogs.[4,33]

INTERPRETATION OF BLOOD GAS DATA

Correct identification of acid-base disturbances may provide a clue to an underlying primary disease process and aids in determining appropriate therapy for the patient. A routine methodical approach to interpretation of blood gas data facilitates the clinician's approach to the patient. The clinician should try to answer the following four questions:

1. Is an acid-base disturbance present?
2. What is the primary disturbance?
3. Is the secondary, or adaptive, response as expected (i.e., is the disturbance simple or mixed)?
4. What underlying disease process(es) is(are) responsible for the acid-base disturbance(s)?

The possibility of an acid-base disturbance should be considered when the history (e.g., vomiting, diarrhea) or the pathophysiology of the patient's disease (e.g., renal failure, diabetes mellitus) is suggestive or when abnormalities in total CO_2 or electrolytes (Na^+, K^+, and Cl^-) are observed in the biochemical profile. Total CO_2 may be increased as a result of metabolic alkalosis or renal adaptation to respiratory acidosis. Total CO_2 may be decreased as a result of metabolic acidosis or renal adaptation to respiratory alkalosis. Thus the acid-base disturbance cannot be classified based on the total CO_2 concentration alone. Objective physical findings suggestive of an acid-base disturbance (e.g., hyperventilation)

are unreliable as indicators of acid-base disturbances and are often not present. Blood gas analysis is required to identify and classify acid-base disorders conclusively.

The clinician should first consider the patient's blood pH. Evaluation of pH often provides the answer to the question of whether an acid-base disturbance is present. If the pH is outside the normal range, an acid-base disturbance is present. If the pH is within the normal range, an acid-base disturbance may or may not be present. If the patient is acidemic and plasma HCO_3^- concentration is decreased, metabolic acidosis is present. If the patient is acidemic and PCO_2 is increased, respiratory acidosis is present. If the patient is alkalemic and plasma HCO_3^- concentration is increased, metabolic alkalosis is present. If the patient is alkalemic and PCO_2 is decreased, respiratory alkalosis is present. These relationships are summarized in Table 9-4. However, complicating acid-base disturbances that would alter pH in the same direction as the primary disturbance cannot be ruled out at this point in the evaluation.

The next step is to calculate the expected compensatory response in the opposing component of the system (e.g., respiratory alkalosis as compensation for metabolic acidosis, metabolic alkalosis as compensation for respiratory acidosis) using the rules of thumb listed in Table 9-5. If the patient's secondary or adaptive response in the compensating component of the system falls within the expected range, a simple acid-base disturbance is probably present. If the adaptive response falls outside the expected range, a mixed disorder may be present (see Chapter 12).

Considering the magnitude of change in pH can help in assessment of mixed disorders. This can be seen by consideration of the Henderson equation:

$$[H^+] = \frac{24 \, PCO_2}{[HCO_3^-]}$$

The effect on extracellular pH of a mixed disorder is minimized if the disorders change PCO_2 and HCO_3^- in the

TABLE 9-6 Blood Gas and Acid-Base Measurements (Mean ± Standard Deviation) in Five Normal Unanesthetized Dogs

Value	Arterial	Mixed Venous	Jugular Venous	Cephalic Venous
pH (U)	7.395 ± 0.028	7.361 ± 0.021	7.352 ± 0.023	7.360 ± 0.022
PCO_2 (mm Hg)	36.8 ± 2.7	43.1 ± 3.6	42.1 ± 4.4	43.0 ± 3.2
PO_2 (mm Hg)	102.1 ± 6.8	53.1 ± 9.9	55.0 ± 9.6	58.4 ± 8.8
HCO_3^- (mEq/L)	21.4 ± 1.6	23.0 ± 1.6	22.1 ± 2.0	23.0 ± 1.4
TCO_2 (mEq/L)	22.4 ± 1.8	24.1 ± 1.7	23.2 ± 2.1	24.1 ± 1.4
BE (mEq/L)	−1.8 ± 1.6	−1.1 ± 1.4	−2.1 ± 1.7	−1.2 ± 1.1
$SHCO_3^-$ (mEq/L)	22.8 ± 1.3	23.0 ± 1.2	22.2 ± 1.3	23.2 ± 1.1

From Ilkiw JE, Rose RJ, Martin ICA: A comparison of simultaneously collected arterial, mixed venous, jugular venous and cephalic venous blood samples in the assessment of blood gas and acid base status in dogs, J Vet Intern Med 5:294, 1991.
BE, *Base excess;* $SHCO_3^-$, *standard bicarbonate.*

TABLE 9-7 Approximate Concentrations of Cations and Anions in Plasma in Normal Dogs and Cats (mEq/L)

Cations	Dog	Cat	Anions	Dog	Cat
Sodium	145	155	Chloride	110	120
Potassium	4	4	Bicarbonate	21	21
Calcium	5	5	Phosphate	2	2
Magnesium	2	2	Sulfate	2	2
Trace elements	1	1	Lactate	2	2
			Other organic acids	4	6
			Protein	16	14
Total:	157	167		157	167

same direction (e.g., respiratory acidosis and metabolic alkalosis) and is maximized if the disorders change PCO_2 and HCO_3^- in opposite directions (e.g., respiratory acidosis and metabolic acidosis). In the former instance, blood pH may remain within the normal range, whereas in the latter instance, blood pH is markedly abnormal. Mixed acid-base disorders are discussed in detail in Chapter 12.

Once the clinician has classified the disturbance as simple or mixed and has defined the type of disturbance(s) present, an attempt should be made to determine whether the acid-base disturbance(s) is(are) compatible with the patient's history and clinical findings. Examples include metabolic acidosis in renal failure, acute diarrhea, ethylene glycol ingestion, or diabetic ketoacidosis; respiratory acidosis in advanced pulmonary disease; metabolic alkalosis in vomiting of stomach contents or loop diuretic administration; and respiratory alkalosis in pulmonary disease or sepsis. The original interpretation of the blood gas data must be questioned if the acid-base disturbance does not fit the patient's history, clinical findings, and other laboratory data. Diagnostic difficulties are most likely in mild acid-base disturbances with blood gas results still within the normal range, in mixed disturbances with counterbalancing components that result in a pH within the normal range, and in acute, rapidly changing disorders without adequate time for achievement of a compensated steady state.

ANION GAP

The major cations of ECF are sodium, potassium, calcium, and magnesium; the major anions are chloride, bicarbonate, plasma proteins, organic acid anions (including lactate), phosphate, and sulfate. The approximate charge contributions of these ions in dogs and cats are listed in Table 9-7. Automated clinical chemistry analyzers provide values for serum sodium, potassium, chloride, and total CO_2 concentrations. Thus the sum of the concentrations of commonly measured cations exceeds the sum of the concentrations of commonly measured anions, and the difference has been called the **anion gap**[18,47]:

$$(Na^+ + K^+) - (Cl^- + HCO_3^-)$$

The serum concentration of potassium varies little, and its charge contribution is small compared with that of sodium. Therefore the anion gap often is defined as:

$$Na^+ - (Cl^- + HCO_3^-)$$

From several reported studies, the normal anion gap calculated as $(Na^+ + K^+) - (Cl^- + HCO_3^-)$ is approximately 12 to 24 mEq/L in dogs* and 13 to 27 mEq/L in cats.[7,11-13] In one study, the anion gap was significantly increased in aged dogs compared with young dogs (16.7 ± 0.7 versus 14.3 ± 0.8 mEq/L). The increase in anion gap was attributed to a slight decrease in serum chloride concentration that was balanced by an increase in the net negative charge associated with plasma proteins and phosphate.[4] In recent studies, the anion gap was calculated to be 18.8 ± 2.9 mEq/L (range, approximately 13 to 25 mEq/L)[16] for dogs and 24.1 ± 3.5 mEq/L (range, approximately 17 to 31 mEq/L) for cats.[45]

In reality, there is no anion gap because the law of electroneutrality must always be satisfied. This can be indicated by including terms for unmeasured cations (UCs) and unmeasured anions (UAs) as follows:

$$Na^+ + K^+ + UC = Cl^- + HCO_3^- + UA$$
$$UA - UC = (Na^+ + K^+) - (Cl^- + HCO_3^-)$$

Thus the anion gap is the difference between UAs and UCs and may be affected by changes in the concentration of either component. However, the magnitude of change in the concentration of any of the UCs (e.g., calcium, magnesium) necessary to cause an appreciable change in the anion gap would probably be incompatible with life.[19] As a result, most discussions of the anion gap focus on changes in UAs.

---

*References 1,8,34,36,39,50,58.

Normally, plasma proteins contribute the majority of UA charge in mEq/L.[35] In humans, albumin contributes 2.0 to 2.8 mEq/L for each gram per deciliter, and globulins contribute 1.3 to 1.9 mEq/L for each gram per deciliter.[19] For each 0.1-U increment in pH, there is an approximate 0.1-mEq/L increase in negative charge on plasma proteins.[19,35,69,71] In dogs, net plasma protein charge at a pH of 7.40 is 16 mEq/L and anion gap is approximately 19 mEq/L, and at a pH of 7.40, the anion gap changes 0.42 mEq/L for every 1 g/L change in albumin and 0.25 mEq/L for every 1 g/L change in total plasma proteins.[16]

Increases in anion gap are much more common than decreases, and the concept of anion gap is usually used as an aid in differentiating the causes of metabolic acidosis (see Chapter 10). In organic acidoses (e.g., diabetic ketoacidosis, lactic acidosis), HCO_3^- is titrated by H^+ ions from organic acids. Theoretically, the ECF HCO_3^- concentration should decrease in reciprocal fashion with the increase in concentration of organic acid anions, and the serum chloride concentration should not change (so-called normochloremic metabolic acidosis). The anion gap in this setting should increase proportionately. In practice, however, the decrement in HCO_3^- concentration rarely equals the increment in anion gap for several reasons. For example, buffers other than HCO_3^- are titrated by hydrogen ions from the organic acid; the volume of distribution of the organic anion may differ from that of HCO_3^-; and the prevailing concentration of the organic anion in ECF is affected by its urinary excretion. Furthermore, the patient's HCO_3^- concentration and anion gap before illness are usually not known, and the changes in HCO_3^- concentration and anion gap must by necessity be calculated from available normal values.

The anion gap may be useful in identifying mixed acid-base disturbances. For example, consider a mixed disturbance characterized by metabolic alkalosis and lactic acidosis (e.g., chronic vomiting severe enough to have caused hypotension and impaired tissue perfusion). The pH in such a setting could be normal if HCl loss from the stomach was exactly counterbalanced by accumulation of lactic acid from anaerobic metabolism. A markedly increased anion gap suggests the presence of the complicating organic acidosis. The usefulness of the anion gap in this situation is hampered by the fact that alkalemia itself can cause an increase in the anion gap by several mechanisms.[19,35] Alkalemia results in loss of protons from plasma proteins and an increase in their net negative charge. Hemoconcentration related to volume depletion increases the concentration of plasma proteins and the concentration of their net negative charge. Finally, alkalemia increases lactic acid generation by stimulating phosphofructokinase. The net effect is an increase in the concentration of UAs (lactate and anionic plasma proteins) and an increase in anion gap. The utility of the anion gap concept is considered further in Chapter 12.

Acidosis resulting from administration of NH_4Cl causes a decrease in HCO_3^- concentration because hydrogen ions are released during ureagenesis. There is a reciprocal increase in serum chloride concentration, and as a result, there is no change in the anion gap (so-called hyperchloremic metabolic acidosis). Gastrointestinal loss of HCO_3^- has the same result because the kidney conserves NaCl in response to volume depletion. The use of the anion gap in the classification of metabolic acidosis is considered further in Chapter 10.

A decreased anion gap may be observed in immunoglobin G (IgG) multiple myeloma because the pI of IgG paraproteins is greater than 7.4. Hypoalbuminemia or dilution of plasma proteins by crystalloid infusion can decrease the anion gap by decreasing the concentration of net negative charge associated with plasma proteins. Hypoalbuminemia may be the most common cause of a decreased anion gap, and each 1.0-g/dL decrease in albumin is associated with an approximately 2.4- to 3.0-mEq/L decrease in anion gap.[19,44]

NONTRADITIONAL APPROACH TO ACID-BASE EVALUATION

The traditional approach to acid-base evaluation focuses on the relationship between pH, HCO_3^-, and PCO_2 as described by the Henderson-Hasselbalch equation. In this approach, pH is shown to be a function of HCO_3^- concentration and PCO_2. The PCO_2 is viewed as the **respiratory** component and is determined by alveolar ventilation, whereas the HCO_3^- concentration is considered the **metabolic** (or nonrespiratory) component and is regulated by the kidneys. This approach may lead to the impression that PCO_2 and HCO_3^- are independent variables. In reality, only PCO_2 is independent. When a primary increase in PCO_2 occurs, proteins (notably hemoglobin) buffer the hydrogen ions that are produced by dissociation of H_2CO_3, and the HCO_3^- concentration increases secondarily. Furthermore, an understanding of the effects of changes in other electrolytes (e.g., Na^+, K^+, Cl^-) and plasma proteins on acid-base balance is not facilitated by the traditional approach. The nontraditional approach allows the clinician to better understand the complexity of the acid-base disturbances in some patients.

Stewart formulated a model of acid-base chemistry in biologic systems governed by three physical laws: (1) maintenance of electroneutrality; (2) satisfaction of dissociation equilibria for incompletely dissociated solutes; and (3) conservation of mass.[63,64] The equations that satisfy these laws were solved simultaneously to identify variables that control [H^+]. Independent variables are those that may be altered from outside the system, whereas dependent variables are internal to the system and change only in response to changes in independent variables. Simultaneous solution of Stewart's equations identified three independent variables: strong ion difference (SID), the total concentration of weak acid (HA + A^-) or $[A_{tot}]$, and PCO_2.

The SID changes if the difference between the sum of strong cations and the sum of strong anions changes. Ions are considered strong if they are almost completely dissociated at the pH of body fluids. The strong cations consist of sodium, potassium, calcium, and magnesium. Of these, only Na^+ is present at high enough concentration in ECF that a change in its concentration is likely to have a substantial effect on SID. The strong anions consist of chloride and several other anions that are not routinely measured clinically, and they collectively are referred to as **unmeasured** strong anions (e.g., lactate, acetoacetate, β-hydroxybutyrate, sulfate). Chloride and some unmeasured strong anions can be sufficiently altered in certain disease states to have a substantial effect on SID. The average concentrations of all cations and anions in the plasma of normal dogs and cats are presented in Table 9-7.

The weak anions in ECF are HCO_3^-, plasma proteins, and phosphate. Of these, plasma proteins and phosphate constitute the independent variable A_{tot}, whereas HCO_3^- is a dependent variable. Hypoproteinemia has been shown to be associated with metabolic alkalosis in critically ill human patients in whom a decrease in serum albumin concentration of 1 g/dL caused an increase in standard BE of +3.7 mEq/L.[44] Serum phosphorus concentration (normally approximately 2 mEq/L) cannot decrease enough to cause alkalosis, but hyperphosphatemia in patients with renal failure can make a substantial contribution to A_{tot} and metabolic acidosis. The nontraditional approach to acid-base evaluation is considered in detail in Chapter 13.

CONCEPT OF EXTERNAL HYDROGEN ION BALANCE

External balance for hydrogen ions is maintained by renal excretion of a number of hydrogen ions equal to that consumed in the diet and produced each day by metabolic processes. The majority of hydrogen ions originate from metabolic processes, and little fixed acid originates as such from the diet. A small amount of base is lost each day from the gastrointestinal tract (primarily as organic anions), and this is equivalent to a gain of fixed acid. These processes result in a net daily gain of 50 to 100 mEq of hydrogen ions. Bicarbonate ions that have been titrated by these hydrogen ions must be regenerated. The kidney is the only **regulated** route for H^+ loss from the body.

Metabolic processes that convert cationic compounds to neutral products generate hydrogen ions, whereas those that convert anionic compounds to neutral products consume hydrogen ions.[15,22,72] The main sources of

acid are oxidation of the sulfur-containing (e.g., cysteine, methionine) and cationic (e.g., lysine, arginine) amino acids and hydrolysis of organic phosphate diesters, such as phospholipids and nucleic acids. Oxidation of the sulfur-containing amino acids is the major source of acid produced each day:

$$C_5H_{11}O_2NS \text{ (methionine)} + 7\tfrac{1}{2}O_2 \rightarrow$$
$$\tfrac{1}{2}CH_4ON_2 \text{ (urea)} + 4\tfrac{1}{2}CO_2 + 3\tfrac{1}{2}H_2O + SO_4^{2-} + 2H^+$$
$$C_3H_7O_2NS \text{ (cysteine)} + 5\tfrac{1}{2}O_2 \rightarrow$$
$$\tfrac{1}{2}CH_4ON_2 \text{ (urea)} + 2\tfrac{1}{2}CO_2 + 1\tfrac{1}{2}H_2O + SO_4^{2-} + 2H^+$$

The main sources of base are metabolism of anionic amino acids (e.g., glutamate, aspartate) and the oxidation or utilization for gluconeogenesis of other organic anions (e.g., lactate, citrate).

WHOLE-BODY REGULATION OF ACID-BASE BALANCE

Acid-base balance requires the cooperation of three major organs: liver, kidneys, and lungs. By the process of alveolar ventilation, the lungs remove the tremendous amount of volatile acid (10,000 to 15,000 mmol CO_2) produced each day by metabolic processes. The liver metabolizes amino acids derived from protein catabolism to glucose or triglyceride and releases NH_4^+ in the process. When urea is synthesized in the liver from NH_4^+ and CO_2, H^+ is produced and HCO_3^- is titrated. Consequently, the liver produces much of the fixed or nonvolatile acid that must be excreted each day. The kidneys excrete NH_4^+ in the urine, thus diverting it from ureagenesis and producing a net gain of HCO_3^- and net loss of H^+.

RENAL REGULATION OF ACID-BASE BALANCE

The kidneys maintain normal ECF HCO_3^- concentration by reabsorbing virtually all filtered HCO_3^- and by regenerating HCO_3^- that has been titrated during the daily endogenous production of fixed, or nonvolatile, acid. The latter process is accomplished by excretion of **titratable acidity** (primarily phosphate salts) and **ammonium** salts. The term **net acid excretion** is defined as the sum of titratable acidity and ammonium minus HCO_3^- in the urine. Normally, there is a negligible amount of HCO_3^- in urine.

All three of the functions described above are accomplished by renal tubular secretion of H^+. Hydrogen ion secretion occurs by means of a luminal Na^+-H^+ antiporter in the proximal tubules and loop of Henle and by a luminal H^+-adenosinetriphosphatase (H^+-ATPase) in all H^+-secreting tubular segments. The H^+,K^+-ATPase found in the luminal membranes of the type A interca-

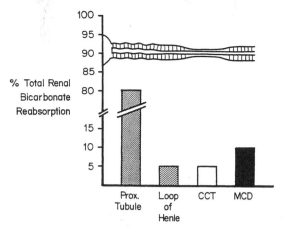

Fig. 9-6 Segmental reabsorption of bicarbonate along the nephron. The major portion of filtered bicarbonate is reabsorbed proximally. Fine-tuning of bicarbonate reabsorption occurs in distal nephron segments, including the medullary and cortical collecting ducts, as well as the thick ascending limb of Henle's loop. (From Kokko JP, Tannen RL: *Fluids and electrolytes*, ed 3, Philadelphia, 1996, WB Saunders, p. 208.)

lated cells of the collecting ducts is quantitatively less important for H^+ secretion but mediates K^+ reabsorption. These transport mechanisms depend on the presence of carbonic anhydrase in tubular cells. Of the filtered HCO_3^-, 90% to 95% is reabsorbed in the first portion of the proximal tubule, and 5% to 10% is reabsorbed in the loop of Henle, distal tubule, and collecting duct (Fig. 9-6).

If secreted H^+ titrates filtered HCO_3^-, HCO_3^- is effectively reabsorbed because one HCO_3^- is added to ECF for each filtered HCO_3^- titrated by a secreted H^+ (Fig. 9-7). This process occurs primarily in the proximal tubules. Net acid excretion and generation of "new" HCO_3^- occur whenever secreted H^+ titrates phosphate in tubular fluid or whenever NH_4^+ is excreted in the urine with Cl^- or in exchange for Na^+ (Figs. 9-8 and 9-9). These processes occur primarily in the distal nephron.

FACTORS AFFECTING RENAL BICARBONATE REABSORPTION

If the glomerular filtration rate (GFR) and ECF volume (ECFV) are constant, the amount of HCO_3^- reabsorbed by the kidneys is equal to the filtered load. Under these conditions, HCO_3^- appears to have a tubular maximum (T_M) of approximately 3 mEq/min and a renal threshold of 25 mEq/L. However, renal reabsorption of HCO_3^- is closely tied to reabsorption of sodium and defense of ECFV. A primary expansion of ECFV leads to natriuresis and a transient decrease in renal HCO_3^- reabsorption. Contraction of the ECFV increases renal tubular reabsorption of sodium and HCO_3^-. When hypovolemia is induced experimentally, renal HCO_3^- reabsorption continues to increase even at extremely high plasma HCO_3^- concentrations.[43,61] Thus the **apparent** T_M for HCO_3^- changes depending on renal sodium avidity, being increased during volume depletion and decreased during volume expansion.

The anionic composition of glomerular ultrafiltrate determines, to a large extent, the effect that sodium

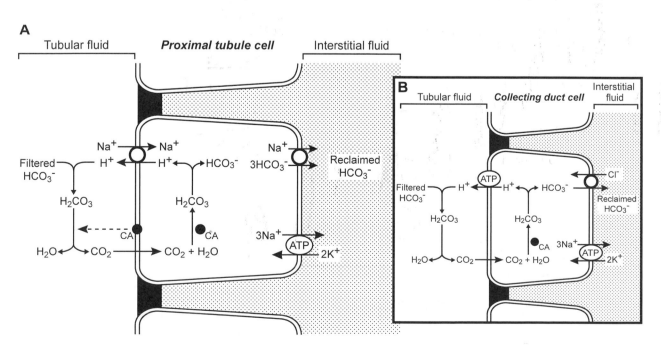

Fig. 9-7 A and **B,** Reabsorption of filtered HCO_3^- by H^+ ion secretion in the proximal tubule. *CA,* Carbonic anhydrase. (Drawing by Tim Vojt.)

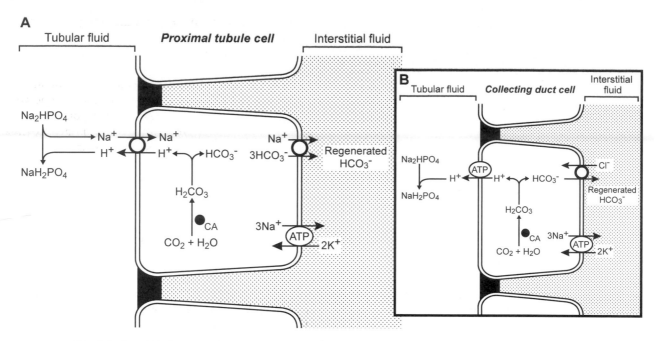

Fig. 9-8 A and **B,** Regeneration of new HCO_3^- by titration of phosphate by secreted H^+ ion in renal tubule. *CA,* Carbonic anhydrase. (Drawing by Tim Vojt.)

avidity has on the electrolyte composition of the reabsorbed tubular fluid. If an adequate amount of chloride is present in the filtrate, the kidney reabsorbs chloride with sodium, and alkalosis does not develop. If there is insufficient chloride in the filtrate, however, sodium is reabsorbed with HCO_3^-, and alkalosis develops. The prevailing acid-base status of the ECF can be viewed as a consequence of factors governing sodium and chloride reabsorption in the kidney.[54] At a given rate of renal sodium reabsorption, a change in the reabsorption of either Cl^- or HCO_3^- must be accompanied by a reciprocal change in reabsorption of the other anion.

Renal HCO_3^- reabsorption is increased by an increase in arterial Pco_2 and decreased by a decrease in arterial

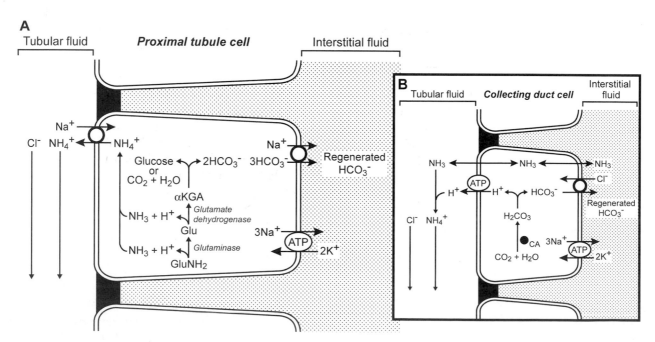

Fig. 9-9 A and **B,** Regeneration of new HCO_3^- by ammonium excretion in renal tubules. *CA,* Carbonic anhydrase. (Drawing by Tim Vojt.)

P_{CO_2}. This effect may be mediated by a decrease (or increase) in pH within renal tubular cells and increased (or decreased) availability of H^+ for secretion. There is an inverse relationship between serum chloride concentration and the rate of renal HCO_3^- reabsorption that results from the requirement for electroneutrality during sodium reabsorption (see preceding paragraph). When serum chloride concentration is reduced, the filtered load of chloride decreases, and the kidneys reabsorb more sodium with HCO_3^-. When serum chloride concentration is increased, the filtered load of chloride increases, and the kidneys reabsorb more sodium with chloride and less with HCO_3^-. The fact that chloride and HCO_3^- are the only important resorbable anions in tubular fluid is important in understanding the pathophysiology of chloride-responsive metabolic alkalosis (see Chapters 4 and 10).

Hyperkalemia is associated with decreased renal HCO_3^- reabsorption in the distal nephron, and hypokalemia is associated with increased HCO_3^- reabsorption. During hypokalemia, transcellular shifting of potassium ions out of renal tubular cells into ECF occurs in exchange for hydrogen ions. This results in greater availability of H^+ for secretion by the tubular cells. When H^+ is secreted into tubular fluid, HCO_3^- is added to ECF. The opposite effect occurs with hyperkalemia, and there are fewer hydrogen ions in tubular cells available for secretion into tubular fluid. Aldosterone increases HCO_3^- reabsorption in the collecting ducts directly by stimulating the luminal H^+-ATPase responsible for H^+ secretion and indirectly by increasing lumen electronegativity by enhancement of sodium reabsorption.

TITRATABLE ACIDITY

Titratable acidity refers to the amount of strong base needed to titrate a 24-hour urine sample back to a pH of 7.40 and represents the amount of H^+ excreted in the urine in combination with weak acid anions, primarily phosphate. When urine pH is very low (e.g., 5.0 to 5.5), other weak acids such as creatinine ($pK_a = 5.0$) and urate ($pK_a = 5.8$) contribute to titratable acidity. Frequently, however, the term titratable acidity is considered synonymous with urinary phosphate ($pK_a = 6.8$). Of the daily 50 to 100 mEq of fixed or nonvolatile acid produced by metabolic processes, approximately 20 to 40 mEq (40%) is excreted as titratable acidity.

The pK_a of a weak acid is the pH at which one half of the buffer is in the salt and one half in the acid form (i.e., the ratio of salt to acid is 1.0), and buffers are most effective within 1.0 pH unit of their pK_a. Phosphate is a very effective urinary buffer because its pK_a (6.8) falls between the pH of distal tubular fluid (6.0) and that of glomerular filtrate (7.4). The amount of phosphate available for buffering tubular fluid is the product of serum phosphorus concentration and GFR (i.e., the filtered load of phosphate). The filtered load of phosphate is relatively constant in a normal individual in phosphorus balance.

AMMONIUM EXCRETION

Excretion of ammonium by the kidney is essential for eliminating the daily fixed acid load and regenerating titrated bicarbonate. Most of the ammonium to be excreted is produced from glutamine in the proximal tubule by action of the enzyme glutaminase[20,21]:

(1) glutamine $\rightarrow$ α-ketoglutarate^{2-} + $2NH_4^+$
(2) α-ketoglutarate^{2-} + $2H^+$ $\rightarrow$ CO_2 + H_2O (oxidation)
or
α-ketoglutarate^{2-} + $2H^+$ $\rightarrow$ glucose (gluconeogenesis)
(3) $2NH_4^+$ + CO_2 $\rightarrow$ urea + $2H^+$ (urea cycle)

It can be seen from these reactions that two H^+ are consumed when the α-ketoglutarate produced from glutamine is either oxidized or converted to glucose. This results in the simultaneous generation of two new bicarbonate ions. If the liver uses an equal number of ammonium ions for urea synthesis, two H^+ are produced, two HCO_3^- are titrated, and there is no net gain of HCO_3^-. If the NH_4^+ is excreted in the urine along with Cl^- or in exchange for Na^+, however, a net gain of HCO_3^- occurs.

The classical theory of ammonium excretion by the kidney suggests that NH_3 diffuses passively through the luminal membrane of the tubular cell into tubular fluid. Hydrogen ions derived from the dissociation of carbonic acid could then combine with NH_3 to form NH_4^+ because the pK_a for this reaction is 9.2. In the pH range of tubular fluid (6.0 to 7.0), only 0.1% to 1% of this buffer pair would exist as NH_3. Thus the associated H^+ is strongly attached to NH_3 by forming NH_4^+ and does not affect urine pH (Fig. 9-10).

The classical theory of ammonium excretion by the kidney was based on diffusion trapping of NH_3 in tubular fluid. According to this theory, the lipid-soluble, nonionized NH_3 diffuses passively into tubular fluid, where it is trapped by combination with H^+ to form less permeant NH_4^+. This theory dictates that diffusion equilibrium occurs for NH_3 and that renal tubular cells do not transport NH_4^+. These assumptions have been questioned.[20]

Several renal transport mechanisms contribute to the ultimate appearance of NH_4^+ in urine. Ammonium arises from the metabolism of glutamine and glutamate, primarily in the proximal tubules. The ammonium ions that are produced substitute for H^+ on the luminal Na^+/H^+ antiporter and are secreted into the tubular lumen. When the α-ketoglutarate resulting from the deamination of glutamine and glutamate is metabolized either to CO_2 and H_2O via the Krebs cycle or to glucose via glycolysis, there is a net gain of $2HCO_3^-$, and these "regenerated" bicarbonate ions are returned to the interstitial fluid via a basolateral $3HCO_3^-/Na^+$ cotransporter. The

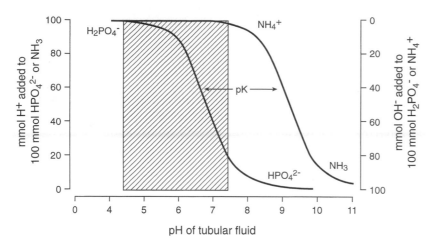

Fig. 9-10 Explanation of how NH_4^+ excretion allows removal of acid without affecting urine pH. (Drawing by Tim Vojt.)

secreted NH_4^+ travels down the lumen of the descending limb of Henle's loop and is reabsorbed in the thick ascending limb by substituting for K^+ in the luminal Na^+-K^+-$2Cl^-$ cotransporter in this nephron segment. The cytoplasm of the tubular cells has a higher pH than the tubular fluid, which allows some NH_3 to form that then can diffuse across the basolateral membranes into the medullary interstitium where it reaches a high concentration. The NH_3 does not escape back across the luminal membranes into the tubular fluid because the luminal membranes of the thick ascending limb are impermeable to NH_3. The interstitial NH_3 then diffuses into segments of the nephron that lack luminal carbonic anhydrase and consequently have the lowest luminal pH (i.e., the S3 segment of the proximal tubule, the cortical collecting duct, and most of the medullary collecting duct). In these segments, the low luminal pH facilitates trapping of NH_3 in the lumen as NH_4^+. In the S3 segment of the proximal tubule, the NH_4^+ that is formed is reabsorbed (i.e., recycled) in the thick ascending limb of Henle's loop. The cell membranes of the collecting ducts are highly permeable to NH_3 (but not NH_4^+), which facilitates diffusion of interstitial NH_3 across the basolateral membranes into the cells and across the luminal membranes into the tubular fluid where it is trapped as NH_4^+. The NH_4^+ trapped in the collecting ducts is excreted in the urine and represents a major avenue for elimination of hydrogen ions from the body and for regenerating titrated bicarbonate ions.

The ability of the kidneys to excrete an acid load despite their inability to reduce urine pH below 5.0 (in dogs and cats) is explained by the high pK_a (9.2) of the NH_3-NH_4^+ buffer pair[68] (see Fig. 9-10). In the normal animal, 30 to 60 of the 50 to 100 (60%) mEq of the fixed or nonvolatile acid produced each day is excreted in the urine as ammonium, either as the chloride salt or in exchange for sodium. The more acidic the urine, the greater the proportion of ammonium that exists as NH_4^+. The kidney can also increase its production of ammonium from glutamine during acidosis. At any given urine pH, the rate of ammonium salt excretion is higher in the presence of acidosis,[68] and renal ammonium excretion can increase five- to ten-fold (from basal ammonium excretion of 30 to 60 mEq to as much as 300 mEq per day) in response to chronic metabolic acidosis (Fig. 9-11).

POTASSIUM AND ACID-BASE BALANCE

The distribution of potassium ions between intracellular fluid and ECF may be affected by acid-base disorders. When HCl was infused acutely into nephrectomized dogs, approximately 50% of the H^+ load was buffered intracellularly.[55,65] Intracellular sodium and potassium ions entered ECF in exchange for the H^+ entering cells, and serum potassium concentration increased. These early animal studies and observations in a small number of human patients[10] led to the prediction that metabolic acidosis would be associated with a 0.6-mEq/L increase in serum potassium concentration for each 0.1-U decrease in pH. A review of animal studies demonstrated that the change in serum potassium concentration observed during acute metabolic acidosis caused by mineral acids (e.g., HCl, NH_4Cl) was variable.[3] Furthermore, an increase in serum potassium concentration does not occur in acute metabolic acidosis caused by organic acids (e.g., lactic acid, ketoacids).* Acute infusion of β-hydroxybutyrate in normal dogs caused an increase in insulin in portal venous blood and hypokalemia, presumably as a result of potassium uptake by cells.[2] Acute infusion of HCl led to hyperkalemia and increased portal vein glucagon concentration.[2] These acute changes in serum potassium concentration are not the result of changes in renal excretion of potassium.[2,49]

The hyperkalemia associated with acute metabolic acidosis caused by mineral acids is transient. In a study of

---

References 2,3,29,48,49,66.

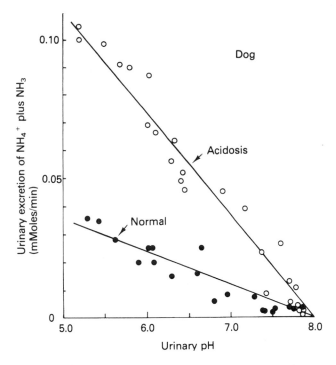

Fig. 9-11 Effect of acidosis on urinary ammonium excretion. (From Valtin H: *Renal function: mechanisms preserving fluid and solute balance in health*, Boston, 1983, Little, Brown & Co., p. 238.)

acute and chronic metabolic acidosis induced in dogs by administration of HCl or NH_4Cl, hyperkalemia was observed after acute infusion of HCl, but hypokalemia developed after 3 to 5 days of NH_4Cl administration.[41] The observed hypokalemia was associated with inappropriately high urinary excretion of potassium and increased plasma aldosterone concentration.[41] Similar findings in rats with chronic metabolic acidosis induced by NH_4Cl have been reported.[53] Acute metabolic acidosis induced by administration of mineral acid decreases renal proximal tubular reabsorption of sodium, leading to volume contraction and increased distal delivery of sodium. Increased Na^+-H^+ and Na^+-K^+ exchange then occurs in the distal nephron, mediated by increased distal tubular fluid flow and hyperaldosteronism. These findings suggest that mild hypokalemia and potassium depletion are likely to develop during chronic metabolic acidosis caused by administration of a mineral acid. The observation of hyperkalemia during chronic metabolic acidosis should prompt consideration of impaired renal potassium excretion or some other cause of hyperkalemia (see Chapter 5).

REFERENCES

1. Adrogue HJ, Brensilver J, Madias NE: Changes in the plasma anion gap during chronic metabolic acid-base disturbances, *Am J Physiol* 235:F291, 1978.
2. Adrogue HJ, Chap Z, Ishida T, et al: Role of the endocrine pancreas in the kalemic response to acute meta-bolic acidosis in conscious dogs, *J Clin Invest* 75:798, 1985.
3. Adrogue HJ, Madias NE: Changes in plasma potassium concentration during acute acid base disturbances, *J Clin Invest* 71:456, 1981.
4. Aguilera-Tejero E, Fernandez H, Estepa JC, et al: Arterial blood gases and acid-base balance in geriatric dogs, *Res Vet Sci* 63:253, 1997.
5. Astrup P: New approach to acid-base metabolism, *Clin Chem* 7:1, 1961.
6. Astrup P, Jorgensen K, Siggaard-Andersen O, et al: Acid-base metabolism: new approach, *Lancet* 1:1035, 1960.
7. Atkins CE, Tyler R, Greenlee P: Clinical, biochemical, acid-base, and electrolyte abnormalities in cats after hyper-tonic sodium phosphate enema administration, *Am J Vet Res* 46:980, 1985.
8. Bleich HL, Berkman PM, Schwartz WB: The response of cerebrospinal fluid composition to sustained hypercapnia, *J Clin Invest* 43:11, 1964.
9. Burnell JM: Changes in bone sodium and carbonate in metabolic acidosis and alkalosis in the dog, *J Clin Invest* 50:327, 1971.
10. Burnell JM, Villamil MF, Uyeno BT, et al: The effect in humans of extracellular pH change on the relationship between serum potassium concentration and intracellular potassium, *J Clin Invest* 35:935, 1956.
11. Chew DJ, Leonard M, Muir WW: Effect of sodium bicar-bonate infusion on serum osmolality, electrolyte concen-trations, and blood gas tensions in cats, *Am J Vet Res* 52:12, 1991.
12. Ching SV, Fettman MJ, Harnar DW, et al: The effect of chronic dietary acidification using ammonium chloride on acid-base and mineral metabolism in the adult cat, *J Nutr* 119:902, 1989.
13. Christopher MM, Eckfeld JH, Eaton JW: Propylene glycol ingestion causes D-lactic acidosis, *Lab Invest* 62:114, 1990.
14. Cohen JJ, Brackett NC, Schwartz WB: The nature of the carbon dioxide titration curve in the normal dog, *J Clin Invest* 43:777, 1964.
15. Cohen RM, Feldman GM, Fernandez PC: The balance of acid, base and charge in health and disease, *Kidney Int* 52:287, 1997.
16. Constable PD, Stämpfli HR: Experimental determination of net protein charge and A_{tot} and K_a of nonvolatile buffers in canine plasma, *J Vet Intern Med* 19:507, 2005.
17. Cornelius LM, Rawlings CA: Arterial blood gas and acid base values in dogs with various diseases and signs of dis-ease, *J Am Vet Med Assoc* 178:992, 1981.
18. Emmett M, Narins RG: Clinical use of the anion gap, *Medicine (Baltimore)* 56:38, 1977.
19. Gabow PA: Disorders associated with an altered anion gap, *Kidney Int* 27:472, 1985.
20. Good DW: New concepts in renal ammonium excretion. In Seldin DW, Giebisch G, editors: *The regulation of acid-base balance*, New York, 1989, Raven Press, p. 169.
21. Halperin ML: How much "new" bicarbonate is formed in the distal nephron in the process of net acid excretion? *Kidney Int* 35:1277, 1989.
22. Halperin ML, Jungas RL: Metabolic production and dis-posal of hydrogen ions, *Kidney Int* 24:709, 1983.
23. Harrington JT, Cohen JJ, Kassirer JP: Introduction to the clinical acid-base disturbances. In Cohen JJ, Kassirer JP, editors: *Acid-base*, Boston, 1982, Little, Brown & Co., p. 119.
24. Haskins SC: An overview of acid-base physiology, *J Am Vet Med Assoc* 170:423, 1977.

25. Haskins SC: Sampling and storage of blood for pH and blood gas analysis, *J Am Vet Med Assoc* 170:429, 1977.

26. Haskins SC: Blood gases and acid-base balance: clinical interpretation and therapeutic implications. In Kirk RW, editor: *Current veterinary therapy VIII,* Philadelphia, 1983, WB Saunders, p. 201.

27. Herbert DA, Mitchell RA: Blood gas tensions and acid-base balance in awake cats, *J Appl Physiol* 30:434, 1971.

28. Hutchison AS, Ralston SH, Drybaugh FJ, et al: Too much heparin: possible source of error in blood gas analysis, *BMJ* 287:1131, 1983.

29. Ilkiw JE, Davis PE, Church DB: Hematologic, biochemical, blood gas, and acid base values in greyhounds before and after exercise, *Am J Vet Res* 50:583, 1989.

30. Ilkiw JE, Rose RJ, Martin ICA: A comparison of simultaneously collected arterial, mixed venous, jugular venous and cephalic venous blood samples in the assessment of blood gas and acid base status in dogs, *J Vet Intern Med* 5:294, 1991.

31. James KM, Polzin DJ, Osborne CA, et al: Effects of sample handling on total carbon dioxide concentrations in canine and feline serum and blood, *Am J Vet Res* 58:343, 1997.

32. Kilborn SH, Bonnett BN, Pook HA: Comparison of three different methods of total carbon dioxide measurement, *Vet Clin Pathol* 24:22, 1995.

33. King LG, Anderson JG, Rhodes WH, et al: Arterial blood gas tensions in healthy aged dogs, *Am J Vet Res* 53:1744, 1992.

34. Madias NE, Adrogue JH, Cohen JJ: Effect of natural variations in $PaCO_2$ on plasma HCO_3^- in dogs: a redefinition of normal, *Am J Physiol* 236:F30, 1979.

35. Madias NE, Ayus JC, Adrogue HJ: Increased anion gap in metabolic alkalosis: the role of plasma protein equivalency, *N Engl J Med* 300:1421, 1979.

36. Madias NE, Bossert WH, Adrogue HJ: Ventilatory response to chronic metabolic acidosis and alkalosis in the dog, *J Appl Physiol* 56:1640, 1984.

37. Madias NE, Cohen JJ: Acid-base chemistry and buffering. In Cohen JJ, Kassirer JP, editors: *Acid-base,* Boston, 1982, Little, Brown & Co., p. 13.

38. Madias NE, Cohen JJ: Acid-base chemistry and buffering. In Cohen JJ, Kassirer JP, editors: *Acid-base,* Boston, 1982, Little, Brown & Co., p. 17.

39. Madias NE, Schwartz WB, Cohen JJ: The maladaptive renal response to secondary hypocapnia during chronic HCl acidosis in the dog, *J Clin Invest* 60:1393, 1977.

40. Madiedo G, Sciacca R, Hause L: Air bubbles and temperature effect on blood gas analysis, *J Comp Pathol* 33:864, 1980.

41. Magner PO, Robinson L, Halperin RM, et al: The plasma potassium concentration in metabolic acidosis: a re-evaluation, *Am J Kidney Dis* 11:220, 1988.

42. Malnic G, Giebisch G: Mechanism of renal hydrogen ion secretion, *Kidney Int* 1:280, 1972.

43. Malnic G, Mellow Aires M: Kinetic study of bicarbonate reabsorption in proximal tubule of the rat, *Am J Physiol* 220:1759, 1971.

44. McAuliffe JJ, Lind LJ, Leith DE, et al: Hypoproteinemic alkalosis, *Am J Med* 81:86, 1986.

45. McCullough SM, Constable PD: Calculation of the total plasma concentration of nonvolatile weak acids and the effective dissociation constant of nonvolatile buffers in plasma for use in the strong ion approach to acid-base balance in cats, *Am J Vet Res* 64:1047-1051, 2003.

46. Middleton DJ, Ilkiw JE, Watson ADJ: Arterial and venous blood gas tensions in clinically healthy cats, *Am J Vet Res* 42:1609, 1981.

47. Oh MS, Carrol JH: The anion gap, *N Engl J Med* 297:814, 1977.

48. Oster JR, Perez GO, Castro A, et al: Plasma potassium response to acute metabolic acidosis induced by mineral and nonmineral acids, *Miner Electrolyte Metab* 4:28, 1980.

49. Oster JR, Perez GO, Vaamonde CA: Relationship between blood pH and potassium and phosphorus during acute metabolic acidosis, *Am J Physiol* 235:F345, 1978.

50. Polzin DJ, Stevens JB, Osborne CA: Clinical evaluation of the anion gap in evaluation of acid-base disorders in dogs, *Compend Contin Educ Pract Vet* 4:102, 1982.

51. Pruden EL, Siggaard-Andersen O, Tietz NW: Blood gases and pH. In Burtis CA, Ashwood ER, editors: *Tietz fundamentals of clinical chemistry,* Philadelphia, 1996, WB Saunders, p. 506.

52. Rodkey WG, Hannon JP, Dramise JG, et al: Arterialized capillary blood used to determine the acid-base and blood gas status of dogs, *Am J Vet Res* 39:459, 1978.

53. Scandling JD, Ornt DB: Mechanism of potassium depletion during chronic metabolic acidosis in the rat, *Am J Physiol* 252:F122, 1987.

54. Schwartz WB, Cohen JJ: The nature of the renal response to chronic disorders of acid-base equilibrium, *Am J Med* 64:417, 1978.

55. Schwartz WB, Orning KJ, Porter R: The internal distribution of hydrogen ions with varying degrees of metabolic acidosis, *J Clin Invest* 36:373, 1957.

56. Schwartz WB, Relman AS: A critique of the parameters used in the evaluation of acid-base disorders. "Whole blood buffer base" and "standard bicarbonate" compared with blood pH and plasma bicarbonate concentration, *N Engl J Med* 268:1382, 1963.

57. Severinghaus JW: Siggard-Andersen and the "Great Transatlantic acid-base debate," *Scand J Clin Lab Invest* 54(suppl 214):99, 1993.

58. Shull RM: The value of anion gap and osmolal gap determinations in veterinary medicine, *Vet Clin Pathol* 7:12, 1978.

59. Siggaard-Andersen O, Engel K, Jorgensen K, et al: A micro method for determination of pH, carbon dioxide tension, base excess and standard bicarbonate in capillary blood, *Scand J Clin Lab Invest* 12:172, 1960.

60. Singer RB, Hastings AB: An improved clinical method for the estimation of disturbances of the acid-base balance of human blood, *Medicine (Baltimore)* 27:223, 1948.

61. Slatopolsky E, Hoffsten P, Purkerson M, et al: On the influence of extracellular fluid volume expansion and of uremia on bicarbonate reabsorption in man, *J Clin Invest* 49:988, 1970.

62. Solter PF, Haskins SC, Patz JD: Comparison of PO_2, PCO_2 and pH in blood collected from the femoral artery and a cut claw of cats, *Am J Vet Res* 49:1882, 1988.

63. Stewart PA: *How to understand acid-base,* New York, 1981, Elsevier.

64. Stewart PA: Modern quantitative acid-base chemistry, *Can J Physiol Pharmacol* 61:1444, 1983.

65. Swan RC, Pitts RF: Neutralization of infused acid by nephrectomized dogs, *J Clin Invest* 34:205, 1955.

66. Tobin RB: Varying role of extracellular electrolytes in metabolic acidosis and alkalosis, *Am J Physiol* 195:687, 1958.

67. Valtin H, Gennari FJ: *Acid-base disorders: basic concepts and clinical management,* Boston, 1987, Little, Brown & Co.

68. Valtin H, Schafer JA: *Renal function,* Boston, 1995, Little, Brown & Co.

69. van Leeuwen AM: Net cation equivalency ("base binding power") of the plasma proteins: a study of ion-protein

interaction in human plasma by means of in vivo ultrafiltration and equilibrium dialysis, *Acta Med Scand* 422(suppl):1, 1964.

70. van Sluijs FJ, de Vries HW, de Bruijne JJ, et al: Capillary and venous blood compared with arterial blood in the measurement of acid-base and blood gas status of dogs, *Am J Vet Res* 44:459, 1983.

71. van Slyke DD, Hastings AB, Hiller A, et al: Studies of gas and electrolyte equilibria in blood. XIV. The amounts of alkali bound by serum albumin and globulin, *J Biol Chem* 79:769, 1920.

72. Walser M: Roles of urea production, ammonium excretion, and amino acid oxidation in acid-base balance, *Am J Physiol* 250:F181, 1986.

73. Whitehair KJ, Haskins SC, Whitehair JG, et al: Clinical applications of quantitative acid-base chemistry, *J Vet Intern Med* 9:1, 1995.

74. Zweens J, Frankena H, van Kampen EJ, et al: Ionic composition of arterial and mixed venous plasma in the unanesthetized dog, *Am J Physiol* 233:F412, 1977.

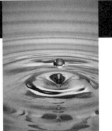

CHAPTER · 10

METABOLIC ACID-BASE DISORDERS

Stephen P. DiBartola

Metabolic disturbances of acid-base balance are associated with many disease states, and identification of the acid-base disturbance may facilitate diagnosis of the underlying disease process. For example, observation of hypochloremic metabolic alkalosis on a serum biochemical profile of a vomiting dog may lead to recognition of gastrointestinal obstruction as the cause. The regulation of normal acid-base balance is considered in detail in Chapter 9.

METABOLIC ACIDOSIS

Metabolic acidosis is characterized by a primary decrease in plasma HCO_3^- concentration, increased $[H^+]$, decreased pH, and a secondary, or adaptive, decrease in P_{CO_2}. In one study, metabolic acidosis was the most common acid-base disturbance in dogs and cats.[53]

Metabolic acidosis can be caused by loss of HCO_3^--rich fluid from the body, addition of fixed acid to the body or its production by metabolism within the body, or failure of renal excretion of fixed acid. Loss of HCO_3^--rich fluid usually occurs via the gastrointestinal tract (e.g., small bowel diarrhea) but also may occur via the kidneys (e.g., carbonic anhydrase inhibitors, proximal renal tubular acidosis). The HCO_3^- concentration of diarrheal fluid exceeds that of plasma, whereas its Cl^- concentration is lower. The loss of such fluid results in a hyperchloremic metabolic acidosis. Examples of the addition of fixed acid to the body include toxins (e.g., ethylene glycol, salicylate) and compounds used therapeutically (e.g., ammonium chloride, cationic amino acids). Examples of metabolic production of fixed acid within the body include lactic acidosis and diabetic ketoacidosis. Renal failure, hypoadrenocorticism, and distal renal tubular acidosis are examples of impaired urinary excretion of fixed acid. Small bowel diarrhea, renal failure, hypoadrenocorticism, diabetic ketoacidosis, and lactic acidosis during cardiovascular collapse are the most common causes of metabolic acidosis in small animal practice.

BODY BUFFER RESPONSE TO AN ACUTE ACID LOAD

When HCl was infused acutely into nephrectomized dogs, approximately 40% of the acid was buffered by extracellular HCO_3^-, 10% by red cell buffers (primarily hemoglobin), and 50% by intracellular buffers of soft tissues and bone (primarily proteins and phosphates).[207] In nonnephrectomized unanesthetized dogs infused intermittently with HCl, intracellular buffers contributed approximately 50% of the buffer response, regardless of the magnitude of the H^+ load.[195] Within a few minutes of an acute fixed acid load, administered H^+ is buffered by HCO_3^- in plasma water. Plasma proteins and phosphates play a minor role in this acute response. Some of the administered acid enters red cells and is buffered by hemoglobin. The CO_2 produced by the combination of the H^+ with HCO_3^- ions is rapidly removed from the body by alveolar ventilation. Within 30 minutes, the acid load has been distributed to the interstitial fluid, where HCO_3^- again plays the dominant role in the acute buffer response. After several hours, H^+ enters intracellular water in exchange for sodium and potassium ions. These hydrogen ions are buffered within cells by proteins and phosphates. In early studies,[195,207] serum potassium concentration increased, but serum sodium concentration decreased after infusion of HCl. The relative roles of these buffers are depicted in Fig. 10-1.

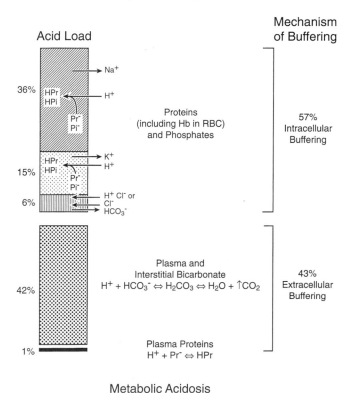

Fig. 10-1 Distribution of buffer response to a fixed acid load. (Drawing by Tim Vojt. Adapted from Pitts RF: *Physiology of the kidney and body fluids*, ed 2, Chicago, 1968, Year Book Medical Publishers, p. 171.)

RESPIRATORY RESPONSE TO AN ACUTE ACID LOAD

A fixed acid load increases $[H^+]$ and thereby stimulates peripheral and central chemoreceptors to increase alveolar ventilation. This effect begins within hours and is complete within 12 to 24 hours. In humans, there is an approximately 1.2-mm Hg reduction in P_{CO_2} for each 1-mEq/L decrement in plasma HCO_3^- concentration to a minimum P_{CO_2} of approximately 10 mm Hg.[88,180] In dogs with uncomplicated metabolic acidosis induced by chronic feeding of HCl, the observed compensatory respiratory response is an approximately 0.7-mm Hg decrement in P_{CO_2} per 1-mEq/L decrement in plasma HCO_3^- concentration.* In these studies, the smallest observed respiratory response was an approximately 0.5-mm Hg decrement in P_{CO_2} per mEq/L decrement in plasma HCO_3^- concentration,[2] and the largest response was a 1.1-mm Hg decrement in P_{CO_2} per mEq/L decrement in plasma HCO_3^- concentration.[58] Data are limited on the respiratory response of cats to metabolic acidosis, but there is some evidence that the cat fails to develop respiratory compensation to the same extent as observed in the dog in spontaneous[219] and NH_4Cl-induced metabolic acidosis.[38,75,123,196,197]

The classical explanation of the respiratory response to metabolic acidosis is that the increase in $[H^+]$ (decrease in pH) stimulates ventilation, and the resultant decrease in P_{CO_2} returns the HCO_3^-/P_{CO_2} ratio and pH toward normal. This is true in acute metabolic acidosis, but the resultant secondary hypocapnia has been observed to decrease plasma HCO_3^- concentration further in chronic metabolic acidosis, presumably by reducing renal HCO_3^- reabsorption. This secondary hypocapnia contributes to 40% of the observed decrease in plasma HCO_3^- concentration during chronic HCl acidosis.[133] Thus chronic metabolic acidosis decreases plasma HCO_3^- concentration by two mechanisms: the effect of the administered HCl on body buffers and a reduction in renal HCO_3^- reabsorption that accompanies secondary hyperventilation. In this study, serum potassium concentration decreased during development of chronic HCl acidosis (contrary to what is typically described for acute metabolic acidosis caused by mineral acids), whereas serum sodium concentration was unchanged.[133]

RENAL RESPONSE TO AN ACUTE ACID LOAD

The role of the kidney is to excrete the fixed acid load imposed by the underlying disease process responsible for metabolic acidosis. The kidney accomplishes this task primarily by augmenting its excretion of NH_4^+. Titratable acidity changes little unless there is a change in the filtered load of phosphate. Chloride ions accompany

---

the NH_4^+ into urine while HCO_3^- is regenerated and reabsorbed into extracellular fluid (ECF) to restore HCO_3^- that was titrated during the acute fixed acid load. Within 48 hours of a fixed acid load, approximately 25% of the added acid has been excreted in the urine, and the remainder is excreted during the next 4 days.[215] The kidney can increase its NH_4^+ excretion as much as five- to ten-fold during chronic metabolic acidosis.[203,218,221] There is some evidence that cats do not adapt to metabolic acidosis by enhanced renal ammoniagenesis.[123] The role of the kidney in regulation of acid-base balance is discussed further in Chapter 9.

CLINICAL FEATURES OF METABOLIC ACIDOSIS

The clinical signs in small animals with metabolic acidosis are more likely to be caused by the underlying disease responsible for metabolic acidosis than by the acidosis itself. In humans, respiratory compensation for metabolic acidosis leads to characteristic hyperventilation, recognized by a deep, rhythmic breathing pattern (i.e., Kussmaul's respirations). Such a characteristic respiratory pattern has not been described in small animal patients, and metabolic acidosis is usually suspected by observation of a low total CO_2 content on a biochemical profile and confirmed by blood gas analysis.

Severe acidosis has serious detrimental effects on cardiovascular function, including decreased cardiac output, decreased arterial blood pressure, and decreased hepatic and renal blood flow.[3] Myocardial contractility is decreased when blood pH falls below 7.20.[147,166] Impaired contractility may result from a decrease in myocardial intracellular pH (pH_i) and displacement of calcium ions from critical binding sites on contractile proteins. Acidosis may predispose the heart to ventricular arrhythmias or ventricular fibrillation. Acidosis has a direct arterial vasodilating effect that is offset by increased release of endogenous catecholamines. However, the inotropic response to catecholamines is impaired, and this may be associated with a reduction in the number of β-adrenergic receptors.[137] Acidosis has a direct vasoconstrictive effect on the venous side of the circulation, which tends to centralize blood volume and predisposes to pulmonary congestion. Acidosis shifts the oxygen-hemoglobin dissociation curve to the right, thus enhancing O_2 release from hemoglobin, but this effect is offset by a decrease in red cell 2,3-diphosphoglycerate, which develops after 6 to 8 hours of acidosis and shifts the curve back to the left.[147]

Acidemia produces insulin resistance that impairs peripheral uptake of glucose and inhibits anaerobic glycolysis by inhibiting phosphofructokinase.[6] During severe acidosis, the liver may be converted from a consumer to a producer of lactate.[130] Severe acidosis also impairs the ability of the brain to regulate its volume, leading to obtundation and coma. Acute mineral acidosis causes hyperkalemia by a transcellular shifting of

potassium from intracellular fluid to ECF in exchange for hydrogen ions. This effect causes a very variable change in serum potassium concentration and is not observed with organic acidosis.[5] Acute reduction in blood pH causes displacement of calcium ions from negatively charged binding sites (e.g., $-COO^-$ groups) on proteins (primarily albumin) as these sites become protonated, and an increase in ionized serum calcium concentration results. Chronic metabolic acidosis leads to release of buffer (mainly calcium carbonate) from bone, and osteodystrophy and hypercalciuria result.

DIAGNOSIS OF METABOLIC ACIDOSIS

Metabolic acidosis is associated with several different diseases and should be considered in any severely ill patient. Often, the diagnosis is first suspected by review of the electrolyte and total CO_2 results on the patient's biochemical profile. It is confirmed by blood gas analysis. The causes of metabolic acidosis may be divided into those associated with a normal anion gap (hyperchloremic metabolic acidosis) and those associated with an increased anion gap (normochloremic metabolic acidosis) (Box 10-1).

Box 10-1 **Causes of Metabolic Acidosis**

Increased Anion Gap (Normochloremic)
Ethylene glycol intoxication
Salicylate intoxication
Other rare intoxications (e.g., paraldehyde, methanol)
Diabetic ketoacidosis*
Uremic acidosis†
Lactic acidosis

Normal Anion Gap (Hyperchloremic)
Diarrhea
Renal tubular acidosis
Carbonic anhydrase inhibitors (e.g., acetazolamide)
Ammonium chloride
Cationic amino acids (e.g., lysine, arginine, histidine)
Posthypocapnic metabolic acidosis
Dilutional acidosis (e.g., rapid administration of 0.9% saline)
Hypoadrenocorticism‡

---

*Patients with diabetic ketoacidosis may have some component of hyperchloremic metabolic acidosis in conjunction with increased anion gap acidosis.[6,8]
†The metabolic acidosis early in renal failure may be hyperchloremic and later convert to typical increased anion gap acidosis.[222]
‡Patients with hypoadrenocorticism typically present with hypochloremia caused by impaired water excretion, absence of aldosterone, impaired renal function, and lactic acidosis. These factors prevent manifestation of hyperchloremia.

The anion gap represents the difference between the commonly measured plasma cations and the commonly measured anions. This concept is discussed in detail in Chapters 9 and 12. The normal electrolyte composition of canine plasma is compared with that in normal (hyperchloremic) and increased (normochloremic) anion gap metabolic acidosis in Fig. 10-2. The anion gap concept is useful in the diagnostic approach to the patient with metabolic acidosis, but it must not be taken literally. In reality, electroneutrality is maintained, and there is no actual anion gap. Normally, the anion gap is made up of the net negative charge on sulfates, phosphates, plasma proteins, and organic anions (e.g., lactate, citrate). Recent studies have shown that in normal dogs and cats, a substantial portion of the anion gap arises from the negative charge on plasma proteins. The net protein charge of plasma at pH 7.40 was calculated to be 16.0 mEq/L in dogs,[52] and this value was determined to be 13.7 mEq/L in cats.[141] Factors other than metabolic acidosis may also affect the value of the anion gap, and these are discussed in Chapter 12.

When the anion gap is calculated as $[(Na^+ + K^+) - (Cl^- + HCO_3^-)]$, normal values in dogs are in the range of 12 to 25 mEq/L.[3,52,176,201] Values for anion gap may be somewhat higher in cats (17 to 31 mEq/L) than in dogs (13 to 25 mEq/L) because of some unaccounted protein and phosphate charge.[52,141] In other studies, the mean anion gap for normal cats (calculated as described above) was approximately 20 mEq/L.[37,40,41] If the observed metabolic acidosis is characterized by a high anion gap, it is assumed to have arisen from an acid that does not contain chloride as its anion. Examples include some inorganic acids (e.g., phosphates, sulfates) or organic acids (e.g., lactate, ketoacids, salicylate, metabolites of ethylene glycol). In this setting, titration of body buffers by the acid results in accumulation of an anion other than chloride. If the observed metabolic acidosis is characterized by a normal anion gap, there is a reciprocal increase in the plasma chloride concentration to balance the decrease in plasma HCO_3^- concentration. In the following discussion, the causes of metabolic acidosis have been divided into those associated with a normal anion gap and those associated with an increased anion gap.

DISORDERS ASSOCIATED WITH A NORMAL ANION GAP

Diarrhea

The concentration of HCO_3^- in intestinal fluid usually is higher than that of plasma, whereas its Cl^- concentration is lower. This results from the addition of alkaline

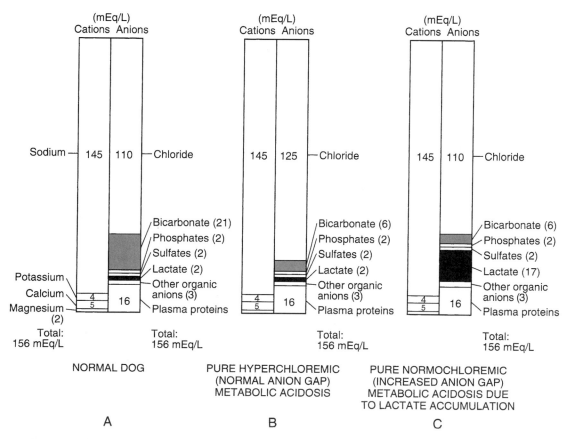

Fig. 10-2 Theoretical examples of electrolyte distribution in **(A)** normal canine plasma, **(B)** a dog with pure hyperchloremic (normal anion gap) metabolic acidosis, and **(C)** a dog with normochloremic (increased anion gap) metabolic acidosis caused by lactate accumulation (i.e., lactic acidosis). (Adapted from Toto RD: Metabolic acid-base disorders. In Kokko JP, Tannen RL, editors: *Fluids and electrolytes*, ed 2, Philadelphia, 1990, WB Saunders, p. 324.)

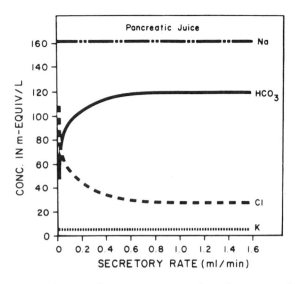

Fig. 10-3 Influence of secretory rate on electrolyte composition of canine pancreatic juice. Note the inverse relationship between Cl^- and HCO_3^- concentrations and the relatively constant concentrations of Na^+ and K^+. (From Cohen JJ, Kassirer JP: *Acid-base.* Boston, 1982, Little, Brown, & Co., p. 135.)

pancreatic and biliary secretions to luminal contents and from secretion of HCO_3^- in exchange for Cl^- in the ileum (Fig. 10 3 and Table 10 1). In some diseases of the small intestine, increased delivery of ileal contents to the colon may overwhelm the considerable capacity of the colon for reabsorption of fluid and electrolytes. As a result, severe acute small bowel diarrhea may cause loss of HCO_3^- in excess of Cl^- with resultant hyperchloremic metabolic acidosis. The acidosis is not purely hyperchloremic but rather is mixed if volume depletion and impaired tissue perfusion lead to lactic acid accumulation.

In one study of 134 dogs with gastroenteritis caused by parvoviral infection, only 13% had low total CO_2 concentrations.[108] In another study of 17 dogs with parvoviral gastroenteritis, 59% had normal pH at presentation.[97] In the animals with abnormal blood gas results, alkalemia (6 of 17) was more common than acidemia (1 of 17). The majority (64%) of the dogs in

this study were presented for both vomiting and diarrhea. Hypochloremia is more common than hyperchloremia in parvoviral gastroenteritis.[97,108] In another study consisting of 25 puppies with parvoviral enteritis, plasma concentrations of sodium, potassium, chloride, and bicarbonate were lower than those of control dogs; however, increases in serum L-lactate concentration were uncommon, and increases in serum D-lactate concentration were not observed.[155] Most dogs in this study had mild compensated metabolic acidosis.

Renal Tubular Acidosis

Renal tubular acidosis (RTA) is characterized by hyperchloremic metabolic acidosis caused by either decreased HCO_3^- reabsorption (proximal RTA) or defective acid excretion (distal RTA) in the presence of a normal glomerular filtration rate (GFR). RTA is uncommonly recognized in small animal practice.

Distal Renal Tubular Acidosis. In distal (**classic** or **type 1**) **RTA,** the urine cannot be maximally acidified because of impaired hydrogen ion secretion in the collecting ducts, and urine pH typically is above 6.0, despite moderately to markedly decreased plasma HCO_3^- concentration. Increased urine pH (>6.0) in the presence of acidosis is the hallmark of distal RTA. Urinary tract infection by a urease-positive organism (e.g., *Proteus* sp., *Staphylococcus aureus*) must be ruled out before considering distal RTA. Urinary net acid excretion is decreased, but bicarbonaturia usually is mild because urinary HCO_3^- concentration is only 1 to 3 mEq/L in the pH range of 6.0 to 6.5. Nephrolithiasis (usually calcium phosphate stones), nephrocalcinosis (resulting from alkaline urine pH and decreased urinary citrate concentration), bone demineralization (resulting from loss of bone buffer stores during chronic acidosis), and urinary potassium wasting with hypokalemia are features of distal RTA in human patients. Mutations in cytosolic carbonic anhydrase, the basolateral Cl^-/HCO_3^- anion exchanger, and luminal H^+-ATPase that affect function of the α-intercalated cells have been associated with inherited forms of distal renal tubular acidosis in humans.[159] Urinary fractional excretion of HCO_3^- is normal (<5%) in distal RTA

TABLE 10-1 Electrolyte Composition of Luminal Fluid at the End of Individual Segments of the Gastrointestinal Tract

Segment End	Na$^+$ (mEq/L)	K$^+$ (mEq/L)	HCO$_3^-$ (mEq/L)	Cl$^-$ (mEq/L)
Duodenum	60	15	15	60
Jejunum	140	6	30	100
Ileum	140	8	70	60
Colon	40	90	30	15*

From Sleisinger MH, Fordtran JS, editors: Gastrointestinal diseases, ed 3, Philadelphia, 1983, WB Saunders, p. 258.
The large anion gap in luminal fluid at the end of the colon is caused by the presence of organic anions resulting from bacterial metabolism. These organic anions represent functional base loss in the stool because they could have been metabolized in the body to yield HCO$_3^-$.

when plasma HCO_3^- concentration is increased to normal by alkali administration.

A diagnosis of distal RTA may be confirmed by an ammonium chloride tolerance test during which urine pH is monitored (using a pH meter) before and at hourly intervals for 5 hours after oral administration of 0.2 g/kg NH_4Cl. Under such conditions, the urine pH of normal dogs decreased to a minimum value of 5.16 at 4 hours after administration of ammonium chloride.[199] Dogs in this study also developed systemic acidosis (pH approximately 7.22 and HCO_3^- approximately 14 mEq/L at 2 hours after ammonium chloride administration). The amount of alkali required to correct the acidosis in human patients with distal RTA is variable but typically less than that required in proximal RTA. The required dosage of alkali in distal RTA may be as little as 1 mEq/kg/day (i.e., that required to offset daily endogenous acid production) or more than 2 to 4 mEq/kg/day. A combination of potassium and sodium citrate (depending on potassium balance) may be the preferred source of alkali.[181]

Proximal Renal Tubular Acidosis. In **proximal (type 2) RTA,** renal reabsorption of HCO_3^- is markedly reduced and urinary fractional excretion of HCO_3^- is increased (>15%) when plasma HCO_3^- concentration is increased to normal. Bicarbonaturia is absent and urine pH is appropriately low when metabolic acidosis is present and plasma HCO_3^- concentration is decreased because distal acidifying ability is intact. When plasma HCO_3^- concentration is decreased, the filtered load of HCO_3^- is reduced, and almost all of the filtered HCO_3^- is reabsorbed in the distal tubules, despite the presence of the proximal tubular defect. Thus proximal RTA can be viewed as a "self-limiting" disorder in which plasma HCO_3^- stabilizes at a lower than normal concentration after the filtered load falls sufficiently that distal HCO_3^- reabsorption can maintain plasma HCO_3^- at a new but lower steady-state concentration. Mutations in renal tubular transport proteins such as the electrogenic basolateral $Na^+/3HCO_3^-$ cotransporter[65] and one of the five forms of the luminal Na^+/H^+ antiporter have been implicated in the pathogenesis of inherited forms of proximal renal tubular acidosis in humans.[105]

Other abnormalities of proximal tubular function typically accompany impaired HCO_3^- reabsorption in proximal RTA, and these include defects in glucose, phosphate, sodium, potassium, uric acid, and amino acid reabsorption. This combination of proximal tubular defects is known as Fanconi's syndrome. Serum potassium concentration usually is normal in affected human patients at the time of diagnosis, but alkali therapy may precipitate hypokalemia and aggravate urinary potassium wasting, presumably by increasing distal delivery of sodium and HCO_3^-.

The diagnosis of proximal RTA is made by finding an acid urine pH (<5.5 to 6.0) in the presence of hyperchloremic metabolic acidosis and normal GFR but an increased urine pH (>6.0) and increased urinary fractional excretion of HCO_3^- (>15%) after plasma HCO_3^- concentration has been increased to normal by alkali administration. If present, the detection of other defects in proximal tubular function (e.g., glucosuria with normal blood glucose concentration) establishes the diagnosis. Correction of metabolic acidosis by alkali therapy is more difficult in proximal RTA than in distal RTA because of the marked bicarbonaturia that occurs when plasma HCO_3^- concentration is increased to normal. Alkali dosages in excess of 10 mEq/kg/day may be required to correct the plasma HCO_3^- concentration, and such therapy may result in frank hypokalemia. Thus potassium citrate may be the preferred source of alkali.

Multiple renal tubular reabsorptive defects resembling Fanconi's syndrome have been reported in young basenji dogs.[23-25,70] Clinical findings included polyuria, polydipsia, weight loss, dehydration, and weakness. Affected dogs had abnormal fractional reabsorption of glucose, bicarbonate, phosphate, sodium, potassium, and urate, and they had isolated cystinuria or generalized aminoaciduria. The renal tubular disorder in affected basenji dogs is thought to be the result of a metabolic or membrane defect affecting sodium movement or increased back leak or cell-to-lumen flux of amino acids. In one study, brush border membranes isolated from basenji dogs with Fanconi's syndrome had decreased sodium-dependent glucose transport but no abnormality of cystine uptake despite the observed reabsorptive defect for cystine.[143] Defective urinary concentrating ability leads to isosthenuria or hyposthenuria, and GFR may be normal initially but decreased later in the course of the disease. Hypokalemia has also been observed late in the course of the disease.[70] Death usually results from acute renal failure and papillary necrosis or acute pyelonephritis. A distinctive renal lesion is hyperchromatic karyomegaly of renal tubular cells.

Fanconi's syndrome has been observed sporadically in other breeds[71,129,142,168,198] and has been reported in association with administration of some drugs.[14,25,146] In one case, Fanconi's syndrome developed in association with primary hypoparathyroidism and resolved after treatment with calcium and calcitriol.[77] Rickets in growing children and osteomalacia in adults are features of Fanconi's syndrome in human patients that usually are not observed in affected dogs. However, congenital Fanconi's syndrome and renal dysplasia were associated with histologic features of rickets in two Border terriers.[56] The skeletal abnormalities in one of the affected dogs resolved after treatment with calcitriol and potassium phosphate. Transient Fanconi's syndrome and proximal renal tubular acidosis also have been reported in a dog with high liver enzyme activities, and toxin exposure was considered as a possible explanation.[103]

In one report, an 8-year-old female German shepherd had hyperchloremic metabolic acidosis, polyuria, polydipsia, isosthenuria, glucosuria with normal blood glucose concentration, and alkaline urine pH (7.46) after oral administration of NH_4Cl.[62] The metabolic acidosis was unresponsive to $NaHCO_3$ administration at dosages up to 4 mEq/kg/day. This dog appeared to have distal (type 1) RTA and renal glucosuria. In another case of apparent distal RTA, a 5-year-old mixed breed dog was presented for evaluation of anorexia and was determined to have alkaline urine pH with hyperchloremic metabolic acidosis.[176] In another report, an 8-year-old female German shepherd was presented for polyuria, polydipsia, weight loss, and lethargy.[21] It had a normal GFR, metabolic acidosis, hyposthenuria, and intermittent glucosuria. Fractional reabsorption of sodium, glucose, and HCO_3^- was decreased, but reabsorption of chloride, phosphate, potassium, urate, and amino acids was normal. The dog gained weight, and its clinical signs were reversed after treatment with $NaHCO_3$ at approximately 10 mEq/kg/day. This dog appeared to have proximal (type 2) RTA.

Distal RTA has been reported in two cats with pyelonephritis caused by *Escherichia coli*.[68,219] Clinical signs included polyuria, polydipsia, anorexia, lethargy, enlarged kidneys, and isosthenuria. In one cat, urine pH was 5.0 at the time pyelonephritis was first diagnosed, but distal RTA was documented at a later time by the presence of hyperchloremic metabolic acidosis, alkaline urine pH, and failure to lower urine pH after oral administration of NH_4Cl.[68] Findings were similar for the other cat, but hyperphosphaturia and persistent hypokalemia also were detected.[219] Distal RTA and hepatic lipidosis were reported in another cat without urinary tract infec-

tion.[26] The clinical features of proximal (type 2) and distal (type 1) RTA are summarized in Table 10-2.

Hyporeninemic hypoaldosteronism, characterized by hyperkalemia with decreased plasma renin and aldosterone concentrations, occurs in some human patients, notably those with diabetes mellitus who also have mild to moderate renal insufficiency.[57] The hyperchloremic metabolic acidosis observed in these patients has been called **type 4 RTA**. This syndrome has not been characterized in veterinary medicine but should be considered in dogs and cats with hyperkalemia and mild to moderate hyperchloremic metabolic acidosis after hypoadrenocorticism has been ruled out by an adrenocorticotropic hormone (ACTH) response test. The diagnosis may be established by finding an inappropriately decreased plasma aldosterone concentration in the presence of hyperkalemia.

Carbonic Anhydrase Inhibitors

Carbonic anhydrase inhibitors, such as acetazolamide, decrease proximal tubular reabsorption of HCO_3^- in the kidney by noncompetitive inhibition of luminal and cellular carbonic anhydrase. Hypokalemia is caused by increased sodium delivery to the distal nephron and its reabsorption there in exchange for potassium. As hyperchloremic metabolic acidosis develops, the filtered load of HCO_3^- decreases and the effect of carbonic anhydrase inhibitors on HCO_3^- reabsorption is limited. Acetazolamide given at 7 to 10 mg/kg three times daily causes self-limiting hyperchloremic metabolic acidosis, mild to moderate hypokalemia, and mild hypocalcemia in dogs.[96,186] The effects of acetazolamide were greatest after 3 days of administration, and blood chemistry results stabilized after 5 days of administration.[186] Acetazolamide is used most commonly in small animal practice for the treatment of glaucoma.

TABLE 10-2   Clinical Features of Proximal and Distal Renal Tubular Acidosis

Clinical Feature	Proximal RTA	Distal RTA
Hypercalciuria	Yes	Yes
Hyperphosphaturia	Yes	Yes
Urinary citrate	Normal	Decreased
Bone disease	Less severe	More severe
Nephrocalcinosis	No	Yes
Nephrolithiasis	No	Yes (calcium phosphate)
Hypokalemia	Mild	Mild to severe
Potassium wasting	Worsened by $NaHCO_3$	Improved by $NaHCO_3$
Alkali required for treatment	>10 mEq/kg/day	<3 mEq/kg/day
Other defects of proximal tubular function*	Yes	No
Reduction in plasma HCO_3^-	Moderate	Variable (can be severe)
$FE_{HCO_3^-}$ at normal plasma HCO_3^- concentration	>15%	<5%
Urine pH during acidemia	<5.5	>6.0
Urine pH after NH_4Cl	<5.5	>6.0

*Decreased fractional reabsorption of sodium, potassium, phosphate, urate, glucose, and amino acids.
FE, *Fractional excretion.*

Ammonium Chloride

Administration of NH_4Cl is equivalent to administration of HCl because the NH_4^+ is converted in the liver to urea and H^+. Ammonium chloride has been used commonly as a urinary acidifier in dogs and cats. A study of cats receiving 800 mg of NH_4Cl per day as powder or tablet showed that venous blood pH and HCO_3^- concentrations were decreased to values at the lower end of the normal range.[196] A combination product supplying 580 mg each of NH_4Cl and D,L-methionine had a more marked effect on venous blood pH and HCO_3^- concentrations than that observed with 800 mg of NH_4Cl alone, but results were still within the reported normal range.[197] In another study of cats, NH_4Cl at 300 mg/kg/day did not significantly alter venous blood pH, PCO_2, or HCO_3^- concentration, but 400 mg/kg/day significantly decreased blood HCO_3^- concentration during the course of the study.[75] Ammonium chloride at a dosage of 535 mg/kg/day administered to dogs over 6 days caused hyperchloremic metabolic acidosis and was associated with hypokalemia, presumably related to increased aldosterone secretion.[136] In another study of dogs, NH_4Cl at 200 mg/kg/day reduced urine pH to approximately 5.0 and produced mild metabolic acidosis without change in serum potassium concentration.[193]

In young, growing and adult dogs, addition of NH_4Cl to the diet leads to demineralization of bone.[29,112] Chronic acid feeding has also been reported to affect bone metabolism in cats. Diets containing 3% NH_4Cl slowed growth of young cats, decreased blood pH and HCO_3^- concentrations, and lowered urine pH. Urinary calcium excretion increased in these cats, and bone demineralization was observed on histologic examination of caudal vertebrae.[28] Adult cats fed 1.5% NH_4Cl for 6 months developed hyperchloremic metabolic acidosis and negative balance for calcium and potassium,[38] but no significant changes in trabecular bone remodeling or bone mineral density were found.[39] In one study, administration of NH_4Cl to cats fed a potassium-restricted diet resulted in hypokalemia, possibly by reducing gastrointestinal absorption of potassium.[67] Results of these studies indicate that NH_4Cl should be used with caution and blood gases should be monitored during therapy.

Infusion of Cationic Amino Acids

Metabolism of cationic amino acids (e.g., lysine, arginine, histidine) results in production of H^+ as the NH_4^+ from these amino acids is converted to urea in the liver. For this reason, amino acid–containing fluids used in total parenteral nutrition can contribute to hyperchloremic metabolic acidosis. Other contributing factors are the presence of sulfur-containing amino acids (e.g., methionine, cysteine) in the fluid and development of hypophosphatemia during refeeding, which may reduce renal excretion of titratable acid.

Posthypocapnic Metabolic Acidosis

During compensation for chronic respiratory alkalosis, renal net acid excretion decreases with consequent reduction in plasma HCO_3^- and increase in plasma Cl^- concentrations. When the stimulus for hyperventilation is removed and PCO_2 increases, pH decreases because it requires 1 to 3 days for the kidneys to increase net acid excretion and to increase plasma HCO_3^- concentration. Until this occurs, a state of "posthypocapnic" metabolic acidosis exists. Recovery is spontaneous as long as sodium and phosphate are available in the diet to allow the appropriate increase in renal net acid excretion.[79]

Dilutional Acidosis

Dilutional acidosis refers to a decrease in plasma HCO_3^- concentration that occurs when extracellular volume is expanded using an alkali-free chloride-containing solution such as 0.9% NaCl. The high chloride concentration of 0.9% NaCl and the highly resorbable nature of the chloride ion in the renal tubules contribute to the decrease in plasma HCO_3^- concentration and the increase in Cl^- concentration. Dilutional acidosis can be corrected by substitution of a solution with a lower chloride concentration (e.g., lactated Ringer's solution, 0.45% NaCl).

Hypoadrenocorticism

Aldosterone increases renal tubular lumen negativity by enhancing sodium reabsorption in the collecting duct and secondarily increases hydrogen ion secretion. It also directly stimulates H^+ secretion by increasing the activity of the luminal H^+-ATPase pump in the medullary collecting duct. These effects allow urinary excretion of H^+ and K^+ when distal delivery of sodium is decreased. Deficiency of aldosterone in hypoadrenocorticism results in metabolic acidosis and hyperkalemia. Metabolic acidosis of variable severity is common in dogs with hypoadrenocorticism.[145,175] In one study, low total CO_2 concentration suggesting the presence of metabolic acidosis was found in 81 of 200 (41%) dogs with hypoadrenocorticism.[175] In a study of 10 cats with hypoadrenocorticism, 3 were reported to have decreased serum total CO_2 concentrations.[174] Treatment of hypoadrenocorticism includes volume expansion with 0.9% NaCl and replacement of deficient mineralocorticoids and glucocorticoids.

DISORDERS ASSOCIATED WITH AN INCREASED ANION GAP

Ethylene Glycol Ingestion

Ethylene glycol (EG) is an organic solvent (molecular mass, 62 daltons) used in commercial antifreeze solutions. Ingestion of antifreeze by dogs and cats is a common cause of oliguric acute renal failure in small animal practice, and mortality exceeds 80% in affected animals.[51,84,211] EG itself is not toxic, but it is converted in the liver to

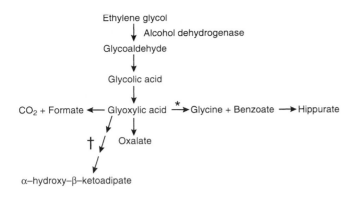

Ethylene glycol

↓ Alcohol dehydrogenase

Glycoaldehyde

↓

Glycolic acid

↓

CO_2 + Formate ← Glyoxylic acid —*→ Glycine + Benzoate → Hippurate

† ↓ ↓ Oxalate

↓

α–hydroxy–β–ketoadipate

* Pyridoxine is a cofactor for this reaction.
† Thiamine is a cofactor for this reaction.

Fig. 10-4 Metabolism of ethylene glycol.

several metabolites that cause severe metabolic acidosis and acute renal failure (Fig. 10-4). It is rapidly absorbed from the gastrointestinal tract and is undetectable in plasma of dogs 48 hours after administration.[161,190]

Pathophysiology. EG is first metabolized in the liver to glycoaldehyde by alcohol dehydrogenase. Glycoaldehyde uncouples oxidative phosphorylation and may contribute to neurologic signs observed early in the course of intoxication. Subsequent steps in metabolism produce glycolic and glyoxylic acids. Glycolic acid is primarily responsible for the severe metabolic acidosis that occurs in animals poisoned by EG.[44] Renal tubular injury results from glycoaldehyde, glycolic acid, and glyoxylic acids, and calcium oxalate crystals are deposited within renal tubules. The observation of these birefringent crystals in the presence of acute tubular nephrosis confirms the diagnosis of EG intoxication.

Vomiting, polydipsia, and polyuria may occur soon after ingestion of EG, but the owners of poisoned animals often do not detect these signs. Within 12 hours of ingestion, neurologic signs (e.g., lethargy, ataxia, stupor, seizures, coma) may develop. Cardiac and pulmonary manifestations (e.g., tachypnea, tachycardia) occur 12 to 24 hours after ingestion but rarely are detected in clinical cases. Oxalate crystals may be detected in the urine as early as 3 to 6 hours after ingestion of EG.[60,61] Renal failure occurs in dogs as early as 24 to 48 hours after ingestion and is manifested by anorexia, lethargy, vomiting, and oliguria or anuria.[86] In cats, azotemia may develop within 12 to 24 hours after ingestion of EG.[60] Unfortunately, most dogs and cats with EG poisoning are presented for veterinary attention after renal failure has already developed.

A severe normochloremic (i.e., high anion gap) metabolic acidosis occurs within 3 hours of EG ingestion and persists for at least 24 hours.[60,61,86,211] Serum hyperosmolality and osmolal gap peak 1 to 6 hours after ingestion and persist for 12 to 24 hours,[60,61,86] but the osmolal gap may be normal in animals presented later in the course of the disease.[211] Calcium oxalate dihydrate crystals ("Maltese cross" or "envelope" forms) may be observed in the urine, but calcium oxalate monohydrate crystals ("picket fence" or "dumbbell" forms) are observed more commonly. Calcium oxalate dihydrate crystals occasionally are found in the urine of normal dogs and cats, whereas calcium oxalate monohydrate crystals rarely are seen except in animals that have ingested EG (Fig. 10-5).[60,211] Crystals previously referred to as hippurates actually are calcium oxalate monohydrate crystals.[120,210] Other laboratory findings include azotemia, isosthenuria, hypocalcemia, hyperphosphatemia, and hyperglycemia.[211] Hyperphosphatemia observed very early in the course of EG intoxication (3 to 12 hours after ingestion) probably is the result of the high phosphorus content of rust-retardant antifreeze preparations.[51,61] Hyperechogenicity of the renal cortex is observed on renal ultrasonography as early as 5 hours after ingestion of EG.[1]

Treatment. The response to treatment depends on the amount of EG ingested and the amount of time that elapses before treatment. In early studies, dogs that ingested less than 10 mL/kg EG were saved if treated within 2 to 4 hours of ingestion,[15,161,190] and cats survived up to 6 mL/kg EG if treated within 4 hours.[172] Treatment consists of inducing vomiting with apomorphine or performing gastric lavage with activated charcoal if ingestion has been recent (<8 hours before presentation). Severe hypocalcemia is corrected with calcium gluconate, and $NaHCO_3$ is administered to combat metabolic acidosis. A $NaHCO_3$ dosage of 1 to 2 mEq/kg may be used empirically. Calcium gluconate and $NaHCO_3$ must not be given simultaneously because calcium carbonate crystals form, and the solution becomes turbid. Attempts to stimulate urine production with furosemide (2 to 4 mg/kg) or mannitol (1 g/kg) usually are futile.

Alcohol dehydrogenase has greater affinity for ethanol than EG. For this reason, 20% ethanol has been administered intravenously to affected dogs at a dosage of 5.5 mL/kg every 4 hours for five treatments and then every 6 hours for four additional treatments.[85] Cats are treated with 20% ethanol at a dosage of 5 mL/kg every 6 hours for five treatments and then every 8 hours for four additional treatments. This treatment is unlikely to be of benefit if more than 12 to 24 hours have elapsed since ingestion of EG. 4-Methylpyrazole (Antizol, Orphan Medical, Minnetonka, MN) is a pharmacologic inhibitor of alcohol dehydrogenase that has become available to treat dogs with EG toxicosis.[59,61] In dogs, it is superior to ethanol because it does not cause central nervous system (CNS) depression, but it must be administered within 8 hours of EG ingestion. The dosage of 4-methylpyrazole used in dogs with EG intoxication is 20 mg/kg

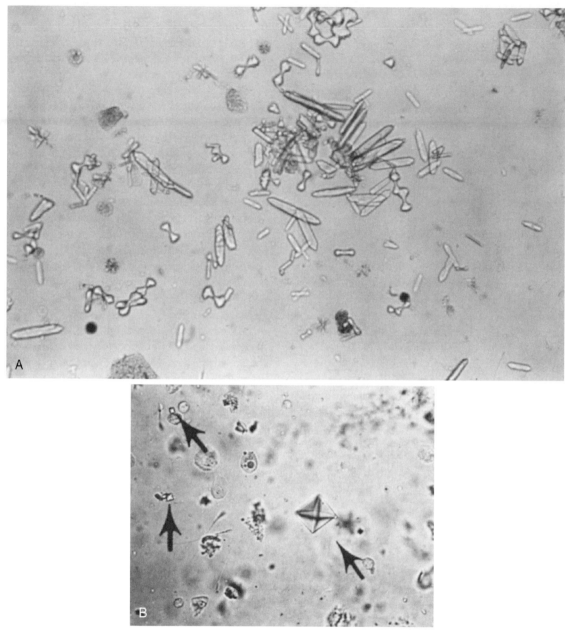

Fig. 10-5 Photomicrographs of **(A)** calcium oxalate monohydrate and **(B)** dihydrate crystals in urine sediment. (From Chew DJ, DiBartola SP: Diagnosis and pathophysiology of renal disease. In Ettinger SJ, editor: *Textbook of veterinary internal medicine,* Philadelphia, 1989, WB Saunders, p. 1907.)

intravenously, followed by 15 mg/kg intravenously at 12 and 24 hours and 5 mg/kg intravenously at 36 hours.[51,59,61] Unfortunately, 4-methylpyrazole is not efficacious in EG-intoxicated cats unless administered at the same time as the EG is consumed. The observed lack of effectiveness of 4-methylpyrazole in EG-intoxicated cats may be related to a shorter half-life of EG in cats (2 to 5 hours) compared with dogs (8 to 10 hours) and more rapid development of acute renal failure in cats or to decreased efficacy of 4-methylpyrazole as an inhibitor of alcohol dehydrogenase in cats.[60] Thiamine promotes conversion of glyoxylate to glycine, and pyridoxine promotes

conversion of glyoxylate to α-hydroxy-β-ketoadipate (see Fig. 10-4). These vitamins may be administered to promote alternative pathways of glyoxylate metabolism, but efficacy has not been demonstrated for such treatment. In one study, all nonazotemic dogs treated with 4-methylpyrazole within 2 to 8.5 hours after EG ingestion survived, whereas only 1 of 21 azotemic dogs treated 8.5 to 38 hours after ingestion survived.[51]

Peritoneal dialysis or hemodialysis is necessary if the animal has anuric or oliguric renal failure at the time of presentation. Early dialysis may also be helpful to remove toxic intermediate metabolites. Despite dialysis, affected dogs may progress to end-stage renal disease and become dependent on dialysis. The prognosis for survival in adult dogs and cats with anuric or oliguric acute renal failure caused by EG intoxication is unfortunately very poor.[51,211]

Salicylate Intoxication

Aspirin (acetylsalicylic acid) is hydrolyzed to salicylic acid ($pK_a' = 3.0$) in the liver. Salicylate intoxication is uncommon in small animal practice and is an example of a mixed acid-base disturbance characterized by metabolic acidosis and respiratory alkalosis. Salicylate intoxication in anesthetized, spontaneously breathing dogs resulted in a mixed respiratory alkalosis and metabolic acidosis.[202] The stimulation of ventilation is caused by a direct effect of salicylate on the medullary respiratory center. Salicylate also uncouples oxidative phosphorylation in mitochondria, and the associated disturbances in carbohydrate metabolism lead to metabolic acidosis characterized by an increased anion gap associated with accumulation of lactic acid, ketoacids, and other organic acids. Salicylate usually makes a minor contribution to the observed increase in unmeasured anions.

Gastric lavage with activated charcoal should be performed if ingestion occurred less than 6 to 12 hours before admission. Administration of $NaHCO_3$ promotes removal of salicylate from tissues and enhances its urinary excretion by the mechanism of **diffusion trapping.** Alkalinization of ECF and urine increases the proportion of drug present in the ionized form and thus favors diffusion of more nonionized salicylic acid from cells into ECF and urine, where it can be trapped as the poorly diffusible ionized form. An attempt should be made to maintain urine pH above 7.5 during alkaline diuresis with $NaHCO_3$, especially if metabolic acidosis is the predominant acid-base disturbance. Alkalinization should be carried out with caution, if at all, when respiratory alkalosis is the predominant acid-base disturbance. Glucose infusion is recommended to prevent reduction in CNS glucose concentration. Hypokalemia may develop during treatment as a result of $NaHCO_3$ administration and diuresis, and parenteral fluids should be supplemented with potassium as needed.

Diabetic Ketoacidosis

Pathophysiology. Overproduction of acetoacetic acid ($pK_a' = 3.58$) and β-hydroxybutyrate ($pK_a' = 4.70$) by the liver occurs in diabetes mellitus because of a deficiency of insulin and relative excess of glucagon. An increase in glucagon and decrease in insulin shift the liver from its normal role in esterification of fatty acids into triglycerides to β-oxidation of fatty acids into ketoacids. At the normal pH of ECF (7.40), these organic acids are completely dissociated, and the hydrogen ions that are released titrate HCO_3^- and other body buffers. Acetone is formed by the nonenzymatic decarboxylation of acetoacetate and does not contribute additional fixed acid. The pathophysiology and treatment of diabetic ketoacidosis are discussed in detail in Chapter 20.

Metabolic acidosis is common in dogs and cats with diabetic ketoacidosis. In one series, mean plasma HCO_3^- concentration in 72 dogs with diabetic ketoacidosis was approximately 11 mEq/L at the time of diagnosis with a range of 4 to 20 mEq/L, whereas the mean HCO_3^- concentration in 20 affected cats was 13 mEq/L with a range of 8 to 22 mEq/L.[73] In an early study of dogs with diabetes mellitus, mean plasma HCO_3^- concentration was 13.7 mEq/L in eight survivors (range, 9.3 to 21.0 mEq/L) and 18.1 mEq/L in five nonsurvivors (range, 13.4 to 30.2 mEq/L).[124] In another study of dogs with diabetic ketoacidosis, mean arterial pH and HCO_3^- concentration were 7.201 (range, 6.986 to 7.395) and 11.1 mEq/L (range, 4.1 to 19.7 mEq/L) before treatment and 7.407 $\pm$ 0.053 and 18.2 $\pm$ 0.7 mEq/L 24 hours after treatment.[128] Only three dogs (those with pH < 7.1) received sodium bicarbonate treatment. Metabolic acidosis with median pH of 7.14 (range, 7.04 to 7.24) and HCO_3^- concentration of 10 mEq/L (range, 6 to 15 mEq/L) was found in 25 of 33 cats evaluated by venous blood gas analysis in a survey of cats with diabetic ketoacidosis.[27] Cats with HCO_3^- concentrations below 14 mEq/L received bicarbonate supplementation of their fluids. In another series of diabetic cats, median total CO_2 was 13 mEq/L in ketoacidotic cats and 15 mEq/L in nonketoacidotic cats.[55] In a study of 116 dogs with diabetes mellitus, 43 (37%) had diabetic ketoacidosis with median venous blood pH of 7.228 (range, 6.979 to 7.374) and median bicarbonate concentration of 10.1 mEq/L (range, 4.0 to 19.3 mEq/L).[69]

The nitroprusside reagent (e.g., Acetest, Bayer, Tarrytown, NY) detects only ketone (−C=O) groups (e.g., acetoacetate, acetone). The concentration of β-hydroxybutyrate typically exceeds that of acetoacetate in uncontrolled diabetic ketoacidosis, and the dipstick reaction underestimates the degree of ketonuria. This problem can be overcome by adding a few drops of hydrogen peroxide to urine, which nonenzymatically converts β-hydroxybutyrate to acetoacetate.[157] When insulin is administered and metabolism of ketones proceeds, there is a shift toward acetoacetate, and the dipstick reaction transiently becomes more strongly positive. This possibility should be recognized by the clinician and should not cause concern. In a study of 116 diabetic dogs (of which 88 had not previously received insulin), all ketotic and ketoacidotic dogs and 21 of 32 (66%) "non-ketotic" dogs (i.e., negative urine dipstick test for ketones) had abnormally high serum β-hydroxybutyrate concentrations (>0.15 mmol/L) at presentation.[69] The increase in unmeasured anions (as reflected in the anion gap) gives a rough estimate of the concentration of ketoanions in serum. However, this estimate is inaccurate if lactic acidosis develops because lactate also is an unmeasured anion.

To some extent, the anions of these ketoacids are excreted in the urine along with sodium and potassium for electroneutrality. These organic anions are lost from the body and cannot be metabolized to HCO_3^- after correction of diabetic ketoacidosis with insulin therapy. Their loss thus contributes to depletion of body buffer and cation stores. Osmotic diuresis is induced by hyperglycemia and also contributes to the whole-body cation deficit. The extent of impairment in renal function may determine whether patients with diabetic ketoacidosis have an increased anion gap metabolic acidosis or hyperchloremic metabolic acidosis at the time of presentation. Patients with severe volume depletion have an increased anion gap because of retention of ketoanions, whereas those without volume depletion have hyperchloremia as a result of increased urinary excretion of the sodium and potassium salts of ketoanions and retention of chloride.[4,8]

Treatment. The best treatment for the acidosis of uncontrolled diabetes mellitus is fluid therapy and insulin. Insulin administration allows glucose utilization by skeletal muscle and adipose tissue, decreases hepatic glucose production, prevents lipolysis and ketogenesis, and permits peripheral metabolism of ketoacids. Several regimens for administration of insulin to ketoacidotic dogs and cats have been described.[74] The particular protocol of insulin administration is probably less crucial to the ultimate outcome than the individualized care provided by the veterinarian during management of the diabetic animal.

Several factors may contribute to a delay in the repair of the HCO_3^- deficit in patients with diabetic ketoacidosis.[89] Ketoacid anions that have been excreted in the urine are lost to the body and cannot be metabolized to HCO_3^-. After treatment with fluids and insulin, recovery may be faster in patients with a high anion gap because the retained ketoanions are metabolized, yielding HCO_3^-.[6,8] Thus withholding alkali may be more rational for diabetic patients with high anion gap metabolic acidosis than for those with hyperchloremic metabolic acidosis. Dilutional acidosis may occur if ECF volume (ECFV) is expanded with alkali-free solutions such as 0.9% saline. If hyperventilation persists, it may impair renal reabsorption of HCO_3^-, and renal acid excretion may require several days to become fully augmented.

The use of $NaHCO_3$ to treat diabetic ketoacidosis is highly controversial, and clear benefits of its use have not been demonstrated in human patients. For example, there was no difference in recovery (based on rate of decrease of blood glucose and ketone concentrations and rate of increase of blood or cerebrospinal fluid [CSF] pH or HCO_3^- concentration) when $NaHCO_3$ was or was not administered to human patients with diabetic ketoacidosis who presented with blood pH values in the range of 6.90 to 7.14.[152] In another study, treatment with $NaHCO_3$ delayed resolution of ketosis in diabetic ketoacidosis.[164]

There are several theoretical arguments against the use of $NaHCO_3$ in diabetic ketoacidosis. Acidosis in the CNS may develop after $NaHCO_3$ administration. The blood-brain barrier is permeable to CO_2 but less permeable to the charged HCO_3^- ion. If $NaHCO_3$ is administered, pH increases in ECF as the HCO_3^-/PCO_2 ratio increases, and compensatory hyperventilation decreases somewhat. As a result, PCO_2 increases and CO_2 diffuses into the CNS. However, bicarbonate diffusion into CNS lags behind that of CO_2. During this time, the HCO_3^-/PCO_2 ratio and pH in the CNS may decrease. This has been referred to as **paradoxical CNS acidosis**.[177] The frequency of occurrence of this complication and its clinical significance are uncertain.[121]

The pathophysiology of diabetic ketoacidosis also affects oxygen delivery to tissues. Chronic acidosis shifts the oxygen-hemoglobin dissociation curve to the right, thus enhancing delivery of oxygen to the tissues. Conversely, phosphorus deficiency in diabetes decreases red cell 2,3-diphosphoglycerate concentration and causes a shift of the oxygen-hemoglobin dissociation curve back to the left. Correction of acidosis with $NaHCO_3$ shifts the curve farther to the left and potentially decreases oxygen delivery to tissues. However, administration of insulin and fluid therapy also lead to correction of the acidosis and should have a similar effect on the oxygen-hemoglobin dissociation curve.

Overzealous therapy with $NaHCO_3$ may contribute to late development of metabolic alkalosis because insulin promotes metabolism of retained ketoacid anions to HCO_3^-. This excess HCO_3^- should be readily excreted in the urine if renal function is adequate. Other potentially detrimental effects of $NaHCO_3$ therapy include aggravation of hyperosmolality as a consequence of the obligatory sodium load, tetany resulting from a sudden decrease in ionized serum calcium concentration, and precipitation of severe hypokalemia as extracellular potassium ions move into cells during administration of insulin and correction of acidosis. For all these reasons, $NaHCO_3$ is not used unless severe acidosis (pH < 7.1 to 7.2) is present and then only in small amounts (see section on Treatment of Metabolic Acidosis).

Uremic Acidosis

Pathophysiology. The metabolic acidosis of chronic renal failure is usually mild to moderate in severity (plasma HCO_3^- concentration, 12 to 15 mEq/L) and may be hyperchloremic early in the course of the disease process.[222] Later in the course of the disease, the anion gap increases because of retention of phosphates, sulfates, and organic anions. Acid-base status is usually well preserved in chronic renal failure until GFR decreases to 10% to 20% of normal. In retrospective studies of small animal patients with chronic renal failure, plasma HCO_3^-

concentrations were less than 16 mEq/L in 40% of dogs with chronic renal failure caused by amyloidosis[64] and less than 15 mEq/L in 63% of cats with chronic renal failure of various causes.[63] A high anion gap was observed in 43% of affected dogs (>25 mEq/L) and in 19% of affected cats (>35 mEq/L) in these studies. In acute renal failure, there has been insufficient time for the kidneys to adapt to the disease state, and the metabolic acidosis of acute renal failure is usually more severe than that observed in chronic renal failure. Complications such as sepsis and marked tissue catabolism may contribute to the severity of metabolic acidosis in acute renal failure.

Delivery of HCO_3^- from the proximal tubules to the distal nephron is increased in chronic renal failure.[218] In dogs with experimentally induced unilateral renal disease, renal HCO_3^- reabsorption was not different in the diseased and control kidneys, but bicarbonaturia developed when the normal kidney was removed, and the contralateral diseased kidney was forced to function in a uremic environment.[151] The osmotic diuresis characteristic of uremia may thus contribute to the increased delivery of HCO_3^- to the distal tubules. Increased parathyroid hormone concentration as a result of renal secondary hyperparathyroidism does not seem to have important adverse effects on HCO_3^- reabsorption in experimentally induced renal disease in dogs.[10,191,192] The ability to lower urine pH maximally is preserved in chronic renal failure.

The main method by which the diseased kidney responds to chronic retention of fixed acid is by enhanced renal ammoniagenesis. Total ammonium excretion decreases during progressive chronic renal disease, but ammonium excretion is observed to be markedly increased when expressed per 100 mL GFR or per remnant nephron.[66,187] On a per-nephron basis, the diseased kidney can increase its ammonium excretion three- to five-fold.[203,218,221] This adaptive mechanism seems to be fully expended when the GFR decreases to less than 20% of normal. At this point, the diseased kidneys can no longer effectively cope with the daily fixed acid load, and a new steady state is established at a lower than normal plasma HCO_3^- concentration. The relatively mild decrease in plasma HCO_3^- concentration that is observed in chronic renal failure has been attributed to the contribution of the large reservoir of buffer (e.g., calcium carbonate) in bone. However, the capacity of the skeleton to buffer the amount of acid that accumulates in long-standing chronic renal failure has been questioned.[163] The decrease in total ammonium excretion that occurs in chronic renal failure may be counterbalanced by decreased urinary excretion of organic anions (e.g., citrate, lactate, pyruvate, ketoanions).[50] Metabolism of these retained organic anions would result in a net gain of HCO_3^- that would offset the decreased excretion of H^+ in the form of NH_4^+.

The amount of phosphate buffer available in urine in chronic renal failure is relatively fixed and likely to be at its maximum because of hyperphosphatemia and the effects of increased plasma parathyroid hormone concentration.[187,203] Furthermore, phosphorus binders and dietary phosphorus restriction are commonly used to treat chronic renal failure and may limit the amount of phosphate that can contribute to titratable acidity. When expressed on a per-nephron basis, however, titratable acidity is increased in chronic renal failure.[150]

Treatment. Whether to treat well-compensated mild to moderate metabolic acidosis in adult patients with chronic renal failure is controversial. The potential benefits of such treatment include minimizing potential depletion of bone buffers, preventing the catabolic effects of uremic acidosis on muscle protein, preventing tubulointerstitial damage resulting from complement activation by ammonia, and improving the patient's ability to combat a superimposed acidotic crisis (e.g., acute diarrhea).[182] Thus treatment with oral $NaHCO_3$ at a dosage of 0.5 to 1.0 mEq/kg/day or an amount sufficient to maintain plasma HCO_3^- concentration at 15 mEq/L or above is reasonable if the patient can tolerate the associated sodium load. One teaspoon of baking soda contains 5 g $NaHCO_3$ (1.3 g of which is sodium). An advantage of using calcium carbonate (e.g., Tums [GlaxoSmithKline, Brentford, UK], Os-Cal [GlaxoSmithKline]) as a phosphorus binder in chronic renal failure is that this compound can serve as both a source of alkali and a source of calcium, if small amounts of calcitriol (2 to 3 ng/kg/day) are also provided. The patient should be monitored for development of hypercalcemia when calcium carbonate and calcitriol are administered concurrently. Potassium and sodium citrate should not be used for alkali therapy in chronic renal failure patients that also are being treated with aluminum-containing phosphorus binders (e.g., aluminum hydroxide, aluminum carbonate) because citrate can increase aluminum absorption from the gastrointestinal tract in this clinical setting.[148]

Lactic Acidosis

Lactic acidosis is characterized by an accumulation of lactate in body fluids and a plasma lactate concentration greater than 5 mEq/L.[130] The pK_a' of lactic acid is 3.86, and it is completely dissociated at the normal pH of ECF (7.40). Lactic acidosis has been divided into two categories (Box 10-2).[49,100,122] In type A (hypoxic) lactic acidosis, mitochondrial function is normal but O_2 delivery to tissues is inadequate. In type B (nonhypoxic) lactic acidosis, there is adequate O_2 delivery to tissues but defective mitochondrial oxidative function and abnormal carbohydrate metabolism. Inborn errors of metabolism affecting gluconeogenesis and mitochondrial oxidative function are documented to cause type B lactic acidosis in humans.

Box 10-2 — Causes of L-Lactic Acidosis*

Type A: hypoxic

Increased oxygen demand
 Severe exercise
 Convulsions
Decreased oxygen availability
 Reduced tissue perfusion
  Cardiac arrest, cardiopulmonary resuscitation
  Shock
  Hypovolemia
  Left ventricular failure
  Low cardiac output
  Acute pulmonary edema
 Reduced arterial oxygen content
  Hypoxemia ($P_{O_2} \leq 30$ mm Hg)
  Extremely severe anemia (packed cell volume < 10%)

Type B: nonhypoxic

Drugs and toxins
 Phenformin
 Salicylates
 Ethylene glycol
 Many others[130]
Diabetes mellitus
Liver failure
Neoplasia (e.g., lymphosarcoma)
Sepsis
Renal failure
Hypoglycemia
Hereditary defects
 Mitochondrial myopathies
 Defects in gluconeogenesis

*D-Lactic acidosis occurs with short bowel syndrome in humans and has been observed in cats fed propylene glycol.[40,41]

Defects in mitochondrial oxidative function are called mitochondrial myopathies and are caused by hereditary defects in specific mitochondrial enzyme systems. A number of case reports suggest that similar defects occur in dogs.[104,165,167,216] Pyruvate dehydrogenase deficiency is suspected to occur in Clumber spaniels.[98,113] This discussion focuses on type A (hypoxic) lactic acidosis.

Normal Physiology. Lactate is a metabolic end product. Its production allows regeneration of cytosolic nicotinamide adenine dinucleotide (NAD^+) during anaerobic metabolism, and its ultimate fate is reoxidation back to pyruvate:

$$CH_3COCOO^- + NADH + H^+ \underset{\text{lactate dehydrogenase}}{\rightleftharpoons} CH_3CHOHCOO^- + NAD^+$$
(pyruvate) → (lactate)

The equilibrium of this reaction is far to the right, and the normal ratio of lactate to pyruvate is 10:1. The main determinants of cytosolic lactate concentration are the concentration of pyruvate and the $NADH/NAD^+$ ratio, both of which are affected by mitochondrial oxidative function.

Pyruvate is produced in the cytosol by anaerobic glycolysis (Embden-Meyerhof pathway). Under aerobic conditions, NADH is oxidized to NAD^+ in the mitochondria and pyruvate enters the mitochondria for conversion to acetylcoenzyme A (CoA) and utilization in the tricarboxylic acid (Krebs) cycle, or it is converted to oxaloacetate and used for gluconeogenesis in the liver and renal cortex. Under anaerobic conditions (e.g., tissue hypoxia), oxidative pathways in the mitochondria are disrupted, and NAD^+ must be replenished by reduction of pyruvate to lactate in the cytosol. Thus lactate accumulation is the price to be paid for maintaining energy production under anaerobic conditions.

At rest, skin, red cells, brain, skeletal muscle, and gut all produce lactate. During tissue hypoxia, skeletal muscle and gut become the major producers of lactate. The liver and kidney are the main consumers of lactate, using it for gluconeogenesis (primarily in the liver) or oxidizing it to CO_2 and water. Protons are consumed when lactate is metabolized:

Gluconeogenesis
$$2CH_3CHOHCOO^- + 2H^+ \rightarrow C_6H_{12}O_6$$
Oxidative metabolism
$$CH_3CHOHCOO^- + H^+ + 3O_2 \rightarrow 3CO_2 + 3H_2O$$

Both of these reactions require normal mitochondrial oxidative function. The protons are consumed when adenosine triphosphate (ATP) is synthesized from adenosine diphosphate (ADP) and when NADH is oxidized to NAD^+ in the mitochondria.[122,130] Protons are released by hydrolysis of ATP to ADP and by reduction of NAD^+ to NADH, reactions that occur mainly in the cytosol. The protons do not arise from dissociation of lactic acid because the anion lactate is the predominant metabolite at normal hepatocyte pH_i (pH_i = 7.00 to 7.20). Thus lactic acidosis reflects imbalance between ATP hydrolysis and synthesis and between reduction and oxidation of NAD^+. The protons produced during anaerobic glycolysis are buffered by bicarbonate and nonbicarbonate buffers. Protons are consumed and the buffers replenished when lactate is metabolized to glucose or oxidized to CO_2 and water.

Pathophysiology. Lactic acidosis occurs when production of lactate by muscle and gut exceeds its utilization by liver and kidney. Both pathways of lactate utilization depend on intact mitochondrial oxidative function, and clinical settings characterized by tissue hypoxia are the most common causes of lactic acidosis (see Box 10-2). Hepatic uptake of lactate is decreased when arterial P_{O_2} decreases to approximately 30 mm Hg.[209] Severe acidosis further impairs hepatic uptake of lactate, and the liver eventually becomes a producer rather than a consumer of lactate.[126]

In an experimental model of hypoxic lactic acidosis (type A) induced by ventilating dogs with 8% O_2, lactate concentration was more than 5 mEq/L, pH was less than 7.2, HCO_3^- concentration was less than 12 mEq/L, P_{O_2} was less than 30 mm Hg, and hepatocyte pH_i was less than 7.00.[9] When a similar degree of acidosis was created by infusing lactic acid into dogs with normal P_{O_2}, hepatocyte pH_i remained greater than 7.00, and hepatic extraction of lactate (as a percentage of the delivered load) was approximately three times higher than that observed in the hypoxic animals. Hypoxemia reduces hepatic O_2 uptake, and hepatocyte pH_i decreases, presumably as a result of CO_2 accumulation within cells. This study demonstrated that impaired hepatic extraction of lactate is related to decreased hepatic O_2 uptake and pH_i but not to arterial pH. During severe hypoxia, increased lactate production by gut and muscle and decreased hepatic extraction of lactate lead to progressive lactic acidosis. Impaired hepatic extraction of lactate and increased splanchnic production also contribute to the lactic acidosis of sepsis in dogs.[42]

Clinical Features. Lactic acidosis may occur in several clinical settings, especially those associated with poor perfusion and tissue hypoxia (e.g., cardiac arrest and cardiopulmonary resuscitation, shock, left ventricular failure). The clinician should strongly consider the possibility of lactic acidosis in such settings (see Box 10-2). Usually, lactic acidosis results from accumulation of the L isomer of lactate. D-Lactic acidosis, characterized by the accumulation of the D isomer, is rare but has been reported in human patients with "short-bowel syndrome" in whom gut bacteria metabolize glucose to D-lactate. D-Lactic acidosis also has been observed in cats fed propylene glycol[40,41] and has been documented in a cat with pancreatic insufficiency presumably as a consequence of intestinal bacterial overgrowth.[169]

Lactic acidosis should be suspected whenever there is an unexplained increase in unmeasured anions (i.e., an unexplained increase in the anion gap). Confirmation requires measurement of plasma lactate concentration, but this has not been performed commonly in small animal practice. Care should be taken to avoid vascular stasis when collecting venous blood for lactate determinations, and blood samples should be centrifuged immediately after collection to avoid a spurious increase in lactate concentration related to anaerobic glycolysis by red cells. Lactate concentrations in dogs have been

reported in many experimental studies.* From results of these studies, normal plasma lactate concentrations in dogs are expected to be less than 2 mEq/L. Control plasma lactate concentrations in cats were 1.46 mEq/L in one study.[11]

Racing caused venous lactate concentrations in greyhounds to increase from 0.57 to 28.93 mEq/L, but lactate concentrations returned to 0.53 mEq/L 3 hours after exercise.[106] Arterial pH decreased from 7.365 to 6.997 and returned to 7.372 3 hours after exercise, and HCO_3^- concentration decreased from 21.1 to 3.1 mEq/L and returned to 20.5 mEq/L 3 hours after exercise. Plasma potassium concentration does not increase in response to organic acidosis as it does in acute mineral acidosis.[5] In the racing greyhounds, there was no change in plasma potassium concentration despite severe lactic acidosis.

Cardiac Arrest and Cardiopulmonary Resuscitation. Oxygen delivery to and CO_2 removal from tissues are dependent on adequate tissue perfusion. Cardiac arrest is an extreme example of impaired tissue perfusion. During cardiopulmonary resuscitation (CPR), reduced tissue perfusion and reduced O_2 delivery cause anaerobic metabolism and lactic acidosis. In dogs, lactate concentrations increased linearly during the time between cardiac arrest and the onset of CPR.[33] Lactate concentrations increased progressively during closed-chest CPR in dogs[34] and remained stable but did not decrease during 30 minutes of open-chest CPR.[33] In this model, closed-chest CPR did not provide adequate tissue perfusion and O_2 delivery to halt anaerobic metabolism.

During CPR, arterial blood gases reflect alveolar-arterial gas exchange, whereas mixed venous blood gases reflect tissue acid-base status and oxygenation.[140] Respiratory alkalosis develops in arterial blood as a result of mechanical ventilation, whereas respiratory acidosis develops in venous blood because of poor tissue perfusion and impaired transport of accumulated CO_2 to the lungs. In one study of human patients undergoing CPR, average arterial pH was 7.41, whereas average mixed venous pH was 7.15.[220] Arterial P_{CO_2} averaged 32 mm Hg and mixed venous P_{CO_2} was 74 mm Hg, whereas arterial and venous HCO_3^- concentrations were similar.

Closed-chest CPR, initiated after 6 minutes of cardiac arrest, was studied in dogs.[189] Sodium bicarbonate (2 mEq/kg) was administered after 20 minutes of cardiac arrest. Administration of $NaHCO_3$ increased both arterial and venous pH. Before $NaHCO_3$, arterial P_{CO_2} was approximately 40 mm Hg, and with CPR it decreased to 20 mm Hg as a result of mechanical ventilation. After $NaHCO_3$, arterial P_{CO_2} increased to 30 mm

---

References 32,47,72,76,78,83,99,101,102,106,108,114, 119,131,139,140,154,179,213,214.

Hg. Venous P_{CO_2} was nearly 50 mm Hg, and it slowly increased during 30 minutes of cardiac arrest to 60 mm Hg in untreated dogs. Bicarbonate treatment caused venous P_{CO_2} to increase transiently to 100 mm Hg, and it decreased to 70 mm Hg 10 minutes after $NaHCO_3$ administration. The pH of CSF was not changed by $NaHCO_3$ administration.

The normal arteriovenous pH gradient in dogs is 0.01 to 0.04.[7,18,138] Reduced cardiac output increases arteriovenous pH and P_{CO_2} gradients as a result of arterial hypocapnia and venous hypercapnia.[7,18,140,220] The ventilation-to-perfusion ratio is increased because of decreased pulmonary blood flow, accounting for the observed arterial hypocapnia. Venous hypercapnia results from anaerobic metabolism and a greater than normal addition of CO_2 to venous blood from hypoperfused tissues and diminished CO_2 excretion in the lungs because of pulmonary hypoperfusion. These increases in arteriovenous pH and P_{CO_2} gradients occur only if pulmonary ventilation continues. Respiratory arrest abolishes arteriovenous pH and P_{CO_2} gradients.[7] In summary, arterial P_{CO_2} is not an accurate reflection of CO_2 removal from tissues during CPR, and analysis of mixed venous P_{CO_2} is recommended.[7,18,138,140,220]

During CPR and ventilation with 100% O_2, arterial P_{O_2} may be normal, but tissue perfusion is low (20% to 25% of normal).[100] After $NaHCO_3$ administration, additional CO_2 is produced, and venous hypercapnia persists if ventilation is inadequate. Improving tissue perfusion is much more important during CPR than is $NaHCO_3$ administration. Effective cardiac compression and adequate perfusion allow delivery of O_2 to and removal of CO_2 from tissues. Conversely, tissue acidosis is aggravated and pH_i is decreased by $NaHCO_3$ administration if the CO_2 generated cannot be removed from the tissues by the lungs. The increase in tissue CO_2 decreases pH_i because CO_2 diffuses more rapidly into cells than does the charged HCO_3^-, thereby lowering the intracellular HCO_3^-/P_{CO_2} ratio. Intracellular acidosis of the myocardium leads to impaired cardiac contractility, decreased cardiac output, and aggravation of lactic acidosis. Thus the main goals of CPR are to provide adequate tissue perfusion by effective cardiac compression and to ventilate the patient with 100% O_2. In one study of short (5 minutes) and prolonged (15 minutes) cardiac arrest in dogs, $NaHCO_3$ administration improved acidosis without a significant increase in P_{CO_2}.[217] The authors concluded that $NaHCO_3$ might be useful to reverse the acidosis of cardiac arrest if ventilation is adequate and $NaHCO_3$ is administered in a reasonable therapeutic window.

Lymphosarcoma in Dogs. Dogs with lymphosarcoma had higher lactate concentrations than control animals, and their lactate concentrations increased significantly 30 minutes after administration of 500 mg/kg dextrose.[214] Blood lactate concentrations were higher before and 1 hour after infusion of lactated Ringer's solution in dogs with lymphosarcoma as compared with control animals.[213] Blood lactate concentration returned to baseline during the second hour of the 6-hour infusion. The authors concluded that dogs with stage III or IV lymphosarcoma might have abnormal carbohydrate metabolism and a transient inability to handle lactate loads. Tumors may produce increased amounts of lactate as a result of excessive anaerobic metabolism and possibly as a result of less than normal hepatic extraction of lactate. Induction of remission with doxorubicin chemotherapy did not improve hyperlactatemia in dogs with lymphosarcoma.[162]

Treatment. The outcome of lactic acidosis depends on the severity and reversibility of the underlying disease process responsible for the acid-base disturbance. If treatment of lactic acidosis is to be successful, prompt diagnosis and correction of the underlying disease state are crucial. Tissue perfusion and oxygen delivery should be improved by aggressive fluid therapy to expand ECFV. Ventilation with O_2 should be considered if the patient's spontaneous ventilation is inadequate. Infections should be treated with appropriate antimicrobial agents, and cardiac output should be improved, if necessary, by administration of inotropic agents. If the underlying disease cannot be corrected, the prognosis for patients with lactic acidosis is very poor. If the underlying disease can be corrected, the accumulated lactate is metabolized, yielding an equivalent amount of HCO_3^-, and the acidosis is reversed.

When the pH of the patient's blood decreases to below 7.1 to 7.2, administration of alkali is justified to prevent the detrimental effects of severe acidosis on the cardiovascular system (e.g., impaired myocardial contractility, impaired cardiovascular responsiveness to catecholamines, increased susceptibility to ventricular arrhythmias). Small doses of $NaHCO_3$ should be administered to increase the patient's pH to 7.2.[3,100,130]

Approximately 10% to 15% of administered $NaHCO_3$ is converted immediately to CO_2.[100] It is essential that ventilation increase to allow removal of accumulated CO_2 from the body. It is probably safe to administer $NaHCO_3$ if the patient can reasonably be expected to increase ventilation spontaneously. If not, administration of $NaHCO_3$ may be detrimental. In any case, $NaHCO_3$ should be administered slowly to minimize the increase in mixed venous P_{CO_2}.

The volume of distribution (V_d) of administered HCO_3^- is variable, depending on the severity of the acidosis.[2] Thus there is no simple way to calculate the dosage of $NaHCO_3$ required to increase the pH to 7.2. Volumes of distribution of 0.21 and 0.5 have been recommended for calculation of the bicarbonate space.[3,100] Sodium bicarbonate should be used cautiously and only in amounts necessary to increase the pH to 7.2. It should be administered slowly over several minutes to a few hours, and at least 30 minutes should be allowed to elapse after the infusion before judging its effect.[3]

The use of $NaHCO_3$ in lactic acidosis is controversial.[156,204] Using the canine model of hypoxic lactic acidosis described above,[9] affected dogs were left untreated, treated with 2.5 mEq/kg $NaHCO_3$, or treated with 2.5 mEq/kg 1 M NaCl.[81,82] Animals treated with bicarbonate showed a greater decrease in pH and HCO_3^- concentration and higher lactate concentration than the other groups. Gut lactate production was greater in dogs that received $NaHCO_3$ than in dogs that received NaCl, and portal vein Pco_2 was higher in the group that received $NaHCO_3$. Arterial blood pressure and cardiac output declined in the untreated group and the group that received $NaHCO_3$ but were higher in the group that received NaCl. Increased portal vein Pco_2 and hepatic accumulation of lactate presumably caused hepatocyte pH_i to decrease. The ability of the liver to extract lactate depends on adequate hepatic blood flow and normal hepatocyte pH_i, both of which are decreased in this model. During hypoxia ($Po_2 < 30$ mm Hg), the liver is unable to increase its lactate extraction, despite an increased load delivered from the ischemic gut. The investigators concluded that use of $NaHCO_3$ during lactic acidosis might not be effective and might even be detrimental.

Dichloroacetate (DCA) stimulates the enzyme pyruvate dehydrogenase, which converts pyruvate to acetyl CoA.[54] In the canine model of hypoxic lactic acidosis described before,[9] DCA was compared with NaCl.[80] DCA increased pH and HCO_3^- concentration and maintained a constant lactate concentration, whereas NaCl treatment was associated with a decrease in pH and HCO_3^- concentration and an increase in lactate concentration. Hepatic lactate extraction increased with DCA, whereas liver and muscle accumulation of lactate decreased. Muscle pH_i increased with DCA, but neither treatment changed arterial blood pressure or cardiac output. DCA was also studied in a cardiac arrest model in dogs.[200] This study compared DCA, DCA and $NaHCO_3$, $NaHCO_3$, and no treatment. Bicarbonate treatment increased arterial pH, but DCA did not. DCA did not decrease lactate concentration or increase pH in either the peripheral circulation or CNS. In a canine model of hemorrhagic shock, DCA administration decreased arterial lactate concentrations but was associated with decreased cardiac stroke volume, decreased myocardial efficiency, and reduced myocardial lactate consumption.[13] Thus there are conflicting results regarding the usefulness of DCA in canine models of lactic acidosis.

Carbicarb is an equimolar mixture of Na_2CO_3 and $NaHCO_3$ that limits the generation of CO_2 during the buffering process:

$$Na_2CO_3 + H_2O + CO_2 \rightarrow 2HCO_3^- + 2Na^+$$

However, some of the HCO_3^- generated from this reaction can buffer H^+ released from nonbicarbonate buffers and generate CO_2 in the presence of carbonic anhydrase:

$$2HCO_3^- + 2H^+ \rightarrow 2H_2CO_3 \rightarrow 2H_2O + 2CO_2$$

In the canine model of hypoxic lactic acidosis described earlier,[9] 2.5 mEq/kg Carbicarb was compared with 2.5 mEq/kg $NaHCO_3$.[19] Arterial pH increased after administration of Carbicarb but decreased after $NaHCO_3$. Mixed venous Pco_2 was unchanged after Carbicarb administration but increased after $NaHCO_3$. Arterial lactate concentration increased after administration of $NaHCO_3$ but stabilized after Carbicarb, whereas lactate utilization by gut, muscle, and liver improved with Carbicarb but decreased after $NaHCO_3$. Hepatocyte pH_i increased after Carbicarb and decreased after $NaHCO_3$. Arterial blood pressure decreased to a lesser extent and cardiac output stabilized with Carbicarb, whereas cardiac output decreased with $NaHCO_3$. It was concluded that Carbicarb had a beneficial effect on myocardial contractility. Myocardial contractility may decrease after $NaHCO_3$ administration as a result of increased venous Pco_2 and decreased myocardial pH_i. Decreased cardiac output follows and leads to decreased blood flow and decreased O_2 delivery to gut, muscle, and liver, resulting in decreased lactate utilization and increased production. Carbicarb improved arterial pH without impairing myocardial contractility, presumably because it did not increase venous Pco_2. This study suggests that Carbicarb is superior to $NaHCO_3$ in the treatment of lactic acidosis in dogs.

In another study, Carbicarb was compared with sodium bicarbonate and hypertonic saline in a canine model of hemorrhagic shock.[17] All dogs received identical sodium loads. Groups that received Carbicarb and sodium bicarbonate experienced similar increases in serum bicarbonate, but arterial Pco_2 increased more in bicarbonate-treated dogs than in those treated with Carbicarb. Hemodynamics, oxygen delivery, and oxygen consumption improved in all three groups, and these effects were attributed to the sodium load. Carbicarb, $NaHCO_3$, and NaCl were compared in a model of hypoxic lactic acidosis in anesthetized, mechanically ventilated dogs.[178] Carbicarb increased arterial pH, base excess, and cardiac index without an increase in lactate. Bicarbonate increased Pco_2, but no adverse effects of $NaHCO_3$ on hemodynamics or pH_i were detected.

A sodium-free 0.3 N solution of tromethamine (THAM) is another CO_2-consuming alkalinizing agent that is capable of buffering both nonvolatile (H^+) and volatile (H_2CO_3 derived from CO_2) acid. THAM and sodium bicarbonate had similar buffering ability when evaluated in dogs with experimentally induced metabolic acidosis.[149] Dogs treated with THAM did not experience the transient hypernatremia and hypercapnia that were observed in bicarbonate-treated dogs.

TREATMENT OF METABOLIC ACIDOSIS

The main goal in treatment of metabolic acidosis is prompt diagnosis and specific treatment of the underlying cause of the acid-base disorder. Correction of the underlying disease that is responsible for the patient's metabolic acidosis may be all that is necessary (e.g., fluids and insulin in diabetic ketoacidosis). In some instances, however, the underlying disease cannot be corrected (e.g., chronic renal failure), and alkali therapy must be considered.

In general, administration of $NaHCO_3$ should be reserved for clinical settings in which the patient's blood pH is less than 7.1 to 7.2, and $NaHCO_3$ should be administered only in amounts necessary to increase the pH to 7.2. Therapy with sodium bicarbonate is less likely to be harmful in animals with simple hyperchloremic metabolic acidosis (normal anion gap) because of the absence of unmeasured organic anions. In patients with normochloremic metabolic acidosis (increased anion gap), unmeasured organic anions (e.g., ketoacids, lactate) are present and can be metabolized to HCO_3^- during recovery. Administration of $NaHCO_3$ in such a setting may result in late development of metabolic alkalosis. This complication should not be serious if renal function is normal because the kidneys can excrete the excess HCO_3^-.

Severe acidosis may lead to life-threatening cardiovascular complications (e.g., impaired cardiac contractility, impaired pressor response to catecholamines, sensitization to ventricular arrhythmias).[147] Thus if blood pH is less than 7.1 to 7.2, judicious treatment with $NaHCO_3$ is justified. The aim of therapy should be to increase the patient's pH to 7.2 ($[H^+]$ = 63 nEq/L), at which point the risk of life-threatening hemodynamic complications is reduced.

For example, consider a 10-kg dog with a pH of 7.000, $[H^+]$ = 100 nEq/L, $[HCO_3^-]$ = 6 mEq/L, and Pco_2 = 25 mm Hg. We assume that normal values are a pH of 7.387, $[H^+]$ = 41 nEq/L, $[HCO_3^-]$ = 21 mEq/L, and Pco_2 = 36 mm Hg and that the normal compensatory respiratory response to metabolic acidosis is a 0.7-mm Hg decrement in Pco_2 per 1.0 mEq/L decrement in $[HCO_3^-]$. How much $NaHCO_3$ must be administered to increase the dog's pH to 7.200 ($[H^+]$ = 63 nEq/L)? This may be determined using the Henderson equation:

$$[H^+] = \frac{24 Pco_2}{[HCO_3^-]}$$

Thus the desired $[HCO_3^-]$ would be 24(25)/63 or 9.5 mEq/L if we assume that the Pco_2 will not change. However, alveolar hyperventilation is likely to subside somewhat as the acidemia is partially corrected. If we assume that the Pco_2 will increase to 28 mm Hg, the required $[HCO_3^-]$ is 24(28)/63 or 10.7 mEq/L. Thus

we want to increase the dog's $[HCO_3^-]$ to 9.5 to 10.7 mEq/L.

We still must determine how much $NaHCO_3$ to administer. This can be calculated using the formula:

$$mEq\ HCO_3^- = V_d \times weight\ (kg) \times HCO_3^-\ deficit/L$$

where V_d is the volume of distribution for HCO_3^-. However, the volume of distribution of HCO_3^- varies inversely with the initial HCO_3^- concentration and changes for at least 90 minutes after HCO_3^- administration to dogs.[2] In this study, dogs with chronic metabolic acidosis and initial plasma HCO_3^- concentrations of 10 mEq/L were given 5 mEq/kg $NaHCO_3$ and had average V_d values of 60% at 30 minutes and 76% at 90 minutes. This increase in V_d represents distribution of administered HCO_3^- from extracellular to intracellular sites. Bicarbonate distributes to ECF within 15 minutes and to intracellular and bone buffers within 2 to 4 hours.[183] Thus it is impossible to assign a single value for the V_d of $NaHCO_3$ administered to dogs with metabolic acidosis. Any dosage recommendations must be considered only rough guidelines to treatment.

The dogs in this study[2] had ECFVs equal to approximately 24.5% of body weight as measured by radiosulfate space. If we arbitrarily choose 0.5, a value approximately twice ECFV:

$$HCO_3^-\ (mEq) = 0.5 \times 10 \times (9.5 - 6) = 17.5\ mEq$$
or
$$HCO_3^-\ (mEq) = 0.5 \times 10 \times (10.7 - 6) = 23.5\ mEq$$

Thus the desired amount of $NaHCO_3$ is between 17.5 and 23.5 mEq. The $NaHCO_3$ should be administered over the first few hours of therapy and blood gases reevaluated before making a decision about additional alkali administration. This amount of $NaHCO_3$ represents a dose of 1.7 to 2.3 mEq/kg, and an empirical dose of 2 mEq/kg could safely have been used.

In patients with severe acidosis, any additional small reduction in plasma HCO_3^- concentration represents a large percentage change and can markedly increase $[H^+]$ (and reduce pH).[184] For example, consider a normal dog with a pH of 7.387, $[H^+]$ = 41 nEq/L, Pco_2 = 36 mm Hg, and $[HCO_3^-]$ = 21 mEq/L that sustains a peracute reduction in $[HCO_3^-]$ of 2 mEq/L (new $[HCO_3^-]$ = 19 mEq/L) before respiratory compensation can develop. The new $[H^+]$ can be calculated from the Henderson equation as 24(36)/19 = 45 nEq/L (pH 7.347). This represents a 0.04-U change in pH and a 4-nEq/L change in $[H^+]$. Now consider a dog with a pH of 7.102, $[H^+]$ = 79 nEq/L, Pco_2 = 23 mm Hg, and $[HCO_3^-]$ = 7 mEq/L that sustains a peracute reduction in $[HCO_3^-]$ of 2 mEq/L (new $[HCO_3^-]$ = 5 mEq/L) before respiratory compensation can develop. The dog's new $[H^+]$ is $24(23)/5 = 110$ nEq/L (pH 6.959). This represents a 0.14-U change in pH and a 31-nEq/L change in $[H^+]$. This change in $[H^+]$ is almost eight times greater than that observed in the previous example. Thus a small change in $[HCO_3^-]$ has a much more dramatic effect on $[H^+]$ and pH when the initial $[HCO_3^-]$ concentration is very low. For this reason, patients with very low plasma HCO_3^- concentrations and pH values less than 7.1 to 7.2 should be treated promptly with small amounts of $NaHCO_3$ to increase their pH to the hemodynamically safe value of 7.2.

Potential complications of $NaHCO_3$ therapy include volume overload caused by administered sodium, tetany resulting from decreased serum ionized calcium concentration caused by increased binding of calcium to plasma proteins, decreased O_2 delivery to tissues because of increased affinity of hemoglobin for O_2, paradoxical CNS acidosis as hyperventilation abates and CO_2 diffuses into CSF, late development of alkalosis as metabolism of organic anions (e.g., ketoanions, lactate) replenishes body HCO_3^- stores, and hypokalemia as potassium ions enter and H^+ ions exit intracellular fluid in response to alkalinization of ECF.[94]

METABOLIC ALKALOSIS

Metabolic alkalosis is characterized by a primary increase in plasma HCO_3^- concentration, decreased $[H^+]$, increased pH, and a secondary or adaptive increase in PCO_2. Metabolic alkalosis was the third most common acid-base disturbance in dogs and cats in one study.[53]

Metabolic alkalosis can be caused by loss of chloride-rich fluid from the body via either the gastrointestinal tract or kidneys or by chronic administration of alkali. In the normal animal, renal excretion of exogenously administered alkali is very efficient, and it is difficult to create metabolic alkalosis by administration of alkali unless there is some factor preventing renal HCO_3^- excretion. Most cases of metabolic alkalosis in small animal practice are caused either by vomiting of stomach contents or by administration of diuretics. In a review of 962 dogs evaluated by blood gas determinations, 20 (2%) were found to be alkalemic.[179] Of these 20 dogs, 13 had metabolic alkalosis and 7 had respiratory alkalosis. Of the 13 dogs with metabolic alkalosis, 10 had a history of gastrointestinal disease.

CLASSIFICATION OF METABOLIC ALKALOSIS

Patients with metabolic alkalosis may be divided into two groups.[90,109,110,185,212] One group has ECFV depletion and avid renal retention of sodium and chloride. These patients respond to chloride administration and are said to have **chloride-responsive metabolic alkalosis.** The other group has normal or increased ECFV, and all sodium chloride ingested on a daily basis is excreted in the urine. These patients do not respond to chloride administration and are said to have **chloride-resistant metabolic alkalosis.**

In most instances of chloride-responsive metabolic alkalosis, the chloride concentration of the fluid lost from the body is greater than that of the ECF, so there has been a disproportionate loss of chloride. For example, the chloride concentration of gastric fluid is approximately 150 mEq/L, whereas serum chloride concentration is approximately 110 mEq/L in the dog and 120 mEq/L in the cat. Chloride-responsive metabolic alkalosis is much more common in small animal practice than is chloride-resistant metabolic alkalosis.

DEVELOPMENT OF CHLORIDE-RESPONSIVE METABOLIC ALKALOSIS

The pathophysiology of chloride-responsive metabolic alkalosis can be understood by considering the events associated with selective removal of gastric HCl.[117,118,158] Loss of H^+ from the stomach is associated, milliequivalent for milliequivalent, with an increase in the concentration of HCO_3^- in ECF. Plasma HCO_3^- concentration and the filtered load of HCO_3^- in the kidneys increase. Natriuresis, kaliuresis, suppression of net acid excretion with bicarbonaturia, increased urine flow rate, and renal water loss follow, but bicarbonaturia is transient and insufficient to return plasma HCO_3^- concentration to normal.[158] These events occurred without any change in GFR in a study of dogs made alkalotic by hemofiltration and replacement of ECF with a solution containing HCO_3^- as the only anion.[20] It is thought that the abatement of bicarbonaturia was caused by renal sodium avidity, engendered by the volume deficit that developed as a result of the initial natriuresis and diuresis. Renal sodium avidity is thus established and contributes to perpetuation of the alkalosis and development of a potassium deficit as long as chloride intake remains deficient. These events constitute the **development phase** of chloride-responsive metabolic alkalosis.

Probably the most important factors in the **maintenance phase** of chloride-responsive metabolic alkalosis are ECFV depletion and the chloride deficit, two factors that are difficult to separate experimentally.[45,87,111,160,188] Other factors that contribute to perpetuation of metabolic alkalosis are the effects of aldosterone and the potassium deficit. Aldosterone concentration is increased by ECFV depletion and results in increased distal renal Na^+-H^+ and Na^+-K^+ exchange. This results in perpetuation of alkalosis and development of a potassium deficit. Potassium depletion leads to a transcellular shift of H^+ from ECF to intracellular fluid in exchange for potassium ions. When this shift occurs in renal tubular cells, it decreases pH_i and enhances H^+ secretion by the renal tubular cells, further aggravating the alkalosis. Hypokalemia also stimulates renal ammoniagenesis, presumably through stimulation of glutaminase via decreased pH_i. The increase in renal ammonium excretion enhances renal acid excretion and contributes to increased plasma HCO_3^- concentration. Hypokalemia also may decrease GFR as a consequence of glomerular hemodynamic changes and may directly impair chloride reabsorption in the distal nephron, resulting in enhanced lumen electronegativity and facilitation of H^+ secretion into tubular fluid.

RESPONSE OF THE BODY TO METABOLIC ALKALOSIS

The body's response to metabolic alkalosis is the reverse of its response to administration of a mineral acid such as HCl. The kidney is more effective in excreting an alkaline load than an acid load, provided that the subject is not sodium avid and sufficient chloride is provided.

Acute Buffer Response

In an early study of the buffer response to alkali, nephrectomized dogs were given 20 mEq/kg $NaHCO_3$ with a resultant increase in plasma HCO_3^- concentration to approximately 60 mEq/L.[206] Of the administered HCO_3^-, almost one third (32%) was titrated by intracellular buffers. Of this 32%, 4% was converted to carbonic acid by H^+ from lactic acid released into ECF from cells. Increased pH_i enhances cellular production of lactic acid by stimulation of phosphofructokinase. Approximately 2% entered red cells in exchange for chloride (so-called chloride shift), and 26% was titrated by H^+ released from intracellular proteins and phosphates while sodium and potassium ions entered cells to maintain electroneutrality. By comparison, intracellular buffers handle approximately 50% of a mineral acid load.[195,207]

Approximately two thirds (68%) of the HCO_3^- load was confined to ECF. In response to the increase in pH, plasma proteins buffered 1% of this HCO_3^-. That is, plasma proteins released hydrogen ions in numbers sufficient to convert 1% of the infused HCO_3^- to carbonic acid. The remaining 67% was retained in the ECF compartment and contributed to the observed increase in plasma HCO_3^- concentration. These buffer reactions are summarized in Fig. 10-6.

Respiratory Response to Metabolic Alkalosis

The decrease in $[H^+]$ that accompanies chronic metabolic alkalosis stimulates chemoreceptors and is responsible for the observed decrease in alveolar ventilation. Secondary or adaptive alveolar hypoventilation protects pH in the presence of increased plasma HCO_3^- concentration (Fig. 10-7). A review of studies of dogs with experimentally induced metabolic alkalosis suggests that for each 1.0-mEq/L increase in plasma HCO_3^- concentration, there is an adaptive 0.55- to 0.77-mm Hg increase in P_{CO_2}.[20,35,131,132,171] This adaptive hypoventilation is associated with some degree of hypoxemia. Arterial P_{O_2} decreased to 60 to 70 mm Hg in dogs made

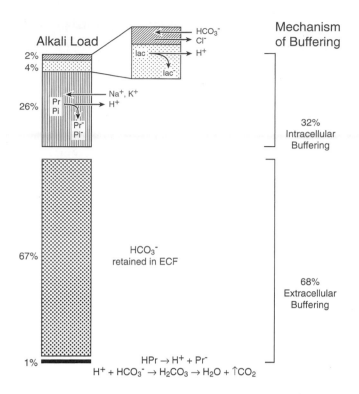

Fig. 10-6 Distribution of buffer response to a fixed alkaline load. (Drawing by Tim Vojt. Adapted from Pitts RF: *Physiology of the kidney and body fluids*, ed 2, Chicago, 1968, Year Book Medical Publishers, p. 173.)

alkalotic by feeding a diet with a chloride deficit and administering furosemide.[171]

The ventilatory response to metabolic alkalosis usually is considered to be less marked than the response to metabolic acidosis (i.e., a 0.6-mm Hg increase in P_{CO_2} for each 1-mEq/L increase in plasma HCO_3^- concentration in metabolic alkalosis as compared with a 1.2-mm Hg decrease in P_{CO_2} for each 1-mEq/L decrease in plasma HCO_3^- concentration in metabolic acidosis). This view has been challenged by a study of the ventilatory response of dogs to HCl acidosis and metabolic alkalosis induced by diuretics, removal of gastric acid, or mineralocorticoid administration.[132] The ventilatory responses to all of these experimental acid-base disturbances were not significantly different from one another, and it was concluded that an average change of 0.74 mm Hg P_{CO_2} can be expected for each 1.0-mEq/L change of plasma HCO_3^- concentration of metabolic origin. In one study, the respiratory compensation for metabolic alkalosis ranged from a 0.4- to 0.6-mm Hg increment in P_{CO_2} for each 1-mEq/L increment in HCO_3^- for arterial, mixed venous, and jugular venous samples in dogs made alkalotic by the administration of furosemide.[107] As a rule, a 1-mEq/L increase in plasma HCO_3^- concentration is expected to be associated with an adaptive 0.7-mm Hg increase in P_{CO_2} in dogs with metabolic alkalosis.

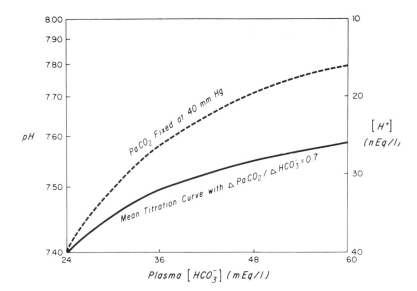

Fig. 10-7 Beneficial effect of respiratory adaptation on [H⁺] and pH. (From Harrington JT, Kassirer JP: Metabolic alkalosis. In Cohen JJ, Kassirer JP, editors: *Acid-base*. Boston, 1982, Little, Brown & Co, p. 237.)

Renal Response to Metabolic Alkalosis

In the normal animal, the kidneys rapidly and effectively excrete administered alkali. Metabolic alkalosis persists only if renal excretion of HCO_3^- is impaired. This may occur if there is reduced GFR (decreased filtered load of HCO_3^-), a continued high rate of alkali administration, or some stimulus for the kidneys to retain sodium in the presence of a relative chloride deficit. In most dogs and cats with metabolic alkalosis, a combination of renal sodium avidity and diminished chloride availability is responsible for perpetuation of the alkalosis. A potassium deficit and hypokalemia develop as the kidneys increase Na^+-K^+ exchange in the distal nephron.

When sodium, chloride, and water are removed in proportion to their concentrations in ECF, sodium avidity develops but alkalosis does not.[91] When the sodium deficit in an alkalotic animal is repaired by infusing a fluid identical in composition to the alkalotic ECF, metabolic alkalosis is corrected by selective retention of chloride.[45] This occurs even when the filtered load of chloride is kept constant during the infusion of fluid.[46] Thus both sodium avidity and decreased chloride availability seem to be necessary for the perpetuation of metabolic alkalosis.

Potassium deficiency does not cause alkalosis but rather is a result of the alkalotic state. In fact, isolated potassium deficiency in dogs leads to mild metabolic acidosis.[30,31] When potassium retention is prevented but sodium chloride is supplied, alkalosis is corrected despite a persisting potassium deficit.[12,117,158] If potassium is supplied but chloride is not, alkalosis cannot be corrected.[116] Administration of potassium chloride leads to complete correction of both alkalosis and the potassium deficit.

The renal response to hypercapnia in metabolic alkalosis was studied in normal unanesthetized dogs made alkalotic by dietary chloride restriction and administration of ethacrynic acid.[131] Adaptive hypercapnia was allowed to develop and then prevented by exposure to hypoxia. During development of metabolic alkalosis, serum sodium concentration remained unchanged, but serum chloride, potassium, and phosphorus concentrations decreased, and lactate and unmeasured anion (i.e., anion gap) concentrations increased. With hypercapnia, plasma HCO_3^- concentration was maintained at 7.7 mEq/L above control values, whereas without hypercapnia it was maintained at 4.5 mEq/L above control values. Thus approximately 60% of the increase in plasma HCO_3^- concentration was caused by the renal response to chloride and volume depletion, whereas 40% of the increase could be attributed to adaptive hypercapnia. This response appeared to be a direct effect of PCO_2 on renal acid excretion and HCO_3^- reabsorption and was not related to any change in extracellular pH because the degree of alkalemia remained unchanged throughout the experiment. This portion of the increase in plasma HCO_3^- concentration (40%) may be considered maladaptive because it contributes to a higher extracellular pH. When metabolic alkalosis persists, this indiscriminate renal response to hypercapnia results in a further increase in plasma HCO_3^- concentration and abrogates the original beneficial effect of the increased plasma HCO_3^- concentration on extracellular pH.

CLINICAL FEATURES OF METABOLIC ALKALOSIS

The clinical features of dogs and cats with metabolic alkalosis are usually those of the underlying disease process. Neurologic signs have been reported in human patients with severe metabolic alkalosis and include agitation, disorientation, stupor, and coma.[92] Muscle twitching and seizures may occur but have been observed rarely in dogs with severe metabolic alkalosis.

Clinical signs also may result from the accompanying potassium depletion. Signs of potassium depletion include muscle weakness of varying severity, cardiac arrhythmias, alterations in renal function (e.g., defective concentrating

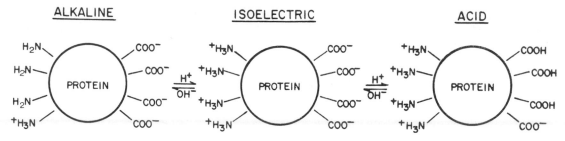

Fig. 10-8 Effect of alkalosis and acidosis on the charge of plasma proteins. (Modified from Pitts RF: *Physiology of the kidney and body fluids*, ed 2, Chicago, 1974, Year Book Medical Publishers, p. 186.)

ability), and gastrointestinal motility disturbances (e.g., ileus). These complications are discussed in Chapter 5.

Muscle twitching may occur as a result of decreased serum ionized calcium concentration because alkalosis increases the number of negative charges on proteins, allowing more calcium ions to be bound (Fig. 10-8). Serum ionized calcium concentration decreases and may account for neuromuscular irritability by rendering the threshold potential of cells more negative (i.e., bringing the resting potential closer to the threshold potential) (Fig. 10-9). Administration of a single dose (4 mEq/kg) of sodium bicarbonate to normal cats resulted in a 10% decrease in serum ionized calcium concentration and an 8% decrease in serum total calcium concentration. These changes persisted for 3 hours, but no clinical signs were observed.[36]

Metabolic alkalosis shifts the oxygen-hemoglobin dissociation curve to the left (Bohr effect) and impairs oxygen release from hemoglobin. This effect probably is not clinically significant because an increase in red cell 2,3-diphosphoglycerate concentration occurs after 6 to 8 hours of metabolic alkalosis and results in a shift of the curve back to the right.[16]

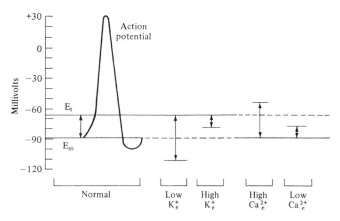

Fig. 10-9 Effect of hypocalcemia on the threshold potential (E_t) of cells. The height of the arrows is equal to the difference between the resting and threshold potentials and represents the excitability of the cell membrane. (From Rose BD: *Clinical physiology of acid-base and electrolyte disorders*, ed 3, New York, 1989, McGraw-Hill Co., p. 704.)

DIAGNOSIS OF METABOLIC ALKALOSIS

Specific clinical manifestations of metabolic alkalosis have not been reported in dogs and cats. The clinician must have a high index of suspicion for this disorder when presented with an animal having compatible clinical signs, usually chronic vomiting of stomach contents. Thus an accurate history is the key to suspecting the diagnosis. Metabolic alkalosis also can be suspected from the results of routine serum biochemical tests. Blood gas analysis should be performed if decreased serum chloride and potassium concentrations are observed and total CO_2 content is increased. Blood gas analysis allows the clinician to determine whether primary metabolic alkalosis is present and whether the magnitude of respiratory compensation is as predicted (see earlier). The concentration of unmeasured anions (i.e., anion gap) in metabolic alkalosis may increase because of loss of hydrogen ions from nonbicarbonate buffers. The increased anion gap is primarily caused by increased numbers of negative charges on proteins and partially the result of the increase in plasma protein concentration that occurs as a consequence of ECFV depletion.[3]

Urine pH is low during the maintenance phase of metabolic alkalosis because of enhanced distal Na^+-H^+ exchange and reabsorption of all filtered HCO_3^-. However, urine pH is alkaline during development of and recovery from metabolic alkalosis. Thus urinary pH is of little diagnostic significance in metabolic alkalosis.

Causes of Metabolic Alkalosis

Metabolic alkalosis can be caused by continuous administration of alkali, disproportionate loss of chloride (chloride-responsive alkalosis), or excessive mineralocorticoid effect (chloride-resistant alkalosis). In some instances, the mechanism of metabolic alkalosis is unknown, and these examples are classified as miscellaneous. Most dogs with gastric dilatation-volvulus have metabolic acidosis or normal blood gas values at presentation,[153,223] but, uncommonly, metabolic alkalosis and hypokalemia have been reported.[115] The causes of metabolic alkalosis are listed in Box 10-3, and the pathophysiology of the major types of metabolic alkalosis is considered further here.

Chloride Responsive
Vomiting of stomach contents
Diuretic therapy
Posthypercapnia

Chloride Resistant
Primary hyperaldosteronism
Hyperadrenocorticism

Alkali Administration
Oral administration of sodium bicarbonate or other
    organic anions (e.g., lactate, citrate, gluconate, acetate)
Oral administration of cation exchange resin with
    nonabsorbable alkali (e.g., phosphorus binder)

Miscellaneous
Refeeding after fasting
High-dose penicillin
Severe potassium or magnesium deficiency

Chloride-Responsive Metabolic Alkalosis

Chronic vomiting of stomach contents and administration of diuretics are the most common causes of chloride-responsive metabolic alkalosis in dogs and cats.

Administration of Alkali. Acute administration of 4 mEq/kg $NaHCO_3$ to normal unanesthetized cats resulted in mild increases in venous blood pH and HCO_3^- concentration lasting 180 minutes.[37] A slight decrease in serum chloride concentration persisted for 30 minutes, whereas a mild increase in PCO_2 persisted for 60 minutes. A solution of $NaHCO_3$ (6.6 mEq/L) infused over 30 minutes into anesthetized dogs caused transient increases in arterial PCO_2, pH, base excess, and standard bicarbonate concentration.[95] Prompt renal excretion of administered $NaHCO_3$ presumably prevented any persistent change in acid-base values in these acute studies. Renal acid excretion decreases, urine pH increases, and administered $NaHCO_3$ is excreted within hours. There is an acute increase in carbonic acid and PCO_2 as body buffers release H^+ to combine with the administered HCO_3^-. The excess $NaHCO_3$ is excreted in the urine, increased ventilation occurs in response to increased PCO_2, and acid-base balance is restored to normal.

When alkali is administered chronically, plasma HCO_3^- concentration becomes a function of the daily dosage administered but returns to normal within a few days after alkali administration is discontinued. If alkali is given to subjects rendered sodium avid by previous dietary salt restriction, smaller dosages of alkali result in greater increases in plasma HCO_3^- concentration than are observed when higher alkali dosages are used in subjects receiving normal amounts of dietary salt.

Sources of alkali other than $NaHCO_3$ may also contribute to metabolic alkalosis. Such organic anions include lactate that has accumulated during lactic acidosis, ketoacids in uncontrolled diabetes mellitus, and citrate in banked blood or that administered in an attempt to prevent recurrence of calcium oxalate urolithiasis. These organic anions yield HCO_3^- when metabolized:

$$Anion^- + O_2 \rightarrow HCO_3^- + CO_2 + H_2O$$

This reaction often serves to replace the HCO_3^- titrated during development of the acidosis (e.g., lactic acidosis, diabetic ketoacidosis). If $NaHCO_3$ has been administered during treatment, however, metabolism of the organic anion after correction of the acidosis can result in metabolic alkalosis. If renal function is normal and volume depletion is not present, the kidneys promptly excrete the excess HCO_3^- and restore normal acid-base balance.

Administration of nonabsorbable alkali (e.g., aluminum hydroxide used as a phosphorus binder in patients with renal failure) usually does not cause metabolic alkalosis. Neutralization of H^+ by $Al(OH)_3$ in the stomach results in the net addition of HCO_3^- to ECF. Combination of Al^{3+} with HCO_3^- secreted by the pancreas produces insoluble $Al_2(CO_3)_3$ in the duodenum, and there is no net increase in HCO_3^- ions in ECF. If, however, $Al(OH)_3$ is administered concurrently with a cationic exchange resin (e.g., polystyrene sulfonate), the resin can bind Al^{3+}, leaving HCO_3^- secreted by the pancreas to be reabsorbed in the small intestine, thus resulting in alkalinization of ECF. When renal failure is present, the kidneys have reduced capacity to excrete retained HCO_3^-, and metabolic alkalosis could result. This sequence of events is most likely to occur in an animal with oliguric renal failure that is treated concurrently with $Al(OH)_3$ for hyperphosphatemia and with polystyrene sulfonate for hyperkalemia.

Gastric Fluid Loss. The H^+ and Na^+ concentrations of gastric fluid are inversely related to one another, whereas the K^+ concentration is relatively stable (approximately 10 mEq/L). The Cl^- concentration is very high (approximately 150 mEq/L) and remains remarkably constant even when hypochloremia develops. Subtracting the sum of the Na^+ and K^+ concentrations of gastric fluid from the Cl^- concentration yields an approximation of the H^+ concentration. The composition of gastric fluid is compared with that of other body fluids in Fig. 10-10. When a dog or cat vomits stomach contents, water is lost along with large amounts of HCl and small amounts of potassium and sodium.

The H^+ produced during gastric acid secretion originates from the dissociation of carbonic acid; thus an equal number of HCO_3^- ions are generated in ECF. In the normal animal, gastric acid secretion does not

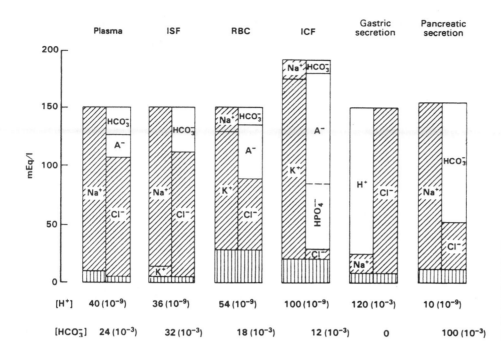

Fig. 10-10 Comparison of electrolyte composition of gastric juice to other body fluids using Gamblegrams. Strong ions are crosshatched. (From Jones NL: *Blood gases and acid-base physiology*, ed 2, New York, 1987, Thieme Medical Publishers, p. 133.)

disturb acid-base balance because the increase in ECF HCO_3^- concentration that accompanies parietal cell H^+ secretion is balanced by pancreatic HCO_3^- secretion in the duodenum, and Cl^- secreted into the stomach is recaptured lower in the gastrointestinal tract. When stomach contents are lost, H^+ and Cl^- are removed from this system, and HCO_3^- secreted into the duodenum by the pancreas is no longer titrated by gastric H^+ but is reabsorbed farther down in the gastrointestinal tract in place of Cl^-. The normal relationship between gastric and pancreatic secretions in the gastrointestinal tract is shown in Fig. 10-11. Continued loss of gastric fluid can result in marked increases in plasma HCO_3^- concentration, and chronic vomiting of stomach contents is the most common cause of metabolic alkalosis in small animal practice.

In studies of gastric alkalosis, experimental subjects are rendered sodium avid by feeding a low-salt diet. Gastric fluid is then continuously removed by nasogastric suction, and fluid and electrolyte losses other than HCl are quantitatively replaced.[117,118,158] The effects of repeated gastric drainage over 3 days on plasma HCO_3^- and chloride concentrations and on potassium, sodium, and chloride balance in experimental dogs are shown in Fig. 10-12. Note that the resulting metabolic alkalosis is corrected by provision of NaCl despite a progressively negative potassium balance. In the clinical setting, persistent vomiting of stomach contents leads to fluid and electrolyte losses (H^+ and $Cl^- > Na^+$ and K^+), and anorexia prevents adequate dietary intake of electrolytes. In patients with pyloric obstruction, gastrin secretion is

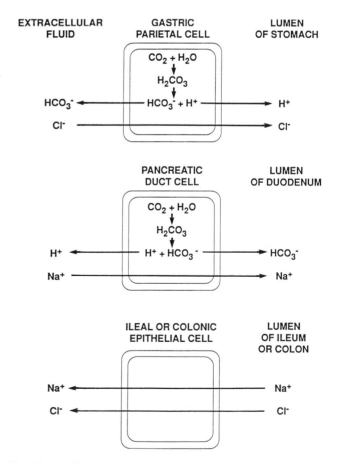

Fig. 10-11 Normal relationship between gastric and pancreatic secretions in the gastrointestinal tract. (Modified from Guyton AC: *Textbook of medical physiology*, ed 7, Philadelphia, 1986, WB Saunders, pp. 775-779.)

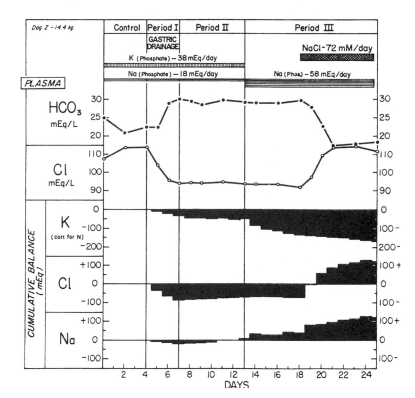

Fig. 10-12 Plasma composition and electrolyte balance in a representative study of selective HCl depletion. (From Needle MA, Kaloyanides GJ, Schwartz WB: The effects of selective depletion of hydrochloric acid on acid-base and electrolyte equilibrium. Reproduced from the *Journal of Clinical Investigation*, 43:1839, 1964, by copyright permission of the American Society for Clinical Investigation.)

enhanced, and gastric acid secretion is stimulated further. Overproduction of gastrin by a gastrin-secreting tumor may also stimulate gastric acid secretion. In one dog with gastrinoma, severe metabolic alkalosis and hypokalemia were associated with a history of chronic vomiting.[205]

Renal avidity for sodium and defense of the ECFV occur because of ongoing fluid and electrolyte losses in the vomiting animal or intake of a low-salt diet and nasogastric suction in the experimental setting. To maintain ECFV, the kidneys must reabsorb sodium by all available mechanisms. Because of ongoing loss of gastric HCl and insufficient dietary intake of salt, there is a chloride deficit; consequently, the kidneys must reabsorb less sodium with chloride and more sodium in exchange for hydrogen and potassium ions. The latter two mechanisms contribute to perpetuation of the metabolic alkalosis and development of potassium depletion as shown in Fig. 10-13. The low urine pH during the maintenance phase reflects increased distal Na^+-H^+ exchange in the sodium-avid state. This observation has led to the term "paradoxical aciduria" to describe the finding of low urine pH in patients with metabolic alkalosis. However, consideration of the relevant pathophysiology shows that this reduction in urine pH is the appropriate renal response under the circumstances. The extent of potassium depletion that develops is related to the severity and chronicity of the metabolic alkalosis.

Provision of chloride as the sodium or potassium salt allows correction of the alkalosis because the kidneys may now preferentially reabsorb sodium with chloride and rely less on Na^+-K^+ and Na^+-H^+ exchange.[12,116,117,158] This allows retained HCO_3^- to be excreted in the urine. Urine pH increases as HCO_3^- is excreted, indicating a favorable response to therapy. Chloride once again appears in the urine when the alkalosis is resolved. *The critical factor in resolution of this form of alkalosis is the provision of chloride as a resorbable anion.* Alkalosis can be corrected without provision of sodium or potassium as long as chloride is provided. Clinically, however, alkalosis is corrected by administering some combination of NaCl and KCl.

Diuretic Administration. Diuretics cause approximately equal losses of sodium and chloride in the urine, but the concentration of chloride in ECF is less than that of sodium by approximately 35 mEq/L. Thus these drugs may cause chloride-responsive metabolic alkalosis by a disproportionate loss of chloride in urine and creation of a relative chloride deficit in ECF. Increased renal sodium avidity is also an important factor in development of the metabolic alkalosis and potassium depletion that may occur during diuretic administration.

Loop diuretics inhibit NaCl reabsorption in the thick ascending limb of Henle's loop by competing with chloride for the Na^+-K^+-$2Cl^-$ luminal carrier. This causes increased delivery of sodium to the distal nephron, where accelerated Na^+-H^+ and Na^+-K^+ exchange occurs as the kidneys attempt to retain more sodium. Increased reliance of the kidneys on these mechanisms for sodium reabsorption contributes to metabolic alkalosis and potassium depletion. These complications are less likely

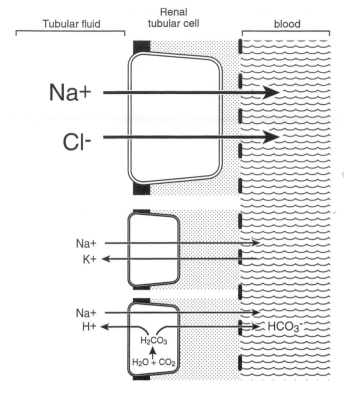

Tubular fluid   Renal tubular cell   blood

Na+

Cl-

Na+
K+

Na+
H+
H_2CO_3
$H_2O + CO_2$
HCO_3^-

Approximate Filtered Loads
(10kg dog with GFR 4ml/min/kg)

Na^+	8352 mEq/day
Cl^-	6336 mEq/day
HCO_3^-	1210 mEq/day
K^+	230 mEq/day

Fig. 10-13 Effects of chloride and potassium depletion on acid-base balance. See text for explanation. (Drawing by Tim Vojt.)

when thiazide diuretics are used. Thiazide diuretics inhibit NaCl transport in the distal tubule and connecting segment. They are less potent than the loop diuretics because their main effect occurs at sites in the nephron distal to those responsible for the majority of sodium reabsorption.

In response to hypokalemia, transcellular shifts of H^+ from ECF into renal tubular cells may occur in exchange for K^+. The resultant increase in intracellular H^+ concentration facilitates renal Na^+-H^+ exchange and aggravates metabolic alkalosis. Stimulation of the renin-angiotensin-aldosterone system by decreased effective circulating volume also favors increased Na^+-H^+ and Na^+-K^+ exchange in the distal nephron. These latter effects are probably important in most forms of chloride-responsive metabolic alkalosis.

Many animals treated with diuretics have congestive heart failure as their primary disease process. If the treatment plan for the animal includes a low-sodium diet, renal sodium avidity is guaranteed and increases the ten-

dency toward metabolic alkalosis and potassium depletion. Complications from diuretic therapy are unlikely if the animal is drinking water and eating a diet with adequate amounts of chloride. However, complications can develop if the animal becomes anorexic.

Posthypercapnia. Blood pH increases rapidly when Pco_2 is suddenly reduced in patients with chronic hypercapnia. This has been called posthypercapnic metabolic alkalosis. In such patients, plasma HCO_3^- concentration has previously been increased by adaptive changes in renal HCO_3^- reabsorption. In response to the lowered Pco_2, it takes several hours for the kidneys to decrease Na^+-H^+ exchange and begin to excrete the previously retained HCO_3^-. It may take several days for the kidneys to excrete all of the excess HCO_3^-, and sufficient chloride must be available during this time for reabsorption with sodium. Chloride deficiency during recovery from chronic hypercapnia plays a role in sustaining posthypercapnic metabolic alkalosis. Provision of chloride allows the alkalosis to be corrected.[194] Posthypercapnic metabolic alkalosis occurs most commonly in human patients with chronic pulmonary disease who are treated by mechanical ventilation. It is important that Pco_2 is decreased slowly and that adequate chloride intake is provided to prevent this complication.

Chloride-Resistant Metabolic Alkalosis

Several disorders in human medicine may cause chloride-resistant metabolic alkalosis. Of these, primary hyperaldosteronism and hyperadrenocorticism may occur in small animal practice. However, chloride-resistant metabolic alkalosis is rare in dogs and cats.

Primary Hyperaldosteronism. In primary hyperaldosteronism, increased secretion of aldosterone, usually by an adrenocortical tumor, results in sodium retention, volume expansion, hypernatremia, mild to moderate hypertension, potassium deficiency, hypokalemia, and metabolic alkalosis resistant to chloride administration. Plasma renin activity is low, but plasma aldosterone concentration is high. Affected human patients are in salt balance at an expanded ECFV and excrete ingested NaCl in the urine. Stimulation of distal nephron Na^+-H^+ and Na^+-K^+ exchange by excess mineralocorticoids is probably the most important pathophysiologic feature of primary hyperaldosteronism.

Several dogs and cats with primary hyperaldosteronism caused by aldosterone-producing adenomas or adenocarcinomas of the adrenal gland have been reported in the veterinary literature. Clinical features in affected animals included polyuria, polydipsia, weakness, hypertension, hypokalemia, hypernatremia, mild metabolic alkalosis, dilute urine, and extremely high serum aldosterone concentrations (for additional information and references see Chapter 5).

Hyperadrenocorticism. Metabolic alkalosis occurs in approximately one third of human patients with Cushing's syndrome.[93] It is more common in patients with adrenocortical carcinomas and in those with ectopic production of ACTH by nonadrenal malignancies than in those with pituitary-dependent hyperadrenocorticism. The frequency of metabolic alkalosis and serum electrolyte disturbances in dogs with hyperadrenocorticism is uncertain. Serum sodium and potassium concentrations often are normal in dogs with hyperadrenocorticism. This may reflect the fact that 80% to 85% of dogs with hyperadrenocorticism have pituitary-dependent disease. In a large group of dogs with hyperadrenocorticism, 21 of 52 (40%) dogs had increased serum sodium concentrations and 25 of 52 (48%) had decreased serum potassium concentrations.[125] The relative frequency of pituitary- and adrenal-dependent disease was not reported in this study. In another study, mild hypernatremia and hypokalemia were observed occasionally in dogs with hyperadrenocorticism, and total CO_2 content was increased in 33% of affected dogs.[173] In another report, hypokalemia was found in only 5% of dogs with pituitary-dependent hyperadrenocorticism but in 45% of those with adrenocortical neoplasia.[144] A high rate of secretion of cortisol and other corticosteroids such as desoxycorticosterone and corticosterone in patients with adrenocortical malignancies could be responsible for hypernatremia, hypokalemia, and metabolic alkalosis in adrenal-dependent hyperadrenocorticism.

Miscellaneous

Large doses of penicillin, ampicillin, or carbenicillin administered as a sodium salt can lead to hypokalemia and metabolic alkalosis in human patients. The drug may increase lumen electronegativity in the distal nephron by acting as a nonresorbable anion and enhancing Na^+-H^+ and Na^+-K^+ exchange. "Refeeding" alkalosis can occur in human patients when glucose is administered after prolonged fasting. The mechanism for this type of alkalosis is unknown. These types of metabolic alkalosis have not been reported in the veterinary literature.

TREATMENT OF METABOLIC ALKALOSIS

Acid-base disturbances are secondary phenomena. Diagnosis and definitive treatment of the responsible disease process are integral to the successful resolution of acid-base disorders. However, it must be remembered that alkalosis persists until chloride is replaced if vomiting of stomach contents or diuretic administration is responsible for the metabolic alkalosis. The goal of treatment in chloride-responsive metabolic alkalosis is to replace the chloride deficit while providing sufficient potassium and sodium to replace existing deficits. Definitive treatment of the underlying disease process (e.g., removal of a gastric foreign body) prevents recurrence of the metabolic alkalosis.

Patients with chronic pulmonary disease that have hypoxemia and hypercapnia are at greater risk from metabolic alkalosis than others because superimposition of metabolic alkalosis can further reduce ventilation and lead to worsening of hypoxemia. Thus metabolic alkalosis should be treated appropriately if present and avoided if not present. Giving oxygen to patients with metabolic alkalosis should also be avoided if possible because this may impair ventilation and further aggravate hypercapnia.

Potassium without chloride (e.g., potassium phosphate) corrects neither the alkalosis nor the potassium deficit because administered potassium is excreted in the urine. A chloride salt must be given for alkalosis to be resolved and potassium retention to occur. Provision of chloride as either the sodium or potassium salt corrects chloride-responsive metabolic alkalosis. This therapy allows the kidneys to reabsorb the sodium the body requires with chloride to maintain electroneutrality. Thus a NaCl solution (0.45% or 0.9%) with added KCl is the fluid of choice for dogs and cats with chloride-responsive metabolic alkalosis. It is best to use solutions containing NaCl and KCl because affected animals typically have been sick long enough to develop clinically significant potassium deficits. Administering 0.9% NaCl without KCl can cause diuresis and increased urinary excretion of potassium, thus worsening any potassium deficit. As shown in Fig. 10-12, provision of NaCl corrects metabolic alkalosis induced in dogs by gastric drainage, but the potassium deficit persists unless potassium is provided. A few days may be required to restore normal electrolyte and acid-base balance, but in nearly all instances, these measures are sufficient to resolve the alkalosis. In human patients with severe metabolic alkalosis or in those with severely impaired renal function, HCl or arginine HCl has been used for rapid correction of metabolic alkalosis, but there is no report of the use of these compounds in animals with metabolic alkalosis, and their use is not recommended.

H2-blocking drugs such as cimetidine, ranitidine, or famotidine may be considered as adjunctive therapy if gastric losses are ongoing because this approach reduces gastric acid secretion. For the patient with heart failure receiving loop diuretics, oral KCl administration is the best way to provide chloride without sodium and prevent further retention of fluid and aggravation of edema. Even in the presence of sodium avidity, provision of chloride lessens Na^+-H^+ and Na^+-K^+ exchange at distal nephron sites and prevents development of alkalosis when loop diuretics are used. Simultaneous use of distal blocking agents such as spironolactone, triamterene, or amiloride may also be considered. These drugs work in the principal cells of the cortical collecting tubule and impair Na^+-H^+ and Na^+-K^+ exchange by inhibiting aldosterone-sensitive sodium channels. In metabolic alkalosis caused by chronic administration of alkali, discontinuation of the source of alkali results in correction of the alkalosis over a few days, provided that renal function is normal.

Chloride-resistant metabolic alkalosis is uncommon in comparison with chloride-responsive metabolic alkalosis. When present, its successful treatment requires that the underlying disease be diagnosed and treated before alkalosis can be resolved. Cases of chloride-resistant metabolic alkalosis are rare in veterinary medicine.

REFERENCES

1. Adams WH, Toal RL, Walker MA, et al: Early renal ultrasonographic findings in dogs with experimentally induced ethylene glycol nephrosis, *Am J Vet Res* 50:1370, 1989.
2. Adrogue HJ, Brensilver J, Cohen J, et al: Influence of steady-state alterations in acid-base equilibrium on the fate of administered bicarbonate in the dog, *J Clin Invest* 71:867, 1983.
3. Adrogue HJ, Brensilver J, Madias NE: Changes in the plasma anion gap during chronic metabolic acid-base disturbances, *Am J Physiol* 235:F291, 1978.
4. Adrogue HJ, Eknoyan G, Suki WK: Diabetic ketoacidosis: role of the kidney in the acid-base homeostasis re-evaluated, *Kidney Int* 25:591, 1984.
5. Adrogue HJ, Madias NE: Changes in plasma potassium concentration during acute acid base disturbances, *J Clin Invest* 71:456, 1981.
6. Adrogue HJ, Madias NE: Management of life-threatening acid-base disorders, *N Engl J Med* 338:26, 1998.
7. Adrogue HJ, Rashad MN, Gorin AB, et al: Arteriovenous acid-base disparity in circulatory failure: studies on mechanism, *Am J Physiol* 257:F1087, 1989.
8. Adrogue HJ, Wilson H, Boyd AE, et al: Plasma acid-base patterns in diabetic ketoacidosis, *N Engl J Med* 307:1603, 1982.
9. Arieff AI, Graf H: Pathophysiology of type A hypoxic lactic acidosis in dogs, *Am J Physiol* 253:E271, 1987.
10. Arruda JAL, Carrasquillo T, Cubria A, et al: Bicarbonate reabsorption in chronic renal failure, *Kidney Int* 9:481, 1976.
11. Atkins CE, Tyler R, Greenlee P: Clinical, biochemical, acid-base, and electrolyte abnormalities in cats after hypertonic sodium phosphate enema administration, *Am J Vet Res* 46:980, 1985.
12. Atkins EL, Schwartz WB: Factors governing correction of the alkalosis associated with potassium deficiency: the critical role of chloride in the recovery process, *J Clin Invest* 41:218, 1962.
13. Barbee RW, Kline JA, Watts JA: Depletion of lactate by dichloroacetate reduces cardiac efficiency after hemorrhagic shock, *Shock* 14:208-214, 2000.
14. Bark H, Perk R: Fanconi syndrome associated with amoxicillin therapy in the dog, *Canine Pract* 20:19, 1995.
15. Beckett SD, Shields RP: Treatment of acute ethylene glycol (antifreeze) poisoning in the dog, *J Am Vet Med Assoc* 158:472, 1971.
16. Bellingham AJ, Detter JC, Lenfant C: Regulatory mechanisms of hemoglobin oxygen affinity in acidosis and alkalosis, *J Clin Invest* 50:700, 1971.
17. Benjamin J, Oropello JM, Abalos AM, et al: Effects of acid-base correction on hemodynamics, oxygen dynamics, and resuscitability in severe canine hemorrhagic shock, *Crit Care Med* 22:1616, 1994.
18. Bergman KS, Harris BH: Arteriovenous pH difference—a new index of perfusion, *J Pediatr Surg* 23:1190, 1988.
19. Bersin RM, Arieff AL: Improved hemodynamic function during hypoxia with Carbicarb, a new agent for the management of acidosis, *Circulation* 77:227, 1988.
20. Borkan S, Northrup TE, Cohen JJ, et al: Renal response to metabolic alkalosis induced by isovolemic hemofiltration in the dog, *Kidney Int* 32:322, 1987.
21. Bovee KC: *Characterization and treatment of isolated renal tubular acidosis in a dog,* Washington, DC, 1984, American College of Veterinary Internal Medicine, p. 48.
22. Bovee KC, Joyce T, Reynolds R, et al: The Fanconi syndrome in basenji dogs: a new model for renal transport defects, *Science* 201:1129, 1978.
23. Bovee KC, Joyce T, Reynolds R, et al: Spontaneous Fanconi syndrome in the dog, *Metabolism* 27:45, 1978.
24. Bovee KC, Joyce T, Blazer-Yost B, et al: Characterization of renal defects in dogs with a syndrome similar to Fanconi syndrome in man, *J Am Vet Med Assoc* 174:1094, 1979.
25. Brown SA, Rackich PM, Barsanti JA, et al: Fanconi syndrome and acute renal failure associated with gentamicin therapy in a dog, *J Am Anim Hosp Assoc* 22:635, 1986.
26. Brown SA, Spyridakis LK, Crowell WA: Distal renal tubular acidosis and hepatic lipidosis in a cat *J Am Vet Med Assoc* 189:1350, 1986.
27. Bruskiewicz KA, Nelson RW, Feldman EC, et al: Diabetic ketosis and ketoacidosis in cats: 42 cases (1980–1995), *J Am Vet Med Assoc* 211:188, 1997.
28. Buffington CA, Cook NE, Rogers QR, et al: The role of diet in feline struvite urolithiasis syndrome. In Burger IH, Rivers JPW, editors: *Nutrition of the dog and cat,* London, 1989, Cambridge University Press, p. 357.
29. Burnell JM: Changes in bone sodium and carbonate in metabolic acidosis and alkalosis in the dog, *J Clin Invest* 50:327, 1971.
30. Burnell JM, Dawbron JK: Acid-base parameters in potassium depletion in the dog, *Am J Physiol* 218:1583, 1970.
31. Burnell JM, Teubner EJ, Simpson DP: Metabolic acidosis accompanying potassium deprivation, *Am J Physiol* 227:329, 1974.
32. Cain SM, Dunn JE: Transient arterial lactic acid changes in unanesthetized dogs at 21,000 feet, *Am J Physiol* 206:1437, 1964.
33. Carden DL, Martin GB, Nowak RM, et al: Lactic acidosis as a predictor of downtime during cardiopulmonary arrest in dogs, *Am J Emerg Med* 3:120, 1985.
34. Carden DL, Martin GB, Nowak RM, et al: Lactic acidosis during closed-chest CPR in dogs, *Ann Emerg Med* 16:1317, 1987.
35. Chazan JA, Appleton FM, London AM, et al: Effects of chronic metabolic acid-base disturbances on the composition of cerebrospinal fluid in the dog, *Clin Sci* 36:345, 1969.
36. Chew DJ, Leonard M, Muir WW: Effect of sodium bicarbonate infusions on ionized calcium and total calcium concentrations in serum of clinically normal cats, *Am J Vet Res* 50:145, 1989.
37. Chew DJ, Leonard M, Muir WW: Effect of sodium bicarbonate infusion on serum osmolality, electrolyte concentrations, and blood gas tensions in cats, *Am J Vet Res* 52:12, 1991.
38. Ching SV, Fettman MJ, Hamar DW, et al: The effect of chronic dietary acidification using ammonium chloride on acid-base and mineral metabolism in the adult cat, *J Nutr* 119:902, 1989.

39. Ching SV, Norrdin RW, Fettman MJ, et al: Trabecular bone remodeling and bone mineral density in the adult cat during chronic dietary acidification with ammonium chloride, *J Bone Miner Res* 5:547, 1990.

40. Christopher MM, Eckfeldt JH, Eaton JW: Propylene glycol ingestion causes D-lactic acidosis, *Lab Invest* 62:114, 1990.

41. Christopher MM, Perman V, White JG, et al: Propylene glycol–induced Heinz body formation and D-lactic acidosis in cats, *Prog Clin Biol Res* 319:69, 1989.

42. Chrusch C, Bands C, Bose D, et al: Impaired hepatic extraction and increased splanchnic production contribute to lactic acidosis in canine sepsis, *Am J Respir Crit Care Med* 161:517-526, 2000.

43. Clark DD, Chang BS, Garella SG, et al: Secondary hypocapnia fails to protect "whole body" intracellular pH during chronic HCl-acidosis in the dog, *Kidney Int* 23:336, 1983.

44. Clay KL, Murphy RC: On the metabolic acidosis of ethylene glycol intoxication, *Toxicol Appl Pharmacol* 39:39, 1977.

45. Cohen JJ: Correction of metabolic alkalosis by the kidney after isometric expansion of extracellular fluid, *J Clin Invest* 47:1181, 1968.

46. Cohen JJ: Selective chloride retention in repair of metabolic alkalosis without increasing filtered load, *Am J Physiol* 218:165, 1970.

47. Cohen JJ, Brackett NC, Schwartz WB: The nature of the carbon dioxide titration curve in the normal dog, *J Clin Invest* 43:777, 1964.

48. Cohen JJ, Madias NE, Wolf CJ, et al: Regulation of acid-base equilibrium in chronic hypocapnia: evidence that the response of the kidney is not geared to the defense of extracellular [H^+], *J Clin Invest* 57:1483, 1976.

49. Cohen RD, Woods RA: *Clinical and biochemical aspects of lactic acidosis,* London, 1976, Blackwell Scientific.

50. Cohen RM, Feldman GM, Fernandez PC: The balance of acid, base and charge in health and disease, *Kidney Int* 52:287, 1997.

51. Connally HE, Thrall MA, Forney SD, et al: Safety and efficacy of 4-methylpyrazole for treatment of suspected or confirmed ethylene glycol intoxication: 107 cases (1983–1995), *J Am Vet Med Assoc* 209:1880, 1996.

52. Constable PD, Stämpfli HR: Experimental determination of net protein charge and A_{tot} and K_a of nonvolatile buffers in canine plasma, *J Vet Intern Med* 19:507, 2005.

53. Cornelius LM, Rawlings CA: Arterial blood gas and acid base values in dogs with various diseases and signs of disease, *J Am Vet Med Assoc* 178:992, 1981.

54. Crabb DW, Young EA, Harris RA: The metabolic effects of dichloroacetate, *Metab Clin Exp* 30:1024, 1981.

55. Crenshaw KL, Peterson ME: Pretreatment clinical and laboratory evaluation of cats with diabetes mellitus: 104 cases (1992–1994), *J Am Vet Med Assoc* 209:943, 1996.

56. Darrigrand-Haag RA, Center SA, Randolph JF, et al: Congenital Fanconi syndrome associated with renal dysplasia in 2 Border terriers, *J Vet Intern Med* 10:412, 1996.

57. DeFronzo RA: Hyperkalemia and hyporeninemic hypoaldosteronism, *Kidney Int* 17:118, 1980.

58. DeSousa RC, Harrington JT, Ricanati ES, et al: Renal regulation of acid-base equilibrium during chronic administration of mineral acid, *J Clin Invest* 53:465, 1974.

59. Dial SM, Thrall M, Hamar DW: 4-Methylpyrazole as treatment for naturally acquired ethylene glycol intoxication in dogs, *J Am Vet Med Assoc* 195:73, 1989.

60. Dial SM, Thrall MAH, Hamar DW: Comparison of ethanol and 4-methylpyrazole as treatments for ethylene glycol intoxication in cats, *Am J Vet Res* 55:1771, 1994.

61. Dial SM, Thrall MAH, Hamar DW: Efficacy of 4-methylpyrazole for treatment of ethylene glycol intoxication in dogs, *Am J Vet Res* 55:1762, 1994.

62. DiBartola SP, Leonard PO: Renal tubular acidosis in a dog, *J Am Vet Med Assoc* 180:70, 1982.

63. DiBartola SP, Rutgers HC, Zack PM, et al: Clinicopathologic findings associated with chronic renal disease in cats: 74 cases (1973–1984), *J Am Vet Med Assoc* 190:1196, 1987.

64. DiBartola SP, Tarr MJ, Parker AT, et al: Clinicopathologic findings in dogs with renal amyloidosis: 59 cases (1976–1986), *J Am Vet Med Assoc* 195:358, 1989.

65. Dinour D, Chang MH, Satoh J, et al: A novel missense mutation in the sodium bicarbonate cotransporter (NBCe1/SLC4A4) causes proximal tubular acidosis and glaucoma through ion transport defects, *J Biol Chem* 279:52238-52246, 2004.

66. Dorhout-Mees EJ, Machado M, Slatopolsky E, et al: The functional adaptation of the diseased kidney. III. Ammonium excretion, *J Clin Invest* 45:289, 1966.

67. Dow SW, Fettman MJ, Smith KR, et al: Effects of dietary acidification and potassium depletion on acid-base balance, mineral metabolism and renal function in adult cats, *J Nutr* 120:569, 1990.

68. Drazner FH: Distal renal tubular acidosis associated with chronic pyelonephritis in a cat, *Calif Vet* 34:15, 1980.

69. Duarte R, Simoes DMN, Franchini ML, et al: Accuracy of serum β-hydroxybutyrate measurements for the diagnosis of diabetic ketoacidosis in 116 dogs, *J Vet Intern Med* 16:411-417, 2002.

70. Easley JR, Breitschwerdt EB: Glucosuria associated with renal tubular dysfunction in three basenji dogs, *J Am Vet Med Assoc* 168:938, 1976.

71. Escolar E, Perezalenza D, Diaz M, et al: Canine Fanconi syndrome, *J Small Anim Pract* 34:567, 1993.

72. Evans GO: Plasma lactate measurements in healthy beagles, *Am J Vet Res* 48:131, 1987.

73. Feldman EC, Nelson RW: *Canine and feline endocrinology and reproduction,* Philadelphia, 1996, WB Saunders p. 400.

74. Feldman EC, Nelson RW: *Canine and feline endocrinology and reproduction,* Philadelphia, 1996, WB Saunders, p. 411.

75. Finco DR, Barsanti JA, Brown SA: Ammonium chloride as a urinary acidifier in cats: efficacy, safety, and rationale for its use, *Mod Vet Pract* 67:537, 1986.

76. Fine A, Brosnan JT, Herzberg GR: Release of lactate by the liver in metabolic acidosis in vivo, *Metabolism* 33:393, 1984.

77. Freeman LM, Breitschwerdt EB, Keene BW, et al: Fanconi's syndrome in a dog with primary hypoparathyroidism, *J Vet Intern Med* 8:349, 1994.

78. Gennari FJ, Goldstein MB, Schwartz WB: The nature of the renal adaptation to chronic hypocapnia, *J Clin Invest* 51:1722, 1972.

79. Gougoux A, Kaehny WD, Cohen JJ: Renal adaptation to chronic hypocapnia: dietary constraints in achieving H^+ retention, *Am J Physiol* 229:1330, 1975.

80. Graf H, Leach W, Arieff AI: Effects of dichloroacetate in the treatment of hypoxic lactic acidosis in dogs, *J Clin Invest* 76:919, 1985.

81. Graf H, Leach W, Arieff AI: Evidence for a detrimental effect of bicarbonate therapy in hypoxic lactic acidosis, *Science* 227:754, 1985.

82. Graf H, Leach W, Arieff AI: Metabolic effects of sodium bicarbonate in hypoxic lactic acidosis in dogs, *Am J Physiol* 249:F630, 1985.

83. Graham TE, Barclay JK, Wilson BA: Skeletal muscle lactate release and glycolytic intermediates during hypercapnia, *J Appl Physiol* 60:568, 1986.

84. Grauer GF, Thrall MA: Ethylene glycol (antifreeze) poisoning in the dog and cat, *J Am Anim Hosp Assoc* 18:492, 1982.

85. Grauer GF, Thrall MA: Ethylene glycol (antifreeze) poisoning. In Kirk RW, editor: *Current veterinary therapy IX.* Philadelphia, 1986, WB Saunders, p. 206.

86. Grauer GF, Thrall MA, Henre BA, et al: Early clinicopathologic findings in dogs ingesting ethylene glycol, *J Am Vet Med Assoc* 45:2299, 1984.

87. Harrington JT: Metabolic alkalosis, *Kidney Int* 26:88, 1984.

88. Harrington JT, Cohen JJ: Metabolic acidosis. In Cohen JJ, Kassirer JP, editors: *Acid-base,* Boston, 1982, Little, Brown & Co., p. 128.

89. Harrington JT, Cohen JJ: Metabolic acidosis. In Cohen JJ, Kassirer JP, editors: *Acid-base,* Boston, 1982, Little, Brown & Co., p. 157.

90. Harrington JT, Kassirer JP: Metabolic alkalosis. In Cohen JJ, Kassirer JP, editors: *Acid-base,* Boston, 1982, Little, Brown & Co., p. 227.

91. Harrington JT, Kassirer JP: Metabolic alkalosis. In Cohen JJ, Kassirer JP, editors: *Acid-base.* Boston, 1982, Little, Brown & Co., p. 232.

92. Harrington JT, Kassirer JP: Metabolic alkalosis. In Cohen JJ, Kassirer JP, editors: *Acid-base.* Boston, 1982, Little, Brown & Co., p. 240.

93. Harrington JT, Kassirer JP: Metabolic alkalosis. In Cohen JJ, Kassirer JP, editors: *Acid-base.* Boston, 1982, Little, Brown & Co., p. 280.

94. Hartsfield SM: Sodium bicarbonate and bicarbonate precursors for treatment of metabolic acidosis, *J Am Vet Med Assoc* 179:914, 1981.

95. Hartsfield SM, Thurmon JC, Corbin JE, et al: Effects of sodium acetate, bicarbonate and lactate on acid-base status in anaesthetized dogs, *J Vet Pharmacol Ther* 4(1):51-61, 1981.

96. Haskins SC, Munger RJ, Helphrey MG, et al: Effect of acetazolamide on blood acid-base and electrolyte values in dogs, *J Am Vet Med Assoc* 179:914, 1981.

97. Heald RD, Jones BD, Schmidt DA: Blood gas and electrolyte concentrations in canine parvoviral enteritis, *J Am Anim Hosp Assoc* 22:745, 1986.

98. Herrtage ME, Houlton JE: Collapsing Clumber spaniels, *Vet Rec* 105:334, 1979.

99. Hetenyi G, Paradis H, Kucharczyk J: Glucose and lactate turnover and gluconeogenesis in chronic metabolic acidosis and alkalosis in normal and diabetic dogs, *Can J Physiol Pharmacol* 66:140, 1988.

100. Hindman BJ: Sodium bicarbonate in the treatment of subtypes of acute lactic acidosis: physiologic considerations, *Anesthesiology* 72:1064, 1990.

101. Honer WG, Jennings DB: Pco_2 modulation of ventilation and HCO_3^- buffer during chronic metabolic acidosis, *Respir Physiol* 54:241, 1983.

102. Hornbein TF, Pavlin EG: Distribution of H^+ and HCO_3^- between CSF and blood during respiratory alkalosis in dogs, *Am J Physiol* 228:1149, 1975.

103. Hostutler RA, DiBartola SP, Eaton KA: Transient proximal renal tubular acidosis and Fanconi syndrome in a dog, *J Am Vet Med Assoc* 224:1611-1614, 2004.

104. Houlton JE, Herrtage ME: Mitochondrial myopathy in the Sussex spaniel, *Vet Rec* 106:206, 1980.

105. Igarashi T, Sekine T, Inatomi J, et al: Unraveling the molecular pathogenesis of isolated proximal renal tubular acidosis, *J Am Soc Nephrol* 13: 2171-2177, 2002.

106. Ilkiw JE, Davis PE, Church DB: Hematologic, biochemical, blood gas, and acid base values in greyhounds before and after exercise, *Am J Vet Res* 50:583, 1989.

107. Ilkiw JE, Rose RJ, Martin ICA: A comparison of simultaneous collected arterial, mixed venous, jugular venous and cephalic venous blood samples in the assessment of blood gas and acid base status in dogs, *J Vet Intern Med* 5:294, 1991.

108. Jacobs RM, Weiser MG, Hall RL, et al: Clinicopathologic findings of canine parvoviral enteritis, *J Am Anim Hosp Assoc* 16:809, 1980.

109. Jacobson HR: Chloride-responsive metabolic alkalosis. In Seldin DW, Gebisch G, editors: *The regulation of acid-base balance,* New York, 1989, Raven Press, p. 431.

110. Jacobson HR: Chloride-resistant metabolic alkalosis. In Seldin DW, Gebisch G, editors: *The regulation of acid-base balance,* New York, 1989, Raven Press, p. 459.

111. Jacobson HR, Seldin DW: On the generation, maintenance, and correction of metabolic alkalosis, *Am J Physiol* 245:F425, 1983.

112. Jaffe HC, Bodansky A, Chandler JP: Ammonium chloride decalcification as modified by calcium intake: the relationship between generalized osteoporosis and osteitis fibrosa, *J Exp Med* 56:823, 1932.

113. Jarvinen A-K, Sankari S: Lactic acidosis in a Clumber spaniel, *Acta Vet Scand* 37:119, 1996.

114. Jennings DB, Davidson JSD: Acid-base and ventilatory adaptations in conscious dogs during chronic hypercapnia, *Respir Physiol* 58:377, 1984.

115. Kagan KG, Schaer M: Gastric dilatation and volvulus in a dog—a case justifying electrolyte and acid-base assessment, *J Am Vet Med Assoc* 182:703, 1983.

116. Kassirer JP, Berkman PM, Lawrenz DR, et al: The critical role of chloride in the correction of hypokalemic alkalosis in man, *Am J Med* 38:172, 1965.

117. Kassirer JP, Schwartz WB: Correction of metabolic alkalosis in man without repair of potassium deficiency: a reevaluation of the role of potassium, *Am J Med* 38:19, 1966.

118. Kassirer JP, Schwartz WB: The response of normal man to selective depletion of hydrochloric acid. Factors in the genesis of persistent gastric alkalosis, *Am J Med* 40:10, 1966.

119. Kazemi H, Valenca LM, Shannon DC: Brain and cerebrospinal fluid lactate concentration in respiratory acidosis and alkalosis, *Respir Physiol* 6:178, 1969.

120. Kramer JW, Bistline D, Sheridan P, et al: Identification of hippuric acid crystals in the urine of ethylene glycol–intoxicated dogs and cats, *J Am Vet Med Assoc* 184:584, 1984.

121. Kreisberg RA: Diabetic ketoacidosis: new concepts and trends in pathogenesis and treatment, *Arch Intern Med* 88:681, 1978.

122. Kreisberg RA: Pathogenesis and management of lactic acidosis, *Annu Rev Med* 35:181, 1984.

123. Lemieux G, Lemieux C, Duplessis S, et al: Metabolic characteristics of cat kidney: failure to adapt to metabolic acidosis, *Am J Physiol* 259:R277, 1990.

124. Ling GV, Lowenstine LJ, Pulley LT, et al: Diabetes mellitus in dogs: a review of initial evaluation, immediate and long-term management, and outcome, *J Am Vet Med Assoc* 170:521, 1977.

125. Ling GV, Stabenfeldt GH, Comer KM, et al: Canine hyperadrenocorticism: pretreatment clinical and laboratory evaluation of 117 cases, *J Am Vet Med Assoc* 174:1211, 1979.

126. Lloyd MH, Iles RA, Simpson BR, et al: The effect of simulated metabolic acidosis on intracellular pH and lactate metabolism in the isolated perfused rat liver, *Clin Sci* 45:543, 1973.

127. Lowance DC, Garfinkel HB, Mattern WD, et al: The effect of chronic hypotonic volume expansion on the renal regulation of acid-base equilibrium, *J Clin Invest* 51:2928, 1972.

128. Macintire DK: Treatment of diabetic ketoacidosis in dogs by continuous low-dose intravenous infusion of insulin, *J Am Vet Med Assoc* 202:1266, 1993.

129. MacKenzie CP, van den Broek A: The Fanconi syndrome in a whippet, *J Small Anim Pract* 23:469, 1982.

130. Madias NE: Lactic acidosis, *Kidney Int* 29:752, 1986.

131. Madias NE, Adrogue HJ, Cohen JJ: Maladaptive renal response to secondary hypercapnia in chronic metabolic alkalosis, *Am J Physiol* 238:F283, 1980.

132. Madias NE, Bossert WH, Adrogue HJ: Ventilatory response to chronic metabolic acidosis and alkalosis in the dog, *J Appl Physiol* 56:1640, 1984.

133. Madias NE, Schwartz WB, Cohen JJ: The maladaptive renal response to secondary hypocapnia during chronic HCl acidosis in the dog, *J Clin Invest* 60:1393, 1977.

134. Madias NE, Wolf CJ, Cohen JJ: Regulation of acid-base equilibrium in chronic hypercapnia, *Kidney Int* 27:538, 1985.

135. Madias NE, Zelman SJ: The renal response to chronic mineral acid feeding: a re-examination of the role of systemic pH, *Kidney Int* 29:667, 1986.

136. Magner PO, Robinson L, Halperin RM, et al: The plasma potassium concentration in metabolic acidosis: a re-evaluation, *Am J Kidney Dis* 11:220, 1988.

137. Marsh JD, Margolis TI, Kim D: Mechanism of diminished contractile response to catecholamines during acidosis, *Am J Physiol* 254:H20, 1988.

138. Martin GB, Carden DL, Nowak RM, et al: Comparison of central venous and arterial pH and Pco_2 during open chest CPR in the canine model, *Ann Emerg Med* 14:529, 1985.

139. Maskrey M, Jennings DB: Ventilation and acid-base balance in awake dogs exposed to heat and CO_2, *J Appl Physiol* 58:549, 1985.

140. Mathias DW, Clifford PS, Klopfenstein HS: Mixed venous blood gases are superior to arterial blood gases in assessing acid-base status and oxygenation during acute cardiac tamponade in dogs, *J Clin Invest* 82:833, 1988.

141. McCullough SM, Constable PD: Calculation of the total plasma concentration of nonvolatile weak acids and the effective dissociation constant of nonvolatile buffers in plasma for use in the strong ion approach to acid-base balance in cats, *Am J Vet Res* 64:1047-1051, 2003.

142. McEwan NA, Macartney L: Fanconi's syndrome in a Yorkshire terrier, *J Small Anim Pract* 28:737, 1987.

143. McNamara PD, Rea CT, Bovee KC, et al: Cystinuria in dogs: comparison of the cystinuric component of the Fanconi syndrome in basenji dogs to isolated cystinuria, *Metabolism* 38:8, 1989.

144. Meijer JC: Canine hyperadrenocorticism. In Kirk RW, editor: *Current veterinary therapy VII,* Philadelphia, 1980, WB Saunders, p. 975.

145. Melian C, Peterson ME: Diagnosis and treatment of naturally-occurring hypoadrenocorticism in 42 dogs, *J Small Anim Pract* 37:268, 1996.

146. Meyer DJ: Temporary remission of hypoglycemia in a dog with an insulinoma after treatment with streptozotocin, *Am J Vet Res* 38:1201, 1977.

147. Mitchell JH, Wildenthal K, Johnson RL: The effects of acid-base disturbances on cardiovascular and pulmonary function, *Kidney Int* 1:375, 1972.

148. Molitoris BA, Froment DH, MacKenzie TA, et al: Citrate: a major factor in the toxicity of orally administered aluminum compounds, *Kidney Int* 36:949-953,1989.

149. Moon PE, Gabor L, Gleed RD, et al: Acid-base, metabolic, and hemodynamic effects of sodium bicarbonate or tromethamine administration in anesthetized dogs with experimentally induced metabolic acidosis, *Am J Vet Res* 58:771, 1997.

150. Morrin PAF, Bricker NS, Kime SW, et al: Observations on the acidifying capacity of the experimentally diseased kidney of the dog, *J Clin Invest* 41:1297, 1962.

151. Morrin PAF, Gedney WB, Newmark LN, et al: Bicarbonate reabsorption in the dog with experimental renal disease, *J Clin Invest* 41:1303, 1962.

152. Morris LR, Murphy MB, Kitabchi AE: Bicarbonate therapy in severe diabetic ketoacidosis, *Ann Intern Med* 105:836, 1986.

153. Muir WW: Acid-base and electrolyte disturbances in dogs with gastric-dilatation volvulus, *J Am Vet Med Assoc* 181:229, 1982.

154. Musch TI, Friedman DB, Haidet GC, et al: Arterial blood gases and acid-base status of dogs during graded dynamic exercise, *J Appl Physiol* 61:1914, 1986.

155. Nappert G, Dunphy E, Ruben D, et al: Determination of serum organic acids in puppies with naturally-acquired parvoviral enteritis, *Can J Vet Res* 66:15-18, 2002.

156. Narins RG, Cohen JJ: Bicarbonate therapy for organic acidosis: the case for its continued use, *Ann Intern Med* 106:615, 1987.

157. Narins RG, Jones ER, Stom MC, et al: Diagnostic strategies in disorders of fluid, electrolyte and acid base homeostasis, *Am J Med* 72:496, 1982.

158. Needle MA, Kaloyandies GJ, Schwartz WB: The effects of selective depletion of hydrochloric acid on acid base and electrolyte equilibrium, *J Clin Invest* 43:1836, 1964.

159. Nicoletta JA, Schwartz GJ: Distal renal tubular acidosis, *Curr Opin Pediatr* 16:194-198, 2004.

160. Norris SH, Kurtzman NA: Does chloride play an independent role in the pathogenesis of metabolic alkalosis? *Semin Nephrol* 8:101, 1988.

161. Nunamaker DM, Medway W, Berg P: Treatment of ethylene glycol poisoning in the dog, *J Am Vet Med Assoc* 159:310, 1971.

162. Ogilvie GK, Vail DM, Wheeler SL, et al: Effects of chemotherapy and remission on carbohydrate metabolism in dogs with lymphoma, *Cancer* 69:233-238, 1992.

163. Oh MS: Irrelevance of bone buffering to acid-base homeostasis in chronic metabolic acidosis, *Nephron* 59:7, 1991.

164. Okuda Y, Adrogue HJ, Field JB, et al: Counterproductive effects of sodium bicarbonate in diabetic ketoacidosis, *J Clin Endocrinol Metab* 81:314, 1996.

165. Olby NJ, Chan KK, Targett MP, et al: Suspected mitochondrial myopathy in a Jack Russell terrier, *J Small Anim Pract* 38:213, 1997.

166. Orchard CH, Kentish JC: Effects of changes of pH on the contractile function of cardiac muscle, *Am J Physiol* 258:C967, 1990.

167. Paciello O, Maiolino P, Fatone G, et al: Mitochondrial myopathy in a German shepherd dog, *Vet Pathol* 40:507-511, 2003.

168. Padrid P: Fanconi syndrome in a mixed breed dog, *Mod Vet Pract* 69:162, 1988.

169. Parker RA, Cohn LA, Wohlstadter DR, et al: D-lactic acidosis secondary to exocrine pancreatic insufficiency in a cat, *J Vet Intern Med* 19:106-110, 2005.

170. Pavlin EG, Hornbein TF: Distribution of H^+ and HCO_3^- between CSF and blood during respiratory acidosis, *Am J Physiol* 228:1145, 1975.

171. Penman RW, Luke RF, Jarboe TM: Respiratory effects of hypochloremic alkalosis and potassium depletion in the dog, *J Appl Physiol* 33:170, 1972.

172. Penumarthy L, Oehme FW: Treatment of ethylene glycol toxicosis in cats, *Am J Vet Res* 36:209, 1974.

173. Peterson M: Hyperadrenocorticism, *Vet Clin North Am* 14:731, 1984.

174. Peterson ME, Greco DS, Orth DN: Primary hypoadrenocorticism in ten cats, *J Vet Intern Med* 3:55, 1989.

175. Peterson ME, Kintzer PP, Kass PH: Pretreatment clinical and laboratory findings in dogs with hypoadrenocorticism—225 cases (1979–1993), *J Am Vet Med Assoc* 208:85, 1996.

176. Polzin DJ, Stevens JB, Osborne CA: Clinical evaluation of the anion gap in evaluation of acid-base disorders in dogs, *Compend Contin Educ Pract Vet* 4:102, 1982.

177. Posner J, Plum F: Spinal fluid pH and neurologic symptoms in systemic acidosis, *N Engl J Med* 277:605, 1967.

178. Rhee KH, Toro LO, McDonald GG, et al: Carbicarb, sodium bicarbonate, and sodium chloride in hypoxic lactic acidosis, *Chest* 104:913, 1993.

179. Robinson EP, Hardy RM: Clinical signs, diagnosis, and treatment of alkalemia in dogs: 20 cases (1982–1984), *J Am Vet Med Assoc* 192:943, 1988.

180. Rose BD: *Clinical physiology of acid-base and electrolyte disorders,* New York, 1994, McGraw-Hill Book Co., p. 542.

181. Rose BD: *Clinical physiology of acid-base and electrolyte disorders,* New York, 1994, McGraw-Hill Co., p. 588.

182. Rose BD: *Clinical physiology of acid-base and electrolyte disorders,* New York, 1994, McGraw-Hill Co., p. 564.

183. Rose BD: *Clinical physiology of acid-base and electrolyte disorders,* New York, 1994, McGraw-Hill Co., p. 591.

184. Rose BD: *Clinical physiology of acid-base and electrolyte disorders,* New York, 1994, McGraw-Hill Co., p. 589.

185. Rose BD: *Clinical physiology of acid-base and electrolyte disorders,* New York, 1994, McGraw-Hill Book Co., p. 515.

186. Rose RJ, Carter J: Some physiological and biochemical effects of acetazolamide in the dog, *J Vet Pharmacol Ther* 2:215, 1979.

187. Sabatini S: The acidosis of chronic renal failure, *Med Clin North Am* 67:845, 1983.

188. Sabatini S, Kurtzman NA: The maintenance of metabolic alkalosis: factors which decrease bicarbonate excretion, *Kidney Int* 25:357, 1984.

189. Sanders AB, Otto CW, Kern KB, et al: Acid-base balance in a canine model of cardiac arrest, *Ann Emerg Med* 17:667, 1988.

190. Sanyer JL, Oehme FW, McGavin MD: Systematic treatment of ethylene glycol toxicosis in dogs, *Am J Vet Res* 34:527, 1973.

191. Schmidt RW, Bricker NS, Gavellas G: Renal bicarbonate reabsorption in experimental uremia in the dog, *Kidney Int* 10:287, 1976.

192. Schmidt RW, Gavellas G: Bicarbonate reabsorption in dogs with experimental renal disease: effects of proportional reduction of sodium or phosphate intake, *Kidney Int* 12:393, 1977.

193. Schober KE: Investigation into intraerythrocytic and extraerythrocytic acid-base and electrolyte changes after long-term ammonium chloride administration in dogs, *Am J Vet Res* 57:743, 1996.

194. Schwartz WB, Hays RM, Pak A, et al: Effects of chronic hypercapnia on electrolyte and acid-base equilibrium. II. Recovery, with special reference to the influence of chloride intake, *J Clin Invest* 40:1238, 1961.

195. Schwartz WB, Orning KJ, Porter R: The internal distribution of hydrogen ions with varying degrees of metabolic acidosis, *J Clin Invest* 36:373, 1957.

196. Senior DF, Sundstrom DA, Wolfson BB: Effectiveness of ammonium chloride as a urinary acidifier in cats fed a popular brand of canned cat food, *Feline Pract* 16:24, 1986.

197. Senior DF, Sundstrom DA, Wolfson BB: Testing the effects of ammonium chloride and DL-methionine on the urinary pH of cats, *Vet Med* 81:88, 1986.

198. Settles EL, Schmidt D: Fanconi syndrome in a Labrador retriever, *J Vet Intern Med* 8:390, 1994.

199. Shaw DH: Acute response of urine pH following ammonium chloride administration to dogs, *Am J Vet Res* 50:1829, 1989.

200. Sheikh A, Fleisher G, Delgado-Paredes C, et al: Effect of dichloroacetate in the treatment of anoxic lactic acidosis in dogs, *Crit Care Med* 14:970, 1986.

201. Shull RM: The value of anion gap and osmolal gap determinations in veterinary medicine, *Vet Clin Pathol* 7:12, 1978.

202. Silva PRM, Fonseca-Costa A, Zin WA, et al: Respiratory and acid-base parameters during salicylic intoxication in dogs, *Braz J Med Biol Res* 19:279, 1986.

203. Simpson DP: Control of hydrogen ion homeostasis and renal acidosis, *Medicine (Baltimore)* 50:503, 1971.

204. Stacpoole PW: Lactic acidosis: the case against bicarbonate therapy, *Ann Intern Med* 105:276, 1986.

205. Straus E, Johnson GF, Yalow RS: Canine Zollinger-Ellison syndrome, *Gastroenterology* 72:380, 1977.

206. Swan RC, Axelrod DR, Seip M, et al: Distribution of sodium bicarbonate infused into nephrectomized dogs, *J Clin Invest* 34:1795, 1955.

207. Swan RC, Pitts RF: Neutralization of infused acid by nephrectomized dogs, *J Clin Invest* 34:205, 1955.

208. Takano N: Blood lactate accumulation and its causative factors during passive hyperventilation in dogs, *Jpn J Physiol* 16:481, 1966.

209. Tashkin DP, Goldstein PJ, Simmons DH: Hepatic lactate uptake during decreased liver perfusion, *Am J Physiol* 223:968, 1972.

210. Thrall MA, Grauer GF, Mero KN: Clinicopathologic findings in dogs and cats with ethylene glycol intoxication, *J Am Vet Med Assoc* 184:37, 1984.

211. Thrall MA, Dial SM, Winder DR: Identification of calcium oxalate monohydrate crystals by X-ray diffraction in urine of ethylene glycol–intoxicated dogs, *Vet Pathol* 22:625, 1985.

212. Toto RD, Alpern RJ: Metabolic acid-base disorders. In Kokko JP, Tannen RL, editors: *Fluids and electrolytes,* Philadelphia, 1996, WB Saunders, p. 201.

213. Vail DM, Ogilvie GK, Fettman MJ, et al: Exacerbation of hyperlactatemia by infusion of lactated Ringer's solution in dogs with lymphoma, *J Vet Intern Med* 4:228, 1990.

214. Vail DM, Ogilvie GK, Wheeler SL, et al: Alterations in carbohydrate metabolism in canine lymphoma, *J Vet Intern Med* 4:8, 1990.

215. Valtin H, Gennari FJ: *Acid-base disorders: basic concepts and management,* Boston, 1987, Little, Brown & Co.

216. Vijayasarathy C, Giger U, Prociuk U, et al: Canine mitochondrial myopathy associated with reduced mitochondrial messenger RNA and altered cytochrome *c* oxidase activities in fibroblasts and skeletal muscle, *Comp Biochem Physiol* 109:887, 1994.

217. Vukmir RB, Bircher NG, Radovsky A, et al: Sodium bicarbonate may improve outcome in dogs with brief or prolonged cardiac arrest, *Crit Care Med* 23:515, 1995.

218. Warnock DG: Uremic acidosis, *Kidney Int* 34:278, 1988.

219. Watson ADJ, Culvenor JA, Middleton DJ, et al: Distal renal tubular acidosis in a cat with pyelonephritis, *Vet Rec* 119:65, 1986.

220. Weil MH, Rackow EC, Trevino R, et al: Difference in acid-base state between venous and arterial blood during cardiopulmonary resuscitation, *N Engl J Med* 315:153, 1986.

221. Welbourne T, Weber M, Bank N: The effect of glutamine administration on urinary ammonium excretion in normal subjects and patients with renal disease, *J Clin Invest* 51:1852, 1972.

222. Widmer B, Gerhard RE, Harrington JT, et al: Serum electrolyte and acid-base composition: the influence of graded degrees of chronic renal failure, *Arch Intern Med* 139:1099, 1979.

223. Wingfield WE, Twedt DC, Moore RW, et al: Acid-base and electrolyte values in dogs with acute gastric dilatation-volvulus, *J Am Vet Med Assoc* 180:1070, 1982.

CHAPTER · 11

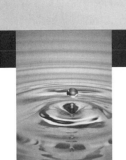

RESPIRATORY ACID-BASE DISORDERS

Rebecca A. Johnson and Helio Autran de Morais

"Life is a struggle, not against sin, not against the Money Power, not against malicious animal magnetism, but against hydrogen ions."

Henry Louis Mencken (1919)

Respiratory acid-base disorders are those abnormalities in acid-base equilibrium initiated by a change in arterial carbon dioxide tension ($Paco_2$). $Paco_2$ is regulated by respiration; a primary increase in $Paco_2$ acidifies body fluids and initiates the acid-base disturbance called respiratory acidosis, whereas a decrease in $Paco_2$ alkalinizes body fluids and is known as respiratory alkalosis. The primary responsibility of the lungs is to exchange gases at the blood-gas interface. In the mammalian lung, oxygen and carbon dioxide move by diffusion from areas of high to low partial pressure. Diffusion of gases is directly proportional to the surface area of the interface and inversely proportional to the thickness of membrane (Fick's law). With a relatively large surface area and a very thin (<1 μm) blood-gas interface, the lungs are well suited for their role in gas exchange.

GAS TRANSPORT DURING RESPIRATION

OXYGEN

Contraction of the diaphragm moves gases down the continually branching airways until they reach the transitional and respiratory bronchioles, alveolar ducts, and alveoli. Within this respiratory zone, alveolar ventilation and gas exchange occur as oxygen moves down its concentration gradient and into the red blood cells. The partial pressure of oxygen in the red blood cells approximates that of alveolar gas within the first third of the lung capillaries, primarily because of the lung's considerable diffusion capabilities. Oxygen then is carried in the blood to meet the oxygen demand of the tissues in two forms: dissolved and combined with hemoglobin. Most of the delivered oxygen is bound by hemoglobin with only a small contribution from the dissolved oxygen (0.003 mL dissolved O_2 per 100 mL of blood per mm Hg Po_2). The maximal amount of oxygen that can be combined with hemoglobin is called the oxygen capacity. Approximately 1.36 mL of O_2 can combine with 1 g of hemoglobin. Assuming 15 g of hemoglobin per 100 mL of blood, this results in approximately 21 mL O_2 per 100 mL blood carried to the tissues. As determined by the oxygen-hemoglobin dissociation curve (Fig. 11-1), at low Po_2, the amount of oxygen carried by hemoglobin increases rapidly with increases in Po_2. However, at higher Po_2 (>60 to 70 mm Hg), the curve flattens off, and little additional hemoglobin loading occurs. Unloading of large amounts of oxygen from hemoglobin is facilitated in the tissues where oxygen pressures are much lower (10 to 60 mm Hg) and the curve is very steep. Several factors shift this curve to the right and aid in the unloading of oxygen to the tissues, including increased H^+ ion and carbon dioxide concentrations (as seen in respiratory acidosis), increased temperature, and increased 2,3-diphosphogycerate (2,3-DPG), a compound that competes with oxygen for its binding site on hemoglobin.

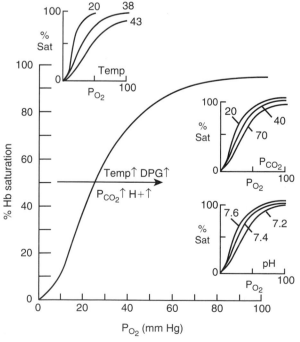

Fig. 11-1 Rightward shift of the O_2 dissociation curve by increase of H^+, Pco_2, temperature, and 2,3-diphosphogylcerate (DPG). (Adapted from West JB: *Respiratory physiology. The essentials,* ed 7, Philadelphia, 2005, Lippincott Williams & Wilkins, p. 79.)

CARBON DIOXIDE

As oxygen is transported to and used by tissues, metabolic processes in the body normally produce approximately 15,000 mmol of carbon dioxide daily. The lungs are responsible for excreting a great deal more carbonic acid (H_2CO_3 and dissolved carbon dioxide) each day than the kidneys.[53] Hence, alveolar ventilation and carbon dioxide removal have a large influence on acid-base balance. Dissolved carbon dioxide is 20 times more soluble than oxygen. It is so diffusible that we can assume complete equilibration of Pco_2 across membranes. As the tissues produce carbon dioxide, equilibrium is achieved rapidly between intracellular and extracellular compartments. Thus CO_2 diffuses rapidly from the tissues into red blood cells. Within the red blood cell, carbonic anhydrase (CA) hydrates CO_2 forming carbonic acid:

$$\overset{\text{CA}}{CO_2 + H_2O \leftrightarrow H_2CO_3 \leftrightarrow H^+ + HCO_3^-} \quad (1)$$

As shown in Fig. 11-2, carbonic acid spontaneously dissociates into H^+ and HCO_3^- at intracellular pH. The HCO_3^- ions diffuse from the red cells into plasma. The cell membrane is relatively impermeable to cations, and chloride (Cl^-) ions diffuse into the red cells from plasma to maintain electroneutrality (so-called "chloride shift"). In the lungs, the shift of chloride out of red cells is facilitated by the high intracellular concentration of chloride (~60 mEq/L) when compared with other cells. Most of the carbon dioxide (~81%) is transported to the lung as bicarbonate. A small amount is transported still dissolved in plasma (~8%), and some is combined with amino groups of blood proteins (~11%), the most important of which is carbaminohemoglobin.[67]

CONTROL OF ALVEOLAR VENTILATION AND CHEMOSENSITIVITY

The drive to breathing originates within respiratory centers of the brainstem (i.e., ventral respiratory group), which comprises a network responsible for respiratory rhythm generation and respiratory pattern formation. These central respiratory areas receive input from chemoreceptors in the periphery and from areas throughout the central nervous system (CNS) while sending efferent signals to the muscles of respiration, such as the diaphragm and accessory muscles (i.e., intercostal and upper airway muscles) (Fig. 11-3).

Inputs from CO_2-, O_2-, and pH-sensitive chemoreceptors alter alveolar ventilation.[6,17,47] The primary stimuli for changes in alveolar ventilation are hypoxemia ($Pao_2 < 60$ mm Hg) and carbon dioxide-induced changes in intracellular and extracellular pH. In the normal animal,

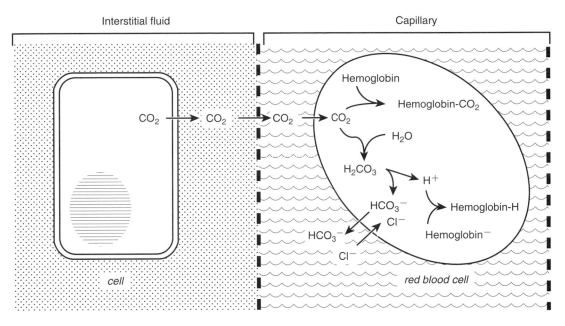

Fig. 11-2 The chloride shift. Increased CO_2 from cell metabolism leaves plasma and enters red blood cells, where it combines with hemoglobin and forms carbaminohemoglobin. The largest amount of CO_2 inside red blood cells is hydrated to form carbonic acid, which dissociates into bicarbonate and hydrogen ions. Bicarbonate diffuses out of the red blood cells into plasma in exchange for chloride ions.

peripheral chemoreceptors primarily are found within the carotid and aortic bodies; these organs are influenced by changes in O_2 and CO_2 and pH. In addition to the periphery, O_2-sensitive chemoreceptors also are present in the CNS, but their contribution to ventilatory responses to hypoxia remains unclear.[62] As a result, peripheral chemoreceptors at the bifurcation of the carotid bodies dominate the hypoxic ventilatory response and are responsible for approximately 90% of the increase in minute ventilation seen with hypoxemia.[12,16] Along with peripheral CO_2 chemoreceptors, CO_2/pH-sensitive receptors also are located centrally throughout the brainstem (i.e., nucleus tractus solitarius, locus ceruleus, midline medullary raphe, rostral ventral respiratory group, fastigial nucleus, retrotrapezoid nucleus; for review, see Putnam et al[54]). Although both peripheral and central chemoreceptors contribute to CO_2-induced ventilatory responses, the central receptors appear to be quantitatively more important for producing changes in ventilation mediated by CO_2; resection of the peripherally located carotid bodies only leads to a small increase in resting $Paco_2$ levels (2 to 4 mm Hg) secondary to a decrease in alveolar ventilation.[37,54] The CO_2-sensitive chemoreceptors are extremely responsive, and small changes in CO_2/pH affect breathing dramatically. For example, in resting awake humans, a 1-mm increase in Pco_2 increases ventilation by approximately 20% to 30%.[17]

The lungs are the only avenue for CO_2 elimination. Carbon dioxide efficiently diffuses across the alveolar capillary wall. Thus under most circumstances, the CO_2 partial pressure is essentially the same in the alveoli ($Paco_2$) and arteries ($Paco_2$). In the steady state, $Paco_2$ is inversely proportional to alveolar ventilation (Va) based on the alveolar ventilation equation:

$$Paco_2 = 0.863 \left(\frac{Vco_2}{Va} \right) \quad (2)$$

where Vco_2 is the metabolic production of carbon dioxide and 0.863 is a constant that equates dissimilar units for Vco_2 and Va.[72] The Va is the fraction of the total minute ventilation (Ve) that is produced at the gas exchange units of the lung. The portion of gas not reaching the gas exchange areas of the lung is termed dead space gas. The dead space to tidal volume ratio (Vd/Vt) refers to the portion of each tidal volume that ventilates dead space and is "wasted." Therefore the alveolar gas equation can be rewritten as:

$$Paco_2 = 0.863 \left(\frac{Vco_2}{Ve \left[1 - (Vd/Vt) \right]} \right) \quad (3)$$

As determined by equations (2) and (3), measuring the $Paco_2$ provides direct information about the adequacy of alveolar ventilation. Many primary respiratory acid-base disorders consequently result from alveolar hypoventilation (increased $Paco_2$) or alveolar hyperventilation (decreased $Paco_2$).

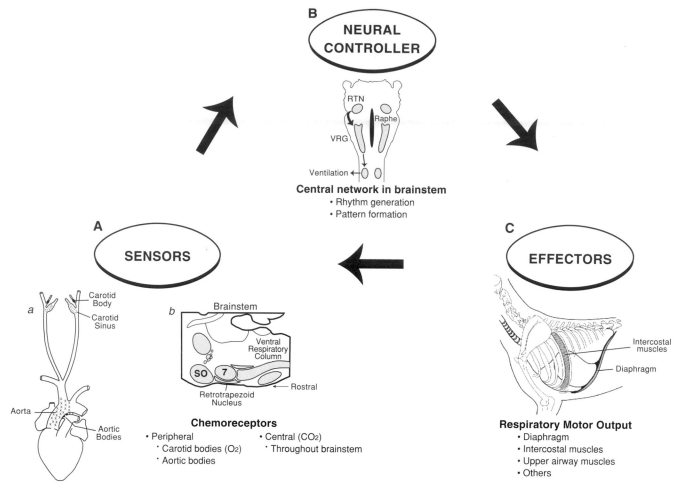

Fig. 11-3 Schematic representation of the respiratory control system. **A,** Sensors. Chemosensory and mechanosensory information originates from peripheral (carotid and aortic bodies) and central receptors (chemosensitive areas throughout the brainstem, **b**). **a,** A representation of peripheral receptors is found in *a*. The carotid bodies located at the bifurcation of the external and internal carotid arteries are responsible for the majority of the hypoxemic ventilatory response in mammals. A stylized view of the lateral aspect of the brainstem is shown in **b**. Chemosensitive areas found throughout the brainstem are the primary receptors mediating the hypercapnic ventilatory response. Many CO_2-sensitive neurons are found in the retrotrapezoid nucleus (RTN) located rostral to the ventral respiratory column, ventral to the facial nucleus (7) and caudal to the superior olive (SO). **B,** Neural controller: a stylized view of the ventral aspect of rat brainstem with RTN neurons is shown. Information from peripheral and central receptors is relayed centrally to ventral brainstem structures. Stimulation of the RTN activates premotor neurons in the ventral respiratory group (VRG), which then activate cranial and spinal motor neurons to modulate respiratory rhythm and pattern of breathing. **C,** Effectors: output from motor neurons reaches the respiratory effector muscles (e.g., diaphragm, intercostal muscles) producing a breath. Information from the effectors feeds back to the sensors to modulate breathing. (**A** redrawn from Mitchell's 2004 adaptation from Alheid GF, Gray PA, Jiang MC, et al: Parvalbumin in respiratory neurons of the ventrolateral medulla of the adult rat, *J Neurocytol* 31:693-717, 2002. **B** redrawn from Mitchell GS: Back to the future: carbon dioxide chemoreceptors in the mammalian brain, *Nat Neurosci* 7:1288-1290, 2004.)

THE ALVEOLAR-ARTERIAL OXYGEN GRADIENT

Frequently, patients with respiratory acidosis or alkalosis also are hypoxemic. When determining management options, it is important to discern between hypoxia from primary lung disease (e.g., ventilation-perfusion mismatching) and alveolar hypoventilation. If breathing room air, the alveolar gas equation dictates that, at steady state, arterial or alveolar (PA_{O_2}) oxygen tension will decrease with an increase in P_{CO_2}:

$$PAO_2 = PIO_2 - \frac{PACO_2}{R} \qquad (4)$$

where R is the respiratory exchange ratio that accounts for the difference between CO_2 production and O_2 consumption at steady state, PIO_2 is the inspired oxygen tension, and $PACO_2$ is the alveolar PCO_2. In normal animals, R is approximately 0.8. Because of the high solubility of CO_2, $PaCO_2$ can be substituted for $PACO_2$ in equation (4) under the assumption that $PaCO_2$ will equal $PACO_2$.

$$PAO_2 = PIO_2 - \frac{PaCO_2}{R} \qquad (5)$$

Thus the difference between PAO_2 and PaO_2 can be calculated as:

$$(A - a)\ O_2\ \text{gradient} = PAO_2 - PaO_2$$
$$= \left[PIO_2 - \left(\frac{PaCO_2}{R} \right) \right] - PaO_2 \qquad (6)$$

Considering R = 0.8, and 1/0.8 = 1.25:

$$(A - a)\ O_2\ \text{gradient} = (PIO_2 - 1.25 PaCO_2) - PaO_2 \qquad (7)$$

At sea level in a patient breathing room air, PIO_2 is approximately 150 mm Hg. This can be substituted in equation (7):

$$(A - a)\ O_2\ \text{gradient} = (150 - 1.25 PaCO_2) - PaO_2 \qquad (7)$$

Values less than 15 mm Hg generally are considered normal.[14] If the $(A - a)\ O_2$ ratio is widened, a component of the hypoxemia results from ventilation-perfusion mismatching. It should be remembered that FIO_2 is dependent on barometric pressure and will be lower at higher altitudes. At an altitude of 500 m (~1640 feet), PIO_2 equals 140 mm Hg, whereas at 1000 m (3280 feet), PIO_2 equals 130 mm Hg. Although it has long been thought that in the hypercapnic patient the alveolar-arterial oxygen difference differentiates hypoxemia caused by pure hypoventilation from hypoxemia in which other lung factors play a role, this idea has been seriously challenged[23,30] because the $(A - a)\ O_2$ gradient may be increased in some patients with extrapulmonary disorders. Clinically, a normal gradient excludes pulmonary disease and suggests some form of central alveolar hypoventilation or an abnormality of the chest wall or inspiratory muscles.[57] To increase the specificity of the test to diagnose ventilation/perfusion mismatch, only patients with $(A - a)\ O_2$ gradient values more than 25 mm Hg[14] should be considered abnormal. These patients are likely to have primary pulmonary disease, but extrapulmonary disorders cannot be completely ruled out.

HYPOXEMIA

Arterial blood gas analysis is not only essential for determining $PaCO_2$ levels and the acid-base condition of a

patient but it also provides information pertaining to a patient's oxygenation status. There are five main reasons for hypoxemia, including low fraction of inspired oxygen, hypoventilation, diffusion impairment, ventilation-perfusion mismatching, and shunt (Box 11-1).

LOW PARTIAL PRESSURE OF INSPIRED O_2 (PIO_2)

Low levels of inspired oxygen produce patient hypoxemia by reductions in mean alveolar oxygen levels (PAO_2), subsequently reducing PaO_2. Although relatively uncommon in veterinary medicine, this type of hypoxemia can result from a decrease in barometric pressure (i.e., residence at high altitudes or nonpressurized airline flights) or improper inhalant anesthetic technique (e.g., administration of N_2O without O_2). In these cases, there is an increase in alveolar ventilation secondary to hypoxemia, which in turn decreases $PaCO_2$. The $(A - a)\ O_2$ difference remains within normal limits because of the concomitant decrease in PIO_2.

HYPOVENTILATION

As previously discussed, the prevailing PAO_2 is determined by the balance between the removal of oxygen by the blood and replenishment of oxygen by alveolar ventilation. According to equations (4) and (5) above, as alveolar ventilation decreases, PAO_2 and PaO_2 decrease, whereas $PACO_2$ and $PaCO_2$ must increase. As a result, the $(A - a)\ O_2$ gradient does not change. If the $(A - a)$ difference is widened, there may be a component of the hypoxemia attributable to primary lung disease such as ventilation-alveolar perfusion mismatching or right-to-left shunting. In addition, the alveolar gas equation also predicts that although increases in alveolar ventilation can change PAO_2 considerably, they can only moderately increase PaO_2. Because of the sigmoid shape of the oxygen-hemoglobin dissociation curve, the effect of increasing alveolar ventilation on arterial oxygen saturation is minimal above a PaO_2 of 55 to 60 mm Hg.[24,41] Clinically important causes of hypoventilation include CNS disease, respiratory depressant drugs, neuromuscular diseases affecting the respiratory muscles, chest wall injury, upper airway obstruction, and severe diffuse pulmonary disease.

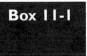

Box 11-1 **Mechanisms of Derangement in Arterial Oxygenation**

Low fraction of inspired oxygen (FIO_2)
Diffusion barrier
Hypoventilation
Ventilation-perfusion mismatch ($\dot{V}\text{-}\dot{Q}$ mismatch)
Right-to-left shunt

DIFFUSION IMPAIRMENT

Diffusion impairment occurs whenever there is incomplete equilibration of alveolar gas and pulmonary end-capillary blood. Equilibration of oxygen between the alveolus and red blood cell is extremely rapid under normal conditions, and this type of hypoxemia infrequently is observed in small animal medicine. However, a diffusion impairment leading to hypoxemia may be seen with thickening of the alveolar-capillary membrane (e.g., "alveolar-capillary block" seen in diffuse pulmonary interstitial disease) or loss of alveolar or capillary surface area (e.g., emphysema or vasculitis). Although hypoxemia caused by a diffusion impairment may occur as a consequence of the aforementioned disease states, it also may be detected under certain circumstances of high cardiac output that markedly decrease transit time of red cells (e.g., exercise). In any case, its contribution to hypoxemia usually is negligible, and a diffusion impairment seldom is the limiting factor in oxygen transfer to arterial blood.

VENTILATION-ALVEOLAR PERFUSION MISMATCH ($\dot{V}$-$\dot{Q}$ MISMATCH)

Despite regional differences in $\dot{V}$-$\dot{Q}$ ratios throughout the mammalian lung, the heterogeneity of individual lung units is relatively limited, resulting in a $\dot{V}$-$\dot{Q}$ ratio of approximately 0.8.[41] This ratio enables mixed venous blood to become fully oxygenated and CO_2 to be eliminated without increases in minute ventilation.[74]

$\dot{V}$-$\dot{Q}$ mismatch is one of the most commonly encountered causes of hypoxemia. It is present in areas of the lung in which perturbations in ventilation or perfusion occur and result in inefficient gas exchange. For example, low $\dot{V}$-$\dot{Q}$ units have low PaO_2 and high alveolar PCO_2, resulting in hypercapnic and hypoxemic blood. In fact, when breathing room air, the blood leaving a gas exchange unit with a $\dot{V}$-$\dot{Q}$ ratio of less than 0.1 is essentially unoxygenated. Low $\dot{V}$-$\dot{Q}$ (poorly ventilated, adequately perfused) units can be found in patients with increased airway resistance (e.g., asthma, bronchitis, chronic obstructive pulmonary disease). High $\dot{V}$-$\dot{Q}$ (poorly perfused, adequately ventilated) units have high PaO_2 and a low $PaCO_2$. In lung areas with $\dot{V}$-$\dot{Q}$ ratios greater than 1, additional increases in ventilation do not improve oxygenation.[50,74] High $\dot{V}$-$\dot{Q}$ ratios are found in diseases with increased compliance (e.g., emphysema) or in low output states (e.g., pulmonary embolism).

Final blood gas tensions are determined by mixing of gas contents from different gas units. Thus $\dot{V}$-$\dot{Q}$ mismatch will produce hypoxemia based on the actual O_2 and CO_2 levels in each lung area and the amount of blood flow to each unit.[50,74] The severity of $\dot{V}$-$\dot{Q}$ mismatch can be assessed using the (A − a) O_2 gradient because both abnormally low and high $\dot{V}$-$\dot{Q}$ ratios increase the gradient. Patients with $\dot{V}$-$\dot{Q}$ mismatch usually are hypoxemic but have normal or decreased $PaCO_2$

because chemoreceptors respond to and minute ventilation is altered by changes in carbon dioxide levels.[49,74] Hypoxemia resulting from $\dot{V}$-$\dot{Q}$ mismatch can be corrected by increasing the fraction of inspired oxygen (FIO_2) by use of 100% O_2.

RIGHT-TO-LEFT SHUNT

Right-to-left shunting is a severe form of $\dot{V}$-$\dot{Q}$ mismatch and results when mixed venous blood completely bypasses ventilated pulmonary alveoli and returns to the arterial circulation. A small amount (2% to 3%) of shunting is present in normal animals through the bronchial and thebesian circulations. In pathologic states, shunt results from perfusion of lung areas that receive no ventilation because of atelectasis or consolidation ($\dot{V}$-$\dot{Q}$ = 0) or from deoxygenated blood flow through anatomic right-to-left channels. Thus shunting is the main cause for hypoxemia in pulmonary edema, atelectasis, pneumonia, and in congenital abnormal cardiac communications between the systemic and pulmonary circulations (e.g., patent ductus arteriosus, ventricular septal defect, atrial septal defect, tetralogy of Fallot) with right-to-left blood flow bypassing the lungs.

Even small amounts of shunt result in clinically relevant hypoxemia because venous blood oxygen content is extremely low and mixed venous blood is being added directly to arterial blood without alveolar gas exchange. Similar to $\dot{V}$-$\dot{Q}$ mismatch, patients with right-to-left shunting have a decreased PaO_2 with normal or decreased $PaCO_2$ and widened (A − a) O_2 gradients. However, one major difference is that the PaO_2 levels in animals with increased shunting fail to return to normal even with 100% O_2 supplementation. In contrast, animals with $\dot{V}$-$\dot{Q}$ mismatch, hypoventilation, or diffusion impairment exhibit pronounced increases in PaO_2 with oxygen enrichment (Table 11-1).

RESPIRATORY ACIDOSIS

Respiratory acidosis, or primary hypercapnia, results when carbon dioxide production exceeds elimination via the lung (for reviews, see Epstein and Singh[15] and Markou et al[41]). Respiratory acidosis almost always is a result of respiratory failure with resultant alveolar hypoventilation and is characterized by an increase in $PaCO_2$, decreased pH, and a compensatory increase in blood HCO_3^- concentration.

METABOLIC COMPENSATION IN RESPIRATORY ACIDOSIS

Acute Respiratory Acidosis

Acute increases in PCO_2 cause intracellular CO_2 levels to increase. An increase in CO_2 concentration shifts the reaction $CO_2 + H_2O \leftrightarrow H_2CO_3 \leftrightarrow HCO_3^- + H^+$ to the right. Bicarbonate and H^+ concentrations slightly increase within 10 minutes because of dissociation of

TABLE 11-1   Theoretical Effect of Breathing 21% and 100% Oxygen on Mean Po_2 Values in Alveolar Gas, Arterial Blood, and Mixed Venous Blood

Fio_2	Ideal Gas Exchange		V̇-Q̇ Mismatch		Right-to-Left Shunt	
	21%	100%	21%	100%	21%	100%
Po_2 (venous in mm Hg)	40	51	40	51	40	42
Po_2 (alveolar in mm Hg)	101	673	106	675	114	677
Po_2 (arterial in mm Hg)	101	673	89	673	59	125
(A − a) Po_2 gradient in mm Hg	0	0	17	2	55	552

From Murray JF: Gas exchange and oxygen transport. In Murray JF, editor: The normal lung, *Philadelphia, 1986, WB Saunders, p. 194.*

H_2CO_3 into HCO_3^- and H^+. Bicarbonate ions are released from erythrocytes in exchange for chloride, increasing plasma strong ion difference (SID). An increase in CO_2 concentration also shifts the general buffer reaction ($A^- + H^+ \leftrightarrow HA$) to the left. Intracellular buffers (e.g., hemoglobin, hemoglobin$^-$ + H^+ $\leftrightarrow$ reduced hemoglobin) play a critical role in acute buffering of hypercapnia, handling 97% of the H^+ load in dogs.[21,39] Only 3% of the H^+ load is handled by extracellular buffers (i.e., plasma proteins). As a result, for each 1-mm Hg increase in Pco_2, these buffers increase HCO_3^- 0.15 mEq/L in dogs[13] and cats[64] (Box 11-2). Presence of moderate hypoxemia does not alter the adaptive response to acute respiratory acidosis.[38]

Box 11-2   Predicted Metabolic Compensations in Respiratory Blood Gas Disorders

Acute Respiratory Acidosis
[HCO_3^-] increases 0.15 mEq/L for every 1-mm Hg increase in Pco_2 in dogs
Same for cats

Chronic Respiratory Acidosis
[HCO_3^-] increases 0.35 mEq/L for every 1-mm Hg increase in Pco_2 in dogs
Degree of compensation is not known for cats

Acute Respiratory Alkalosis
[HCO_3^-] decreases 0.25 mEq/L for every 1-mm Hg decrease in Pco_2 in dogs
Same for cats

Chronic Respiratory Alkalosis
[HCO_3^-] decreases 0.55 mEq/L for every 1-mm Hg decrease in Pco_2 in dogs
Degree of compensation is not known for cats, but pH is usually normal or slightly alkalemic

---

Chronic Respiratory Acidosis

If hypercapnia persists, renal compensation occurs to stabilize plasma HCO_3^- at a higher concentration within 5 days.[31,52,59,68] Chronic hypercapnia causes intracellular H^+ to increase in the renal tubular cells. Up-regulation of the Na^+-H^+ antiporter of the renal brush border occurs,[65] and hydrogen ions are exchanged for sodium and then excreted largely as $NH_4^+Cl^-$.[57,69] Intracellular HCO_3^- is reabsorbed and exchanged for Cl^-, resulting in an increase in plasma SID, chloruresis, and negative chloride balance.[18] The chloride lost in the urine decreases urine SID because the chloride is accompanied by NH_4^+ rather than sodium ions. A new steady state is reached when the increased filtered load of HCO_3^- resulting from the increased plasma concentration of HCO_3^- is balanced by increased renal reabsorption of HCO_3^-. The net effect is buffering of the respiratory acidosis and hypochloremic hyperbicarbonatemia caused by chronic hypercapnia. For each 1-mm Hg increase in Pco_2, HCO_3^- will increase 0.35 mEq/L in dogs (see Box 11-2).[13] The renal response to chronic hypercapnia is not altered by moderate hypoxemia, dietary sodium or chloride restriction, alkali loading, or adrenalectomy.[38] The renal compensation in chronic respiratory acidosis typically is considered to be incomplete, not returning pH completely to normal.[75] In stable human patients with chronic respiratory acidosis, however, a 0.51-mEq/L increase in [HCO_3^-] is expected for each 1-mm Hg increase in Pco_2.[42] Thus arterial pH appears to remain near reference ranges in human patients with long-standing respiratory acidosis.[4] Similar results have been observed in dogs with chronic respiratory acidosis and no identifiable reason for the increase in HCO_3^- concentration other than renal compensation (Goodman and de Morais, unpublished observations).[26] These observations suggest that the kidneys may be able to bring arterial pH back to normal in dogs with longstanding (>30 days) respiratory acidosis. Renal compensation in cats with chronic respiratory acidosis is not known. Cats do not increase renal ammoniagenesis during experimental metabolic acidosis.[34] Cats may not be able to compensate adequately in chronic respiratory acidosis because an increase in ammoniagenesis is the most adaptive factor.

Hypochloremia is a common finding in dogs with experimentally induced chronic hypercapnia.[40,52,59,68] During recovery from chronic hypercapnia, chloride restriction hinders the return of plasma HCO_3^- concentration to normal. Thus the kidney needs chloride to preferentially resorb chloride with sodium, excrete excess HCO_3^- in the urine, and reestablish normal SID in the plasma.

CAUSES OF RESPIRATORY ACIDOSIS

Respiratory acidosis and hypercapnia can occur with any disease process involving the neural control of ventilation, mechanics of ventilation, or alveolar gas exchange resulting in hypoventilation, ventilation-perfusion mismatches, or both. **Acute respiratory acidosis** usually results from sudden and severe primary parenchymal (e.g., fulminant pulmonary edema), airway, pleural, chest wall, neurologic (e.g., spinal cord injury), or neuromuscular (e.g., botulism) disease.[15] **Chronic respiratory acidosis** results in sustained hypercapnia and has many etiologies including alveolar hypoventilation, abnormal respiratory drive, abnormalities of the chest wall and respiratory muscles, and increased dead space.[15] In patients with neuromuscular disease leading to muscular weakness, the degree of hypercapnia appears to be out of proportion to the severity of muscle disease and may be underestimated without blood gas analysis. In these patients, muscle weakness and elastic load are responsible for modulation of central respiratory output. This results in a rapid shallow breathing pattern that leads to chronic CO_2 retention.[43] A more detailed list of causes of respiratory acidosis is found in Box 11-3.

As determined by the alveolar gas equations (1) and (2) above, hypercapnia can result from a decrease in alveolar ventilation (either through a decrease in total minute ventilation or increase in the dead space to tidal volume ratio) or an increase in metabolic production of carbon dioxide. In small animal clinical practice, increased CO_2 production infrequently results in hypercapnia. In normal circumstances (e.g., exercise), an increase in CO_2 production usually is matched by an increase in CO_2 elimination via the lung.[71] However, if CO_2 production is increased with impaired or fixed alveolar ventilation that is unable to effectively remove CO_2, acute respiratory acidosis may develop, as is observed in a few conditions such as heat stroke and malignant hyperthermia.[10,63]

Decreased alveolar ventilation produces hypercapnia from either a reduction in total minute ventilation (also termed global hypoventilation) or abnormal ventilation-perfusion ratios in the lung. In global hypoventilation,

---

Box 11-3 | **Causes of Respiratory Acidosis**

Large Airway Obstruction
Aspiration (e.g., foreign body, vomitus)
Mass (e.g., neoplasia, abscess)
Tracheal collapse
Chronic obstructive pulmonary disease
Asthma
Obstructed endotracheal tube
Brachycephalic syndrome
Laryngeal paralysis/laryngospasm

Respiratory Center Depression
Drug induced (e.g., narcotics, barbiturates, inhalant anesthesia)
Neurologic disease (e.g., brainstem or high cervical cord lesion)

Increased CO_2 Production with Impaired Alveolar Ventilation
Cardiopulmonary arrest
Heatstroke
Malignant hyperthermia

Neuromuscular Disease
Myasthenia gravis
Tetanus
Botulism
Polyradiculoneuritis
Tick paralysis
Electrolyte abnormalities (e.g., hypokalemia)
Drug induced (e.g., neuromuscular blocking agents, organophosphates, aminoglycosides with anesthetics)

Restrictive Extrapulmonary Disorders
Diaphragmatic hernia
Pleural space disease (e.g., pneumothorax, pleural effusion)
Chest wall trauma/flail chest

Intrinsic Pulmonary and Small Airway Diseases
Acute respiratory distress syndrome
Chronic obstructive pulmonary disease
Asthma
Severe pulmonary edema
Pulmonary thromboembolism
Pneumonia
Pulmonary fibrosis
Diffuse metastatic disease
Smoke inhalation

Ineffective Mechanical Ventilation (e.g., Inadequate Minute Ventilation, Improper CO_2 Removal)

Marked Obesity (Pickwickian Syndrome)

CO_2 is delivered to the lung but ventilation is inadequate, and hypercapnia and hypoxemia develop. Global hypoventilation results from either an abnormal ventilatory drive or alterations in respiratory pump mechanics.

In normal animals, carbon dioxide is a marked stimulus for ventilation that subsequently increases central respiratory drive to offset any potential increase in blood CO_2 levels. However, animals with profound reductions in their drive to breathe do not respond to such stimuli and become hypercapnic. Conditions that may result in central hypoventilation include CNS trauma, neoplasia, infection, general anesthesia, narcotics, and cerebral edema. Global hypoventilation also results from failure of respiratory mechanics. In these cases, the respiratory muscles, chest wall, or both are ineffective in maintaining adequate ventilation, and the central respiratory drive usually is increased. Examples of diseases that affect respiratory mechanics are severe obesity, spinal cord injury, and myasthenia gravis.

Maintaining normal ventilation to alveolar perfusion ratios is essential for preserving eucapnia and normoxemia.[73] Areas of lung that are ventilated but ineffectively perfused increase the dead space to tidal volume ratio (V_D/V_T). When a normal breathing pattern shifts to a pattern consisting of very fast respiratory rates and small, inadequate tidal volumes (as seen in some patients with acute respiratory distress syndrome), V_D/V_T increases. In some disease states (e.g., shock), there may be areas of the lung with minimal or no alveolar perfusion. The normal lung has great reserve capabilities, and additional alveoli usually can compensate to keep the Pa_{CO_2} within normal limits. However, if other alveolar units cannot be hyperventilated to remove the CO_2, an increased dead space will result in hypercapnia. Disorders resulting in this type of respiratory acidosis include pulmonary thromboembolism, emphysema, and fibrosis.

DIAGNOSIS AND CLINICAL FEATURES OF RESPIRATORY ACIDOSIS

Most clinical signs in animals with respiratory acidosis reflect the underlying disease process responsible for hypercapnia rather than the hypercapnia itself, and subjective clinical evaluation of the patient alone is not reliable in making a diagnosis of respiratory acidosis. In fact, patients with chronic, compensated respiratory acidosis may have very mild clinical signs. One should consider respiratory acidosis in a patient presented with a disorder likely to be associated with hypercapnia (see Box 11-3). Definitive diagnosis of respiratory acidosis is established by arterial blood gas analysis.

In extremely acute hypoventilation (e.g., cardiopulmonary arrest, airway obstruction), hypoxemia is the immediate threat to life, and a laboratory diagnosis of acute respiratory acidosis is not made in small animal practice. Frequently, the patient dies from hypoxemia before hypercapnia can become severe. Abrupt cessation

of ventilation is fatal within 4 minutes, whereas severe hypercapnia would not develop for 10 to 15 minutes in such a setting.[39] Many small animals presented to veterinarians have been ill long enough to develop a chronic steady state (i.e., 2 to 5 days), and their blood gas results reflect adaptation to chronic hypercapnia. However, if a patient with chronic respiratory acidosis acutely decompensates, life-threatening consequences may develop, and the patient may die quickly.

Although many clinical signs are subtle, especially in chronic respiratory acidosis, investigations in humans and experimental animals show that cardiovascular, metabolic, and neurologic consequences arise after acute hypercapnic acidemia.[69] Hypercapnia stimulates the sympathetic nervous system and causes release of catecholamines.[9,36] Tachyarrhythmias (including ventricular fibrillation) are common and result from increased sympathetic tone, electrolyte fluctuations, associated hypoxemia, and acidemia.[15,32,51] In experimental canine models, acute respiratory acidosis increases heart rate and cardiac output but decreases myocardial contractility and systemic vascular resistance with no change in blood pressure.[70] Thus on physical examination of the patient, one sees a hyperdynamic state, with an increased heart rate and cardiac output, increased or normal blood pressure, and "flushed" or "brick-red" mucous membranes associated with vasodilatation. Hypercapnia also causes a rightward shift of the oxygen-hemoglobin dissociation curve (see Fig. 11-1), promoting unloading of oxygen at the tissues and enhancing oxygen delivery and carrying capacity.[55]

Metabolic consequences of acute hypercapnia include retention of both sodium and water, possibly as a result of increased antidiuretic hormone release, increased cortisol secretion, and activation of the renin-angiotensin system.[39] Respiratory, as well as metabolic, acidosis also may lead to gastroparesis by altering gastric muscle activity and fundic tone.[66]

The nature of the neurologic signs seen depends on the magnitude of hypercapnia, rapidity of change in CO_2 and pH, and amount of concurrent hypoxemia. Acute hypercapnia causes cerebral vasodilatation, subsequently increasing cerebral blood flow and intracranial pressure.[3,33,46,76] Clinically, the CNS effects of hypercapnia can result in signs ranging from anxiety, restlessness, and disorientation to somnolence and coma, especially when P_{CO_2} approaches 70 to 100 mm Hg.[2,39,49,69]

TREATMENT OF RESPIRATORY ACIDOSIS

The most effective treatment of respiratory acidosis consists of rapid diagnosis and elimination of the underlying cause of alveolar hypoventilation. For example, airway obstruction should be identified and relieved, and medications that depress ventilation should be discontinued if possible. Pleurocentesis should be performed to remove fluid or air when pleural effusion or pneumothorax is present. Although at times it is not possible to remove the underlying cause of hypoventilation (e.g., chronic pulmonary disease), appropriate treatment of the primary disease should be initiated along with supportive therapeutic measures. The primary goal is to remove the CO_2, and consequently mechanical ventilation often is necessary.

According to the alveolar gas equation, a patient breathing room air at sea level (PIO_2, ~150 mm Hg) will develop life-threatening hypoxia (PaO_2 < 55 to 60 mm Hg) before life-threatening hypercapnia. Thus supplemental oxygen and assisted ventilation are needed in treating acute respiratory acidosis. Although oxygen therapy may aid in the treatment of acute respiratory acidosis, oxygen may suppress the drive for breathing in patients with chronic hypercapnia. In chronic hypercapnia, the central chemoreceptors become progressively insensitive to the effects of CO_2, and O_2 becomes the primary stimulus for ventilation. As a result, oxygen therapy may further suppress ventilation, worsening respiratory acidosis. If oxygen is administered, PaO_2 should be kept between 60 and 65 mm Hg because the hypoxic drive to breathing remains adequate up to this level.[57]

In respiratory acidosis, the goals of treatment are to ensure adequate oxygenation and to provide adequate alveolar ventilation. Patients approaching respiratory muscle fatigue or respiratory failure or those experiencing progressive acidemia or hypoxemia will need mechanical or assisted ventilation to accomplish these objectives. Respiratory failure in the face of concurrent hypoxemia is diagnosed when $PaCO_2$ is more than 50 mm Hg in a nonsedated or nonanesthetized patient, when PaO_2 is less than 50 mm Hg with a FIO_2 of 0.21, or when a poor response of PaO_2 is less than 50 mm Hg with a FIO_2 of more than 0.5.[8] When mechanical or assisted ventilation is begun, care must be taken to decrease $PaCO_2$ slowly. In human patients, rapid decreases in PCO_2 can result in cardiac arrhythmias, decreased cardiac output, and reduced cerebral blood flow.[39] A sudden decrease in blood PCO_2 also may result in posthypercapnic metabolic alkalosis and rapid diffusion of CO_2 from cerebrospinal fluid into blood, thus quickly increasing cerebrospinal pH.

Therapy with $NaHCO_3$ or other alkalinizing solutions is not indicated in respiratory acidosis. Administration of $NaHCO_3$ increases SID and may decrease [H^+] and ventilatory drive, thus worsening hypoxemia. The resulting decrease in respiratory drive as a result of $NaHCO_3$ administration additionally may increase CO_2 and worsen respiratory failure, especially if alveolar ventilation cannot be increased to balance out the increased CO_2 production. $NaHCO_3$ itself is not innocuous. $NaHCO_3$ may alter hemodynamics, causing hypotension, decreased contractility, and cardiac arrest,[48] as well as decreased cerebral blood flow and cerebrovenous oxygen tension.[5] Thus $NaHCO_3$ treatment is not warranted. In addition, the use of the strong organic base tris(hydroxymethyl)

aminomethane (THAM) has been investigated.[15] THAM promotes CO_2 removal as HCO_3^- is generated. However, the amount of CO_2 removed is very small, and thus THAM has marginal clinical benefit at best.

Administration of a parenteral solution with adequate amounts of Cl^- facilitates recovery from chronic hypercapnia and prevents development of metabolic alkalosis after $PaCO_2$ has returned to normal. Dogs recovering from chronic hypercapnia and receiving a low-salt diet had persistently increased plasma HCO_3^- concentrations.[60] Addition of sodium or potassium chloride to the diet allowed full correction of the acid-base disturbances. Provision of sufficient Cl^- allows the kidney to reabsorb Na^+ in conjunction with Cl^- and to excrete the excess HCO_3^- retained during compensation for chronic hypercapnia.

RESPIRATORY ALKALOSIS

Respiratory alkalosis or primary hypocapnia is characterized by decreased PCO_2, increased pH, and a compensatory decrease in HCO_3^- concentration in the blood. Respiratory alkalosis occurs whenever the magnitude of alveolar ventilation exceeds that required to eliminate the CO_2 produced by metabolic processes in the tissues.

METABOLIC COMPENSATION IN RESPIRATORY ALKALOSIS

Acute Respiratory Alkalosis

When PCO_2 is acutely decreased, CO_2 leaves the cells to achieve a new equilibrium point. Chloride ions leave red blood cells in exchange for HCO_3^-, causing a decrease in plasma HCO_3^- concentration. This results in decreased plasma SID and increases intracellular SID. Furthermore, H^+ translocation into the extracellular space in exchange for sodium and potassium also decreases plasma SID. As in respiratory acidosis, intracellular phosphates and proteins are the major buffers in the acute adaptive response. Extracellular buffering by release of H^+ from plasma proteins constitutes only 1% of the acute response, whereas intracellular buffering accounted for the remaining 99%.[21] In dogs and cats, a compensatory decrease of 0.25 mEq/L in HCO_3^- concentration for each 1-mm Hg decrease in PCO_2 is expected (see Box 11-2).[13,25]

Chronic Respiratory Alkalosis

During chronic respiratory alkalosis, a 0.55-mEq/L decrease in HCO_3^- is expected for each 1-mm Hg decrease in PCO_2 in dogs (see Box 11-2).[13] This represents effective compensation, and the pH is normal or near normal in dogs with chronic respiratory alkalosis. However, normalization of pH may take up to 4 weeks to be achieved.[11] Cats chronically exposed to a hypoxic environment (FIO_2 = 10%) for 28 days also were able to maintain a normal arterial pH.[7] Expected compensation in cats cannot be inferred from this study, but based on the ability to maintain a normal pH, it may be reasonable to assume that cats can compensate to chronic respiratory alkalosis, as well as dogs and humans. As a result, abnormal P_{CO_2} and HCO_3^- concentration with normal pH does not necessarily imply a mixed acid-base disorder in both dogs and cats.

CAUSES OF RESPIRATORY ALKALOSIS

Common causes of respiratory alkalosis include stimulation of peripheral chemoreceptors by hypoxemia, primary pulmonary disease, direct activation of the brainstem respiratory centers, overzealous mechanical ventilation, and situations that cause pain, anxiety, or fear. In addition, respiratory alkalosis can occur during recovery from metabolic acidosis because hyperventilation persists for 24 to 48 hours after correction of metabolic acidosis. A more detailed list of causes is found in Box 11-4.

When P_{O_2} decreases to less than 60 mm Hg, the peripheral chemoreceptors mediate an increase in rate and depth of breathing, resulting in hypocapnia. Decreased oxygen delivery also results in hypocapnia (e.g., severe anemia, cardiovascular shock). The effect of the resulting hypocapnia and decreased $[H^+]$ on the central chemoreceptors is to negatively feedback on the respiratory control system and blunt this initial hyperventilation. As renal compensation occurs, plasma HCO_3^- decreases, $[H^+]$ increases, and central inhibition of further hyperventilation is removed. A steady state results when the peripherally mediated hypoxemic drive to ventilation is balanced by the central effect of the alkalemia resulting from renal adaptation to hypocapnia. If P_{CO_2} is held constant in the presence of hypoxemia (as seen in patients with pulmonary disease), the dampening effect of hypocapnia does not occur, and a lesser degree of hypoxemia may stimulate ventilation.

Pulmonary diseases such as pneumonia, diffuse interstitial lung disease, and thromboembolism may cause respiratory alkalosis. The hyperventilation seen with primary lung disease may be a result, at least in part, of the concurrent hypoxemia. However, pulmonary diseases may cause hyperventilation without hypoxemia as a result of stimulation of stretch receptors and nociceptive receptors.[20,58] The stretch receptors are located in the smooth muscle of the tracheobronchial tree. The nociceptive receptors include irritant receptors in the epithelium of small airways and juxtacapillary receptors (J receptors) lining capillaries in the interstitium. These receptors respond to stimuli such as irritants, interstitial edema, fibrosis, or pulmonary capillary congestion.

DIAGNOSIS AND CLINICAL FEATURES OF RESPIRATORY ALKALOSIS

It is difficult to attribute specific clinical signs to respiratory alkalosis in the dog and cat. The clinical signs usually

| Box 11-4 | Causes of Respiratory Alkalosis |

Hypoxemia (Stimulation of Peripheral Chemoreceptors by Decreased Oxygen Delivery)
Right-to-left shunting
Decreased P_{IO_2} (e.g., high altitude)
Congestive heart failure
Severe anemia
Severe hypotension
Decreased cardiac output
Pulmonary diseases with ventilation-perfusion mismatch
   Pneumonia
   Pulmonary thromboembolism
   Pulmonary fibrosis
   Pulmonary edema
   Acute respiratory distress syndrome

Pulmonary Disease (Stimulation of Stretch/nociceptors Independent of Hypoxemia)
Pneumonia
Pulmonary thromboembolism
Interstitial lung disease
Pulmonary edema
Acute respiratory distress syndrome

Centrally Mediated Hyperventilation
Liver disease
Hyperadrenocorticism
Gram-negative sepsis
Drugs
   Salicylates
   Corticosteroids
   Progesterone (pregnancy)
   Xanthines (e.g., aminophylline)
Recovery from metabolic acidosis
Central neurologic disease
   Trauma
   Neoplasia
   Infection
   Inflammation
   Cerebrovascular accident
Exercise
Heatstroke

Muscle Metaboreceptor Overactivity
Heart failure

Overzealous Mechanical Ventilation

Situations Causing Pain, Fear, or Anxiety

are caused by the underlying disease process and not by the respiratory alkalosis itself. However, in humans, headache, light-headedness, confusion, paresthesias of the extremities, tightness of the chest, and circumoral numbness have been reported in acute respiratory alkalosis.[1,20] In any case, clinical signs in small animals are uncommon because of efficient metabolic compensation, and tachypnea may be the only clinical abnormality found, especially with chronic hypocapnia.

If the pH exceeds 7.6 in respiratory alkalosis, neurologic, cardiopulmonary, and metabolic consequences may arise.[1] Such a pH only can be achieved in acute respiratory alkalosis before renal compensation ensues. Alkalemia results in arteriolar vasoconstriction that can decrease cerebral and myocardial perfusion. In addition, hyperventilation (P_{CO_2} < 25 mm Hg) causes decreased cerebral blood flow, potentially resulting in clinical signs such as confusion and seizures.

Hypocapnia decreases blood pressure and cardiac output in anesthetized but not awake subjects, possibly because anesthetics blunt reflex tachycardia. For example, in anesthetized dogs, acute hypocapnia decreased blood pressure as a result of reduced cardiac output together with an ineffective increase in total peripheral resistance and no change in heart rate.[35,44] Although alkalemia exerts a small positive inotropic effect on the isolated heart, alkalemia also predisposes to refractory supraventricular and ventricular arrhythmias, especially in patients with preexisting cardiac disease.[1]

Acute alkalemia shifts the oxygen-hemoglobin dissociation curve to the left, reducing the release of oxygen to the tissues by increasing affinity of hemoglobin for oxygen (see Fig. 11-1).[28] However, chronic alkalemia negates this effect by increasing the concentration of 2,3-DPG in red cells.[20,27,56]

Hypokalemia may occur as a result of the translocation of potassium into cells and renal and extrarenal losses in patients with acute respiratory alkalosis.[20,27,56] In anesthetized, hyperventilated dogs, potassium is expected to decrease 0.4 mEq/L for each 10-mm Hg decrease in P_{CO_2}.[44] Similar changes (0.6 mEq/L for each 10-mm Hg decrease in P_{CO_2}) were observed in awake dogs with acute respiratory acidosis induced by hypoxemia[29] or by simulating a high altitude environment (30,000 feet).[61] Hypokalemia can result in neuromuscular weakness, sensitization to digitalis-induced arrhythmias, polyuria, and increased ammonia production that amplifies the effects of hepatic encephalopathy.[1] However, the hypokalemia induced by respiratory alkalosis is mild and short-lived. Hypokalemia is not present in patients with chronic respiratory alkalosis.[2a,19,22]

TREATMENT OF RESPIRATORY ALKALOSIS

Treatment should be directed toward relieving the underlying cause of the hypocapnia; no other treatment is effective. Respiratory alkalosis severe enough to cause clinical consequences for the animal is uncommon. Hypocapnia itself is not a major threat to the well-being of the patient. Thus the underlying disease responsible for hypocapnia should receive primary therapeutic attention.

SUMMARY

Respiratory acid-base disorders and derangements in arterial blood gases are common entities that may lead to increased morbidity and mortality in small animal patients. Early and proper diagnosis of these disease states is essential in providing correct and effective therapy. Recent, more widespread availability of "bedside" portable blood gas analyzers in small animal practice has allowed the practitioner to monitor the acid-base and oxygenation status of the patient, thus providing more efficient, high quality care for the compromised small animal patient.

REFERENCES

1. Adrogué HJ, Madias NE: Management of life-threatening acid-base disorders (first of two parts), *N Engl J Med* 338:26-34, 1998.
2. Adrogué HJ, Madias NE: Management of life-threatening acid-base disorders (second of two parts), *N Engl J Med* 338:107-111, 1998.
2a. Adrogué HJ, Madias NE: Changes in plasma potassium concentration during acute acid-base disturbances, *Am J Med* 71:456-467, 1981.
3. Alberti E, Hoyer S, Hamer J, et al: The effect of carbon dioxide on cerebral blood flow and cerebral metabolism in dogs, *Br J Anaesth* 47:941-947, 1975.
4. Alfaro V, Torras R, Ibáñez J, et al: A physical-chemical analysis of the acid-base response to chronic obstructive pulmonary disease, *Can J Physiol Pharmacol* 74:1229-1235, 1996.
5. Arvidsson S, Haggendal E, Winso I: Influence on cerebral blood flow of infusion of sodium bicarbonate during respiratory acidosis and alkalosis in the dog, *Acta Anaesthesiol Scand* 25:146-152, 1981.
6. Ballantyne D, Scheid P: Central chemosensitivity of respiration: a brief overview, *Respir Physiol* 129:5-12, 2001.
7. Barnard P, Andronikou S, Pokorski M, et al: Time-dependent effect of hypoxia on carotid body chemosensory function, *J Appl Physiol* 63:685-691, 1987.
8. Bateman SW: Ventilating the lung injured patient: what's new? In *Proceedings of the American College of Veterinary Surgeons Symposium*, Chicago, 2001, pp. 562-565.
9. Brofman JD, Leff AR, Munoz NM, et al: Sympathetic secretory response to hypercapnic acidosis in swine, *J Appl Physiol* 69:710-717, 1990.
10. Brunson DB, Hogan KJ: Malignant hyperthermia: a syndrome not a disease, *Vet Clin North Am Small Anim Pract* 34:1419-1433, 2004.
11. Bureau M, Bouverot P: Blood and CSF acid-base changes and rate of ventilatory acclimatization of awake dogs to 3,550 m, *Respir Physiol* 24:203-216, 1975.
12. Caruana-Montaldo B, Gleeson K, Zwillich CW: The control of breathing in clinical practice, *Chest* 117:205-225, 2000.
13. de Morais HAS, DiBartola SP: Ventilatory and metabolic compensation in dogs with acid-base disturbances, *J Vet Emerg Crit Care* 1:39-49, 1991.
14. DiBartola SP, de Morais HAS: Respiratory acid-base disorders. In DiBartola SP, editor: *Fluid therapy in small animal practice*, Philadelphia, 1992, WB Saunders, pp. 258-275.

15. Epstein SK, Singh N: Respiratory acidosis, *Respir Care* 46:366-383, 2001.

16. Feldman JL: Neurophysiology of breathing in mammals. In Bloom FE, Mountcastle VB, editors: *Handbook of physiology. Section I, the nervous system, vol. 4, Intrinsic regulatory systems of the brain*, Bethesda, 1986, American Physiological Society, pp. 463-524.

17. Feldman JL, Mitchell GS, Nattie EE: Breathing: rhythmicity, plasticity, chemosensitivity, *Annu Rev Neurosci* 26:239-266, 2003.

18. Galla JH, Luke RG: Chloride transport and disorders of acid-base balance, *Annu Rev Physiol* 50:141-158, 1988.

19. Gennari FJ, Goldstein MB, Schwartz WB: The nature of the renal adaptation to chronic hypocapnia, *J Clin Invest* 51:1722-1730, 1972.

20. Gennari FJ, Kassirer JP: Respiratory alkalosis. In Cohen JJ, Kassirer JP, editors: *Acid-base.* Boston, 1982, Little, Brown & Co., pp. 349-376.

21. Giebisch G, Berger L, Pitts RF: The extrarenal response to acute acid-base disturbances of respiratory origin, *J Clin Invest* 34:231-245, 1955.

22. Gougoux A, Kaehny WD, Cohen JJ: Renal adaptation to chronic hypocapnia: dietary constraints to achieving H+ retention, *Am J Physiol* 229:1330-1337, 1975.

23. Gray BA, Blalock JM: Interpretation of the alveolar-arterial oxygen difference in patients with hypercapnia, *Am Rev Respir Dis* 143:4-8, 1991.

24. Greene KE, Peters JI: Pathophysiology of acute respiratory failure, *Clin Chest Med* 15:1-12, 1994.

25. Hampson NB, Jöbsis-VandlerVliet FF, Piantadosi CA: Skeletal muscle oxygen availability during respiratory acid-base disturbances in cats. *Respir Physiol* 70:143-158, 1987.

26. Hara Y, Nezu Y, Harada Y, et al: Secondary chronic respiratory acidosis in a dog following the cervical cord compression by an intradural glioma, *J Vet Med Sci* 64:863-866, 2002.

27. Harrington JT, Kassirer JP: Metabolic alkalosis. In Cohen JJ, Kassirer JP, editors: *Acid-base.* Boston, 1982, Little, Brown & Co., pp.227-306.

28. Hodgkin JE, Soeprono FF, Chan DM: Incidence of metabolic alkalemia in hospitalized patients, *Crit Care Med* 8:725-728, 1980.

29. Höhne C, Boemke W, Schleyer N, et al: Low sodium intake does not impair renal compensation of hypoxia-induced respiratory alkalosis, *J Appl Physiol* 92:2097-2104, 2002.

30. Hughes JMB: Pulmonary gas exchange. In Hughes JMB, Pride NB, editors: *Lung function tests. Physiological principles and clinical applications*, ed 1, Philadelphia, 1999, WB Saunders, pp. 75-92.

31. Jennings DB, Davidson JS: Acid-base and ventilatory adaptation in conscious dogs during chronic hypercapnia, *Respir Physiol* 58:377-393, 1984.

32. Kerber RE, Pandian NG, Hoyt R, et al: Effect of ischemia, hypertrophy, hypoxia, acidosis, and alkalosis on canine defibrillation, *Am J Physiol* 244:H825-H831, 1983.

33. Kontos HA, Raper AJ, Patterson JL: Analysis of vasoactivity of local pH, P_{CO_2} and bicarbonate on pial vessels, *Stroke* 8:358-360, 1977.

34. Lemieux G, Lemieux C, Duplessis S, et al: Metabolic characteristics of cat kidney: failure to adapt to metabolic acidosis, *Am J Physiol* 259:R277-R281, 1990.

35. Little RC, Smith CW: Cardiovascular response to acute hypocapnia due to overbreathing, *Am J Physiol* 206:1025-1030, 1964.

36. Low JM, Gin T, Lee TW, et al: Effect of respiratory acidosis and alkalosis on plasma catecholamine concentrations in anesthetized man, *Clin Sci (Lond)* 84:69-72, 1993.

37. Lugliani R, Whipp BJ, Seard C, et al: Effect of carotid-body resection on ventilatory control at rest and during exercise in man, *N Engl J Med* 285:1105-1111, 1971.

38. Madias NE, Adrogué HJ: Cross-talk between two organs: how the kidney responds to disruption of acid-base balance by the lung, *Nephron Physiol* 93:61-66, 2003.

39. Madias NE, Cohen JJ: Respiratory acidosis. In Cohen JJ, Kassirer JP, editors: *Acid-base*, Boston, 1982, Little, Brown & Co., pp. 307-348.

40. Madias NE, Wolf CJ, Cohen JJ: Regulation of acid-base equilibrium in chronic hypercapnia, *Kidney Int* 27:538-543, 1985.

41. Markou NK, Myrianthefs PM, Baltopoulos GJ: Respiratory failure: an overview, *Crit Care Nurs Q* 27:353-379, 2004.

42. Martinu T, Menzies D, Dial S: Re-evaluation of acid-base prediction rules in patients with chronic respiratory acidosis, *Can Respir J* 10:311-315, 2003.

43. Misuri G, Lanini B, Gigliotti F, et al: Mechanism of CO_2 retention in patients with neuromuscular disease, *Chest* 117:447-453, 2000.

44. Muir WW, Wagner AE, Buchanan C: Effects of acute hyperventilation on serum potassium in the dog, *Vet Surg* 19:83-87, 1990.

45. Murray JF: Gas exchange and oxygen transport. In Murray JF, editor: *The normal lung*, Philadelphia, 1986, WB Saunders, p. 194.

46. Nakahata K, Kinoshita H, Hirano Y, et al: Mild hypercapnia induces vasodilation via adenosine triphosphate-sensitive K+ channels in parenchymal microvessels of the rat cerebral cortex, *Anesthesiology* 99:1333-1339, 2003.

47. Nattie EE: CO_2, brainstem chemoreceptors and breathing, *Prog Neurobiol* 59:299-331, 1999.

48. Nishikawa T: Acute haemodynamic effects of sodium bicarbonate in canine respiratory and metabolic acidosis, *Br J Anaesth* 70:196-200, 1993.

49. Nunn JF: Changes in the carbon dioxide tension. In *Nunn's applied respiratory physiology*, ed 5, Edinburgh, 2000, Butterworth-Heinemann, pp. 460-471.

50. Nunn JF: Distribution of pulmonary ventilation and perfusion. In *Nunn's applied respiratory physiology*, ed 5, Edinburgh, 2000, Butterworth-Heinemann, pp. 163-199.

51. Orchard CH, Kentish JC: Effects of changes of pH on the contractile function of cardiac muscle, *Am J Physiol* 258:C967-C981, 1990.

52. Polak A, Haynie GD, Hays RM, et al: Effects of chronic hypercapnia on electrolyte and acid-base equilibrium. I. Adaptation, *J Clin Invest* 40:1223-1237, 1961.

53. Porcelli RJ: Pulmonary hemodynamics. In Parent RA, editor: *Treatise on pulmonary toxicology. Vol 1. Comparative biology of the normal lung*, Boca Raton, FL, 1992, CRC Press, pp. 241-270.

54. Putnam RW, Filosa JA, Ritucci NA: Cellular mechanisms involved in CO_2 and acid signaling in chemosensitive neurons, *Am J Physiol Cell Physiol* 287:C1493-C1526, 2004.

55. Ramirez J, Totapally BR, Hon E, et al: Oxygen-carrying capacity during 10 hours of hypercapnia in ventilated dogs, *Crit Care Med* 28:1918-1923, 2000.

56. Rimmer JM, Gennari FJ: Metabolic alkalosis, *J Intensive Care Med* 2:137-150, 1987.

57. Rose BD, Post TW: Respiratory acidosis. In Rose BD, Post TW, editors: *Clinical physiology of acid-base and electrolyte disorders*, ed 5, New York, 2001, McGraw-Hill, pp. 647-672.

58. Rose BD, Post TW: Respiratory alkalosis. In Rose BD, Post TW, editors: *Clinical physiology of acid-base and electrolyte disorders,* ed 5, New York, 2001, McGraw-Hill, pp. 673-681.

59. Schwartz WB, Brackett NC, Cohen JJ: The response of extra-cellular hydrogen ion concentration to graded degrees of chronic hypercapnia: the physiologic limits of the defense of pH, *J Clin Invest* 44:291-301, 1965.

60. Schwartz WB, Hays RM, Polak A, et al: Effects of chronic hypercapnia on electrolyte and acid-base equilibrium. II. Recovery, with special reference to the influence of chloride intake, *J Clin Invest* 40:1238-1249, 1961.

61. Smith DC, Barry JQ, Gold AJ: Respiratory alkalosis and hypokalemia in dogs exposed to simulated high altitude, *Am J Physiol* 202:1041-1044, 1962.

62. Solomon IC, Edelman NH, O'Neal MH: CO_2/H^+ chemoreception in the cat pre-Bötzinger complex in vivo. *J Appl Physiol* 88:1996-2007, 2000.

63. Sprung CL, Portocarrero CJ, Fernaine AV, et al: The metabolic and respiratory alterations of heat stroke, *Arch Intern Med* 140:665-669, 1980.

64. Szlyk PC, Jennings BD: Effects of hypercapnia on variability of normal respiratory behavior in awake cats, *Am J Physiol* 252:R538-R547, 1987.

65. Talor Z, Yang WC, Shuffield J, et al: Chronic hypercapnia enhances Vmax of Na^+-H^+ antiporter of renal brush-border membranes, *Am J Physiol* 253:F394-F400, 1987.

66. Tournadre JP, Allaouchiche B, Malbert CH, et al: Metabolic acidosis and respiratory acidosis impair gastro-pyloric motility in anesthetized pigs, *Anesth Analg* 90:74-79, 2000.

67. Valtin H, Gennari FJ: *Acid base disorders: basic concepts and clinical management,* Boston, 1987, Little, Brown & Co., pp. 7-10.

68. van Ypersele de Strihou C, Gulyassy PF, Schwartz WB: Effects of chronic hypercapnia on electrolyte and acid-base equilibrium. III. Characteristics of the adaptive and recovery process as evaluated by provision of alkali, *J Clin Invest* 41:2246-2253, 1962.

69. Wall RE: Respiratory acid-base disorders, *Vet Clin North Am Small Anim Pract* 31:1355-1367, 2001.

70. Walley KR, Lewis TH, Wood LD: Acute respiratory acidosis decreases left ventricular contractility but increases cardiac output in dogs, *Circ Res* 67:628-635, 1990.

71. Wasserman K, Hansen JE, Sue DY, et al: *Principles of exercise testing and interpretation,* Philadelphia, 1987, Lea & Febiger.

72. Weinberger SE, Schwartzstein RM, Weiss JW: Hypercapnia, *N Engl J Med* 321:1223-1231, 1989.

73. West JB: Causes of carbon dioxide retention in lung disease, *N Engl J Med* 284:1232-1236, 1971.

74. West JB: Ventilation-perfusion relationships, *Am Rev Respir Dis* 116:919-943, 1977.

75. West JB: *Respiratory physiology: the essentials,* ed 7, Philadelphia, 2004, Lippincott Williams & Wilkins, pp. 75-89.

76. Williams G, Roberts PA, Smith S, et al: The effect of apnea on brain compliance and intracranial pressure, *Neurosurgery* 29:242-246, 1991.

CHAPTER · 12

MIXED ACID-BASE DISORDERS

Helio Autran de Morais and Andrew L. Leisewitz

"A patient will have as many diseases as he/she pleases."

Anonymous

A mixed acid-base disturbance is characterized by the presence of two or more separate primary acid-base abnormalities occurring in the same patient. An acid-base disturbance is said to be simple if it is limited to the primary disturbance and the expected compensatory response. Box 12-1 shows a classification of mixed acid-base disorders.

Recognition of a mixed acid-base disorder is important from a diagnostic and a therapeutic point of view. It permits early detection of complications (e.g., the

Box 12-1	Classification of Mixed Acid-Base Disorders

Disorders with Neutralizing Effects on pH

Mixed Respiratory-metabolic Disorders
Respiratory acidosis and metabolic alkalosis
Respiratory alkalosis and metabolic acidosis

Mixed Metabolic Disorders
Metabolic acidosis and metabolic alkalosis

Disorders with Additive Effects on pH

Mixed Respiratory-metabolic Disorders
Respiratory acidosis and metabolic acidosis
Respiratory alkalosis and metabolic alkalosis

Mixed Metabolic Disorders
Normal plus high-anion gap metabolic acidosis
Mixed high-anion gap metabolic acidosis
Mixed normal-anion gap metabolic acidosis

Triple Disorders
Metabolic acidosis, metabolic alkalosis, and respiratory acidosis
Metabolic acidosis, metabolic alkalosis, and respiratory alkalosis

presence of metabolic acidosis and respiratory alkalosis in a dog with parvovirus gastroenteritis may indicate sepsis), provides orientation for treatment (e.g., $NaHCO_3$ is contraindicated in the majority of patients with metabolic acidosis and respiratory acidosis), and allows detection of complications associated with therapy (e.g., a patient with chronic respiratory acidosis that develops metabolic alkalosis after treatment with diuretics experiences further compromise of ventilation by the metabolic process).

In approaching mixed acid-base disturbances, a proper understanding of the terms **acidosis, alkalosis, acidemia,** and **alkalemia** is crucial. **Acidosis** and **alkalosis** refer to the pathophysiologic processes that cause net accumulation of acid or alkali in the body, whereas **acidemia** and **alkalemia** refer specifically to the pH of extracellular fluid. In acidemia, the extracellular fluid pH is less than normal and the $[H^+]$ is higher than normal. In alkalemia, the extracellular fluid pH is higher than normal and the $[H^+]$ is lower than normal. For example, a patient with chronic respiratory alkalosis may have a blood pH value that is within the normal range. Such a patient has alkalosis but does not have alkalemia.

COMPENSATION

The definition of a simple acid-base disturbance includes both the primary process causing changes in Pco_2 or $[HCO_3^-]$ and the compensatory mechanisms affecting these measurements. A primary increase or decrease in one component (e.g., Pco_2 or $[HCO_3^-]$) is associated with a predictable compensatory change in the same direction in the other component (Table 12-1). Lack of appropriate compensation is evidence of a mixed acid-base disorder. Unfortunately, the magnitude of expected compensation in a given clinical situation is not known with certainty, and data in dogs have been derived mainly from experiments using normal dogs[16] (Table 12-2). Compensatory rules for cats should be used with caution because values are derived from a limited number of normal cats with experimentally induced acid-base disorders. The reader is referred to Chapters 9, 10, and 11 for further discussion of compensation.

RESPIRATORY COMPENSATION IN METABOLIC PROCESSES

Metabolic acidosis is characterized by an increase in $[H^+]$, a decrease in serum $[HCO_3^-]$ and blood pH, and a secondary decrease in Pco_2 as a result of secondary hyperventilation. The expected decrease in Pco_2 in dogs with metabolic acidosis may be estimated as 0.7 mm Hg for each 1-mEq/L decrease in $[HCO_3^-]$.[16] Cats with experimentally induced metabolic acidosis consistently show a lack of ventilatory compensation. In one study in which cats were chronically fed a diet containing NH_4Cl, significant decreases in pH and $[HCO_3^-]$ were observed, but there was no change in Pco_2.[9] Similar results were obtained in another study also adding NH_4Cl to the diet[31] and with dietary phosphoric acid supplementation.[19] Contrary to what happens in dogs and humans, the feline kidney apparently is unable to adapt to metabolic acidosis and does not increase production of ammonia or glucose from glutamine during acidosis.[31] Based on these studies, cats may not compensate for metabolic acidosis to the same extent (if at all) as do dogs and humans. Thus formulas for dogs or humans should not be extrapolated for use in cats. The clinical finding of metabolic acidosis and normal Pco_2 in a cat should not be interpreted as evidence of a mixed process until more data are available about respiratory compensation in cats.

TABLE 12-1 Primary and Secondary Changes in Simple Acid-Base Disorders

Disorder	Primary Change	Compensatory Response
Metabolic acidosis	↓ HCO_3^-	↓ Pco_2
Metabolic alkalosis	↑ HCO_3^-	↑ Pco_2
Respiratory acidosis	↑ Pco_2	↑ HCO_3^-
Respiratory alkalosis	↓ Pco_2	↓ HCO_3^-

TABLE 12-2 Compensatory Response in Simple Acid-Base Disturbances in Dogs and Cats*

Disturbance	Primary Change	Clinical Guide for Compensation	
		Dogs	**Cats†**
Metabolic acidosis	Each 1 mEq/L ↓ HCO_3^-	P_{CO_2} ↓ by 0.7 mm Hg	P_{CO_2} does not change
Metabolic alkalosis	Each 1 mEq/L ↑ HCO_3^-	P_{CO_2} ↑ by 0.7 mm Hg	P_{CO_2} ↑ by 0.7 mm Hg
Respiratory acidosis			
Acute	Each 1 mm Hg ↑ P_{CO_2}	HCO_3^- ↑ by 0.15 mEq/L	HCO_3^- ↑ by 0.15 mEq/L
Chronic	Each 1 mm Hg ↑ P_{CO_2}	HCO_3^- ↑ by 0.35 mEq/L	Unknown
Long-standing‡	Each 1 mm Hg ↑ P_{CO_2}	HCO_3^- ↑ by 0.55 mEq/L	Unknown
Respiratory alkalosis			
Acute	Each 1 mm Hg ↓ P_{CO_2}	HCO_3^- ↓ by 0.25 mEq/L	HCO_3^- ↓ by 0.25 mEq/L
Chronic	Each 1 mm Hg ↓ P_{CO_2}	HCO_3^- ↓ by 0.55 mEq/L	Similar to dogs§

Data in dogs from de Morais and DiBartola.[16] See text for references in cats.
†Data from cats are derived from a very limited number of cats.
‡More than 30 days.
§Exact degree of compensation has not been determined, but cats with chronic respiratory alkalosis maintain normal arterial pH.

Metabolic alkalosis is characterized by a decrease in $[H^+]$, an increase in serum $[HCO_3^-]$ and blood pH, and a secondary increase in P_{CO_2} as a result of compensatory hypoventilation. As a rule of thumb, a 1.0-mEq/L increase in plasma $[HCO_3^-]$ is expected to be associated with an adaptive 0.7-mm Hg increase in P_{CO_2} in dogs with metabolic alkalosis.[16] Little is known about respiratory compensation in cats with metabolic alkalosis. In one study with 12- to 14-week-old kittens made alkalotic by selective dietary chloride depletion, a 1.0-mEq/L increase in plasma $[HCO_3^-]$ concentration was associated with a 0.7-mm Hg increase in P_{CO_2}.[62] This value is remarkably similar to that observed in humans and dogs, but care should be exercised when extrapolating data from normal kittens to sick adult cats.

Time is an important consideration when assessing compensation. Even in the experimental setting in which sudden changes in $[HCO_3^-]$ can be achieved, the respiratory response to acute metabolic acidosis in dogs occurs slowly, and it often takes 17 to 24 hours for maximal respiratory compensation to develop.[16] Thus using the formulas within the first 24 hours of onset of metabolic acidosis may lead to an underestimation of the ventilatory response and the erroneous assumption that a mixed metabolic and respiratory disorder is present.

METABOLIC COMPENSATION IN RESPIRATORY PROCESSES

Respiratory acidosis is that acid-base disorder resulting from a primary increase in carbon dioxide tension (P_{CO_2}) in the blood. It is synonymous with **primary hypercapnia** and is characterized by increased P_{CO_2}, increased $[H^+]$, decreased pH, and a compensatory increase in

$[HCO_3^-]$ in blood. **Respiratory alkalosis** is that acid-base disorder resulting from a primary decrease in P_{CO_2} in the blood. It is synonymous with the term **primary hypocapnia** and is characterized by decreased P_{CO_2}, decreased $[H^+]$, increased pH, and a compensatory decrease in $[HCO_3^-]$ in blood.

Adaptive changes in plasma $[HCO_3^-]$ occur in two phases. In respiratory acidosis, the first phase represents titration of nonbicarbonate buffers, whereas in respiratory alkalosis, the first phase represents release of H^+ from nonbicarbonate buffers within cells. This response is completed within 15 minutes (see Chapter 11). The second phase reflects renal adaptation and consists of increased net acid excretion and increased HCO_3^- reabsorption (decreased Cl^- reabsorption) in respiratory acidosis and a decrease in net acid excretion in respiratory alkalosis. Experimentally, renal adaptation requires 2 to 5 days for a chronic steady state to be established.[21,46,51]

During **acute respiratory acidosis,** a compensatory increase of 0.15 mEq/L in $[HCO_3^-]$ for each 1-mm Hg increase in P_{CO_2} should be expected in dogs.[16] There is a lack of data for compensation in cats with acute respiratory acid-base disorders, but values appear to be similar to those observed in dogs. In anesthetized, artificially ventilated cats made hypercapnic by exposure to increasing CO_2 levels, the average compensatory increase in $[HCO_3^-]$ was 0.07 to 0.1 mEq/L for each 1-mm Hg increase in P_{CO_2}.[24,54] In three awake cats exposed to an FI_{CO_2} of 4%,[53] $[HCO_3^-]$ increased 0.16 mEq/L for each 1-mm Hg increase in P_{CO_2}, a value very similar to the one observed in dogs. During **acute respiratory alkalosis,** a compensatory decrease of 0.25 mEq/L in $[HCO_3^-]$ for each 1-mm Hg decrease in P_{CO_2} should be expected in dogs.[16] Compensation to hyperventilation has only been studied in anesthetized cats. The $[HCO_3^-]$ decreased an average 0.26 mEq/L for each 1-mm Hg decrease in P_{CO_2}, a value similar to that obtained in dogs.[24]

In dogs with **chronic respiratory alkalosis,** a decrease of 0.55 mEq/L in $[HCO_3^-]$ is expected for each 1-mm Hg decrease in P_{CO_2}.[2,16] It is interesting to note that even in severe chronic respiratory alkalosis, the pH usually is normal. However, the normalization of pH in a clinical setting may take longer than 5 to 7 days. In humans with sustained respiratory alkalosis, the pH may not return to normal for 2 or more weeks.[40] Cats chronically exposed to a hypoxic environment (FI_{O_2} = 10%) for 28 days also were able to maintain a normal arterial pH.[4] Expected compensation in cats cannot be inferred from this study, but based on the ability to maintain a normal pH, it may be reasonable to assume that cats can compensate to chronic respiratory alkalosis as well as dogs and humans. In dogs with **chronic respiratory acidosis,** serum $[HCO_3^-]$ increases 0.35 mEq/L for each 1-mm Hg increase in P_{CO_2}.[16] Similar rules have been used in humans with chronic respiratory acidosis, but these rules have been shown to work well in unstable, but not in stable, patients with long-standing respiratory acidosis.[35] In this latter group of patients, a 0.51-mEq/L increase in $[HCO_3^-]$ is expected for each 1-mm Hg increase in P_{CO_2}.[35] Thus arterial pH appears to remain near reference ranges in human patients with long-standing respiratory acidosis.[3] Similar results have been observed in dogs with chronic respiratory acidosis and no other identifiable reason for increased $[HCO_3^-]$ concentration other than renal compensation.[22,25] Increases of 0.45[25] to 0.57 mEq/L[22] $[HCO_3^-]$ for each 1-mm Hg increase in P_{CO_2} have been observed in dogs with chronic respiratory acidosis, suggesting that renal compensation in dogs with long-standing respiratory acidosis may return arterial pH to normal in stable patients.

CLINICAL APPROACH

The first step is a careful history to search for clues that may lead the clinician to suspect the presence of acid-base disorders, followed by a complete physical examination. Urinalysis, routine serum chemistries, and electrolyte concentrations are useful, but confirmation of a mixed acid-base disorder requires blood gas analysis. After identifying the primary acid-base disorder (respiratory or metabolic), the expected compensation of the opposing parameter ($[HCO_3^-]$ in a respiratory process; P_{CO_2} in a metabolic process) should be calculated using the formulas in Table 12-2. A mixed acid-base disorder should be suspected when inappropriate compensation for the primary disorder is demonstrated. Compensation is said to be inappropriate if a patient's P_{CO_2} differs from expected P_{CO_2} by more than 2 mm Hg in a primary metabolic process or if a patient's $[HCO_3^-]$ differs from the expected $[HCO_3^-]$ by more than 2 mEq/L in a respiratory acid-base disorder.[2,16]

An example illustrates how compensation can be estimated. Consider a dog that presents with diarrhea caused by a parvovirus infection with the following arterial blood gas results: pH = 7.35, $[HCO_3^-]$ = 13 mEq/L, and P_{CO_2} = 24 mm Hg. The pH in the low normal range with decreased $[HCO_3^-]$ indicates that the primary process is a metabolic acidosis. The expected compensation is estimated assuming P_{CO_2} = 36 mm Hg and $[HCO_3^-]$ = 21 mEq/L as midpoint values. The change in $[HCO_3^-]$ ($\Delta[HCO_3^-]$) is:

$$\Delta[HCO_3^-] = \text{midpoint } [HCO_3^-] - \text{patient } [HCO_3^-]$$
$$= 21 \text{ mEq/L} - 13 \text{ mEq/L} = 8 \text{ mEq/L}$$

Knowing that for each mEq/L decrease in $[HCO_3^-]$ in a metabolic acidosis, P_{CO_2} decreases 0.7 mm Hg (see Table 12-2), the expected compensatory change in P_{CO_2} is estimated as:

$$P_{CO_{2expected}} = \text{midpoint } P_{CO_2} - \Delta P_{CO_2}$$

where

$$\Delta P_{CO_2} = \Delta[HCO_3^-] \times 0.7 = 5.6 \text{ mm Hg}$$

Thus

$$P_{CO_{2expected}} = \text{midpoint } P_{CO_2} - \Delta[HCO_3^-] \times 0.7$$
$$= 36 \text{ mm Hg} - 5.6 = 30.4 \text{ mm Hg}$$

Because the expected compensation has an error margin of ±2,

$$P_{CO_{2expected}} = 30.4 \pm 2, \text{ or } 28.4 \text{ to } 32.4 \text{ mm Hg}$$

This patient has a P_{CO_2} (24 mm Hg) that is more than 2 mm Hg lower than the minimal value for the expected P_{CO_2} (28.4 mm Hg), indicating the presence of respiratory alkalosis in addition to metabolic acidosis. A similar line of thinking can be applied to calculate the expected compensation in other primary acid-base disorders. Some guidelines for adequate use of compensatory rules from Table 12-2 are expressed in Box 12-2. Some useful guidelines for quickly detecting mixed acid-base disorders in selected patients are shown in Box 12-3, whereas potential technical problems that may lead to misdiagnosing a mixed acid-base disorder are shown in Box 12-4.

EVALUATION OF THE METABOLIC COMPONENT OF THE ACID-BASE DISORDER

Metabolic alkalosis can result from an increase in the strong ion difference (SID) caused by hypochloremia or by decrease in the concentration of total plasma weak acids $[A_{tot}]$ caused by hypoalbuminemia. Metabolic acidosis can be caused by a decrease in SID as a result of hyperchloremia or increased concentration of other strong anions (e.g., lactate, sulfate, β-hydroxybutyrate), or by an increase in $[A_{tot}]$ as a result of hyperphosphatemia. See Chapter 13 for further discussion of the role of albumin and phosphate in acid-base disorders.

Chloride Changes

Chloride is the most important extracellular strong anion. Increases in chloride lead to metabolic acidosis by decreasing SID, whereas decreases in chloride cause metabolic alkalosis by increasing SID. Therefore plasma $[Cl^-]$ and $[HCO_3^-]$ have a tendency to change in opposite directions in hypochloremic alkalosis and hyperchloremic acidosis. The contribution of $[Cl^-]$ to changes in base excess (BE) and $[HCO_3^-]$ can be estimated by calculating the chloride gap, the chloride/sodium ratio, and the sodium-chloride difference (Table 12-3).

Chloride gap is calculated as:

$$[Cl^-]gap = [Cl^-]normal - [Cl^-]corrected$$

or

$$[Cl^-]gap = [Cl^-]normal - [Cl^-]patient \times [Na^+]normal / [Na^+]patient$$

Normal values may vary among laboratories, but using midpoint values from Chapter 4, chloride gap can be estimated for dogs as:

$$[Cl^-]gap = 110 - [Cl^-]patient \times 146 / [Na^+]patient$$

and for cats as:

$$[Cl^-]gap = 120 - [Cl^-]patient \times 156 / [Na^+]patient$$

Values greater than 4 mEq/L are associated with hypochloremic alkalosis, whereas values less than −4 mEq/L are associated with hyperchloremic acidosis. A shorter way to evaluate chloride contribution is to use the chloride/sodium ratio.[18] Reference values have not been adequately established for dogs and cats, but experience with limited number of cases suggests that values greater than 0.78 in dogs and more than 0.80 in cats are associated with hyperchloremic metabolic acidosis, whereas values less than 0.72 in dogs and less than 0.74 in cats are associated with hypochloremic alkalosis. Whenever sodium concentration is normal, the difference between the sodium and chloride concentrations ($[Na^+] - [Cl^-]$) can be used. Normally, $[Na^+] - [Cl^-]$ is approximately 36 mEq/L in dogs and cats. Values greater than 40 mEq/L are an indication of hypochloremic alkalosis, whereas values less than 32 mEq/L are associated with hyperchloremic acidosis.[15]

It is always important to remember that the renal adaptation to respiratory disorders is accomplished by changing SID by varying the amount of chloride or bicarbonate that is reabsorbed with sodium. Thus in chronic respiratory acidosis, there is a compensatory hypochloremic alkalosis, whereas in chronic respiratory alkalosis, there is a compensatory hyperchloremic acidosis. In fact, all change in bicarbonate concentration can be explained by the changes in chloride during chronic respiratory acidosis.[3]

Increase in Unmeasured Anions

Unlike chloride, most other strong anions (e.g., ketoanions, lactate, anions of renal failure) are not routinely measured and need to be estimated. Three methods combining blood gas results with electrolyte and protein data will be considered here: anion gap (AG), BE algorithm, and strong ion gap (SIG). The AG is further discussed in Chapters 9 and 10, whereas the BE algorithm and the SIG are further discussed in Chapter 13.

The **anion gap** is a helpful tool in the differentiation between hyperchloremic and high-AG metabolic acidoses. Chemically, there is no AG because the law of electroneutrality must be maintained. The AG is the difference between the unmeasured anions (UA^-) and unmeasured cations (UC^+). Following the electroneutrality law, we obtain:

$$([Na^+] + [K^+] + [UC^+]) - ([Cl^-] + [HCO_3^-] + [UA^-])$$

or

$$AG = ([Na^+] + [K^+]) - ([Cl^-] + [HCO_3^-])$$
$$= ([UA^-] - [UC^+])$$

Thus every time there is an increase in $[Cl^-]$ or $[UA^-]$, $[HCO_3^-]$ decreases to maintain electroneutrality. The AG estimates all unmeasured anions, making no distinction between unmeasured strong anions (e.g., lactate, ketoanions) that can change pH and weak anions (e.g., negatively charged phosphate ions and proteins) that do not affect pH or $[HCO_3^-]$. In acidosis resulting from a decrease in SID caused by an increase in $[Cl^-]$, $[HCO_3^-]$ decreases and the difference ($[UA^-] - [UC^+]$) and consequently the AG remain constant (hyperchloremic or normal AG acidosis). When the SID decreases because of an increase in an unmeasured strong anion (e.g., lactate), $[HCO_3^-]$ decreases, $[Cl^-]$ is unchanged, and the difference ($[UA^-] - [UC^+]$) increases; thus the AG also increases (normochloremic or high AG acidosis).

Except for some relatively uncommon circumstances, an increase in the AG implies an accumulation of organic acids in the body.[40] Unfortunately, the AG is not very sensitive in detecting increases in unmeasured strong anions, especially in lactic acidosis. In addition, the AG in normal dogs and cats is mostly a result of the net negative charge of proteins and thus is heavily influenced by protein concentration, especially albumin.[12,36] In fact, hypoalbuminemia probably is the only impor-

tant cause of a decrease in the AG. At plasma pH of 7.4 in dogs, each decrease of 1 g/dL in albumin concentration is associated with a decrease of 4.1 mEq/L in the AG, whereas each decrease of 1 g/dL in total protein concentration is associated with a decrease of 2.5 mEq/L in the AG.[12] Similar data are not available for cats.

Because many critically ill patients with increased unmeasured strong anions also have hypoalbuminemia, the AG may be artificially normal because of the decrease in $[UA^-]$ resulting from hypoalbuminemia. The AG can be corrected for changes in protein concentration in dogs by using the following formulas[12]:

$$AG_{Alb\text{-}adjusted} = AG + 4.2 \times (3.77 - [alb])$$

or

$$AG_{TP\text{-}adjusted} = AG + 2.5 \times (6.37 - [TP])$$

where [alb] is albumin concentration in g/dL and [TP] is total protein concentration in g/dL.

Although the contribution of serum phosphate concentration to the AG is negligible in normal dogs and cats, hyperphosphatemia also can increase the AG in the absence of an increase in strong unmeasured anions. The AG can be adjusted for an increase in phosphate concentration by expressing phosphate in mEq/L (see Chapter 7) and assuming plasma pH to be 7.4 as:

$$AG_{alb\text{-}phosph\text{-}adjusted} = AG + 4.2 \times (3.77 - [alb])$$
$$+ (2.52 - 0.58 \times [Phosph])$$

$$AG_{TP\text{-}phosph\text{-}adjusted} = AG + 0.25 \times (6.37 - [TP])$$
$$+ (2.52 - 0.58 \times [Phosph])$$

where [Phosph] is the concentration of phosphorus in mg/dL.

The **base excess algorithm** is another method to estimate unmeasured strong ions that has been adapted for use in dogs and cats[14] and applied in clinical cases.[17,30,59] It accounts first for the effects of changes in free water, chloride, protein, and phosphate concentrations in the BE. Any remaining BE is attributed to presence of unmeasured strong anions. Formulas to use with the BE algorithm are presented in Chapter 13 (see Box 13-4). Values less than −5 mmol/L are suggestive of an increase in unmeasured strong anions.[14] The BE algorithm is a useful clinical tool despite a few shortcomings. There are theoretical limitations in extrapolating traditional BE calculations for use in dogs and cats. In addition, protein influence on BE is estimated based on data for human albumin, which behaves differently than canine[12] and feline albumin.[36]

The **strong ion gap** is the difference between all unmeasured strong anion charge and all unmeasured strong cation charge.[11] The SIG has been simplified ($SIG_{simplified}$) to be estimated based on $[A_{tot}]$, the total concentration of nonvolatile weak acids in plasma (see Chapter 13).[11] Albumin is used to estimate $[A_{tot}]$ in the $SIG_{simplified}$ because albumin is the most important buffer in plasma. Assuming a plasma pH of 7.4, $SIG_{simplified}$ can be calculated in dogs as[12]:

$$SIG_{simplified} = [alb] \times 4.9 - AG$$

In cats, at a plasma pH of 7.35, $SIG_{simplified}$ is estimated as[36]:

$$SIG_{simplified} = [alb] \times 4.58 - AG + 9$$

Increase in unmeasured strong anions is suspected whenever $SIG_{simplified}$ is less than −5 mEq/L. In patients with hyperphosphatemia, however, AG should be corrected for the presence of hyperphosphatemia $[AG_{phosph-adjusted} = AG + (2.52 - 0.58 \times [Phosph])]$ before calculating $SIG_{simplified}$. The $SIG_{simplified}$ has not been adequately tested in dogs and cats, but its derivation is sound, and it is superior to the AG to detect increases in unmeasured strong anions in horses.[11]

A stepwise approach should be followed in all patients with suspected mixed acid-base disorders (Fig. 12-1):

1. Perform electrolyte and blood gas analysis.
2. Determine the pH and the nature of the primary disorder.
3. Calculate the expected compensation: Is it a simple or mixed disorder?
4. Calculate the chloride contribution to metabolic disorder ($[Cl^-]$gap, $[Cl^-]/[Na^+]$ ratio, $[Cl^-] - [Na^+]$; see Table 12-3).
5. Estimate the concentration of the unmeasured strong anions (AG, BE algorithm, or $SIG_{simplified}$).
6. Compare the chloride contribution with the presence of unmeasured strong anions: Is there a mixed metabolic disorder? (Table 12-4)
7. Consider other laboratory data (e.g., creatinine, glucose, and so on).
8. Correlate the clinical and laboratory findings.
9. Plan individualized therapy.

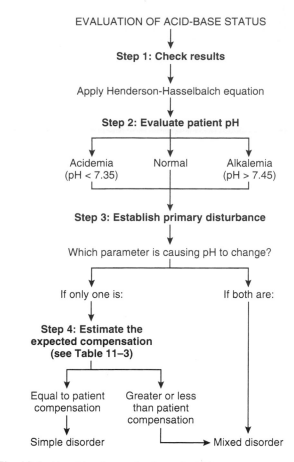

Fig. 12-1 Algorithm for evaluation of acid-base status in patients with suspected mixed acid-base disorders.

MIXED ACID-BASE DISTURBANCES

DISORDERS WITH NEUTRALIZING EFFECTS ON pH

Patients with mixed disorders composed of primary problems with an offsetting effect on pH may be presented with normal, low, or high pH. When pH is abnormal, however, because of the counterbalancing effect of

---

TABLE 12-3 Chloride Contribution in Metabolic Acid-Base Disorders

Test	Hyperchloremic Acidosis	Normal	Hypochloremic Alkalosis
$[Cl^-]$gap	<−4 mEq/L	−4-4 mEq/L	>4 mEq/L
$[Cl^-]/[Na^+]$ ratio			
Dogs	<0.72	0.72-0.78	>0.78
Cats	<0.74	0.74-0.8	>0.8
$[Na^+] - [Cl^-]$	<32 mEq/L	32-40 mEq/L	>40 mEq/L

TABLE 12-4 Evaluation of Mixed Metabolic Disorders

Chloride Contribution*	Unmeasured Strong Anion Contribution	
	NORMAL AG or SIG$_{simplified}$ >−5 mEq/L or UA$_{strong}$ >−5 mmol/L	↑ AG or SIG$_{simplified}$ <−5 mEq/L or UA$_{strong}$ <−5 mmol/L
↓ [Cl⁻]gap, ↓ [Cl⁻]/[Na⁺] or ↓ [Na⁺] − [Cl⁻]	Hyperchloremic acidosis	Hyperchloremic acidosis and ↑ unmeasured strong anion acidosis
Normal [Cl⁻]gap, Normal [Cl⁻]/[Na⁺] or Normal [Na⁺] − [Cl⁻]	Normal	↑ Unmeasured strong anion acidosis
↑ [Cl⁻]gap, ↑ [Cl⁻]/[Na⁺] or ↑ [Na⁺] − [Cl⁻]	Hypochloremic alkalosis	Hypochloremic alkalosis and ↑ unmeasured strong anion acidosis

AG, *Anion gap;* SIG$_{simplified}$, *simplified strong ion gap;* UA$_{strong}$, *unmeasured strong anions estimated using the base excess algorithm;*
[Cl⁻]gap, *chloride gap;* [Cl⁻]/[Na⁺], *chloride to sodium ratio;* [Na⁺] − [Cl⁻], *sodium to chloride difference.*
Metabolic compensation in chronic respiratory acid-base disturbances can also change chloride concentration.

the second primary disorder, changes tend not to be pronounced. Box 12-5 shows examples of potential causes of counterbalancing mixed acid-base disorders.

Respiratory Acidosis and Metabolic Alkalosis

This is an uncommon clinical situation and in human medicine usually occurs in patients with chronic lung disease who develop vomiting or are treated with diuretics.[6] It may occur in acute situations in dogs with gastric dilatation-volvulus that can present with metabolic alkalosis caused by loss of gastric acid and respiratory acidosis resulting from diaphragmatic compression caused by the distended stomach.[2] The P_{CO_2} and $[HCO_3^-]$ are high, and pH tends to be normal or only slightly abnormal. It is important to remember that dogs with long-standing respiratory acidosis can have normal arterial pH.[22] When the mixed disorder is confirmed, treatment should be directed at correcting the most life-threatening underlying disease process first. No therapy is necessary to correct pH if pH is normal or near normal. Patients with chronic pulmonary disease that have hypoxemia and hypercapnia are at greater risk from metabolic alkalosis than are others because superimposition of metabolic alkalosis can further reduce ventilation and lead to worsening of hypoxemia.[49] Therefore metabolic alkalosis should not be overlooked if the patient has a chronic lung disease.

Respiratory Alkalosis and Metabolic Acidosis

Many clinical situations can lead to this mixed disorder, usually with high-AG metabolic acidosis. These patients have low P_{CO_2} and low $[HCO_3^-]$, and their pH tends to be nearly normal. It is important to remember that chronic respiratory alkalosis is a simple acid-base disturbance, and affected patients can be presented with normal pH. Thus in the presence of a normal pH, low P_{CO_2},

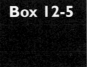

Box 12-5 **Examples of Potential Causes of Counterbalancing Mixed Acid-Base Disorders**

Mixed Respiratory and Metabolic Disorders
Respiratory Acidosis and Metabolic Alkalosis
  Pulmonary edema and diuretics
  Gastric dilatation-volvulus

Respiratory Alkalosis and Metabolic Acidosis
  Hypoadrenocorticism-like syndrome in dogs with gastrointestinal disease
  Septic shock
  Salicylate toxicity
  Heat stroke
  Gastric dilatation-volvulus
  Liver disease (RTA and impaired metabolism of lactate)
  Pulmonary edema with hypoxemia or low cardiac output
  Parvovirus gastroenteritis and sepsis
  Severe exercise
  Acute tumor lysis syndrome
  Severe canine babesiosis caused by *Babesia canis rossi*
  Cardiopulmonary resuscitation (only in arterial blood)

Mixed Metabolic Disorders
Metabolic Acidosis and Metabolic Alkalosis
  Gastric dilatation-volvulus
  Renal failure with vomiting
  Vomiting and lactic acidosis
  Renal failure and loop diuretics
  Diabetic ketoacidosis with vomiting
  Severe canine babesiosis caused by *B. canis rossi*
  Liver disease (hypoproteinemia, diuretics, vomiting, RTA, and impaired metabolism of lactate)

RTA, Renal tubular acidosis.

and low $[HCO_3^-]$, the clinician must decide whether the patient has simple respiratory alkalosis or metabolic acidosis associated with respiratory alkalosis. In this situation, the history can provide important clues. The presence of hypoxemia with increased hematocrit suggests chronic respiratory alkalosis. An increase in unmeasured strong anions is helpful because the majority of metabolic acidoses associated with respiratory alkalosis are normochloremic, whereas compensation for chronic respiratory alkalosis is characterized by corrected hyperchloremia.

Diseases associated with metabolic acidosis and respiratory alkalosis are shown in Box 12-5. In some conditions such as sepsis, patients may be presented initially with respiratory alkalosis, and metabolic acidosis (usually caused by lactic acidosis) only develops later.[23,26] Sepsis complicating any disease known to cause metabolic acidosis can result in a metabolic acidosis superimposed on respiratory alkalosis. Exercise also can cause a mixed disorder that begins with respiratory alkalosis. In mild exercise (35% of maximal O_2 consumption), mild respiratory alkalosis occurs.[38] When dogs are maximally exercised, lactic acidosis is superimposed on the initial respiratory alkalosis.[27,38,45] Dogs with heat stroke also present initially with respiratory alkalosis and later develop mixed respiratory alkalosis and metabolic acidosis.[50] Salicylate toxicity in dogs and cats causes hyperventilation initially, but metabolic acidosis then develops.[42] The hyperventilation associated with salicylate toxicity is caused by central stimulation, and only a small portion of the hyperventilation can be attributed to hyperthermia.[52] In human patients with salicylate intoxication, metabolic acidosis is caused by accumulation of organic acids, including lactate and ketoacids.[49] This also may be true in small animals.[42]

Gastric dilatation-volvulus complex has been associated with respiratory alkalosis and metabolic acidosis in dogs,[37] in which the respiratory alkalosis may be the result of pain,[37] sepsis,[2] or restriction of pulmonary expansion. Patients with liver disease may develop a wide variety of acid-base disturbances. Hyperventilation is common and appears to be multifactorial.[8] Metabolic acidosis also has been associated with liver disease in dogs.[13] Human patients with cirrhosis demonstrate enhanced proximal renal tubular sodium reabsorption that may limit distal H^+ secretion[5] and lead to hyperchloremic acidosis. Type B lactic acidosis also can develop in patients with liver failure because liver disease can decrease liver uptake and metabolism of lactate.[40] Distal renal tubular acidosis has been associated with hepatic lipidosis in a cat presenting with normal AG acidosis.[7]

Special considerations apply to cardiopulmonary resuscitation. Arterial blood gases may indicate respiratory alkalosis because gas exchange is occurring in blood that traverses the pulmonary circulation. Mixed venous P_{CO_2} has been shown to be significantly higher than arterial P_{CO_2} during cardiopulmonary resuscitation in dogs.[32] In this setting, arterial values reflect the adequacy of ventilatory support, whereas mixed venous values may correlate better with tissue pH.[58]

In patients with mixed metabolic acidosis and respiratory alkalosis, pH tends to be normal, and specific treatment to correct pH usually is not necessary. Treatment should be directed at the underlying causes of the metabolic acidosis and respiratory alkalosis.

Metabolic Acidosis and Metabolic Alkalosis

This mixed disorder usually is seen in patients with long-standing high-AG metabolic acidosis (e.g., chronic renal failure, uncomplicated ketoacidosis) that begin vomiting and develop hypochloremic alkalosis. Because albumin is a weak acid, a decrease in albumin concentration is associated with metabolic alkalosis. Superimposition of hypoalbuminemia on chronic metabolic acidosis also can lead to this mixed acid-base disorder. Alternatively, this mixed metabolic disorder can begin as metabolic alkalosis with subsequent development of severe volume depletion resulting in hypoperfusion and lactic acidosis. Depending on the relative severity of the two opposing disorders, pH and $[HCO_3^-]$ can be increased, normal, or decreased. Recognition of both disturbances in this setting is very important because treatment of one without attention to the other permits the unattended abnormality to emerge unopposed. Information in Table 12-4 can be used to help diagnose mixed metabolic acidosis and metabolic alkalosis. Mixed hyperchloremic metabolic acidosis and hypochloremic metabolic alkalosis can theoretically coexist (e.g., patients with vomiting and diarrhea), but because these disturbances have offsetting effects on $[Cl^-]$ and $[HCO_3^-]$, only the prevailing disorder can be identified. Diseases associated with mixed metabolic acidosis and metabolic alkalosis are shown in Box 12-5. The pH usually is normal in these settings, and treatment of stable patients should be directed at resolving the underlying disease processes. Patients with lactic acidosis and severe volume depletion need more aggressive therapy.

DISORDERS WITH ADDITIVE EFFECTS ON pH

Mixed disorders composed of primary problems with an additive effect on pH always have abnormal pH. Depending on the combination of primary problems, the pH can be dangerously high or low and requires immediate attention. Box 12-6 shows examples of potential causes of additive mixed acid-base disorders.

Respiratory Acidosis and Metabolic Acidosis

This combination of acid-base disturbances may occur in a variety of settings usually in patients with acute severe respiratory compromise (e.g., thoracic trauma, pulmonary edema, cardiopulmonary arrest, acute neuromuscular junctional disruption such as with toxic or metabolic or

Box 12-6   Examples of Potential Causes of Additive Mixed Acid-Base Disorders

Mixed Respiratory and Metabolic Disorders

Respiratory Acidosis and Metabolic Acidosis

Hypoadrenocorticism-like syndrome in dogs with gastrointestinal disease
Cardiopulmonary arrest
Severe pulmonary edema
Thoracic trauma with hypovolemic shock
Low cardiac output heart failure with pulmonary edema
Advanced septic shock ($\dot{V}/\dot{Q}$ mismatch)
Gastric dilatation-volvulus
Acute tumor lysis syndrome
Gastrointestinal endoscopy*
Venom of the scorpion *Leiurus quinquestriatus*
Neurotoxic poisons and metabolic conditions disrupting neuromuscular junction function

Respiratory Alkalosis and Metabolic Alkalosis

Gastric dilatation-volvulus
Hyperadrenocorticism with pulmonary thromboembolism
Respirator-induced mixed alkalosis (correction of P_{CO_2} too rapidly)
Congestive heart failure and diuretics
Hepatic disease and diuretics, vomiting, or hypoproteinemia
Severe canine babesiosis caused by *Babesia canis rossi*
Parvovirus gastroenteritis and sepsis

Mixed Metabolic Disorders

Hyperchloremic and High-anion Gap Metabolic Acidoses

Renal failure
Resolving diabetic ketoacidosis
Diarrhea complicating high-anion gap acidosis
Severe canine babesiosis caused by *Babesia canis rossi*

Mixed High-anion Gap Acidoses

Diabetic ketoacidosis and renal failure
Diabetic ketoacidosis and lactic acidosis
Ethylene glycol intoxication with lactic acidosis
Uremic acidosis and other high-anion gap acidosis

Mixed Normal-anion Gap Metabolic Acidosis

Fluid therapy with fluids rich in chloride (e.g., lactated Ringer's solution, 0.9% NaCl) in a patient with hyperchloremic acidosis
Diarrhea and parenteral nutrition

*pH is usually only slightly acidemic, and most patients do not require therapy.[28]

junctionopathies) that also have lactic acidosis as a result of hypoxemia, shock, or poor cardiac output (see Box 12-6). Thus metabolic acidosis usually is caused by an increase in unmeasured strong ions. There is an additive effect lowering the pH because the normal compensation for metabolic acidosis is impaired because of pulmonary disease. The $[HCO_3^-]$ is low; P_{CO_2} is normal or high; and the resultant pH can be dangerously low.

Dogs, cats, and human patients with cardiopulmonary arrest typically develop lactic acidosis as a result of low cardiac output and hypoventilation.[32,39,58] During resuscitation, however, arterial blood gases may indicate a normal pH with mixed metabolic acidosis and respiratory alkalosis and not reflect the ongoing marked reduction in mixed venous and tissue pH. Mixed venous blood should be used for analysis in this setting.[58] In addition to being better for assessing global tissue perfusion and cardiac output, venous pH and P_{CO_2} will change earlier and to a greater extent than arterial values during periods of circulatory insufficiency.[44] Patients with pulmonary edema may develop hypoxemia and lactic acidosis.[57] The situation is worse in patients in which pulmonary edema is secondary to heart failure. Low cardiac output compromises tissue perfusion, worsening the lactic acidosis.[40] Dogs in septic shock usually demonstrate respiratory alkalosis and metabolic acidosis. Later in the course of the disease process, however, patients may develop respiratory acidosis because of ventilation-perfusion ($\dot{V}/\dot{Q}$) mismatch.[23,26] Dogs with gastric dilatation-volvulus complex also can present with metabolic acidosis caused by lactic acidosis and respiratory acidosis resulting from diaphragmatic compression by the distended stomach.[37]

Systemic pH is very low in patients with combined metabolic and respiratory acidosis, and specific therapy must be initiated quickly.[6] In those patients in which lactic acidosis is the cause of metabolic acidosis, tissue hypoxia is the most likely underlying cause, and therapeutic measures should be taken to augment oxygen delivery to the tissues and to reestablish cardiac output.[33] Patients should be artificially ventilated if necessary. This will reduce P_{CO_2} and increase pH. Sodium bicarbonate is not indicated to treat patients with metabolic acidosis that also have respiratory acidosis because they cannot excrete the CO_2 generated by $NaHCO_3$ administration. The CO_2 will diffuse into the cells and further decrease intracellular pH. Sodium bicarbonate may be considered in ventilated patients with $[HCO_3^-]$ less than 5 mEq/L because at this concentration even a small decrease in serum bicarbonate is associated with a large decrease in serum pH.[20] In this situation, small titrated doses of $NaHCO_3$ are used as a temporizing measure to maintain $[HCO_3^-]$ greater than 5 mEq/L while attempts to improve oxygenation are continued. (See Chapter 10 for further discussion of lactic acidosis.)

Respiratory Alkalosis and Metabolic Alkalosis

This mixed disorder is commonly present in human patients with hepatic failure or in those with congestive heart failure and pulmonary edema who are treated with diuretics. These patients have low P_{CO_2}, high $[HCO_3^-]$, and high pH, and their alkalemia may be severe. Similar clinical conditions also occur in small animal medicine (see Box 12-6), but severe alkalemia is not common. Mixed respiratory and metabolic alkalosis was not observed in study of 20 dogs with alkalemia identified from 962 dogs in which blood gas analysis was performed.[48] In dogs with experimental metabolic alkalosis, superimposition of chronic respiratory alkalosis causes a decrease in $[HCO_3^-]$, sufficient not only to prevent development of significant alkalemia but also to offset entirely the effect of hypocapnia on plasma $[H^+]$.[34] In dogs, mixed metabolic alkalosis and respiratory alkalosis are more common in patients with chronic respiratory disease placed on diuretics. Severe alkalemia is only likely to occur in dogs with long-standing respiratory acidosis and a compensatory increase in $[HCO_3^-]$ that are placed on a ventilator. This maneuver acutely lowers P_{CO_2}, whereas $[HCO_3^-]$ remains high for approximately 24 hours.[22] Severe alkalemia also was observed in dogs with severe canine babesiosis caused by *Babesia canis rossi*.[30]

Because most patients with this mixed disorder have metabolic alkalosis superimposed on chronic metabolic alkalosis, therapy usually is directed at correcting the metabolic alkalosis. In addition, compensation for simple chronic respiratory alkalosis is so effective that pH usually is normal. Therefore correction of the metabolic alkalosis will be associated with normalization of pH even if the chronic respiratory alkalosis cannot be treated. The goal of treatment in metabolic alkalosis is to replace the chloride deficit while providing sufficient potassium and sodium to replace existing deficits. Dehydrated patients should be rehydrated accordingly. Definitive treatment of the underlying disease process prevents recurrence of the metabolic alkalosis.

Hyperchloremic and High-AG Metabolic Acidoses

This mixed disorder usually is seen in patients with renal failure, in the resolving phase of ketoacidosis, or in patients with high-AG acidosis that develop diarrhea or receive fluid therapy (see Box 12-6). The pH and $[HCO_3^-]$ are low, and the diagnosis is suggested by an increase in unmeasured anions and a chloride gap of less than −4 mEq/L (see Table 12-4).

Human patients with chronic renal failure (serum creatinine concentration of 2 to 4 mg/dL) initially develop hyperchloremic acidosis. With progression of the disease (serum creatinine concentration of 4 to 14 mg/dL), metabolic acidosis progresses, but the further decrease in total CO_2 is associated with an increase in unmeasured strong ions (e.g., sulfate, acetate) and hyperphosphatemia, whereas hyperchloremia remains unchanged.[60] However, human patients with advanced renal failure sometimes may have a simple acid-base disorder, either hyperchloremic or high-AG acidosis.[47,56] Patients with diabetes mellitus may have a mixed high-AG and hyperchloremic acidosis because of development of diarrhea or in the resolving phase of the ketoacidotic crisis.[47,56] Hyperchloremia in the recovery phase develops for at least three reasons: (1) large volumes of saline are administered; (2) KCl is infused in large doses; and (3) ketones are lost in the urine, and NaCl is reabsorbed by the kidneys.[40] As discussed earlier, human patients with chronic hepatic disease may have enhanced proximal renal tubular sodium reabsorption that may limit distal H^+ secretion.[5] This may lead to hyperchloremic acidosis, decreased lactate metabolism, and development of a high-AG acidosis. Severe canine babesiosis caused by *B. canis rossi* also has been shown to cause this combination of disturbances.[30] The treatment in mixed hyperchloremic and high AG acidoses should be directed at the primary disorders responsible for metabolic acidosis. Treatment with $NaHCO_3$ may be necessary in selected patients with low pH and severe corrected hyperchloremia or renal failure. Limitations of $NaHCO_3$ treatment for lactic acidosis were discussed earlier. Sodium bicarbonate is not indicated in diabetic patients even if pH is less than 7.0.[43,55]

Mixed High-AG Metabolic Acidosis

Two different causes of high-AG metabolic acidosis may coexist in the same patient, and this usually is a result of lactic or uremic acidosis superimposed on another cause of high-AG acidosis. The pH and $[HCO_3^-]$ are low in affected patients with increased unmeasured ions and normal chloride gap (see Table 12-4). It is not possible to differentiate between simple and mixed high-AG metabolic acidosis if only blood gases and serum electrolytes are assessed. Serum creatinine concentration, blood urea nitrogen (BUN), and plasma lactate concentration must be measured to confirm the presence of this mixed disorder.[40]

Patients with ketoacidosis may develop lactic acidosis because of decreased tissue perfusion or impaired lactate utilization caused by decreased insulin activity. In this circumstance, lactic acidosis promotes conversion of acetoacetate to β-hydroxybutyrate, which does not react with nitroprusside in the urinalysis dipstrip reagent pad, thereby masking the ketoacidosis.[40] It has been suggested that adding a few drops of hydrogen peroxide to the urine specimen would nonenzymatically convert β-hydroxybutyrate to acetoacetate, which then would be detected by the nitroprusside reagent.[41] However, this method has been shown to be ineffective in converting β-hydroxybutyrate to acetoacetate in dogs.[10]

Treatment in this mixed disorder should be directed toward resolving the primary disorder causing metabolic acidosis and toward stabilizing the patient. The use and limitations of $NaHCO_3$ in lactic acidosis, uremic acidosis, and ketoacidosis have been discussed previously.

Patients with severe acidosis (pH, <7.1) and renal failure may benefit from small, titrated doses of $NaHCO_3$.

Mixed Hyperchloremic Metabolic Acidosis

This is a very rare disorder in veterinary medicine because the only clinical situation that commonly causes hyperchloremic acidosis is diarrhea. The pH and $[HCO_3^-]$ are decreased in these patients, and the AG is normal with corrected hyperchloremia (see Table 12-4). Fluid therapy with lactated Ringer's solution or 0.9% NaCl solution with or without KCl supplementation is a common cause of hyperchloremic acidosis in hospitalized patients. In patients with a preexisting hyperchloremic acidosis, fluid therapy will induce a mixed hyperchloremic metabolic acidosis. Parenteral nutrition in patients with diarrhea also could cause a mixed hyperchloremic metabolic acidosis because of addition of cationic amino acids (e.g., lysine HCl, arginine HCl). Treatment should be directed toward resolving the primary disease responsible for the acidosis. Treatment with $NaHCO_3$ is safer in hyperchloremic acidoses and should be used if pH is less than 7.10 or the $[HCO_3^-]$ is less than 10 mEq/L. The potential causes of mixed metabolic disorders are summarized in Box 12-6.

TRIPLE DISORDERS

Metabolic Acidosis, Metabolic Alkalosis, and Respiratory Acidosis or Alkalosis

Triple disorders occur whenever a respiratory disturbance complicates a mixed metabolic acidosis and metabolic alkalosis. The pH and $[HCO_3^-]$ may be normal, decreased, or increased, and PCO_2 is greater than expected when the mixed metabolic disturbance is complicated by respiratory acidosis and lower than expected when it is complicated by respiratory alkalosis. Patients with low-output heart failure treated with diuretics may develop lactic acidosis and hypochloremic alkalosis. If such a patient develops interstitial pulmonary edema, there is a decrease in compliance, and stimulation of ventilation causes PCO_2 to decrease and respiratory alkalosis to develop.[1] With increasing severity of the edema, hypoventilation with respiratory acidosis may occur.[1] However, dogs have good collateral ventilation, and hypercapnia occurs only in fulminant pulmonary edema.[57]

Patients with gastric dilatation-volvulus can present with metabolic alkalosis and lactic acidosis.[29,37,61] These patients also can develop respiratory alkalosis as a result of a pain-induced increase in ventilation[37] or sepsis.[2] Respiratory acidosis also can develop if ventilation is impaired by a grossly overdistended stomach.[37] Severe babesiosis in dogs infected with *B. canis rossi* also can cause triple disorders with respiratory alkalosis as a result of a systemic inflammatory response syndrome (in a sepsis-like state), lactic acidosis, and hyperchloremic acidosis.[30] It is not known why dogs with this disease develop hyperchloremic acidosis. Other potential causes of triple disorders are outlined in Box 12-7. The treatment of triple disorders should be directed at stabilizing the patient's clinical condition and resolving the underlying disease process. In the majority of these cases, the metabolic acidosis is caused by lactic acid accumulation. Therefore the principles discussed under mixed respiratory acidosis with lactic acidosis are valid here.

TREATMENT

When treating a patient with a mixed disorder, always prioritize the order in which the abnormalities are managed:

1. Treat the most life-threatening disorder that the body cannot address itself first (e.g., decompress the dilated stomach of a patient with gastric dilatation-volvulus while aggressively supporting intravascular volume before trying to manipulate ventilatory volume or rate or correct electrolyte disturbances; manage the metabolic components [carbohydrate and fluid abnormalities] of the acid-base abnormalities in the patient with diabetic ketoacidosis before concerning yourself with the respiratory abnormalities). Correcting these priority disorders will allow the body the opportunity to address the lesser abnormalities itself.
2. Treat the most treatable disorder next.
3. Direct manipulation of blood pH is rarely required and more often than not may be contraindicated.
4. Take into consideration the systemic pH of the patient. For example, if a dog has a pH of 7.35 and $[HCO_3^-]$ of 12 mEq/L, no attempts should be made to correct this relatively normal pH. The exception to the rule is the patient with $[HCO_3^-]$ of 5 mEq/L or less. In these patients, a small decrease in $[HCO_3^-]$ is associated with a large decrease in pH.
5. Do not overlook the second disorder. The effect that treating one disorder has on the second disorder must

---

Box 12-7 | **Examples of Potential Causes of Triple Disorders**

Metabolic Acidosis, Metabolic Alkalosis, and Respiratory Acidosis
Low-output heart failure with pulmonary edema and diuretics
Gastric dilatation-volvulus

Metabolic Acidosis, Metabolic Alkalosis, and Respiratory Alkalosis
Low-output heart failure with pulmonary edema and diuretics
Gastric dilatation-volvulus
Parvovirus gastroenteritis (vomiting, diarrhea, and sepsis)
Severe canine babesiosis caused by *Babesia canis rossi*

be anticipated, and both processes ought to be assessed simultaneously.

The potential complications of treatment also should be anticipated (e.g., overshoot metabolic alkalosis after $NaHCO_3$ treatment), and iatrogenic mixed acid-base disorders should be avoided (e.g., administration of drugs that suppress ventilation in patients with metabolic acidosis). The reader is referred to chapters on the individual acid-base disorders for further discussion of treatment (see Chapters 10 and 11). However, bear in mind that mixed disturbances that cause additive effects on pH (e.g., respiratory and metabolic acidosis) require more aggressive therapy than those with neutralizing effects (e.g., respiratory alkalosis and metabolic acidosis).

REFERENCES

1. Aberman A, Fulop M: The metabolic and respiratory acidosis of acute pulmonary edema, *Ann Intern Med* 76:173-178, 1972.
2. Adams LG, Polzin DJ: Mixed acid-base disorders, *Vet Clin North Am Small Anim Pract* 19:307-326, 1989.
3. Alfaro V, Torras R, Ibáñez J, et al: A physical-chemical analysis of the acid-base response to chronic obstructive pulmonary disease, *Can J Physiol Pharmacol* 74:1229-1235, 1996.
4. Barnard P, Andronikou S, Pokorski N, et al: Time-dependent effect of hypoxia on carotid body chemosensory function, *J Appl Physiol* 63:685-691, 1987.
5. Better O, Goldschmid Z, Chaimowitz C, et al: Defect in urinary acidification in cirrhosis, *Arch Intern Med* 130:77-82, 1972.
6. Bia M, Thier SO: Mixed acid-base disturbances: a clinical approach, *Med Clin North Am* 65:347-361, 1981.
7. Brown SA, Spyridakis LK, Crowell WA: Distal renal tubular acidosis and hepatic lipidosis in a cat, *J Am Vet Med Assoc* 189:1350-1352, 1986.
8. Center SA: Pathophysiology and laboratory diagnosis of liver disease. In Ettinger SJ, editor: *Textbook of veterinary internal medicine: diseases of dog and cat*, ed 3, Philadelphia, 1989, WB Saunders, pp. 1421-1478.
9. Ching SV, Fettman MJ, Hamar DW, et al: The effect of chronic dietary acidification using ammonium chloride on acid-base and mineral metabolism in the adult cat, *J Nutr* 119:902-915, 1989.
10. Christopher M, Pereira J, Brigmon R, et al: Automated determination of β-hydroxybutyrate for the assessment of ketoacidosis. *Proc Am Coll Vet Intern Med*, New Orleans, LA, 1991, p. 903.
11. Constable PD, Hinchcliff KW, Muir WW: Comparison of anion gap and strong ion gap as predictors of unmeasured strong ion concentration in plasma and serum from horses, *Am J Vet Res* 59:881-887, 1998.
12. Constable PD, Stämpfli HR: Experimental determination of net protein charge and A_{tot} and K_a of nonvolatile buffers in canine plasma, *J Vet Intern Med* 19:507-514, 2005.
13. Cornelius LM, Rawlings CA: Arterial blood gas and acid-base values in dogs with various diseases and signs of disease, *J Am Vet Med Assoc* 178:992-995, 1981.
14. de Morais HSA: A nontraditional approach to acid-base disorders. In DiBartola SP, editor: *Fluid therapy in small animal practice*, Philadelphia, 1992, WB Saunders, pp. 297-320.
15. de Morais HSA: Mixed acid-base disorders. In DiBartola SP, editor: *Fluid therapy in small animal practice*, ed 2, Philadelphia, 2000, WB Saunders, pp. 251-261.
16. de Morais HSA, DiBartola SP: Ventilatory and metabolic compensation in dogs with acid-base disturbances, *J Vet Emerg Crit Care* 1:39-49, 1991.
17. DiBartola SP, de Morais HSA: Appendix: clinical cases. In DiBartola SP, editor: *Fluid therapy in small animal practice*, Philadelphia, 1992, WB Saunders, pp. 599-688.
18. Durward A, Skellett S, Mayer S, et al: The value of the chloride:sodium ratio in differentiating the aetiology of metabolic acidosis, *Intensive Care Med* 27:828-835, 2001.
19. Fettman MJ, Coble JM, Hamar DW, et al: Effect of dietary phosphoric acid supplementation on acid-base balance and mineral and bone metabolism in adult cats, *Am J Vet Res* 53:2125-2135, 1992.
20. Gauthier PM, Szerlip HM: Metabolic acidosis in the intensive care unit, *Crit Care Clin* 18:298-308, 2002.
21. Gennari FJ, Goldstein MB, Schwartz W: The nature of the renal adaptation to chronic hypocapnia, *J Clin Invest* 51:1722-1730, 1972.
22. Goodman LA, de Morais HSA: Unpublished observation 2005.
23. Goodwin J-K, Schaer M: Septic shock, *Vet Clin North Am Small Anim Pract* 19:1239-1258, 1990.
24. Hampson NB, Jöbsis-VandlerVliet FF, Piantadosi CA: Skeletal muscle oxygen availability during respiratory acid-base disturbances in cats, *Respir Physiol* 70:143-158, 1987.
25. Hara Y, Nezu Y, Harada Y, et al: Secondary chronic respiratory acidosis in a dog following the cervical cord compression by an intradural glioma, *J Vet Med Sci* 64:863-866, 2002.
26. Hauptman JG, Tvedten H: Osmolal and anion gaps in dogs with acute endotoxic shock, *Am J Vet Res* 47:1617-1619, 1986.
27. Ilkiw JE, Davis PE, Church DB: Hematological, biochemical, blood-gas, and acid-base values in greyhounds before and after exercise, *Am J Vet Res* 50:583-586, 1989.
28. Jergens AE, Riedesel DH, Ries PA, et al: Cardiopulmonary responses in healthy dogs during endoscopic examination of the gastrointestinal tract, *Am J Vet Res* 56:215-220, 1995.
29. Kagan KG, Schaer M: Gastric dilatation and volvulus in a dog—a case justifying electrolyte and acid-base assessment, *J Am Vet Med Assoc* 183:703-705, 1983.
30. Leisewitz AL, Jacobson LS, de Morais HSA, et al: The mixed acid-base disturbances of severe canine babesiosis, *J Vet Intern Med* 15:445-452, 2001.
31. Lemieux G, Lemieux C, Duplessis S, et al: Metabolic characteristics of cat kidney: failure to adapt to metabolic acidosis, *Am J Physiol* 259:R277-R281, 1990.
32. Lippert AC, Evans AT, White BC, et al: The effect of resuscitation technique and pre-arrest state of oxygenation on blood-gas values during cardiopulmonary resuscitation in dogs, *Vet Surg* 17:283-290, 1988.
33. Madias NE: Lactic acidosis, *Kidney Int* 29:752-774, 1986.
34. Madias NE, Cohen JJ, Adrogué HJ: Influence of acute and chronic respiratory alkalosis on preexisting chronic metabolic alkalosis, *Am J Physiol* 258:F479-F485, 1990.
35. Martinu T, Menzies D, Dial S: Re-evaluation of acid-base prediction rules in patients with chronic respiratory acidosis, *Can Respir J* 19:311-315, 2003.
36. McCullough SM, Constable PD: Calculation of the total plasma concentration of nonvolatile weak acids and the effective dissociation constant of nonvolatile buffers in plasma for use in the strong ion approach to acid-base balance in cats, *Am J Vet Res* 64:1047-1051, 2003.

37. Muir WW III: Acid-base and electrolyte disturbances in dogs with gastric dilatation-volvulus, *J Am Vet Med Assoc* 181:229-231, 1982.

38. Musch TI, Friedman DB, Haidet GC, et al: Arterial blood gases and acid-base status of dogs during graded dynamic exercise, *J Appl Physiol* 61:1914-1919, 1986.

39. Nakakimura K, Fleischer JE, Drummond JC, et al: Glucose administration before cardiac arrest worsens neurologic outcome in cats, *Anesthesiology* 72:1005-1011, 1990.

40. Narins RG, Emmett M: Simple and mixed acid-base disorders: a practical approach, *Medicine* 59:161-187, 1980.

41. Narins RG, Jones ER, Stom MC, et al: Diagnostic strategies in disorders of fluid, electrolyte and acid-base abnormalities, *Am J Med* 72:46-52, 1982.

42. Oehme FW: Aspirin and acetaminophen. In Kirk RW, editor: *Current veterinary therapy IX*, Philadelphia, 1986, WB Saunders, pp. 188-190.

43. Okuda Y, Adrogue HJ, Field JB, et al: Counterproductive effects of sodium bicarbonate in diabetic ketoacidosis, *J Clin Endocrinol Metab* 81:314-320, 1996.

44. Oropello JM, Manasia A, Hannon E, et al: Continuous fiberoptic arterial and venous blood gas monitoring in hemorrhagic shock, *Chest* 109:1049-1055, 1996.

45. Pieschl RL, Toll PW, Leith DE, et al: Acid-base changes in the running greyhound: contributing variables, *J Appl Physiol* 73:2297-2304, 1992.

46. Polak A, Haynie GD, Hays RM, et al: Effects of chronic hypercapnia on electrolyte and acid-base equilibrium. I. Adaptation, *J Clin Invest* 40:1223-1237, 1961.

47. Ray S, Piraino B, Chong TK, et al: Acid excretion and serum electrolyte patterns in patients with advanced chronic renal failure, *Miner Electrolyte Metab* 16:355-361, 1990.

48. Robinson EP, Hardy RM: Clinical signs, diagnosis, and treatment of alkalemia in dogs: 20 cases (1982-1984), *J Am Vet Med Assoc* 7:943-949, 1988.

49. Rose BD: *Clinical physiology of acid-base and electrolyte disorders*, ed 3, New York, 1989, McGraw-Hill.

50. Schall WD: Heat stroke. In Kirk RW, editor: *Current veterinary therapy VII*, Philadelphia, 1980, WB Saunders, pp. 195-197.

51. Schwartz WB, Brackett NC, Cohen JJ: The response of extracellular hydrogen ion concentration to graded degrees of chronic hypercapnia: the physiologic limits of defense of pH, *J Clin Invest* 44:291-301, 1965.

52. Silva PR, Fonseca-Costa A, Zin WA, et al: Respiratory and acid-base parameters during salicylic intoxication in dogs, *Braz J Med Biol Res* 19:279-286, 1986.

53. Szlyk PC, Jennings BD: Effects of hypercapnia on variability of normal respiratory behavior in awake cats, *Am J Physiol* 252:R538-R547, 1987.

54. Torbati D, Mokashi A, Lahiri S: Effects of acute hyperbaric oxygenation on respiratory control in cats, *J Appl Physiol* 67:2351-2355, 1989.

55. Viallon A, Zeni F, Lafond P, et al: Does bicarbonate therapy improve the management of severe diabetic ketoacidosis? *Crit Care Med* 27:2690-2693, 1999.

56. Wallia R, Greenberg A, Piraino B, et al: Serum electrolyte patterns in end-stage renal disease, *Am J Kidney Dis* 8:98-104, 1986.

57. Ware WA, Bonagura JD: Pulmonary edema. In Fox PR, editor: *Canine and feline cardiology*, New York, 1988, Churchill Livingstone, pp. 205-217.

58. Weil MH, Rackow EC, Trevino R, et al: Difference in acid-base state between venous and arterial blood during cardiopulmonary resuscitation, *N Engl J Med* 315:153-156, 1986.

59. Whitehair KJ, Haskins SC, Whitehair JG, et al: Clinical application of quantitative acid-base chemistry, *J Vet Intern Med* 9:1-11, 1995.

60. Widmer B, Gerhardt RE, Harrington JT, et al: Serum electrolyte and acid-base composition: the influence of graded degrees of chronic renal failure, *Arch Intern Med* 139:1099-1102, 1979.

61. Wingfield WE, Twedt DC, Moore RW, et al: Acid-base and electrolyte values in dogs with acute gastric dilatation-volvulus, *J Am Vet Med Assoc* 180:1070-1072, 1982.

62. Yu S, Morris JG: Chloride requirement of kittens for growth is less than current recommendations, *J Nutr* 129:1909-1914, 1999.

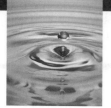

CHAPTER · 13

STRONG ION APPROACH TO ACID-BASE DISORDERS

Helio Autran de Morais and Peter D. Constable

"Assumptions can be dangerous, especially in science. They usually start as the most plausible or comfortable interpretation of the available facts. But when their truth cannot be immediately tested and their flaws are not obvious, assumptions often graduate to articles of faith, and new observations are forced to fit them. Eventually, if the volume of troublesome information becomes unsustainable, the orthodoxy must collapse."

John S. Mattick, Sci Am Oct 2004

Determination of the mechanisms underlying acid-base disturbances has been an important clinical goal for more than 100 years. Landmark advancements in the clinical diagnosis and treatment of acid-base disturbances have included the Henderson-Hasselbalch equation (1916), the base excess (BE) concept (1960), calculation of the anion gap (AG) (1970s),[33] introduction of the strong ion approach,[39] and development of the strong ion gap (SIG) concept.[4,23,24]

The two main goals of acid-base assessment are to identify and quantify the magnitude of an acid-base disturbance and to determine the mechanism for the acid-base disturbance by identifying changes in variables that **independently** alter acid-base balance.[10] Independent variables influence a system from the outside and cannot be affected by changes within the system or by changes in other independent variables. In contrast, dependent variables are influenced directly and predictably by changes in the independent variables. Singer and Hastings proposed in 1948 that plasma pH was determined by two independent factors, P_{CO_2} and net strong ion charge, equivalent to the strong ion difference (SID, or the difference in charge between fully dissociated strong cations and anions in plasma). Stewart suggested in 1983 that a third variable, $[A_{tot}]$ or the total plasma concentration of nonvolatile weak buffers (e.g., albumin, globulins, and phosphate), also exerted an independent effect on plasma pH. One of Stewart's major contributions to clinical acid-base physiology was his proposal that plasma pH was determined by three independent factors: P_{CO_2}, SID, and $[A_{tot}]$ (Fig. 13-1). An understanding of the three independent variables (P_{CO_2}, SID, A_{tot}) is required to apply the strong ion approach to acid-base disorders in dogs and cats.

P_{CO_2}: Carbon dioxide tension can be changed by alveolar ventilation, which has a profound effect on $[HCO_3^-]$ and pH. Approximately 50% of the daily variability of $[HCO_3^-]$ in normal dogs can be attributed to changes in P_{CO_2} alone. Because arterial P_{CO_2} (Pa_{CO_2}) is inversely proportional to the alveolar ventilation, measurement of Pa_{CO_2} provides the clinician with direct information about the adequacy of alveolar ventilation. Increase in P_{CO_2} or respiratory acidosis is caused by and synonymous with hypoventilation, whereas a decrease in P_{CO_2} or respiratory alkalosis is caused by and synonymous with hyperventilation.

SID: Simple ions in plasma can be divided into two main types: nonbuffer ions (strong ions or strong electrolytes) and buffer ions. Strong ions are fully dissociated at physiologic pH and therefore exert no buffering effect. However, strong ions do exert an electrical effect because the sum of completely dissociated cations does not equal the sum of completely dissociated anions. Stewart termed this difference the SID. Because strong ions do not participate in chemical reactions in plasma at physiologic pH, they act as a collective positive unit of charge (SID). The quantitatively most important strong ions in plasma are Na^+, K^+, Ca^{2+}, Mg^{2+}, Cl^-, lactate, β–hydroxybutyrate, acetoacetate, and SO_4^{2-}. The influence of strong ions on pH and $[HCO_3^-]$ can always be summarized in terms of the SID. Changes in SID of a magnitude capable of altering acid-base balance usually occur as a result of increasing concentrations of Na^+, Cl^-, SO_4^{2-}, or organic anions or decreasing concentrations of Na^+ or Cl^-. An increase in SID (by decreasing $[Cl^-]$ or increasing $[Na^+]$) will cause a strong ion (metabolic) alkalosis, whereas a decrease in SID (by decreasing $[Na^+]$ or increasing $[Cl^-]$, $[SO_4^{2-}]$, or organic anions) will cause a

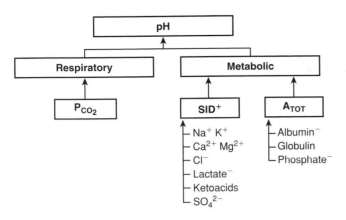

Fig. 13-1 Determinants of plasma pH at 37° C as assessed by the simplified strong ion model. Both [SID$^+$] and [A$_{tot}$] provide independent measures of the nonrespiratory (metabolic) component of plasma pH. (From Constable PD: Clinical assessment of acid-base status: comparison of the Henderson-Hasselbalch and strong ion approaches, *Vet Clin Pathol* 29:115-128, 2000.)

strong ion (metabolic) acidosis. A Gamblegram of normal plasma (Fig. 13-2) shows the relationship between strong cations, strong anions, and buffer ions (HCO$_3^-$ and the nonvolatile weak acids, A$^-$). A graphic representation of SID and the AG also is shown in Fig. 13-2.

[A$_{tot}$]: In contrast to strong ions, buffer ions are derived from plasma weak acids and bases that are not fully dissociated at physiologic pH. The conventional dissociation reaction for a weak acid (HA) and its conjugated base (A$^-$) pair is HA $\leftrightarrow$ H$^+$ + A$^-$. At equilibrium, an apparent dissociation constant (K_a) can be calculated. For a weak acid to act as an effective buffer, its pK_a (defined as the negative logarithm of the weak acid dissociation constant K_a) lies within the range of pH ±1.5.

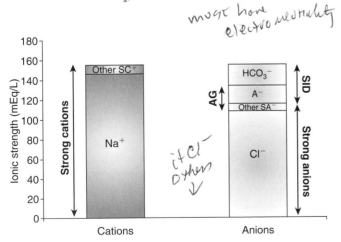

Fig. 13-2 Gamblegram of normal plasma showing cations: sodium (Na$^+$), and other strong cations (SC$^+$) in one column, and anions: chloride (Cl$^-$), other strong anions (SA$^-$), net charge of nonvolatile buffers (A$^-$), and bicarbonate (HCO$_3^-$) in the second column.

Because normal plasma pH is approximately 7.4, substances with a pK_a between 5.9 and 8.9 can act as buffers. The main nonvolatile plasma buffers act as weak acids at physiologic pH (e.g., phosphate, imidazole [histidine] groups on plasma proteins). Also known as the non-HCO$_3^-$ buffer system, they form a closed system containing a fixed quantity of buffer. The non-HCO$_3^-$ buffer system is composed of a diverse and heterogeneous group of plasma buffers that can be modeled as a single buffer pair (HA and A$^-$). An assumption in Stewart's strong ion model is that HA and A$^-$ do not take part in plasma reactions that result in the net destruction or creation of HA or A$^-$. When HA dissociates, it ceases to be HA (therefore decreasing plasma [HA]) and becomes A$^-$ (therefore increasing plasma [A$^-$]). The total amount of A, or A$_{tot}$, is the sum of A in dissociated [A$^-$] and undissociated [HA] forms. It remains constant according to the law of conservation of mass.

The great advantage of Stewart's strong ion approach is that it provides a mechanistic view as to why pH is changing and fully integrates electrolyte and acid-base physiology. However, his approach is heavily mathematical. The so-called Stewart equation is a fourth order polynomial that cannot be solved using a pocket calculator. With that in mind, this chapter will focus on the concepts behind the Stewart approach, emphasizing the relationship between weak and strong ions and acid-base balance and developing an understanding of why pH and [HCO$_3^-$] are changing. Frameworks adapting Stewart's approach to clinical uses also will be reviewed. The mathematical and physicochemical background of this approach is described in detail elsewhere.* A comparison of diagnostic approaches using routine screening (total CO$_2$), the Henderson-Hasselbalch approach, and the simplified strong ion approach is shown in Table 13-1.

Because clinically important acid-base derangements result from changes in P$_{CO_2}$, SID, or A$_{tot}$, the strong ion approach distinguishes six primary acid-base disturbances (respiratory, strong ion, or nonvolatile buffer ion acidosis and alkalosis; Fig. 13-3) instead of the traditional four primary acid-base disturbances (respiratory or metabolic acidosis and alkalosis) characterized by the Henderson-Hasselbalch equation.[5,8,10] Acidemia results from an increase in P$_{CO_2}$ and nonvolatile buffer concentrations (albumin, globulin, phosphate) or from a decrease in SID. Alkalemia results from a decrease in P$_{CO_2}$ and nonvolatile buffer concentration or from an increase in SID.

DISORDERS OF P$_{CO_2}$

Increases in P$_{CO_2}$ are associated with **respiratory acidosis,** whereas decreases in P$_{CO_2}$ lead to **respiratory alkalosis.** There are no differences between the Henderson-

---

References 7,8,11,37,39,43,44.

TABLE 13-1 Diagnostic Approaches to Acid-Base Disturbances*

Diagnostic Approach	Parameters Measured	Type of Disorder	Abnormal Parameter	Acidosis	Alkalosis
Routine screening Henderson-Hasselbalch	Total CO_2 pH, PCO_2; calculate BE_{ECF}†	Metabolic Respiratory	Abnormal total CO_2 Abnormal PCO_2	↓total CO_2 ↑PCO_2	↑total CO_2 ↓PCO_2
		Metabolic	Abnormal BE_{ECF}	↓BE_{ECF} (preferred) or ↓HCO_3^-	↑BE_{ECF} (preferred) or ↑HCO_3^-
Simplified strong ion	pH, PCO_2, Na^+, K^+, Cl^-, lactate, albumin and inorganic phosphate‡	Respiratory	Abnormal PCO_2	↑PCO_2	↓PCO_2
		Metabolic (SID)	Abnormal SID^+	↓SID^+	↑SID^+
		Metabolic (A_{TOT})	Abnormal A_{TOT}	↑[phosphate]	↓[albumin]

*BE_{ECF} indicates extracellular base excess; SID, strong ion difference; A_{TOT} total plasma concentration of nonvolatile weak buffers.
†The anion gap is calculated to determine whether unmeasured anions are present (requires measurement of three other parameters: Na^+, K^+, Cl^-).
‡The strong ion gap is calculated to determine if unmeasured strong ions are present.
Adapted from Constable PD: Clinical assessment of acid-base status: comparison of the Henderson-Hasselbalch and strong ion approaches, Vet Clin Pathol 29:115-128, 2000.

Hasselbalch approach and the strong ion approach in relation to PCO_2. See Chapter 11 for further discussion on respiratory acid-base disorders.

DISORDERS OF [A_{TOT}]

Albumin, globulins, and inorganic phosphate are nonvolatile weak acids and collectively are the major contributors to [A_{tot}]. Consequently, changes in their concentrations will directly change pH, and this represents a major philosophical difference between the strong ion and Henderson-Hasselbalch approaches.

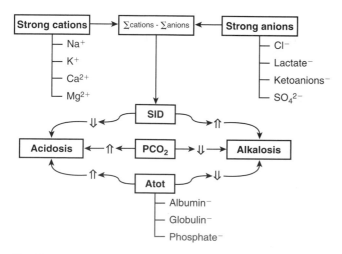

Fig. 13-3 Mechanisms leading to alkalosis and acidosis.

There are three general mechanisms by which A_{tot} can change: (1) a change in the free water content of plasma; (2) an increase in plasma albumin, phosphate, or globulin concentrations; and (3) a decrease in plasma albumin, phosphate, or globulin concentrations.

Values for the total plasma concentration of nonvolatile weak acids and the effective dissociation constant (K_a) for plasma nonvolatile buffers are species specific. Values for A_{tot} and K_a have been experimentally determined in the plasma of humans,[38] cats,[29] and dogs[3] and theoretically determined for the plasma of humans.[5] Canine and feline plasma proteins have a greater net negative charge than human plasma proteins because their albumin contributes proportionally more to net protein charge, has a different amino acid composition, and carries a greater net negative charge at physiologic pH. These characteristics explain the higher AG in dogs and cats because the AG in healthy dogs and cats essentially reflects the total protein concentration. A_{tot} in dogs is 17.4 mmol/L (equivalent to 0.27 mmol/g of total protein or 0.47 mmol/g of albumin), whereas K_a is 0.17 × 10^{-7} (pK_a = 7.77).[3] A_{tot} in cats is 24.3 mmol/L (equivalent to 0.35 mmol/g of total protein or 0.76 mmol/g of albumin), whereas K_a is 0.67 × 10^{-7} (pK_a = 7.17).[29]

The contribution of proteins to A_{tot} has been determined in vitro for dogs.[3] The net protein charge of canine plasma at pH = 7.40 is approximately 16 mEq/L, equivalent to 0.25 mEq/g of total protein or 0.42 mEq/g of albumin. The overall effect of a 1-g/dL increase in total protein concentration is a decrease in pH of 0.047.

The contribution of phosphate to A_{tot} can be estimated by first converting phosphate concentration to mmol/L and then multiplying by its valence. One millimole (atomic weight in milligrams) of phosphate has 31 mg of elemental phosphorus. Thus the phosphate concentration in mg/dL can be converted to mmol/L by dividing by 3.1. The valence of phosphate changes with pH, but at a pH of 7.4, it is 1.8. Thus a phosphorus concentration of 5 mg/dL is equivalent to 1.6 mmol/L and 2.88 mEq/L at a pH of 7.4.

NONVOLATILE BUFFER ION ALKALOSIS

Hypoalbuminemia

The fact that hypoalbuminemia tends to increase pH and cause metabolic alkalosis was first identified in people in 1986 by McAuliffe et al.[28] Phosphate is the second most important component of $[A_{tot}]$ and normally is present in plasma at a low concentration (<4 mmol/L). Therefore hypophosphatemia does not cause metabolic alkalosis. The effects of a decrease in A_{tot} (A_{tot} alkalosis) on $[HCO_3^-]$ are shown in a Gamblegram in Fig. 13-4. Hypoproteinemic alkalosis has been identified clinically in dogs and cats.[13,24,40] In vitro, a 1-g/dL decrease in albumin concentration is associated with an increase in pH of 0.093 in cats[29] and 0.047 in dogs.[3] It is not clear whether the increase in pH secondary to hypoalbuminemia is associated with ventilatory compensation. Recently, the effect of hypoproteinemia on acid-base equilibrium was evaluated in human patients, and results suggest that compensatory hypoventilation does occur in patients with hypoalbuminemic alkalosis.[24] However, this study was based on critically ill patients, a population that may have several simultaneous acid-base alterations, making it difficult to estimate some of the compensatory changes. Increased PCO_2 in patients with hypoalbumine-

mia also has been observed in another study,[28] whereas hyperventilation and consequently decreased PCO_2 were identified by Rossing et al.[35] The latter study included patients with congestive heart failure and cirrhosis, and hyperventilation may have been induced by the underlying diseases and not by the metabolic acid-base disorder. However, good correlation between arterial PCO_2 and albumin concentration was observed in that study. Metabolic compensation with decreased SID caused by an increase in chloride concentration seems to occur in human patients with hypoproteinemic alkalosis.[28,42] Data are not currently available regarding compensation for nonvolatile buffer ion alkalosis in dogs or cats.

The most common causes of hypoproteinemic alkalosis are shown in Box 13-1. Hypoalbuminemic alkalosis is common in the critical care setting.[17] Presence of hypoalbuminemia complicates identification of increased unmeasured anions (e.g., lactate, ketoanions) because hypoproteinemia not only increases pH but also decreases AG.[14,18a,21] Thus the severity of the underlying disease leading to metabolic acidosis may be underesti-

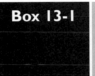

Box 13-1 **Principal Causes of Nonvolatile Ion Buffer ($[A_{tot}]$) Acid-Base Abnormalities**

Nonvolatile Ion Buffer Alkalosis (decreased $[A_{tot}]$)
Hypoalbuminemia
Decreased production
    Chronic liver disease
    Acute phase response to inflammation
    Malnutrition/starvation
Extracorporeal loss
    Protein-losing nephropathy
    Protein-losing enteropathy
Sequestration
    Inflammatory effusions
    Vasculitis

Nonvolatile Ion Buffer Acidosis (increased $[A_{tot}]$)
Hyperalbuminemia
Water deprivation

Hyperphosphatemia
Translocation
    Tumor cell lysis
    Tissue trauma or rhabdomyolysis
Increased intake
    Phosphate-containing enemas
    Intravenous phosphate
Decreased loss
    Renal failure
    Urethral obstruction
    Uroabdomen

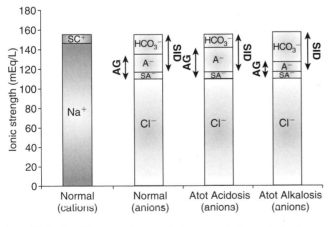

Fig. 13-4 Gamblegram of normal plasma and change in ionic strength of weak anions with increased (A_{tot} acidosis) and decreased (A_{tot} alkalosis) concentration of nonvolatile weak acids. SID does not change, but anion gap (AG) is increased in A_{tot} acidosis and decreased in A_{tot} alkalosis. *Na+*, Sodium; *SC+*, other strong cations; *Cl-*, chloride; *SA-*, other strong anions; *A-*, net charge of nonvolatile buffers; *HCO3-*, bicarbonate.

mated if the effects of hypoalbuminemia on pH, [HCO_3^-], and AG are not considered. Treatment for hypoalbuminemic alkalosis should be directed at the underlying cause and the decreased colloid oncotic pressure.

NONVOLATILE BUFFER ION ACIDOSIS

Hyperphosphatemia

Hyperphosphatemia, especially if severe, can cause a large increase in [A_{tot}], leading to metabolic acidosis (see Box 13-1). Although extremely rare, an increase in albumin concentration also can lead to metabolic acidosis.[36] A Gamblegram representing A_{tot} acidosis is shown in Fig. 13-4. The most important cause of hyperphosphatemic acidosis is renal failure. Metabolic acidosis in patients with renal failure is multifactorial but mostly is caused by hyperphosphatemia and increases in unmeasured strong anions.[32,34] Hyperphosphatemic acidosis also has been observed after hypertonic sodium phosphate enema administration in cats.[1] In experimental cats that have been given hypertonic sodium phosphate enemas, serum phosphate concentration changed from a mean of 2.8 mEq to 8.1 mEq/L within 15 minutes after a 60-mL dose and from 2.3 mEq/L to 8.8 mEq/L within 30 minutes with a 120-mL dose.[1] In both groups, the increase in [SID] was enough to offset the increase in lactate concentration, whereas protein concentration did not change. Because P_{CO_2} also did not change, the metabolic acidosis could be caused by an increase in unmeasured anions or phosphate, but an increase in any organic acid other than lactate would have been unlikely. Using the data from this study, a strong correlation can be found between changes in phosphate and changes in BE ($r = 0.95$ with the 60-mL dose, and $r = 0.96$ with the 120-mL dose). More than 90% of the change in the AG in the first 4 hours can be explained entirely by changes in lactate and phosphate. Clinically, hyperphosphatemic acidosis also occurred in a cat that received a phosphate-containing urinary acidifier.[19] Treatment for hyperphosphatemic acidosis should be directed at the underlying cause. Sodium bicarbonate administered intravenously shifts phosphate inside cells and may be used as adjunc-tive therapy in patients with hyperphosphatemic acidosis.[2]

DISORDERS OF SID

Changes in SID usually are recognized by changes in [HCO_3^-] or BE from their reference values. It is important to understand that the change in SID from normal is equivalent to the change in [HCO_3^-] or BE from normal whenever the plasma concentrations of nonvolatile buffer ions (albumin, phosphate, globulin) are normal. In other words, the Henderson-Hasselbalch and strong ion approaches are equivalent whenever plasma albumin, phosphate, and globulin concentrations are within their reference ranges.

A decrease in SID is associated with metabolic acidosis, whereas an increase in SID is associated with metabolic alkalosis. There are three general mechanisms by which SID can change (Table 13-2): (1) a change in the free water content of plasma; (2) a change in [Cl^-]; and (3) an increase in the concentration of other strong anions.

SID ALKALOSIS

There are two general mechanisms by which SID can increase, leading to metabolic alkalosis: an increase in [Na^+] or a decrease in [Cl^-]. Strong cations other than sodium are tightly regulated, and changes of a magnitude that could affect SID clinically either are not compatible with life or do not occur. Conversely, chloride is the only strong anion present in sufficient concentration to cause an increase in SID when its concentration is decreased. Common causes of SID alkalosis are presented in Box 13-2.

Concentration Alkalosis

Concentration alkalosis develops whenever a deficit of water in plasma occurs and is recognized clinically by the presence of hypernatremia or hyperalbuminemia. Solely decreasing the content of water increases the plasma concentration of all strong cations and strong anions and thus increases SID (Fig. 13-5). This decrease in water

---

TABLE 13-2   Mechanisms for SID Changes

Disorder	Mechanism	Clinical Recognition
SID acidosis		
⇓ In strong cations	⇑ Free water (⇓ Sodium)	Dilutional acidosis
⇑ In strong anions	⇑ Chloride	Hyperchloremic acidosis
	⇑ Unmeasured strong anions	Organic acidosis
SID alkalosis		
⇑ In strong cations	⇓ Free water (⇑ Sodium)	Concentration alkalosis
⇓ In strong anions	⇓ Chloride	Hypochloremic alkalosis

Box 13-2   Principal Causes of SID Alkalosis in Dogs and Cats

Concentration Alkalosis (⇑ [Na⁺])

Pure Water Loss
Inadequate access to water (water deprivation)
Diabetes insipidus

Hypotonic Fluid Loss
Vomiting
Nonoliguric renal failure
Postobstructive diuresis

Hypochloremic Alkalosis (⇓ [Cl⁻] corrected)

Excessive Gain of Sodium Relative to Chloride
Isotonic or hypertonic sodium bicarbonate administration

Excessive Loss of Chloride Relative to Sodium
Vomiting of stomach contents
Therapy with thiazides or loop diuretics

---

content also increases A_{tot}, but the increase in SID has a greater effect on pH. A decrease in extracellular fluid (ECF) volume alone will not alter acid-base status because such a decrease in volume does not change any of the independent variables and therefore cannot change acid-base status (see Chapter 4 for more information). However, if the decrease in ECF volume is associated with a relatively greater loss of free water as in diabetes insipidus or hypotonic losses in animals with diarrhea, vomiting, or osmotic diuresis, then an acid-base change (concentration alkalosis) will result because

of the increase in SID. Hypernatremia also can be associated with sodium gain in animals with hyperadrenocorticism or in those treated with hypertonic saline or $NaHCO_3$. Hypernatremia is further discussed in Chapter 3. Therapy for concentration alkalosis should be directed at treating the underlying cause responsible for the change in [Na⁺]. If necessary, [Na⁺] and osmolality should be corrected (see Chapter 3).

Hypochloremic Alkalosis

If there is no change in the water content of plasma, plasma [Na⁺] will be normal. Other strong cations (e.g., Mg^{2+}, Ca^{2+}, K⁺) are regulated for purposes other than acid-base balance, and their concentrations never change sufficiently to substantially affect SID. Consequently, when water content is normal, SID changes only as a result of changes in strong anions. If [Na⁺] remains constant, decreases in [Cl⁻] can increase SID (so-called hypochloremic alkalosis; Fig. 13-6). Primary decreases in [Cl⁻] unrelated to increases in plasma water content are recognized by the presence of a low corrected chloride concentration (see Chapter 4). Hypochloremic alkalosis may be caused by an excessive loss of chloride relative to sodium or by administration of substances containing more sodium than chloride as compared with normal ECF composition. Excessive loss of chloride relative to sodium as compared with normal ECF composition can occur in the urine after administration of diuretics that cause chloride wasting (e.g., furosemide) or when the fluid lost has a low or negative SID as in the case of vomiting of stomach contents. The administration of substances containing more sodium

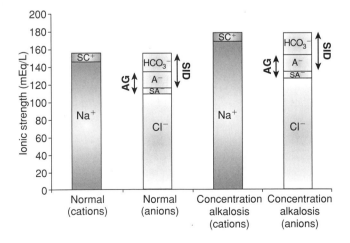

Fig. 13-5 Gamblegram of normal plasma and change in ionic strength of anions and cations secondary to a decrease in free water content in plasma (concentration alkalosis). All anions and cations, as well as SID and anion gap (AG), increase proportionally in patients with concentration alkalosis. *Na⁺*, Sodium; *SC⁺*, other strong cations; *Cl⁻*, chloride; *SA⁻*, other strong anions; *A⁻*, net charge of nonvolatile buffers; *HCO₃⁻*, bicarbonate.

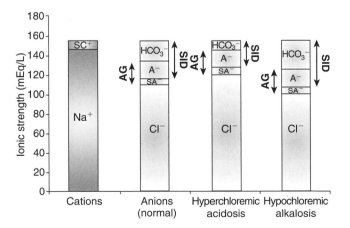

Fig. 13-6 Gamblegram of normal plasma and change in ionic strength of anions secondary to increases (hyperchloremic acidosis) or decrease (hypochloremic alkalosis) in chloride (Cl⁻) content in plasma. SID is decreased in hyperchloremic acidosis and increased in hypochloremic alkalosis, whereas anion gap (AG) remains constant during primary chloride changes. *Na⁺*, Sodium; *SC⁺*, other strong cations; *SA⁻*, other strong anions; *A⁻*, net charge of nonvolatile buffers; *HCO₃⁻*, bicarbonate.

than chloride (e.g., $NaHCO_3$) also increases SID, causing metabolic alkalosis.

A particular type of hypochloremic alkalosis that does not respond to chloride administration alone (as NaCl) is called chloride-resistant metabolic alkalosis and usually is caused by hyperadrenocorticism or hyperaldosteronism. Increased concentrations of cortisol or aldosterone cause sodium retention by activating the type I renal mineralocorticoid receptors.[41] Experimentally, administration of desoxycorticosterone acetate (DOCA) twice daily in sodium-supplemented dogs caused a significant increase in $[Na^+]$ and $[HCO_3^-]$ with no change in $[Cl^-]$.[27] When $NaHCO_3$ was added to the diet instead of NaCl, $[Na^+]$ and $[HCO_3^-]$ increased significantly, but $[Cl^-]$ decreased.[27] Approximately 30% of dogs with hyperadrenocorticism have mild hypernatremia.[26,30] In a study of 117 dogs with hyperadrenocorticism,[26] only 12 had $[Cl^-]$ less than 105 mEq/L. However, 25 of these dogs had hypernatremia, and the $[Cl^-]$, although within the normal range, could have been low relative to the $[Na^+]$ (i.e., corrected hypochloremia). The mean $[Na^+]$ was 150 mEq/L; the mean $[Cl^-]$ was 108 mEq/L; and the mean $[Cl^-]$ after correcting for changes in free water was 105 mEq/L. The corrected hypochloremia that occurs in the presence of high mineralocorticoid or glucocorticoid concentrations likely is responsible for the mild metabolic alkalosis observed in these patients. The lack of response to NaCl can be explained by a resetting of the regulatory mechanism and associated increased urinary loss of chloride.[22] Thus in so-called chloride-resistant metabolic alkalosis, something (e.g., excessive mineralocorticoid activity) prevents chloride retention, and consequently SID cannot be lowered by chloride administration.

Therapy of chloride-responsive hypochloremic alkalosis is directed at correcting the SID with a solution containing chloride (e.g., 0.9% NaCl, lactated Ringer's solution, KCl-supplemented fluids). In cases in which expansion of extracellular volume is desired, intravenous infusion of 0.9% NaCl is the treatment of choice. Corrected hypochloremia and hypochloremic alkalosis are further discussed in Chapters 4 and 10.

SID ACIDOSIS

Three general mechanisms can cause SID to decrease, resulting in SID (metabolic) acidosis: (1) a decrease in $[Na^+]$; (2) an increase in $[Cl^-]$; and (3) an increased concentration of other strong anions (e.g., L-lactate, β-hydroxybutyrate). Common causes of SID acidosis are presented in Box 13-3.

Dilutional Acidosis

Dilutional acidosis occurs whenever there is an excess of water in plasma and is recognized clinically by the presence of hyponatremia. Increasing the water content of plasma decreases the concentration of all strong cations and strong anions, and thus SID (Fig. 13-7). The

---

| **Box 13-3** | **Principal Causes of SID Acidosis in Dogs and Cats** |

Dilution Acidosis ($\Downarrow$ [Na⁺])
With Hypervolemia (gain of hypotonic fluid)
Severe liver disease
Congestive heart failure
Nephrotic syndrome

With Normovolemia (gain of water)
Psychogenic polydipsia
Hypotonic fluid infusion

With Hypovolemia (loss of hypertonic fluid)
Vomiting
Diarrhea
Hypoadrenocorticism
Third space loss
Diuretic administration

Hyperchloremic Acidosis ($\Uparrow$ [Cl⁻] corrected)
Excessive Loss of Sodium Relative to Chloride
Diarrhea

Excessive Gain of Chloride Relative to Sodium
Fluid therapy (e.g., 0.9% NaCl, 7.2% NaCl, KCl–
  supplemented fluids)
Total parenteral nutrition

Chloride Retention
Renal failure
Hypoadrenocorticism

Organic Acidosis ($\Uparrow$ unmeasured strong anions)
Uremic Acidosis
Diabetic Ketoacidosis
Lactic Acidosis
Toxicities
Ethylene glycol
Salicylate

---

increase in water content also decreases A_{tot}, but the decrease in SID has a greater effect on pH. An increase in ECF volume alone will not alter acid-base status because such an increase in volume does not change any of the independent variables (see Chapter 4). However, if the increase in ECF volume is associated with a relatively greater addition of free water, then an acid-base change (dilutional acidosis) will result because of the decrease in SID.

Large increases in free water are necessary to cause an appreciable decrease in SID. It has been estimated that in dogs and cats, a decrease in $[Na^+]$ by 20 mEq/L is associated with a 5-mEq/L decrease in BE.[11] Dilutional acidosis has been associated with congestive heart failure, hypoadrenocorticism, third space loss of sodium, and hypotonic fluid administration. However, hyponatremia in dogs most commonly is caused by gastrointestinal

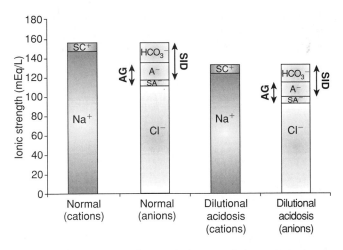

Fig. 13-7 Gamblegram of normal plasma and change in ionic strength of anions and cations secondary to an increase in free water content in plasma (dilution acidosis). All anions and cations, as well as SID and anion gap (AG), decrease proportionally in patients with dilution acidosis. Na^+, Sodium; SC^+, other strong cations; Cl^-, chloride; SA^-, other strong anions; A^-, net charge of nonvolatile buffers; HCO_3^-, bicarbonate.

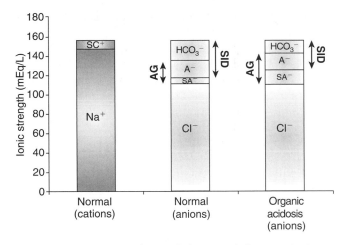

Fig. 13-8 Gamblegram of normal plasma and change in ionic strength of anions secondary to increases in unmeasured strong anions (organic acidosis) in plasma. SID is decreased in organic acidosis, whereas anion gap (AG) is increased because of increase in unmeasured strong anions. Na^+, Sodium; SC^+, other strong cations; SA^-, other strong anions; A^-, net charge of nonvolatile buffers; HCO_3^-, bicarbonate.

loss of sodium. Hyponatremia is further discussed in Chapter 3. Therapy for dilutional acidosis should be directed at the underlying cause of the change in $[Na^+]$. If necessary, $[Na^+]$ and osmolality should be corrected (see Chapter 3).

Hyperchloremic Acidosis

Increases in $[Cl^-]$ can substantially decrease SID, leading to so-called hyperchloremic acidosis (see Fig. 13-6). Hyperchloremic acidosis may be caused by chloride retention (e.g., early renal failure, renal tubular acidosis), excessive loss of sodium relative to chloride (e.g., diarrhea), or by administration of substances containing more chloride than sodium as compared with normal ECF composition (e.g., administration of KCl, 0.9% NaCl). Administration of 0.9% NaCl is a common cause of hyperchloremic acidosis in hospitalized patients[12] and is the classic example of strong ion acidosis.[9] Treatment of hyperchloremic acidosis should be directed at correction of the underlying disease process. Special attention should be given to plasma pH. Bicarbonate therapy can be instituted whenever plasma pH is less than 7.2. Corrected hyperchloremia and hyperchloremic acidosis are further discussed in Chapters 4 and 10.

SID Acidosis Caused by an Increase in Unmeasured Strong Anions (Organic Acidosis)

Accumulation of metabolically produced organic anions (e.g., L-lactate, acetoacetate, citrate, β-hydroxybutyrate) or addition of exogenous organic anions (e.g., salicylate, glycolate from ethylene glycol poisoning, formate from methanol poisoning) will cause metabolic acidosis because these strong anions decrease SID (Fig. 13-8).

Accumulation of some inorganic strong anions (e.g., SO_4^{2-} in renal failure) will resemble organic acidosis because these substances decrease SID. The pK values for the clinically most important organic anions are as follows: lactate = 3.9, acetoacetate = 3.6, citrate = 4.3, and β-hydroxybutyrate = 4.4. Thus the pK values of these ions are at least 3 pH units below normal plasma pH, and at a pH of 7.4, the concentrations of their dissociated forms are at least 1000 times greater than the concentrations of the nondissociated forms. For example, at a pH of 7.4 for each molecule of lactic acid, there are approximately 3200 molecules of lactate. Thus it can be assumed that these organic acids are completely dissociated within the pH range of body fluids compatible with life and consequently behave as strong ions. The most frequently encountered causes of organic acidosis in dogs and cats are renal failure (uremic acidosis), diabetic ketoacidosis, lactic acidosis, and ethylene glycol toxicity. Management of organic acidosis should be directed at stabilization of the patient and treatment of the primary disorder. Sodium bicarbonate may help patients in renal failure with acidosis but not patients with lactic acidosis or ketoacidosis. The efficacy of $NaHCO_3$ therapy in renal failure partly is related to the shift of phosphate inside the cell with consequent amelioration of the hyperphosphatemic acidosis. Sodium bicarbonate should be used cautiously because metabolism of accumulated organic anions will normalize SID and increase $[HCO_3^-]$. The initial goal in acidemic patients with renal failure is to increase systemic pH to more than 7.2. Organic acidoses are further discussed in Chapter 10.

CLINICAL APPROACH

Three simplified approaches have been developed to allow the clinical use of Stewart's strong ion approach: the effective SID method also know as the Stewart-Figge's methodology,[18] the BE approach or Fencl-Stewart's algorithm,[16] and Constable's simplified strong ion model.[8]

EFFECTIVE SID MODEL

Figge et al[18] developed and successfully tested in humans a mathematical approach to evaluate metabolic acid-base disorders. Unmeasured strong ions (XA^-) are estimated by subtracting the "effective SID" (SID_{eff}), an approximation of the "real" SID, from the "apparent SID" (SID_{app}) as $XA^- = SID_{app} - SID_{eff}$. The SID_{app} is calculated using electrolytes measured in the serum ($SID_{app} = [Na^+] + [K^+] + [Mg^{2+}] + [Ca^{2+}] - [Cl^-]$), and SID_{eff} is a satisfactory approximation of the "real SID." Despite being a very promising model for assessment of metabolic acid-base disorders, the Stewart-Figge's model was developed using protein behavior based on human albumin and has not been tested in dogs or cats. In addition, calculation of SID_{eff} is not simple and may be clinically impractical.

BASE EXCESS ALGORITHM

BE has been used to assess changes in the metabolic component because SID is synonymous with buffer base. BE is a measurement of the deviation of buffer base (and therefore SID) from normal values, assuming nonvolatile buffer ion concentrations (albumin, phosphate, globulin) are normal. However, it should be pointed out that Siggaard-Andersen studied human blood with a constant protein concentration. A BE nomogram has been developed for dogs[15] using Siggaard-Andersen's approach. However, the canine nomogram has rarely been used because blood gas analyzers were developed for the human medical market and therefore assume that human blood is being analyzed.

The BE has been used clinically for more than a decade to assess the metabolic acid-base status in human patients[42] and has been adapted for use in dogs and cats.[11,13] This approach attempts to take into account the effect that changes in sodium (i.e., dilutional acidosis and concentration alkalosis), chloride (i.e., hypochloremic alkalosis and hyperchloremic acidosis), phosphate (i.e., hyperphosphatemic acidosis), and plasma protein (i.e., hypoproteinemic alkalosis and hyperproteinemic acidosis) concentrations exert on plasma pH, purportedly facilitating identification and quantification of unmeasured strong ions (i.e., organic acidosis) in plasma. Values less than −5 mmol/L are suggestive of an increase in unmeasured strong anions.[11] Formulas to estimate changes in BE resulting from changes in SID and A_{tot} are presented in Box 13-4. A complete description of the

derivation of these formulas, as well as their limitations, can be found elsewhere.[7] The BE algorithm is a useful clinical tool despite a few shortcomings. These formulas were helpful in understanding complex acid-base disorders in dogs and cats.[13,24,40] Unfortunately, no controlled clinical studies have been performed in dogs and cats

---

Box 13-4	Estimation of Change in Base Excess Caused by Changes in [SID] and [A_{tot}]

Changes in Base Excess Caused by Changes in [A_{tot}]
Albumin Contribution (Δ Albumin in mEq/L)
$$\Delta \text{ Albumin} = 3.7 \, ([alb]_{normal} - [alb]_{patient})$$

Phosphate Contribution (Δ Phosphate in mEq/L)
If phosphate concentration is in mMol/L:
$$\Delta \text{ Phosphate} = 1.8 \, [\text{Phosphate}]_{patient}$$

If phosphate concentration is in mg/dL:
$$\Delta \text{ Phosphate} = 0.58 \, [\text{Phosphate}]_{patient}$$

Changes in Base Excess Caused by Changes in [SID]
Contribution from Changes in Free Water in mEq/L
$$\Delta \text{ Free water} = 0.25 \, ([Na^+]_{patient} - [Na^+]_{normal})$$

Chloride Contribution in (Δ Chloride in mEq/L)
$$\Delta \text{ Chloride} = [Cl^-]_{normal} - [Cl^-]_{corrected}$$

Contribution from Unidentified Strong Anions (Δ [XA^-] in mEq/L)
$$\Delta \, [XA^-] = [BE]_{patient} - (\Delta \text{ Albumin} + \Delta \text{ Phosphate} + \Delta \text{ Free water} + \Delta \text{ Chloride})$$

SID, Strong ion difference; [A_{tot}], total plasma concentration of nonvolatile weak buffers; [alb]$_{normal}$, normal albumin concentration (midpoint) in g/dL; [alb]$_{patient}$, patient's albumin concentration in g/dL; [Phosphate]$_{patient}$, patient's inorganic phosphorus concentration in mMol/L or mg/dL; [Na+]$_{patient}$, patient's sodium concentration in mEq/L; [Na+]$_{normal}$, normal sodium concentration (midpoint) in mEq/L; [Cl-]$_{normal}$, normal chloride concentration (midpoint) in mEq/L; [Cl-]$_{corrected}$, patient's corrected chloride concentration in mEq/L; [BE]$_{patient}$, patient's base excess in mEq/L. Reference values for the author's laboratory: [alb]$_{normal}$ = 3.1 g/dL; [Na+]$_{normal}$ = 156 mEq/L for cats and 146 mEq/L for dogs; [Cl-]$_{normal}$ = 120 mEq/L for cats and 110 mEq/L for dogs.

Adapted from de Morais HSA, Muir WW: Strong ions and acid-base disorders. In Bonagura JD, editor: *Kirk's current veterinary therapy XII*, ed 12, Philadelphia, 1995, WB Saunders, pp. 121-127.

with acid-base disturbances to assess the accuracy of these formulas, and there are theoretical limitations in extrapolating traditional BE calculations for use in dogs and cats.[12a] In addition, the influence of protein on BE is estimated based on data for human albumin, which behaves differently than canine and feline albumin.

SIMPLIFIED STRONG ION MODEL

The simplified strong ion model assumes that plasma ions act as strong ions, volatile buffer ions (HCO_3^-), or nonvolatile buffer ions (A^-).[8] Therefore plasma contains three types of charged entities: SID, HCO_3^-, and A^-. The requirement for electroneutrality dictates that at all times the SID equals the sum of bicarbonate buffer ion activity (HCO_3^-) and nonvolatile buffer ion activity (A^-), such that $SID^+ = HCO_3^- + A^-$. This approach obviously assumes that all ionized entities in plasma can be classified as a strong ion, a volatile buffer ion, or a nonvolatile buffer ion (A^-). This assumption forms the basis for the simplified strong ion model. A complete description of the mathematical background of the simplified strong ion model, as well as its limitations, can be found elsewhere.[7,8]

The simplified strong ion approach is a quantitative, mechanistic acid-base model. Unlike Stewart's strong ion model, the simplified strong ion model uses hydrogen ion activity (pH) instead of concentration, provides a practical experimental method for determining species-specific values for K_a and A_{tot} (CO_2 tonometry of plasma), and simplifies to the Henderson-Hasselbalch equation when applied to aqueous nonprotein solutions (where A_{tot} = 0 mEq/L and SID = $[HCO_3^-]$).[7] The simplified strong ion model also explains many of the anomalies of the Henderson-Hasselbalch equation. It explains why the apparent value for pK_1' in plasma is dependent on pH, protein concentration, and sodium concentration and also provides a mechanistic explanation for the temperature dependence of plasma pH.[7] The simplified strong ion model shares two of the disadvantages of Stewart's strong ion model: (1) difficulty in accurately determining SID; and (2) mathematical complexity when compared with the traditional Henderson-Hasselbalch equation. It is unlikely that the simplified strong ion approach will replace the traditional Henderson-Hasselbalch approach clinically and in descriptive experimental studies because two (pH and PCO_2) of the three (pH, PCO_2, and $[HCO_3^-]$) unknowns in the Henderson-Hasselbalch equation can be measured accurately and easily in plasma, whereas only two (pH and PCO_2) of the four unknowns in the simplified strong ion approach (pH, PCO_2, SID, and A_{tot}) can be measured easily and accurately. However, in mechanistic experimental studies, the simplified strong ion model is preferred because it conveys on a fundamental level the mechanisms underlying acid-base disturbances.

STRONG ION GAP

The SIG concept is a modification of the simplified strong ion model that overcomes one of the limitations of this model, namely, algebraic complexity. SIG is the difference in charge between all unmeasured strong anions and all unmeasured strong cations.[4] Because there are more strong cations than strong anions, normal SIG is positive:

$$SIG = [UC_{strong}^+] - [UA_{strong}^-]$$

where $[UC_{strong}^+]$ is the sum of all unmeasured strong cations (e.g., ionized calcium, ionized magnesium), whereas $[UA_{strong}^-]$ is the sum of all unmeasured strong anions (e.g., ketoanions, lactate, sulfate). The calculated value of the SIG will change depending on the strong ions measured. The most important strong cations in plasma based on their concentration are Na^+ and K^+, whereas the most prevalent strong anion is Cl^-. Thus SIG can be defined in its simplest form when only these three strong ions are measured as:

$$SIG = [Na^+] + [K^+] - [Cl^-] = [UC_{strong}^+] - [UA_{strong}^-]$$

where $[UC_{strong}^+]$ is the sum of all strong cations other than $[Na^+]$ and $[K^+]$, and $[UA_{strong}^-]$ is the sum of all strong anions other than $[Cl^-]$. Electroneutrality must be maintained in plasma, and the excess of positive charges from the SIG is balanced by the negative charges of HCO_3^- and the nonvolatile buffers $[A^-]$. Thus electroneutrality can be expressed as:

$$SIG + [Na^+] + [K^+] - [Cl^-] - [HCO_3^-] - [A^-] = 0$$

because

$$AG = [Na^+] + [K^+] - [Cl^-] - [HCO_3^-],$$
$$SIG + AG - [A^-] = 0$$

or

$$SIG = [A^-] - AG$$

Based on the relationship above, the SIG has been simplified ($SIG_{simplified}$) so as to allow estimation based on $[A_{tot}]$ (the sum of $[A^-]$ and its weak acid pair $[HA]$) and AG.[4] Albumin is used to estimate $[A_{tot}]$ in the $SIG_{simplified}$ because albumin is the most important buffer in plasma. At a normal plasma pH of 7.4, $SIG_{simplified}$ can be calculated in dogs as[3]:

$$SIG_{simplified} = [alb] \times 4.9 - AG$$

TABLE 13-3 Comparison of the Traditional Henderson-Hasselbalch Approach to Acid-Base Disturbances to the Strong Ion Model

System	Advantages	Disadvantages	Errors and Limitations
Henderson-Hasselbalch approach ($[HCO_3^-]$ or base excess and anion gap)	Widely and routinely used Easy to calculate	Descriptive Anion gap lacks sensitivity and specificity Does not account for changes caused by protein and phosphorus	Does not explain effects of temperature on pH Does not explain dependence on pK_1' on pH States that there is a linear relationship between pH and log P_{CO_2} Can only accurately be applied to plasma at normal temperature, pH, and protein and sodium concentration
Strong ion model	Mechanistic Explains effects of protein and phosphorus on pH	True SID can only be estimated Algebraic complexity	Uses hydrogen ion concentration instead of pH Stewart's strong ion equation does not algebraically simplify to the Henderson-Hasselbalch equation in an aqueous solution with no proteins

$[HCO_3^-]$, *Bicarbonate concentration*; pK_1', *negative logarithm of the apparent dissociation constant for plasma carbonic acid.*

In cats, at a normal plasma pH of 7.35, $SIG_{simplified}$ can be calculated as[29]:

$$SIG_{simplified} = [alb] \times 7.4 - AG$$

An increase in unmeasured strong anions is suspected whenever $SIG_{simplified}$ is less than -5 mEq/L. In patients with hyperphosphatemia, however, AG should be corrected for the presence of hyperphosphatemia $\{AG_{phosphate-adjusted} = AG + (2.52 - 0.58 \times [Phosphate])\}$ before calculating $SIG_{simplified}$. The $SIG_{simplified}$ offers a more accurate approach to identifying unmeasured strong ions in plasma than does the AG. The critical difference between the AG and $SIG_{simplified}$ is that the $SIG_{simplified}$ provides an estimate of the difference between unmeasured strong cations and strong anions, whereas AG provides an estimate of the difference between unmeasured cations and anions (including strong ions and nonvolatile buffer ions such as albumin, globulins, and phosphate). Therefore a change in $SIG_{simplified}$ provides a more specific method for detecting a change in unmeasured strong ions (such as lactate) than does a change in AG. The $SIG_{simplified}$ has not been adequately tested in dogs and cats, but its derivation is sound, and it is superior to the AG in detecting increases in unmeasured strong anion concentration in horses[4] and cattle.[6]

CONCLUSION

The traditional approach for evaluation of acid-base status using pH, P_{CO_2}, and $[HCO_3^-]$ has several clinically relevant limitations. It does not give a complete assessment of the sources of pathophysiologic changes in the metabolic component ($[HCO_3^-]$); it may lead to the conclusion that changes in electrolytes are only secondarily related to acid-base status; and it does not recognize changes in pH caused by changes in protein or inorganic phosphate concentrations. The strong ion model is compared with the traditional Henderson-Hasselbalch approach to acid-base disturbances in Table 13-3. Using the strong ion model, the relationship between electrolytes and acid-base status becomes clear, and it becomes apparent that they should no longer be viewed as separate entities. The end result is a better understanding of how acid-base disorders develop and how they should be treated. It is hoped that improved patient care will follow enhanced understanding of the pathophysiologic principles underlying acid-base disturbances. Clearly, the strong ion approach is more time consuming than are conventional methods, and therefore it is less convenient in daily practice.[31] This argument is particularly true in patients with normal protein and phosphate concentrations, in which the traditional Henderson-Hasselbalch approach in conjunction with an estimation of unmeasured anions works well as a first approximation of a more complex system and is therefore the preferred method. In critically ill patients or patients with multiple problems, the Stewart approach provides a more comprehensive evaluation of acid-base status and greater insight into their possible causes and most appropriate therapy.

REFERENCES

1. Atkins CE, Tyler R, Greenlee F: Clinical, biochemical, acid-base, and electrolyte abnormalities in cats after hypertonic sodium phosphate enema administration, *Am J Vet Res* 46:980-988, 1985.
2. Barsotti G, Lazzeri M, Cristofano C, et al: The role of metabolic acidosis in causing uremic hyperphosphatemia, *Miner Electrolyte Metab* 1986;12:103-106.

3. Constable PD, Stämpfli HR: Experimental determination of net protein charge and A_{tot} and K_a of nonvolatile buffers in canine plasma, *J Vet Intern Med* 19:507-514, 2005.

4. Constable PD, Hinchcliff KW, Muir WW: Comparison of anion gap and strong ion gap as predictors of unmeasured strong ion concentration in plasma and serum from horses, *Am J Vet Res* 59:881-887, 1998.

5. Constable PD: Total weak acid concentration and effective dissociation constant of nonvolatile buffers in human plasma, *J Appl Physiol* 91:1364-1371, 2001.

6. Constable PD: Calculation of variables describing plasma nonvolatile weak acids for use in the strong ion approach to acid-base balance in cattle, *Am J Vet Res* 63:482-490, 2002.

7. Constable PD: Clinical assessment of acid-base status: comparison of the Henderson-Hasselbalch and strong ion approaches, *Vet Clin Pathol* 29:115-128, 2000.

8. Constable PD: A simplified strong ion model for acid-base equilibria: application to horse plasma, *J Appl Physiol* 83:297-311, 1997.

9. Constable PD: Hyperchloremic acidosis: the classic example of strong ion acidosis, *Anesth Analg* 96:919-922, 2003.

10. Corey HE: Stewart and beyond: new models of acid-base balance, *Kidney Int* 64:777-787, 2003.

11. de Morais HSA : A nontraditional approach to acid-base disorders. In DiBartola SP, editor: *Fluid therapy in small animal practice,* Philadelphia, 1992, WB Saunders, pp. 297-320.

12. de Morais HSA: Chloride disorders: hyperchloremia and hypochloremia. In DiBartola SP, editor: *Fluid therapy in small animal practice,* ed 2, Philadelphia, 2000, WB Saunders, pp. 73-82.

12a. de Morais HSA: Has Stewart finally arrived in the clinic? *J Vet Intern Med* 19:489-490, 2005.

13. DiBartola SP, de Morais HSA: Case examples. In DiBartola SP, editor: *Fluid therapy in small animal practice,* Philadelphia, 1992, WB Saunders, pp. 599-688.

14. Durward A, Mayer A, Skellett A, et al: Hypoalbuminemia in critically ill children: incidence, prognosis, and influence in the anion gap, *Arch Dis Child* 88:419-422, 2003.

15. Emuakpor DS, Maas AHJ, Ruigrok TJC, et al: Acid-base curve nomogram for dog blood, *Pflugers Archiv* 363:141-147, 1976.

16. Fencl V, Leith DE: Stewart's quantitative acid-base chemistry: applications for biology and medicine, *Respir Physiol* 91:1-16, 1993.

17. Fencl V, Jabor A, Kazda A, et al: Diagnosis of metabolic acid-base disturbances in critically ill patients, *Am J Respir Crit Care Med* 162:2246-2251, 2000.

18. Figge J, Rossing TH, Fencl VL The role of proteins in acid-base equilibria, *J Lab Clin Med* 117:453-467, 1991.

18a. Figge J, Jabor A, Kazda A, et al: Anion gap and hypoalbuminemia, *Crit Care Med* 26:1807-1810, 1998.

19. Fulton R, Fruechte L: Poisoning induced by administration of a phosphate-containing urinary acidifier in a cat, *J Am Vet Med Assoc* 198:8-12, 1991.

20. Gilfix BM, Bique M, Magder S: A physical chemical approach to the analysis of acid-base balance in the clinical setting, *J Crit Care* 8:187-197, 1993.

21. Hatherill M, Waggie Z, Purves L, et al: Correction of anion gap for albumin in order to detect occult tissue anions in shock, *Arch Dis Child* 87:526-529, 2002.

22. Jones NL: *Blood gases and acid base physiology,* ed 2, New York, 1987, Thieme Medical Publishers.

23. Kellum JA, Kramer DJ, Pinsky MR: Strong ion gap: a methodology for exploring unexplained anions, *J Crit Care* 10:51-55, 1995.

24. Leisewitz AL, Jacobson LS, de Morais HSA, et al: The mixed acid-base disturbances of severe canine babesiosis, *J Vet Intern Med* 15:445-452, 2001.

25. Leith DE: The new acid-base: power and simplicity. Proc ACVIM Forum, Washington, DC, 449-455 1990.

26. Ling G, Stabenfeldt OH, Comer KM, et al: Canine hyper-adrenocorticism: pretreatment clinical and laboratory evaluation of 117 cases, *J Am Vet Med Assoc* 174:1211-1215, 1979.

27. Madias NE, Bossert WH, Adrogué HJ: Ventilatory response to chronic metabolic acidosis and alkalosis in the dog, *J Appl Physiol* 56:1640-1646, 1984.

28. McAuliffe JJ, Lind LJ, Leith DE, et al: Hypoproteinemic alkalosis, *Am J Med* 81:86-90, 1986.

29. McCullough SM, Constable PD: Calculation of the total plasma concentration of nonvolatile weak acids and the effective dissociation constant of nonvolatile buffers in plasma for use in the strong ion approach to acid-base balance in cats, *Am J Vet Res* 64:1047-1051, 2003.

30. Meijer JC: Canine hyperadrenocorticism. In Kirk RW, editor: *Current veterinary therapy VII,* ed 7, Philadelphia, 1980, WB Saunders, pp. 974-978.

31. Moviat M, van Haren F, van der Hoeven H: Conventional or physicochemical approach to intensive care unit patients with metabolic acidosis, *Crit Care* 7:R41-R45, 2003.

32. Naka T, Bellomo R: Bench-to-bedside review: treating acid-base abnormalities in the intensive care unit—the role of renal replacement therapy, *Crit Care* 8:108-114, 2004.

33. Oh MS, Carroll HJ: Current concepts. The anion gap, *N Engl J Med* 297:814-817, 1977.

34. Rocktaeschel J, Morimatsu H, Uchino S, et al: Acid-base status of critically ill patients with acute renal failure: analysis based on Stewart-Figge methodology, *Crit Care* 7:R60-R63, 2003.

35. Rossing TH, Boixeda D, Maffeo H, et al: Hyperventilation with hypoproteinemia, *J Lab Clin Med* 112:553-559, 1988.

36. Rossing TH, Maffeo N, Fencl V: Acid-base effects of altering plasma protein concentration in human blood in vitro, *J Appl Physiol* 61:2260-2265, 1986.

37. Sirker AA, Rhodes A, Grounde RM, et al: Acid-base physiology: the traditional and the modern approaches, *Anesthesia* 57:348-356, 2002.

38. Stämpfli HR, Constable PD: Experimental determination of net protein charge and A_{tot} and K_a of nonvolatile buffers in human plasma, *J Appl Physiol* 95:620-630, 2003.

39. Stewart PA: Modern quantitative acid-base chemistry, *Can J Physiol Pharmacol* 61:1444-1461, 1983.

40. Whitehair KJ, Haskins SC, Whitehair JG, et al: Clinical application of quantitative acid-base chemistry, *J Vet Intern Med* 9:1-11, 1995.

41. Whitworth JA, Mangos GJ, Kelly JJ: Cushing, cortisol, and cardiovascular disease, *Hypertension* 36:912-916, 2000.

42. Wilkes P: Hypoproteinemia, strong-ion difference, and acid-base status in critically ill patients, *J Appl Physiol* 84:1740-1748, 1998.

43. Wooten EW: Calculation of physiological acid-base parameters in multicompartment systems with application to human blood, *J Appl Physiol* 95:2333-2344, 2003.

44. Wooten EW: Science review: quantitative acid-base physiology using Stewart Model, *Crit Care* 8:448-452, 2004.

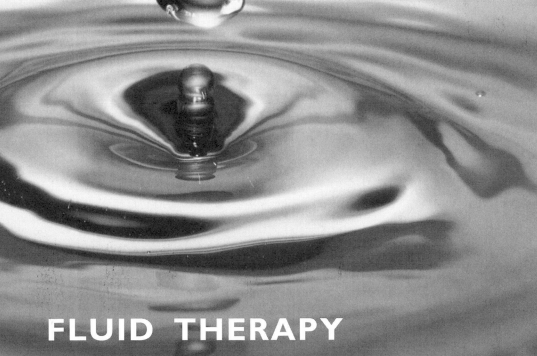

SECTION

IV

FLUID THERAPY

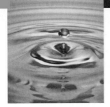

CHAPTER 14

INTRODUCTION TO FLUID THERAPY

Stephen P. DiBartola and Shane Bateman

She had apparently reached the last moments of earthly existence, and now nothing could injure her—indeed, so entirely was she reduced, that I feared I should be unable to get my apparatus ready ere she expired. Having inserted a tube into the basilic vein, cautiously—anxiously, I watched the effects; ounce after ounce was injected, but no visible change was produced. Still persevering, I thought she began to breathe less laboriously, soon the sharpened features, and sunken eye, and fallen jaw, pale and cold, bearing the manifest impress of death's signet, began to glow with returning animation; the pulse which had long ceased, returned to the wrist; at first small and quick, by degrees it became more and more distinct, fuller, slower, and firmer, and in the short space of half an hour, when six pints had been injected, she expressed in a firm voice that she was free from all uneasiness, actually became jocular, and fancied that all she needed was a little sleep; her extremities were warm, and every feature bore the aspect of comfort and health.

Thomas Latta, describing the first use of intravenous fluid therapy
in a human patient with cholera in a letter to the Lancet, *1832.*

Fluid therapy is supportive. The underlying disease process that caused the fluid, electrolyte, and acid-base disturbances in the patient must be diagnosed and treated appropriately. Normal homeostatic mechanisms allow the clinician considerable margin for error in fluid therapy, provided that the heart and kidneys are normal. This is fortunate because estimation of the patient's fluid deficit is difficult and may be quite inaccurate. The purpose of this chapter is to provide an overview of the principles of fluid therapy. The composition and distribution of body fluids are discussed in Chapter 1, and the technical aspects of vascular access are discussed in Chapter 15. Fluid therapy potentially consists of three phases: resuscitation, rehydration, and maintenance. Most patients in shock (see Chapter 23) require rapid administration of a large volume of crystalloid, colloid, or other fluid to expand the intravascular space and correct perfusion deficits. Dehydrated patients also require sustained administration of crystalloid fluids for 12 to 36 hours to replace fluid losses from the interstitial and intracellular spaces. Patients with normal hydration unable to consume sufficient water to sustain fluid balance require maintenance fluid therapy with crystalloid solutions. In formulating and implementing a fluid therapy plan, eight questions should be considered[10,28]:

1. Is the patient suffering from a shock syndrome that requires immediate fluid administration?
2. Is the patient dehydrated?
3. Can the patient consume an adequate volume of water to sustain normal fluid balance?
4. What type of fluid should be given?
5. By what route should the fluid be given?
6. How rapidly should the fluid be given?
7. How much fluid should be given?
8. When should fluid therapy be discontinued?

IS THE PATIENT SUFFERING FROM A SHOCK SYNDROME THAT REQUIRES IMMEDIATE FLUID ADMINISTRATION?

Shock patients (see Chapter 23) urgently require fluid therapy. The presence of altered mental status and cool extremities in association with tachycardia or severe bradycardia, mucous membrane pallor, prolonged or absent capillary refill time, reduced or absent peripheral pulses, and hypotension are among the most common physical examination findings in patients in shock. Such physical examination findings in association with a compatible clinical history are the basis for the decision to institute a resuscitation phase of fluid therapy. Some forms of shock may be associated with variations in these physical examination findings, and it is crucial to understand the different shock syndromes. (See Chapter 23 for more information on shock.)

The shock syndromes most likely to respond to marked volume expansion of the intravascular space are hypovolemic and distributive shock states. Obstructive forms of shock often respond favorably to moderate volume expansion. Fluid administration is contraindicated in patients with predominantly cardiogenic forms of shock.

Regardless of their underlying disease, severely dehydrated patients can be in shock and require a resuscitation phase of fluid therapy before initiating the rehydration phase. However, not all patients in shock are dehydrated and thus may or may not require a rehydration phase of therapy. The rapidity and volume of loss from both the intravascular and extravascular fluid compartments in conjunction with the extent of any compensatory response will determine whether the patient is in shock or is dehydrated.

IS THE PATIENT DEHYDRATED?

The need for a rehydration phase is dependent on the underlying condition of the patient. For surgical patients, there are additional indications for fluid therapy, such as maintenance of venous access for emergencies and establishment of diuresis to maintain renal perfusion during anesthesia (see Chapter 17). For medical patients, the answer to this question depends on an assessment of the animal's state of hydration. The hydration status of the animal is estimated by careful evaluation of the history, physical examination findings, and the results of a few simple laboratory tests.[7,11]

In its most narrow sense, dehydration refers to loss of pure water. However, the term dehydration usually is used to include hypotonic, isotonic, and hypertonic fluid losses. The type of dehydration is classified by the tonicity of the fluid remaining in the body (e.g., a hypotonic loss would result in hypertonic dehydration). Isotonic and hypotonic losses are most common in small animal practice. Isotonic fluid loss can result in volume depletion and nonosmotic stimulation of antidiuretic hormone (ADH) release, thus preventing effective excretion of consumed water and resulting in hypotonic dehydration. Types of dehydration are depicted in Fig. 3-1 and are discussed in detail in Chapter 3.

FLUID BALANCE

Normal sources of fluid input are water consumed in food, water that is drunk, and water produced in the body as a result of metabolism. Nutrient oxidation produces approximately 0.1 g of water per kilocalorie of energy released.[2] Maintenance water and electrolyte needs parallel caloric expenditure,[20,22,23] and normal daily losses of water and electrolytes include respiratory, fecal, and urinary losses. Estimated daily caloric and water requirements for dogs and cats are shown in Tables

14-1 and 14-2[23] and in Fig. 14-1.[20] Respiratory loss of fluid can be important in dogs because panting has been adapted for thermoregulation in this species. Pyrexic patients also can lose fluid by this route. Normally, cutaneous losses are unimportant in dogs and cats because eccrine sweat glands are limited to the foot pads and do not play an important role in thermoregulation in these species. Sympathetic stimulation as a result of heat stress in the cat may result in increased secretion of saliva, and a small volume of fluid may be lost by this route.

In disease states, decreased fluid intake results from anorexia, and increased fluid loss may occur by urinary (e.g., polyuria) and gastrointestinal (e.g., vomiting, diarrhea) routes. Other less common routes of loss include skin (e.g., extensive burns), respiratory tract, and salivary secretions, as described before. Third-space loss of fluid occurs when effective circulating volume is decreased, but the fluid lost remains in the body. Examples include intestinal obstruction, peritonitis, pancreatitis, and effusions or hemorrhage into body cavities. Decreased fluid intake and increased loss often coexist (e.g., anorexia, vomiting, and polyuria in a uremic animal).

HISTORY

Historical information about the route of fluid loss may suggest the affected fluid compartment or compartments, as well as the patient's electrolyte and acid-base derangements. The time period over which fluid losses have occurred and an estimate of their magnitude should be determined. Information about food and water consumption, gastrointestinal losses (e.g., vomiting, diarrhea), urinary losses (i.e., polyuria), and traumatic losses (e.g., blood loss, extensive burns) should be obtained from the owner. Excessive insensible water losses (e.g., increased panting, pyrexia) and third-space losses may be determined from the history and physical examination. In addition, the clinician's knowledge of the suspected disease can aid in predicting the composition of the fluid lost (e.g., vomiting caused by pyloric obstruction leads to loss of hydrogen, chloride, potassium, and sodium ions and development of metabolic alkalosis, whereas small bowel diarrhea typically leads to loss of bicarbonate, chloride, sodium, and potassium ions and development of metabolic acidosis) (Table 14-3).

PHYSICAL EXAMINATION

The physical findings associated with fluid losses of 5% to 15% of body weight vary from no clinically detectable changes (5%) to signs of hypovolemic shock and impending death (15%) (Table 14-4).[7,11,20] The clinician may estimate the hydration deficit by evaluating skin turgor or pliability, the moistness of the mucous membranes, the position of the eyes in their orbits, heart rate, character of peripheral pulses, capillary refill time, and extent of peripheral venous distention (e.g., inspection of jugular veins). A decrease in the volume of the inter-

Average weights for breeds are shown

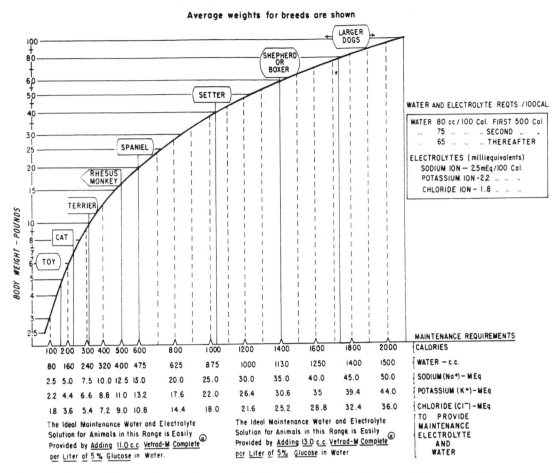

Fig. 14-1 Daily water, calorie, and electrolyte requirements for dogs and cats. (From Harrison JB, Sussman HH, Pickering DE: Fluid and electrolyte therapy in small animals, *J Am Vet Med Assoc* 137:638, 1960.)

stitial compartment leads to decreased skin turgor and dryness of the mucous membranes. A decrease in plasma volume leads to tachycardia, alterations in peripheral pulses, and collapse of peripheral veins. When these cardiovascular signs are present, the patient is in shock and should be resuscitated promptly before correction of the hydration deficit. Typically, such signs of hypovolemic shock appear with loss of at least 10% to 12% of the patient's body weight. The fluid deficit in a given patient is difficult to determine with accuracy because of the subjectivity of skin turgor evaluation and the possibility of undetected ongoing (contemporary) losses. Thus a crude clinical estimate of hydration status and the patient's response to fluid administration become important tools in evaluating the extent of dehydration that was present and in formulating ongoing fluid therapy.

Skin turgor is dependent on the amount of subcutaneous fat and elastin and on interstitial volume. Detection of dehydration by skin turgor is dependent on the animal's skin turgor before dehydration developed, the position of the animal (e.g., standing, recumbent) when the skin is checked, the site used for evaluation,

and the amount of subcutaneous fat.[19] Skin pliability should be tested over the lumbar region with the dog in a standing position. When evaluated by skin turgor, obese animals may appear well hydrated owing to excessive subcutaneous fat despite being dehydrated. Conversely, emaciated animals and older animals may appear more dehydrated than they actually are because of lack of subcutaneous fat and elastin. A false impression of dehydration also may occur with persistent panting, which may dry the oral mucous membranes. The urinary bladder should be small in a dehydrated animal with normal renal function. A large, urine-filled bladder in a severely dehydrated patient indicates failure of the normal renal concentrating mechanism.

Body weight recorded on a serial basis traditionally has been thought to be the best indicator of hydration status, especially when fluid loss has been acute and previous body weight has been recorded. Loss of 1 kg of body weight indicates a fluid deficit of 1 L. Unfortunately, previous body weight is often unknown in animals presented for treatment. However, records from previous routine hospital visits may provide this information.

TABLE 14-1 Daily Water and Calorie Requirements for the Dog*

Body Weight (kg)	Total kcal/day or Water mL/day	/kg	/hr
1	132	132	6
2	214	107	9
3	285	95	12
4	348	87	15
5	407	81	17
6	463	77	19
7	515	74	21
8	566	71	24
9	615	68	26
10	662	66	28
11	707	64	29
12	752	63	31
13	795	61	33
14	837	60	35
15	879	59	37
16	919	57	38
17	959	56	40
18	998	55	42
19	1037	55	43
20	1075	54	45
21	1112	53	46
22	1149	52	48
23	1185	52	49
24	1221	51	51
25	1256	50	52
26	1291	50	54
27	1326	49	55
28	1360	49	57
29	1394	48	58
30	1427	48	59
35	1590	45	66
40	1746	44	73
45	1896	42	79
50	2041	41	85
55	2182	40	91
60	2319	39	97
70	2583	37	108
80	2836	35	118
90	3080	34	128
100	3316	33	138

From Haskins SC: A simple fluid therapy planning guide, Semin Vet Med Surg (Small Anim) 3:232, 1988.
*132 kcal/kg$^{0.75}$; Nutritional requirements of the dog, *National Research Council*, 1985, Bethesda, MD.

TABLE 14-2 Daily Water and Calorie Requirements for the Cat*

Body Weight (kg)	Total kcal/day or Water mL/day	/kg	/hr
1.0	80	80	3
1.5	108	72	5
2.0	135	67	6
2.5	159	64	7
3.0	182	61	8
3.5	205	58	9
4.0	226	57	9
4.5	247	55	10
5.0	268	53	11

From Haskins SC: A simple fluid therapy planning guide, Semin Vet Med Surg (Small Anim) 3:232, 1988.
*80 kcal/kg$^{0.75}$; Nutritional requirements of the cat, *National Research Council*, 1987, Bethesda, MD.

muscle mass and fluid loss. An anorexic animal may lose 0.1 to 0.3 kg of body weight per day per 1000 kcal energy requirement.[13] Losses in excess of this amount indicate fluid loss. Another factor that must be considered in evaluating body weight is the possibility of third-space loss. Fluid lost into a third space does not decrease body weight.[23]

LABORATORY FINDINGS

The hematocrit or packed cell volume (PCV), total plasma protein concentration (TPP), and urine specific gravity (USG) are simple laboratory tests that can aid in the evaluation of hydration. It is important to obtain these values before initiating fluid therapy. The PCV and TPP should be evaluated together to minimize errors in interpretation. The PCV and TPP increase with all types of fluid losses excluding hemorrhage, whereas serum sodium concentration increases, decreases, or remains unchanged depending on the loss (e.g., hypotonic, hypertonic, isotonic). The effects of the different types of dehydration on the serum sodium concentration are discussed in Chapter 3. Table 14-5 shows possible interpretations of various combinations of PCV and TPP values. The PCV alone may be an unreliable indicator of hemoconcentration in water-deprived dogs, and although TPP increases, test results may not be above the upper limit of the normal range.[19] In one study of dogs and cats admitted to an intensive care unit, baseline measurements of PCV and TPP were not abnormally high in animals judged clinically to be dehydrated, and fluid therapy with crystalloids in dogs had no significant effect on PCV, although TPP decreased slightly.[18] The USG before fluid therapy is helpful in the preliminary evaluation of renal function. USG should be high (>1.045)

Despite conventional reasoning, clinician estimates of hydration in dogs and cats admitted to a veterinary teaching hospital intensive care unit did not reliably predict changes in weight after 24 to 48 hours of fluid therapy.[18] Loss of weight in chronic diseases includes loss of

TABLE 14-3 Potential Fluid, Electrolyte, and Acid-Base Disturbances in Various Diseases and Suggested Crystalloid Solutions

Abnormality	Type of Dehydration	Electrolyte Balance	Acid-Base Status	Fluid Therapy
Simple dehydration, stress, exercise	Hypertonic	—	—	Half strength or balanced electrolyte solution; 5% dextrose solution
Heat stroke	Hypertonic	K⁺ variable, Na⁺ variable	Metabolic acidosis	Half strength electrolyte solution followed by balanced electrolyte solution
Anorexia	Isotonic	K⁺ loss	Mild metabolic acidosis	Balanced electrolyte solution; KCl
Starvation	Isotonic	K⁺ loss	Mild metabolic acidosis	Half strength or balanced electrolyte solution; KCl; calories
Vomiting	Isotonic or hypertonic	Na⁺, K⁺, and Cl⁻ loss	Metabolic alkalosis; metabolic acidosis chronically	Ringer's solution; 0.9% saline with KCl supplementation
Diarrhea	Isotonic or hypertonic	Na⁺ loss, K⁺ loss chronically	Metabolic acidosis	Balanced electrolyte solution; HCO₃⁻; KCl (if chronic)
Diabetes mellitus	Hypertonic	K⁺ loss	Metabolic acidosis	Balanced electrolyte solutions; KCl
Hyperadrenocorticism	Isotonic	K⁺ loss	Occasionally mild metabolic alkalosis	Balanced electrolyte solutions; KCl
Hypoadrenocorticism	Isotonic or hypertonic	Na⁺ loss, K⁺ retention	Metabolic acidosis	0.9% saline followed by balanced electrolyte solutions
Urethral obstruction	Isotonic or hypertonic	K⁺ retention; Na⁺, Cl⁻ variable	Metabolic acidosis	0.9% saline followed by balanced electrolyte solutions; KCl postobstruction
Acute renal failure	Isotonic or hypertonic (with vomiting)	K⁺ retention; Na⁺, Cl⁻ variable	Metabolic acidosis	Balanced electrolyte solutions
Chronic renal failure	Isotonic or hypertonic (with vomiting)	Na⁺, K⁺, Cl⁻ variable	Metabolic acidosis	Balanced electrolyte solutions
Congestive heart failure	Plethoric (Na⁺, H₂O retention early; hypotonic chronically)	Na⁺ retention (but dilutional hyponatremia)	Metabolic acidosis (chronically)	5% dextrose solution
Hemorrhagic shock	Isotonic		Metabolic acidosis	Balanced electrolyte solutions; blood
Endotoxic shock	Isotonic		Metabolic acidosis	Balanced electrolyte solutions; 0.9% saline

From Muir WW, DiBartola SP: Fluid therapy. In Kirk RW, editor: Current veterinary therapy VIII. *Philadelphia, 1983, WB Saunders, p 31.*

in a dehydrated dog or cat if renal function is normal. This may not be true if other disorders affecting renal concentrating ability, such as medullary washout of solute, are present. Furthermore, previous administration of corticosteroids or furosemide can decrease urinary concentrating ability. After fluid therapy has been initiated, USG falls into the isosthenuric range if rehydration has been achieved.

CAN THE PATIENT CONSUME AN ADEQUATE VOLUME OF WATER TO SUSTAIN NORMAL FLUID BALANCE?

Hospitalized patients that have been volume resuscitated and rehydrated may not have recovered to the extent that appetite and ability to consume water have returned to

TABLE 14-4 Physical Findings in Dehydration

Percent Dehydration	Clinical Signs
<5	Not detectable
5-6	Subtle loss of skin elasticity
6-8	Definite delay in return of skin to normal position
	Slight prolongation of capillary refill time
	Eyes possibly sunken in orbits
	Possibly dry mucous membranes
10-12	Tented skin stands in place
	Definite prolongation of capillary refill time
	Eyes sunken in orbits
	Dry mucous membranes
	Possibly signs of shock (tachycardia, cool extremities, rapid and weak pulses)
12-15	Definite signs of shock
	Death imminent

From Muir WW, DiBartola SP: Fluid therapy. In Kirk RW, editor: Current veterinary therapy VIII, Philadelphia, 1983, WB Saunders, p 33.

normal. Such patients require administration of adequate amounts of fluid to meet their needs. The needs of partially or completely anorexic hospitalized dogs and cats are not well understood. Most predictions about maintenance fluid requirements are extrapolated from studies of normal nonanorexic animals. Absorption of nutrients into the bloodstream and their subsequent metabolism produces solutes that must be excreted in urine. Sensible fluid losses and urine production are decreased during fasting in normal animals because less solute requires excretion. Thus the maintenance fluid requirements of partially or completely anorexic patients are difficult to predict. Typically fluids are administered to veterinary patients in volumes predicated on the needs of animals that are not anorexic. Careful observation of urine production in such patients is warranted. If the patient is expected to have normal urinary concentrating ability and is urinating large volumes of dilute urine frequently, excessive fluid administration may be a contributing factor. Careful reduction of fluid administration and subsequent observation are warranted in such patients.

WHAT TYPE OF FLUID SHOULD BE GIVEN?

A fluid is said to be **balanced** if its composition resembles that of extracellular fluid (ECF; e.g., lactated Ringer's solution, Normosol-R [Abbott Laboratories, Abbott Park, IL], Plasma-Lyte 148 [Baxter Healthcare, Deerfield, IL]) and **unbalanced** if it does not (e.g., normal saline). Fluid preparations may be further classified as crystalloids or colloids. **Crystalloids** are solutions containing electrolyte and nonelectrolyte solutes capable of entering all body fluid compartments (e.g., 5% dextrose, 0.9% saline, lactated Ringer's solution). Crystalloids exert their effects primarily on the interstitial and intracellular compartments. **Colloids** are large-molecular-weight substances that are restricted to the plasma compartment in patients with an uncompromised intact endothelium and include plasma, dextrans, hydroxyethyl starch

TABLE 14-5 Interpretation of Hematocrit and Total Plasma Protein Concentrations

PCV (%)	Total Plasma Proteins (g/dL)	Interpretation
Increased	Increased	Dehydration
Increased	Normal or decreased	Splenic contraction
		Polycythemia
		Dehydration with preexisting hypoproteinemia
Normal	Increased	Normal hydration with hyperproteinemia
		Anemia with dehydration
Decreased	Increased	Anemia with dehydration
		Anemia with preexisting hyperproteinemia
Decreased	Normal	Nonblood loss anemia with normal hydration
Normal	Normal	Normal hydration
		Dehydration with preexisting anemia and hypoproteinemia
		Acute hemorrhage
		Dehydration with secondary compartment shift
Decreased	Decreased	Blood loss
		Anemia and hypoproteinemia
		Overhydration

From Muir WW, DiBartola SP: Fluid therapy. In Kirk RW, editor: Current veterinary therapy VIII, Philadelphia, 1983, WB Saunders, p 34.

(hetastarch), and hemoglobin-based oxygen-carrying (HBOC) fluids (e.g., Oxyglobin, Biopure Corporation, Cambridge, MA). Colloids exert their primary effect on the intravascular compartment.

Some types of colloids may be used in patients with shock and in those with severe hypoalbuminemia (i.e., albumin < 1.5 g/dL). A major limitation to the use of plasma as a colloid is the rapid disappearance of albumin from the vascular space. Dextran 70 is a polymer of glucose that has an average molecular weight of 70,000. Its use in humans has been associated with coagulopathies. Hetastarch has an average molecular weight of 480,000. In humans, coagulopathies also have been associated with the use of hetastarch but typically only when standard dosage recommendations have been exceeded. The main advantages of colloids are that more of the administered solution remains in the plasma compartment and there generally is thought to be less risk of edema in patients with an intact endothelium. Colloids are discussed in detail in Chapter 27.

Crystalloid solutions are equally effective in expanding the plasma compartment, but 2.5 to 3.0 times as much crystalloid solution must be given (compared with a colloid solution) because the crystalloid is distributed to other sites (e.g., interstitial compartment, intracellular compartment).[26,27,39] Pulmonary capillaries normally are more permeable to protein, resulting in a higher interstitial concentration of protein and more resistance to leakage of fluid from capillaries.[30] Peripheral edema is more likely to occur after crystalloid administration because muscle and subcutaneous capillaries are less permeable to protein.

Crystalloid solutions also can be classified as **replacement** or **maintenance** solutions. The composition of **replacement solutions** (e.g., lactated Ringer's, Normosol-R, Plasma-Lyte 148) resembles that of ECF (Fig. 14-2). **Maintenance solutions** (e.g., Normosol-M, Plasma-Lyte 56) contain less sodium (40 to 60 mEq/L) and more potassium (15 to 30 mEq/L) than replacement fluids. A simple maintenance solution can be formulated by mixing one part 0.9% NaCl with two parts 5% dextrose and adding 20 mEq KCl per liter of final solution. The approximate composition of such a fluid would be 51 mEq/L sodium, 20 mEq/L potassium, 71 mEq/L chloride, and 33.5 g/L dextrose. It would provide 133 kcal/L and have an osmolality of 328 mOsm/kg. An alternative maintenance solution may be made by mixing one part lactated Ringer's solution with two parts 5% dextrose and adding 20 mEq KCl per liter of final solution. This solution has the following approximate composition: 43 mEq/L sodium, 21 mEq/L potassium, 56 mEq/L chloride, 1 mEq/L calcium, 9 mEq/L lactate, and 33.5 g/L dextrose. It would provide 133 kcal/L and have an osmolality of 317 mOsm/kg.

Another commonly used crystalloid is 5% dextrose. Administering 5% dextrose is equivalent to giving water because the glucose is oxidized to CO_2 and water. In fact, the main reason for giving 5% dextrose is to correct a pure water deficit. Except in very small animals, administration of 5% dextrose cannot be relied on to maintain daily caloric needs because 5% dextrose contains only 200 kcal/L. Consider a normal, active 10-kg dog. Its

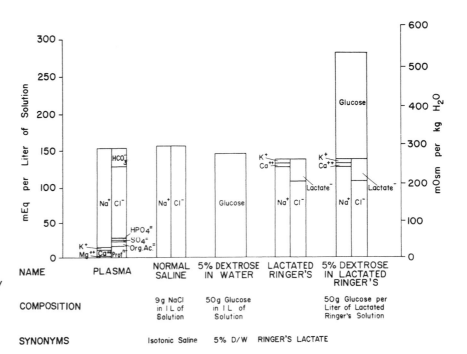

Fig. 14-2 Comparison of electrolyte composition of plasma with that of commonly used crystalloid solutions. (From Muir WW, DiBartola SP: Fluid therapy. In Kirk RW, editor: *Current veterinary therapy VIII,* Philadelphia, 1983, WB Saunders, p. 30.)

maintenance energy requirement (MER) is approximately 740 kcal:

$$\text{MER (kcal)} = 60 \times \text{body weight (kg)} + 140$$

To provide this number of kilocalories from 5% dextrose (200 kcal/L), almost 4 L of fluid must be administered per day. Such a volume is almost seven times more than the daily maintenance requirement for fluid in this dog. Administration of 4 L of 5% dextrose over a 24-hour period would initiate a diuresis that would impair utilization of the administered dextrose and cause increased urinary losses of electrolytes.

The veterinary practitioner can manage most animals requiring fluid therapy with a limited number of crystalloid and additive solutions. The most useful crystalloid solutions for routine use are a balanced replacement solution (e.g., lactated Ringer's solution, Normosol-R, Plasma-Lyte 148), 0.9% saline, and 5% dextrose in water. The solute composition of these fluids is compared with that of ECF in Fig. 14-2, and the electrolyte composition of several commercially available solutions is summarized in Table 14-6.

Supplementation of crystalloid solutions with KCl may be necessary when body fluid losses have included large amounts of potassium. An empirical scale has been devised to estimate the amount of potassium to add to parenterally administered fluids (Table 14-7).[17] This protocol has not been evaluated experimentally in dogs or cats but has been used successfully in clinical veterinary patients during the past 30 years. Potassium supplementation is discussed in Chapter 5.

Other additive solutions include 50% dextrose, calcium chloride, calcium gluconate, potassium phosphate, 8.4% sodium bicarbonate, and water-soluble B vitamins. Thiamine supplementation may be particularly important in cats because their requirement for this vitamin may be higher than that of dogs. Phosphate rarely is used as an additive but often is required in patients with diabetic ketoacidosis during insulin therapy.[40] Phosphate supplementation is discussed in Chapter 7. Theoretically, sodium bicarbonate should not be added to solutions containing calcium (e.g., lactated Ringer's solution, Plasmalyte-R) because of the risk of forming insoluble calcium carbonate crystals. Despite this concern, no adverse consequences have been observed when small amounts of sodium bicarbonate have been added to lactated Ringer's solution.[22,23]

When additives are used, the clinician must keep in mind that the final osmolality of the fluid may be higher than anticipated. The final osmolality may be approximated by adding the number of milliequivalents per liter of electrolyte and millimoles per liter of nonelectrolyte solutes found in the solution. The final osmolality of the solution also may differ depending on how the solution was formulated. For example, if 500 mL of lactated Ringer's solution is mixed with 500 mL of 5% dextrose to create a replacement solution with 2.5% dextrose, the resulting solution has an approximate osmolality of 275 mOsm/kg (virtually the same as that of lactated Ringer's solution). Conversely, if 50 mL of 50% dextrose is added to 1 L of lactated Ringer's solution, the resulting solution contains 2.5% dextrose but has an approximate osmolality of 391 mOsm/kg, which is substantially higher.

The choice of fluid to administer is dependent on the nature of the disease process and the composition of the fluid lost. Underlying acid-base and electrolyte disturbances should be taken into consideration when choosing the type of fluid to administer. The clinician should attempt to replace losses with a fluid that is similar in volume and electrolyte composition to that which has been lost from the body (see Table 14-3). If clinical assessment of the patient suggests a fluid-responsive type of shock, the resuscitation phase of fluid therapy should be instituted. If the patient has abnormally low oncotic pressure or an underlying disease condition for which a low-volume resuscitation strategy may prove advantageous, synthetic colloids should be considered as the primary fluid choice for resuscitation (see Chapters 23 and 27). If neither of these considerations applies, resuscitation with a balanced crystalloid solution is indicated. If there are no clinical signs of hypovolemia, the hydration deficit and maintenance needs may be combined and administered during the next 24 hours.

Persistent vomiting caused by pyloric obstruction would be expected to result in losses of hydrochloric acid, potassium, sodium, and water, potentially producing hypokalemia, hypochloremia, and metabolic alkalosis. The initial fluid of choice in this setting is 0.9% NaCl with 20 to 30 mEq KCl per liter. Except in the case of vomiting of stomach contents, lactated Ringer's is a good first choice for fluid therapy while awaiting laboratory results. Normal saline (0.9% NaCl) is less ideal because it is not a balanced solution. It contains chloride in greater concentration than body fluids (154 mEq/L versus 110 mEq/L in dogs and 120 mEq/L in cats), and as a result of displacement of bicarbonate with chloride in ECF and initiation of natriuresis, it has a mild acidifying effect.[32] Examples of fluid therapy in specific diseases are listed in Table 14-3.

In one study, five different solutions were administered to unanesthetized dogs during a 1-hour period: 0.9% NaCl, 0.9% NaCl with 5% dextrose, lactated Ringer's solution, Normosol-R, and Normosol-R with 2% dextran.[32] The approximate composition of these fluids is presented in Table 14-8. The fluids were warmed to body temperature, and no decreases in rectal temperature were observed. Laboratory variables were measured after 1 hour of infusion. Fluids were administered at 76 mL/kg/hr except for Normosol-R with dextran, which was administered at a rate of 31.5 mL/kg/hr.

Most of the fluids increased heart rate, diastolic arterial pressure, and central venous pressure (CVP), and all

TABLE 14-6 Electrolyte Composition of Commercially Available Fluids

Fluid	Glucose* (g/L)	Na+ (mEq/L)	Cl- (mEq/L)	K+ (mEq/L)	Ca2+ (mEq/L)	Mg2+ (mEq/L)	Buffer† (mEq/L)	Osmolarity (mOsm/L)	Cal/L	pH
				Dextrose and Electrolyte Solution Composition						
5% dextrose	50	0	0	0	0	0	0	252	170	4.0
10% dextrose	100	0	0	0	0	0	0	505	340	4.0
2.5% dextrose in 0.45% NaCl	25	77	77	0	0	0	0	280	85	4.5
5% dextrose in 0.45% NaCl	50	77	77	0	0	0	0	406	170	4.0
5% dextrose in 0.9% NaCl	50	154	154	0	0	0	0	560	170	4.0
0.45% NaCl	0	77	77	0	0	0	0	154	0	5.0
0.9% NaCl	0	154	154	0	0	0	0	308	0	5.0
3% NaCl	0	513	513	0	0	0	0	1026	0	5.0
Ringer's solution	0	147.5	156	4	4.5	0	0	310	0	5.5
Ringer's lactated solution	0	130	109	4	3	0	28 (L)	272	9	6.5
2.5% dextrose in Ringer's lactated solution	25	130	109	4	3	0	28 (L)	398	94	5.0
5% dextrose in Ringer's lactated solution	50	130	109	4	3	0	28 (L)	524	179	5.0
2.5% dextrose in half-strength Ringer's lactated solution	25	65.5	55	2	1.5	0	14 (L)	263	89	5.0
Normosol-M in 5% dextrose‡	50	40	40	13	0	3	16 (A)	364	175	5.5
Normosol-R‡	0	140	98	5	0	3	27 (A) 23 (G)	296	18	6.4
Plasma-Lyte§	0	140	103	10	5	3	47 (A) 8 (L)	312	17	5.5
Plasma-Lyte M in 5% dextrose§	50	40	40	16	5	3	12 (A) 12 (L)	376	178	5.5
Plasma	1	145	105	5	5	3	24 (B)	300	—	7.4
				Additives and Special Solutions						
20% mannitol	200 (M)	0	0	0	0	0	0	1099	0	
7.5% NaHCO3	0	893	0	0	0	0	893	1786	0	
8.4% NaHCO3	0	1000	0	0	0	0	1000 (B)	2000	0	
10% CaCl2	0	0	2720	0	1360	0	0	4080	0	
14.9% KCl	0	0	2000	2000	0	0	0	4000	0	
50% dextrose	500	0	0	0	0	0	0	2780	1700	4.2

From Chew DJ, DiBartola SP: Manual of Small Animal Nephrology and Urology. New York, 1986 Churchill-Livingstone, p. 308.

All glucose, with one exception: M, mannitol.

†Buffers used: A, acetate; B, bicarbonate; G, gluconate; L, lactate.

‡CEVA Laboratories. Overland Park, KS.

§Travenol Laboratories, Deerfield, IL.

TABLE 14-7 Sliding Scale for Potassium Supplementation

Serum Potassium (mEq/L)	mEq KCl to Add to 250 mL Fluid	Maximal Fluid Infusion Rate* (mL/kg/hr)
<2.0	20	6
2.1-2.5	15	8
2.6-3.0	10	12
3.1-3.5	7	16

From Muir WW, DiBartola SP: Fluid therapy. In Kirk RW, editor: Current veterinary therapy VIII, Philadelphia, 1983, WB Saunders, p 38.
So as not to exceed 0.5 mEq/kg/hr.

of them decreased hematocrit, hemoglobin, and total protein concentrations by 21% to 25%. All solutions except for Normosol-R and Normosol-R with 2% dextran caused an increase in serum chloride concentration, and the saline solutions decreased pH and bicarbonate concentration. All solutions except Normosol-R caused a decrease in serum potassium concentration. The causes of the decreased serum potassium concentrations in these dogs presumably included dilution and increased distal tubular flow rate with enhanced urinary excretion of potassium. The presence of 5% dextrose in two of the solutions resulted in significantly lower serum potassium concentrations, suggesting movement of potassium into cells with glucose.

Serum sodium concentrations were similar despite differences in the sodium concentrations of the various fluids, demonstrating effective natriuresis in normal dogs receiving sodium-containing crystalloid solutions. Serum chloride concentration increased with administration of the saline solutions containing 154 mEq/L chloride, and mild metabolic acidosis developed. Serum chloride concentration also increased slightly with administration of lactated Ringer's solution (112 mEq/L chloride), but there was no change in acid-base balance. The increased serum chloride concentration and alterations in acid-base balance could have resulted from decreased reabsorption of bicarbonate with sodium in the kidney during natriuresis and decreased strong ion difference.[37,38] Expansion acidosis is an unlikely explanation because all fluids administered presumably expanded the ECF volume.

Anions such as acetate, gluconate, and lactate are added to crystalloid solutions as a source of base because their oxidative metabolism in the body yields bicarbonate. The alkalinizing effect of the metabolism of these anions and that of citrate is as follows:

Acetate
$$NaC_2H_3O_2 + 2O_2 \rightarrow CO_2 + H_2O + Na^+HCO_3^-$$

Citrate
$$K_3C_6H_5O_7 + 4\tfrac{1}{2}O_2 \rightarrow 3CO_2 + H_2O + 3K^+HCO_3^-$$
Gluconate
$$NaC_6H_{11}O_7 + 5\tfrac{1}{2}O_2 \rightarrow 5CO_2 + 5H_2O + Na^+HCO_3^-$$
Lactate
$$NaC_3H_5O_3 + 3O_2 \rightarrow 2CO_2 + 2H_2O + Na^+HCO_3^-$$

Most lactate is produced in muscle and gut and metabolized to either glucose (via cytosolic gluconeogenesis) or CO_2 and water (via mitochondrial oxidation) in the liver. Normally, gluconeogenesis predominates. Acetate is metabolized primarily in muscle. The alkalinizing effect of these anions is delayed because of the requirement for metabolism. In one study, equivalent doses of acetate, bicarbonate, and lactate had similar alkalinizing effects in anesthetized dogs 45 minutes after infusion.[21] The effect of bicarbonate occurred earliest because metabolism was not necessary.

Lactate originally was introduced for the treatment of acidosis because of technical difficulties in preparation of bicarbonate solutions suitable for intravenous use.[5,36] These technical difficulties have been overcome, but crystalloid solutions containing lactate as a source of base (e.g., lactated Ringer's solution) still are widely used for fluid therapy in clinical practice. Most patients treated with lactate-containing replacement solutions respond well, probably as a result of ECF volume expansion and improved tissue perfusion.

Whether it is converted to glucose or oxidized to CO_2 and water, the metabolism of lactate consumes hydrogen ions and has an alkalinizing effect:

Gluconeogenesis
$$2CH_3CHOHCOO^- + 2H^+ \rightarrow C_6H_{12}O_6$$
Oxidative metabolism
$$CH_3CHOHCOO^- + H^+ + 3O_2 \rightarrow 3CO_2 + 3H_2O$$

There has been some concern that lactate in lactated Ringer's solution may be harmful to patients with poor tissue perfusion and severe metabolic acidosis (pH, <7.1 to 7.2). Administration of lactate as a salt cannot contribute directly to metabolic acidosis. Rather, the ability of the liver to metabolize lactate and the potentially detrimental effect of lactate on myocardial contractility have been debated. During severe hypoxia, increased lactate production in gut and muscle and decreased hepatic extraction of lactate led to progressive lactic acidosis. In moderate metabolic acidosis, administration of lactated Ringer's solution probably is beneficial because any tendency toward lactate accumulation is likely to be offset by improved hepatic perfusion and oxygen delivery as a result of ECF volume expansion.

Newer commercially available balanced crystalloid solutions contain approximately twice the amount of

TABLE 14-8 Composition of Fluids Administered to Awake Dogs

Solution	Na (mmol/L)	K (mmol/L)	Ca (mmol/L)	Mg (mmol/L)	Cl (mmol/L)	Lactate (mmol/L)	Acetate (mmol/L)	Gluconate (mmol/L)	Glucose (mmol/L)	pH
0.9% sodium chloride	154				154					5.4
0.9% sodium chloride plus 5% dextrose	154				154				277.5	4.2
Hartmann's solution*	131	5	2		112	28				6.3
Normosol-R	140	5		1.5	98		27	23		5.7
Normosol-R plus 2% dextran	140	5		1.5	98		27	23		6.4

From Rose RJ: Some physiological and biochemical effects of the intravenous administration of five different electrolyte solutions in the dog, J Vet Pharmacol Ther 2:281, 1979.
Lactated Ringer's solution.

bicarbonate precursors when compared with lactated Ringer's solution. As a result, these solutions generally are thought to be more efficient than lactated Ringer's solution in treatment of metabolic acidosis, provided that metabolic conversion of the precursors to bicarbonate occurs quickly. There is some concern that such fluids may contribute to the development of metabolic alkalosis, but this does not occur in animals with relatively normal renal function because the kidneys can efficiently excrete the excess bicarbonate.

Crystalloid solutions with preservatives must be avoided in cats. Benzoic acid derivatives (e.g., benzyl alcohol, methylparaben, propylparaben, ethylparaben) have been added to some solutions for their antimicrobial effect. Clinical signs in cats receiving fluids with such preservatives have included behavioral changes, hypersalivation, ataxia, muscle fasciculations, seizures, dilated nonresponsive pupils, coma, and death.[3,9,33] Young cats may be at increased risk for these complications.

BY WHAT ROUTE SHOULD FLUIDS BE GIVEN?

The route of fluid therapy depends on the nature of the clinical disorder, its severity, and its duration.

INTRAVENOUS

The intravenous route is preferred when the patient is very ill, when there has been severe fluid loss, or when the fluid loss has been acute. This route also is used during anesthesia to maintain renal perfusion and vascular access for emergencies. The intravenous route provides rapid dispersion of water and electrolytes and allows precise dosage. A large volume can be given rapidly, and hypertonic fluids can be given safely via a large vein. This route requires vascular access and close monitoring during infusion to avoid complications such as overhydration, infection, thrombosis, phlebitis, embolism, and impaired fluid delivery (e.g., obstruction of the catheter by a change in the patient's limb position).

The veins available for vascular access include the jugular, cephalic, lateral saphenous, and femoral veins. There are advantages and disadvantages of each, but the jugular vein is most useful because it allows delivery of large volumes, administration of hypertonic or potentially irritating solutions, measurement of CVP, and repeated venous blood sampling. The cephalic vein also is commonly used, but fluid delivery can be hindered by flexion of the elbow, and extremely hypertonic or irritating solutions should not be used. Intravenous catheter function and the catheter-skin interface should be monitored routinely to detect complications. Catheters that remain clean and free of complications need not be replaced at some routine interval. The types of catheters used and their placement are discussed in Chapter 15.

SUBCUTANEOUS

The subcutaneous route is convenient for maintenance fluid therapy in small dogs and cats. The subcutaneous space in dogs and cats can accommodate relatively large volumes of fluid, and potassium can be used in concentrations up to 30 to 35 mEq/L without irritation.[13] Approximately 10 mL/kg or 50 to 200 mL may be administered per site.[34] Fluid is administered under the skin along the back from the area of the scapulae to the lumbar region. Volume overload is unlikely to occur when fluids are administered subcutaneously in patients with no underlying cardiac insufficiency. Furthermore, some owners can use subcutaneous administration to give fluids at home to animals with chronic disease problems (e.g., chronic renal failure).

The subcutaneous route is not adequate for patients with acute and severe losses (e.g., shock) and is not recommended for extremely dehydrated or hypothermic animals because peripheral vasoconstriction may reduce absorption and dispersion of the administered fluid in these settings. The volume that may be given is limited by skin elasticity, and this route is not useful in larger animals requiring large volumes of fluids. Irritating or hypertonic solutions must not be used subcutaneously; only isotonic fluids are recommended. Isotonic fluids containing bicarbonate precursors other than lactate also are not recommended for subcutaneous administration. Although not harmful, they appear to cause mild local discomfort and are not well tolerated by veterinary patients. The subcutaneous administration of 5% dextrose in water should be avoided because equilibration of ECF with a pool of electrolyte-free solution may lead to temporary aggravation of electrolyte imbalance.

ORAL

The oral route is most physiologic, and fluids with a wide variety of compositions may be given. Oral fluid therapy is useful for administering hypertonic fluids with high caloric density. Fluid can be administered rapidly with minimal adverse effects, and caloric needs can be met. However, this route should not be used in the presence of gastrointestinal dysfunction (e.g., vomiting, diarrhea). The oral route also is inadequate in animals that have had acute or extensive fluid losses because dispersion and utilization of the administered fluid and electrolytes are not sufficiently rapid. In anorexic animals without vomiting or diarrhea, fluid can be administered orally using a number of different techniques (e.g., nasogastric tube, esophagostomy tube, gastrostomy tube).

INTRAPERITONEAL

Intraperitoneal administration of fluid allows moderately rapid absorption of large volumes. Only isotonic fluids can be used because administration of hypertonic fluids results in further contraction of the extracellular compartment as water enters the peritoneal space by osmosis. Peritonitis also is a potential complication of this route. The intraperitoneal route is not used commonly except to perform peritoneal dialysis as described in Chapter 28.

INTRAOSSEOUS (INTRAMEDULLARY)

The intraosseous, or intramedullary, route is useful in very young or small animals in which venous access is difficult. The procedure has been available for many years[6] and has received renewed attention.[14,16,29] This route provides rapid vascular access via bone marrow sinusoids and medullary venous channels and allows rapid dispersion of fluid. The bone marrow does not collapse when the patient is hypovolemic, and access to the marrow is simple. For some clinicians, this technique may be accomplished more rapidly than performing a venous cutdown. Sites that can be used for intraosseous administration of fluid include the tibial tuberosity, trochanteric fossa of the femur, wing of the ilium, and greater tubercle of the humerus. The periosteum should be anesthetized by infiltration with 1% lidocaine solution to avoid pain during needle placement. The potential risks include osteomyelitis and pain on administration of fluid. However, pain was not observed clinically in two studies.[16,29]

HOW FAST MAY FLUIDS BE GIVEN?

Poiseuille's law governs the flow of fluids through a catheter:

$$\text{Flow} = \frac{\pi(P_1 - P_2)r^4}{8\eta L}$$

where $P_1 - P_2$ represents the pressure differential on the fluid, η is the viscosity of the fluid, r is the radius of the catheter, and L is the length of the catheter. Thus the diameter of the catheter is of primary importance in establishing a rapid rate of flow. The choice of catheter length sometimes is affected by factors other than flow rate (e.g., use of jugular catheters to monitor CVP). In a study of gravity flow of lactated Ringer's solution, in vivo flow rates averaged 7% less than in vitro flow rates, presumably because of tissue pressure.[15] Fluid flow rate increased by 50% when the pressure differential was increased by raising the fluid bag from 0.91 to 1.75 m. Flow rate increased linearly with increasing catheter radius rather than geometrically as predicted by Poiseuille's law.

The rate of fluid administration is dictated by the magnitude and rapidity of the fluid loss. The patient with fluid-responsive shock syndrome requires aggressive fluid administration. Fluid administration rates may vary, depending on the type of fluid or combination of types that has been chosen. One approach is to calculate a "shock fluid dose" and administer it as rapidly as possible in divided aliquots until a stable and sustainable cardiovascular endpoint has been achieved (see Chapter 23). Clinical evaluation of the patient should occur after administration of each aliquot using a "titrate to effect" approach. The shock dosage of synthetic colloids is 20 mL/kg for dogs and 10 to 15 mL/kg for cats. The shock dosage of isotonic crystalloids is 80 to 90 mL/kg for dogs and 40 to 60 mL/kg for cats. In experimental studies, crystalloid fluids administered at 90 mL/kg/hr did not cause pulmonary edema in normal dogs and cats.[4,8]

Anesthetized cats receiving lactated Ringer's solution at a rate of 225 mL/kg for 1 hour developed serous nasal discharge, chemosis, ascites, diarrhea, and fluid exudation from catheter sites. At necropsy, these cats had ascites, pancreatic edema, and accumulation of free fluid in the trachea. Body temperature decreased and CVP and left atrial pressure increased in cats receiving 225 mL/kg/hr, whereas hematocrit, total protein concentration, and colloidal osmotic pressure decreased in cats receiving both 90 and 225 mL/kg/hr.[4]

Lactated Ringer's solution was administered to unanesthetized, dehydrated dogs at rates of 90, 225, and 360 mL/kg for 1 hour.[8] At rates of 90 and 225 mL/kg/hr, some dogs had serous nasal discharge, mild coughing, and slight chemosis. At 360 mL/kg/hr, marked serous nasal discharge, restlessness, coughing, dyspnea, pulmonary crackles, ascites, polyuria, chemosis, protrusion of eyes, and diarrhea were observed. These signs resolved when fluid administration was discontinued. Hematocrit, TPP, and serum potassium concentration decreased during fluid administration. In this study, body temperature decreased despite the fact that fluids were warmed to 37° C. Serum sodium concentration remained unchanged, but pulse rate, respiratory rate, and systemic arterial pressure increased slightly. Pulmonary capillary wedge pressure (PWP) and CVP increased, and these measurements correlated well with one another. It was concluded that lactated Ringer's solution at 90 mL/kg/hr was tolerated safely. CVP should be monitored if fluids must be administered at rates in excess of 90 mL/kg/hr.

Contemporary losses must also be considered when adjusting the rate of fluid administration. Severe ongoing losses (e.g., vomiting and diarrhea in a patient with acute gastroenteritis) may necessitate rapid administration to keep pace with contemporary fluid loss. When fluids are given rapidly, it is necessary to monitor cardiovascular and renal function.

It usually is not necessary or desirable to replace the hydration deficit rapidly in chronic disease states. Instead, the hydration deficit may be calculated, the daily maintenance requirement of fluid added to this amount, and the total volume administered over 24 hours.[35] Ongoing or contemporary losses also must be considered and taken into consideration when estimating the patient's fluid requirements for a 24-hour period. This approach allows adequate time for equilibration of fluid and electrolytes with the intracellular compartment and avoids potential complications (e.g., edema or effusion related to increased hydrostatic pressure, diuresis, and loss of administered electrolytes in urine). It is the method most commonly used for medical patients at the Ohio State University Veterinary Teaching Hospital.

Whenever possible, intravascular volume deficits should be replaced before anesthesia and surgery. Ideally, such patients also should be rehydrated depending on the urgency of their underlying condition. During induction and maintenance of anesthesia, prevention of hypovolemia and maintenance of renal perfusion are essential. Induction of diuresis in this setting may be an important factor in prevention of intraoperative acute renal failure. A basal fluid administration rate of 5 to 10 mL/kg/hr is recommended during anesthesia and surgery. During major surgery (e.g., exploratory laparotomy, thoracotomy), fluid administration at twice this basal rate is recommended. Fluid therapy during anesthesia and surgery is discussed in more detail in Chapter 17.

Most administration sets designed for adult human patients deliver 10 to 20 drops/mL, whereas pediatric administration sets deliver 60 drops/mL.[35] This information is used to calculate the drip rate:

Adult administration set:

$$mL/hr \times 1\ hr/60\ min \times 10\ drops/mL$$

or

$$(mL/hr)/6 = drops/min$$

Pediatric administration set:

$$mL/hr \times 1\ hr/60\ min \times 60\ drops/mL$$

or

$$mL/hr = drops/min$$

Fluid orders should be written so that the volume to be administered is recorded as mL/day, mL/hr, and drops/min. This allows personnel to detect errors in calculations. The clinician should not assume that the animal has received the volume of fluid ordered, and the volume actually received should be noted in the record by nursing personnel. All additives should be clearly listed on the bottle, and adhesive labels for this purpose are available (Fig. 14-3). Infusion pumps are available for clinical use (e.g., Heska, Baxter) and provide a highly accurate record of the volume infused (Fig. 14-4). These pumps also have alarm systems that can alert personnel when flow is obstructed. The availability of affordable electronic fluid pumps has resulted in widespread incorporation of such equipment into veterinary practice. Although use of infusion pumps makes fluid administration safer and more accurate, the equipment must be

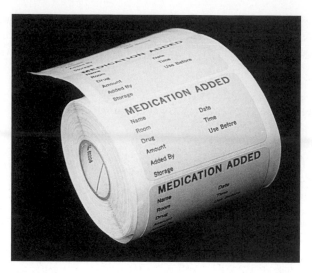

Fig. 14-3 Adhesive label for fluid additives. (From Chew DJ: Parenteral fluid therapy. In Sherding RG, editor: *The cat: diseases and clinical management,* New York, 1989, Churchill Livingstone, p. 50.)

used appropriately, maintained in good working order, and tested regularly for accuracy. Mistakes in fluid administration still can occur as a consequence of human error or equipment failure. For practices that do not routinely use electronic fluid pumps, several management practices may assist in accurately and safely delivering fluid therapy. A strip of adhesive tape can be attached to the bottle and marked appropriately to provide a quick visual estimate of the volume of fluid received (Fig. 14-5). In the Buretrol system (Baxter, Deerfield, IL), a reservoir allows a predetermined volume of fluid to be delivered over a given period (Fig. 14-6). This approach prevents infusion of excessive volumes of fluid to small animals. The technical aspects of fluid therapy are discussed in detail in Chapter 15.

HOW MUCH FLUID SHOULD BE GIVEN?

The purpose of fluid therapy is to increase tissue perfusion, repair fluid deficits, supply daily fluid needs, and replace ongoing losses. It has been emphasized: "the aim of therapy is not to administer fluids but to induce positive fluid balance."[31]

COMPONENTS OF FLUID THERAPY

The volume requirements of patients with fluid-responsive shock syndromes can vary widely. Ultimately, the goal of reestablishing widespread effective tissue perfusion should dictate the volume of fluid administered. In general, the same cardiovascular parameters used to characterize the patient's shock syndrome should return to normal or to the extent they are able to do so given the limitations of the patient's underlying disease

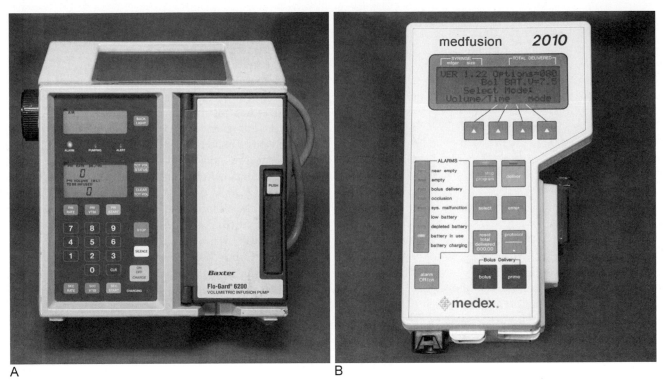

Fig. 14-4 A and **B,** Fluid infusion pumps. **A,** Baxter Flo-Gard 6200 Volumetric Infusion Pump (Baxter Health Care, Deerfield IL). **B,** Medex Medfusion 2010 Syringe Infusion Pump (Medex, Carlsbad CA).

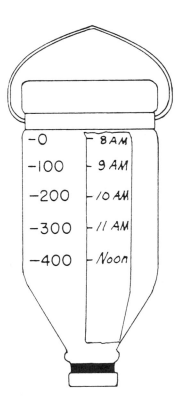

Fig. 14-5 Use of labeled adhesive tape to monitor rate of fluid administration. (From Chew DJ: Parenteral fluid therapy. In Sherding RG, editor: *The cat: diseases and clinical management,* New York, 1989, Churchill Livingstone, p. 54.)

condition. For example, a severely dehydrated dog with tachycardia, pale mucous membranes, prolonged capillary refill time, and hypotension should receive a volume of fluid sufficient to return these cardiovascular parameters to normal, and these parameters should not deviate from normal when the rate of fluid administration is decreased and rehydration of the patient begun. In patients not experiencing ongoing loss of fluids from the intravascular compartment or other more complex cardiovascular derangements, response to fluid resuscitation should be rapid and complete.

The initial assessment of hydration determines the volume of fluid needed to replace the **hydration deficit (replacement requirement).**[12,20] The hydration deficit is calculated as the percentage dehydration (estimated by physical examination) times the patient's body weight in kilograms. The resultant value is the fluid deficit in liters. During the rehydration phase of therapy, this volume is administered for 24 hours in conjunction with maintenance fluid requirements and replacement of ongoing or contemporary losses that are occurring.

Coincident with or after replacement of the animal's hydration deficit, the **maintenance fluid requirement** must be administered.[12,20] The maintenance fluid requirement is the volume needed per day to keep the animal in balance (i.e., no net change in body water). Daily fluid requirements (mL/kg/day) parallel energy requirements (kcal/kg/day).[20,22,23]

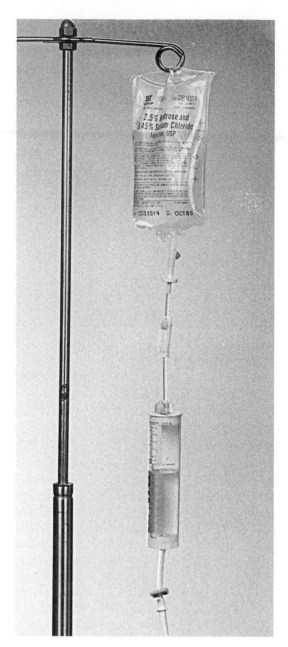

Fig. 14-6 Buretrol device. (From Chew DJ: Parenteral fluid therapy. In Sherding RG, editor: *The cat: diseases and clinical management,* New York, 1989, Churchill Livingstone, p. 53.)

The **basal energy requirement** (BER) is that of a resting animal in a thermoneutral environment 12 to 18 hours after eating.[24] In dogs, BER is not a linear function of body weight but rather is related to body surface area by the following equation[1]:

$$BER \ (kcal/day) = 97 \, W^{0.655}$$

where W is body weight in kilograms. This relationship is plotted in Fig. 14-7 so that BER may be determined from body weight.

The **maintenance energy requirement** (MER) is that of a moderately active adult animal in a nonthermoneutral environment. The MER in sedentary animals is approximately 1.5 to 2.0 BER.

In domestic cats, the relationship of basal heat production to body weight is almost linear because of the small size and relatively narrow normal range of body weight in this species.[25] Based on available data, BER in cats may be estimated as 50 to 60 kcal/kg/day. However, the question remains whether daily energy requirements approximate daily fluid requirements. Daily fluid requirements of anorexic dogs and cats in a hospital environment and the relationship of these fluid requirements to the daily urinary solute load are areas deserving future clinical study.

At the Ohio State University Veterinary Teaching Hospital, the maintenance fluid requirement for dogs and cats is determined from reference charts that use the above formulas to calculate accurate daily fluid requirements based on caloric needs. Although estimates of 40 to 60 mL/kg/day frequently are used to calculate maintenance fluid requirements, it is important to recognize that such estimates are only accurate for some veterinary patients. Cats, very small dogs, and very large dogs are not well served by the use of such estimates, and these patients likely will benefit from more accurate assessment of their fluid requirements. Approximately two thirds of the maintenance requirement represents **sensible** (i.e., easy to measure) losses of fluid (urine output), and one third represents **insensible** (i.e., difficult to measure) losses (primarily fecal and respiratory water loss). Thus daily maintenance for a 10-kg dog may be 600 mL, with 400 mL representing sensible loss and 200 mL representing insensible loss.

Some clinicians multiply maintenance fluid requirements by some factor between 1 and 3 to estimate a patient's 24-hour fluid needs. Assuming 60 mL/kg/day to represent the maintenance rate of fluid administration, the information in Table 14-9 can be used to quickly determine the implied hydration deficit and actual rate of fluid administration using this approach.

In addition to the hydration deficit (replacement requirement) and maintenance requirement, **contemporary (ongoing) losses** must be considered. These are not always easily determined or quantitated in small animals but can be very important in fluid therapy. An attempt should be made to estimate ongoing losses, which may include losses related to vomiting, diarrhea, polyuria, large wounds or burns, drains, peritoneal or pleural losses, panting, fever, and blood loss. During surgical procedures, careful attention should be given to the amount of blood lost, drying of exposed tissues, and effusions removed by suction. Blood lost at surgery should be estimated, and 3 mL of crystalloid solution should be administered for each milliliter of blood lost. Each 4 × 4-inch gauze sponge, when saturated with

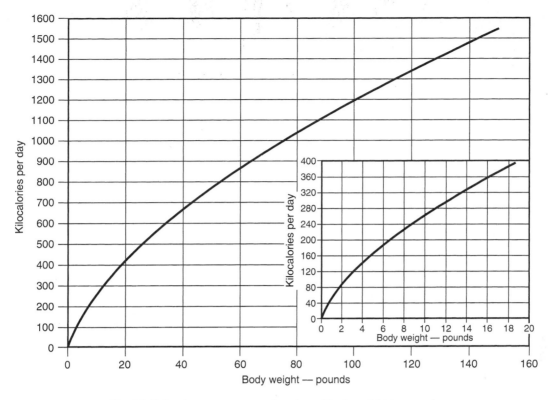

Fig. 14-7 Basal energy rate as a function of body weight in pounds.

blood, represents a blood loss of 15 mL.[28] Contemporary losses must be estimated and carefully replaced along with the maintenance volume of fluid. Box 14-1 summarizes the components of fluid therapy and their calculation.

FAILURE TO ACHIEVE REHYDRATION

Repeated assessment of the patient by observation of clinical signs and determinations of body weight, urine output, PCV, TPP, and USG is mandatory in making appropriate readjustments of fluid therapy. Reasons for

TABLE 14–9 Maintenance and Dehydration Fluid Volume Requirements*

Maintenance (M) + Dehydration (%)	mL/kg/day	Factor × Maintenance
M + 1	70	1.17
M + 2	80	1.33
M + 3	90	1.50
M + 4	100	1.67
M + 5	110	1.83
M + 6	120	2.00
M + 7	130	2.17
M + 8	140	2.33
M + 9	150	2.50
M + 10	160	2.67

From Chew DJ, Kohn CW, DiBartola SP: Disorders of fluid balance and fluid therapy. In Fenner WR, edition: Quick reference to veterinary medicine, ed. 2, Philadelphia, 1991, JB Lippincott, p. 570.
Maintenance defined as 60 mL/kg/day.

Box 14-1 Calculation of Replacement Requirement (Hydration Deficit)

1. Hydration deficit (replacement requirement)
   a. Body weight (lbs) × % dehydration as a decimal × 500* = deficit in milliliters
   b. Body weight (kg) × % dehydration as a decimal = deficit in liters
2. Maintenance requirement (40-60 mL/kg/day)
   a. Sensible losses (urine output): 27-40 mL/kg/day
   b. Insensible losses (fecal, cutaneous, respiratory): 13-20 mL/kg/day
3. Contemporary (ongoing) losses (e.g., vomiting, diarrhea, polyuria)

From Muir WW, DiBartola SP: Fluid therapy. In Kirk RW, editor: *Current veterinary therapy VIII*, Philadelphia, 1983, WB Saunders, p. 35.
*500 mL = 1 lb.

failure to achieve satisfactory rehydration include calculation errors, underestimation of the initial hydration deficit, contemporary losses larger than first appreciated (e.g., vomiting, diarrhea), infusion of fluid at an excessively rapid rate with consequent diuresis and obligatory urinary loss of fluid and electrolytes, administered fluid not reaching the extracellular compartment (e.g., technical problems with the intravenous catheter, third-space loss), sensible losses larger than appreciated (e.g., polyuria), and insensible losses larger than appreciated (e.g., panting, fever). Failure to achieve successful hydration is an indication to increase the volume of fluid administered if the heart and kidneys are functioning adequately. As a rule, the daily fluid volume may be increased by an amount equivalent to 5% of body weight if the initial infusion fails to restore hydration. Finally, the possibility must be considered that the animal was not dehydrated at presentation (e.g., abnormal skin turgor related to old age or emaciation). This should be considered if the animal does not gain weight despite several days of fluid therapy.

MONITORING FLUID THERAPY

It is important to remember that the hydration deficit as estimated by history and physical examination is only an **estimate**, and fluid therapy must be tailored to physical (e.g., body weight) and laboratory (e.g., PCV, TPP) findings during the first few days of fluid therapy.

PHYSICAL AND LABORATORY FINDINGS

A complete physical examination, including evaluation of skin turgor and careful thoracic auscultation, should be performed once or twice daily for animals receiving fluid therapy. Hematocrit, TPP, and body weight should be monitored. Serial body weight has been considered one of the most important variables to follow, and animals receiving continuous fluid therapy should be weighed once or twice daily **using the same scale**. A gain or loss of 1 kg can be considered an excess or deficit of 1 L of fluid because lean body mass is not quickly gained or lost. A dehydrated patient should gain weight as rehydration is achieved, and afterward weight should remain relatively constant. However, weight may increase without restoration of effective circulating volume in patients with severe third-space losses. Despite these traditional principles, one study of dogs and cats hospitalized in an intensive care unit showed that clinical estimates of dehydration did not reliably predict changes in body weight after 24 to 48 hours of fluid therapy.[18]

URINE OUTPUT

The clinician should observe the animal's urine output carefully after fluid therapy has begun. Oliguria should be strongly suspected in patients with acute renal failure, especially those with possible ethylene glycol ingestion.

Urine output should be monitored when fluids are administered intravenously at a rapid rate and renal function is in question. Normal urine output is 1 to 2 mL/kg/hr. As the patient becomes rehydrated, physiologic oliguria should resolve, and urine output should increase while USG decreases. If oliguria that was present at admission persists after the hydration deficit has been replaced, it is prudent to divide daily fluid therapy into six 4-hour intervals if the status of renal function is uncertain. The calculated insensible volume plus a volume equal to the urine output of the previous 4 hours is administered during each 4-hour period (known as measuring "ins and outs"). The risk of overhydration is minimized, and fluid therapy keeps pace with urine output even if oliguria is present when this technique is used. If oliguria persists, an increase in the daily fluid volume by an amount equal to 5% of body weight is justified on the assumption that the initial clinical estimate of dehydration was inaccurate. If oliguria does not respond to mild volume expansion, administration of increased volumes of fluid may result in pulmonary edema.

CENTRAL VENOUS PRESSURE

Measurement of CVP with a jugular catheter positioned at the level of the right atrium allows the cardiovascular response to fluid administration to be monitored. Normal CVP is 0 to 3 cm H_2O. CVP increases from below normal into the normal range when fluids are administered to a dehydrated animal. A progressive increase in CVP above normal during fluid therapy is an indication to decrease the rate of fluid administration or to stop fluid therapy temporarily. A sudden and sustained increase in CVP may indicate failure of the cardiovascular system to handle the fluid load effectively and could result in pulmonary edema caused by left-sided heart failure. In addition to the volume of fluid administered, other factors that may affect CVP include heart rate, vascular capacity, and cardiac contractility. A reduction in any of these three parameters could cause an increase in CVP.

The Frank-Starling curve (Fig. 14-8) relates stroke volume (SV) to left ventricular end-diastolic pressure (LVEDP). If there is no obstruction across the mitral valve, left atrial pressure (LAP) should equal LVEDP, a measure of cardiac function. PWP measured with a Swan-Ganz catheter is an estimate of LAP. Generally, there is a direct relationship between right atrial pressure (RAP) and LAP. Thus measuring CVP gives an indirect indication of LVEDP. Without cardiac dysfunction, CVP correlates well with PWP and LAP. In one study, pulmonary artery diastolic pressure and PWP increased before CVP in dogs receiving an infusion of lactated Ringer's solution.[8]

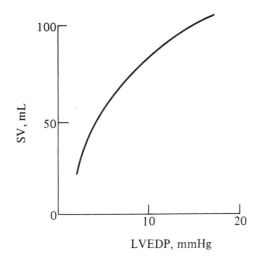

Fig. 14-8 Frank-Starling law of the heart relating stroke volume (SV) to left ventricular end-diastolic pressure (LVEDP). (From Rose BD: *Clinical physiology of acid-base and electrolyte disorders,* ed 3, New York, 1989, McGraw-Hill, p. 369, with permission of the McGraw-Hill Companies.)

COMPLICATIONS OF FLUID THERAPY

Signs of overhydration occur when fluid is administered too rapidly. These may include serous nasal discharge, chemosis, restlessness, shivering, tachycardia, cough, tachypnea, dyspnea, pulmonary crackles and edema, ascites, polyuria, exophthalmos, diarrhea, and vomiting.[8] Expected laboratory abnormalities include a reduction in PCV and TPP and an increase in body weight.

When the intravenous route is chosen for fluid therapy, the clinician has made a commitment to careful, aseptic catheter placement and proper maintenance (see Chapter 15). The animal should be checked daily for cleanliness of the catheter site, local pain or swelling, fever, or cardiac murmurs. If any of these signs are observed, the catheter should be removed, its tip cultured, the patient started on appropriate antibiotic therapy, and a new catheter placed in another vein. Complications related to catheter placement include bacterial endocarditis, thrombophlebitis, thromboembolism, and migration of a catheter fragment. When not in use, the catheter should be irrigated with a small volume (<1 mL) of a solution containing between 1 and 5 U of heparin per milliliter of 0.9% NaCl ("heparinized saline"). The complications of fluid therapy are discussed further in Chapter 16.

WHEN SHOULD FLUID THERAPY BE DISCONTINUED?

Ideally, fluid therapy is discontinued when hydration is restored and when the animal can maintain fluid balance on its own by oral intake of food and water. As the animal recovers, fluid therapy usually is tapered by decreasing the volume of fluid administered by 25% to 50% per day. If an animal remains anorexic for more than 3 to 5 days, enteral or parenteral nutritional therapy must be considered. Parenteral nutrition is discussed in Chapter 25.

REFERENCES

1. Abrams JT: The nutrition of the dog. In Rechcigl M, editor: *CRC handbook series in nutrition and food. Section G: diets, culture media, and food supplements,* Boca Raton, FL, 1977, CRC Press, p. 1.
2. Anderson RS: Water balance in the dog and cat, *J Small Anim Pract* 23:588, 1982.
3. Bedford PGC, Clark EGC: Experimental benzoic acid poisoning in the cat, *Vet Rec* 90:53, 1972.
4. Bjorling DE, Rawlings CA: Relationship of intravenous administration of Ringer's lactate solution to pulmonary edema in halothane-anesthetized cats, *Am J Vet Res* 44:1000, 1983.
5. Cohen RD, Simpson R: Lactate metabolism, *Anesthesiology* 43:661, 1975.
6. Corley EA: Intramedullary transfusion in small animals, *J Am Vet Med Assoc* 142:1005, 1963.
7. Cornelius LM: Fluid therapy in small animal practice, *J Am Vet Med Assoc* 176:110, 1980.
8. Cornelius LM, Finco DR, Culver DH: Physiologic effects of rapid infusion of Ringer's lactate solution into dogs, *Am J Vet Res* 39:1185, 1978.
9. Cullison RF, Menard PD, Buck WB: Toxicosis in cats from the use of benzyl alcohol in lactated Ringer's solution, *J Am Vet Med Assoc* 182:61, 1983.
10. DiBartola SP: Disorders of fluid, acid-base, and electrolyte balance. In Sherding RG, editor: *Medical emergencies (contemporary issues in small animal practice),* New York, 1985, Churchill Livingstone, p. 137.
11. Finco DR: Fluid therapy—detecting deviations from normal, *J Am Anim Hosp Assoc* 8:155, 1972.
12. Finco DR: A scheme for fluid therapy in the dog and cat, *J Am Anim Hosp Assoc* 8:178, 1972.
13. Finco DR: Fluid therapy. In Kirk RW, editor: *Current veterinary therapy VI,* Philadelphia, 1977, WB Saunders, p. 8.
14. Fiser DH: Intraosseous infusion, *N Engl J Med* 322:1579, 1989.
15. Fulton RB, Hauptman JG: In vitro and in vivo rates of fluid flow through catheters in peripheral veins of dogs, *J Am Vet Med Assoc* 198:1622, 1991.
16. Garvey MS: Fluid and electrolyte balance in critical patients, *Vet Clin North Am Small Anim Pract* 19:1021, 1989.
17. Greene RW, Scott RC: Lower urinary tract disease. In Ettinger SJ, editor: *Textbook of veterinary internal medicine,* Philadelphia, 1975, WB Saunders, p. 1572.
18. Hansen B, DeFrancesco T: Relationship between hydration estimate and body weight change after fluid therapy in critically ill dogs and cats, *J Vet Emerg Crit Care* 12:235, 2002.
19. Hardy RM, Osborne CA: Water deprivation test in the dog: maximal normal values, *J Am Vet Med Assoc* 174:479, 1979.
20. Harrison JB, Sussman HH, Pickering DE: Fluid and electrolyte therapy in small animals, *J Am Vet Med Assoc* 137:637, 1960.

21. Hartsfield SM, Thurmon JC, Corbin JE, et al: Effects of sodium acetate, bicarbonate and lactate on acid-base status in anesthetized dogs, *J Vet Pharmacol Ther* 4:51, 1981.

22. Haskins SC: Fluid and electrolyte therapy, *Compend Contin Educ Pract Vet* 6:244, 1984.

23. Haskins SC: A simple fluid therapy planning guide, *Semin Vet Med Surg* 3:227, 1988.

24. Kleiber M: *The fire of life,* Huntington, NY, 1975, Robert E. Krieger Publishing Co.

25. McDonald ML, Rogers QR, Morris JG: Nutrition of the domestic cat, a mammalian carnivore, *Annu Rev Nutr* 4:521, 1984.

26. Monafo W: Expensive salt water, *Surgery* 89:525, 1981.

27. Moss GS, Lowe RJ, Jilek J, et al: Colloid or crystalloid in the resuscitation of hemorrhagic shock: a controlled clinical trial, *Surgery* 89:434, 1981.

28. Muir WW, DiBartola SP: Fluid therapy. In Kirk RW, editor: *Current veterinary therapy VIII,* Philadelphia, 1983, WB Saunders, p. 28.

29. Otto CM, McCal-Kauffman G, Crowe DT: Intraosseous infusion of fluids and therapeutics, *Compend Contin Educ Pract Vet* 11:421, 1989.

30. Rose BD: *Clinical physiology of acid base and electrolyte disorders,* New York, 1994, McGraw-Hill, p. 455.

31. Rose BD: *Clinical physiology of acid base and electrolyte disorders,* New York, 1994, McGraw-Hill, p. 409.

32. Rose RJ: Some physiological and biochemical effects of the intravenous administration of five different electrolyte solutions in the dog, *J Vet Pharmacol Ther* 2:279, 1979.

33. Ryan CP: Toxicity associated with lactated Ringer's solution containing preservatives, *J Am Vet Med Assoc* 12:7, 1982.

34. Schaer M: General principles of fluid therapy in small animal medicine, *Vet Clin North Am Small Anim Pract* 19:203, 1989.

35. Schall WD: General principles of fluid therapy, *Vet Clin North Am* 12:453, 1982.

36. Schwartz WB, Waters WC: Lactate versus bicarbonate, *Am J Med* 32:831, 1962.

37. Stewart PA: *How to understand acid-base,* New York, 1981, Elsevier.

38. Stewart PA: Modern quantitative acid-base chemistry, *Can J Physiol Pharmacol* 61:1444, 1983.

39. Virgilio RW, Rice CL, Smith DE, et al: Crystalloid versus colloid resuscitation: is one better? *Surgery* 85:129, 1979.

40. Willard MD, Zerbe CA, Schall WD, et al: Severe hypophosphatemia associated with diabetes mellitus in six dogs and one cat, *J Am Vet Med Assoc* 190:1007, 1987.

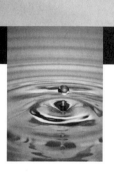

CHAPTER · 15

TECHNICAL ASPECTS OF FLUID THERAPY

Bernard D. Hansen

Fluid therapy is an indispensable component of veterinary medical practice. As the role of fluid therapy in veterinary emergency and critical care practice has become more sophisticated, there has been increased interest in identifying optimal techniques of fluid therapy delivery. Nevertheless, there have been only a few reports of clinical studies comparing therapies or identifying complications in veterinary patients, and many of the principles described in this chapter are based on interpretation of human medical practice. Whenever possible, the guidelines offered here are based on clinical studies in veterinary patients, experimental work using animal models, the author's personal experience, and a bit of common sense.

ROUTES OF FLUID ADMINISTRATION

The most frequently used routes of parenteral therapy are intravenous, intraosseous, and subcutaneous. Intraperitoneal administration of fluids is potentially hazardous and offers no significant advantages over other routes; therefore it is not discussed further. The route of parenteral fluid administration is chosen based on the underlying disorder and its severity, therapeutic goals, fluid composition, and characteristics of the patient, including species, size, age, and accessibility of veins.

SUBCUTANEOUS

Subcutaneous fluid administration (hypodermoclysis) is a convenient and inexpensive route of maintenance fluid therapy for patients that do not require vascular access for other purposes. It should be reserved for relatively stable animals because peripheral vasoconstriction in illness may limit absorption of fluids and prevents successful use of the subcutaneous route. The fluid should be nearly isotonic (200 to 400 mOsm) to limit discomfort and complications. Although sodium-free or low-sodium fluids are tolerated by many human patients, the composition of fluid administered subcutaneously should ideally be comparable with that of extracellular fluid because electrolyte-free or hypertonic fluids are associated with higher complication rates.[2,23,61] The potential for pain, inflammation, and electrolyte imbalances from a large volume of subcutaneous electrolyte-free fluid may be a realistic concern in small animals; therefore it is prudent to avoid large volumes of low-sodium fluids in cats and small dogs. In humans, subcutaneous fluids can be supplemented with potassium at a concentration up to 40 mEq/L.[63] Other potential complications include infection resulting in subcutaneous cellulitis and skin necrosis from caustic or hypertonic fluids or fluids administered under high pressure into an unyielding subcutaneous space.

The volume administered at any single site is limited by the distensibility of subcutaneous tissue. Therefore fluids are usually administered in the subcutaneous space over the dorsal neck and cranial trunk, where loose connective tissue is abundant. Although the addition of hyaluronidase to fluids for hypodermoclysis therapy in humans increases the rate of absorption of fluid, there is no evidence that the addition of this enzyme improves patient tolerance.[12,61] However, it may be of value in dogs and cats with limited distensibility of their subcutaneous tissue when rapid administration is necessary because of time constraints. The fluid should be warmed to body temperature before administration to limit the patient's discomfort and enhance local blood flow and absorption. The skin should be cleansed with a cotton ball and alcohol to remove debris from the surface. Fluid may be administered with a syringe and 22-gauge needle in small animals or by gravity flow with a fluid administration set through a 20- to 18-gauge needle in larger animals. One company markets a subcutaneous catheter (Endo-Sof, Global Veterinary Products, New Buffalo, MI) designed to be implanted for repeated use. Although the catheter material is inert and can stay in place for a long time, failure to adhere to strict aseptic technique will result in bacterial contamination.

INTRAVENOUS

Intravenous administration is the route of choice when blood volume expansion is desired. It is clearly superior to subcutaneous administration for any critically ill patient with poor perfusion of tissues. Indications for vein cannulation include administration of fluids, drugs, total parenteral nutrition, blood products, intravenous anesthetics, and as a precaution against the need for venous access in the event of an emergency.

INTRAOSSEOUS

Intraosseous fluid administration provides access to the vascular space via the capillary beds of the medullary vascular system. It is an excellent alternative to the intravenous route in neonates, in whom vascular access is technically difficult. This route is best suited for rapid, short-term administration of fluids, blood products, or drugs in emergency situations.

INTRAVENOUS CATHETERS

Catheter products currently available include wing tip needle, over the needle, through the needle, and those placed through an introducer or over a guide wire (Table 15-1). Selection is influenced by operator experience, availability, cost, and patient requirements. The catheters most often used for routine fluid administration are the over-the-needle and through-the-needle types. Smaller diameter catheters made of soft material are less traumatic to veins than large or stiff catheters. For routine maintenance therapy, the smallest gauge catheter that provides adequate flow should be used. If rapid administration of fluid is required, the largest gauge size possible should be used (Table 15-2). The maximal fluid flow rate increases as the radius of the catheter lumen is increased. For small catheters (<14 gauge), this relationship is linear, whereas for larger catheters, flow rate increases geometrically with size and is proportional to the lumen radius raised to the fourth power (r^4).[24] Short over-the-needle catheters are preferred for rapid intravenous access in emergencies because they can be inserted rapidly and are available in sizes up to 8.5 French.

WINGED NEEDLE CATHETERS

Winged needle catheters are designed for short-term (single dose) administration of fluid or drugs into a peripheral vein. They are available in needle sizes of 27 to 16 gauge and with various lengths of plastic tubing connecting the needle to a Luer adapter. Plastic wings at the needle hub facilitate handling and securing the needle. The risk of needle puncture of the vessel wall and subsequent extravasation is high because the sharp

TABLE 15-1   Intravenous Catheter Design

Style	Advantages	Disadvantages
Winged steel needle	Can be inserted rapidly with little to no skin prep	Will not remain in place very long High risk of extravasation
Over-the-needle (OTN)	Well suited for peripheral vein Inexpensive Technically easy to use Multiple veterinary distributors	Most brands cannot be used for central access Cannot be tunneled very far subcutaneously Stiff materials more damaging to veins Unreliable for aspirating blood
Over-the-needle with guide wire	Can be inserted into small/difficult veins Arterial catheters useful for dorsal pedal artery	Same as OTN More expensive than OTN
Through-the-needle (TTN)	Can be used for central access Useful for repeated blood collection Can be tunneled subcutaneously Made of softer/less irritating material Less likely to produce thrombophlebitis over time	Technically more difficult to insert Greater potential for hemorrhage than OTN type More expensive than OTN
Through introducer sheath with or without guide wire	Can be used to achieve central venous access Can insert relatively large/multilumen catheter Can create a long subcutaneous tunnel Catheter material may be very soft (silicone, polyurethane) Can be placed in veins too difficult for TTN-style catheter	Same as TTN, plus: Requires drape/sterile field/sterile gloves

needle bevel is left exposed within the lumen of the vein. Therefore these catheters are best used only for collection of blood or for single infusions of nonirritating drugs or fluids under direct supervision. They are usually positioned in the cephalic vein, where there is less risk of displacement by patient movement. They must be located sufficiently distal to the elbow that joint flexion will not displace the needle through the vessel wall. Although these have little use in long-term fluid administration, they have two major advantages for emergency or critical care patients: (1) they may be inserted rapidly

with little or no skin preparation; and (2) in many operators' experience they are the most effective device to obtain percutaneous venous access in cats (and occasionally small dogs) via cannulation of the medial cutaneous saphenous vein.

OVER-THE-NEEDLE CATHETERS

Over-the-needle catheters are well suited for easy insertion into peripheral veins in companion animals. The wide range of available gauge sizes allows flexibility in vein selection and maximal flow rates. Some are designed for arterial cannulation (Arrow Radial Artery catheter, Arrow International, Reading, PA) and incorporate a wire guide stylet that facilitates placement. Multilumen catheters (Arrow Twin Cath, Arrow International) allow infusion of incompatible solutions through a single catheter. In the past decade, there has been an industry-wide move toward catheters that incorporate safety mechanisms to limit the risk of operator injury and exposure to patient blood. Safety catheters irreversibly retract or cover the needle during an insertion attempt and can be used for only one attempt.

Over-the-needle catheters are useful for short procedures such as anesthesia and for intravenous fluid administration for 48 to 72 hours. These catheters are usually positioned in the cephalic, accessory cephalic, medial and lateral saphenous, or femoral veins. Any accessible superficial vein may be satisfactory (e.g., ear veins in rabbits or dogs with pendulous ears).

TABLE 15-2   Suggested Intravenous Catheter Gauges

Weight	Jugular Vein (Through-the-Needle)	Limb Vein (Over-the-Needle)
Maintenance Therapy		
<5 kg	22	24-20
5-15 kg	22-19	22-18
>15 kg	19-16	20-18
Resuscitation		
<5 kg	22-19	22-18
5-15 kg	19-16	18-14
>15 kg	16-14	16-10

There are several disadvantages associated with over-the-needle catheters. They may fray or splinter at the tip during insertion and cause excessive injury to the vein with a high risk of thrombosis. They are difficult to secure adequately and may slide in and out of the skin during a patient's movement. This action facilitates entry of skin surface bacteria through the catheter wound and into the vein. When they are located in distal limb veins, fluid flow through these catheters is often affected by limb position (e.g., elbow flexion often stops gravity flow of fluids through a cephalic vein catheter). Several brands of these catheters are composed of stiff Teflon or irritating polypropylene and are not suited for extended dwell periods in an external jugular vein or in veins that cross a joint where motion enhances catheter-induced vessel trauma.

THROUGH-THE-NEEDLE CATHETERS

Through-the-needle catheters are long (6 to 36 inches) and are often used to gain deep or central venous access from peripheral sites. These catheters are generally known as midline catheters in human medicine because they are designed to obtain access to proximal limb veins from distant venipuncture sites. Because of the anatomy of the external jugular and lateral saphenous veins in companion animals, these catheters work well to obtain central venous access. This allows the catheter tip to be positioned in a large central vein with rapid blood flow, allowing safe administration of viscous or hypertonic solutions. It is often difficult to thread these catheters past the elbow and axillary regions of the forelimb; thus they are of limited usefulness in cephalic veins. Body position and movement do not affect the rate of fluid flow through a deep or central venous catheter. Multiple blood samples may be withdrawn easily from these catheters. They may be anchored securely to the skin and tunneled extensively through subcutaneous tissue and are therefore less likely to conduct surface bacteria into a vein than are shorter catheters.[44,50] Small vein cannulation is often more difficult than with over-the-needle catheterization, and the risk of catheter or air embolization during catheterization is greater.

GUIDED CATHETERS AND PERIPHERALLY INSERTED CENTRAL CATHETERS

Central venous catheters designed for insertion into a human internal jugular or subclavian vein almost always use a guide wire placement technique to increase the likelihood of successful cannulation. Because they are composed of soft material, they either incorporate a wire stylet or are threaded over a preplaced guide wire using the technique of Seldinger.[65] Some of the catheters marketed for use in humans are suitable for use in dogs and cats (e.g., Arrow Pediatric Central Venous Catheterization Sets, Arrow International). Some guide wire catheters are marketed specifically for use in dogs and cats (Mila International, Florence KY; Global Veterinary Products). The guide wire technique allows central vein access via insertion into veins that may not be successfully cannulated otherwise. Other peripherally inserted central catheters (PICCs; Mila International, Global Veterinary Products) are inserted through a short, larger introducer sheath with or without a guide wire. A major advantage of these catheter designs is the availability of double or even triple lumen products that allow greater vascular access through a single catheter.

CATHETER COMPOSITION

Catheter composition affects handling characteristics during insertion and influences the potential for thrombosis and phlebitis. Widely used catheter materials include polyvinyl chloride (PVC), polyethylene, polypropylene, polyurethane, silicon elastomer (Silastic), tetrafluoroethylene (TFE Teflon), and fluoroethylene-propylene (FEP Teflon) (Table 15-3). These materials are chemically inert, but leaching of plasticizers and stabilizing agents from some plastics probably contributes to the development of phlebitis, especially in small veins with low blood flow.[55,68,78] Silicone elastomer catheters are the most chemically inert, whereas PVC, polypropylene, and polyethylene are the most reactive. Teflon and polyurethane are intermediate in reactivity. Some catheters composed of more irritating material are coated with silicone elastomer to reduce their reactivity.

TABLE 15-3 Catheter Materials

Material	Reactivity	Stiffness	Thrombogenicity
Teflon	++	++++	++
Polyether-based polyurethane	+	++	+
Polyester-based polyurethane	++	+++	++
Polyvinyl chloride	++++	+++	+++
Polyethylene	+++	+++	+++
Polypropylene	+++	+++	+++
Silicone elastomer	+	+	+

Relative values for each material: +, minimal; ++, mild; +++, moderate; ++++, high.

Catheter thrombogenicity is related not only to chemical reactivity but also to the stiffness of the material and the smoothness of its surface.[17,31] Teflon is the stiffest material; polypropylene, PVC, and polyethylene are more flexible. Stiff catheters are easier to pass through the skin and subcutaneous tissues but are more prone to kinking and more likely to damage vessel walls and cause thrombophlebitis. Polyurethane elastomer (e.g., Vialon, Becton Dickinson, Franklin Lakes, NJ; others) and silicone elastomer catheters are much softer and more flexible. Silicone elastomer catheters are so flexible that they are difficult to introduce into a vein without a stylet or guide wire.

Many brands of catheters are made radiopaque by the addition of heavy metal salts (barium or bismuth) to the plastic. When mixed uniformly into the material, these salts increase the roughness of the catheter surface and increase the risk of thrombosis.[31] If embedded within the wall of the catheter, or if the catheter is coated with another, less thrombogenic material (e.g., silicon elastomer), this risk is lower. Heparin coating may significantly reduce catheter thrombus formation for 1 to 2 days.[60,67] Some manufacturers have developed antibiotic-coated catheters that appear to reduce the risk of catheter-associated sepsis.[40] Examples of antiseptics either coated onto or impregnated into catheters include chlorhexidine and silver sulfadiazine.[6]

VEIN SELECTION

Catheter site selection depends on several factors, including operator experience, accessibility, therapeutic goals, risk of infection, risk of damage to the catheter, and risk of thrombosis.

ACCESSIBILITY

Peripheral vein cannulation is most often performed in the cephalic and accessory cephalic veins of the thoracic limbs and the lateral saphenous vein of the pelvic limbs. Other suitable veins include the medial saphenous (cats), the femoral veins (in some cats and dogs), and the ear veins in dogs with pendulous ears. These veins may fill very slowly in animals with poor peripheral perfusion and can be difficult to visualize or palpate. In this setting, the saphenous veins may be superior (lateral in dogs, medial in cats) because the relatively thin skin overlying them allows better visualization and control over catheter insertion. Catheterization may be facilitated by the vascular access procedures described in the following sections.

THERAPEUTIC GOALS

Short-term administration of fluids may be accomplished using any vein, and choice of vein in this setting depends primarily on operator experience and catheter design. Central venous catheterization is preferred in patients that require long-term fluid administration or parenteral nutrition, administration of hypertonic solutions or irritating drugs, frequent blood sampling, or central venous pressure (CVP) monitoring. Central venous access is most easily accomplished by cannulation of the external jugular or saphenous veins. The right external jugular is preferred over the left because this vein joins the cranial cava in a straighter line through the brachycephalic trunk than does the left, facilitating catheter passage into the cranial vena cava.

RISK OF INFECTION

The risk of infection is increased in the presence of bandage contamination. Catheters inserted into peripheral veins that are likely to be soiled by vomiting, diarrhea, or urine pose a greater threat. Therefore the saphenous veins are not ideal choices in animals with diarrhea or polyuria, and the cephalic vein is not a good choice in an animal with frequent vomiting. There is a greater threat of infection of catheters inserted through a cut-down incision or through skin that is wounded or infected. Therefore unhealthy skin is avoided, and catheters inserted through incisions are removed as soon as possible, ideally within 6 hours.

RISK OF DAMAGE TO THE CATHETER

Catheters located in limb veins are particularly accessible to the animal's teeth, and some animals chew at and damage or remove the catheter. Catheters located in an ear vein may prompt scratching and head shaking that eventually dislodge the device. Some form of restraint, such as an Elizabethan collar, may be necessary to prevent damage to catheters located at these sites. The risk of catheter damage is considerably lower when the jugular vein is used and bandaged adequately. Surprisingly, most sick dogs and cats do not disturb properly positioned, carefully bandaged intravenous catheters. Animals that chew or scratch at their catheters frequently do so because of excessive irritation. Catheters and bandages that were tolerated initially and subsequently provoke chewing or scratching should be carefully inspected for evidence of tightness, wetness, or infection.

RISK OF THROMBOSIS

There is a risk of thrombosis whenever a vein is cannulated. Thrombosis is more likely in small veins with low blood flow or when the intravascular portion of the catheter traverses a mobile joint. Some specific diseases such as preexisting phlebitis, glomerulonephritis, protein-losing enteropathy, autoimmune hemolytic anemia, and any disorder that causes systemic inflammation are complicated by increased risk of serious thrombosis and pulmonary thromboembolism.[20,34,38] Intravenous catheterization in these animals is probably accompanied by a higher risk of clinically significant thrombosis than in other diseases. It may be advisable to avoid venous catheterization in these animals whenever possible. When catheterization is unavoidable, one should use short, soft, small diameter catheters that are removed as soon as possible. Compared with catheterization of peripheral veins, catheterization of the jugular vein in companion animals is probably not an independent risk factor for venous thrombosis and pulmonary thromboembolism, but the consequences of thrombosis in that location are more apparent and severe. Cats with aortic saddle thrombi have poor blood flow to their pelvic limbs and devitalization of those tissues. Pelvic limb vein catheterization in these animals is associated with a high risk of venous thrombosis and infection and must be avoided.

CATHETER PLACEMENT

SKIN PREPARATION

Healthy animals undergoing short-term catheterization for elective procedures (e.g., anesthesia for ovariohysterectomy) rarely develop phlebitis or sepsis from sloppy technique during catheter placement. In contrast, sick animals with compromised immunity may not tolerate even a minor breach of aseptic technique, and intravenous catheters may quickly become colonized and serve as a point source for bacteremia and septic phlebitis. With the exception of emergency venous access, these patients require careful aseptic technique for skin preparation and catheter insertion. If an intravenous catheter is to remain in place for more than a few hours, the skin must be prepared as for any surgical procedure. Every effort must be made to be thorough but gentle because abraded or scarified skin is not healthy and will support colonization by pathogenic bacteria. Key points include avoiding clipper burn and avoiding rough cotton gauze for skin cleansing:

1. A wide clip centered on the intended venipuncture site is performed. A no. 40 blade is used to obtain a close cut. The clipper blade must be well lubricated and held **parallel** to the skin (not raked across it) to limit clipper burn, and the coat is clipped sufficiently far from the point of insertion so there is no risk the catheter will touch hair during the procedure. If it is not possible to clip a sufficiently wide area, consider wrapping the appendage or neck with a temporary bandage to hold down the haircoat and keep it out of contact with the catheter.

2. Wash your hands and apply a germicidal lotion (e.g., Avagard [3M, St. Paul, MN], Citrus II [Beaumont Products, Kennasaw, GA], IC Lotion [R&R Lotion, Scottsdale, AZ], or Purell [GOJO Industries, Akron, OH]). Don a clean examination glove on the dominant hand using a "no touch" technique. Treat this glove as though it were sterile, and do not touch its fingers with your bare hand when removing it from the container.

3. Local anesthesia with subcutaneous lidocaine often facilitates catheterization. Although some animals react to the transient sting of injected lidocaine, this is often less stressful than the sensation produced by a large-gauge catheter being forced through the skin. Local anesthesia also provides the option of making a facilitation incision at the venipuncture site (see the section on Percutaneous Facilitation Procedure). If local anesthesia is desired, it should be done immediately after clipping to allow time to take effect while the skin is prepared. The skin is wiped once with an alcohol-soaked cotton ball, and the venipuncture site is anesthetized with 0.1 to 0.5 mL of lidocaine/bicarbonate 9:1 mixture administered subcutaneously. By mixing nine parts of lidocaine with one part of sodium bicarbonate solution, the sting of lidocaine is reduced.[46,56] If made in advance, the lidocaine/bicarbonate mixture should be used within 1 month because the lidocaine in this mixture degrades at a rate of approximately 11% per week.[75]

4. The skin must be cleaned for at least 2 and preferably 3 minutes with cotton balls freshly soaked with the surgical scrub of choice. Do not use containers of premade antiseptic-soaked gauze or cotton balls; people reaching into the container with their bare hands contaminate these. Most antiseptic soaps require **continuous wet contact** for that entire time to be effective. This means that there is **no rinsing with alcohol or water between scrubs until the full 2 to 3 minutes have elapsed.** Frequent changing of the cotton balls facilitates removal of surface debris. The following antiseptic agents are useful:

    a. Chlorhexidine gluconate 4% (Hibiclens, G.C. America, Alsip, IL; Chlorhexiderm, DVM Pharmaceuticals, Miami, FL), chlorhexidine diacetate 2% (Nolvasan, Fort Dodge Animal Health, Overland Park, KS): Chlorhexidine is active against a broad spectrum of gram-positive and gram-negative bacteria. It is more effective than povidone-iodine at preventing catheter-related infection in humans.[10,42] Its activity is not diminished by the presence of organic matter such as blood and is not appreciably degraded by alcohol, and there is considerable residual activity after a single application. The Food and Drug Administration does not recommend chlorhexidine soap as a surgical scrub for cats.

    b. Povidone-iodine (Betadine 7.5% scrub [Perdue, Stamford, CT], Poviderm 7.5% scrub [Vetus/Burns Veterinary Supply, Farmer's Branch, TX]): This formulation of iodine supplies the antiseptic activity of iodine in a form that is less irritating and less staining than iodine or tincture of iodine. The antiseptic activity is reduced in the presence of organic matter, and this formulation is more likely to cause skin irritation than is chlorhexidine.[52,53] It is the preferred antiseptic for use on cats.

c. Two percent iodine, tincture of iodine: Iodine is bactericidal at very low concentrations. In the absence of organic matter, a 1% solution kills most surface bacteria within seconds and is more effective than povidone-iodine.[37,69] It discolors hair and skin and frequently causes skin irritation.

d. Ethyl alcohol, isopropyl alcohol: These agents are typically used as 70% solutions. By themselves, they are reasonable germicidal agents for initial skin preparation, but they do not kill spores, require wet contact for at least 2 minutes, and have no residual activity.[8,71] Hence, they are not particularly useful patient skin antiseptics when the goal is to limit skin colonization at an insertion site under a catheter dressing.[7] They are commonly used to remove excess surgical scrub from the prepared skin site during catheterization. The germicidal activities of iodine, povidone-iodine, and chlorhexidine are increased in the presence of ethyl alcohol. There appears to be no advantage to using isopropyl alcohol over sterile saline as a final rinse to remove residual antiseptic soap.[53] Isopropyl alcohol causes vasodilatation at the site of application and may promote cutaneous bleeding during venipuncture. This effect may be even more pronounced when using rubbing alcohols, some of which have added rubefacients. If the patient's skin is abraded, an alcohol rinse should be avoided altogether in favor of sterile saline.

5. Residual scrub solution is removed from the skin and surrounding hair with cotton balls or gauze sponges soaked in alcohol, hydrogen peroxide, sterile water, or sterile saline solution. Soap left on the skin and coat will cause dermatitis—remove all of it!

6. If desired, the skin may be painted with a povidone-iodine solution or an iodine tincture. The solution is allowed to dry before catheter insertion.

PERCUTANEOUS CATHETERIZATION

Winged Needle Catheters

Materials Needed

1. Appropriate catheter
2. Two clean latex examination gloves
3. One roll of 1-inch white tape
4. One catheter injection cap, intravenous tubing set, syringe filled with drug or intravenous solution, catheter "T" piece, or other needleless injection site device (e.g., Interlink connectors, Baxter Healthcare, Deerfield, IL; CLAVE or CLC 2000 connectors, ICU Medical, San Clemente, CA; Abbott Laboratories, Abbott Park, IL) (Fig. 15-1)
5. Single dose of povidone-iodine ointment applied on a sterile gauze sponge (if the needle is to remain in place unobserved)

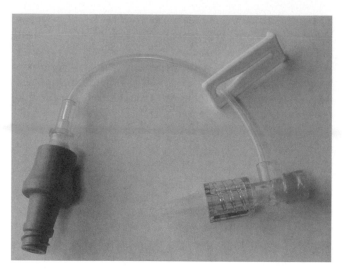

Fig. 15-1 An example of a needleless connector device (CLAVE connectors [ICU Medical, San Clemente, CA; Abbott Laboratories, Abbott Park, IL) attached to a catheter "T" piece.

Procedure

1. Because this device is intended for short infusions and because the stainless steel needle may be less likely to drag surface contamination into the wound, skin preparation may be minimal. Although not essential, clipping the hair at the injection site facilitates visualization of the vein for needle placement. Whether the coat is clipped, wipe the area once with alcohol-soaked cotton balls or gauze to remove dander and flatten the coat.

2. Wash your hands, and put on clean examination gloves.

3. Flush the catheter with intravenous fluid or drug solution to purge air from the system. Disconnect the syringe from the tubing, and hold the catheter by its "wings" in your dominant hand. To prevent fluid from draining out of the system, hold the tubing coiled in the same hand, with the Luer end held level with the needle tip.

4. After an assistant occludes the vein, tense the skin slightly with the opposite hand to stabilize. Do not touch the needle shaft or the skin at the intended point of insertion.

5. Hold the catheter by the plastic wing(s) with the bevel facing up, and push it through the skin and into the vein. There are two technique options:

   a. Direct puncture: Visualize the vein, and position the needle tip directly over it, pointed in the direction of blood flow. While holding the needle at a 30-degree angle with respect to the long axis of the vein, advance the needle through the skin and vessel wall in a single rapid motion.

   b. Indirect method: Visualize the vein, and penetrate the skin on either side (but not directly over) of it. Push the needle through the skin at a

45-degree angle, and advance it subcutaneously for 0.5 cm (1/4 inch) parallel to the vein. At that point, redirect the needle at a shallower angle into the vein.

6. Blood flows into the catheter tubing when the vein is entered. Advance the needle fully into the vein. Lift the needle slightly as it is advanced, a technique that is important for any venipuncture, to minimize the risk of penetrating the vessel wall (Fig. 15-2).

7. The assistant should immediately release the pressure on the vein.

8. Attach the syringe with drug solution or intravenous fluid to the tubing, and fill the catheter with solution. Alternatively, an intravenous fluid line may be attached if immediate fluid administration is desired. Examine the skin near the end of the catheter for any evidence of extravasation at the start of the infusion.

9. If the catheter has two pliable wings, lay them flat on the skin surface, and wrap a single piece of white tape over them and around the limb. This tape should be applied snugly but not tightly enough to occlude the vein. The tape does not cover the point of entry.

10. If the needle is to remain in place and unobserved, it may be prudent to apply a gauze sponge with antiseptic ointment to the skin penetration site, and secure this to the limb with a second piece of 1-inch white tape.

11. Coil the tubing, and secure the Luer end to the limb with another piece of tape. This coil helps prevent movement of the catheter if traction is applied to the tubing.

Over-the-Needle Style Catheters

Materials Needed

1. Appropriate catheter
2. Two clean latex examination gloves

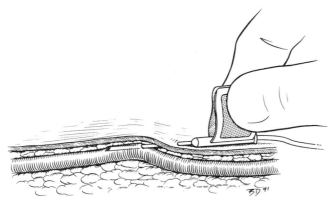

Fig. 15-2 Technique for placement of a needle into a superficial vein. Once the vein has been entered, the bevel remains oriented toward the skin, and the shaft of the needle is lifted up against the superficial wall of the vessel as the needle is advanced. The needle bevel functions like the curved tip of a ski and prevents the point from catching on the vessel wall.

3. One roll 1-inch waterproof white tape
4. One roll each of appropriately sized stretch gauze, stretch bandaging material, and cast padding
5. One catheter injection cap, catheter "T" piece, or needleless connection device
6. Syringe with heparinized saline solution, 1 to 2 U/mL
7. Sterile gauze sponges
8. Single dose of povidone-iodine ointment
   All materials are arranged ready for use on a clean tray or Mayo stand:
1. Antiseptic ointment applied onto a gauze sponge
2. Syringe with heparinized saline attached to "T" piece and the air flushed out (if using an injection cap or needleless connector, purge the air out of that device)
3. Catheter opened and ready for use
4. Tape strips made as needed

Procedure

1. Prepare the venipuncture site aseptically as described previously.
2. Wash your hands, apply germicidal skin lotion (if not already done), and don new clean examination gloves.
3. A small incision through the skin facilitates insertion of large-gauge catheters (Fig. 15-3, *A*) or placement of the catheter through tough skin (see the section on Percutaneous Facilitation Procedure). The techniques for direct and indirect insertion are the same as noted previously. **Indirect catheterization is strongly preferred** because this forms a subcutaneous tunnel between the point of entry through the skin and the point of entry into the vein that serves as a barrier to bacterial migration.[45,49]

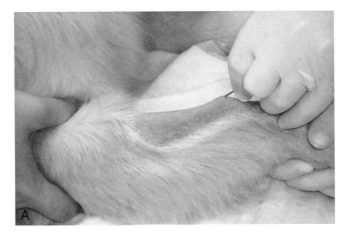

Fig. 15-3 Catheterization of the cephalic vein with an over-the-needle style catheter. **A,** The skin has been clipped widely, the insertion site blocked with a 9:1 lidocaine/bicarbonate mixture, and the skin has been aseptically prepared as described in the text. An 18-gauge injection needle is used to create a facilitation incision in the skin. The skin at that site must never be touched.

(Continued)

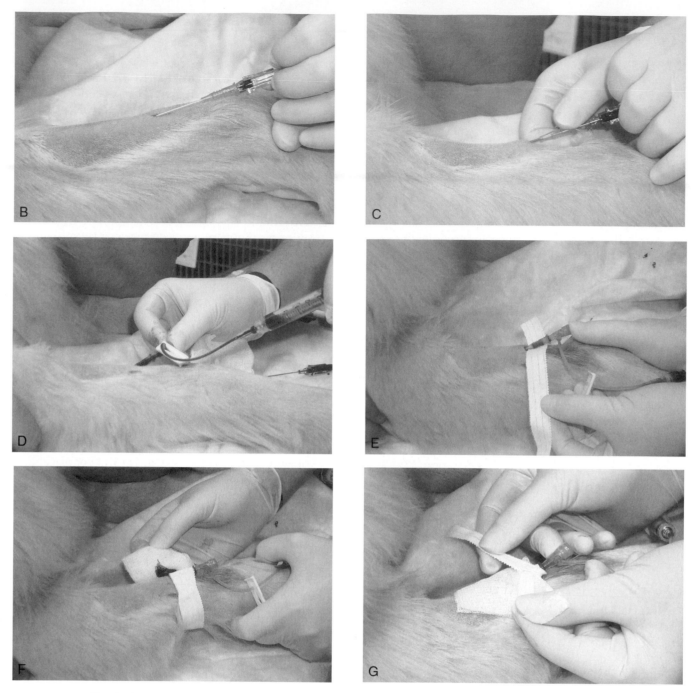

Fig. 15-3 cont'd B, The tip of the needle-catheter assembly is advanced into the skin puncture and proximally, parallel to the long axis of the vein, through the subcutis as far as practical before entering the vein. The catheter shaft is not allowed to contact the distal limb hair. The catheter is angled toward the vein and advanced into it. The goal should be to "snag" the outer layer of the vein with the needle tip. The flow of blood into the clear needle hub depicted here confirms venipuncture. **C,** The needle is held stationary, and the catheter is advanced fully to the Luer hub, or as deeply as possible without crossing a joint. **D,** The needle is removed, and an injection plug or "T" piece is connected to the Luer fitting. Any air is aspirated, and the system is purged with heparinized saline. **E,** The end of a 1-cm-wide (½ inch) strip of white porous tape is secured around the catheter hub, and then the remainder of the tape is wrapped firmly, but loosely, around the limb. **F,** A 5 × 5-cm (2 × 2-inch) gauze with antiseptic ointment is laid over the skin insertion site and secured with more porous white tape. **G,** In this example, a ½-inch-wide (1-cm) strip is applied as a "yoke" around the hub, with the long ends directed proximally. Incorporation of those ends into the bandage will help prevent the catheter from becoming partially withdrawn.

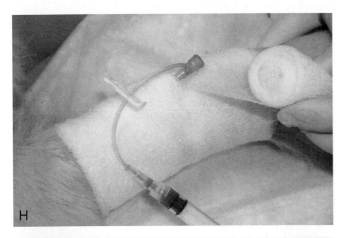

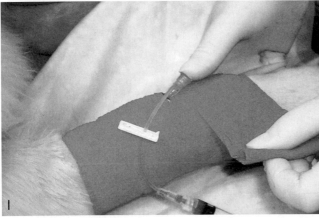

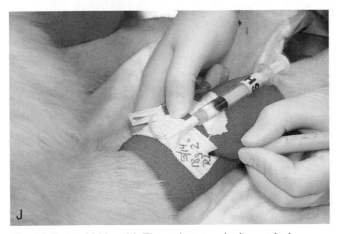

Fig. 15-3 cont'd H and **I,** The catheter and adjacent limb are wrapped with 5- to 8-cm-wide (2 to 3-inch) cotton cast padding, applied heavily enough to provide some support to the catheter and prevent a tourniquet effect. A layer of stretch gauze is applied more snugly over the cast padding. A final layer of stretch bandaging material (with or without adhesive) is applied, more snugly still, over the stretch gauze. The "T" piece extension is secured to the stretch bandage material with white tape to prevent any traction on the Luer connection. It may be connected to an intravenous administration set, needleless connector, or a new locking Luer syringe filled with heparinized saline. **J,** The bandage is initialed and dated.

4. An assistant restrains the animal and occludes the proximal vein. Grasp the catheter firmly at the junction of the needle and catheter hubs, ensuring that the catheter does not loosen and partially slide off the needle during manipulation. **Never touch the skin at the point of insertion, and never touch the needle/catheter shaft.** The needle bevel is directed up during the procedure. Advance the needle, first subcutaneously and then into the vein. Penetration of the vein often is heralded by a distinct "pop" as the needle punctures the tough vessel wall and by the flow of blood into the needle hub (Fig. 15-3, *B*).

5. Advance the needle and catheter as a unit for another 3 to 5 mm. This ensures that both the needle and catheter tips are within the lumen of the vein. During this maneuver, hold the needle shaft as parallel to the long axis of the vein as practical, and lift the catheter tip away from the deep wall of the vein (as described for winged needle catheterization, see Fig. 15-2). Once the catheter tip has entered the vessel, slide the catheter off the needle and into the lumen of the vein (Fig. 15-3, *C*). If the catheter material is very soft and flexible, an alternative technique is to retract the needle 5 mm back into the catheter and advance the catheter and needle in unison all the way into the vein.

6. Your assistant should now release the vein compression, and the needle is withdrawn.

7. Attach the catheter injection cap, "T" piece, or needleless connector device, and flush the catheter with heparinized saline solution (Fig. 15-3, *D*).

8. Remove any blood or fluid on the catheter hub and surrounding skin with sterile or clean gauze sponges.

9. If a cephalic or lateral saphenous vein is cannulated, wrap the catheter hub with a strip of 1.5- to 2.5-cm (½ or 1 inch) white tape, and extend this strip around the limb. The tape should be pressed tightly onto the catheter hub but loosely anchored to the limb (Fig. 15-3, *E* to *G*). The goal is to secure it to the limb, yet avoid wrapping it too tightly. When cannulating the medial saphenous or femoral vein (or any vein at a large, flat surface), the catheter hub should be anchored to the skin with a suture to limit in-and-out movement during flexion and extension of the limb. To provide a secure anchor without strangulating skin, place a single loop of suture material through the skin under the catheter hub, and create a slightly loose loop incorporating skin only by tying a secure square knot. Then tie the free ends of this anchor tightly around the catheter hub with a surgeon's knot.

10. Cover the point of insertion with antiseptic ointment on a sterile gauze sponge (Fig. 15-3, *F*).

11. If the catheter is to remain in place for more than 6 hours, it should be covered with a short, light band-

age that extends 6 to 12 cm (2 to 4 inches) above and below the point of insertion (Fig. 15-3, *G* to *J*).

Through-the-Needle Intermediate-Style Catheters

Materials Needed for Placement in the External Jugular Vein

1. Appropriate catheter: the ideal length will result in the tip of the catheter within the cranial vena cava just cranial to the right atrium
2. Two clean latex examination gloves
3. 00 or 000 monofilament nylon, needle holders, suture scissors
4. 22-gauge needle
5. One roll each 2.54 cm (1 inch) waterproof white tape and porous white tape
6. One roll each of appropriately sized stretch gauze, cast padding, and adhesive (Elastikon, Johnson & Johnson, New Brunswick, NJ) or coadhesive (Vetrap, 3M, St. Paul, MN) wrap
7. One catheter injection cap, catheter "T" piece, or needleless connection device
8. Syringe with heparinized saline solution, 1 to 2 U/mL
9. Sterile gauze sponges
10. Single dose of povidone-iodine ointment
11. Tube of cyanoacrylate adhesive (DURO superglue, Loc Tite Corp., Cleveland, OH) (optional)

All materials are arranged ready for use on a clean tray or Mayo stand:

1. Antiseptic ointment applied onto a gauze sponge
2. "T" piece, injection cap, or needleless connection device purged with saline solution
3. Catheter opened and ready for use
4. Tape strips made as needed

Procedure

1. Prepare the venipuncture site as described previously.
2. Wash your hands, apply germicidal lotion (if not already done), and put on clean examination gloves.
3. Proper positioning is critical for successful cannulation of the external jugular vein. In animals with thin skin and large, easily distended veins, the procedure is easily accomplished with the animal restrained in lateral recumbency. In this position, the external jugular vein is usually located directly lateral to the trachea. Sternal recumbency or a sitting position is preferred in animals that resist being restrained on their side and in those with thick skin or small, poorly distensible veins. In both the sternal and sitting positions, the animal should be held with its pelvic limbs directed away from the side chosen for venipuncture (Fig. 15-4, *A*). This maneuver makes the neck more convex on that side and reduces the depth of the jugular furrow. An assistant elevates the head, and the nose should be initially held in a horizontal position and directed away from the intended site at a 30- to 45-degree angle with the median plane. If the animal has abundant loose skin on the neck, elevating the nose tenses the skin and facilitates identification of the vein. It is helpful to experiment with different head and nose positions until the optimal position is found. If you are right handed, occlude the vein at the thoracic inlet with the thumb of the left hand, and use your left index finger to palpate the vein. The patient's right external jugular vein is preferred because it may be easier to advance the catheter into the cranial vena cava from this side. The puncture site should be 1 to 2 cm (about ½ to ¾ inch) lateral to the vein and in the cranial half of the neck.

4. As with over-the-needle catheters, a small skin incision facilitates insertion of large-gauge catheters and eases access through tough skin (Fig. 15-4, *B*). The techniques for direct and indirect insertion are the same as noted previously. **Indirect insertion is strongly preferred** because this forms a subcutaneous tunnel between the point of entry through the skin and the point of entry through the vein that serves as a barrier to bacterial migration. **Never touch the skin at the point of insertion, and never touch the needle/catheter shaft.**

5. Fully retract the catheter into the sterile sheath so that it is not visible at the needle bevel. Grasp the device firmly at the hub of the needle, and penetrate the skin with the bevel of the needle facing away from the skin surface. When possible, advance the needle subcutaneously parallel to the vein for at least 2 cm (¾ inch) before introducing it into the vein (Fig. 15-4, *C*). Penetration of the vein is usually heralded by a distinct pop as the needle punctures the tough wall of the vessel. A flashback of blood entering the needle hub is usually, but not always, seen (Fig. 15-4, *D*). The catheter may then be manipulated through the sterile sheath and advanced through the needle.

6. If you suspect successful venipuncture but do not see a flashback, try advancing the catheter through the needle. If the catheter is not easily advanced, it is likely that the catheter has entered subcutaneous tissue. In that case, withdraw the entire assembly in unison. Do not pull the catheter back through the needle until the needle is withdrawn because of the risk of shearing on the needle bevel. Inspect the needle and catheter for damage; if none is present, it may be used for another attempt. Any subsequent attempts can be made through the original skin wound.

7. Because the needle forms a hole in the vessel wall that is larger in diameter than the catheter, post-catheterization hemorrhage is occasionally a problem. This can be minimized by holding the

venipuncture site above the level of the heart to reduce venous pressure, such as by performing jugular vein cannulation with the animal in a sitting position. Accurate needle positioning minimizes laceration of the vein, and rapid application of a sterile dressing and bandage provides direct compression and tamponade.

8. Depending on the brand of catheter used, the needle is split off the catheter or is covered with a plastic needle guard as directed by the manufacturer (Fig. 15-4, *E*).

9. Remove the wire stylet (Fig. 15-4, *F*).

10. Attach the "T" piece, injection cap, or needleless connection device to the Luer hub. If using a "T" piece, first attach a syringe with heparinized saline solution to it, and purge all air from the lumen. If you use an injection cap, purge the air from its dead space by filling it with sterile solution. Attach the device, aspirate any air from the catheter, and confirm catheter patency by successful aspiration of blood. Purge the catheter with the solution (Fig. 15-4, *G*).

11. If the catheter was inserted completely, withdraw it 1 to 2 cm (½ to ¾ inch) from the skin, and dry this exposed section with a sterile gauze sponge. Wrap a 2.5- to 5-cm (1 to 2 inches) "butterfly" of waterproof white tape around the catheter and needle guard. This piece of tape should bridge the needle guard and the exposed portion of catheter to where it enters the skin (Fig. 15-4, *H*). Through-the-needle catheters frequently fail because of kinking at the point of exit from the needle guard or the point of entry into the skin. The tape prevents this by forming a protective "sandwich" around the catheter as it exits the needle guard or hub.

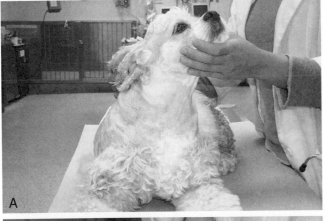

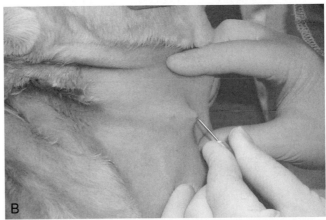

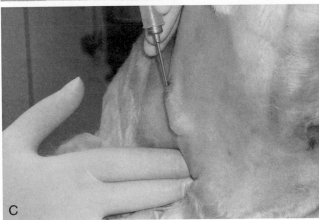

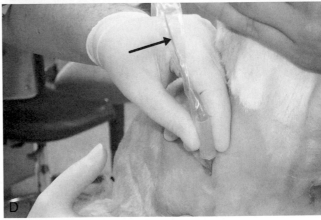

Fig. 15-4 Procedure for jugular vein catheterization using a 19-gauge 20-cm (8-inch) Intracath (Becton Dickenson). **A,** Proper positioning in sternal recumbency, with the nose and rear legs directed away from the side to be catheterized. **B,** Following blockade with a 9:1 mixture of lidocaine/bicarbonate and sterile prep, a facilitation incision is made in the skin lateral and cranial to the point of entry into the vein. **C,** The device is grasped firmly at the hub of the needle, and the skin wound is penetrated with the bevel of the needle facing away from the neck. The needle is advanced subcutaneously parallel to the vein and with the bevel oriented away from the neck for at least ¾ inch (2 cm) before introduction into the vein. **D,** Penetration of the vein is often heralded by a distinct pop as the needle punctures the tough wall of the vessel. A flashback of blood entering the catheter (arrow) is often seen. Note that the needle has been advanced subcutaneously nearly to the hub before venipuncture.

(Continued)

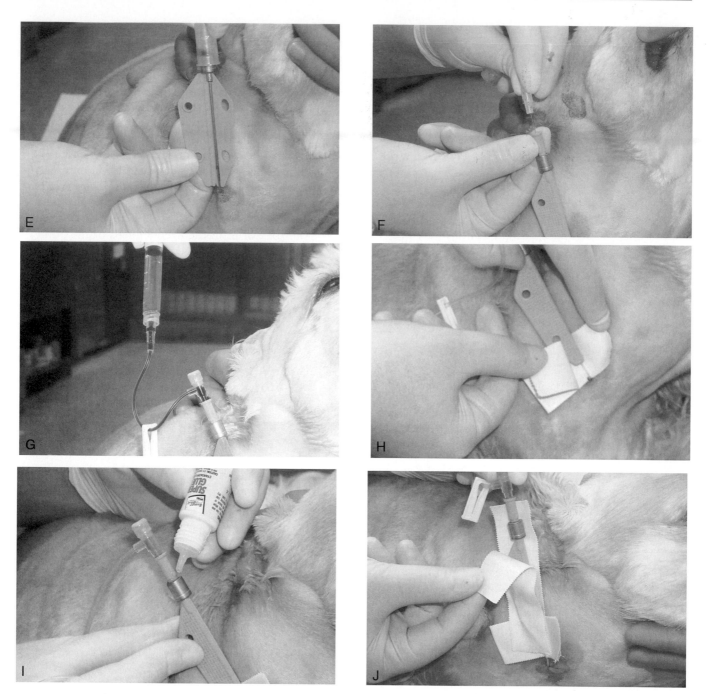

Fig. 15-4 cont'd E, A plastic needle guard is applied over the needle. **F,** The catheter wire stylet is removed while holding the catheter hub steady. **G,** The injection plug should be applied quickly to avoid air embolization. The syringe and "T" piece have been applied and air aspirated back into the syringe. The blood is then purged back through the catheter and the catheter filled with heparinized saline. **H,** A "butterfly" of waterproof 2.5 cm (1 inch) white tape is applied to bridge the end of the needle guard and the first 1 cm (½ inch) of catheter. **I,** If desired, the friction connection between the catheter hub and needle hub may be secured with cyanoacrylate adhesive. **J,** A "sandwich" of 2.5-cm (1-inch) waterproof white tape is applied to the long axis of the needle guard, catheter hub, and original "butterfly" of tape.

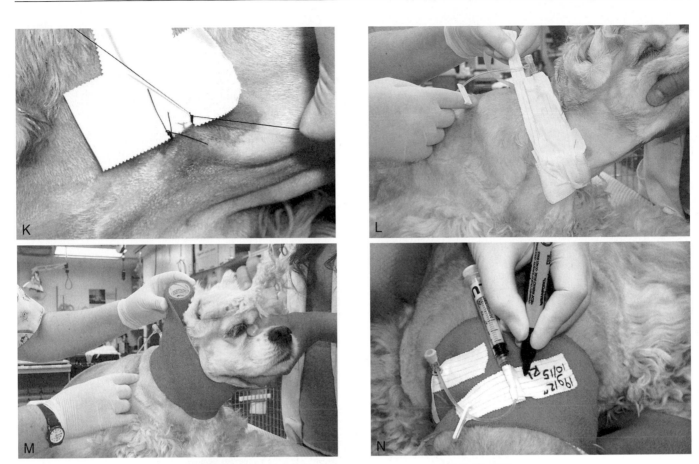

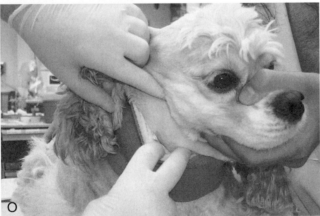

Fig. 15-4 cont'd K, This provides a secure connection between the catheter assembly and skin sutures. **L,** The point of insertion is covered with povidone-iodine impregnated gauze, and the catheter is loosely anchored to the neck with porous 2.5-cm (1-inch) white cloth tape. In this example, the tape has been split down the middle to the last 13 cm (5 inches), which has been applied directly to the original "sandwich" of waterproof tape. One of the strip halves was wrapped down and around the dog's neck, and the other was wrapped upward in the opposite direction. **M,** Sequential layers of 5-cm (2-inch) cast padding, stretch gauze, and coadhesive stretch bandage material are applied, rolling up the neck on the catheter side. During the application the animal's nose should be oriented down in a natural head position. **N,** A piece of split tape is applied to hold the bandage material down around the exposed hub of catheter, and the Luer end of the "T" piece is anchored with another piece of tape, which is labeled with a description of the catheter, the date, and the operator initials. **O,** With the animal's nose pointed down, the front of the ventral aspect of the bandage is checked for tightness. If it is too snug, it is partially split with scissors.

12. If the catheter was too long, leave an appropriate length outside the skin, and incorporate it into a "sandwich" of white tape as described previously. If there is sufficient length, it may be coiled into a loop that is completely encased between the two layers of tape.

13. Dry the Luer connection at the junction of the needle and catheter hubs with a sterile gauze sponge, and compress them together firmly. If desired, a drop of cyanoacrylate adhesive may be applied to the surfaces before forcing them together (Fig. 15-4, *I*). This connection may also be bridged with a "sandwich" created by two strips of 1-inch white tape that cover the first "butterfly" strip of tape and extend from the suture site all the way to the injection cap (Fig. 15-4, *J*).

14. Suture the tape "sandwich" to the skin at points on both sides of the catheter within 0.5 cm (0.2 inch) of the penetration site (Fig. 15-4, *K*).

15. Cover the point of insertion with the antiseptic-treated gauze sponge.

16. Anchor the catheter with a strip of porous white tape. If a jugular vein is cannulated, firmly apply the tape to the base of the needle guard, and then wrap it in a manner that pulls the catheter in a dorsal direction on the ipsilateral side to help prevent the catheter from slipping ventrally later (Fig. 15-4, *L*). The goal is to secure the catheter to the skin, not to wrap it on tightly.

17. Apply layers of cast padding, stretch gauze, and elastic bandage material, wrapping up (dorsally) on the ipsilateral side in the case of a jugular vein catheter. While wrapping the catheter bandage, hold the limb or neck in a natural position (partially flexed limb or nose pointed down) to prevent binding (Fig. 15-4, *M* to *O*).

Guidewire Placement of Central Venous Catheters

Materials Needed

1. Commercial guide wire-style central venous catheter (e.g., Arrow Two-Lumen Central Venous Catheterization Set, Arrow International). Most commercial products are sold as a kit with a sterile drape.

2. Sterile surgical gloves

3. 00 or 000 monofilament nylon, needle holders, suture scissors

4. 22-gauge needle

5. One roll each 1-inch waterproof white tape and porous white tape

6. One roll each of appropriately sized stretch gauze, cast padding, and adhesive (Elastikon, Johnson & Johnson) or coadhesive (Vetrap, 3M) wrap

7. One catheter injection cap, catheter "T" piece, or needleless connection device

8. Syringe with heparinized saline solution, 1 to 2 U/mL

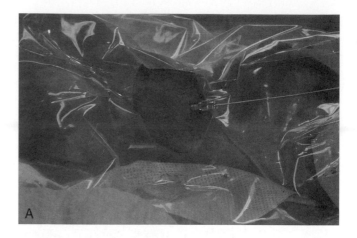

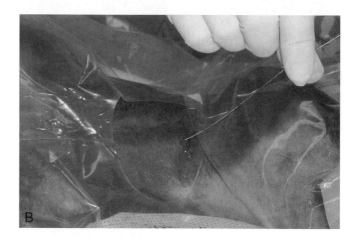

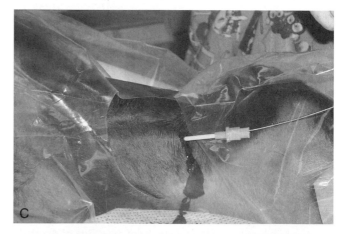

Fig. 15-5 Seldinger technique for jugular vein cannulation. The dog is in left lateral recumbency with its head to the right. **A,** An 18-gauge over-the-needle style catheter has been inserted into the right jugular vein through a small skin incision, and the central catheter's guide wire has been threaded approximately 4 inches into the vein. **B,** The 18-gauge catheter has been removed, leaving the guide wire in place. **C,** A vein dilator has been threaded over the needle and advanced into the vein. It helps to rotate the dilator back and forth while pushing it into the vessel. The dilator is rigid and functions to tear a hole in the vessel wall the same diameter as the central catheter.

(Continued)

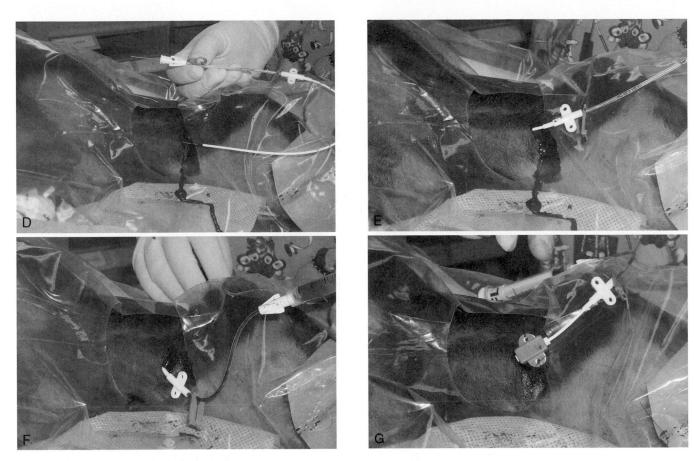

Fig. 15-5 cont'd D, The dilator has been removed and the catheter threaded over the exposed portion of the guide wire. It is essential to confirm that the end of the guide wire is visible beyond the Luer catheter connection before advancing the catheter into the vein. **E,** Once confirmed, the guide wire is held stationary, and the catheter is advanced into the vein. **F,** The wire is removed, and a syringe and "T" piece assembly have been attached to the catheter, and all air has been aspirated out. **G,** The catheter has been partially withdrawn to the ideal depth, and a catheter collar has been attached and is securely sutured to the skin at the insertion site. The catheter is then bandaged as for through-the-needle catheters.

9. Sterile gauze sponges
10. Single dose of povidone-iodine ointment

Procedure

Many animated and graphical instructional resources for the Seldinger guide wire technique are available on the Internet.

1. Prepare the skin as described previously.
2. The catheter set is opened, and sterile gloves are worn.
3. The catheterization site is draped with a sterile field drape.
4. A facilitation incision is created at the skin insertion site with a no. 11 blade. The incision should be no wider than the diameter of the catheter. As with through-the-needle catheters, the skin insertion site is as far away from the vein penetration site as practical.

5. The vein is cannulated with either a guide needle or an over-the-needle style catheter supplied with the kit.
6. A flexible guide wire is threaded through the introducer catheter several inches into the vein, taking care to avoid threading it into the heart (Fig. 15-5, *A*).
7. The guide wire is held stationary, and the introducer catheter is removed over it (Fig. 15-5, *B*).
8. A vein dilator is threaded over the guide wire into the vein (Fig. 15-5, *C*). The dilator tears an opening in the vein to the same diameter as the central catheter.
9. The vein dilator is removed, and the central venous catheter is threaded over the guide wire. Be sure that the guide wire protrudes from the Luer fitting at the end of the catheter (Fig. 15-5, *D*).
10. The catheter is passed along the guide wire to a depth calculated to place the tip near the right atrium in the cranial vena cava (Fig. 15-5, *E*).

11. All air is aspirated from the catheter, and then it is purged with heparinized saline solution (Fig. 15-5, *F*).
12. If the catheter is not fully seated, a suture collar is placed around it and anchored to the skin at the insertion site (Fig. 15-5, *G*).
13. The catheter is wrapped as previously described.

VASCULAR ACCESS PROCEDURES

These techniques aid catheterization when direct percutaneous access is difficult. They are especially helpful in emergencies when cannulation with a large-gauge catheter is required.[14,30]

Percutaneous Facilitation Procedure

A facilitation incision is a small cut made just through the skin at the intended point of entry, directly over or just to the side of the vein. This incision is easily made with the bevel edge of an 18-gauge needle or with the tip of a no. 11 Bard-Parker blade. In the conscious patient, inject a lidocaine/bicarbonate 9:1 mixture subcutaneously at the site at least 2 to 3 minutes before performing the procedure. Hold the needle (or blade) like a pencil, and incise the skin to the subcutis parallel to, but not directly over, the vein, creating a wound just large enough for the catheter to pass through. This incision reduces the resistance encountered as the catheter traverses the skin and provides greater control of the venipuncture when compared with forcing the catheter through unbroken skin. The catheter should be tunneled subcutaneously as far parallel as practical before it enters the vein. As long as the wound is no larger than the catheter diameter, the dermis will form a tight seal around the catheter shaft to limit bacterial migration from the skin.

Minicut-down Procedure

This approach is the same as the facilitation procedure, but the incision is sufficiently extended so that the vessel's sides and superficial surface are visible. The vessel may then be catheterized under direct visualization, or it is carefully dissected free of surrounding tissue, elevated from the wound, incised with the bevel of a 20-gauge needle, and then catheterized. This procedure is best done on any superficial vessel that has not been previously traumatized by percutaneous attempts. It is a reliable technique when direct percutaneous catheterization is difficult because of vascular collapse. However, the resultant skin wound promotes bacterial migration along the outer surface of the catheter. Therefore the catheter should be removed as soon as possible.

Emergency Cut-down Procedure

An emergency cut down is used to cannulate a vein when attempts at percutaneous catheterization have failed or are likely to fail in a patient that requires immediate venous access. *This is an essential skill for emergency clinicians that should be considered for any patient requiring*
immediate venous access. Any vein may be used, but the author prefers the lateral saphenous vein in dogs (Fig. 15-6, *A*) because the thin skin overlying this vein facilitates access, and the vein may be successfully and rapidly isolated with shaking hands. With practice, you should be able to catheterize this vein within 30 to 60 seconds.

1. If time permits, clip the hair and cleanse the skin. This step may be omitted in patients with short hair coats that require immediate access; if the hair coat is long or matted, it is worth the time and effort to clip it first. Relatively stable conscious animals should receive local anesthesia with a 1% to 2% lidocaine/bicarbonate 9:1 mixture.
2. Create a ¾- to 2-inch (1.3 to 5 cm) incision with a no. 11 Bard-Parker blade cranial and parallel to (not directly over) the vein. Orient the cutting edge of the blade **away** from the leg; poke the tip through a fold of elevated (tented) skin over the lateral tibia; and lift the blade as you advance it up the leg in a sweeping motion (Fig. 15-6, *B*).
3. Retract the wound to expose the vein, and push against the vein from underneath the leg with an index finger to elevate it from the wound (Fig. 15-6, *C*).
4. Vigorously push the closed jaw tips of a curved mosquito forceps directly down on the vein, and then open the jaws along the long axis of the vessel to strip perivascular fascia away from the vein (Fig. 15-6, *D* and *E*). Lift the forceps from the wound; close the jaws; and repeat this step three to five times to completely free up the vein. This is critical to allow rapid, reliable access to the vein lumen in the next step.
5. Close the forceps jaws; pass the instrument tip under the cranial edge of the vein; and advance it caudally to stretch the vein over the handles at the finger holds (Fig. 15-6, *F*).
6. **If your hands are steady,** you can attempt direct catheterization of the vein with an over-the-needle style catheter. This is more difficult than it may first appear because the fascia around the vein no longer anchors it, and if your hands tremble, there is a high chance you will lacerate the vein and lose your chance for success.
   a. Grasp the mosquito forceps handle with your nondominant hand, and pull the vein toward the foot to stretch and stabilize it.
   b. With the needle bevel oriented away from the vein, puncture the tough superficial wall with the tip directly over the distal handle arm, and advance it sufficiently to drag the catheter tip within the vessel lumen.
   c. Once the catheter tip is within the lumen, pull the forceps handle toward the foot to straighten the vein, and slide the catheter off the needle and up the vein all the way to the catheter hub.

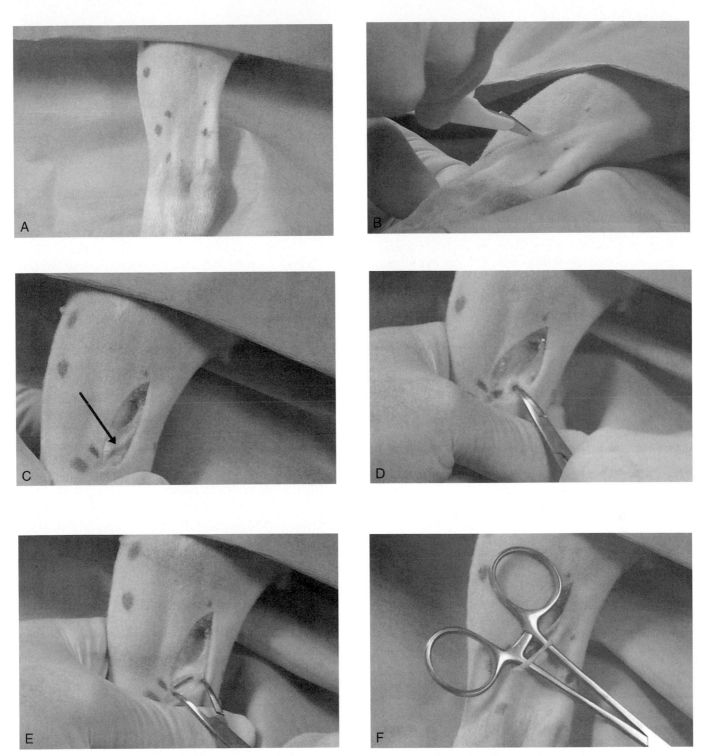

Fig. 15-6 Emergency venous cut down on a canine lateral saphenous vein **(A). B,** A no. 11 B-P blade is poked through the skin on the lateral aspect of the tibia 1 cm ($^1/_2$ inch) proximal to the saphenous vein and is lifted as it is advanced through the skin for about 4 cm (1 $^3/_4$ inches) parallel to the vein. **C,** The distal aspect of the skin wound is retracted to expose the vein (arrow). **D,** The index finger of the hand holding the leg is pushed up under the vein, and the closed jaws of a 4-inch mosquito forceps is forced onto the vein directly over the fingertip. **E,** The jaws of the forceps are opened along the long axis of the vein while firmly pushing the forceps into it and against the finger underneath. **F,** All perivascular fascia should be stripped away within three to five repeats of step E. The forceps jaws are closed, and the forceps are slid under the vein in a cranial-to-caudal direction. Once pushed all the way to the finger holds, the weight of the hinge end will prevent the forceps from falling off the leg. The vein is now elevated from the wound and occluded proximally and distally by the forceps handles.

(Continued)

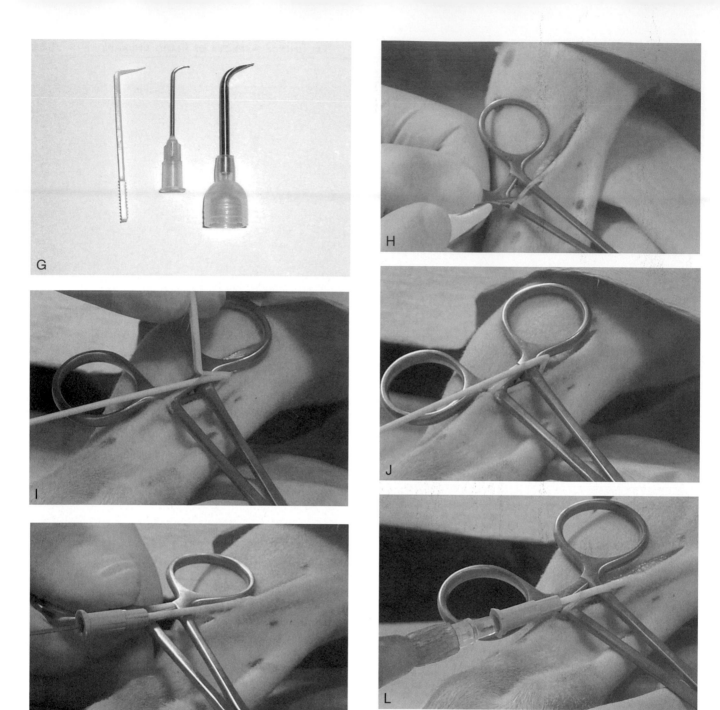

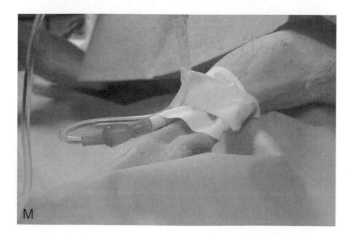

Fig. 15-6 cont'd G, A catheter introducer will be used to facilitate entry of the catheter into the vein. It may be purchased (plastic introducer at left) or fashioned from the bent and dulled tip of a suitable size needle. **H,** The no. 11 blade is held upside down to make a venotomy incision directly over the distal handle. **I,** The venotomy wound is opened with the catheter introducer, and the needle is partially withdrawn from the tip of the catheter and is advanced into the wound until it lodges where the vein makes a 90-degree turn into the wound. **J,** The catheter introducer is then set aside. **K,** The forceps are pulled toward the hock to straighten out the vein, and the catheter is advanced off of the needle up the vein. **L,** An intravenous fluid line is connected immediately. **M,** The wound margins are pulled together, and the entire area is wrapped with waterproof white tape. The tape should securely anchor a loop of fluid administration set tubing.

7. **If your hands are trembling,** it is safer to use a catheter introducer. These may be purchased (Catheter Introducer [part 6999], Becton Dickinson) or made from an injection needle for cats and small dogs or from a microchip implantation needle for large dogs (Fig. 15-6, *G*).

   a. Use the no. 11 blade to create a small venotomy incision directly over the distal handle. It helps to hold the blade upside down for this step as well, poke it through the superficial vessel wall, and lift it up away from the vein as it is advanced (ever so slightly) up the vessel (Fig. 15-6, *H*).

   b. Insert the catheter introducer into the wound, and lift it to expose the vessel lumen. If it does not easily advance to its elbow, you have probably not entered the vessel lumen and are dissecting perivascular fascia instead.

   c. Use a large-bore, over-the-needle catheter with the needle pulled back from the tip of the catheter so that the needle tip is not visible. Introduce the catheter into the vessel lumen (Fig. 15-6, *I*), and advance it to the level of the proximal forceps handle, at which point it will travel no further because the vessel bends at a 90-degree angle as it courses down into the wound (Fig. 15-6, *J*).

   d. Remove the catheter introducer; pull the forceps toward the paw to straighten and stretch the vein; and advance the catheter off the needle all the way to the hub (Fig. 15-6, *K*).

8. Set the needle aside, and connect an intravenous fluid line directly to the catheter (Fig. 15-6, *L*). Draw the wound edges together over the catheter, and wrap the entire area with white tape to close the wound temporarily, protect it from contamination, and secure the catheter and fluid line to the limb (Fig. 15-6, *M*).

9. When the patient has been stabilized, an elective, sterile catheter should be inserted into a different limb and the cut down catheter removed.

   a. Remove the tape, and flush the wound liberally with a sterile irrigant solution. If the hair coat was not clipped, fill the wound with sterile water-soluble lubricant, clip the coat, and flush the lubricant and clipped hair away. Fill the wound with fresh lubricant, and perform a surgical scrub of the surrounding skin.

   b. Compress the venotomy site with sterile 4 × 4-inch gauze sponges, and remove the catheter. Hold gentle pressure over the area for 2 to 5 minutes; this usually stops any bleeding unless the wound in the vessel wall was large.

   c. Remove the sponges, and carefully continue to irrigate the wound. If the venotomy incision continues to bleed, partial or complete ligation may be necessary. Once you are satisfied that the wound is clean, close the proximal two thirds to three fourths of the skin incision with monofilament

nylon suture, leaving the distal section free to drain. Cover the wound with a light dressing, and change the dressing at least daily until healing is advanced, usually 3 to 5 days.

Intraosseous Vascular Access

This route is useful for emergency administration of fluids, blood products, and drugs to neonates and occasionally to older animals with difficult access because of vascular collapse or small size.[21,54] Older and larger animals are generally best treated with venous cut down. The intraosseous technique is best suited for puppies and kittens using the intertrochanteric fossa of the femur, the tibial tuberosity, the medial surface of the proximal tibia 1 to 2 cm (½ to ¾ inch) distal to the tibial tuberosity or the greater tubercle of the humerus.

Materials Needed

1. One to two milliliters of 2% lidocaine/bicarbonate 9:1 mixture
2. No. 11 Bard-Parker scalpel blade
3. Needle:
   a. 16- to 20-gauge bone marrow needle (dogs, cats)
   b. 18- to 22-gauge spinal needle (cats, young dogs)
   c. 18- to 25-gauge hypodermic needle (neonates of any species)
   d. Commercial intraosseous needle (disposable intraosseous needles, Global Veterinary Products)
4. 12-mL syringe
5. Heparinized saline solution in a 3- to 6-mL syringe
6. Antiseptic ointment on a sterile gauze sponge
7. Limb stocking material
8. Bandaging material

Procedure

1. When time permits, clip the site, and prepare it aseptically. In the conscious animal, anesthetize the skin and periosteum with a lidocaine/bicarbonate 9:1 mixture.
2. Create a stab incision through the skin with the blade; introduce the needle into the wound; and advance it to the periosteum. Seat the needle into the cortex by pushing the needle lightly into the bone while rotating it about its long axis back and forth over 30-degree turns.
3. When the needle is seated in the cortex, apply increasing pressure to it as you rotate back and forth to force it through the cortex. A sudden reduction in resistance is often felt as the cortex is breached. If using a threaded commercial intraosseous needle, screw it through the cortex as soon as you gain purchase into it, and drill it into the marrow.
4. The position of the needle may be tested by flicking it with a finger. If the needle is firmly seated in bone, it will not wobble when struck. When the limb is moved, the needle should move solidly with the bone.

5. Attach the 12-mL syringe, and apply vacuum. If the needle tip is within the bone marrow, some marrow elements should enter the syringe. If an injection needle without a stylet was used, the needle may be obstructed with a "core" of cortical bone. This may sometimes be expelled by forceful injection of saline with a 1-mL syringe. If no marrow elements are aspirated, try rotating the needle 90 degrees, or advance it a bit further.

6. Flush the needle with a small amount of the saline solution. Only modest resistance to injection is encountered unless the bone is very small. Fluid delivered by gravity flow should flow freely (although slowly). Begin the fluid infusion, and frequently palpate the surrounding tissue for any evidence of fluid leakage from the bone. Leakage usually occurs when the needle has penetrated the opposite cortex and the tip is outside the bone or when excessive rocking motion was used during insertion, leaving a large hole in the cortical bone surrounding the needle through which fluid escapes.

7. Once the needle is properly positioned, anchor it by passing a suture through the periosteum and tying it to the hub of the needle or to a tape butterfly secured to the hub.

8. Cover the entry site with antiseptic ointment. A "doughnut" of limb stocking material can be placed around the needle. It should be thick enough to be level with the top of the needle hub. Secure this padding to the patient with bandaging material.

BANDAGING

All intravenous catheters must be adequately secured to the body. Catheters left in place for more than 6 hours should be covered with a sterile dressing and a bandage that provides protection against traction, damage, and contamination. The bandage should be heavy enough to protect the catheter but should not be completely occlusive so that moisture can evaporate from the skin and dressing. The point of entry should be covered with povidone-iodine ointment on a sterile gauze sponge. Single-dose packets of ointment are preferred over jars that become contaminated with repeated use, and povidone-iodine is preferred over triple antibiotic ointments, which support growth of fungi and resistant bacteria.[48,81] Catheters used for short procedures may be dressed with a small amount of ointment at the entry site and secured to the neck or limb with white tape. White tape is inelastic and must be wrapped loosely (with the neck or limb held in a natural position) to prevent binding, venous occlusion, and edema. Additional stability is achieved by suturing the catheter hub to the skin before wrapping. The catheter should be anchored securely enough to minimize any in-and-out movement through the skin. This allows the skin to close around the catheter and form a natural barrier to bacterial migration.

Interestingly, there is little evidence from human patients that any type of dressing reduces the incidence of catheter infection compared with catheters left exposed and kept clean and dry.[51] Newer transparent "breathable" dressings appear to offer little advantage for human patients over gauze dressings[26] and do not adhere as well to animal skin. If the catheter is to remain in place for longer periods, a layer of cast padding thick enough to provide some physical support to the entire bandage is applied. A layer of stretch gauze may be wrapped around the padding; this should be applied snugly enough to create a firm unit of material but not tightly enough to occlude venous return. The outermost layer may be an adhesive or coadhesive bandaging material. This material is also wrapped on snugly but not tightly enough to occlude venous return. If the animal is prone to peripheral edema, a limb bandage may be extended distally to the paw. However, this is not routinely necessary in an ambulatory animal with a properly applied catheter bandage. A heavy full limb bandage may be used (with or without a rigid splint) if the indwelling catheter crosses a joint. Immobilization of the joint in this setting helps reduce endothelial trauma and may help prevent venous thrombosis secondary to mechanical injury by the catheter.

CATHETER MAINTENANCE

The need for an intravenous catheter should be reviewed daily and the catheter removed when it is no longer therapeutically necessary. Until then, the vein and the limb or face should be examined at least twice daily for evidence of infection or edema. Regional lymph nodes should be palpated for signs of swelling or tenderness. If any evidence of inflammation or thrombosis is found, the catheter should be removed. If the bandage is too tight, it should be loosened or completely replaced. When distal edema is evident, the culprit is usually white tape that was applied too tightly.

Based on rates of phlebitis in humans and personal observations, over-the-needle catheters should be routinely removed by no later than 72 to 96 hours.[50] The dressing covering a through-the-needle catheter should be routinely replaced at 48 hours or more frequently if it appears wet or soiled. At this time, the skin and vein are examined and palpated for evidence of inflammation or thrombosis. If either is suspected, the catheter is removed. If the catheter and vein appear in good condition, the skin surrounding the entry site is cleansed with an antiseptic scrub and cotton balls. Disruption of the entry wound or any in-and-out movement of the catheter through the wound is avoided. The skin is allowed to dry completely; fresh antiseptic ointment on sterile gauze is applied; and the catheter is rewrapped. Removal of percutaneously inserted through-the-needle catheters is routinely considered after 4 days; however, they may be safely left in place for longer periods if they were inserted using a long subcutaneous tunnel and are carefully maintained.[41] If intravenous therapy is to be continued, a new catheter is inserted before the old one is removed whenever possible. Intraosseous catheters are removed when they are no longer needed, when fluid begins leaking into surrounding tissue or by 48 hours, whichever comes first. Surgically inserted catheters made of inert materials and with long subcutaneous tunnels may be left in place for days to months.

Catheters in use for continuous fluid therapy probably do not need to be flushed periodically to prevent catheter obstruction with a clot. Continuous infusion of central venous and arterial catheters with solutions containing 1 U/mL of heparin prolongs the life of those catheters in human patients.[16,35,60] In contrast, the value of intermittent flushing of catheters with heparin solutions is less clear, with some recent studies showing that use of heparinized saline prolongs catheter patency and others showing no benefit from intermittent heparin solutions compared with saline alone.[47,59,60] These discrepancies may be partly because of study differences in training nursing staff to properly flush catheters (Fig. 15-7) or disparities in data analysis.[64] No objective studies have addressed this issue in veterinary patients. Based on human practice and observations of veterinary patients, catheters that are not being used may be filled once daily with concentrated heparin (100 to 1000 U/mL). Catheters used only for intermittent administration of drugs should be flushed with sterile saline (with or without heparin) and locked with a more concentrated heparin solution immediately after drug administration. Frequent flushing with higher concentrations of heparin in cats and small dogs may produce systemic anticoagulation and should be avoided.

Sterility of the infusion system must be maintained. Only new sterile administration sets should be attached to a new catheter (unless it is used for just a few hours, e.g., as for intraoperative fluid therapy), and disconnections are made only when essential. Hands should be washed and disposable gloves worn for setting up a new system, making disconnections, injecting medications, or withdrawing blood. When fluids are to be administered, a "T" piece or needleless connection device should be used at the catheter, and locking Luer connections should be used between the administration set, extension sets (if used), and the patient catheter. Needleless connection devices that allow blood withdrawal, intravenous administration set disconnections, and drug administration minimize contamination of catheter connection when compared with opening the tubing system to attach a syringe directly.[5] The patient's end of fluid administration tubing must be anchored to the catheter bandage with a piece of white tape to relieve traction on the catheter connector ("T" piece or similar device) and prevent separation. If the animal needs to be moved,

avoid disconnecting the fluid line whenever possible. If a needleless connector is not used, the fluid line should be clamped at the "T" piece and the fluid bag and line carried with the patient.

All intravenous tubing and containers are changed every 72 hours or sooner if contamination is suspected. Injection ports and needleless connection devices should be cleaned carefully with 70% isopropanol before needle puncture. Injection port caps are replaced if they are observed to leak or if they have been penetrated more than approximately 20 times.

COMPLICATIONS OF INTRAVENOUS THERAPY

EXTRAVASATION

Extravasation of fluid and infiltration of surrounding tissue occur when a catheter is displaced out of the vein. Needle catheters and stiff plastic catheters are more likely to perforate the vessel wall than softer polyurethane or silicone catheters. Extravasation at a peripheral vein site is heralded by swelling and tenderness. Cooling of the skin over the catheter tip may be palpated as a high-pressure pocket of fluid impairs circulation, especially if room temperature fluids are being administered. If the intravenous solution contains irritating drugs such as thiobarbiturates or thiacetarsamide, swelling may be accompanied by increasing pain, heat, redness, and induration followed by necrosis and sloughing of skin and perivascular tissues. Signs of central vein extravasation may be absent until large quantities of fluid are administered. Complications of central venous extravasation include mediastinal or pleural fluid accumulation resulting in dyspnea. This may be documented by evaluation of physical signs, thoracic radiographs, and fluid analysis. Penetration of the right atrium may occur with a catheter positioned too deeply in the chest, resulting in accumulation of blood and fluid in the pericardial sac and cardiac tamponade.

Extravasation of a short catheter at a peripheral site may be detected early by frequent inspection of the vein. Catheter positioning and patency should be evaluated before injecting any irritating substance. This may be accomplished by aspirating blood and administering a test injection of sterile saline while observing the perivascular area. To aspirate blood without disconnecting a fluid administration line, lower the fluid container below the level of the catheter tip. Gravity flow pulls blood back until it is visible at the catheter hub or administration set tubing. Other recommendations to minimize the risk of extravasation include the following: (1) avoid winged needle catheters for prolonged infusions; (2) use the smallest and softest catheter that will perform adequately; (3) select a large vein at a location well away from a joint; and (4) limit movement of peripheral vein

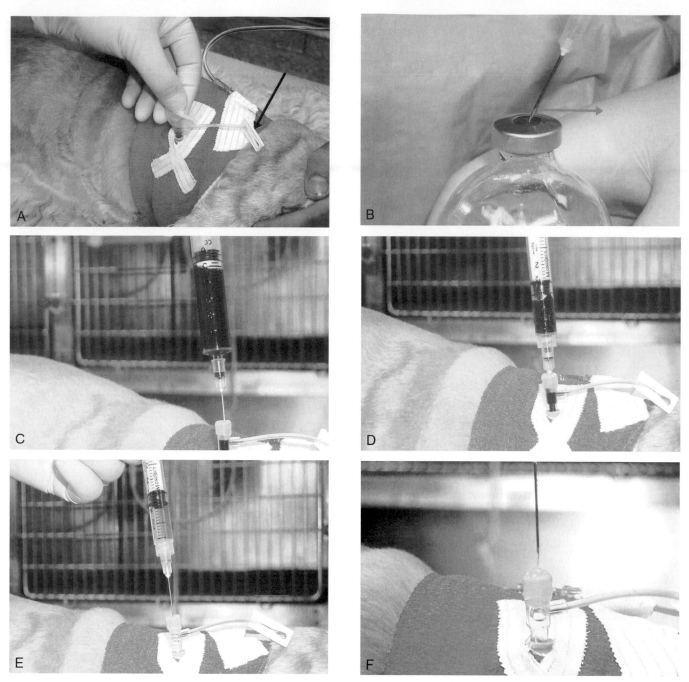

Fig. 15-7 Proper injection and blood collection technique. **A,** Using a conventional "T" piece (the principles are the same if using an injection cap), fluid administration has been interrupted, and the extension tube on the "T" piece has been clamped (arrow). The rubber diaphragm of the injection port is cleaned with alcohol and allowed to air dry. **B,** Proper needle insertion for injection ports and medication bottles. After the needle tip contacts the rubber surface, the needle is dragged slightly, *away* from the bevel orifice (in the direction of the arrow). This stretches the rubber surface at the injection point and reduces the likelihood of "coring" the rubber with the needle during insertion. When the needle is withdrawn, the rubber will return to its original conformation and seal the needle tract. **C,** Use needles less than 20 gauge to inject or aspirate through the injection ports. A 3- to 6-mL purge sample is collected by inserting a 22-gauge needle *just inside* the rubber diaphragm. This purges the dead space of the injection port and the catheter. After the purge sample is collected, the needle is withdrawn from the injection port, capped, and set aside. **D,** The syringe used for sample collection is attached to a new 22-gauge needle that is inserted *all the way to the hub.* This allows the needle to bypass the injection port dead space during sample collection. **E,** After sample collection, the purge sample is returned by injection. A 3-mL syringe with (heparinized) saline flush with a 22-gauge injection needle is used to flush the purge sample completely into the animal. The needle is advanced *just inside* the rubber diaphragm, and 0.5 to 2.0 mL of flush is injected. **F,** The injection of flush is continued *as the needle is completely withdrawn.* If the injection ceases before needle withdrawal, removal of the needle will create a vacuum that pulls blood back into the tip of the catheter, creating a potential obstruction with a clot. When removed, a fully seated 22-gauge injection needle will pull blood into the distal 5 cm (2 inches) of a 22-gauge intravenous catheter.

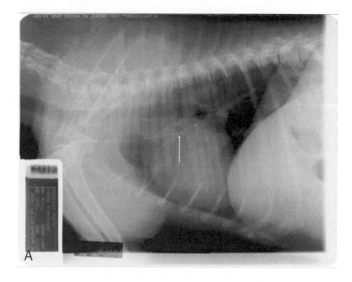

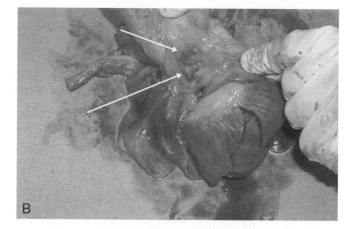

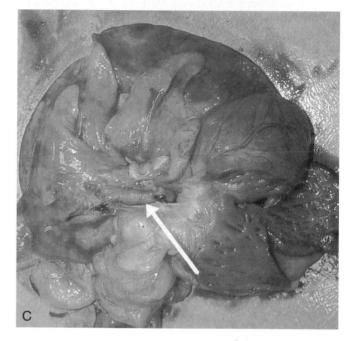

Fig. 15-8 Catheter-related thrombosis. **A,** A 19-gauge through-the-needle style central catheter was placed too deeply into the external jugular vein of this patient and terminates within the right atrium (arrow). **B,** Contact damage to the right atrial wall has resulted in cellular proliferation on the endothelial surface (arrows). **C,** A large catheter-associated thrombus was stripped off of the catheter during removal and immediately killed the patient. The thrombus obstructs the main pulmonary artery (arrow).

catheters located near joints by immobilizing the limb with a heavy bandage or splint.

THROMBOSIS

Thrombosis is a common complication of indwelling catheters. Catheters left in place for more than a few hours are covered with a fibrin sheath and platelets. Within days, cells from the injured vessel wall invade this sheath. If left in place for a week or longer, this process yields a sheath composed of smooth muscle and collagen and covered by endothelium.[79] This sheath strips away from the catheter surface during catheter removal and either is incorporated in the vessel wall or embolizes the pulmonary arteries. When small in mass, these emboli usually go unnoticed, but some fibrin sheaths extend to a larger thrombus hanging freely from the end of the catheter and may embolize the lung (Fig. 15-8).[70,80] Another, potentially more damaging type of thrombus usually forms at contact points between the catheter and

the vessel or atrial wall.[4] Endothelial injury at these points results in local inflammation and thrombus formation.[43] These thrombi are more likely to develop when stiff or reactive catheter materials are used, on long catheters that cross a joint or enter the right atrium, and on catheters with frayed tips. Mural thrombi may grow progressively and eventually obliterate the vessel lumen. Complications of these thrombi may be both obvious and serious.[17,67,78] Heparin-bonded catheters result in less fibrin deposition on catheters used experimentally in dogs and reduce the incidence of catheter-associated thrombosis in humans, at least for a few days.[32,58]

THROMBOPHLEBITIS

Thrombophlebitis represents the most severe end of the spectrum of catheter-related vessel damage and may be caused by mechanical, chemical, or infectious processes. Damage to the endothelial lining of the vein initiates both inflammation (phlebitis) and thrombus formation on the vessel wall. Early signs of thrombophlebitis include tenderness and erythema of the skin over the vessel and palpable induration of the vessel itself. If left untreated, these early signs progress, and the vessel may become completely thrombosed. This is recognized as severe hardening of the vessel and may be accompanied by complete occlusion and inability to infuse fluids. Purulent discharge may be noted from the catheter site. Systemic signs of inflammation including fever and leukocytosis may be present, although some animals develop severe local reactions in the absence of systemic signs.

Mechanical damage is minimized by selecting small catheters and large veins; by using soft, inert catheter materials; and by securely anchoring the catheter to the skin to minimize in-and-out motion. If an indwelling catheter crosses a joint, the limb should be immobilized to limit trauma to the vascular endothelium. Irritating drugs should be administered after adequate dilution and only into central veins with high blood flow rates to minimize local endothelial injury. Hypertonic solutions should be administered only into central veins whenever possible.

INFECTION

Any intravenous catheter supports infection, and there are multiple routes for possible exogenous catheter contamination. In humans and experimental animal models, catheter colonization has been documented from the skin at the exit site,[3,13,33,66] contamination of the hub connection,[15,62] and the hands of nursing staff.[57] In addition, the catheter may be colonized by blood-borne bacteria originating from remote locations. In humans receiving intravenous fluid therapy, infection arising from contamination of the catheter hub and fluid administration set connections is comparatively less likely if sterile technique is strictly followed.[9] Veterinary patients that chew, disconnect, and defecate on their administration sets are probably at higher risk for this source of contamination. The prevalence of positive bacteriologic cultures from catheters at the time of removal ranged from 10.7% to 26% in three small surveys of veterinary patients.[7,36,41] Signs of infection may be identical to those of sterile thrombophlebitis. There is normally a small (1 to 5 mm) diameter zone of inflammation surrounding the skin puncture site, and inflammation extending beyond this range is suspect.[30] Systemic signs including fever and leukocytosis may develop in bacteremic animals. Some may develop organ infection at remote sites (endocarditis, abscessation), and some develop sepsis syndrome.[7] However, other animals develop catheter-related bacteremia with minimal clinical signs. Catheter infection should always be suspected in animals developing clinical evidence of infection while an indwelling catheter is present. If catheter infection is suspected, the catheter should be removed immediately.

Bacteriologic culture of the catheter tip assists in the diagnosis of catheter infection. Before removal, the skin is scrubbed with antiseptic solution and carefully cleaned with alcohol. When the alcohol has dried, the catheter is removed aseptically, and the catheter tip is cut off with a sterile blade and dropped into a tube of culture medium broth for bacteriologic evaluation. If the catheter is suspected to be the cause of infection in a bacteremic animal but the catheter cannot be easily replaced (e.g., catheters inserted surgically in animals with limited venous access), differential bacteriologic culture may be performed. In this procedure, cultures are performed on blood drawn simultaneously through a peripheral vein and through the catheter. In humans, if the catheter blood sample shows a sevenfold increase in identical bacterial colonies compared with the peripheral vein blood culture, the catheter is probably the source of the bacteremia.[19] Prevention of infection is assisted by using sterile technique during catheterization, tunneling the catheter subcutaneously before venipuncture, using needleless connection devices, avoiding tubing disconnections, properly maintaining the catheter dressing, and carefully managing injection ports and fluid containers.[41,50,73] Antibiotic therapy does not appear to alter the risk of catheter infection but is used to treat infections after catheter removal.

CATHETER EMBOLISM

Catheter embolism occurs when a fragment of the catheter becomes free and is carried by blood flow until it lodges in the heart or a pulmonary artery. This may occur in any of the following circumstances:

1. The catheter is accidentally cut during bandage removal.
2. A through-the-needle catheter is advanced, then pulled back into the needle shaft and sheared off by the needle bevel.
3. The needle within an over-the-needle catheter is partially withdrawn and then reinserted while the catheter tip is still within the vein. If the flexible catheter tip is bent to the side, the needle catches on the catheter shaft and amputates the end of the catheter.
4. The catheter shaft disconnects from the catheter hub.

If catheter amputation is observed, a tourniquet is immediately applied proximal to the venipuncture site to hold the embolus and prevent further migration. If the catheter is made of radiopaque material, the area is radiographed to identify the embolus position, and it is removed surgically if possible. Long fragments that have migrated to the right ventricle may be removed with a transvenous loop snare under fluoroscopic guidance.[22] Catheter embolization is best prevented by careful technique during catheter insertion and removal. A misplaced catheter is never withdrawn while the needle is left in place; instead, the catheter and needle are withdrawn together as a unit.

AIR EMBOLISM

Air embolism may occur whenever a catheter is within a vein. The risk of air embolism is highest during insertion of central venous catheters. When the catheter enters the thoracic cavity, the catheter tip is exposed to negative intrathoracic pressure, and air embolism occurs if the free end of the catheter is exposed to the atmosphere. This risk may be higher in dogs with extrathoracic airway obstruction (e.g., brachycephalic breeds) because increased inspiratory effort can produce markedly negative intrathoracic pressure. Air embolism during catheterization is avoided by completing the procedure and sealing the Luer end as rapidly as possible. Air embolism may also result from disconnections or the presence of air within the fluid administration system. The risk of air embolism is higher when using vented fluid administration sets. This risk may be reduced substantially by using collapsible plastic containers and nonvented administration sets. The practice of injecting air into glass containers to increase the rate of fluid delivery is extremely hazardous and should be avoided.

Small air emboli are trapped in the pulmonary vasculature and usually go unnoticed. Larger emboli markedly increase pulmonary vascular resistance and cause respiratory distress and pulmonary edema.[28] A slow infusion of air into the vascular space of dogs increases pulmonary artery and CVPs and produces a progressive decrease in arterial blood pressure. Ultimately, arterial blood pressure is markedly reduced, and cardiovascular collapse occurs. Administration of a bolus of air produces an air lock in the right ventricular outflow tract and circulatory obstruction.

The best treatment for air embolism is to aspirate the air immediately from the right atrium and ventricle if a central venous catheter is in place. If this is not possible, the animal may be positioned in left lateral recumbency to trap gas in the right ventricular apex and allow blood to flow through the right ventricular outflow tract. However, one group found that no one position was better than another to resuscitate dogs with air embolism.[25] Standard cardiopulmonary resuscitation procedures should be instituted if the animal develops respiratory or cardiac arrest.[72]

EXSANGUINATION

Exsanguination is possible whenever the unobserved animal disconnects the catheter or administration tubing. Metal floor grates pose a unique threat: they can snag and separate tubing connection sites, and during the resulting hemorrhage, blood dripping to the cage floor underneath the grate may be difficult to see. Disconnections are particularly likely in dogs that change position frequently. Blood loss may be most severe through cephalic vein

catheters when an animal is in sternal recumbency with its elbows flexed. Anchoring the patient's end of the administration tubing to the catheter bandage helps prevent disconnection at the catheter. Use of locking Luer connections (as opposed to slip-Luer connections) is the best way to reduce the likelihood of an accidental disconnection. Those junctions may also be bridged with waterproof white tape to further reduce that risk.

FLUID ADMINISTRATION AND MONITORING

The many different types of available fluid administration sets and connection devices offer considerable flexibility in intravenous fluid administration. Multiple port flow connectors allow simultaneous infusion of compatible solutions through a single catheter. In-line volume control sets (Buretrol, Baxter Healthcare) permit accurate delivery of small volumes of fluids. A variety of different tubing lengths, diameters, and connections allow many different configurations and combinations of fluids to be delivered to a single catheter. Fluid administration sets are available from several manufacturers. The two basic types are vented and nonvented; these are available in several lengths. All administration sets use an in-line drip chamber to estimate the rate of flow. Depending on the brand, the drip sizes are calibrated so that 1 mL = 10, 15, 20, or 60 drops. Drops per minute are calculated from the formula:

$$\text{Drops per minute} = \frac{\text{total infusion volume} \times \text{drops/mL}}{\text{Total infusion time (min)}}$$

For example, to administer 2000 mL over 24 hours using a basic solution set (10 drops = 1 mL):

$$\frac{2000 \text{ mL} \times 10 \text{ drops/mL}}{1440 \text{ min}} = 14 \text{ drops/min}$$

The rate of flow is regulated by tightening or releasing the intravenous tubing clamp while watching and counting the drip rate. Fluid administration rate may also be controlled by in-line flow regulators (Stat 2 Pumpette, ConMed Corp., Utica, NY) or, more accurately, by electronic fluid pumps or rate controllers. In-line flow regulators are calibrated tubing clamps. Accurate use of these devices depends on unimpeded flow through short catheters 20 gauge or larger and on maintaining a minimum height of about 75 cm (30 inches) between the drip chamber and the level of the heart.

Fluid pumps are available from many manufacturers. All are either peristaltic or metered cassette in design (Fig. 15-9). Peristaltic pumps typically use standard intravenous administration sets, although some devices are restricted to certain brands of tubing. This pump

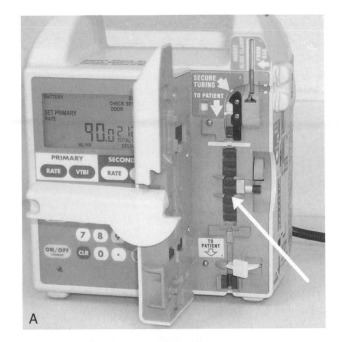

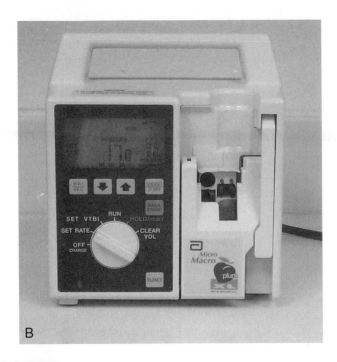

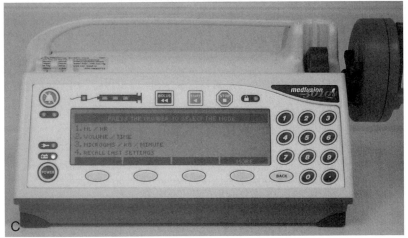

Fig. 15-9 Fluid pumps. **A,** A peristaltic pump, with its fluid path exposed to show the peristalsis mechanism (arrow), which massages fluid through the tubing set. **B,** A volumetric pump that requires a specific in-line cassette that snaps into the drive mechanism. **C,** A syringe pump useful for administration of drugs and very slow administration of fluids.

design uses a continuous peristalsis mechanism to continuously drive fluid at a constant rate. Cassette-style pumps require an in-line fluid path pump mechanism (cassette) as an integral component of an intravenous fluid administration set that works only with a specific model(s) of pump. When fluids need to be given at a very constant rate from moment to moment, peristaltic pumps are generally better than cassette designs, which alternate between pulling fluid from the bag and pushing it to the patient. Peristaltic pumps are less accurate over time, and their accuracy also depends on using an approved intravenous tubing set and changing the tubing position within the pump at regular intervals. Metered cassette pumps are volumetric and are used to deliver prescribed volumes of fluid accurately over longer units of time (many minutes to hours). The rate-constant peristaltic type of fluid pump (or a screw mechanism syringe pump for small volumes) is useful for infusions of fluid with drug additives that require a constant flow rate (e.g., minute to minute amounts of norepinephrine), whereas the volumetric pumps are preferred for accurate administration of prescribed volumes of fluid over longer units of time (e.g., day to day). Pumps marketed specifically for use in animals are available (e.g., Vet/IV, Heska, Fort Collins, CO).

All pumps deliver fluid under pressure. This pressure can overcome resistance to flow from viscous solutions, filters, and partially occluded veins. It also increases the risk to the patient in the case of extravasation because fluid is pumped into the perivascular tissues under pressure. To prevent this, most modern pumps are equipped with pressure monitoring circuitry and can be adjusted to produce an occlusion alarm at preset values.

Intravenous solution containers should be numbered consecutively and clearly labeled with the date, time, and patient's name. Any additives should be clearly identified as to type, quantity added, date and time added, and by whom. Do not use an indelible marker to write directly on the bag because the solvents in the ink may leach through the plastic into the solution inside. When not using a volumetric pump that tracks cumulative fluid administered, a calibrated timing label should be applied to the container and is used to monitor and verify the rate of flow over time. All patients receiving intravenous fluid therapy should be weighed at least daily. Abnormal fluid losses through the urinary tract, nasogastric suction, or cavity drainage should be measured and replaced with equal volumes of appropriate intravenous replacement fluids at frequent intervals. Fluid losses in animals with vomiting or diarrhea may be monitored by knowing the average dry weight of cage paper used in the clinic and subtracting this from the weight of soiled cage papers. The difference (in grams) is converted to milliliters of water and replaced with appropriate intravenous replacement fluid. Monitoring of the PCV and total plasma solids is an inaccurate (PCV) and insensitive (total plasma solids) indicator of hydration status in sick dogs and should not be relied upon as sole measures of hydration.[29] Finding a high urine specific gravity in animals capable of concentrating their urine assists in detection of inadequate circulating blood volume (in animals being treated for shock or extracellular fluid losses) or inadequate administration of water (in animals receiving maintenance fluid therapy).

CENTRAL VENOUS PRESSURE MONITORING

CVP measurement is a useful diagnostic procedure for hemodynamic assessment and management of fluid therapy in critically ill animals. It can be used in a variety of situations to assist in diagnosis and optimal fluid therapy management. It is important to obtain CVP measurements in as technically precise a manner as possible and to obtain consecutive measurements with the patient in the same position each time. As with any monitoring tool, CVP measurements must be interpreted in light of other diagnostic findings, and the pitfall of relying too heavily on a single test must be avoided.

The CVP is the blood pressure within the intrathoracic portions of the cranial or caudal vena cava. CVP is measured clinically for two reasons: (1) to gain information about cardiac function, and (2) to gain information about intravascular blood volume. The CVP is slightly higher than the mean right atrial pressure (RAP), and the two terms, CVP and RAP, are sometimes used interchangeably. However, in some circumstances, the mean RAP may vary independently of CVP.[74] The CVP (or RAP) affects, and is affected by, cardiac output. RAP is quantitatively similar to the pressure in the right ventricle at the end of diastole. As RAP and right ventricular end-diastolic pressure (EDP) increase, right ventricular

end-diastolic volume (EDV) increases. The relationship between ventricular EDP and EDV is not linear (Fig. 15-10). At low ventricular volumes, an increase in EDV does not increase ventricular EDP significantly. At high ventricular volumes when the limit of ventricular distention is reached, small increases in EDV increase both ventricular EDP and atrial pressure substantially. Clinically, if EDV is increased by administration of intravenous fluids, there is little initial increase in EDP (steep portion of curve, Fig. 15-10) until the limit of ventricular expansion is reached. At that point, administration of more fluids no longer increases EDV substantially, but EDP and atrial pressure increase rapidly (plateau portion of curve, Fig. 15-10). Ventricular EDV is an important determinant of stroke volume and cardiac output. The relationship between EDV and stroke volume is nearly linear in normal animals; as EDV increases, stroke volume and cardiac output increase according to the Frank-Starling law of the heart. In many situations (e.g., shock states) it is desirable to increase both stroke volume and cardiac output maximally to optimize oxygen transport to tissues. This is accomplished most effectively by increasing ventricular EDV.

EDV is not easily measured clinically. However, CVP can be monitored to make inferences about possible changes in ventricular EDV or cardiac output. Just as the relationship between EDP and EDV is not linear, the relationship between CVP or RAP and cardiac output is not linear (Fig. 15-11). At low pressures, a small increase in CVP/RAP generates a large increase in cardiac output. At higher pressures, a large increase in RAP does not substantially increase cardiac output (plateau phase of Frank-Starling curves; see Fig. 15-11).

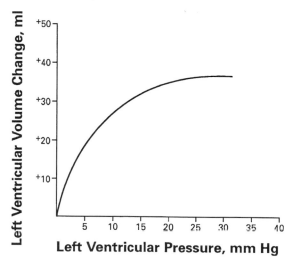

Fig. 15-10 Graph depicting the relationship between left ventricular diastolic pressure and left ventricular volume gain in the dog. As pressure increases from zero, diastolic volume increases rapidly until the limit of the ventricular distention is reached. At that point, even large increases in pressure will not increase ventricular volume substantially.

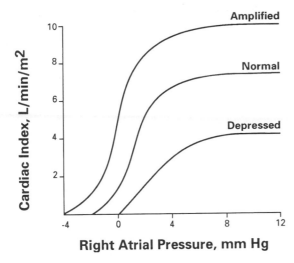

Fig. 15-11 Family of Starling curves plotting the relationship of right atrial pressure (RAP) (or right ventricular end-diastolic pressure) with cardiac index (CI). In the normal heart, small increments in RAP within the normal range (0 to 4 mm Hg) yield large increases in CI. This response is augmented in dogs with endogenous sympathetic cardiac stimulation or in dogs receiving inotropic drugs ("amplified" curve) and is depressed in dogs with myocardial failure ("depressed" curve).

As stated earlier, the CVP also reflects venous blood volume and venous return to the heart. The venous system accommodates small changes in volume with minimal change in venous pressure. However, if a fluid challenge is rapidly administered, both venous return to the heart and CVP increase. If the intravascular volume is substantially reduced, say because of hemorrhage, the CVP decreases, although it may remain in the normal range. Within minutes, circulatory reflexes, including capacitance vein tone, return venous pressure and flow toward normal.

The relationship between CVP, RAP, EDV, cardiac output, and the vascular system is complex and dynamic. Consequently, a single measurement of CVP has no relationship with cardiac output or vascular blood volume. Indeed, even when used to evaluate hemodynamic response to fluid challenge, the CVP can be misleading, particularly when the fluid challenge is administered slowly.[35,77] Although there is a general trend for animals with reduced blood volume to have a low CVP, a dog or cat could experience lethal blood loss and yet have a normal CVP. Nevertheless, repeated measurements during fluid therapy can give important clues about the compliance of the cardiovascular system. When these results are interpreted in light of other clinical findings, valuable information about hemodynamic status may be obtained.

MEASUREMENT

A central venous catheter must be in place. The catheter tip should ideally reside within the thorax just outside the right atrium. A catheter placed in the lateral saphe-

nous vein and positioned so that the tip resides in the caudal vein cava may be an acceptable substitute.[1,39,76] Materials necessary for CVP measurement using a water manometer include:

1. Central venous catheter in place
2. Water manometer (Pharmaseal manometer tray, American Pharmaseal Company, Irwindale, CA; Medex manometer set, Smiths Medical, London, UK)
3. One 30-inch intravenous extension tubing set if needed
4. Three-way stopcock if needed
5. 20-mL syringe filled with saline solution
6. 20-gauge needle

The manometer and tubing are primed with saline solution, and the column is filled to a level well above the anticipated CVP of the patient. The animal is positioned in sternal or lateral recumbency with lateral recumbency preferred. The stopcock at the bottom of the manometer should rest on the table or cage floor. When the stopcock is turned to connect the column of saline with the catheter, the hydrostatic pressure in the column forces fluid through the catheter. The saline column continues to fill until the hydrostatic pressure of the column reaches equilibrium with the hydrostatic pressure of the blood at the end of the catheter. When it has reached equilibrium and has stopped decreasing, the height of the saline column above the catheter tip, expressed as centimeters of water, reflects the blood pressure within the vessel at the catheter tip. Therefore it is important to know approximately where the catheter tip lies in relation to the manometer fluid column. When the animal is in lateral recumbency, the cranial vena cava lies near the midline, and the sternum is a good reference point. In sternal recumbency, the cranial vena cava is approximately level with the point of the shoulder (scapulohumeral) joint.

When the appropriate external anatomic landmark is found, the manometer column is positioned with the stopcock resting on the table surface immediately next to the landmark, and the centimeter mark nearest that point is labeled. This mark is now the zero reference point on the manometer, and all subsequent measurements are read as the distance from that mark. Measurements can be made with the manometer located anywhere nearby that is convenient, as long as the stopcock rests on the same horizontal surface as the animal (Fig. 15-12). If the animal is in a cage, the manometer may be taped to the wall of the cage and used there.

INTERPRETATION

When obtaining a CVP measurement, rhythmic fluctuations in the height of the saline column meniscus are usually seen. These oscillations are caused by two factors: large ones occur with respiration, and smaller ones occur

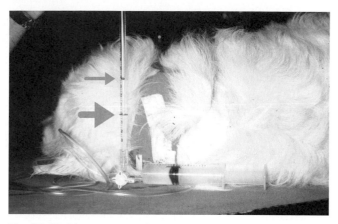

Fig. 15-12 Measurement of central venous pressure (CVP) using a saline column manometer. The dog is positioned in lateral recumbency, and the manometer rests on the table surface. The location of the patient's midline was estimated to be level with the "0" mark on the column, and the marker ring has been slid to that point (large arrow). The saline column stopped falling, and the ball floating on the top of the saline column rests at 4.5 cm at the end of expiration (small arrow). Therefore this patient's CVP is read as 4.5 − 0 = 4.5 cm water.

with each heartbeat. Fluctuations in the column synchronized with respirations are usually easily seen. As the patient inhales, the intrathoracic pressure and CVP decrease; the reverse occurs during exhalation. These excursions are exaggerated in animals with upper airway obstruction and are reversed by positive pressure ventilation. With regard to the cardiac cycle, CVP increases steadily until atrial contraction, jumps up a bit during atrial contraction, and then decreases rapidly at the beginning of diastole (Fig. 15-13). The response of the fluid column in the manometer is too slow to show all of the peaks and valleys of these pressure changes accu-

rately. When using a water column manometer, the best method is to measure the CVP just before inspiration and at the lowest diastolic swing. This value correlates best with real CVP.[11] If the rhythmic fluctuations are absent, malpositioning of the catheter should be suspected: either it is too short or too long and the tip is not within the thoracic cavity, or the tip is butted up against a vessel wall or the right atrial wall. Obstruction of the catheter tip can be confirmed by aspirating blood from the catheter: blood flows rapidly and with little resistance if it is floating freely within the lumen of the vessel. A high CVP or the presence of large fluctuations synchronous with the heartbeat suggests that the catheter tip is in the lumen of the right ventricle; if this is the case, it should be partially withdrawn to the proper level. Dorsal recumbency, abdominal compartment syndrome, or pleural effusion will increase the CVP and may lead to erroneous assumptions about the cardiovascular system if the pressure influence of those syndromes is not taken into consideration.[18,27]

Water manometers tend to overestimate CVP by 0.5 to 5 cm H_2O; this overestimation varies from patient to patient and from measurement to measurement in the same patient, even when positioning is done as carefully as possible.[11] This variation can be important when following a critically ill animal that requires aggressive fluid support and in animals that are hyperventilating, dyspneic, or being treated with positive pressure ventilation. A calibrated electronic pressure transducer connected to the catheter with a short, stiff tube is more accurate in these patients.

Measurement of CVP in animals during fluid challenge yields important information about cardiovascular status. As intravenous fluids are administered and the intravascular blood volume expands, venous return and

Fig. 15-13 Tracing from a patient monitor screen with simultaneous display of the electrocardiogram (top) and right atrial pressure (RAP, bottom). The RAP trace is characterized by the positive a-, c-, and v-waves and by the two negative depressions termed the x- and y-descents. The a-wave represents the increase in RAP during atrial contraction; the c-wave represents the slight increase in atrial pressure as the tricuspid valve bulges into the right atrium during early ventricular contraction; and the v-wave represents the increase in pressure that occurs as blood flows into the atrium while the tricuspid valve is still closed. The x-descent corresponds to the period of ventricular ejection when blood is emptied from the heart. The y-descent represents the decrease in atrial pressure that follows opening of the tricuspid valve and rapid blood flow into the ventricle. The mean RAP is 3 mm Hg, and the electrocardiograph-derived heart rate is 86 beats/min.

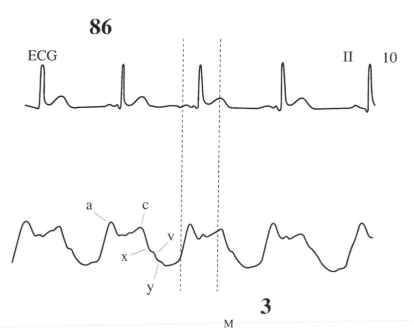

CVP begin to increase. A rapid infusion of 20 mL/kg of crystalloid or 5 mL/kg of colloid into a euvolemic animal with normal cardiac function results in a modest increase in CVP (2 to 4 cm H_2O) that returns to baseline within 15 minutes. A minimal increase or no increase in CVP implies that the vascular volume is markedly reduced. A CVP that increases and returns to baseline rapidly (<5 minutes) implies that there is reduced vascular volume and that the initial volume load has been accommodated by rapid changes in vasomotor tone. A large increase in CVP (>4 cm H_2O) implies reduced cardiac compliance or increased venous blood volume or both. A slow (15 minute) return toward baseline indicates that blood volume is close to normal. A very prolonged return to baseline (>30 minutes) suggests that the intravascular blood volume is elevated relative to cardiac performance.

When administering fluids to treat a dog or cat with noncardiogenic shock, an immediate therapeutic goal may be to administer an intravenous fluid challenge rapidly enough to increase the CVP significantly, by about 2 to 4 cm H_2O, within the first few minutes of therapy. The magnitude of initial increase and the subsequent rate of decrease of the CVP are interpreted in light of the effect of the maneuver on heart rate, pulse profile, mucous membrane color, capillary refill time, blood pressure, and skin temperature to make inferences about venous return relative to cardiac performance. If the impact on those vital signs is modest and the CVP returns to baseline rapidly, another fluid challenge is administered, and the process is repeated. If necessary, repeated fluid boluses may be given until the CVP takes 10 to 15 minutes to decrease to baseline. Once this condition is met, it is likely that blood volume and venous return are nearly optimal relative to cardiac performance and that further increases in CVP are unlikely to yield significant increases in cardiac output. In animals with normal right heart function and normal pleural and intraabdominal pressures, the CVP should not be pushed higher than about 10 to 12 mm Hg. When that pressure is reached, it is likely that pulmonary venous pressure is above 12 to 15 mm Hg (assuming that the left and right ventricles are functioning symmetrically), increasing the likelihood of pulmonary edema. When this limit has been reached, giving more fluids will not help cardiac output (because it will no longer increase EDV) but will only make the patient congested. If there is a need to further increase cardiac output or blood pressure, positive inotropic agents such as dobutamine and/or vasoactive drugs such as norepinephrine or vasopressin are administered.

CVP monitoring is also useful in less critical situations. When administering fluids to an animal with oliguria or congestive heart failure, the CVP can be used to monitor therapy and help prevent inadvertent overadministration of fluids. In that setting, the baseline CVP is measured before fluid therapy is begun and subsequently measured at intervals frequent enough to minimize the risk of fluid overload, usually every 2 to 8 hours. During chronic (slow) fluid administration, significant increases in CVP will not occur until the venous system's volume capacity has been reached, typically after the onset of physical signs of edema or congestion. Therefore any observed increase merits evaluation.

REFERENCES

1. Anter AM, Bondok RS: Peripheral venous pressure is an alternative to central venous pressure in paediatric surgery patients, *Acta Anaesth Scand* 48:1101-1104, 2004.
2. Arinzon Z, Feldman J, Fidelman Z, et al: Hypodermoclysis (subcutaneous infusion) effective mode of treatment of dehydration in long-term care patients, *Arch Gerontol Geriatr* 38:167-173, 2004.
3. Bjornson HS, Colley R, Bower RH, et al: Association between microorganism growth at the catheter insertion site and colonization of the catheter in patients receiving total parenteral nutrition, *Surgery* 92:720-727, 1982.
4. Borow M, Crowley JG: Evaluation of central venous catheter thrombogenicity, *Acta Anaesth Scand Suppl* 81:59-64, 1985.
5. Brown JD, Moss HA, Elliott TS: The potential for catheter microbial contamination from a needleless connector, *J Hosp Infect* 36:181-189,1997.
6. Brun-Buisson C, Doyon F, Sollet JP, et al: Prevention of intravascular catheter-related infection with newer chlorhexidine-silver sulfadiazine-coated catheters: a randomized controlled trial, *Intensive Care Med* 30:837-843, 2004.
7. Burrows CF: Inadequate skin preparation as a cause of intravenous catheter-related infection in the dog, *J Am Vet Med Assoc* 180:747-749, 1982.
8. Calfee DP, Farr BM: Comparison of four antiseptic preparations for skin in the prevention of contamination of percutaneously drawn blood cultures: a randomized trial, *J Clin Microbiol* 40:1660-1665,2002.
9. Cercenado E, Ena J, Rodríguez-Créixems M, et al: A conservative procedure for the diagnosis of catheter-related infections, *Arch Intern Med* 150:1417-1420, 1990.
10. Chaiyakunapruk N, Veenstra DL, Lipsky BA, et al: Chlorhexidine compared with povidone-iodine solution for vascular catheter-site care: a meta-analysis, *Ann Intern Med* 136:792-801, 2002.
11. Clayton DG: Inaccuracies in manometric central venous pressure measurement, *Resuscitation* 16:221-230, 1988.
12. Constans T, Dutertre JP, Froge E: Hypodermoclysis in dehydrated elderly patients: local effects with and without hyaluronidase, *J Palliat Care* 7:10-12,1991.
13. Cooper GL, Hopkins CC: Rapid diagnosis of intravascular catheter-associated infection by direct Gram staining of catheter segments, *N Engl J Med* 312:1142-1147, 1985.
14. Crowe DT: Practical life-saving surgical procedures involving the cardiovascular system, Proceedings of the First International Emergency and Critical Care Symposium, 1998, San Antonio, TX, pp. 32-37.
15. de Cicco M, Panarello G, Chiaradia V, et al: Source and route of microbial colonisation of parenteral nutrition catheters, *Lancet* 2:1258-1261, 1989.
16. de Neef M, Heijboer H, van Woensel JB, et al: The efficacy of heparinization in prolonging patency of arterial

and central venous catheters in children: a randomized double-blind trial, *Pediatr Hematol Oncol* 19:553-560, 2002.

17. Di Costanzo J, Sastre B, Choux R, et al: Mechanism of thrombogenesis during total parenteral nutrition: role of catheter composition, *JPEN J Parenter Enteral Nutr* 12:190-194, 1988.

18. Drellich S: Intraabdominal pressure and abdominal compartment syndrome, *Comp Cont Educ Pract Vet* 22:764-769, 2000.

19. Fan ST, Teoh-Chan CH, Lau KF: Evaluation of central venous catheter sepsis by differential quantitative blood culture, *Eur J Clin Microbiol Infect Dis* 8:142-144, 1989.

20. Faust SN, Heyderman RS, Levin M: Coagulation in severe sepsis: a central role for thrombomodulin and activated protein C, *Crit Care Med* 29:S62-S67, 2001.

21. Fiser DH: Intraosseous infusion, *N Engl J Med* 322:1579-1581, 1990.

22. Fox PR, Sos TA, Bond BR: Nonsurgical removal of a catheter embolus from the heart of a dog, *J Am Vet Med Assoc* 187:275-276, 1985.

23. Frisoli JA, de Paula AP, Feldman D, et al: Subcutaneous hydration by hypodermoclysis. A practical and low cost treatment for elderly patients, *Drugs Aging* 16:313-319,2000.

24. Fulton RB, Hauptman JG: In vitro and in vivo rates of fluid flow through catheters in peripheral veins of dogs, *J Am Vet Med Assoc* 198:1622-1624, 1991.

25. Geissler HJ, Allen SJ, Mehlhorn U, et al: Effect of body repositioning after venous air embolism. An echocardiographic study, *Anesthesiology* 86:710-717, 1997.

26. Gillies D, O'Riordan L, Carr D, et al: Gauze and tape and transparent polyurethane dressings for central venous catheters, *Cochrane Database Syst Rev* 4, 2003.

27. Gookin JL, Atkins CE: Evaluation of the effect of pleural effusion on central venous pressure in cats, *J Vet Intern Med* 13:561-563,1999.

28. Hall JE, Hofman WF, Ehrhart IC: Venous occlusion pressure and vascular permeability in the dog lung after air embolization, *J Appl Physiol* 65:34-40, 1988.

29. Hansen B, DeFrancesco T: Relationship between hydration estimate and body weight change after fluid therapy in critically ill dogs and cats. Intraabdominal pressure and abdominal compartment syndrome, *J Vet Emerg Crit Care* 12:235-243, 2002.

30. Haskins SC: Emergency anesthesia and critical care procedures, Proceedings of the First International Emergency and Critical Care Symposium, San Antonio, TX, pp. 153-157.

31. Hecker JF, Scandrett LA: Roughness and thrombogenicity of the outer surfaces of intravascular catheters, *J Biomed Mater Res* 19:381-395, 1985.

32. Idezuki Y, Watanabe H, Hagiwara M, et al: Mechanism of antithrombogenicity of a new heparinized hydrophilic polymer: chronic in vivo studies and clinical application 3, *Trans Am Soc Artif Intern Organs* 21:436-449, 1975.

33. Kelsey MC, Gosling M: A comparison of the morbidity associated with occlusive and non-occlusive dressings applied to peripheral intravenous devices, *J Hosp Infect* 5:313-321, 1984.

34. Klein MK, Dow SW, Rosychuk RA: Pulmonary thromboembolism associated with immune-mediated hemolytic anemia in dogs: ten cases (1982-1987), *J Am Vet Med Assoc* 195:246-250, 1989.

35. Kumar A, Anel R, Bunnell E, et al: Pulmonary artery occlusion pressure and central venous pressure fail to predict ventricular filling volume, cardiac performance, or the response to volume infusion in normal subjects, *Crit Care Med* 32:691-699, 2004.

36. Lippert AC, Fulton RB, Parr AM: Nosocomial infection surveillance in a small animal intensive care unit, *J Am Anim Hosp Assoc* 24:627-636, 1988.

37. Little JR, Murray PR, Traynor PS, et al: A randomized trial of povidone-iodine compared with iodine tincture for venipuncture site disinfection: effects on rates of blood culture contamination, *Am J Med* 107:119-125, 1999.

38. Littman MP, Dambach DM, Vaden SL, et al: Familial protein-losing enteropathy and protein-losing nephropathy in soft coated Wheaten terriers: 222 cases (1983-1997), *J Vet Intern Med* 14:68-80, 2000.

39. Machon RG, Raffe MR, Robinson EP: Central venous pressure measurements in the caudal vena cava of sedated cats, *J Vet Emerg Crit Care* 5:121-129, 1995.

40. Marin MG, Lee JC, Skurnick JH: Prevention of nosocomial bloodstream infections: effectiveness of antimicrobial-impregnated and heparin-bonded central venous catheters, *Crit Care Med* 28:3332-3338, 2000.

41. Mathews KA, Brooks MJ, Vallient AE: A prospective study of intravenous catheter contamination, *J Vet Emerg Crit Care* 6:33-43, 1996.

42. Mermel LA: Prevention of intravascular catheter-related infections, *Ann Intern Med* 132:391-402, 2000.

43. Mesfin GM, Higgins MJ, Brown WP, et al: Cardiovascular complications of chronic catheterization of the jugular vein in the dog, *Vet Pathol* 25:492-502, 1988.

44. Murphy LM, Lipman TO: Central venous catheter care in parenteral nutrition: a review, *J Parenter Enteral Nutr* 11:190-201, 1987.

45. Nahum E, Levy I, Katz J, et al: Efficacy of subcutaneous tunneling for prevention of bacterial colonization of femoral central venous catheters in critically ill children, *Pediatr Infect Dis J* 21:1000-1004, 2002.

46. Nakayama M, Munemura Y, Kanaya N, et al: Efficacy of alkalinized lidocaine for reducing pain on intravenous and epidural catheterization, *J Anesth* 15:201-203, 2001.

47. Niesen KM, Harris DY, Parkin LS, et al: The effects of heparin versus normal saline for maintenance of peripheral intravenous locks in pregnant women, *J Obstet Gynecol Neonat Nurs* 32:503-508, 2003.

48. Norden CW: Application of antibiotic ointment to the site of venous catheterization—a controlled trial, *J Infect Dis* 120:611-615, 1969.

49. O'Grady NP: Applying the science to the prevention of catheter-related infections, *J Crit Care* 17:114-121, 2002.

50. O'Grady NP, Alexander M, Dellinger EP, et al: Guidelines for the prevention of intravascular catheter-related infections, *Am J Infect Contr* 30:476-489, 2002.

51. Olson K, Rennie RP, Hanson J, et al: Evaluation of a no-dressing intervention for tunneled central venous catheter exit sites, *J Infus Nurs* 27:37-44, 2004.

52. Osuna DJ, DeYoung DJ, Walker RL: Comparison of three skin preparation techniques in the dog. Part 1: Experimental trial, *Vet Surg* 19:14-19, 1990.

53. Osuna DJ, DeYoung DJ, Walker RL: Comparison of three skin preparation techniques. Part 2: Clinical trial in 100 dogs, *Vet Surg* 19:pp. 20-23, 1990.

54. Otto CM, Kaufman GM, Crowe DT: Intraosseous infusion of fluids and therapeutics, *Comp Cont Educ Pract Vet* 11:421-430, 1989.

55. Otto CW: Central venous pressure monitoring. In Blitt CD, editor: *Monitoring in anesthesia and critical care*

medicine, ed 2, New York, 1990, Churchill Livingstone, pp. 169-210.

56. Palmon SC, Lloyd AT, Kirsch JR: The effect of needle gauge and lidocaine pH on pain during intradermal injection, *Anesth Analg* 86:379-381, 1998.

57. Pearson ML: Guideline for prevention of intravascular device-related infections. Hospital Infection Control Practices Advisory Committee, *Infect Contr Hosp Epidemiol* 17:438-473, 1996.

58. Pierce CM, Wade A, Mok Q: Heparin-bonded central venous lines reduce thrombotic and infective complications in critically ill children, *Intensive Care Med* 26:967-972, 2000.

59. Rabe C, Gramann T, Sons X, et al: Keeping central venous lines open: a prospective comparison of heparin, vitamin C and sodium chloride sealing solutions in medical patients, *Intensive Care Med* 28:1172-1176, 2002.

60. Randolph AG, Cook DJ, Gonzales CA, et al: Benefit of heparin in peripheral venous and arterial catheters: systematic review and meta-analysis of randomised controlled trials, *BMJ* 316:969-975, 1998.

61. Rochon PA, Gill SS, Litner J, et al: A systematic review of the evidence for hypodermoclysis to treat dehydration in older people, *J Gerontol A Biol Sci Med Sci* 52:M169-M176, 1997.

62. Salzman MB, Isenberg HD, Shapiro JF, et al: A prospective study of the catheter hub as the portal of entry for microorganisms causing catheter-related sepsis in neonates, *J Infect Dis* 167:487-490, 1993.

63. Sasson M, Shvartzman P: Hypodermoclysis: an alternative infusion technique, *Am Fam Physician* 64:1575-1578, 2001.

64. Schultz AA, Drew D, Hewitt H: Comparison of normal saline and heparinized saline for patency of IV locks in neonates, *Appl Nurs Res* 15:28-34, 2002.

65. Seldinger SI: Catheter replacement of the needle in percutaneous arteriography; a new technique, *Acta Radiol* 39:368-376, 1953.

66. Snydman DR, Gorbea HF, Pober BR, et al: Predictive value of surveillance skin cultures in total-parenteral-nutrition-related infection, *Lancet* 2:1385-1388, 1982.

67. Solomon DD, Arnold WL, Martin ND, et al: An in vivo method for the evaluation of catheter thrombogenicity, *J Biomed Mater Res* 21:43-57, 1987.

68. Spilezewski KL, Anderson JM, Schaap RN, et al: In vivo biocompatibility of catheter materials, *Biomaterials* 9:253-256, 1988.

69. Strand CL, Wajsbort RR, Sturmann K: Effect of iodophor vs iodine tincture skin preparation on blood culture contamination rate, *J Am Med Assoc* 269:1004-1006, 1993.

70. Suojanen JN, Brophy DP, Nasser I: Thrombus on indwelling central venous catheters: the histopathology of "Fibrin sheaths 1", *Cardiovasc Intervent Radiol* 23:194-197, 2000.

71. Swaim SF, Riddell KP, Geiger DL, et al: Evaluation of surgical scrub and antiseptic solutions for surgical preparation of canine paws, *J Am Vet Med Assoc* 198:1941-1945, 1991.

72. Thayer GW, Carrig CB, Evans AT: Fatal venous air embolism associated with pneumocystography in a cat, *J Am Vet Med Assoc* 176:643-645, 1980.

73. Timsit JF, Sebille V, Farkas JC, et al: Effect of subcutaneous tunneling on internal jugular catheter-related sepsis in critically ill patients: a prospective randomized multicenter study, *J Am Med Assoc* 276:1416-1420, 1996.

74. Tkachenko BI, Evlakhov VI, Poyasov IZ: Relationship between venous return and right-atrial pressure, *Bull Exp Biol Med* 131:421-423, 2001.

75. Trissel LA: *Handbook on injectable drugs*, ed 11, Bethesda, MD, 2001, American Society of Health-System Pharmacists, Inc.

76. Tugrul M, Camci E, Pembeci K, et al: Relationship between peripheral and central venous pressures in different patient positions, catheter sizes, and insertion sites, *J Cardiothorac Vasc Anesth* 18:446-450, 2004.

77. Wagner JG, Leatherman JW: Right ventricular end-diastolic volume as a predictor of the hemodynamic response to a fluid challenge, *Chest* 113:1048-1054, 1998.

78. Wistbacka JO, Nuutinen LS: Catheter-related complications of total parenteral nutrition (TPN): a review, *Acta Anaesthiol Scand* 29:84-88, 1985.

79. Xiang DZ, Verbeken EK, Van Lommel AT, et al: Composition and formation of the sleeve enveloping a central venous catheter, *J Vasc Surg* 28:260-271, 1998.

80. Xiang DZ, Verbeken EK, Van Lommel AT, et al: Sleeve-related thrombosis: a new form of catheter-related thrombosis, *Thromb Res* 104:7-14, 2001.

81. Zinner SH, Denny-Brown BC, Braun P, et al: Risk of infection with intravenous catheters: Effect of application of antibiotic ointment, *J Infect Dis* 120:616-619, 1969.

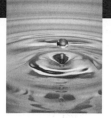

CHAPTER · 16

MONITORING FLUID THERAPY AND COMPLICATIONS OF FLUID THERAPY

Karol A. Mathews

Intravenous administration of fluids to veterinary patients is very common, and placement of an intravenous catheter is one of the most common invasive procedures performed in veterinary practice. Monitoring the patient's response to fluid therapy and considering the potential for complications arising from these products and the presence of a vascular access catheter are fundamental features of treatment.

Intravenous fluids are "drugs" and fluid therapy a "prescription" and should be considered as such to avoid potential complications resulting from inappropriate selection, underdosing, and overdosing.[42] Selection of fluid type and volume is a major component of the therapeutic plan and should include careful assessment of tissue and intravascular losses, acid-base and electrolyte status, age and species of the animal, nature of illness or injury, acute or chronic history, hematocrit and serum albumin concentration, coagulation status, and cardiorespiratory function. The animal's illness or injury is a dynamic event, and selection of fluid type and volume may change according to the patient's response to fluid therapy and with improvement or deterioration of the underlying problem. Therefore constant monitoring to achieve desired endpoints is required. This chapter will introduce the various monitoring techniques frequently used in veterinary practice, the potential for misinterpretation, and complications associated with fluid therapy and catheters.

The patient's history must be considered when formulating a fluid therapy plan. Rapid loss of intravascular fluid such as occurs in sepsis associated with third-space sequestration requires judicious fluid selection and rapid replacement, whereas chronic loss in a patient with adequate perfusion can be afforded a less aggressive approach to prevent excessive diuresis and iatrogenic electrolyte disturbances. The history must include the patient's age and previously diagnosed organ dysfunction. Fluid administration to geriatric patients or those with heart disease must be more cautious than administration to young otherwise healthy individuals. Physical examination should identify the compartment most affected by the fluid deficit: intravascular volume depletion with perfusion deficit, tissue water loss (dehydration) with normal perfusion, or depletion of both compartments (perfusion deficits and dehydration) indicating a large deficit of total body water.

Intravascular volume (perfusion) deficits are managed and monitored differently than are tissue water deficits. Unless severe total body water loss is present, the dehydrated animal may still have adequate tissue perfusion as indicated by normal acid-base status, normal blood lactate concentration, adequate urine production and appropriate concentrating ability, and normal renal and hepatic function (unless primary problems are known to exist with these organs). However, hypoxia resulting from anemia may contribute to end-organ dysfunction or injury despite adequate perfusion.

A thorough physical examination must accompany monitoring using the various technical devices available. Although monitoring central venous pressure (CVP), systemic arterial blood pressure (SABP), pulmonary capillary wedge pressure (PCWP), and cardiac output (CO) provides very useful (and sometimes essential) information, monitoring the patient by physical examination and biochemical evaluation of organ function also are very important, with improvement being the ultimate endpoints for achieving success with fluid therapy. As with the various monitoring devices, standard guidelines for assessing fluid deficits and overload by physical examination exist. However, there are many caveats, and interpretation is not necessarily clear-cut nor can it be assumed that absolute numbers or specific findings are related to fluid volume alone (Tables 16-1 through 16-3). Each patient must be assessed individually based on history, physical findings, and laboratory data.

MONITORING

Assessment of the volume of fluid required to correct fluid deficits in all compartments cannot be accurately derived. Therefore our therapy always is empirical and based on history, physical examination, and laboratory

TABLE 16-1 Physical Signs Associated with Dehydration

Percent Dehydration	Physical Signs
<5	Not detectable
5-6	Mild loss of skin elasticity
6-8	Definite loss of skin elasticity
	May have dry mucous membranes
	May have depressed globes within orbits
8-10	Persistent skin tent with slow return because of loss of skin elasticity
10-12	Persistent skin tent because of loss of skin elasticity
	Depressed globes within orbits
	Dry mucous membranes
	Signs of perfusion deficits (CRT > 2 sec, tachycardia)
12-15	Signs of shock
	Death

Note: The association between % dehydration and circulatory compromise must also be considered with rate of fluid loss. Chronic fluid loss may result in severe dehydration, but perfusion may be adequate; however, fluid loss occurring acutely will result in circulatory collapse at an estimated lower level of hydration. Therefore perfusion status cannot consistently be used to assess hydration status.

CRT, Capillary refill time.

findings. We derive our therapeutic plan using mathematical formulas based on an estimated percentage of intravascular or tissue loss. Our assessment may not be accurate, and therefore the volume of fluid given should be titrated to the patient's needs and the physiological responses to the fluid administered. The extent and invasiveness of monitoring used to assess these responses are dependent on the severity of illness and stability of the patient, other therapies administered, the interrelation-

TABLE 16-2 Confounding Factors of Physical Findings Associated with Dehydration

Assessment	Confounding Factors
Skin turgor ("tent")	Young animal with subcutaneous fat
	Obese animals with subcutaneous fat
	Cachectic animals
	Geriatric animals with loss of tissue elasticity
Mucous membranes	
Dry	Panting, tachypnea, dyspnea
Moist	Nauseated, vomiting, drinking
Position of the globe	Cachexia
Perfusion status	Affected by rate of fluid loss; chronic loss may not affect perfusion parameters until a large volume is lost

TABLE 16-3 Physical Findings Associated with Inadequate Tissue Perfusion

Assessment	Confounding Factors
Mucous Membranes	
Pale pink	Vasoconstriction caused by pain or anxiety
Pale	Volume loss overestimated because of vasoconstriction caused by pain or anxiety
Dark pink or red	Vasodilatation and may be interpreted as normal volume
	Hemodilution and may be interpreted as normal volume
Capillary Refill Time	
	<1 sec may be considered adequate perfusion
	Difficult to interpret if peripherally vasoconstricted because of pain or anxiety

ship among variables affecting the hemodynamic profile (e.g., anemia and perfusion, CVP and mechanical ventilation), the availability of various monitoring devices, and level of expertise of the clinician and support staff. This latter point is very important because interpretation of an isolated result, especially when monitoring devices are not frequently used, can complicate treatment regimens.

ENDPOINTS OF FLUID RESUSCITATION

During administration of any fluid, basic monitoring techniques should be performed, including heart rate (HR), respiratory rate (RR), pulse pressure, capillary refill time (CRT), mucous membrane (MM) color, mentation, and temperature and color of the digits. Although abnormalities in these parameters may not be sensitive indicators of hypovolemia,[44] a general goal for endpoints of resuscitation should be values within the normal range for the size and species of animal with recovery to normal mentation and warm, pink digits. Monitoring urine production with a goal of 0.5 to 1.0 mL/kg/hr also is a useful assessment of adequate volume, and 1.0 to 2.0 mL/kg is considered optimal with normal renal function. When administering fluids to critically ill animals, measuring preload, stroke volume, or CO, targeted to specific values, is superior to measuring systemic blood pressure. Central venous and PCWP are surrogate markers of preload, but use of the pulmonary artery catheter (PAC) to measure the PCWP recently has been shown to be inconsistent and of questionable value in human medicine and is being used less frequently.[29] The CVP and SABP measurements frequently are used in veterinary medicine to guide fluid resuscitation. Measurement of CVP and SABP are associated with major pitfalls (see section on Arterial Blood Pressure and

Central Venous Pressure discussed below), but are still of value when used in conjunction with the physical examination. Suggested measurements for conditions requiring optimal resuscitation include 5 to 8 mm Hg (6.5 to 10.5 cm H_2O) CVP, 80 to 100 mm Hg mean arterial pressure (MAP), and 100 to 120 mm Hg systolic blood pressure (SBP), and for patients in which the goal is adequate resuscitation (i.e., those with ongoing noncompressible hemorrhage), a MAP of 65 mm Hg and an SBP of 90 to 95 mm Hg are acceptable until hemorrhage is controlled either spontaneously or surgically. Pulmonary contusions and other pulmonary conditions predisposing to capillary leak with increased hydrostatic pressure are additional indications for cautious adequate resuscitation. The patient's base deficit or blood lactate concentration also may be used to assess perfusion. The goal should be to achieve an adjusted base excess of 0 to + 4 mEq/L and a lactate concentration less than 1.4 mmol/L in cats and 2.0 mmol/L in dogs.

Intravascular Volume

Blood is composed of plasma and red cells and is separated from the interstitial and intracellular compartments by the vascular walls. Measurements of pressure within this system, such as CVP, MAP, or SBP, are used as indirect assessments of blood volume. However, various physiological or pathophysiological conditions may lead to an increase or decrease in pressure with or without loss or gain of fluid.

CENTRAL VENOUS PRESSURE

The CVP is a measure of the hydrostatic pressure within the intrathoracic vena cavae.[1,20] The CVP is slightly higher than the right atrial pressure (RAP), and RAP is quantitatively similar to right ventricular pressure at end diastole[20] or preload.[8] However, CVP does not reliably predict right ventricular end-diastolic volume.[47] Accurate placement of the catheter and consistency in positioning of the animal are extremely important in interpretation of results and determination of trends.[20] CVP measurements may be obtained from the caudal vena cava in cats.[36] Keeping in mind potential pitfalls, measurement of the CVP during a fluid challenge, such as would be administered in hypovolemia or acute renal failure, can be valuable in assessing the effect of therapy. In the hypovolemic patient, for example, if no appreciable increase in CVP (Box 16-1)[20] is observed after a fluid bolus, additional fluid or colloid should be administered. It has been the author's experience that a rapid infusion of 20 mL/kg of a crystalloid may not be "tolerated" in some patients regardless of cardiovascular status (Table 16-4). Nausea, vomiting, shivering, and restlessness are frequently noted in these individuals. The reason for the observed signs may be associated with a vagally mediated baroreceptor reflex secondary to atrial stretch. Should CVP increase above an acceptable range after such a

| Box 16-1 | Signs Associated with Overhydration |

- Shivering
- Nausea (swallowing and licking lips)
- Vomiting (may be early or late)
- Restlessness
- Polyuria (patient dependent)
- Serous nasal discharge
- Tachypnea (early or late)
- Cough (late)
- Chemosis (late)
- Dyspnea (late)
- Diarrhea (late)
- Ascites (late)
- Exophthalmos (late)
- Depressed mentation (late)
- Tachycardia (followed by bradycardia when severely overloaded)
- Subcutaneous edema (especially hock joint and intermandibular space) (late)
- Pulmonary crackles and edema (late)

challenge in an animal with acute renal failure, fluid administration should be curtailed or stopped. These are general recommendations, and CVP does not reliably predict whether administration of a fluid bolus will or will not significantly increase CO under all conditions.[49,50] Factors other than intravascular volume that influence CVP measurements include cardiac function (e.g., systolic or diastolic dysfunction), pulmonary hypertension (e.g., pulmonary thromboembolic disease), venous compliance (e.g., increased systemic vascular resistance), and intrathoracic pressure (e.g., pleural effusion, pneumothorax, pericardial effusion, mechanical ventilation). Although mechanical ventilation affects CVP, threshold values of CVP in ventilated patients still may be of value to predict hemodynamic instability when assessed in response to increasing airway pressure induced by positive end-expiratory pressure (PEEP).[28] In this study of patients with acute lung injury, subjects with CVP less than 10 mm Hg usually had decreased CO when challenged with increasing PEEP, whereas those with CVP greater than 10 mm Hg had increased, decreased, or unchanged CO.

ARTERIAL BLOOD PRESSURE

Although systemic blood pressure is not an absolute measure of volume, it is frequently monitored during periods of bolus fluid administration when managing shock. When extensive monitoring is required, direct arterial pressure measurements should be obtained. However, on presentation, it may not be possible to successfully perform arterial catheterization, and pressures may be obtained with oscillometric or Doppler

TABLE 16-4 Interpretation of CVP Values in Response to a Rapid Infusion of 20 mL/kg Crystalloid or 5 mL/kg Colloid[20]

Interpretation of Response	Response to Infusion
Euvolemia and normal cardiac function	2-4 cm H_2O increase from baseline returning to baseline in 15 min
Increased venous blood volume, reduced cardiac compliance, or both	An increase in CVP maintained >4 cm H_2O above baseline
Normal blood volume	A slow (15 min) return to baseline
Increased blood volume relative to cardiac performance	A prolonged (>30 min) return to baseline
Markedly reduced intravascular volume; requires further resuscitation	Minimal to no increase in CVP
Reduced intravascular volume and accommodation of fluid within the intravascular space and subsequent reduction in vascular tone; requires further resuscitation	An increase in CVP with rapid (<5 min) return to baseline
Further resuscitation	Raise CVP by 2-4 cm H_2O within first few minutes of bolus therapy. If falls rapidly to baseline, repeat bolus therapy until CVP 5-10 cm H_2O (3-7 mm Hg) requiring 10-15 min to fall; at this point, blood volume and venous return are optimal relative to cardiac performance.
CVP ~7-9 cm H_2O (10-12 mm Hg) with normal intrapleural and intraabdominal pressures	Higher volume may predispose to pulmonary edema; continued fluid resuscitation probably will not improve cardiac output

monitors. However, when the limbs are poorly perfused or the patient is cold, the oscillometric and Doppler methods are insensitive, and it is difficult to obtain accurate measurements, especially in small animals. In the author's experience, the coccygeal artery, with the cuff positioned as far proximal as possible, tends to be more reliable in this instance. The MAP is dependent on CO and systemic vascular resistance (SVR), according to the equation MAP = CO × SVR. Therefore adequate MAP does not necessarily indicate adequate CO if SVR is increased as may occur in a compensatory sympathetic response. During acute blood loss, especially in otherwise young healthy animals, the compensatory response can be quite dramatic and result in nearly normal or normal MAP. If resuscitation is based on normal MAP or SBP alone, inadequate resuscitation with continued poor perfusion likely will occur until the patient decompensates. However, if normal MAP or SBP is accompanied by a physical examination (see section on Physical Findings) that indicates the presence of a sympathetic response, the clinician will be aware of the requirement for additional resuscitation or analgesics. In this setting, it is difficult to know how much blood has been lost and the contribution of pain and anxiety. Pain, anxiety, and hypothermia also contribute to the sympathetic response, and the findings observed may be more a result of these factors than of fluid and blood loss. In this setting, intravascular volume loss may be overestimated, resulting in excessive fluid administration. Therefore fluid requirements and monitoring progress should be assessed based on several factors in addition to pressure

measurements. These considerations include a relatively pain-free patient and an improvement in physical findings (see section on Physical Findings).

CARDIAC OUTPUT MEASUREMENTS

Several techniques are available to measure CO, but most are technically challenging. Recently lithium dilution cardiac output (LiDCO) and PulseCO (both from LiDCO, London, UK) have been investigated for use in humans[29] and in large[33] and small animals.[41] Briefly, isotonic lithium chloride is injected as a bolus via a central or peripheral vein, and a concentration-time curve is generated by an arterial ion-selective electrode attached to an arterial manometer system. The CO is calculated from the lithium dose and the area under the concentration time curve before recirculation. The PulseCO hemodynamic monitor was developed for use in conjunction with the LiDCO to give a beat-by-beat estimate of CO that is derived from analysis of the arterial trace. Although these systems have limitations, their use in veterinary research indicates potential value in clinical practice in anesthetized animals or nonmoving critically ill animals. Movement, flexion, and extension of the catheterized limb contribute to erroneous results (personal observations). A great advantage of this system is that a central catheter is not required, and continuous CO can be measured. Measuring CO during fluid resuscitation has definite advantages over determination of SABP because the former is a more accurate measure of volume. Predetermined goals for CO, stroke volume, and oxygen delivery can be set and monitored with this system.

PHYSICAL FINDINGS

As previously mentioned, SABP may be normal in patients with hypovolemia caused by blood loss, and therefore the physical examination must be considered in conjunction with SABP when assessing adequate resuscitation. Cool limbs, rectal temperature below normal, increased HR and RR, paler than normal MM color, prolonged CRT, and depressed mentation all indicate poor perfusion, regardless of blood pressure readings. If SABP is normal and the patient is free of pain but HR and RR are high and MMs still pale, a compensated stage of shock may exist, and further resuscitation is required. When assessing response to fluid therapy in animals with pain, an opioid analgesic (preferably oxymorphone, hydromorphone, or fentanyl) should be administered to control pain. The sympathetic response associated with pain and anxiety will be reduced, allowing the clinician to assess cardiovascular dynamics solely associated with the blood loss. Administration of these opioids does not compromise the cardiovascular system[35] and will allow better assessment of the patient because the effect of the sympathetic response to pain will be eliminated from consideration. Hypothermia may be a result of poor perfusion caused by low circulating volume or a primary cause that may interfere with achieving resuscitation goals; clinical impression suggests this may be especially so in cats. Marked hypothermia results in bradycardia and decreased CO[46]; therefore warming during resuscitation is necessary. Increased RR also may be associated with pulmonary injury, disease, or fluid overload. An improvement in attitude (i.e., improved cerebral perfusion) should be noted with adequate fluid resuscitation. The CRT and MM color, pulse pressure, and urine production also should improve. Palpation of the bladder and monitoring urine produced by assessing bladder size can be useful when urinary bladder catheterization cannot be performed.

PACKED CELL VOLUME AND TOTAL SOLIDS (OR PROTEIN)

It is essential to obtain baseline packed cell volume (PCV) and total solids (TS) or total protein concentration on admission. During a traumatic event, sympathetic stimulation results in splenic contraction, especially in the dog, increasing the PCV and potentially giving the impression that hemorrhage has not occurred. A normal PCV may be observed after trauma even with clinically relevant blood loss. The TS in this setting will be lower than normal (6.0 to 8.0 g/dL), confirming blood loss. Monitoring these tests as frequently as every 15 minutes during resuscitation may be necessary to evaluate ongoing blood loss and the requirement for administration of oxygen-carrying products. A definitive recommendation regarding transfusion of blood products has not been established in veterinary patients, but

the use of packed red blood cells (PRBCs), whole blood, or hemoglobin-based oxygen carriers (HBOCs) is suggested when the PCV decreases to less than 25% in the dog or less than 20% in the cat, especially when ongoing resuscitation is required. The use of HBOCs may be an effective adjunct to limited resuscitation from hemorrhagic shock[38] while reducing complications of aggressive fluid therapy. Administration of a colloid has been recommended when the TS is less than 4.0 g/dL (less than 40 g/L) to avoid a clinically relevant decrease in colloid osmotic pressure (COP),[37] which may predispose to tissue and pulmonary edema, especially when additional crystalloid fluids are to be administered. The refractometer reading for hetastarch is 4.5 g/dL (45 g/L) and that for pentastarch is 7.5 g/dL (75 g/L). After these colloids are administered, the TS measurement is difficult to interpret and cannot be extrapolated to a COP measurement. Response to administration of colloids must be assessed by direct COP measurement, CO determination, or improvement in clinical signs.

URINE PRODUCTION

During hypovolemia and dehydration, renal blood flow is decreased. When blood volume is decreased by hemorrhage, the decreased pressures result in activation of the sympathetic nervous system, including renal sympathetic nerves. Sodium and water are conserved by constriction of the glomerular arterioles, decreased glomerular filtration rate (GFR), increased tubular reabsorption of salt and water, and activation of the renin angiotensin aldosterone system. Decreased arterial pressure also results in secretion of antidiuretic hormone (ADH).[18] Together, these actions serve to replenish the intravascular space and return blood volume toward normal. As a consequence of these effects, a very small volume of hypertonic urine is produced. In addition to renal blood flow and GFR, urine volume also is dependent on the concentrating ability of the kidneys. If underlying renal tubular dysfunction is present, increased urine volume may not reflect adequate renal perfusion and GFR. When renal function is otherwise normal, however, urine production and specific gravity are useful parameters to monitor when assessing intravascular volume. Urine output has been referred to as the "poor man's cardiac output." Intravenous fluid therapy also will expand the intravascular space and consequently increase urine volume.

Assessment of Urine Output

Careful monitoring is necessary to ensure that urine production is maintained by adequate fluid replacement. Normal urine production is between 0.5 and 2 mL/kg/hr but varies with the concentrating ability of the kidneys. The goal is to maintain urine output of 1 to 2 mL/kg/hr with a urine specific gravity of approximately 1.026 (dog) and 1.035 (cat). However, if there is loss of concentrating ability (e.g., renal tubular injury, *Escherichia coli* pyelonephritis), urine output can be extremely high (25 to 40 mL/kg/hr), and specific gravity may be in the hyposthenuric or isosthenuric range, hence the importance of measuring of urine output and specific gravity. If urine output is decreased, the patient should be assessed for possible third-space loss, capillary leak, increased temperature, vomiting, diarrhea, salivation, or inadequate resuscitation as causes. Calculating appropriate fluid requirement is important because administering an excessive volume of fluids will result in diuresis, medullary washout, and electrolyte disturbances (especially potassium). Ongoing diuresis may require a prolonged hospital stay for correction of resulting fluid and electrolyte imbalances. Measurement of urine volume can be accomplished by:

1. Collection of urine when the animal voids
2. Use of a metabolic cage
3. Intermittent or continuous urinary bladder catheterization
4. Placing preweighed towels or pads under the animal and weighing them after voiding. Any increase in towel or pad weight over baseline, unless otherwise soiled, is assumed to be the result of urine. The volume of urine voided can be estimated by assuming 1000 mL equals 1000 g (1 kg or 2.2 lb). This technique underestimates urine produced because some urine may remain in the cage.

Weighing the animal several times a day will assist in estimating fluid loss or gain. If the animal's weight declines despite fluid therapy, it is assumed that ongoing losses such as high urine output, vomiting, diarrhea, salivation, or evaporative losses caused by fever or hyperthermia are in excess of fluids administered. A weight loss of 0.1 to 0.3 kg body weight per 1000 kcal energy requirement (approximate caloric requirement for a caged 20-kg dog) per day is anticipated in an anorexic animal. Third-space losses must be assessed by other means because weight loss will not be evident. After urine flow has been established, regardless of the underlying problem, ongoing fluid requirements are calculated as follows:

1. Divide the day into six 4-hour intervals, four 6-hour intervals, or three 8-hour intervals.
2. Determine urine produced during each time interval, and add the estimated insensible and ongoing losses for that period.
3. Determine ongoing losses in vomitus, diarrhea, and saliva for the period selected.
4. Determine insensible loss at 20 mL/kg/day. In addition, for each degree Celsius above 38.5° C, add 10% of normal daily maintenance fluid requirement (i.e., if the normal daily requirement is 1 L and temperature is 40.5° C, then 200 mL should be added). Divide this total amount by 6, 4, or 3 depending on the interval selected above.

5. This volume of fluid, in addition to the amount determined by urine produced and ongoing losses, is to be delivered during the next period. Daily weight is advised in all hospitalized patients because unnoticed polyuria or inadequate intravenous or oral fluids for an individual patient may result in weight loss, and excessive intravenous fluid administration may result in unnecessary weight gain.

PERFUSION

LACTATE

The blood lactate concentration may be used as an indicator of perfusion to monitor resuscitation and is discussed further in Chapter 10. Strict adherence to collection (i.e., blood should be collected in heparin) and processing (i.e., immediate) of blood samples is required. Lactate measurements can be performed on arterial or venous samples.[25,32] Normal blood lactate concentrations are less than 2.0 mmol/L in dogs, with 3 to 5 mmol/L representing a mild increase, 5 to 8 mmol/L a moderate increase, and more than 8 mmol/L a severe increase. Normal blood lactate concentrations are less than 1.46 mmol/L in cats. When inadequate oxygen delivery to tissues occurs, cells revert to anaerobic metabolism, and lactate production increases. Monitoring lactate concentrations will provide information about the state of oxygen delivery and adequacy of resuscitation. With restoration of adequate perfusion and oxygen delivery, aerobic metabolism is resumed with a reduction in lactate production. The most common cause of hyperlactatemia is hypoperfusion and tissue hypoxia (type A), but increased lactate concentrations also may be caused by increased production secondary to alkalosis, hypoglycemia, various drugs, and systemic illness (type B).[6] As an example, in those with acute liver failure and sepsis, hyperlactatemia is not necessarily associated with hypoxia. In this situation, the liver becomes a net producer of both lactate and pyruvate.[5] Similarly, in those with sepsis, hyperlactatemia is a consequence of enhanced glycolysis and increased release of lactate from the intestine and the periphery. Therefore hypermetabolism must be considered as a cause for hyperlactatemia when no other indications of inadequate perfusion or tissue hypoxia are present.[5] Type A hyperlactatemia also includes relative hypoxia, in which energy requirements exceed demand such as may occur in strenuous exercise and in extreme muscle activity (e.g., seizures, trembling, struggling).[24] This effect resolves rapidly after cessation of the activity.

Acid-Base Status

Many illnesses and trauma are associated with acid-base disturbances, often, metabolic acidosis. Hypoperfusion and tissue hypoxia result in metabolic acidemia unless a comorbid condition results in metabolic alkalosis, generating a mixed disturbance in which blood pH may be within normal limits. In one study, 95% of animals referred to a tertiary referral center were diagnosed with metabolic acidosis.[30] Knowing the metabolic status of a patient is an extremely important part of the overall assessment of the animal and provides information about the potential origin of the abnormality and the appropriate fluid to select. Eliminating the underlying problem ultimately will correct the abnormal metabolic status, but until it can be resolved, providing optimal therapy to improve outcome is essential. When blood gas analysis is not available, acidemic patients with HCO_3^- loss usually can be identified as having increased serum chloride concentration, decreased total CO_2, and normal anion gap, information that can be obtained from a serum biochemistry profile. If acidemia is caused by the addition of an unmeasured anion (e.g., lactate, glycolate), the serum chloride concentration usually is normal, but the anion gap is increased. Alkalemic patients often are hypochloremic. Monitoring acid-base status provides additional information about improved perfusion and resolution of the illness, as well as the potential need for a change in fluid therapy as the disease process changes. For example, a dog presented with vomiting caused by pyloric obstruction commonly will exhibit a hypochloremic metabolic alkalosis and hyponatremia. 0.9% Sodium chloride is the fluid of choice. Once the underlying problem is resolved and alkalosis has been corrected, continuing with 0.9% sodium chloride may result in hyperchloremic acidosis; therefore a change to a balanced electrolyte solution typically is recommended.

HYDRATION

Physical findings used to assess hydration are skin turgor, position of the globes within the orbits, and moistness of mucous membranes (see Table 16-2).[7] Assessment of these findings should be noted on admission, but causes of these physical findings other than hydration status must be considered (see Table 16-3) when calculating volume requirements to avoid overestimates and underestimates. However, frequent monitoring of these findings is useful when monitoring response to therapy and fluid requirements for ongoing management. Weight gain has been recommended as a monitor of hydration after fluid therapy, and in the author's experience, weighing the animal has proved to be a useful adjunct of fluid management. However, weight gain cannot always be predicted.[21]

FLUID AND ELECTROLYTE DISTURBANCES

SERUM ELECTROLYTE CONCENTRATIONS

Serum electrolyte concentrations require frequent monitoring in a patient with a dynamic illness. In the patient with hypochloremic alkalosis and hyponatremia described previously, caution is required when increasing the sodium content of the fluids administered. An increase of more than 0.5 mEq/L/hr may result in a development of central nervous system lesions. Similar concerns exist when attempting to decrease serum sodium concentration in patients with hypernatremia. Serum potassium concentration is influenced by acidosis, alkalosis, and the underlying illness, and hyperkalemia or hypokalemia may contribute substantially to morbidity. Potassium supplementation often is required in many illnesses, but the need for potassium supplementation should be carefully evaluated and not assumed. Although abnormalities in serum calcium concentration are not as frequent, hypocalcemia and hypercalcemia also have diagnostic and therapeutic implications. Hyperchloremia and hypochloremia can affect the acid-base status of the patient and warrant vigilance and correction as necessary. Hypomagnesemia is a common finding in critical care patients with many underlying illnesses. The electrocardiogram (ECG) may be a useful monitoring tool when electrolyte disturbances exist (e.g., hyperkalemia, hypocalcemia) and result in dysrhythmias; however, one cannot rely on the ECG to diagnose electrolyte abnormalities.

COLLOID OSMOMETRY

Under normal conditions, blood volume and extracellular fluid volume are controlled in parallel to each other. However, there are situations in which the distribution of extracellular fluid between the interstitial space and blood can vary. The principal factors that can cause accumulation of fluid in the interstitial space include (1) increased capillary hydrostatic pressure, (2) decreased plasma COP (oncotic pressure), (3) increased permeability of the capillaries, and (4) obstruction of the lymphatic vessels.[18] With the exception of lymphatic obstruction, these conditions frequently are preexistent in critically ill small animal patients or may develop as a consequence of fluid administration. The endothelium represents a semipermeable membrane that normally prevents loss of proteins.

The COP of whole blood obtained from normal dogs is 19.95 ± 2.1 (range, 15.3 to 26.3) mm Hg and for plasma is 17.5 ± 3.0 mm Hg. In whole blood obtained from normal cats, COP is 24.7 ± 3.7 (range, 17.6 to 33.1) mm Hg and in plasma 19.8 ± 2.4 mm Hg.

COMPLICATIONS

POTENTIAL COMPLICATIONS ASSOCIATED WITH SELECTION OF FLUIDS

Crystalloid Solutions

As previously mentioned, crystalloid fluids should be considered drugs because their various compositions will influence many ionic interactions and shifts in plasma. The type of fluid selected will influence resolution of alkalosis or acidosis. Alkalemia and acidemia will affect the pathologic condition experienced by the animal. If an inappropriate selection is made, such as 0.9% sodium chloride in a patient with hyperchloremia and decreased strong ion difference or in another condition resulting in acidosis, acidosis will worsen, and acidosis has been shown to increase morbidity.[53] Likewise, in a patient with alkalosis, administration of an alkalinizing solution potentially will contribute to morbidity as electrolyte composition of plasma is altered (e.g., hypokalemia, ionized hypocalcemia, hyperammonemia), and a shift of the oxyhemoglobin dissociation curve to the left, with associated problems, occurs. Administration of dextrose also can alter the electrolyte composition of plasma. Intracellular shifts of phosphorus and potassium may occur during dextrose infusions, and careful monitoring and supplementation of these ions are required in patients with hypophosphatemia and hypokalemia. The addition of dextrose makes the solution more acidic because of the oxidation of the sugar. The physiological acid-base effect of an infusion of 5% dextrose also will be a trend toward acidosis because of the effective free water infusion and the effects of glucose metabolism under different patient conditions.[59] Another potential concern with the administration of 5% dextrose in water is the generation of free water when additional water is not needed. Dextrose-containing solutions may be indicated for specific situations (i.e., pure water loss).

Lactated Ringer's solution contains lactate as a bicarbonate precursor. Lactate is metabolized in the liver, and it has been suggested that administration of this fluid may increase lactate concentration in animals with severe liver disease. However, the clinical importance of this effect must be determined on an individual basis. Mild hyperlactatemia has been noted in dogs with lymphosarcoma receiving lactated Ringer's solution.

Because of the calcium content of lactated Ringer's solution, blood transfusions should not be given through the same fluid administration set. Lactated Ringer's solution will result in microscopic clot formation in blood products.[51]

Acetated polyionic solutions (Plasma-Lyte 148, Plasma-Lyte A, Baxter Corp, Mississauga, Ontario, Canada) (Normosol-R, Abbott Laboratories Ltd., Montreal, Quebec, Canada) contain acetate as the alkalinizing component. Acetate is metabolized in muscle cells, and therefore specific organ dysfunction (e.g., kidney disease, liver disease) is not a contraindication for its use. It has been suggested that these solutions not be administered to animals with diabetic ketoacidosis (DKA) because acetate is a ketone precursor and may promote ketone production. This concern appears to be theoretical because concurrent treatment for DKA with insulin prevents further ketone production. Many patients with DKA are acidemic, and crystalloid solutions containing acetate have been the author's choice for fluid therapy for several years. Rapid administration of polyionic acetate solutions may precipitate vasodilatation and hypotension in animals that already are hypovolemic.[48] Although this is a rare event, monitoring blood pressure during administration of acetated crystalloid solutions is recommended. Hypertonic saline solutions have been recommended for various conditions and have several positive attributes. However, rate of infusion is important, and rapid infusions may result in bronchoconstriction and shallow breathing.[54]

Colloid Solutions

Synthetic colloid solutions are recommended for many clinical situations, and the commonly used synthetic colloid solutions are formulated in 0.9% sodium chloride. The primary acid-base effect of the colloid solutions on plasma is acidification. The electrolyte preparations that accompany these macromolecules (e.g., 0.9% saline) also have an important effect on acid-base equilibrium after infusion.[34]

Considering the frequency of use of these products in veterinary practice, very little has been published with regard to complications after their administration. A clinical study evaluating the safety and efficacy of hetastarch after a total dosage of between 9 and 59 mL/kg in dogs with varying problems and associated hypoalbuminemia reported minor hetastarch-associated changes in coagulation tests that were of little clinical relevance.[56] However, none of these dogs had preexisting coagulopathies. A potential complication of colloid administration is hemorrhage, if a preexisting condition exists, in a patient with a moderate coagulopathy. Hemorrhage associated with administration of synthetic colloids has been reported in some human patients.[2] Synthetic colloids are eliminated primarily by renal excretion, and caution must be used when administering these products as rapid volume expanders to patients with oliguria unless oliguria is determined to be caused by hypovolemia or hypotension. These products should not be administered to patients with anuric renal failure or congestive heart failure because of concern about volume overload. Interference with renal function has been reported in human patients receiving synthetic colloids, and most commonly this observation has been associated with use of dextran 40.[11] A reduction in GFR also has been noted in human surgical and trauma patients receiving synthetic colloids.[3] The frequency of renal dysfunction associated with administration of synthetic colloids in veterinary patients is not known.

Another potential complication that may occur is leakage of the small molecules (<50,000 daltons) contained in the currently used synthetic colloid solutions (e.g., hetastarch and pentastarch) into the pulmonary interstitium when administered to animals with capillary leak syndrome.[22,45] A recent review of fluid therapy in sepsis with capillary leakage concluded that additional studies including patients with specific diseases, considering various aspects of the colloids administered, and with specific endpoints for fluid resuscitation should be conducted before definitive recommendations can be made for colloid administration.[40] In the meanwhile, appreciating potential adverse effects, selecting appropriate patients, and monitoring during treatment should reduce the morbidity associated with administration of these solutions.

POTENTIAL COMPLICATIONS ASSOCIATED WITH THE VOLUME OF FLUIDS ADMINISTERED

Diuresis and Electrolyte Losses

The volume of fluids administered tends to be empirically derived, and response to therapy must serve to guide ongoing requirements. Excessive administration serves no therapeutic benefit and frequently results in patient morbidity. A mechanism conserved across species through evolution is the renal-body fluid system for arterial pressure control. Urine output can double when intravascular volume and pressure increase even a few millimeters of mercury above normal, a response termed pressure diuresis. In addition to water loss, a concomitant sodium loss occurs.[13] If this diuresis goes undetected, an excess of all electrolytes is excreted in the urine because of decreased reabsorption in the proximal and distal renal tubules.[14] In some instances, resultant hypokalemia can be quite profound, especially in cats.

The ability to concentrate urine relies on the high osmolarity of the renal medullary interstitial fluid, which provides the osmotic gradient necessary for water reabsorption. Transport of sodium, potassium, chloride, and other ions into the medullary interstitium, along with urea, maintains this osmotic gradient. Increased medullary blood flow, which can occur with excessive fluid administration, will wash out the hyperosmotic interstitium, thereby reducing renal concentrating ability.[16] A vicious cycle then is established in which fluid loss occurs because of lack of concentrating ability. When this occurs, gradual fluid reduction is required to reestablish the hyperosmotic gradient and maintain hydration.

Edema

Administration of fluids can lead to interstitial and pulmonary edema when the patient's illness is associated with inflammation, anuric or oliguric renal failure, cardiac insufficiency, hypoalbuminemia, or with administration of a large overdose of fluids resulting in hypervolemia and a subsequent increase in interstitial hydrostatic pressure.

Interstitial Edema. Under normal conditions there is a slight negative pressure (−3 mm Hg) in most loose subcutaneous tissues of the body. This negative pressure holds the tissues together and offers some resistance to fluid flux caused by the low compliance of the tissue. With small increases in interstitial fluid volume, a large increase in hydrostatic pressure occurs, resisting additional filtration across the capillary. However, with large increases in intravascular hydrostatic pressure and further capillary filtration, the interstitial volume will increase. When the colloid osmotic gradient fails and the lymphatic system is overloaded, the tissue safety factors are overcome with little resistance to further fluid loss. When the interstitial pressure reaches 0 mm Hg, the compliance of the tissue is reduced, facilitating larger volumes of fluid to accumulate in the tissues with little change in interstitial hydrostatic pressure. This effect is called stress relaxation. The proteoglycan meshwork within the interstitium is disrupted as the increased volume of fluid pushes the brush pile of proteoglycans apart, allowing the fluid to flow freely through the tissues.[17] When this occurs, pitting edema is detected by pressing on an area of skin and noting pitting for several seconds until the fluid flows back into the area. Edema also may occur in patients with moderate to severe capillary leak after administration of moderate volumes of crystalloid solutions. Assessing interstitial tissue edema is an essential component of monitoring during fluid administration. Three body regions that are useful to evaluate are the hock because nonedematous animals, regardless of the amount of body fat, have well-defined lateral saphenous veins, Achilles tendons, and bony prominences; the mandibles and intermandibular space because these areas also are well defined in most animals; and the movement of the skin and subcutaneous tissues over the torso. With the development of interstitial edema, these anatomical regions become less defined, and a "jelly-like" appearance of the skin develops. If these findings are generalized, overhydration resulting from excessive fluid administration or capillary leak can be assumed. These regions should always be examined for baseline assessment before fluid administration. Chemosis also may occur with overhydration, but this finding tends to occur later than those previously mentioned. Bandages placed around the neck to secure a catheter into the jugular vein may cause edema of the head and chemosis unassociated with overhydration. Likewise, edema of a distal limb may occur if it is the dependent limb or a bandage is placed above the hock or carpus. Although body weight did not change in the majority of animals treated for dehydration during a 24- to 48-hour period,[21] body weight should be monitored because an increase above that calculated to treat dehydration may indicate fluid overload if confirmed by other physical findings. Fluid losses into third spaces will increase body weight without improvement in overall fluid repletion.

When edema is noted in subcutaneous tissues, it is likely that a similar degree of edema also exists in body organs. It has been this author's observation at necropsy that edema of the brain, gastrointestinal tract, heart, liver, and kidney coexists with subcutaneous edema. This finding may account for some of the clinical signs observed, including depression, vomiting, cardiac arrhythmias, coagulopathy, and oliguria.

Pulmonary Edema. Pulmonary interstitial fluid dynamics differ from those of other tissues. Pulmonary capillary pressure is lower (approximately 7 mm Hg); interstitial fluid pressure in the lung is more negative (−8 to −5 mm Hg) than that of peripheral subcutaneous tissue; and the pulmonary capillaries are relatively permeable to protein molecules, rendering the COP of the pulmonary interstitial fluid approximately 14 mm Hg. These differences favor fluid movement from the alveoli into the interstitium and lymphatics.[15] Pulmonary edema occurs in the same manner as does edema elsewhere in the body. Therefore the conditions discussed above can result in pulmonary edema after an excessive volume of crystalloid, and potentially colloid, is administered. As pulmonary interstitial pressure increases into the positive pressure range and the lymphatics are unable to remove this fluid, it leaks into the alveolar space. In the absence of capillary leak disorders, when the pulmonary capillary pressure exceeds 25 mm Hg (~18 mm Hg above normal) in normal dogs, fluid accumulates in the lungs. Experiments performed on dogs showed that pulmonary capillary pressure must increase to a value at least equal to the COP of the plasma inside the capillaries before clinically relevant pulmonary edema occurs.[15] The COP of normal dogs is 19.95 ± 2.1 (range, 15.3 to 26.3) mm Hg, and measuring COP in addition to evaluating physical findings helps guide fluid management. This information applies to normal dogs and not dogs with capillary leak conditions or those that are hypoproteinemic. When COP is decreased, as in patients with hypoproteinemia, edema formation may occur even at lower hydrostatic pressures. In experimental models, edema begins to form at 11 mm Hg when COP is decreased.[19]

Monitoring physical signs (see Table 16-4) can be effective in assessing potential fluid overload. The author has observed shivering, restlessness, nausea (as indicated by swallowing and licking the lips), and rarely vomiting in some animals as a response to an excessive rate of infusion of a balanced electrolyte solution. These signs stopped within 1 or 2 minutes after discontinuing or reducing the fluid rate for a short period, and the observed behavior was reproduced when a high rate of fluid administration was reestablished. These animals did not have identifiable cardiac disease. While monitoring CVP in one animal with oliguric renal failure that demonstrated this behavior, CVP rapidly increased from 1 cm H_2O to 11 cm H_2O. The fluids were discontinued, but when restarted, the same behavior occurred when

CVP reached 10 to 11 cm H_2O again. The fluid rate in this instance was reestablished at a more reasonable level for this dog. The reason for the observed signs may be associated with a vagally mediated baroreceptor reflex secondary to atrial stretch. Monitoring respiratory rate and effort is simple, and a slight but consistent increase can be an early clue to fluid overload and development of pulmonary edema. A slight but consistent reduction in oxygen saturation (SpO_2) over a few minutes as detected by pulse oximetry may be another indication of pulmonary edema. Confirmation by a reduction in PaO_2 on arterial blood gases may be warranted to confirm the SpO_2 readings. Radiographic assessment of the pulmonary vasculature can be used to monitor fluid administration. In animals, the width of the pulmonary vein should be less than 1.5 times the width of the pulmonary artery, and fluid overload should be considered if the measured difference exceeds this value. In human patients, changes in vascular pedicle width has proven to be a valuable method for monitoring fluid balance in the intensive care unit.[39] The radiographic appearance of pulmonary edema, increased lung sounds such as crackles, and cyanosis indicate a late stage of edema with severe patient compromise. Capillary permeability is increased during systemic inflammatory conditions, endothelial injury, pneumonia, and pancreatitis, and capillary leak would be expected to occur with administration of smaller fluid volumes. Monitoring in affected animals must be diligent with even slight changes being a potential warning sign of pulmonary edema. Pancreatitis is a relatively common problem in cats and dogs requiring fluid therapy. In humans, approximately 33% of pancreatitis patients will develop acute lung injury and acute respiratory distress syndrome.[26] This complication is caused by changes in the pulmonary endothelium associated with the systemic inflammatory process, liberation of pancreatic digestive enzymes (especially elastase), and damage by neutrophils that results in enhanced capillary leak.[9,27] These changes also occur in small animals.[23]

Effusions. When edema occurs in tissues, effusion may occur in potential spaces (e.g., pleural cavity, pericardial cavity, peritoneal cavity, joint cavities). The extent to which effusion occurs will depend on the severity of the fluid overload and capillary leak. Fluid pressure in these potential spaces in the normal state is negative and similar to that of subcutaneous tissue. The interstitial hydrostatic pressure normally is −7 to −8 mm Hg in the pleural cavity, −3 to −5 mm Hg in the joint spaces, and −5 to −6 mm Hg in the pericardial cavity.[12] The abdominal cavity is prone to effusion (i.e., ascites). Pleural and peritoneal effusions may be present because of the disease process even before fluids are administered, and both often are present in patients with moderate to severe pancreatitis. Small volumes of fluid in the peritoneal and pleural cavity are difficult to detect on physical examination. Baseline assessment of the chest should be made by auscultation and thoracic radiography, and gentle ballottement and radiography or ultrasonography can be used to assess the abdomen. Further monitoring may be required during fluid therapy, and a change in the type of fluid administered may be required. With increasing effusion and decreased COP, a colloid should be considered.

Blood Loss

Potentially deleterious effects of aggressive fluid therapy to treat patients after trauma before full assessment can increase morbidity and mortality. After trauma, the term "shock" frequently is used to describe a patient that is tachycardic, tachypneic, and has weaker than normal pulses, paler than normal MMs, and CRT of more than 2 seconds. However, mentation also is an important part of the assessment. If the patient has depressed mentation of varying degree but without known brain injury, this finding suggests clinically important blood loss and shock. However, if the patient still is alert, the physical findings may be the result of a sympathetic response caused by pain and fright and not necessarily associated with blood loss. The initial clinical response, in the latter case, is to immediately institute aggressive fluid therapy to treat presumed shock. One must consider the potential role of the neuroendocrine response in producing these clinical signs with or without blood loss. As an example relating blood loss to clinical signs, a 30-kg blood donor normally can donate 450 mL blood (i.e., 20% of blood volume) without obvious clinical signs. However, it is prudent to consider that a traumatized patient or one with a coagulopathy is bleeding and consider all potential sites of ongoing hemorrhage. If hemorrhage is present, one must determine its severity based on clinical signs, physical examination findings, and serial monitoring of physiological and laboratory test results. Crystalloids, colloids, or blood products should be administered at calculated rates based on clinical signs, physical examination findings, and laboratory data. Immediate compression of an area of hemorrhage should be performed. When compression is not feasible (i.e., within the abdomen or thorax), a careful and skilled approach to volume resuscitation must be conducted. Trauma patients also may have pulmonary contusions. Aggressive fluid therapy in these patients may cause pulmonary edema, and pulmonary status must be evaluated and monitored. If pulmonary contusions are noted, judicious fluid administration to adequate endpoints should be carried out. It should not be assumed that these patients are necessarily hypovolemic. On many occasions, intravenous fluid therapy is not required, and the need for fluid therapy must be assessed on an individual basis.

Noncompressible Hemorrhage. Laboratory studies performed in the 1950s and 1960s set guidelines for the standard approach to resuscitation of patients with hypotensive hemorrhagic shock[60] and focused on early, aggressive administration of crystalloid solutions and blood products. The goal was to restore intravascular volume and vital signs toward normal as quickly as possible regardless of the site of hemorrhage. These guidelines recently have come into question. Early laboratory studies used controlled hemorrhage models, whereas hemorrhage occurring in the clinical setting as a result of blunt or penetrating trauma is uncontrolled until definitive therapy controls bleeding. More recent hemorrhage models have demonstrated that aggressive fluid resuscitation may be harmful and may result in increased hemorrhage and mortality. Using splenic injury models, aggressive fluid therapy significantly increased hemorrhage and mortality.[31,57] Availability of blood products in veterinary practice is limited, and ongoing hemorrhage will be fatal. Other studies demonstrated that achieving a MAP of 40 to 60 mm Hg improved survival compared with a MAP of 80 mm Hg.[58] By achieving a MAP of 40 mm Hg and allowing hemostasis and clot formation with a gradual increase in MAP over several hours, survival was significantly increased when compared with immediate resuscitation to a MAP of 80 mm Hg.[4] Although a clot is formed immediately, it tends to be soft and "jellylike" and inadequate to maintain vascular integrity at high pressures. Allowing time for the clot to become a more rigid hemostatic plug facilitates hemostasis.[55] Clinical trials in human patients are underway to further investigate this strategy. A recent review found no evidence to suggest that prehospital intravenous fluid resuscitation was beneficial and found some evidence that it may be harmful.[10] However, this evidence was not conclusive. A U.K. Consensus Statement suggests a more cautious approach to fluid management than previously advocated and concludes that further research is required on hypotensive (i.e., cautious) resuscitation versus delayed or no fluid replacement, especially in those with blunt trauma.[10] In the author's experience, a more cautious approach to resuscitation in blunt abdominal trauma patients with blood pressure correction to a MAP of 65 mm Hg (i.e., systolic pressure ~95 mm Hg) with resulting physiological parameters of decreased HR, decreased RR, and improvement in MM color and CRT has proved successful. In patients in which physiological parameters do not improve, surgical exploration is warranted. Unnecessary aggressive fluid therapy in a slightly hypotensive or normotensive animal before adequate clot formation could increase blood pressure and disrupt a clot on a lacerated vein or on a splenic or hepatic fracture. Minimum resuscitation to that required to afford adequate perfusion until such time as the hemorrhage is controlled makes more sense clinically. Volume resuscitation should be aggressive when the patient's condition is life threatening. These patients are easily identified, and rapid resuscitation to an *adequate hemodynamic state* (MAP, ~65 mm Hg; systolic, ~90 to 95 mm Hg) until hemorrhage is controlled surgically or spontaneously stops is warranted. With blood volume loss of more than 30%, transfusion of whole blood, packed cells, and plasma or colloids is required in addition to crystalloids. Many abdominal trauma patients can be managed this way if blood products are readily available. However, surgical intervention may be necessary when resuscitative efforts are not successful. The clinician must remember that abdominocentesis will be negative if hemorrhage into the retroperitoneal space has occurred. Conversely, blood loss into the pericardial space resulting in tamponade requires aggressive fluid therapy while preparing the patient for pericardiocentesis. In the acute setting, only very small volumes of blood within the pericardial space are required to cause tamponade.

Compressible Hemorrhage. When hemorrhage is compressible (i.e., that occurring from a limb), pressure is easily applied and hemorrhage stopped. Fluid resuscitation then can occur to optimal requirements without concern of further blood loss.

Autotransfusion of Blood. Autotransfusion of blood from the thorax or abdomen can be lifesaving in an exsanguinating animal if no other source of hemoglobin is available. However, serious complications will arise if blood is autotransfused from abdominal hemorrhage that has occurred as a result of neoplasia. Frequently, hemorrhage associated with neoplasia does not represent a single episode of bleeding but rather one of several with some episodes of hemorrhage occurring days to weeks previously. Various metabolic products in this accumulated blood are triggers for disseminated intravascular coagulation even when filtered. The potential for facilitating metastatic spread of the tumor also is frequently debated.

Approach to Fluid Selection and Volume to Avoid Complications. The volume of fluid to be administered is dependent on the situation at hand. The cause and severity of the hypovolemic state are important factors in fluid (e.g., crystalloid, colloid, blood products) selection and volume of resuscitation. It is important to ascertain whether fluids are required. Traumatized patients do not always have blood loss. When an intravascular volume deficit is confirmed, it is useful to construct a mental algorithm when managing patients with hypovolemia. It is best to start with the question, "Is there hemorrhage or not?" If "yes," "is the hemorrhage compressible or noncompressible?" If it is compressible, the patient should be managed to an optimal goal of resuscitation. If it is noncompressible, the patient should be resuscitated to an *adequate hemodynamic state* as described in the section on End-Points of Fluid Resuscitation. Other questions include "Is there hemorrhage associated with pulmonary contusions?" If so, the patient should be resuscitated to adequate perfusion (see section on End-Points of Fluid Resuscitation). "Is surgical intervention required?" If so, the patient should be resuscitated to an adequate hemodynamic state and then to optimal perfusion when hemorrhage controlled (see section on End-Points of Fluid Resuscitation). "If hemorrhage is not present, is capillary leak present or not? If capillary leak is not present, is COP normal or not?" If COP is normal, the patient should be resuscitated to optimal perfusion (see section on End-Points of Fluid Resuscitation). Crystalloids frequently are adequate. If not, a synthetic or natural colloid may be required. If capillary leak is present, fluid selection is crucial, and different types of fluids frequently are necessary. Resuscitation to optimal perfusion should be attempted, but resuscitation to adequate perfusion frequently is all that can be attained until the underlying illness is resolved.

Recognizing the underlying etiology of hypovolemia and the appropriate type of fluid to administer is important. Being aware of associated problems that will necessitate cautious fluid selection, volume, and rate of administration is key to success. The difference between optimal and adequate perfusion endpoints must be understood. Continued monitoring appropriate for the condition being managed will reduce the frequency of complications that can be associated with administration of fluids. There is no single method to monitor the adequacy of fluid resuscitation. Using a combination of methods and appreciating the limitations of each under the various conditions that are being used will assist the clinician in making the best possible assessment.

COMPLICATIONS ASSOCIATED WITH ROUTES OF FLUID ADMINISTRATION

Fluids can be delivered by several routes: enteral, subcutaneous, intraosseous, intraperitoneal, and most commonly, intravenous. Complications associated with intravenous catheters are discussed in detail in Chapter 15.

Enteral Route

The enteral route can be used effectively to rehydrate otherwise stable veterinary patients, assuming enteral routes of fluid loss (e.g., vomiting, diarrhea) are not present. A nasoesophageal tube is easily placed, and a maintenance electrolyte solution (Normosol-M®, Plasma-Lyte 56®) can be delivered via a fluid administration set.[42] Potential complications with the enteral route include positioning of the tube within the airway, vomiting if the administration rate is too high, and hyperkalemia if potassium supplementation is excessive.

Subcutaneous Route

This route of administration is very commonly used in veterinary practice. However, it is not recommended for animals with moderate to severe dehydration or for those with circulatory compromise. Circulation to the skin is reduced in volume-depleted animals, resulting in slow absorption. If absorption is poor or an excessive volume of fluid is administered, pooling of the fluid may occur in the subcutaneous tissues, and then fluid may gravitate ventrally. Pooling of fluid results in discomfort and lowers body temperature. Lactated Ringer's solution and 0.9% saline are fluids of choice for the subcutaneous route. Acetated polyionic solutions (Plasma-Lyte 148, Plasma-Lyte A, and Normosol-R) appear to cause severe discomfort when administered subcutaneously. The author has observed excessive vocalization and other painful behavior after subcutaneous administration of Plasmalyte 148. These effects may be associated with the acetate itself because the pH 6 of this solution is comparable with that of lactated Ringer's solution and is greater than that of 0.9% sodium chloride. Dextrose-containing solutions should not be administered via this route. Abscess formation and cellulitis also may be complications of this route if aseptic technique is not followed carefully.

Intraosseous

The bone marrow of the femur and humerus occasionally is more easily accessed than small collapsed veins in neonatal and pediatric small animal patients. Strict aseptic technique is required to avoid infection resulting in abscess formation and sepsis. This procedure is painful, and lidocaine should be infiltrated through the skin, subcutaneous tissue, and to the periosteum before attempting catheter placement. Iatrogenic injury to the regional nerves also may occur. Although this route is frequently advocated for our very young and small patients, this has rarely, if ever, been performed at the Ontario Veterinary College because placement of a 2-inch peripheral intravenous catheter into the jugular vein is preferred.

Intraperitoneal

This route is rarely used, but relatively rapid absorption of crystalloid solutions occurs from this site.[52] Concerns using this route include pathological conditions of the abdomen and the risk of peritonitis should contamination occur. Solutions containing acetate (e.g., Plasma-Lyte, Normosol products) should be avoided because they appear to be very painful when introduced into the abdomen. Lactated Ringer's solution and 0.9% saline are advised for this route.

Intravenous

The most common route for fluid administration is the intravenous route. Catheters are placed in peripheral veins (e.g., saphenous, cephalic) or a jugular vein. Strict aseptic technique is required. Complications may occur if surgical preparation of the venipuncture site is not performed. Inflammation at the venipuncture site may indicate infection or phlebitis caused by movement of the

catheter or the rigid material of the catheter (Teflon). In a study in which Violon catheters (Insyte, Becton Dickinson, Franklin Lakes, NJ) were placed after strict aseptic skin preparation, catheter dwell time could be extended up to 10 days with peripheral catheters and longer with jugular catheters.[43] These catheters become very flexible and soft when warmed to body temperature, and catheter replacement every 72 hours is not necessary when using these methods. Reduced inflammation associated with Violon catheters appears to result in minimal discomfort for the animal, and rarely do dogs and cats attempt to remove the catheter. At the Ontario Veterinary College, catheters only are removed when inflammation or fever of unknown origin occurs, or if the catheter is grossly contaminated. Such catheter tips are submitted for culture, and rarely (approximately one annually) is bacterial contamination identified. Inflammation of the catheter insertion site tends to occur at 72 hours in patients with vasculitis (e.g., immune-mediated hemolytic anemia).[43] Vasculitis may also predispose to thrombosis (e.g., immune-mediated hemolytic anemia, pancreatitis). Jugular vein catheterization should be avoided if possible in such animals, but many require frequent blood sampling or parenteral nutrition or both, often necessitating a central catheter. Heparin administration may reduce the potential for thrombosis.

Extravasation of fluids can be a serious complication if the fluid is hyperosmolar (e.g., amino acids, >5% dextrose in electrolyte solutions), contains vasoconstrictive drugs (e.g., epinephrine, norepinephrine), or contains certain chemotherapeutic agents. To reduce or avoid phlebitis associated with hyperosmolar solutions, a central vein should be used to deliver these solutions. If a peripheral vein must be used, a 24- to 22-gauge catheter rather than 20- to 18-gauge catheter should be selected. The area of catheter placement routinely should be assessed each time the veterinarian or technician examines the patient. The bandage does not have to be removed, but the limb should be palpated for heat, swelling, and discomfort. If infusion pumps are used and the alarm signals occlusion, the catheter and entry site should be examined carefully.

Destruction of the catheter or administration set will occur if the animal bites it, and hemorrhage may be a complication if this event is not witnessed. Serious hemorrhage also may occur if the connector on an arterial catheter becomes dislodged and may require blood transfusion if a large amount of blood loss occurs.

REFERENCES

1. Aldrich J, Haskins S: Monitoring the critically ill patient. In Bonagura JD, Kirk RW, editors: *Current veterinary therapy XII*, Philadelphia, 1995, WB Saunders, pp. 98-105.
2. Baldassarre S, Vincent JL: Coagulopathy induced by hydroxyethylstarch, *Anesth Analg* 84:451-453, 1997.

3. Boldt J: Hydroxyethylstarch as a risk factor for acute renal failure: is a change of clinical practice indicated? *Drug Saf* 25:837-846, 2002.

4. Burris D, Rhee P, Kaufmann C, et al: Controlled resuscitation for uncontrolled hemorrhagic shock, *J Trauma* 46:216-223, 1999.

5. Clemmesen O, Ott P, Larsen FS: Splanchnic metabolism in acute liver failure and sepsis, *Curr Opin Crit Care* 10:152-155, 2004.

6. Cohen RD, Woods RF: *Clinical and biochemical aspects of lactic acidosis*, Boston, 1976, Blackwell Scientific, p. 42.

7. Cornelius LM: Fluid therapy in small animal practice, *J Am Vet Med Assoc* 176:110-114, 1980.

8. de Laforcade AM, Rozanski A: Central venous pressure and arterial blood pressure measurements, *Vet Clin North Am Small Anim Pract* 31:1163-1174, 2001.

9. Downey GP, Dong O, Kruger J: Regulation of neutrophil activation in acute lung injury, *Chest* 116(suppl 1):46S-54S, 1999.

10. Dretzke J, Sandercock J, Bayliss S, et al: Clinical effectiveness and cost-effectiveness of prehospital intravenous fluids in trauma patients, *Health Technol Assess* 8:iii, 1-103, 2004.

11. Ferraboli R, Malheiro PS, Abdulkader RC, et al: Anuric acute renal failure caused by dextran-40 administration, *Ren Fail* 19:303-306, 1997.

12. Guyton AC, Hall JE: Body fluid compartments. In Guyton AC, Hall JE, editors: *Textbook of medical physiology,* ed 10, Philadelphia, 2000, WB Saunders, p 264.

13. Guyton AC, Hall JE: Dominant role of the kidney in long-term regulation of arterial pressure and in hypertension: the integrated system for pressure control. In Guyton AC, Hall JE, editors: *Textbook of medical physiology,* ed 10, Philadelphia, 2000, WB Saunders, p. 195.

14. Guyton AC, Hall JE: Integration of renal mechanisms for control of blood volume and extracellular fluid volume; and renal regulation of potassium, calcium, phosphate and magnesium. In Guyton AC, Hall JE, editors: *Textbook of medical physiology,* ed 10, Philadelphia, 2000, WB Saunders, p. 329.

15. Guyton AC, Hall JE: Pulmonary circulation, pulmonary edema, pleural fluid. In Guyton AC, Hall JE, editors: *Textbook of medical physiology,* ed 10, Philadelphia, 2000, WB Saunders, pp. 444-451.

16. Guyton AC, Hall JE: Regulation of extracellular fluid osmolarity and sodium concentration. In Guyton AC, Hall JE, editors: *Textbook of medical physiology,* ed 10, Philadelphia, 2000, WB Saunders, p. 313.

17. Guyton AC, Hall JE: The body fluid compartments: extracellular and intracellular fluids; interstitial fluid and edema. In Guyton AC, Hall JE, editors: *Textbook of medical physiology,* ed 10, Philadelphia, 2000, WB Saunders, p. 264.

18. Guyton AC, Hall JE: The kidneys and body fluids. In Guyton AC, Hall JE, editors: *Textbook of medical physiology,* ed 10, Philadelphia, 2000, WB Saunders pp. 332-335.

19. Guyton AC, Lindsey AW: Effect of elevated left atrial pressure and decreased plasma protein concentration on the development of pulmonary edema, *Circ Res* 7:649-657, 1959.

20. Hansen B: Technical aspects of fluid therapy: catheters and monitoring of fluid therapy. In DiBartola S, editor: *Fluid therapy in small animal practice,* ed 2, Philadelphia, 2000, WB Saunders, pp. 300-305.

21. Hansen B, DeFrancesco T: Relationship between hydration estimate and body weight change after fluid therapy in critically ill dogs and cats, *J Vet Emerg Crit Care* 12:235-243, 2002.

22. Holbeck S, Grande P: Effects on capillary fluid permeability and fluid exchange of albumin, dextran, gelatin and hydroxyethyl starch in cat skeletal muscle, *Crit Care Med* 28:1089-1095, 2000.

23. Holm JL, Chan DL, Rozanski EA: Acute pancreatitis in dogs, *J Vet Emerg Crit Care* 13:201-213, 2003.

24. Hughes D: Lactate measurement: diagnostic, therapeutic, and prognostic implications. In Bonagura JD, editor: *Kirk's current veterinary therapy XIII,* Philadelphia, 2000, WB Saunders, pp. 112-116.

25. Hughes D, Drobatz KJ: Comparison of plasma lactate concentration from cephalic, jugular, and femoral arterial blood samples in normal dogs, *J Vet Emerg Crit Care* 6:115, 1996.

26. Jacobs ML, Daggett WM, Civette JM: Acute pancreatitis: analysis of factors influencing survival, *Ann Surg* 185:43-51, 1977.

27. Jaffray C, Yang J, Carter G: Pancreatic elastase activates pulmonary nuclear factor kappa B and inhibitory kappa B, mimicking pancreatitis-associated adult respiratory distress syndrome, *Surgery* 128:225-231, 2000.

28. Jellinek H, Krafft P, Fitzgerald RD, et al: Right atrial pressure predicts hemodynamic response to apneic positive airway pressure, *Crit Care Med* 28:672-678, 2000.

29. Jonas MM, Tanser SJ: Lithium dilution measurement of cardiac output and arterial pulse waveform analysis: an indicator dilution calibrated beat-by-beat system for continuous estimation of cardiac output, *Curr Opin Crit Care* 8:257-261, 2002.

30. Kilborn S, Pook H, Bonnett B: Comparison of three different methods of total carbon dioxide measurement, *Vet Clin Pathol* 24:22-27, 1995.

31. Krausz MM, Bashenko Y, Hirsh M: Crystalloid or colloid resuscitation of uncontrolled hemorrhagic shock after moderate splenic injury, *Shock* 13:230-236, 2000.

32. Lagutchik MS, Ogilvie GK, Wingfield WE: Lactate levels in critically ill and injured dogs, *J Vet Emerg Crit Care* 6:119, 1996.

33. Linton RA, Young LE, Marlin DJ, et al: Cardiac output measured by lithium dilution, thermodilution and transesophageal Doppler echocardiography in anesthetized horses, *Am J Vet Res* 61:731-737, 2000.

34. Liskaser F, Story DA: The acid-base physiology of colloid solutions, *Curr Opin Crit Care* 5:440-442, 1999.

35. Machado CEG, Dyson DH, Mathews KA: Evaluation of oxymorphone/diazepam and hydromorphone/diazepam induction and transfer to isoflurane in experimentally induced hypovolemic dogs, *Am J Vet Res* (in press).

36. Machon RG, Raffe MR, Robinson EP: Central venous pressure measurements in the caudal vena cava of cats, *J Vet Emerg Crit Care* 5:121-129, 1995.

37. Mandell DC, King LG: Fluid therapy in shock, *Vet Clin North Am Small Anim Pract* 28:623-644, 1988.

38. Manning JE, Katz LM, Brownstein MR, et al: Bovine hemoglobin-based oxygen carrier (HBOC-210) for resuscitation of uncontrolled, exsanguinating liver injury in swine, *Shock* 13:152-159, 2000.

39. Martin GS, Ely W, Carroll FE, et al: Findings on the portable chest radiograph correlates with fluid balance in critically ill patients, *Chest* 122:2087-2095, 2002.

40. Marx G: Fluid therapy in sepsis with capillary leakage, *Eur J Anaesthesiol* 20:429-442, 2003.

41. Mason DJ, O'Grady M, Woods JP, et al: Comparison of a central and a peripheral (cephalic v) injection site for the measurement of cardiac output using the lithium-dilution cardiac output technique in anesthetized dogs, *Can J Vet Res* 66:207-210, 2002.

42. Mathews KA: The various types of parenteral fluids and their indications, *Vet Clin North Am Small Anim* 28:483-513, 1998.

43. Mathews KA, Brooks M, Valliant AE: A prospective study of intravenous catheter contamination, *J Vet Emerg Crit Care* 6:33-37, 1996.

44. McGee A, Abernethy WB III, Simel DL: The rational clinical examination. Is this patient hypovolemic? *JAMA* 281:1022-1029, 1999.

45. Mishler JM: Synthetic plasma volume expanders: their pharmacology, safety and clinical efficacy, *Clin Haematol* 13:75-92, 1984.

46. Moon PF, Ilkiw JE: Surface-induced hypothermia in dogs: 19 cases (1987-1989), *J Am Vet Med Assoc* 202:437-444, 1993.

47. Nelson L: The new pulmonary artery catheter: continuous venous oximetry, right ventricular ejection fraction and continuous cardiac output, *New Horiz* 5:251-258, 1997.

48. Pascoe PJ: Perioperative management of fluid therapy. In DiBartola S, editor: *Fluid therapy in small animal practice,* ed 2, Philadelphia, 2000, WB Saunders, pp. 307.

49. Pinsky MR: Functional hemodynamic monitoring, *Intensive Care Med* 28:386-388, 2002.

50. Reuter DA, Felbinger TW, Schmidt C, et al: Stroke volume variations for assessment of cardiac responsiveness to volume loading in mechanically ventilated patients after cardiac surgery, *Intensive Care Med* 28:392-398, 2002.

51. Ryden SE, Oberman HA: Compatibility of common intravenous solutions with CPD blood, *Transfusion* 15:250-255, 1975.

52. Schaer M: General principles of fluid therapy in small animal medicine, *Vet Clin North Am Small Anim Pract* 19:203-210, 1989.

53. Scheingraber S, Rehm M, Sehmisch C, et al: Rapid saline infusion produces hyperchloremic acidosis in patients undergoing gynecologic surgery, *Anesthesiology* 90:1265-1270, 1999.

54. Schertel ER, Tobias TA: Hypertonic fluid therapy. In DiBartola SP, editor: *Fluid therapy in small animal practice,* Philadelphia, 1992, WB Saunders, p. 471.

55. Sixma JJ, Wester J: The hemostatic plug, *Semin Hematol* 14:265-299, 1977.

56. Smiley LE, Garvey MS: The use of hetastarch as adjunct therapy in 36 dogs with hypoalbuminemia: a phase two clinical trial, *J Vet Intern Med* 8:195-200, 1994.

57. Solomonov E, Hirsh M, Yahiya A: The effect of vigorous fluid resuscitation in uncontrolled hemorrhagic shock after massive splenic injury, *Crit Care Med* 28:749-754, 2000.

58. Stern SA, Kowalenko T, Younger J: Comparison of the effects of bolus vs slow infusion of 7.5% NaCl/6% Dextran-70 in a model of near-lethal uncontrolled hemorrhage, *Shock* 14:616-622, 2000.

59. Story DA, Bellomo R: The acid-base physiology of crystalloid solutions, *Curr Opin Crit Care* 5:436-439, 1999.

60. Wiggers CJ: *Physiology of shock,* New York, 1950, Commonwealth Fund, p 121-143.

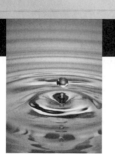

CHAPTER · 17

PERIOPERATIVE MANAGEMENT OF FLUID THERAPY

Peter J. Pascoe

The normal mechanisms of fluid homeostasis are disturbed when an animal undergoes anesthesia and surgery. Consequently, animals should receive fluids during the perioperative period to maintain proper fluid balance. Anesthetized animals should receive fluids:

1. To establish and maintain venous access. A minimal rate of fluid administration is necessary (e.g., 3 mL/hr) and will ensure rapid access to the circulation in the event of an emergency in the perioperative period.

2. To counter the physiologic changes that are associated with anesthetics. Most of the drugs and techniques that are used to anesthetize animals have some effect on the circulation.

3. To replace fluids lost during anesthesia and surgery. During the procedure, the animal cannot drink and its metabolic rate is reduced (decreased production of metabolic water). At the same time, the animal continues to produce urine, salivate, secrete fluid into the gastrointestinal tract, and lose water by evaporation from the respiratory tract. The aim should be at least to replace the expected insensible fluid losses.

4. To correct fluid losses caused by disease and to replace ongoing losses attributed to the procedure. The volume of fluid lost or gained depends on the type of surgical procedure, the skill of the surgeon, the preoperative state of the animal, and the equipment used by the anesthetist. Trauma and surgery are associated with increased secretion of vasopressin, and additional secretion may occur as a result of hypotension or hypovolemia. Other stress hormones (e.g., cortisol, catecholamines, renin) released during the procedure also may play a role in upsetting normal fluid homeostasis and warrant perioperative fluid therapy.

PREOPERATIVE PREPARATION OF THE PATIENT

The animal's fluid balance should be as close to normal as possible before anesthesia. Almost all anesthetics have some effects on circulatory and renal function, and it is important that the patient's circulating volume be optimal so that these effects are not exacerbated. Disturbances that require attention may be classified by their urgency. Some can be corrected acutely (e.g., hypovolemia); some require more time to correct (e.g., hypernatremia); and a few require completion of the procedure before correction of the problem can occur (e.g., hypervolemia associated with acute renal failure in a patient being prepared for hemodialysis).

CHANGES IN VASCULAR VOLUME

HYPOVOLEMIA

Hypovolemia may be caused by fluid loss directly from the vascular space (e.g., hemorrhage), a more general loss (e.g., dehydration), or changes in vascular tone. In all cases, fluid should be given to replace the loss. For a simple loss in which the composition of the vascular space is relatively normal, the loss can be replaced effectively using an isotonic crystalloid, a hypertonic crystalloid, an artificial colloid, or a blood product. The fluid used depends on the severity of the loss and the financial resources of the client. Acute blood loss of up to 30% of blood volume can be replaced adequately using a crystalloid solution (assuming normal hematocrit and total protein concentration before therapy), whereas a loss of 50% of blood volume or more will probably require blood component therapy and possibly additional crystalloid or colloid support. Occasionally, fluid therapy is not sufficient, and surgical management is required to stop bleeding (e.g., ruptured vena cava). In these instances, it is crucial to have one or more large-gauge venous catheters in place in an attempt to keep pace with the loss. In cats and dogs weighing less than 5 kg, it usually is feasible to place an 18-gauge catheter in the jugular vein. In many dogs of 5 to 15 kg, it is feasible to place a 16-gauge catheter in a cephalic vein, whereas in dogs more than 15 kg, a 14-gauge catheter normally may be placed. After the catheter has been placed, the animal should be anesthetized using a technique that induces minimal disturbances in volume status and cardiovascular function. Some investigators advocate withholding fluids from trauma patients with major vessel rupture before surgical intervention. In one study of human patients, a marginal benefit was demonstrated using this approach.[13] Others have advocated resuscitation to lower than normal blood pressures to minimize the chance of dislodging a fragile clot or increasing the rate of hemorrhage.[47] It is likely to be a realistic approach only when blood loss is rapid and surgery can be performed immediately. In patients with major blood loss but no central vessel rupture, it is more appropriate to replace the volume deficit before anesthetizing the animal.

If the patient is expected to lose a large volume of blood during an anticipated elective surgery, the animal can donate blood in advance so as to have autologous blood available. The animal can donate one unit of blood and then return 3 weeks later, at which time the first unit of blood can be returned to the animal and two units of blood drawn. This procedure can be repeated to collect several units from the same animal. This approach usually is not possible because of the lead time needed to complete these multiple collections, but a single donation technique has been reported for cats undergoing partial craniectomy.[55] Another alternative in an animal with relatively normal hematocrit and total protein concentration is to use acute normovolemic hemodilution, collect blood immediately before surgery, and replace it with three times the volume of crystalloid or the same volume of colloid. The expectation is that the animal will lose less protein and red cell volume during the surgery because of hemodilution, and the collected blood will be available for transfusion when it is needed after surgery. The formula for calculating the hemodilution was originally described by Bourke and Smith[18]:

$$\text{Exchangeable blood volume} = \text{Actual blood volume} \times \ln\left(\frac{Hb_0}{Hb_t}\right)$$

where Hb_0 is the original hemoglobin concentration, and Hb_t is the target value. This formula tends to overestimate the exchangeable blood volume, and a more accurate iterative formula has been published that uses a more sophisticated calculation technique.[107]

Although these techniques may be beneficial under special circumstances, they have been evaluated in human medicine and have been found to be very expensive and to provide little benefit to the patient.[19,32,64,88,137] Nevertheless, the American Society of Anesthesiologists (ASA) published guidelines for the use of packed red cells that include the following statements[67]:

1. When appropriate, preoperative autologous blood donation, intraoperative and postoperative blood recovery, acute normovolemic hemodilution, and measures to decrease blood loss (deliberate hypotension and pharmacologic agents) may be beneficial.

2. The indications for transfusion of autologous red blood cells (RBCs) may be more liberal than for allogeneic RBCs because of the lower (but still significant) risks associated with the former.

HYPERVOLEMIA

Hypervolemia is likely to be either iatrogenic or the result of oliguric renal failure or heart failure. In the former situation, it may simply be sufficient to monitor the patient carefully until its fluid volume status has normalized. In the case of oliguric renal failure, it is difficult to reduce the blood volume without dialysis. The primary risk of hypervolemia is related to hypertension and an increase in myocardial work, which could lead to failure in a heart with marginal reserve. Hypervolemia also may lead to pulmonary edema, in which case the circulating volume should be reduced by administration of a diuretic (if renal function is normal) or by phlebotomy if necessary.

CHANGES IN CONTENT

Occasionally, changes in vascular volume do not affect the composition of blood, but in many cases changes in composition also occur and require attention.

ANEMIA

The major concern with anemic patients is the supply of oxygen to the tissues after the animal has been anesthetized with drugs that may impair cardiovascular function. In the chronically anemic animal, some compensation already has occurred to facilitate delivery of oxygen to the tissues. This compensation usually occurs as a result of an increase in cardiac output and a change in the affinity of hemoglobin for oxygen. When the animal is anesthetized, especially using drugs such as α_2 agonists or inhalants, cardiac output is decreased, which reduces the delivery of oxygen to the tissues.

Administration of 100% oxygen increases the amount of oxygen in solution (0.3 mL per 100 mL of blood per 100 mm Hg pressure), but this effect provides little compensation for the decline in cardiac output. Fig. 17-1 illustrates the relationship between hemoglobin concentration and cardiac index assuming a constant saturation of hemoglobin (99%) to deliver oxygen at a given rate (15 mL/kg/min). The second line shows the same relationship for a PaO_2 of 500 mm Hg assuming a hemoglobin saturation of 100%. In acute anemia, the animal may have been able to increase cardiac output, but there has not been sufficient time for changes in hemoglobin affinity to occur, and the delivery of oxygen is likely to be decreased further. What is a "critical" hemoglobin concentration? In many experiments, carried out in dogs, the critical hemoglobin concentration is defined as the point at which oxygen delivery fails to keep up with tissue oxygen demand. In the healthy, lightly anesthetized dog, this concentration appears to be approximately 3 g/dL but varies with the anesthetic used and increases substantially at deeper planes of anesthesia.[158,159] Many human patients are anesthetized and survive with hemoglobin concentrations as low as 3 to 4 g/dL, but anesthesia is not recommended in this situation unless great care is taken to ensure that the patient has adequate cardiovascular reserve and unless techniques can be used that minimize reduction in cardiac output.[7,28] The ASA guidelines are based on the available literature in human medicine.[67] The ASA recommendations for use of packed red cells include the following:

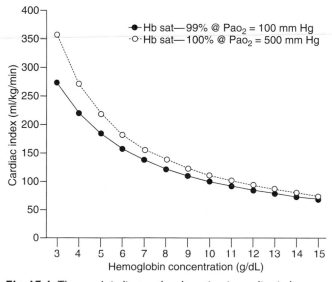

Fig. 17-1 The graph indicates the alteration in cardiac index needed to provide an oxygen delivery of 15 mL/kg/min when the PaO_2 is increased from 100 to 500 mm Hg, assuming that hemoglobin saturation increases from 99% to 100%. Note that the increased PaO_2 begins to make a difference only when the hemoglobin decreases below about 5 g/dL.

1. Transfusion is rarely indicated when the hemoglobin is greater than 10 g/dL and is almost always indicated when it is less than 6 g/dL, especially when the anemia is acute.
2. The determination of whether intermediate hemoglobin concentrations (6 to 10 g/dL) justify or require RBC transfusion should be based on the patient's risk for complications of inadequate oxygenation.
3. The use of a single hemoglobin "trigger" for all patients and other approaches that fail to consider all important physiologic and surgical factors affecting oxygenation are not recommended.

A review in the Cochrane database examined the use of restrictive versus liberal transfusion practices and could identify no adverse effects of the use of transfusion triggers in the 7 to 9 g/dL range.[76] Although hemoglobin concentration is reported on the complete blood count, it is more common for veterinarians to evaluate the hematocrit, which usually is approximately three times the hemoglobin concentration (g/dL). A scoring system for the rational use of packed RBCs in dogs was developed in an attempt to decrease unnecessary use.[90] However, this scoring system did not account for blood transfusions under conditions of rapid blood loss and failure to maintain blood pressure. It is important to assess anemic dogs and cats carefully and to estimate the likelihood of blood loss during the procedure. A dog with a hematocrit of 18% and a healthy cardiovascular system about to undergo a noninvasive diagnostic procedure may be a candidate for anesthesia without previous transfusion. A patient with the same hematocrit but with clinically relevant mitral regurgitation and about to undergo an exploratory laparotomy for an undefined abdominal mass would be more likely to require a preoperative blood transfusion.

POLYCYTHEMIA

Patients with polycythemia are at risk for complications because of the increased viscosity of their blood. High viscosity increases myocardial work and may lead to inadequate flow in some capillary beds, especially if the animal becomes hypotensive.[8] The hematocrit should be reduced to at least 65% by removal of blood and replacement with an isotonic crystalloid before the polycythemic patient is anesthetized. Animals with polycythemia caused by chronic hypoxia (e.g., tetralogy of Fallot) must be monitored carefully for signs of inadequate oxygen delivery when such hemodilution is undertaken.

HYPOPROTEINEMIA

Many drugs given during anesthesia are highly protein bound, and hypoproteinemia may result in a greater fraction of the anesthetic being available. More profound depression thus may occur from a given dose in the hypoproteinemic patient. Most drugs bind to albumin, and it is this fraction of the proteins that is of greatest importance. However, if the drug is titrated to effect, the increased free fraction of drug is accounted for by close monitoring of anesthetic induction. Thus concerns about hypoproteinemia are greater when using intramuscular injection or bolus dose techniques.

Hypoproteinemia also may affect the balance between hydrostatic and colloid oncotic pressure, leading to increased loss of fluid from the capillaries. This effect is of particular concern to the anesthetist because it may increase the likelihood of pulmonary edema formation. Clinically, this effect is of limited importance unless there is a strong possibility that left atrial pressure is increased (e.g., low oncotic pressure in an animal with mitral regurgitation).

HYPERPROTEINEMIA

Increased plasma protein concentration is of concern only as a sign of hypovolemia. In normally hydrated dogs and cats with hyperproteinemia, it is the globulins that are increased, and this fraction has less impact on protein binding of drugs and oncotic pressure than does albumin. However, hyperproteinemia may be a cause of pseudohyponatremia if the total protein concentration exceeds 10 g/dL.

HYPONATREMIA

Rapid correction of hyponatremia may be necessary to treat cerebral edema (usually only when serum sodium is <130 mEq/L). With acute hyponatremia, rapid correction may not cause any complications in the brain, but with chronic hyponatremia, a rapid change in serum sodium concentration can lead to an osmotic demyelination syndrome or myelinolysis occurring one to several days after therapy.[99,114] In both acute and chronic situations, the rate of change should be approximately 0.5 to 1 mEq/hr unless the patient is manifesting signs of cerebral edema, in which case initial therapy with 3% saline may be used to increase serum sodium concentration by 5 to 6 mEq/L over 2 to 3 hours. Ideally, hyponatremia should be corrected before surgery; however, given the required time frame, this is not always possible. Therefore the anesthetist must be prepared to monitor changes in serum sodium concentration carefully to prevent myelinolysis. It may be necessary to administer a diuretic to facilitate excretion of free water. See Chapter 3 for more information.

HYPERNATREMIA

Rapid correction of hypernatremia can lead to acute cerebral edema. If the patient is severely hypovolemic, it is important to correct that deficit using a solution with a sodium concentration similar to that of the patient. If the animal is not severely dehydrated and the serum sodium exceeds 165 mEq/L, correction should proceed slowly to achieve a rate of change of 0.5 to 1 mEq/hr using 0.45% NaCl or 5% dextrose. In dogs, administration of 5% dextrose at 3.7 mL/kg/hr should decrease the serum sodium concentration by 1 mEq/hr. Hypernatremia may increase the minimum alveolar concentration of inhalants, and a higher dose may be required to maintain anesthesia.[152]

HYPOKALEMIA

Hypokalemia can lead to muscle weakness, cardiac arrhythmias, hypotension, and renal insufficiency with associated metabolic acidosis in dogs and cats. In patients with mild hypokalemia but no clinical signs and no identifiable underlying cause, it probably is unnecessary to treat the animal. The patient with hypokalemia that is likely to have a whole-body deficit of potassium should be treated to correct this deficit if possible. The usual recommendation is to correct the deficit at a maximal rate of 0.5 mEq/kg/hr, although higher rates can be used if a severe deficit of total body potassium is suspected (up to 1.0 mEq/kg/hr). If the hypokalemic patient must be anesthetized, it is important to monitor for cardiac arrhythmias and to recognize that the heart will be refractory to class I antiarrhythmic drugs (e.g., quinidine, procainamide, lidocaine) and more sensitive to the toxic effects of digitalis glycosides. Hypotension may occur because there is a decrease in systemic vascular resistance possibly related to decreased sensitivity to angiotensin II.[57] The pressor response to norepinephrine is normal. If muscle relaxants are to be used, it is prudent to start with a dose that is 30% to 50% lower than the normal dose and titrate the final dose to effect. Care should be taken administering glucose, sodium bicarbonate, or β_2 agonists because they tend to decrease serum potassium concentration. If a potassium-supplemented solution is to be used during anesthesia to correct the deficit, it should be used in conjunction with a solution containing a normal concentration of potassium (4 to 5 mEq/L), and the two solutions should be clearly labeled. If the animal requires a bolus of fluid during anesthesia, the solution with normal potassium concentration should be used, thus reducing the risk of iatrogenic hyperkalemia. Solutions containing more than 60 mEq/L of potassium should be given via a central vein.

HYPERKALEMIA

Hyperkalemia also is associated with muscle weakness and cardiac arrhythmias. If these signs are present, it is crucial to reduce the effects of hyperkalemia even though it is not possible to reduce total body potassium content without treating the primary condition (e.g., oliguric renal failure, urethral obstruction). Animals with moderate hyperkalemia (6 to 7 mEq/L) are more likely to develop arrhythmias during anesthesia even if they have not demonstrated electrocardiographic abnormalities earlier. Therapy for hyperkalemia includes administration of calcium to alter the threshold potential of cells, sodium bicarbonate to alter the flux of potassium across the cell membrane, and glucose to facilitate movement of potassium into cells. Insulin may be used with glucose to avoid hyperglycemia, but the blood glucose concentration must be monitored. β-Adrenergic agonists such as albuterol and salbutamol have been used to manage hyperkalemia, and their activity may be enhanced with the use of insulin.[5,101] One study in dogs documented the effect of epinephrine and ritodrine in reducing hyperkalemia.[53] After the animal is anesthetized, ventilation should be monitored and controlled if necessary because hypercapnia may decrease pH and facilitate potassium efflux from cells. Depolarizing muscle relaxants (e.g., succinylcholine) should be avoided because they may cause release of potassium from cells. Nondepolarizing relaxants should be used cautiously (50% to 70% of the normal dose) to avoid prolonged effects. The patient should be monitored carefully by electrocardiography and frequent measurements of serum glucose, potassium, and ionized calcium concentrations and acid-base status. See Chapter 5 for more information.

HYPOCALCEMIA

Decreased calcium concentrations are associated with increased neuromuscular excitability. In the heart, this may manifest itself as a prolonged QT interval and other arrhythmias (e.g., ventricular premature contractions, ventricular fibrillation). As with the other electrolytes, the rate of change is an important factor in the type of clinical signs seen. It is important to treat a patient with hypocalcemia and clinical signs before anesthesia. This can be achieved rapidly while the electrocardiogram is monitored for signs of overly rapid correction (bradycardia). Hyperthermia associated with hypocalcemic seizure activity also should be treated before anesthesia. Hypocalcemic patients are at increased risk from the toxic manifestations of digoxin therapy, and this risk should be taken into consideration when preparing cardiac patients for anesthesia.

HYPERCALCEMIA

Signs of muscle weakness also may be seen with hypercalcemia, but arrhythmias are relatively uncommon. When they do occur, cardiovascular manifestations include bradycardia with prolonged PR interval, wide QRS complex, and shortened QT interval. Hypercalcemia is difficult to treat acutely and usually requires treatment for at least 24 hours before anesthesia. See Chapter 6 for more information.

HYPEROSMOLALITY

Hyperosmolality usually is associated with hypernatremia, hyperglycemia, ketoacidosis, uremia, or the presence of exogenous toxins (e.g., ethylene glycol). In some cases, it may be impossible to reverse the hyperosmolar state adequately before anesthesia because therapy (e.g., hemodialysis) may require an invasive procedure. Hyperosmolality may be associated with disruption of the blood-brain barrier leading to greater uptake of some drugs.[170] This is unlikely to affect most anesthetics because they readily cross the blood-brain barrier normally. The hyperosmolar state associated with hypernatremia may increase the dose of inhalant required for anesthesia.[152]

HYPOOSMOLALITY

This invariably is associated with an excess of free water and hyponatremia and should be managed as described before.

HYPOGLYCEMIA

Hypoglycemia in an awake patient usually is manifested by somnolence progressing to coma. In the anesthetized animal, there may be no outward signs, and unless blood glucose concentration is being monitored, it is unlikely that hypoglycemia would be detected. Hence, it is important to recognize and manage hypoglycemia preoperatively. Most animals regulate their blood glucose concentration closely, but this may not be the case in very young animals, those with insulinomas, and animals with portosystemic shunts. It usually is unnecessary to remove very young animals from their dam until the time of premedication if they are receiving a liquid diet only. If they have been orphaned or are ill and have not been taking in fluids, it is best to check blood glucose concentration before anesthesia and treat accordingly. If blood is difficult to obtain, the animal can be given some oral glucose in the form of Karo syrup (ACH Food Companies, Inc., Memphis, TN) or some other clear dextrose-containing fluid.[50] Intraoperatively, it may be best to use a 2.5% to 5% glucose solution intravenously. Postoperatively, these patients should be monitored carefully or given additional Karo syrup until they can return to their previous feeding regimen. Animals with insulinomas can have resting blood glucose concentrations of 30 to 40 mg/dL and may tolerate these low glucose concentrations quite well. If exogenous glucose is administered as a bolus to an animal with hyperinsulinism, massive release of insulin may trigger a hypoglycemic crisis. Therefore it is important to use relatively dilute solutions of glucose and administer them as an infusion rather than as a bolus. We typically administer 2.5% glucose to these patients the night before surgery at 1 to 1.5 times the normal maintenance rate. Intraoperatively, blood glucose concentration is monitored carefully, and glucose infusions are continued as necessary. After the tumor is removed, blood glucose concentration usually returns rapidly to the normal range. Animals with portosystemic shunts may become hypoglycemic, and glucose supplementation may be needed in the perioperative period. In one retrospective series, 2 of 13 dogs with portosystemic shunts were reported to have developed hypoglycemia intraoperatively.[92]

HYPERGLYCEMIA

Hyperglycemia typically occurs in diabetic dogs and cats and in stressed cats. Hyperglycemia itself may not be dangerous; however, if blood glucose concentration exceeds 400 mg/dL, it may contribute to a hyperosmolar diuresis with subsequent dehydration. With diabetic animals, it is ideal if anesthesia can be postponed until blood glucose concentration can be better regulated. If this is not feasible, the animal should be treated with insulin and glucose to stabilize blood glucose concentration between 200 and 300 mg/dL. In patients with brain trauma or those suffering from focal or global brain ischemia during surgery, hyperglycemia may be detrimental to neurologic outcome.[51,139,140,163] In animal models, blood glucose concentrations as low as 150 to 200 mg/dL have been shown to have negative effects on outcome, but the threshold for cerebral damage seems to be approximately 200 mg/dL.[103,140] In a study of dogs, dextrose administration was associated with greater renal damage after an ischemic insult than lactated Ringer's solution (LRS).[112] It is thought that increased intracellular glucose contributes to lactic acidosis in the cell, decreasing the chance of cell survival.

METABOLIC ACIDOSIS

Dogs and cats generally tolerate moderate acidosis reasonably well. However, severe acidosis is likely to lead to reduced activity of enzyme systems in the body with subsequent alterations in energy production and metabolism of drugs. Acidosis also may alter the activity of some anesthetic drugs because more of the un-ionized active form of anionic drugs is available at lower pH values. In patients with acidosis arising from insufficient oxygen delivery to tissues because of inadequate circulating volume, correction of the volume deficit may reverse acidosis without need for further therapy. Dogs and cats with diabetic ketoacidosis rarely require exogenous alkali if fluid therapy and insulin administration are managed appropriately. In cases in which the underlying condition is difficult to reverse (e.g., hypoxemia related to airway pathology, heart failure, pheochromocytoma), it is important to manage the acidosis before anesthesia. This is normally done using sodium bicarbonate, but Carbicarb and tromethamine may also be used (see Chapter 10 for more information). Sodium bicarbonate usually is available as an 8.4% solution with 1 mEq bicarbonate per mL and an osmolality of 2000 mOsm/L. In animals that are hyperosmolar or hypernatremic, it may be advisable to dilute bicarbonate to an isosmotic solution to prevent further exacerbation of the animal's condition. An osmolality of 300 mOsm/L can be achieved by diluting 1.5 mL of the 8.4% solution in 8.5 mL of sterile water. Sodium bicarbonate also should not be administered through the same intravenous line as catecholamines because it inactivates them (Table 17-1). Care should be taken when administering sodium bicarbonate to patients with respiratory depression because it increases the production of CO_2. If the animal is unable to increase its ventilation in response to increased production of CO_2, there may be little overall change in pH.

METABOLIC ALKALOSIS

Conditions that cause metabolic alkalosis may be associated with a high mortality rate, and 10 of 20 dogs with primary alkalemia died in one study.[128] Induction of anesthesia in an alkalotic patient may be associated with an increased dose requirement because of a decreased amount of un-ionized drug. In most cases, management of metabolic alkalosis requires the administration of chloride-containing solutions. This normally is achieved using 0.9% NaCl supplemented with KCl. Mild alkalosis may be caused by hypoalbuminemia, and correction of serum albumin concentration may be sufficient to correct the alkalosis.

CHANGES IN DISTRIBUTION

DEHYDRATION

Dehydration reduces vascular volume and results in changes in the volume of the intracellular space. The type and extent of change in the various compartments depend on the type of fluid lost. With pure water loss, volume contraction occurs in the intracellular compartment, whereas with hypotonic dehydration, an increase in the volume of the intracellular compartment may occur. With hypotonic loss, it is relatively simple to replace the circulating volume, but it takes longer to replenish the volume lost from the rest of the body. These concepts are discussed further in Chapter 3.

PERIPHERAL EDEMA

Peripheral edema usually is a reflection of poor circulation, leaky capillaries, or low oncotic pressure. Peripheral edema may have little impact on the course of anesthesia and surgery, but edema in certain locations may make induction and maintenance of anesthesia difficult for the anesthetist. If the limbs are edematous, it may be difficult to achieve venous or arterial access. In such cases, it may be necessary to use the jugular vein to place an intravenous catheter because the neck usually is less affected than are the limbs. Occasionally, dogs suffer damage to or occlusion of the jugular veins that can be associated with edema of the head and neck, potentially including the airway. Great care should be taken when intubating edematous animals because the affected tissue often is very fragile. It may be necessary to create a tracheostomy if the upper airway becomes obstructed and there is no way to improve venous drainage. Therapy aimed at improving local (e.g., hot packs, massage) and general (e.g., positive inotropes) circulation or increasing colloid oncotic pressure may reduce peripheral edema.

PULMONARY EDEMA

Pulmonary edema is of great concern to the anesthetist because it impairs gas exchange in the lungs and potentially reduces uptake of inhaled anesthetics. Formation of edema in the pulmonary circulation is a result of

TABLE 17-1 Compatibility of Intravenous Solutions with Other Drugs That Might Be Administered During Anesthesia

Solution	Comments
5% Dextrose	The pH of the solution ranges from 3.5 to 6.5, so alkaline solutions may precipitate.
Lactated Ringer's	Slightly acidic and contains calcium. Do not administer with blood products. Sodium bicarbonate may also react with the calcium and form calcium carbonate.
Acetated polyionic	If it contains no calcium, can be used with blood products and sodium bicarbonate.
Sodium chloride 0.9%	Usually slightly acidic but is compatible with most intravenous solutions; may cause precipitation if added to mannitol.
Sodium bicarbonate	Alkaline solution—incompatible with dobutamine, dopamine, isoproterenol, norepinephrine, and epinephrine. May react with calcium in solution (e.g., lactated Ringer's, acetated Ringer's, some polygelatins).
Dextrans	Slightly acidic—may degrade acid-labile drugs and may form drug complexes but appear to be compatible with most intravenous solutions.
Hetastarch	May be incompatible with some antibiotics—crystals formed with amikacin, cefamandole, cefoperazone, and tobramycin.
Polygelatins	Some preparations contain calcium, and these should not be used with blood products or sodium bicarbonate.
Blood and plasma	Do not administer through the same line as calcium salts.

increased hydrostatic pressure, decreased colloid oncotic pressure, or damage to the endothelium allowing leakage of fluid. Increased hydrostatic pressure may be caused by absolute (e.g., volume overload) or relative (e.g., redistribution of blood to the pulmonary circulation) hypervolemia, increased pulmonary venous pressure (e.g., left ventricular failure, mitral regurgitation), or increased pulmonary flow (e.g., left-to-right shunt, anemia). Volume overload should be treated with diuretics or phlebotomy as described earlier (hypervolemia). In animals with left ventricular failure or mitral regurgitation, the aim of therapy is to promote forward flow by using vasodilators or positive inotropes. In the acute setting, dobutamine is a suitable positive inotrope because it increases myocardial contractility while tending to decrease systemic vascular resistance. Nitroprusside or nitroglycerin can be used to decrease peripheral vascular resistance and can be titrated to effect. Ideally, therapy should be monitored using a catheter that allows measurement of pulmonary capillary wedge pressure (PCWP).

A decrease in colloid oncotic pressure rarely causes pulmonary edema acutely in dogs and cats, but it is important to take low colloid oncotic pressure into account when designing an anesthetic regimen because pulmonary edema may occur with smaller increases in pulmonary hydrostatic pressure. Both ketamine and large doses of oxymorphone have been shown to increase pulmonary vascular pressures.[35,74] If it is thought that low colloid oncotic pressure is contributing to pulmonary edema, therapy should be instituted to increase colloid oncotic pressure (e.g., plasma, dextrans, hetastarch [HES], polygelatins). In the case of pulmonary edema related to leaky membranes, therapy should be aimed at reducing pulmonary vascular pressure (e.g., nitroprusside, diuretics) and providing supportive care for the animal. Supportive care involves provision of oxygen, suction of froth from the airway, and institution of positive-pressure ventilation if necessary. Mechanical ventilation may improve gas exchange in patients with pulmonary edema. Positive-pressure ventilation with the addition of positive end-expiratory pressure (PEEP) or continuous positive airway pressure (CPAP) may not reduce lung water but may increase access to previously collapsed regions of the lung and may increase the capacity of the interstitium to hold fluid.

PLEURAL FLUID

Pleural fluid acts as a space-occupying lesion and impairs ventilation. In most cases, pleural fluid should be drained before anesthetizing the animal. If there appears to be a continuous air leak from the lung, it is best to place a chest drain before anesthesia or place a large-gauge catheter (e.g., 14 gauge) that can be aspirated rapidly to remove any accumulated air. In cases of hemothorax, blood is defibrinated during its residence in the pleural space. Accumulated blood can be aspirated from the pleural space and given back to the animal intravenously without providing additional anticoagulants. Autotransfusion should only be performed if there is minimal risk of bacterial contamination of the blood and no risk of the blood containing cancer cells that could metastasize to other areas of the body. The blood should be passed through a filter to remove clots before it is autotransfused. Cats with pleuritis appear to be in great pain and often are very fractious. It may be beneficial to provide sedation and analgesia (e.g., oxymorphone) and oxygen before attempting to drain the chest.

PERITONEAL FLUID

A large volume of fluid in the abdomen can increase intraabdominal pressure (so-called abdominal compartment syndrome) and should be drained before anesthesia if feasible. Abdominal compartment syndrome is associated with a number of physiologic changes, including hypoventilation with reduced pulmonary compliance; tachycardia; low cardiac output; and increased central venous pressure (CVP), mean pulmonary artery pressure, and PCWP. In the abdomen, the increased pressure reduces urine output and decreases blood flow to the abdominal wall and the splanchnic vascular beds. Intraabdominal hypertension also may increase intracranial pressure (ICP) with a decrease in cerebral perfusion pressure.[83]

Drainage of the abdomen usually is achieved by placing a catheter in the abdominal cavity and drawing off the fluid with a syringe. It is helpful if the catheter has additional side holes cut in it before insertion so that there is less likelihood of the catheter being obstructed by the omentum. Most affected animals have greater respiratory distress lying on their backs, and the catheter usually is inserted with the animal on its side. The author usually places the catheter about halfway between the last rib and the ischium, 1 to 4 inches off the ventral midline. Draining fluid in this manner can take a long time, but this is actually advantageous because rapid removal can result in mesenteric vasodilatation and cardiovascular collapse.[83] In the case of hemoabdomen, the blood may have been defibrinated, but it is best to collect it in an anticoagulant (e.g., heparin, citrate). Collected blood should be used only if there is no gross contamination of the abdomen and no risk of neoplasia. The blood should be passed through a filter to remove clots before it is autotransfused. In cases of massive trauma, it may be better to leave the blood in the abdomen until the surgeon is ready to stop the bleeding. Although the accumulated blood may compromise ventilation during this time, the increased intraabdominal pressure may reduce the rate of hemorrhage.

INCREASED INTRACRANIAL PRESSURE

Increased ICP requires careful management in terms of fluid balance. The cranial vault is a relatively fixed cavity, and any accumulated fluid tends to increase the pressure. An increase in the fluid content of the brain or in the volume of blood or cerebrospinal fluid in the cranial vault promotes an increase in ICP. In situations in which the cause is medically reversible (e.g., hyponatremia), therapy should be carried out before anesthesia. In cases in which the diagnosis or treatment requires anesthesia, the preoperative assessment of the patient must include a detailed examination of fluid balance. Animals with an acute increase in ICP caused by trauma also may be hypovolemic because of other injuries. Judicious use of hypertonic resuscitation fluids is appropriate for these patients because such fluids promote a reduction in ICP while restoring circulating volume.[168] Patients with chronically increased ICP often have had decreased food and water intake for some time and may have been treated with diuretics to reduce ICP. Consequently, such patients often are dehydrated and may have electrolyte disturbances. Whenever possible, preoperative assessment should include examination of the animal for signs of dehydration, an assessment of the cause of increased ICP, an evaluation of renal function, and measurement of serum electrolytes, hematocrit, total proteins, osmolality, and colloid oncotic pressure. If the animal clearly is dehydrated, it should be given fluids before anesthesia to increase its circulating volume. If plasma osmolality is less than 320 mOsm/kg, it may be beneficial to treat the animal with mannitol (0.25 to 1 g/kg).

INCREASED INTRAOCULAR PRESSURE

Patients with glaucoma often are treated similarly to patients with an increased ICP (i.e., diuretics), but they also are given carbonic anhydrase inhibitors (e.g., methazolamide, Teva, Sellersville, PA), which can cause metabolic acidosis over the course of 12 to 24 hours. Although correction of the acidosis may not be essential in many of these animals, treatment with sodium bicarbonate may decrease the risk associated with anesthesia. The combination of dehydration and acidosis may substantially reduce the dose of thiopental required for induction, and care should be taken to titrate this drug to effect in these patients.

AGE

As animals get older, body water and cardiovascular reserve decrease. These changes make older animals more susceptible to fluid overload in the perioperative period. Geriatric patients admitted to the hospital several days before anesthesia and surgery may not have been drinking well (i.e., low tolerance for a new environment) and may be dehydrated.

PREGNANCY

Pregnancy is associated with many changes in fluid balance. In women, the typical changes associated with pregnancy include hyponatremia; decreased blood urea

nitrogen and creatinine concentrations; respiratory alkalosis; decreased serum calcium, magnesium, and protein concentrations; and decreased hematocrit. Similar changes have been documented in dogs. Serum protein concentrations tend to decrease during pregnancy, with the most marked change being a decrease in serum albumin concentration.[25] Hematocrit decreases with a proportionately greater decrease with increasing numbers of fetuses.[4,87] The pregnant dog has a decreased baroreceptor response to hypotension and is more susceptible to hypotension with blood loss.[21,22] Thus the pregnant animal may be more susceptible to the negative circulatory effects of anesthetics and may require an increased volume of fluids during a surgical procedure. In bitches and queens that have been in labor for some time, dehydration and endotoxemia also may be present and add to circulatory instability. Affected patients may benefit from fluid therapy before anesthesia.

CHANGES IN FUNCTION

CARDIOVASCULAR DISEASE

If the heart is failing, it may not tolerate an increased fluid load. Increased preload in this setting may not result in increased cardiac output because of changes in the Frank-Starling curve. Conversely, even a failing heart does not function optimally if preload is allowed to decrease too much. In a prospective study of human patients, it was found that the frequency of postoperative heart failure was highest in patients who had received less than 500 mL/hr of fluids intraoperatively.[29] The most common cause of congestive heart failure in dogs is mitral insufficiency. This condition is characterized by excessive retrograde flow with an increasing volume load on the heart. Treatment often involves use of vasodilators (e.g., nitroglycerin, hydralazine, angiotensin-converting enzyme inhibitors) to decrease afterload and diuretics and salt restriction to decrease circulating volume. Consequently, cardiac patients have the potential to be hypovolemic. The diagnosis of relative hypovolemia in these patients is based on clinical signs such as skin turgor, mucous membrane color, capillary refill time (CRT), and jugular venous distension. Evaluation of renal function (including urine output) may assist in deciding whether the animal is adequately hydrated. Thoracic radiographs can be used to help assess pulmonary venous distension (i.e., lack of pulmonary venous distension implies lower left atrial pressure and hence lack of excessive preload). The most useful measurement in these patients is PCWP. PCWP is obtained by inserting a balloon-tipped catheter into the pulmonary vein from either the jugular or femoral vein. Such invasive monitoring certainly is warranted in some cardiac patients and provides the best guide to fluid therapy. If the animal has right-sided heart failure, monitoring CVP provides similar information. In one study, use of CVP or PCWP was associated with more aggressive fluid therapy (>500 mL/hr), which in turn was associated with a lower risk of postoperative congestive heart failure.[29] In the past, it has been recommended that fluids containing low concentrations of sodium be administered to cardiac patients (e.g., 0.45% saline in 2.5% dextrose). Most of these patients have an increase in total body sodium and an increase in total body water. The latter tends to exceed the former, and affected patients may be hyponatremic.[6] Thus it seems illogical to give a solution that contains additional free water. If such a patient is hypovolemic, it is more appropriate to use a balanced electrolyte solution. If the patient is not hypovolemic or it already has excessive volume, fluids may not be needed.

In other myocardial diseases, it also is important to assess the patient preoperatively for signs of dehydration and heart failure (e.g., distended jugular veins, slow jugular emptying, jugular pulses, ascites, pulmonary edema, pleural effusion). Invasive monitoring as described earlier may be necessary to optimize fluid therapy during anesthesia and surgery. Blood may flow best at a hematocrit of 25% to 30%, but it may be necessary to maintain higher values to maintain optimal tissue oxygenation. If an animal with heart failure also is anemic, consideration should be given to preloading the animal with packed red cells to optimize oxygen delivery.

COAGULATION DEFECTS

Any coagulation defect that is likely to increase intraoperative blood loss should be corrected before surgery if possible. If an animal has a known coagulation defect (e.g., hemophilia, hepatic failure, coumarin poisoning, von Willebrand's disease), it should be given fresh frozen plasma, cryoprecipitate, fresh plasma or fresh whole blood, and vitamin K in the case of coumarin poisoning. These treatments should be given within a few hours of surgery because the half-lives of most clotting factors are relatively short. Although fresh frozen plasma and fresh plasma may have sufficient clotting factors to reverse the coagulation defect, such therapy often fails in animals with severe defects. In dogs with von Willebrand's disease, infusion of cryoprecipitate is a more effective treatment than fresh frozen plasma alone.[30,147] Therapy with plasma from donors receiving desmopressin (DDAVP) may be more effective than plasma from untreated donors.[85] When DDAVP is given to dogs with type 1 von Willebrand's disease, there is a measurable increase in the binding of von Willebrand factor to collagen, suggesting an improvement in clotting ability during surgery.[84] Cryoprecipitate often is prepared from a number of donors and therefore has the potential to provide greater antigenic stimulation or transmit disease. Cryoprecipitate contains 10 to 20 times the normal amount of clotting factors and can be given in a small

volume. Thus it may be useful in animals in which volume overload may be a concern (e.g., Doberman pinschers with von Willebrand's disease and cardiomyopathy). The author has not used cryoprecipitate and has successfully managed dogs with von Willebrand's disease using fresh frozen plasma in mildly affected dogs or by treating both the plasma donor and recipient with DDAVP (1 μg/kg subcutaneously) in more severely affected dogs. Recommendations for the dosage of fresh frozen plasma range from 6 to 30 mL/kg and for cryoprecipitate from 1 U/5 to 15 kg.[147]

Animals with thrombocytopenia or dysfunctional platelets may require platelet infusion before surgery. Platelet life span in immune-mediated thrombocytopenia is considerably shortened, and platelet infusions may be effective for only a matter of hours. Although it is commonplace for platelet-rich plasma to be prepared for affected people, this is relatively rare in veterinary medicine. Platelet preparations have a short half-life (12 to 24 hours), and so they generally are prepared for individual patients in veterinary medicine. Consequently, most patients that are thrombocytopenic or have platelet dysfunction are treated with fresh whole blood. The amount of blood needed (TV) depends on the platelet count of the patient (P_E), the platelet count of the donor blood (P_D), the target platelet count (P_T), and the blood volume (BV) of the patient:

$$BV \times P_E + TV \times P_D = (BV + TV) \times P_T$$

Note: Volumes must be expressed in the same units (i.e., blood volume in microliters if platelet count is per microliter or platelet count/L if blood volume is in liters.)

The ASA guidelines for infusion of platelets are as follows[67]:
1. Prophylactic platelet transfusion is rarely indicated when thrombocytopenia is caused by increased platelet destruction (e.g., idiopathic thrombocytopenic purpura).
2. Prophylactic platelet transfusion is rarely indicated when thrombocytopenia is caused by decreased platelet production when the platelet count is greater than 100×10^9/L and is usually indicated when the platelet count is less than 50×10^9/L. The determination of whether patients with intermediate platelet counts (50 to 100×10^9/L) require therapy should be based on the risk of bleeding.
3. Surgical and obstetric patients with microvascular bleeding usually require platelet transfusion if the platelet count is less than 50×10^9/L and rarely require therapy if it is greater than 100×10^9/L. With intermediate platelet counts (50 to 100×10^9/L), the determination should be based on the patient's risk for more significant bleeding.

4. Operative procedures ordinarily associated with insignificant blood loss may be undertaken in patients with platelet counts less than $50 \times 10^9/L$.

5. Platelet transfusion may be indicated despite an apparently adequate platelet count if a known platelet dysfunction and microvascular bleeding are present.

More recent guidelines also suggest that platelet numbers should not be allowed to decrease to less than $50 \times 10^9/L$ during massive transfusion and should be greater than $100 \times 10^9/L$ in patients with multiple trauma or central nervous system injury.[20]

Patients with disseminated intravascular coagulation (DIC) may need surgical intervention to correct the initiating cause of the DIC. Restoration of circulating volume with fresh whole blood or fresh frozen plasma is the mainstay of preoperative therapy for patients with DIC. If heparin is used, it should be given at a dosage that does not cause significant prolongation of bleeding time (e.g., 75 U/kg every 8 hours subcutaneously). If heparin is added to the blood or plasma (same dosage), the activated partial thromboplastin time (APTT) should be determined before surgery to ensure that it is not excessively prolonged (i.e., not more than twice normal).

RENAL DISEASE

Patients with chronic renal insufficiency are at risk for having their disease exacerbated by the hemodynamic changes during anesthesia and surgery. Affected animals should be managed carefully during the perioperative period. They should be allowed access to water until the time of premedication. Any dehydration present should be corrected before anesthesia.

Patients with severe oliguric renal insufficiency are of concern because they have severely limited ability to excrete an extra fluid load and may already be hypervolemic and hypertensive. If possible, it is advantageous to monitor CVP as a guide to fluid therapy in these animals. Monitoring CVP provides information on how well the heart is able to pump the existing circulating volume and allows the anesthetist to watch the response to fluid therapy in the perioperative period.

HEPATIC DISEASE

Mild hepatic insufficiency rarely causes clinically relevant disturbances in fluid balance, but substantial alterations occur as the severity of hepatic injury progresses. The liver synthesizes many proteins, and hypoalbuminemia and deficiencies of clotting factors may occur as hepatic insufficiency progresses. These alterations are managed as described earlier. Blood ammonia concentrations are increased in patients with portosystemic shunts and in those with hepatic failure. Consequently, it is important not to administer additional ammonia by the use of stored blood products that may have increased ammonia content.

ENDOCRINE DISEASE

DIABETES INSIPIDUS

Animals with diabetes insipidus must be monitored carefully during the preoperative period to be sure they continue to drink water. Animals with complete central diabetes insipidus can become markedly dehydrated within a matter of hours (5% dehydration may occur after 4 hours of water deprivation). Consequently, affected animals should have access to water until the time of premedication, and intraoperative management should take into account the actual urine production of that animal so it is best to place a urinary catheter and use a closed collection system to monitor urine volumes.

HYPERADRENOCORTICISM

Animals with hyperadrenocorticism are polyuric and polydipsic and should have access to water until the time of premedication. Some dogs with hyperadrenocorticism have mildly increased serum sodium and mildly decreased serum potassium concentrations, but these rarely are of sufficient magnitude to be of concern. Animals with hyperadrenocorticism tend to be hypertensive, which may exacerbate underlying cardiac disease (e.g., mitral regurgitation), and they may have increased sensitivity to vasoconstrictive drugs. They also bruise easily, and special care should be taken when placing intravenous catheters. If the affected animal is being anesthetized for major surgery, hypercoagulability and increased risk of pulmonary thromboembolism are concerns. Prophylactic therapies for hypercoagulability may include the use of regular or low molecular weight heparins, plasma, and HES.

HYPOADRENOCORTICISM

Hyponatremia, hypochloremia, hyperkalemia, hypovolemia, hypoglycemia, metabolic acidosis, and azotemia commonly are associated with hypoadrenocorticism. These abnormalities are associated with hypotension and decreased sensitivity to positive inotropes and vasoconstrictive drugs. The fluid of choice for managing these animals is 0.9% NaCl, which tends to correct all of the preceding abnormalities except the hypoglycemia and metabolic acidosis, which should be monitored during therapy and corrected as necessary by administration of glucose and sodium bicarbonate. Hypotension can be especially difficult to manage in these patients intraoperatively, and steroid replacement should be started before induction of anesthesia.

DIABETES MELLITUS

In controlled diabetes, there rarely is any major concern about fluid balance preoperatively. The animal's normal feeding regimen and insulin dose are used on the day before surgery. On the morning of surgery, the animal receives one third to one half of its daily dose of insulin, and blood glucose concentration is monitored throughout the procedure.[94] The animal is treated with glucose, insulin, or some combination of these as determined by serial blood glucose measurements. Animals with uncontrolled diabetes may be dehydrated and may require fluid therapy before anesthesia.

HYPOTHYROIDISM

Patients with hypothyroidism rarely have any electrolyte disturbances but can be hypotensive and have a poor response to positive inotropes and vasoconstrictors. If possible, the animal should be adequately treated for hypothyroidism for at least 1 to 2 weeks before it is anesthetized.

HYPERTHYROIDISM

Animals with hyperthyroidism tend to be in a hyperdynamic state and are at risk for fatal, catecholamine-mediated arrhythmias when anesthetized. It is best if the animal is treated with an agent that antagonizes the action of thyroxine (e.g., methimazole) for at least 2 weeks before anesthesia.[120]

ACCESS TO THE CIRCULATION

The technical aspects of fluid administration are covered in Chapter 15. In the perioperative period, access to the circulation via the intravenous or intraosseous route should be available so that fluids can be given rapidly should the need arise. As discussed earlier, the diameter of the catheter should be sufficient to allow fluids to be administered rapidly enough for the expected deficits. It also is important that the connections to the animal be set up carefully and that they are secure. If the fluid line becomes disconnected with the animal draped for surgery, it may not be detected quickly, and the animal may experience substantial blood loss from the catheter. When the patient is prepared for a surgical procedure, the anesthetist should make sure to set up the fluid lines so that an injection port is accessible without the need to reach under the drapes. The animal also should be positioned in such a way that the fluids can flow easily. Drugs added to the fluids and administered through the same line must be compatible (see Table 17-1). If an animal will be receiving several drugs, it may be necessary to create additional access sites to prevent incompatible drugs from being administered through the same line. Consideration also must be given to the site of access. In cats undergoing declawing of the front paws, it is advisable to place the catheter in the hind leg so that it does not interfere with the surgery. In patients in which the caudal vena cava is to be occluded during surgery, it is important to have the catheter in the forelimb or neck so that fluids reach the remaining circulation during the occlusion. In an emergency in an anesthetized animal with no venous access, the most visible vessel usually is the sublingual vein. This vein can be catheterized rapidly if necessary.

THERMODYNAMIC CONSIDERATIONS

Infusion of fluids with temperatures less than normal body temperature requires that the animal warms the fluid, and this effect cools the animal. If we assume that the specific heat of water (and most of the crystalloid solutions used in fluid therapy) is 1 kcal/kg/° C, it would cost the animal 18 kcal to increase the temperature of 1 L of fluid from 20 to 38° C. If the specific heat of the body is 0.83 kcal/kg/° C, 1 L of fluid at 20° C would cool a 21.7-kg dog by 1° C.[59] Stated in another way, a fluid infusion rate of 10 mL/kg/hr at 20° C would cost the patient 0.18 kcal/hr and would tend to cool the body by approximately 0.2° C/hr. These losses are relatively minor in comparison with the body heat lost via radiation but may become more important when massive fluid volumes are required or the infused fluid is much colder (e.g., stored blood products).

EFFECTS OF ANESTHESIA

Some drugs may alter sympathetic activity and thus affect blood volume and the distribution and excretion of body fluids. Acepromazine is a potent α_1 antagonist, and even low dosages of the drug (0.001 mg/kg) induce this effect. In the healthy patient, this effect is associated with minor decreases in arterial blood pressure and hematocrit.[38] In an animal with increased sympathetic tone, however, the administration of acepromazine may result in profound hypotension. Acepromazine also is a dopamine antagonist and may inhibit the effect of dopamine to increase renal blood flow. Such an effect has been demonstrated with chlorpromazine, but no studies have been carried out with acepromazine.[23] The α_2 agonists have profound effects on the circulation and on renal function. In dogs and cats, administration of these drugs, even at low doses, causes a substantial decrease in cardiac output (40% to 60%). They also have a direct effect on the kidney, the end result of which is marked diuresis (urine output increases 3- to 10-fold). The mechanism for this effect appears to be related to antagonism of vasopressin, and this dehydrating effect may be even more relevant in a patient that is avidly conserving water. The opioids have a variety of actions. The μ agonists (e.g., morphine, oxymorphone, meperidine) have an antidiuretic effect, whereas the κ agonists (e.g., butorphanol, pentazocine, nalbuphine) tend to promote diuresis. The antidiuresis associated with the μ agonists may be the result of stimulation of vasopressin release. Release of vasopressin may be stimulated in the awake patient, but there is a reduction in the release of vasopressin in anesthetized patients receiving large doses of potent opioids (causing a reduced stress response).[42] The dissociative drugs (e.g., ketamine, tiletamine) tend to decrease urine output despite increases in cardiac output and blood pressure.[52] These drugs also tend to decrease baroreceptor responses, and this may be important in the anesthetized patient with relative hypovolemia that undergoes changes in body position.

Drugs that are used for the induction and maintenance of anesthesia all tend to decrease urine output, mainly through their hemodynamic effects.[82] Thiopental has been shown to alter renal sodium resorption, leading to increased sodium and water losses in dogs, but in human patients there is either no change or a decrease in urine output.[56,82] Thiopental also decreases hematocrit (which may be important in an anemic patient), but it has little effect on plasma volume.[156] Propofol causes hypotension if given rapidly, and it may cause some reduction in glomerular filtration rate and urine flow.[119] In normal sheep, there was minimal effect on renal function, but there was a significant detrimental effect during sepsis.[17] Etomidate preserves circulation better than most other drugs administered intravenously for induction, but it may alter renal function by virtue of the base in which it is constituted. Etomidate usually is supplied in propylene glycol, which can induce renal failure if enough is given. This would be unlikely with an induction dose of the drug, but continuous infusion might be associated with nephrotoxicity from the propylene glycol or the hemolysis that is likely to occur. Severe renal insufficiency was reported in dogs after an infusion of etomidate.[109] All of the inhalants are associated with a decrease in renal function, but this effect can be prevented to some extent by preloading the animals with fluids. Methoxyflurane has long been associated with nephrotoxicity in people, but this effect has not been reported in dogs and cats. There is some concern that sevoflurane can react with soda lime or baralyme, releasing a polyvinyl compound (Compound A) that is nephrotoxic, but this has not yet been seen to be a clinically important issue.

Positive-pressure ventilation has been associated with changes in renal function. A reduction in urine output occurs with the institution of positive-pressure ventilation, with CPAP or PEEP.[86] The techniques of PEEP and CPAP increase CVP, mean pulmonary artery pressure, and PCWP.[106] The increase in CVP tends to increase renal vein pressure, which may alter interstitial pressure within the kidney.[130] The use of intermittent positive-pressure ventilation (IPPV) and PEEP or CPAP is associated with an increase in vasopressin secretion, but it is likely that increased renal interstitial pressure has a more important effect because the decrease in urine output can be seen without changes in vasopressin.[129]

Regional anesthetic techniques also may result in volume-responsive hypotension. This is particularly true with epidural or intrathecal techniques. In people, the spinal cord ends at vertebral level L1/L2, and it is necessary to inject enough drug to extend high into the thoracic region to block enough spinal segments for abdominal surgery. As a result, there is a significant block of sympathetic outflow from the thoracic and lumbar spinal cord segments, which can result in hypotension. The cord ends at vertebral level L6/L7 in dogs and at S1/S2 in cats. Thus it is feasible to achieve an effective abdominal block in dogs and cats without substantial loss of sympathetic tone. However, hypotension can occur with this technique, and the animal should be monitored accordingly.

Intraoperative blood loss is affected by blood pressure and body temperature. In some situations in which it is difficult to control blood loss, it may be possible to reduce the loss by maintaining pressure at a lower than normal value for the period of concern. It would be advantageous to be able to monitor lactate concentrations to ensure that global perfusion was not being adversely affected by this approach. Hypothermia has been shown to alter coagulation. The mechanism for this effect appears to be mainly related to platelet function until body temperature decreases to less than 33° C when the effects on enzymes become manifest.[167] In dogs, it has been noted that platelet counts decrease by 70% between 37 and 32° C because of splenic sequestration, but the defective release of thromboxane A_2, down-regulation of platelet glycoprotein Ib-IX, and up-regulation of platelet surface protein GMP-140 also alter platelet aggregation.[75,108] Several studies in humans have shown increased blood loss during procedures normally associated with hemorrhage, even with small changes in body temperature (e.g., 30% greater loss with intraoperative temperature differences of <2° C).[134,166] Other studies in humans have not been able to repeat these findings, and there are no similar studies in dogs and cats.[69,121]

MONITORING FLUID THERAPY

Determining the best fluid regimen and judging the adequacy of therapy are dependent on monitoring the patient. Unfortunately, clinical signs are crude guides at best, and technology has not provided techniques to monitor all of the necessary information. Nevertheless, we can obtain a reasonable amount of information and integrate it into a picture that helps guide our therapy.

MONITORING CHANGES IN VOLUME

Methods for monitoring intravascular volume are not available in routine practice. Most of the techniques that have been used in the laboratory involve dye dilution and require sophisticated measuring techniques and calculations to determine intravascular volume. Even if such information was available, it is unlikely that absolute values for vascular volume would be of much use because it is unlikely that a normal volume measurement for the animal in question would be available before the procedure. However, trends over time may be helpful. Devices that measure changes in blood volume are available on sophisticated hemodialysis machines and provide a guide to therapy in situations in which blood volumes can change rapidly. In general, however, changes in blood volume must be inferred from clinical signs.

Loss of skin turgor is a helpful sign when present, but in many animals skin turgor changes little until volume depletion is severe.[72] Radiographic signs of hypovolemia include microcardia and a decrease in the size of the caudal vena cava and pulmonary vessels. CRT is used to monitor the microcirculation and, if prolonged, implies poor tissue perfusion. Poor tissue perfusion may be the result of hypovolemia, heart failure, vasoconstriction, or endotoxemia. This clinical sign has been examined carefully in humans and was found to be a poor predictor of volume status.[136] CRT is significantly affected by body temperature and ambient temperature.[9,65] CRT also can appear normal immediately after cardiac arrest. In dogs and cats, it is usual to use the mucous membranes of the mouth for testing capillary refill, and this technique may avoid some of the changes occurring in people as a result of alterations in ambient temperature because the temperature of the mouth remains relatively constant. The ability to assess CRT accurately is affected by the presence of pigment in the mucous membranes of some animals, making it impossible to obtain a result in these individuals.

Heart rate increases in response to hypovolemia but is a nonspecific sign. In anesthetized animals that develop unexplained tachycardia, the author often gives a fluid bolus to determine whether the animal is hypovolemic. A decreased heart rate after fluid infusion without resumption of tachycardia is indicative of preexisting hypovolemia.

Low CVP, PCWP, and systemic blood pressure all can imply low circulating volume but also can change for other reasons. The CVP and PCWP probably are better measurements of volume status because they are affected by cardiac preload, which is largely dependent on blood volume. In dogs and cats receiving IPPV and direct arterial pressure monitoring, systolic pressure may vary because of the effect of intrathoracic pressure changes on venous return. Although not totally predictable, significant decreases in systolic pressures associated with ventilation are indicative of hypovolemia (assuming ventilation pressure is 10 to 20 cm H_2O). In one study, the systolic pressure variation was approximately 6% with a 5% loss of blood volume and increased linearly to approximately 11% with 30% loss of blood volume.[118] Systolic pressure variation was much less in hypotension without hypovolemia.[122] The PCWP was a better predictor of responders to a fluid bolus than was the systolic pressure variation in one study in human cardiac patients.[11]

Cardiac output tends to decrease with hypovolemia, but this is a relatively nonspecific change because cardiac output also decreases with increased systemic vascular resistance or myocardial failure. Evaluation of cardiac output in conjunction with pressure measurements allows the clinician to interpret volume status more readily. Determination of cardiac output and PCWP can be carried out by placement of a thermistor and pressure port in the pulmonary artery and taking the measurements with sophisticated and expensive equipment. Placement of these catheters in small patients (<5 kg) is particularly difficult and makes it virtually impossible to obtain such readings in a clinical setting. A newer, simpler technique uses access to a vein and an artery with injection of lithium into a vein and withdrawal of blood from the artery while measuring lithium concentration (LiDCO, Cambridge, UK). This method can provide a limited number of cardiac output measurements in medium- to large-sized dogs. A method for providing continuous cardiac output measurements based on pulse contour analysis also has been developed, but clinical utility still is being evaluated (PulseCO, Cambridge, UK).

Urine output decreases with hypovolemia but also decreases with hypotension or low cardiac output. If urine output remains relatively normal, it is unlikely that the animal is hypovolemic. Measurement of urine volume requires time, and it is difficult to obtain accurate measurements at shorter time intervals than every hour. Consequently, measurement of urine volume cannot be used to monitor acute changes in circulating volume. The only available method for the measurement of urine output involves the insertion of a urinary catheter, and this involves some risk of introducing a urinary tract infection (UTI).[116,125,145,165] The risk of UTI with catheterization is greater in female dogs than in male dogs.[14] If monitoring urine output is necessary, a sterile urinary catheter should be inserted aseptically and immediately connected to a closed drainage system.[100] The reservoir of the urinary collection system should be maintained below the level of the patient. If the animal is being moved, it is best to clamp the drainage system so that urine cannot reflux up the tubing into the bladder. The urinary catheter should be left in the patient for the shortest duration possible because the risk of a UTI increases with every day the catheter is left in place. Ideally, the animal should not receive antibiotics while the catheter is in place (unless the UTI already has been diagnosed) because use of antibiotics increases the likelihood of antibiotic-resistant UTI. Withholding antibiotics may not be feasible in a surgical setting, and it is important to monitor for development of UTI using urinalysis and urine culture.

MONITORING CHANGES IN COMPOSITION

Blood samples must be obtained to monitor changes in the composition of the blood. The results of sodium, potassium, chloride, calcium, bicarbonate, pH, carbon dioxide tension (Pco_2), Po_2, osmolality, colloid oncotic pressure, hematocrit, protein, glucose, urea, and creatinine determinations may affect fluid therapy decisions. When a patient requires monitoring of the composition of blood, it is important to determine how blood samples are to be obtained intraoperatively. It often is difficult to obtain samples from peripheral venous catheters (particularly in small patients), and other sites must be used. Samples can be obtained from the jugular vein with relative ease, and a jugular catheter should be placed if several samples are likely to be required. If it is not necessary to measure CVP, a short intravenous catheter can be used (1.5 to 2 inches). Also useful in the anesthetized patient are the lingual veins. These vessels usually are readily accessible during anesthesia and can be sampled several times without the insertion of a catheter. All of these measurements can be obtained using such samples, but care must be taken with interpretation of Po_2. Single arterial samples can be obtained from the lingual, femoral, ulnar, auricular, or dorsal pedal arteries. If several samples will be required and it is advisable to know the Pao_2, an arterial catheter should be placed. In most dogs and cats, the most accessible vessel for this purpose is the dorsal pedal artery over the metatarsal area. If this vessel is inaccessible (e.g., bilateral tibial fractures) or cannot be catheterized, it is feasible to use the other vessels mentioned. If a femoral arterial catheter is placed, great care is needed because it is relatively easy for such catheters to pull out of the vessel while still attached to the skin. Unless a long stiff catheter has been placed in the femoral artery, it is not advisable to allow the animal to recover with the catheter still in place. The ulnar artery is difficult to catheterize because the shape of the limb makes it difficult to approach the site at a sufficiently narrow angle. The auricular arteries are useful in dogs with large ears (e.g., spaniels, dachshunds) and can be used in the postoperative period, although there is some risk of ischemia with prolonged catheterization. A catheter can be placed in the lingual artery after induction of anesthesia, but it must be removed before the end of surgery and the vessel held off for 15 minutes after the catheter has been removed to prevent the formation of a sublingual hematoma. Care must be taken when flushing auricular and lingual arterial catheters to prevent the injection of air because air could be introduced into the carotid arteries, resulting in air embolism of the cerebral arteries.

The electrocardiogram is used to presumptively identify changes in serum electrolyte concentrations. The electrocardiogram is useful in this regard because the magnitude of electrocardiographic changes is dependent both on the rate of change and on the actual serum concentration of electrolyte.

MONITORING CHANGES IN DISTRIBUTION

Dehydration is monitored using the clinical signs described earlier. The presence or absence of peripheral edema and ascites should be readily apparent. In some cases, it may be helpful to measure limb or abdominal circumference to determine whether the fluid accumulation is increasing or decreasing. Measuring the size of the abdomen is particularly difficult but still may be of use in individual patients. An indelible marker can be used to identify the site of measurement for future reference and thus improve accuracy. Pleural fluid accumulation can be monitored only by thoracic radiography or by draining the fluid on an intermittent or continuous basis.

ICP can be measured and can play a crucial role in the management of patients with increased ICP. The catheter is inserted into the cranial vault and attached to a measuring device. The simplest approach is to use a fluid-filled catheter, which can provide sensitive measurements of ICP and also allow measurement of intracranial compliance. The latter can be helpful because it can provide an estimate of the risk of brain herniation. A fiberoptic catheter that measures pressure indirectly can be inserted directly into the brain. The objective measurement of intraocular pressure with a Schiøtz or applanation tonometer may help guide fluid therapy in patients with high intraocular pressure.

INTRAOPERATIVE FLUID MANAGEMENT

Intraoperative fluid management depends on:
1. How well the patient has been prepared beforehand
2. How much fluid loss occurs normally (insensible loss)
3. How much fluid loss occurs because of the equipment used (e.g., dry gas causes greater water loss than humidified gas)
4. Changes in vascular tone and cardiac output
5. The amount and nature of the tissue exposed during surgery
6. The amount of blood lost

In most patients, crystalloid solutions are used first, and colloids and blood products are added as required.

CRYSTALLOIDS

The anesthetized animal has ongoing fluid losses of approximately $132 \times BW^{0.75}$ mL/day for the dog and $80 \times BW^{0.75}$ mL/day for the cat, where BW is body weight in kilograms. It is likely that losses will be less than predicted by these formulas because the metabolic rate of most anesthetized animals is less than in the awake resting state. A maintenance solution would be appropriate merely to replace this loss. However, it is expected that fluid losses will increase during anesthesia because of increased loss from the respiratory tract and that there will be changes in hemodynamics that will require fluid therapy (see section on Effects of Anesthesia). Consequently, it has been traditional to use isotonic replacement solutions during anesthesia and expect that the kidneys will excrete any excess sodium in the postoperative period. Replacement solutions do not contain high concentrations of potassium and can be given rapidly if necessary without risk of potassium toxicity.

The rate of administration often is set arbitrarily at 10 mL/kg/hr. This rate of administration is based on research in humans in the 1960s suggesting that this rate was appropriate for losses occurring during major abdominal surgery. The author has used this approach in many dogs and cats with few adverse effects. In the original studies, blood volume was measured using radioactive tracers.[138,160] These techniques are accurate in a steady state but may not be accurate when volumes are changing during fluid infusion. Later studies evaluated the dilution of hemoglobin or albumin or the change in blood water content to assess acute changes in blood volume.[71,144,149] Although these initial studies were performed in healthy human volunteers, they provide some useful information. In one study, infusions were carried out at different rates using two different volumes.[71] The interstitial fluid space is roughly twice the volume of the intravascular space, and isotonic replacement solutions redistribute, leaving approximately 33% of the infused volume in the vascular space. In this study, the volume retained in the vascular space 15 minutes after the end of the infusion was approximately 20%, and it was approximately 15% after 30 minutes, indicating rapid redistribution of crystalloid solutions. The volume of distribution for the balanced electrolyte solution was similar to the expected plasma volume but only 50% to 70% of the expected volume for the interstitial space. Regions of the interstitial space with poor blood supply or rigid structure (e.g., bone) may be less likely to take up fluid, and this may account for the difference in calculated volumes. Studies in sheep have examined the redistribution of 0.9% NaCl during isoflurane anesthesia, and the results showed a similar rate of redistribution away from the vascular space, but there was much greater retention in the interstitial space when compared with the awake animal.[34] This observation was accounted for by a dramatic reduction in urine output during isoflurane anesthesia. These data suggest that fluid may accumulate in the interstitium during anesthesia to the detriment of the patient.[123] Further work by this group in elderly trauma patients suggests that excretion of fluid also is decreased in the postoperative period.[150] Careful measurement of respiratory function in awake 59- to 67-year-old people showed some impairment of respiratory function when they were given 40 mL/kg LRS over 3 hours.[78]

The authors of these volume-kinetic studies proposed that their data could be used to calculate infusion rates that would expand the plasma compartment (bolus) and maintain it at this volume (infusion). To increase blood volume by 5%, the patient would receive 36 mL/kg/hr for 20 minutes and an ongoing infusion of 15 mL/kg/hr.[149] In another study, nomograms were presented for men and women showing the infusion rate and time required to achieve a specific blood volume expansion and the infusion rate required to maintain this expansion.[71] Whether these data apply to anesthetized animals is uncertain, but the results suggest that a fluid rate of 10 mL/kg/hr is relatively conservative.

In a study of healthy dogs undergoing elective ovariohysterectomy or castration, the rate of polyionic fluid administration was examined to determine how it affected hematocrit, total protein concentration, glucose concentration, and systolic blood pressure.[58] The authors tested an acetated polyionic solution given at 0, 5, 10, and 15 mL/kg/hr for 1 to 2 hours. They saw no differences among groups, suggesting that there was no advantage to fluid therapy for these cases. Cardiac output and renal function were not evaluated, and so it is not possible to say whether fluids affected these functions. Crystalloid fluid administration at 11 mL/kg/hr for 60 minutes to halothane-anesthetized cats did not result in any changes in packed cell volume or total protein concentration.[15] These cats had undergone thoracotomy for placement of catheters and did not start the study with normal values (packed cell volume = 25%, total proteins = 4.9 g/dL, colloid oncotic pressure = 10.2 mm Hg) and thus may be regarded as similar to compromised animals in a clinical situation.

Even after deciding that 10 mL/kg/hr of an isotonic fluid is a good starting point for intraoperative fluid therapy, a decision still must be made about which solution to use. Common crystalloids available include normal saline (0.9% NaCl), a lactated polyionic fluid (LRS), an acetated polyionic fluid (e.g., acetated Ringer's solution, Normosol-R, Plasma-Lyte 148, Isolyte S, Polyionic R), or 5% dextrose in water, saline, or polyionic solutions.

NORMAL SALINE

Normal saline is used widely as a replacement solution intraoperatively. It is the solution of choice for patients with hypercalcemia or hypochloremic alkalosis. This solution contains higher amounts of chloride than plasma and tends to decrease the strong ion difference, leading to acidosis. In classical terms, it dilutes the concentration of bicarbonate and provides large amounts of chloride for reabsorption from the glomerular filtrate, thus leading to hyperchloremic acidosis. The degree of acidosis is not likely to be a problem in the healthy patient but may exacerbate acidosis in a compromised patient.

LACTATED RINGER'S SOLUTION (HARTMANN'S SOLUTION)

LRS is a balanced electrolyte solution containing lactate that contributes to the correction of acidosis and is the author's fluid of choice for most anesthetized patients. Potential disadvantages of this solution are as follows:

1. It contains calcium, and because blood products generally are stored using a compound that chelates calcium, it is not ideal to administer LRS through the same intravenous line as blood products. A 1:10 mixture of blood and LRS resulted in clot formation within 2 minutes at 37° C (see Table 17-1).[132]

2. It contains less sodium than plasma, which could lead to greater loss of fluid into the intracellular compartment, which in turn may be detrimental in patients with cerebral edema. In models of traumatic brain injury, infusion of LRS was associated with an increase in ICP.[124,169] In a model of closed-head trauma in rats, use of LRS did not affect neurologic outcome or formation of brain edema.[51]

3. It contains lactate, which mostly is metabolized in the liver (~56% of normal lactate metabolism occurs in the liver). In some LRS, the lactate is in the form of L-lactate (e.g., the lactate in Baxter's product is derived from fermentation), whereas in others, a racemic mixture with equal amounts of the D- and L-lactate is used (e.g., the lactate in Hospira's product is derived from chemical production of lactate). The L-form is more readily metabolized than is the D-form.[73] It is stated on the bag of LRS that it should not be used in patients with a lactic acidosis, but infusion of LRS was not associated with an increase in blood lactate concentrations even when there was considerable impairment of hepatic function.[43,62] However, hepatic removal of lactate is a saturable process, and infusion of lactate in patients with severe hyperlactatemia (>9 mmol/L) may result in an increase in blood lactate concentration.[113] However, at concentrations of lactate greater than 9 mmol/L, the peripheral tissues remove more lactate than the liver, and peripheral metabolism of lactate is not saturable.[113] In clinical patients with initial lactate concentrations greater than 10 mmol/L, infusion of LRS and other volume support was always associated with a decrease in blood lactate concen-

trations.[27] Some patients with cancer may be hyperlactatemic and have increased ability to recycle lactate to glucose.[164] In some patients with cancer cachexia, concern has been expressed that the metabolism of lactate consumes energy and thus lactated solutions should not be used. It has been shown that dogs with lymphoma have a transient inability to cope with the lactate load imposed by infusion of LRS.[157] Although this finding may be valid in unusual cases, the amount of lactate provided with LRS at 10 mL/kg/hr is approximately 36% of the basal production or utilization rate, and it is likely that any negative effect is transient.[2]

The metabolism of lactate is either by gluconeogenesis or by oxidation, and hydrogen ions are consumed in both instances. It takes approximately 30 minutes for this alkalinizing effect to be accomplished.[73] The alkalinizing effect is not as great as that seen with acetate (~50%).

ACETATED POLYIONIC SOLUTIONS

It is thought that acetate is metabolized rapidly throughout the body, and the alkalinizing effect of this solution is more readily available. As with lactate, the effect takes approximately 30 minutes to be evident.[73] In some commercial solutions, gluconate also is used. There is little information on the effects of gluconate, but it does appear to cause a slight increase in pH.[91] Acetated Ringer's solution suffers from the same disadvantage as LRS in terms of its sodium content. Many of the commercial solutions are calcium free and can be given through the same line as blood products. The main disadvantage of solutions containing acetate is the vasodilatation that can occur with rapid administration.[66,81] In a normal healthy patient, a bolus of acetated polyionic solution usually results in an increase in heart rate but little change in blood pressure, but in a patient that is already hypovolemic, dramatic decreases in blood pressure can be seen (Fig. 17-2).[133] Acetate-containing solutions also are contraindicated in patients with diabetic ketoacidosis because they tend to increase blood ketone concentrations.[3]

5% DEXTROSE

Five percent dextrose in water contains no electrolytes, and only water remains when the dextrose is metabolized. Five percent dextrose may be the solution of choice for patients that have suffered from pure water loss, but it is rarely indicated as the prime replacement solution during anesthesia and surgery. Apart from the fact that the volume of distribution of the 5% dextrose is likely to be larger than that of a balanced electrolyte solution (which would result in a diminished ability to maintain circulating volume), the glucose itself may be detrimental in certain circumstances.[127] In both acute renal and acute cerebral injury, high concentrations of

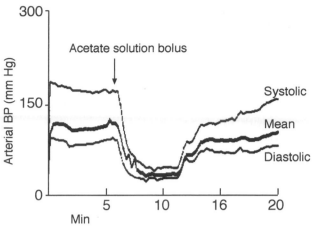

Fig. 17-2 Administration of an acetated solution (Plasma-Lyte 148) to a 16-kg dog being anesthetized for cataract surgery. The 50-mL bolus was given before the start of surgery. Hypotension occurred, and the dog was given 0.5 μg/kg of epinephrine intravenously when the mean pressure had leveled off at 33 mm Hg (~10 minutes).

glucose may be detrimental.[96,103,112] Concentrations of glucose more than 200 mg/dL may be of concern in animals with cerebral ischemia.[96,103]

2.5% Dextrose in Half-Strength Ionic Solution

Dextrose (5%) can be mixed with any of the preceding ionic solutions in a 1:1 ratio to halve the ionic strength. Such solutions may be of use in the management of patients with hypernatremia. These solutions are designed to increase the free-water content of the body, and it is important to monitor electrolyte concentrations to ensure that excessive dilution does not occur.

Hypertonic Solutions

These solutions may provide rapid resuscitation in the preoperative period but are seldom used intraoperatively. They may be needed in special circumstances such as for an animal with rapid hemorrhage when blood products are unavailable, an animal with a high ICP, or a patient with hyponatremia. Most of these solutions have very high sodium concentrations, and it is important to monitor serum sodium concentrations before and after their administration. Maintenance with an isotonic crystalloid usually is required after administration of these solutions. See Chapter 25 for more information about hypertonic solutions.

COLLOIDS

Dextrans, HES, polygelatins, and plasma are the main colloid solutions available. They are used to correct hypovolemia, provide colloid oncotic pressure, and, in

the case of fresh frozen plasma, provide clotting factors. The synthetic colloids are polydisperse colloids that, by definition, contain particles of several different molecular weights. In the past, the average molecular weight (M_w) of such solutions was described, but this approach favors the high molecular weight particles. It now is common to describe the solution according to the number molecular weight (M_n), which is the total weight of all the molecules divided by the number of molecules. In the case of dextran 70, the M_w is 70,000, but the M_n is 41,000 (Table 17-2). Use of M_n allows recognition of the smaller molecular weight particles in the solution. The terms have clinical significance because the oncotic pressure exerted by the solution depends on the number of particles present, whereas the duration of effect depends on the size of the particles present. The duration of effect of a colloid is short if the particles rapidly leak through the endothelium.

Dextrans

The dextran molecule is a linear polysaccharide produced by certain strains of *Leuconostoc* bacteria growing in sucrose-containing media. Dextrans are supplied in low and high molecular weight forms (dextran 40 and 70, respectively) with plasma half-lives estimated at 1 to 3 and 2 to 6 hours.[154] In dogs with normal renal function, 70% of a dose of dextran 40 and 40% of a dose of dextran 70 are excreted unchanged in the urine within 24 hours. The remaining molecules are metabolized slowly to glucose by dextranase in the liver. Some of these molecules may be present in the body weeks after their administration. The plasma volume expansion achieved per gram of dextran is roughly the same, regardless of molecular weight (~20 to 25 mL water/g dextran).[77] Clinically, however, dextran 40 has a greater concentration per milliliter and provides greater plasma volume expansion initially.

Concerns about the use of dextrans include effects on hemostasis and allergic reactions. Dextrans tend to prolong bleeding times by interfering with fibrin clot formation, reducing factor VIII and von Willebrand's factor, diluting clotting factors, and interfering with platelet function. In dogs, rapid infusion of dextran 70 caused a decrease in von Willebrand's factor antigen and factor VIII activity and increases in APTT and buccal mucosal bleeding time.[33,61] Dextrans and HES also alter the structure of the fibrin clot, giving it a weaker, more chaotic appearance.[63] These effects suggest that dextrans may not be the best choice for fluid therapy when major surgery is planned. Clinically, it seems that infusions of dextrans have been associated with increased bleeding, but no studies have documented increased blood loss when dextrans have been used. Allergic reactions have been reported in human patients, but the frequency appears to be less than 0.1%, and such reactions have not been reported in dogs or cats.

TABLE 17-2 Physicochemical Properties of the Artificial Colloids

Colloid	M$_w$ (kDa)	M$_n$ (kDa)	Colloid (g/L)	pH	Relative Viscosity	Na (mmol/L)	Cl (mmol/L)	Ca (mmol/L)	K (mmol/L)	Osmolality (mOsm/L)	Colloid Oncotic Pressure (mm Hg)
Dextran 40, NaCl	40	26	100	3.5-7	5.1-5.4	154	154	0	0	310	NM*
Dextran 40, dextrose	40	26	100	3-7		0	0	0	0	255	NM*
Dextran 70, NaCl	70	41	60	5.1-5.7	3.4-4	154	154	0	0	310	59*
Oxypolygelatin (Vetaplasma, Gelifundol)	30	23.3	55			145	100	2	0	200	45-47
Succinylated gelatin (Gelofusine)	35	22.6	40	7.4		154	125	0.4	0.4	279	34
Urea-linked gelatin (Haemaccel)	35	24.5	35	7.2-7.3	1.7-1.8	145	145	6.26	5.1	310	NM* 25.5-28.5†

NM, Not measurable because of diffusion of smaller molecules.
*Data from Tønnessen T, Tollofsrud S, Kongsgaard UE, et al: Colloid osmotic pressure of plasma replacement fluids, Acta Anaesthesiol Scand 37:424-426, 1993.
†Data from Evans PA, Garnett M, Boffard K, et al: Evaluation of the effect of colloid (Haemaccel) on the bleeding time in the trauma patient, J R Soc Med 89:101P-104P, 1996.

In humans, dextran 40 has been used to reduce the occurrence of deep vein thrombosis. It is thought that this effect is caused by decreased viscosity of blood after dextran administration. There also is some evidence that low molecular weight dextrans alter red cell aggregation and decrease clumping of red cells in the microcirculation. Use of dextran 70 also reduced the frequency of fatal postoperative pulmonary embolism from 2.0% to 0.35%. In these studies, dextrans were given on the day of surgery. The only common conditions in dogs and cats complicated by pulmonary thromboembolism are hyperadrenocorticism and the nephrotic syndrome, and the use of dextrans has not been investigated in these settings in veterinary medicine.

A number of reports have linked dextrans to renal failure. This complication has been attributed to increased viscosity of the glomerular filtrate associated with early excretion of low molecular weight particles.[95,171] Experimental studies in dogs identified changes in proximal tubular cells but no effect on renal function. Affected human patients have received large doses of dextrans and have had an associated increase in oncotic pressure. Treatment by exchange transfusion to lower oncotic pressure has been successful, suggesting that the renal changes are not structural but functional.[162,171] There are no reports of renal failure after dextran administration in dogs or cats.

HETASTARCH

HES is a synthetic polymer of glucose (amylopectin) that closely resembles glycogen and contains predominantly α-1,4 linkages. Starch normally is metabolized by amylases, and by adding hydroxyethyl groups to positions 2, 3, or 6 on the glucose molecules, the rate of metabolism can be reduced. Metabolic breakdown is slower with increased substitution and a higher ratio of C2:C6 substitution. This understanding has led to development of different molecules that are described by their molecular weight, the proportion of substitution, and their C2:C6 ratio (Table 17-3).[45] In the literature, the molecular weight and substitution ratio usually are used to define the product. For example, HES 200/0.5 represents HES with an average molecular weight of 200 kDa and a molar substitution ratio of 5 hydroxyethyl groups per 10 molecules of glucose. It would be preferable to include the C2:C6 ratio of the molecule because HES 200/0.5 with a substitution ratio of 13.4:1 behaved very differently than HES 200/0.5 with a C2:C6 substitution ratio of 5.7:1.[155] The original commercially available preparation of HES has an average molecular weight (M_w) of 450 kDa with a number molecular weight (M_n) of 69 kDa. This solution was made up in normal saline. A newer high molecular weight HES (Hextend, BioTime, Inc., Emeryville, CA) is made up in a balanced electrolyte solution so that infusion is less likely to be associated with hyperchloremic acidosis, and the presence of calcium may reduce the occurrence of clotting abnormalities. The newer HESs have even lower molecular weights, and HES 130/0.4 (Voluven, Fresenius Kabi Austria GmbH, Graz, Austria) is thought to have close to ideal properties because it does not remain in plasma as long as bulkier molecules, but it also does not interfere with coagulation as much. In any of these solutions, the smaller molecules (molecular weight, <59 kDa) are excreted by the kidneys or pass through the vascular endothelium into the interstitial space. Molecules that reach the interstitial space are taken up by macrophages and slowly metabolized by cellular lysozymes. The larger molecules are slowly broken down by α-amylases. Dogs have approximately three times as much amylase as do humans, and HES 450/0.7 is broken down faster. In dogs, 31.5% of administered HES was excreted in the urine, and 38% remained in plasma after 24 hours.[154] The half-life of HES 450/0.7 in humans varies with time after administration and dose (e.g., the half-life is 1.5 to 3.6 days during the first 3 days after administration and 13 to 17 days between 7 and 42 days after administration). After three consecutive daily doses, the excretion of 41% to 46% of this HES took 168 hours compared with 48 hours after a single dose. This dependence on time and dose has not been demonstrated in dogs.[142] In hypoalbuminemic dogs, the administration of HES 450/0.7 was associated with an increase in colloid oncotic pressure and a reduction in peripheral edema in most treated patients. There was no apparent correlation between the dose of HES 450/0.7 or the change in colloid oncotic pressure and resolution of edema. A few dogs showed prolongation of APTT and a decrease in platelet numbers, but it was unclear whether this effect was caused by the HES treatment. Some dogs with abnormal hemostasis before treatment actually became normal after treatment.[143] In another trial using HES in 30 hypoalbuminemic dogs, there was an increase in colloid oncotic pressure with the administration of 7.7 to 43.9 mL/kg, but this effect lasted less than 12 hours. It was suggested that maintenance of colloid oncotic pressure would require additional HES or administration of other colloids.[110]

As with dextrans, there has been concern about the effect of HES on coagulation.[148] In early experiments in dogs, infusion of 10 mL/kg was not associated with increased blood loss or any change in bleeding time. With infusions of 20 to 30 mL/kg, however, bleeding time and quantity of blood lost increased. These effects were more pronounced with dextrans than with HES 450/0.7.[89] Factor VIII complex consistently is decreased after HES 450/0.7 administration, and it is advised that HES 450/0.7 not be given to dogs with known or suspected von Willebrand's disease.[142] In a study in which very large doses (110 to 120 mL/kg) of HES 450/0.7 were used, prolonged bleeding times were identified. Platelets appeared swollen and shiny

TABLE 17-3 Physicochemical Properties of Hetastarch Solutions

Colloid	M$_w$ (kDa)	M$_n$ (kDa)	Molar Substitution	C2:C6 Ratio	Colloid (g/L)	pH	Na (mmol/L)	Cl (mmol/L)	Ca (mmol/L)	K (mmol/L)	Lactate (mmol/L)	Osmolality (mOsm/L)	Colloid Oncotic Pressure (mm Hg)
Hetastarch 670 (Hextend)	670		0.75	4-5:1	60	5.9	143	124	5	3	28*	307	31.3 ± 0.6†
Hetastarch 450	450	69	0.7	4.6:1	60	5.5	154	154	0	0	0	310	29-32‡
Hetastarch 264 (Pentaspan)	264	63	0.45		100	5	154	154	0	0	0	326	
Hetastarch (Pentalyte)	264	63	0.45		60		143	124	5	3	28*		32.2 ± 1†
Hetastarch 200 (Expahes)	200		0.5	5:1	100	4-7	154	154	0	0	0	300	65
Hetastarch 200 (haes-steril)	240		0.4-0.55	5:1	60 or 100	3.5-6	154	154	0	0	0	308	
Hetastarch 200 (Elohäst)	200		0.6-0.66	5:1	100	4-7	154	154	0	0	0	308	25
Hetastarch 130 (Voluven)	130		0.4	9:1	60	4-5.5	154	154	0	0	0	308	
Hetastarch 70 (Expafusion)	70		0.5	4:1	60	6	138	125	1.5	4	20	290	

*Hextend and Pentalyte also contain 0.45 mmol/L of magnesium and 99 mg/dL of dextrose.

†Data from Nielsen VG, Baird MS, Brix AE, et al: Extreme, progressive isovolemic hemodilution with 5% human albumin, PentaLyte, or Hextend does not cause hepatic ischemia or histologic injury in rabbits, Anesthesiology 90:1428-1435, 1999.

‡Data from Tonnessen T, Tollofsrud S, Kongsgaard UE, et al: Colloid osmotic pressure of plasma replacement fluids, Acta Anaesthesiol Scand 37:424-426, 1993.

and had decreased adhesion.[102] Clots were friable and had weak tensile strength. These effects were presumably caused by more than just hemodilution, and these findings should be borne in mind when using HES 450/0.7 at the time of surgery. Studies in humans undergoing surgery have not documented any increase in blood loss associated with the administration of HES 450/0.7.[12,161] The lower molecular weight HESs are associated with fewer alterations in coagulation. HES 130/0.4 causes fewer effects on coagulation than HES 200/0.5 and may reduce the need for blood transfusions in human orthopedic patients.[98] The author has not seen increased bleeding tendency in dogs given HES 450/0.7, but the dosage used has not exceeded 20 mL/kg.

Other concerns with HESs are their effects on renal and hepatic function. Renal function appears to be minimally affected if it was normal initially, but septic patients may be at increased risk for renal injury after HES administration.[135] Hepatic failure has been noted in some human patients who have had repeated infusions of high molecular weight HES, but such usage does not appear to be a major risk factor in the perioperative period in veterinary patients.[31] Serum amylase concentrations are expected to increase after the use of HES. Pruritus is another consequence of HES infusion and appears to be related to dose rather than HES type. If pruritus occurs, it can be of major concern to the patient and is refractory to treatment.[10]

HES may be beneficial to the patient by reducing the inflammatory response to surgery. In human patients undergoing abdominal surgery, concentrations of interleukin-6 and -8 and intercellular adhesion molecule-1 were lower when HES 130/0.4 was used for intravascular volume replacement instead of LRS.[97] The effect on adhesion molecules also may alter the capillary leak that can occur in trauma and sepsis. The idea that HES may protect against vascular leakage is supported by a study showing that HES 200/0.5 did not appear in cerebrospinal fluid in patients with an impaired blood-brain barrier.[45]

HES administration increases plasma volume by 71% to 172% of the administered volume and generally increases plasma volume by at least the volume administered.[142] The degree of expansion depends largely on the concentration of HES. Greater blood volume expansion (e.g., 130%) is seen with 10% as compared with 6% solutions. In this regard, HES is about equivalent to dextran 70 but has a slightly longer duration of action. In one study in dogs, 25 mL/kg of dextran 70 or HES 450/0.7 gave an almost identical increase in plasma volume compared with the volume infused (~140%), but at 12 hours the dextran effect had decreased to 18%, whereas the HES effect had decreased to 38%. By 24 hours, the dextran effect had further decreased to 1%, whereas HES still caused a 16% increase in plasma volume compared

with the volume infused.[154] The incidence of anaphylactoid reactions with HES use in people is similar to that recorded for dextrans. Whereas antibodies to dextrans have been found in humans, no antibodies to HES have been found in dogs, cats, or humans even after chronic use. The frequency of life-threatening reactions appears to be lower for HES than for other colloids.[142] No anaphylactoid reactions to HES have been reported in dogs or cats.

GELATIN SOLUTIONS

Gelatin solutions are prepared by degradation of bovine collagen and come in several forms. The process involves exposure of the raw material to hydrochloric acid for several days, to saturated calcium hydroxide for several weeks, and finally to a temperature of at least 138° C. The three currently used preparations are oxypolygelatin (Vetaplasma/Geloplasma, Institut Merieux Benelux, Brussels, Belgium), succinylated gelatin (Gelofusine, B Braun Medical, Bethlehem, PA), and urea-linked gelatin (Haemaccel, Intervet, Milton Keynes, UK). Oxypolygelatin was available in the United States, and the other two forms have been used extensively in Europe. The main advantages of these solutions are that they have lower molecular weights than the other colloids (and hence are excreted rapidly), they appear to be minimally antigenic, and they have minimal effects on coagulation.[105] In one report, the use of more than 79,000 units of succinylated gelatin in humans was summarized.[105] The infusion of a solution of succinylated gelatin was associated with an increase in plasma volume equal to or approximately 10% less than the volume infused; hence there is little risk of volume overload. Of the infused volume, approximately 50% was present in the circulation after 4 to 5 hours, although it has been stated that the plasma half-life is approximately 8 hours.[105] The plasma half-life of oxypolygelatin is 2 to 4 hours. The majority of the gelatin is excreted by the kidneys, with 71% of the urea-linked gelatin and 62% of the succinylated gelatin being found in the urine in people within 24 hours. In chimpanzees, 66% of a dose of oxypolygelatin was found in the urine within 24 hours. Mechanisms for the metabolism of the remaining molecules are not well defined, but it is thought that they are metabolized by proteolytic enzymes in the liver with some of the end products being excreted in the feces (~15% of the total dose).[105]

Anaphylactoid reactions to gelatin solutions are rare. It is uncertain whether these reactions represent an immunologic response or are caused by histamine release. An overall incidence of allergic reactions to gelatins was reported to be 0.115%, with the highest incidence reported for oxypolygelatin (0.617%).[126] In this report, it was also noted that the severity of the reactions was greater with the gelatins than with other colloids (0.038% versus 0.008% for dextrans and 0.006% for HES). In a study of the release of histamine associated with use of urea-linked gelatin in anesthetized patients, a 26% incidence of histamine release was reported with 4 of 57 patients exhibiting life-threatening signs.[104] Patients with malignant disease were twice as likely to release histamine and were seven times more likely to have a life-threatening episode. Pretreatment of patients with histamine blockers (H_1 and H_2) reduced the incidence of clinical signs to 0%.[104] The gelatin solution (500 mL) in this study was given over 20 minutes (~20 to 25 mL/kg/hr), and it has been recommended that these solutions be administered slowly.

In the early reports of gelatin infusion, minimal effects on coagulation were identified.[105] However, subsequent studies showed that the effects are somewhat similar to those observed with other colloids but of lesser magnitude. An increase in bleeding time was recorded in healthy people and in trauma victims and was attributed to a decrease in von Willebrand's factor activity.[41,49] In studies using thromboelastography to measure the dynamics of clot formation, dilution with gelatins resulted in more rapid onset of clot formation, more rapid strengthening of the clot, and some decrease in the maximal strength obtained.[48,111] In both of these studies, gelatin was compared with hydroxyethyl starch, and the latter induced greater changes than did the gelatin solution. In one study, 50% dilution with dextran 40 prolonged most coagulation parameters to such an extent as to be unmeasurable.[111] In a clinical study examining the use of gelatin as a priming solution before cardiopulmonary bypass, ristocetin-induced platelet agglutination was significantly impaired, and this effect was not corrected by the use of aprotinin as compared with the control group (albumin prime).[151] There also was a direct correlation between postoperative blood loss and the amount of gelatin used during the operation with the greatest blood loss occurring in patients receiving more than 3.5 L of gelatin (~45 mL/kg).[151] In another study evaluating human patients undergoing orthopedic surgery, no major differences were noted between patients receiving similar volumes of 6% HES or 3% gelatin (<33 mL/kg/day) for colloid replacement.[12] Despite these findings, gelatin infusions often are given rapidly to veterinary patients before or during surgery with little evidence of adverse effects on coagulation or histamine release.

PLASMA PROTEIN

Plasma protein is available either as a fresh or frozen preparation or as liquid or frozen plasma that has been harvested during the collection and storage of blood. Fresh plasma may be prepared so that it contains platelets (platelet-rich plasma) and clotting factors. It must be used within 4 hours of preparation because of the risk of bacterial contamination at the recommended room temperature storage. Fresh frozen plasma contains clotting factors, which are destroyed if the unit has been thawed for more than 8 hours, but contains no platelets.

Fresh frozen plasma can be used in any situation in which blood volume must be expanded, hematocrit is within an acceptable range, and no allergic reaction to foreign protein is anticipated. If there is no major concern about dilution of existing clotting factors, the stored form of the plasma can be used. The infusion of plasma tends to increase colloid oncotic pressure and increase both serum albumin and globulin concentrations. The main concerns about the use of plasma intraoperatively are cost and the potential for allergic reactions. Commercially, plasma is more expensive than any of the other colloids, but its use is justified in animals with marginal coagulation (e.g., use of fresh frozen plasma in a patient with low plasma protein concentration related to hepatic dysfunction) or in surgical cases in which there is concern about dilutional coagulopathy. Life-threatening allergic reactions to plasma infusions are not common, but urticaria may be observed. The author has not seen any episodes of profound hypotension associated with plasma infusions but has seen considerable swelling of the head and limbs develop. If such a reaction occurs, the plasma infusion should be stopped immediately and the animal treated with antihistamines (H_1 and H_2 blockers). Corticosteroids also may be administered if warranted by the severity of the reaction. This type of therapy rarely reverses the clinical signs but may prevent exacerbation of the condition. A note should be made in the patient's medical record to ensure that it does not receive infusions of plasma products in the future. In dogs and cats with portosystemic shunts, there is concern about the ammonia content of stored plasma because it tends to increase with time. Clinical signs of encephalopathy in these patients are related in part to blood ammonia concentration, and it is advisable not to burden them with an additional source of ammonia.

PACKED RED BLOOD CELLS

Packed red cells are used primarily in patients with low hematocrits before surgery or in patients that are likely to have low tolerance for a decreased hematocrit that develops during surgery (e.g., a patient with minimal cardiovascular reserve). It is advisable to crossmatch both dogs and cats before transfusion. Crossmatching requires some time, and it is important to plan for the use of packed red cells by having the crossmatch results available before the animal requires transfusion. The indications for packed red cells are given in the earlier section on Anemia. Administration of packed red cells can be difficult because of the viscosity of the solution and can be facilitated by diluting the cells with warm normal saline, by using adult rather than pediatric administration sets, and by using the largest venous access possible (ideally >20 gauge). Smaller needles (<20 gauge) tend to impede the flow of the blood and may lead to hemolysis if external pressure is applied for the administration.

WHOLE BLOOD

Ideally, whole blood is used when the animal needs all of the components present in whole blood. Practically, whole blood often is used because it is more convenient than individual component therapy. Fresh whole blood contains all of the normal clotting factors and active platelets. Clotting factors and platelets deteriorate within the first 24 hours, and stored whole blood is ineffective at restoring normal coagulation. Whole blood typically is used in patients that are bleeding actively or have already lost a large volume of blood and are likely to become severely hemodiluted if other fluids are used. Some concern has been expressed about the effect of blood transfusion on immune function. A beneficial effect was first noticed in renal transplant patients. Patients who had received blood transfusions in association with renal transplantation were less likely to reject the grafted organ.[115] Additional studies in human patients showed an increased frequency of infections in patients receiving allogeneic blood transfusions.[46] These included wound infections, UTIs, and respiratory tract infections, and the frequency of infection increased with the number of units of blood received.[93,153] Patients receiving their own blood did not have such an increase in infection rate, and studies have focused on reducing the white cell count in transfused blood to determine whether this will alter the infection rate.[16] This approach seems to have met with success, but further analysis is required before its efficacy is understood.[79] Another effect of immunosuppression caused by blood transfusions is its effect on cancer development. In several animal models, allogeneic infusions have been associated with increased tumor growth, but the results of studies in humans are not clear.[16,54,131] Leukocyte removal before transfusion may reduce the effect on cancer growth.[16] Leukoreduction has been used in collecting blood from dogs, but this procedure has not been reported with regard to its effect on cancer recurrence.[24]

Another concern with the administration of blood products is that citrate present in stored blood will decrease the availability of calcium in the recipient. In normal humans, the amount of citrate found in one unit of blood (~32 mg/kg) can be metabolized in 3 to 5 minutes without the person developing hypocalcemia. However, the rate of metabolism of citrate decreases with decreased hepatic perfusion (e.g., shock), decreased hepatic function, and hypothermia. In these settings, plasma citrate concentration may increase rapidly. This effect is of concern mainly when blood is given rapidly (>30 mL/kg/hr), and calcium salts may be given when rapid transfusion of blood or plasma is required.[1] Calcium must be given through a separate intravenous line because it may cause the transfused blood to clot in the line if it is given concurrently. Calcium chloride should be given at a dosage of 5 to 10 mg/kg and calcium gluconate at 18 to 35 mg/kg for an equivalent effect.[36] The patient is less likely to have a hypotensive response if calcium can be given before or during the rapid administration of citrate-containing blood products.[37] If serum ionized calcium concentration can be measured, sufficient calcium should be given to return the ionized calcium concentration to normal, but the animal should be treated only if serum ionized calcium concentration is decreased. If blood is not being given rapidly or is not needed on a continuous basis, it rarely is necessary to administer calcium because the serum calcium concentration will be corrected rapidly by the animal as a result of changes in parathyroid hormone concentration and by mobilization of calcium stores in the body.[1,141]

Stored blood usually is kept at 4° C and is more likely to cause arrhythmias and decreased cardiac output if administered without being warmed first. A 250-mL unit of blood at 4° C requires 7.2 kcal of heat to warm it to 38° C. Stated differently, an infusion of 25 to 30 mL/kg of blood at 4° C can decrease body temperature by as much as 1° C. Given these facts, it is best if blood can be warmed before it is given. This can be achieved by placing the blood in warm water (up to 42° C but no higher) before infusion or by running the blood through a warming device as it is being infused. Warming can be as simple as running the line through a container of warm water or as sophisticated as using a device specifically designed to heat blood safely as it is being infused. The effectiveness of these techniques depends on the length of line exposed to the heat and the rate of infusion. Most of the commercial devices that are designed for this purpose require the addition of an extra length of line that conforms to the heating device. Such devices further increase the cost of blood or blood component therapy.

HEMOGLOBIN SOLUTIONS

Various hemoglobin solutions have been tested over the years, but only one has been licensed for veterinary use.[40] Oxyglobin (Biopure Corporation, Cambridge, MA) is an ultrapure glutaraldehyde polymerized hemoglobin of bovine origin made up in a modified LRS. This hemoglobin solution has a P50 (oxygen tension at 50% saturation) of 35 mm Hg, a molecular weight of 64 to 500 kDa, and a colloid oncotic pressure of approximately 20 mm Hg.[117] It comes as a purple-colored solution and contains 13 mg/dL of hemoglobin. The solution may be stored at room temperature and has a shelf life of 24 months. This latter feature makes it an attractive product for veterinarians who use canine or feline blood infrequently and who do not have access to blood donors of known status. When given to a patient, it acts as a colloidal solution but has the added advantage of providing oxygen-carrying capacity. It can be given intraoperatively in any situation in which blood would normally be used except in circumstances requiring clotting factors or platelets. Administration leads to jaundice and hematuria in many patients, and interference with a number of biochemical tests (e.g., sodium, potassium, chloride, blood urea) may occur.[26] Monitoring the patient by use of pulse oximetry reflects changes in arterial hemoglobin saturation, but measurement of hematocrit alone no longer provides an accurate indication of hemoglobin content.[80] Measurement of total protein concentration using a refractometer also will be affected because of the presence of free hemoglobin. The recommended rate of administration for Oxyglobin is 10 mL/kg/hr in dogs and 5 mL/kg/hr in cats, but boluses of 1 to 2 mL/kg may be used in animals suffering from acute hypovolemia. Special care needs to be taken when giving Oxyglobin to cats because pulmonary edema has been reported in a number of cats and is probably related to acute circulatory overload.[60] Some degree of systemic vasoconstriction may occur with Oxyglobin administration because of the scavenging effect of free hemoglobin on nitric oxide. This effect may be of benefit in some severely hypotensive and hypovolemic patients in which an immediate increase in blood pressure would be desirable. Oxyglobin also would be very useful in an animal that fails to crossmatch to existing donors and yet needs increased oxygen-carrying capacity intraoperatively.[39] Experimentally, it has been shown that Oxyglobin results in a more rapid increase in muscle tissue oxygenation than occurs with the infusion of a similar dose of stored packed cells.[146] This observation suggests that animals with severe shock, anemia, or ischemia may benefit from an infusion of Oxyglobin as an initial treatment that could then be followed by more Oxyglobin or the use of blood products.

POSTOPERATIVE FLUID MANAGEMENT

The patient will continue to lose fluids over time and may have decreased food and water intake after surgery. Consequently, it is essential to consider fluid therapy in the postoperative period. The choice of fluid is governed by factors similar to those used before and during surgery. A main factor to consider is when the animal is likely to be able to regulate its own fluid balance. With minor surgical procedures, this may be almost immediately after surgery, but with procedures in which recovery is slow or oral intake is contraindicated, it is necessary to continue fluid therapy. Continuing fluid therapy may be particularly important in geriatric patients because they often are unwilling to drink in the hospital environment and may be at greater risk because of marginal renal function.

REFERENCES

1. Abbott TR: Changes in serum calcium fractions and citrate concentrations during massive blood transfusions and cardiopulmonary bypass, *Br J Anaesth* 55:753-759, 1983.
2. Adrogue HJ, Tannen RL: Ketoacidosis, hyperosmolar states, and lactic acidosis. In Kokko JP, Tannen RL, editors: *Fluids and electrolytes*, ed 3, Philadelphia, 1996, WB Saunders, pp. 643-674.
3. Akanji AO, Sacks S: Effect of acetate on blood metabolites and glucose tolerance during haemodialysis in uraemic non-diabetic and diabetic subjects, *Nephron* 57:137-143, 1991.
4. Allard RL, Carlos AD, Faltin EC: Canine hematological changes during gestation and lactation, *Comp Anim Pract* 19:3-6, 1989.
5. Allon M, Copkney C: Albuterol and insulin for treatment of hyperkalemia in hemodialysis patients, *Kidney Int* 38:869-872, 1990.
6. Anand IS, Ferrari R, Kalra GS, et al: Edema of cardiac origin. Studies of body water and sodium, renal function, hemodynamic indexes, and plasma hormones in untreated congestive cardiac failure, *Circulation* 80:299-305, 1989.
7. Asao Y, Hirasaki A, Matsushita M, et al: A patient who recovered successfully from severe anemia which continued for one hour, *Masui* 46:700-703, 1997.
8. Baer RW, Vlahakes GJ, Uhlig PN, et al: Maximum myocardial oxygen transport during anemia and polycythemia in dogs, *Am J Physiol* 252:H1086-H1095, 1987.
9. Baraff LJ: Capillary refill: is it a useful clinical sign? *Pediatrics* 92:723-724, 1993.
10. Barron ME, Wilkes MM, Navickis RJ: A systematic review of the comparative safety of colloids, *Arch Surg* 139:552-563, 2004.
11. Bennett-Guerrero E, Kahn RA, Moskowitz DM, et al: Comparison of arterial systolic pressure variation with other clinical parameters to predict the response to fluid challenges during cardiac surgery, *Mt Sinai J Med* 69:96-100, 2002.
12. Beyer R, Harmening U, Rittmeyer O, et al: Use of modified fluid gelatin and hydroxyethyl starch for colloidal volume replacement in major orthopaedic surgery, *Br J Anaesth* 78:44-50, 1997.
13. Bickell WH, Wall MJ, Pepe PE, et al: Immediate versus delayed fluid resuscitation for hypotensive patients with penetrating torso injuries, *N Engl J Med* 331:1105-1109, 1994.
14. Biertuempfel PH, Ling GV, Ling GA: Urinary tract infection resulting from catheterization in healthy adult dogs, *J Am Vet Med Assoc* 178:989-991, 1981.
15. Bjorling DE, Rawlings CA: Relationship of intravenous administration of Ringer's lactate solution to pulmonary edema in halothane-anesthetized cats, *Am J Vet Res* 44:1000-1006, 1983.
16. Blajchman MA: Immunomodulation and blood transfusion, *Am J Ther* 9:389-395, 2002.
17. Booke M, Armstrong C, Hinder F, et al: The effects of propofol on hemodynamics and renal blood flow in healthy and in septic sheep, and combined with fentanyl in septic sheep, *Anesth Analg* 82:738-743, 1996.
18. Bourke DL, Smith TC: Estimating allowable hemodilution, *Anesthesiology* 41:609-612, 1974.
19. Brecher M, Rosenfeld M: Mathematical and computer modeling of acute normovolemic hemodilution, *Transfusion* 34:176-179, 1994.
20. British Committee for Standards in Haematology, Blood Transfusion Task Force: Guidelines for the use of platelet transfusions, *Br J Haematol* 122:10-23, 2003.

21. Brooks VL, Keil LC: Changes in the baroreflex during pregnancy in conscious dogs: heart rate and hormonal responses, *Endocrinology* 135:1894-1901, 1994.

22. Brooks VL, Keil LC: Hemorrhage decreases arterial pressure sooner in pregnant compared with nonpregnant dogs: role of baroreflex, *Am J Physiol* 266:H1610-H1619, 1994.

23. Brotzu G: Inhibition by chlorpromazine of the effects of dopamine on the dog kidney, *J Pharm Pharmacol* 22:664-667, 1970.

24. Brownlee L, Wardrop KJ, Sellon RK, et al: Use of a prestorage leukoreduction filter effectively removes leukocytes from canine whole blood while preserving red blood cell viability, *J Vet Intern Med* 14:412-417, 2000.

25. Cairoli F, Colombo G, Arrighi S: Variazioni di alcune componente ematiche nella cagna di razza Beagle durante la gravidanza ed il puerperio, *Clin Vet (Milano)* 103:267-283, 1980.

26. Callas DD, Clark TL, Moreira PL, et al: In vitro effects of a novel hemoglobin-based oxygen carrier on routine chemistry, therapeutic drug, coagulation, hematology, and blood bank assays, *Clin Chem* 43:1744-1748, 1997.

27. Canizaro PC, Prager MD, Shires GT: The infusion of Ringer's lactate solution during shock. Changes in lactate, excess lactate, and pH, *Am J Surg* 122:494-501, 1971.

28. Carson JL, Poses RM, Spence RK, et al: Severity of anaemia and operative mortality and morbidity, *Lancet* 1:727-729, 1988.

29. Charlson M, MacKenzie C, Gold J, et al: Risk for postoperative congestive heart failure, *Surg Gynecol Obstet* 172:95-104, 1991.

30. Ching YNLH, Meyers KM, Brassard JA, et al: Effect of cryoprecipitate and plasma on plasma von Willebrand factor multimeters and bleeding time in Doberman Pinschers with type-I von Willebrand's disease, *Am J Vet Res* 55:102-110, 1994.

31. Christidis C, Mal F, Ramos J, et al: Worsening of hepatic dysfunction as a consequence of repeated hydroxyethyl-starch infusions, *J Hepatol* 35:726-732, 2001.

32. Clugston P, Fitzpatrick D, Kester D, et al: Autologous blood use in reduction mammaplasty: is it justified? *Plast Reconstr Surg* 95:824-828, 1995.

33. Concannon KT, Haskins SC, Feldman BF: Hemostatic defects associated with two infusion rates of dextran 70 in dogs, *Am J Vet Res* 53:1369-1375, 1992.

34. Connolly CM, Kramer GC, Hahn RG, et al: Isoflurane but not mechanical ventilation promotes extravascular fluid accumulation during crystalloid volume loading, *Anesthesiology* 98:670-681, 2003.

35. Copland V, Haskins S, Patz J: Oxymorphone: cardiovascular, pulmonary, and behavioral effects in dogs, *Am J Vet Res* 48:1626-1630, 1987.

36. Cote CJ, Drop LJ, Daniels AL, et al: Calcium chloride versus calcium gluconate: comparison of ionization and cardiovascular effects in children and dogs, *Anesthesiology* 66:465-470, 1987.

37. Cote CJ, Drop LJ, Hoaglin DC, et al: Ionized hypocalcemia after fresh frozen plasma administration to thermally injured children: effects of infusion rate, duration, and treatment with calcium chloride, *Anesth Analg* 67:152-160, 1988.

38. Coulter DB, Whelan SC, Wilson RC: Determination of blood pressure by indirect methods in dogs given acetylpromazine maleate, *Cornell Vet* 71:76-84, 1981.

39. Crystal MA, Mott J, Van Der Veldt P: Blood loss and no matching donor, *Vet Forum* 16:55-57, 1999.

40. Day TK: Current development and use of hemoglobin-based oxygen-carrying (HBOC) solutions, *J Vet Emerg Crit Care* 13:77-93, 2003.

41. de Jonge E, Levi M, Berends F, et al: Impaired haemostasis by intravenous administration of a gelatin-based plasma expander in human subjects, *Thromb Haemost* 79:286-290, 1998.

42. de Lange S, Boscoe MJ, Stanley TH, et al: Antidiuretic and growth hormone responses during coronary artery surgery with sufentanil-oxygen and alfentanil-oxygen anesthesia in man, *Anesth Analg* 61:434-438, 1982.

43. Didwania A, Miller J, Kassel D, et al: Effect of intravenous lactated Ringer's solution infusion on the circulating lactate concentration: part 3. Results of a prospective, randomized, double-blind, placebo-controlled trial [see comments], *Crit Care Med* 25:1851-1854, 1997.

44. Dieterich HJ: Recent developments in European colloid solutions, *J Trauma* 54:S26-30, 2003.

45. Dieterich HJ, Reutershan J, Felbinger TW, et al: Penetration of intravenous hydroxyethyl starch into the cerebrospinal fluid in patients with impaired blood-brain barrier function, *Anesth Analg* 96:1150-1154, table of contents, 2003.

46. Duffy G, Neal K: Differences in post-operative infection rates between patients receiving autologous and allogeneic blood transfusion: a meta-analysis of published randomized and nonrandomized studies, *Transfus Med* 6:325-328, 1996.

47. Dutton RP, Mackenzie CF, Scalea TM: Hypotensive resuscitation during active hemorrhage: impact on in-hospital mortality, *J Trauma* 52:1141-1146, 2002.

48. Egli GA, Zollinger A, Seifert B, et al: Effect of progressive haemodilution with hydroxyethyl starch, gelatin and albumin on blood coagulation, *Br J Anaesth* 78:684-689, 1997.

49. Evans PA, Garnett M, Boffard K, et al: Evaluation of the effect of colloid (Haemaccel) on the bleeding time in the trauma patient, *J R Soc Med* 89:101P-104P, 1996.

50. Faggella AM, Aronsohn MG: Anesthetic techniques for neutering 6- to 14-week-old kittens, *J Am Vet Med Assoc* 202:56-62, 1993.

51. Feldman Z, Zachari S, Reichenthal E, et al: Brain edema and neurological status with rapid infusion of lactated Ringer's or 5% dextrose solution following head trauma, *J Neurosurg* 83:1060-1066, 1995.

52. Fischer D, Omlor D, Kreuscher D: Influence of ketamine anaesthesia on renal and cardiovascular functions in mongrel dogs, *Int Urol Nephrol* 11:271-277, 1979.

53. Follett DV, Loeb RG, Haskins SC, et al: Effects of epinephrine and ritodrine in dogs with acute hyperkalemia, *Anesth Analg* 70:400-406, 1990.

54. Francis DM, Shenton BK: Blood transfusion and tumour growth: evidence from laboratory animals, *Lancet* 2:871, 1981.

55. Fusco JV, Hohenhaus AE, Aiken SW, et al: Autologous blood collection and transfusion in cats undergoing partial craniectomy, *J Am Vet Med Assoc* 216:1584-1588, 2000.

56. Gagnon JA, Felipe I, Nelson LD: Influence of thiopental anesthesia on renal sodium and water excretion in the dog, *Am J Physiol* 243:F265-F270, 1982.

57. Galvez OG, Bay WH, Roberts BW, et al: The hemodynamic effects of potassium deficiency in the dog, *Circ Res* 40(suppl 1):I-11-I-16, 1977.

58. Gaynor JS, Wertz EM, Kesel LM, et al: Effect of intravenous administration of fluids on packed cell volume,

blood pressure, and total protein and blood glucose concentrations in healthy halothane-anesthetized dogs, *J Am Vet Med Assoc* 208:2013-2015, 1996.

59. Gentilello LM, Moujaes S: Treatment of hypothermia in trauma victims: thermodynamic considerations, *J Intensive Care Med* 10:5-14, 1995.

60. Gibson GR, Callan MB, Hoffman V, et al: Use of a hemoglobin-based oxygen-carrying solution in cats: 72 cases (1998-2000), *J Am Vet Med Assoc* 221:96-102, 2002.

61. Glowaski MM, Moon-Massat P, Erb H, et al: Effects of oxypolygelatin and dextran 70 on hemostatic variables in dogs, *Vet Anaesth Analg* 30:230-238, 2003.

62. Goldstein SM, MacLean LD: Ringer's lactate infusion with severe hepatic damage: effect on arterial lactate level, *Can J Surg* 15:318-321, 1972.

63. Gollub S, Schaefer C: Structural alteration in canine fibrin produced by colloid plasma expanders, *Surg Gynecol Obstet* 127:783-793, 1968.

64. Goodnough L, Grishaber J, Monk T, et al: Acute preoperative hemodilution in patients undergoing radical prostatectomy: a case study analysis of efficacy, *Anesth Analg* 78:932-937, 1994.

65. Gorelick MH, Shaw KN, Baker MD: Effect of ambient temperature on capillary refill in healthy children, *Pediatrics* 92:699-702, 1993.

66. Graefe U, Milutinovich J, Follette WC, et al: Less dialysis-induced morbidity and vascular instability with bicarbonate in dialysate, *Ann Intern Med* 88:332-336, 1978.

67. Gunter P: Practice Guidelines for Blood Component Therapy: a report by the American Society of Anesthesiologists Task Force on Blood Component Therapy, *Anesthesiology* 85:1219-1220, 1996.

68. Guidelines for the use of platelet transfusions, *Br J Haematol* 122:10-23, 2003.

69. Guest JD, Vanni S, Silbert L: Mild hypothermia, blood loss and complications in elective spinal surgery, *Spine J* 4:130-137, 2004.

70. Hahn RG, Drobin D, Ståhle L: Volume kinetics of Ringer's solution in female volunteers, *Br J Anaesth* 78:144-148, 1997.

71. Hahn RG, Svensen C: Plasma dilution and the rate of infusion of Ringer's solution, *Br J Anaesth* 79:64-67, 1997.

72. Hardy RM, Osborne CA: Water deprivation test in the dog: maximal normal values, *JAMA* 174:479-483, 1979.

73. Hartsfield SM, Thurmon JC, Corbin JE, et al: Effects of sodium acetate, bicarbonate and lactate on acid-base status in anaesthetized dogs, *J Vet Pharmacol Ther* 4:51-61, 1981.

74. Haskins SC, Farver TB, Patz JD: Ketamine in dogs, *Am J Vet Res* 46:1855-1860, 1985.

75. Hessel EA 2nd, Schmer G, Dillard DH: Platelet kinetics during deep hypothermia, *J Surg Res* 28:23-34, 1980.

76. Hill SR, Carless PA, Henry DA, et al: Transfusion thresholds and other strategies for guiding allogeneic red blood cell transfusion, *Cochrane Database Syst Rev* 2:CD002042, 2002.

77. Hint H: Relationships between the chemical and physicochemical properties of dextrans and its pharmacological effects. In Derrick JR, Guest MR, editors: *Dextrans. Current concepts of basic actions and clinical applications*, ed 1, Springfield, IL, 1971, Charles C. Thomas, pp. 3-26.

78. Holte K, Jensen P, Kehlet H: Physiologic effects of intravenous fluid administration in healthy volunteers, *Anesth Analg* 96:1504-1509, 2003.

79. Houbiers JG, van de Velde CJ, van de Watering LM, et al: Transfusion of red cells is associated with increased incidence of bacterial infection after colorectal surgery: a prospective study, *Transfusion* 37:126-134, 1997.

80. Hughes GS, Francom SF, Antal EJ, et al: Effects of a novel hemoglobin-based oxygen carrier on percent oxygen saturation as determined with arterial blood gas analysis and pulse oximetry, *Ann Emerg Med* 27:164-169, 1996.

81. Iseki K, Onoyama K, Maeda T, et al: Comparison of hemodynamics induced by conventional acetate hemodialysis, bicarbonate hemodialysis and ultrafiltration, *Clin Nephrol* 14:294-298, 1980.

82. Ishihara H, Ishida K, Oyama T, et al: Effects of general anaesthesia and surgery on renal function and plasma ADH levels, *Can Anaesth Soc J* 25:312-318, 1978.

83. Ivatury RR, Diebel L, Porter JM, et al: Intra-abdominal hypertension and the abdominal compartment syndrome, *Surg Clin North Am* 77:783-800, 1997.

84. Johnstone IB: Desmopressin enhances the binding of plasma von Willebrand factor to collagen in plasmas from normal dogs and dogs with type I von Willebrand's disease, *Can Vet J* 40:645-648, 1999.

85. Johnstone IB, Crane S: The effects of desmopressin on hemostatic parameters in the normal dog, *Can J Vet Res* 50:265-271, 1986.

86. Kaczmarczyk G: Pulmonary-renal axis during positive-pressure ventilation, *New Horiz* 2:512-517, 1994.

87. Kaneko M, Nakayama H, Igarashi N, et al: Relationship between the number of fetuses and the blood constituents of Beagles in late pregnancy, *J Vet Med Sci* 55:681-682, 1993.

88. Kanter M, van Maanen D, Anders K, et al: Preoperative autologous blood donations before elective hysterectomy, *JAMA* 276:798-801, 1996.

89. Karlson KE, Garzon AA, Shaftan GW, et al: Increased blood loss associated with administration of certain plasma expanders: dextran 75, dextran 40, and hydroxyethyl starch, *Surgery* 62:670-678, 1967.

90. Kerl ME, Hohenhaus AE: Packed red blood cell transfusions in dogs: 131 cases 1989, *J Am Vet Med Assoc* 202:1495-1499, 1993.

91. Kirkendol PL, Starrs J, Gonzalez FM: The effects of acetate, lactate, succinate and gluconate on plasma pH and electrolytes in dogs, *Trans Am Soc Artif Intern Organs* 26:323-327, 1980.

92. Komtebedde J, Forsyth SF, Breznock EM, et al: Intrahepatic portosystemic venous anomaly in the dog: perioperative management and complications, *Vet Surg* 20:37-42, 1991.

93. Koval K, Rosenberg A, Zuckerman J, et al: Does blood transfusion increase the risk of infection after hip fracture? *J Orthop Trauma* 11:260-265, 1997.

94. Kronen PWM, Moon-Massat PF, Ludders JW, et al: Comparison of two insulin protocols for diabetic dogs undergoing cataract surgery, *Vet Anaesth Analg* 28:146-155, 2001.

95. Kurnik BR, Singer F, Groh WC: Case report: dextran-induced acute anuric renal failure, *Am J Med Sci* 302:28-30, 1991.

96. Lam AM, Winn HR, Cullen BF, et al: Hyperglycemia and neurological outcome in patients with head injury, *J Neurosurg* 75:545-551, 1991.

97. Lang K, Suttner S, Boldt J, et al: Volume replacement with HES 130/0.4 may reduce the inflammatory response in patients undergoing major abdominal surgery, *Can J Anaesth* 50:1009-1016, 2003.

98. Langeron O, Doelberg M, Ang ET, et al: Voluven, a lower substituted novel hydroxyethyl starch (HES 130/0.4), causes fewer effects on coagulation in major orthopedic surgery than HES 200/0.5, *Anesth Analg* 92:855-862, 2001.

99. Laureno R, Karp B: Myelinolysis after correction of hyponatremia, *Ann Intern Med* 126:57-62, 1997.

100. Lees G: Use and misuse of indwelling urethral catheters, *Vet Clin North Am Small Anim Pract* 26:499-505, 1996.

101. Lens XM, Montoliu J, Cases A, et al: Treatment of hyperkalaemia in renal failure: salbutamol v. insulin, *Nephrol Dial Transplant* 4:228-232, 1989.

102. Lewis JH, Szeto ILF, Bayre WL, et al: Severe hemodilution with hydroxyethyl starch and dextrans, *Arch Surg* 93:941-950, 1966.

103. Li LPA, Shamloo M, Katsura KI, et al: Critical values for plasma glucose in aggravating ischaemic brain damage: correlation to extracellular pH, *Neurobiol Dis* 2:97-108, 1995.

104. Lorenz W, Duda D, Dick W, et al: Incidence and clinical importance of perioperative histamine release: randomized study of volume loading and antihistamines after induction of anaesthesia, *Lancet* 343:933-940, 1994.

105. Lundsgaard-Hansen P, Tshirren B: Modified fluid gelatin as a plasma substitute, *Prog Clin Biol Res* 19:227-257, 1978.

106. Matsumura LK, Ajzen H, Chacra AR, et al: Effect of positive pressure breathing on plasma antidiuretic hormone and renal function in dogs, *Braz J Med Biol Res* 16:261-270, 1983.

107. Meier J, Kleen M, Habler O, et al: New mathematical model for the correct prediction of the exchangeable blood volume during acute normovolemic hemodilution, *Acta Anaesthesiol Scand* 47:37-45, 2003.

108. Michelson AD, MacGregor H, Barnard MR, et al: Reversible inhibition of human platelet activation by hypothermia in vivo and in vitro, *Thromb Haemost* 71:633-640, 1994.

109. Moon PF: Acute toxicosis in two dogs associated with etomidate-propylene glycol infusion, *Lab Anim Sci* 44:590-594, 1994.

110. Moore LE, Garvey MS: The effect of hetastarch on serum colloid oncotic pressure in hypoalbuminemic dogs, *J Vet Intern Med* 10:300-303, 1996.

111. Mortier E, Ongenae M, De Baerdemaeker L, et al: In vitro evaluation of the effect of profound haemodilution with hydroxyethyl starch 6%, modified fluid gelatin 4% and dextran 40 10% on coagulation profile measured by thromboelastography, *Anaesthesia* 52:1061-1064, 1997.

112. Moursi M, Rising CL, Zelenock GB, et al: Dextrose administration exacerbates acute renal ischemic damage in anesthetized dogs, *Arch Surg* 122:790-794, 1987.

113. Naylor JM, Kronfeld DS, Freeman DE, et al: Hepatic and extrahepatic lactate metabolism in sheep: effects of lactate loading and pH, *Am J Physiol* 247:E747-E755, 1984.

114. O'Brien D, Kroll R, Johnson G, et al: Myelinolysis after correction of hyponatremia in two dogs, *J Vet Intern Med* 8:40-48, 1994.

115. Opelz G, Sengar DP, Mickey MR, et al: Effect of blood transfusions on subsequent kidney transplants, *Transplant Proc* 5:253-259, 1973.

116. Palacios A, Martainez M, Costela J, et al: Postoperative infection and anesthesia: analysis of various risk factors, *Rev Esp Anestesiol Reanim* 42:87-90, 1995.

117. Paradis NA: Dose-response relationship between aortic infusions of polymerized bovine hemoglobin and return of circulation in a canine model of ventricular fibrillation and advanced cardiac life support, *Crit Care Med* 25:476-483, 1997.

118. Perel A, Pizov R, Cotev S: Systolic pressure variation is a sensitive indicator of hypovolemia in ventilated dogs subjected to graded hemorrhage, *Anesthesiology* 67:498-502, 1987.

119. Petersen J, Shalmi M, Christensen S, et al: Comparison of the renal effects of six sedating agents in rats, *Physiol Behav* 60:759-765, 1996.

120. Peterson ME: Feline hyperthyroidism, *Vet Clin North Am Small Anim Pract* 14:809-826, 1984.

121. Pit MJ, Tegelaar RJ, Venema PL: Isothermic irrigation during transurethral resection of the prostate: effects on peri-operative hypothermia, blood loss, resection time and patient satisfaction, *Br J Urol* 78:99-103, 1996.

122. Pizov R, Ya'ari Y, Perel A: Systolic pressure variation is greater during hemorrhage than during sodium nitroprusside-induced hypotension in ventilated dogs, *Anesth Analg* 67:170-174, 1988.

123. Prien T, Backhaus N, Pelster F, et al: Effect of intraoperative fluid administration and colloid osmotic pressure on the formation of intestinal edema during gastrointestinal surgery, *J Clin Anesth* 2:317-323, 1990.

124. Ramming S, Shackford SR, Zhuang J, et al: The relationship of fluid balance and sodium administration to cerebral edema formation and intracranial pressure in a porcine model of brain injury, *J Trauma* 37:705-713, 1994.

125. Rebollo M, Bernal J, Llorca J, et al: Nosocomial infections in patients having cardiovascular operations: a multivariate analysis of risk factors, *J Thorac Cardiovasc Surg* 112:908-913, 1996.

126. Ring J, Messmer K: Incidence and severity of anaphylactoid reactions to colloid volume substitutes, *Lancet* i:466-469, 1977.

127. Roberts JP, Roberts JD, Skinner C, et al: Extracellular fluid deficit following operation and its correction with Ringer's lactate: a reassessment, *Ann Surg* 202:1-8, 1985.

128. Robinson EP, Hardy RM: Clinical signs, diagnosis, and treatment of alkalemia in dogs: 20 cases (1982-1984), *J Am Vet Med Assoc* 192:943-949, 1988.

129. Rossaint R, Jorres D, Nienhaus M, et al: Positive end-expiratory pressure reduces renal excretion without hormonal activation after volume expansion in dogs, *Anesthesiology* 77:700-708, 1992.

130. Rossaint R, Krebs M, Forther J, et al: Inferior vena caval pressure increase contributes to sodium and water retention during PEEP in awake dogs, *J Appl Physiol* 75:2484-2492, 1993.

131. Rusthoven JJ: Blood transfusion and cancer: clinical studies. In Singal DP, editor: *Immunological effects of blood transfusion*, ed 1, Boca Raton, FL, 1994, CRC Press, pp. 85-110.

132. Ryden SE, Oberman HA: Compatibility of common intravenous solutions with CPD blood, *Transfusion* 15:250-255, 1975.

133. Saragoca MA, Bessa AM, Mulinari RA, et al: Sodium acetate, an arterial vasodilator: haemodynamic characterisation in normal dogs, *Proc Eur Dial Transplant Assoc Eur Ren Assoc* 21:221-224, 1985.

134. Schmied H, Kurz A, Sessler DI, et al: Mild hypothermia increases blood loss and transfusion requirements during total hip arthroplasty, *Lancet* 347:289-292, 1996.

135. Schortgen F, Lacherade JC, Bruneel F, et al: Effects of hydroxyethylstarch and gelatin on renal function in severe sepsis: a multicentre randomised study, *Lancet* 357:911-916, 2001.

136. Schriger DL, Baraff LJ: Capillary refill—is it a useful predictor of hypovolemic states? *Ann Emerg Med* 20:601-605, 1991.

137. Segal JB, Blasco-Colmenares E, Norris EJ, et al: Preoperative acute normovolemic hemodilution: a meta-analysis, *Transfusion* 44:632-644, 2004.

138. Shires T, Williams J, Brown F: Acute changes in extracellular fluids associated with major surgical procedures, *Ann Surg* 154:803-810, 1961.

139. Sieber FE: The neurologic implications of diabetic hyperglycemia during surgical procedures at increased risk for brain ischemia, *J Clin Anesth* 9:334-340, 1997.

140. Sieber FE, Traystman RJ: Special issues: glucose and the brain, *Crit Care Med* 20:104-114, 1992.

141. Silberstein LE, Naryshkin S, Haddad JJ, et al: Calcium homeostasis during therapeutic plasma exchange, *Transfusion* 26:151-155, 1986.

142. Smiley LE: The use of hetastarch for plasma expansion, *Probl Vet Med* 4:652-667, 1992.

143. Smiley LE, Garvey MS: The use of hetastarch as adjunct therapy in 26 dogs with hypoalbuminemia: a phase two clinical trial, *J Vet Intern Med* 8:195-202, 1994.

144. Ståhle L, Nilsson A, Hahn RG: Modeling the volume of expandable body fluid spaces during i.v. fluid therapy, *Br J Anaesth* 78:138-143, 1997.

145. Stamm W: Infections related to medical devices, *Ann Intern Med* 89:764-769, 1978.

146. Standl T, Freitag M, Burmeister MA, et al: Hemoglobin-based oxygen carrier HBOC-201 provides higher and faster increase in oxygen tension in skeletal muscle of anemic dogs than do stored red blood cells, *J Vasc Surg* 37:859-865, 2003.

147. Stokol T, Parry B: Efficacy of fresh-frozen plasma and cryoprecipitate in dogs with von Willebrand's disease or hemophilia A, *J Vet Intern Med* 12:84-92, 1998.

148. Strauss RG: Review of the effects of hydroxyethyl starch on the blood coagulation system, *Transfusion* 21:299-302, 1981.

149. Svensén C, Hahn RG: Volume kinetics of Ringer solution, dextran 70, and hypertonic saline in male volunteers, *Anesthesiology* 87:204-212, 1997.

150. Svensen C, Ponzer S, Hahn RG: Volume kinetics of Ringer solution after surgery for hip fracture, *Can J Anaesth* 46:133-141, 1999.

151. Tabuchi N, de Haan J, Gallandat Huet RC, et al: Gelatin use impairs platelet adhesion during cardiac surgery, *Thromb Haemost* 74:1447-1451, 1995.

152. Tanifuji Y, Eger EI: Brain sodium, potassium, and osmolality: effects on anesthetic requirement, *Anesth Analg* 57:404-410, 1978.

153. Tartter PI: Blood transfusion and bacterial infections: clinical studies. In Singal DP, editor: *Immunological effects of blood transfusion*, ed 1, Boca Raton, FL, 1994, CRC Press, pp. 111-126.

154. Thompson WL, Fukushima T, Rutherford RB, et al: Intravascular persistence, tissue storage, and excretion of hydroxyethyl starch, *Surg Gynecol Obstet* 131:965-972, 1970.

155. Treib J, Haass A, Pindur G, et al: HES 200/0.5 is not HES 200/0.5. Influence of the C2/C6 hydroxyethylation ratio of hydroxyethyl starch (HES) on hemorheology, coagulation and elimination kinetics, *Thromb Haemost* 74:1452-1456, 1995.

156. Usenik EA, Cronkite EP: Effects of barbiturate anesthesia on leukocytes in normal and splenectomized dogs, *Anesth Analg* 44:167-170, 1965.

157. Vail DM, Ogilvie GK, Fettman MJ, et al: Exacerbation of hyperlactatemia by infusion of lactated Ringer's solution in dogs with lymphoma, *J Vet Intern Med* 4:228-232, 1990.

158. Van der Linden P, De Hert S, Mathieu N, et al: Tolerance to acute isovolemic hemodilution. Effect of anesthetic depth, *Anesthesiology* 99:97-104, 2003.

159. Van der Linden P, Schmartz D, Gilbart E, et al: Effects of propofol, etomidate, and pentobarbital on critical oxygen delivery, *Crit Care Med* 28:2492-2499, 2000.

160. Virtue RW, LeVine DS, Aikawa JK: Fluid shifts during the surgical period: RISA and S35 determinations following glucose, saline or lactate infusion, *Ann Surg* 163:523-528, 1965.

161. Vogt NH, Bothner U, Lerch G, et al: Large-dose administration of 6% hydroxyethyl starch 200/0.5 total hip arthroplasty: plasma homeostasis, hemostasis, and renal function compared to use of 5% human albumin, *Anesth Analg* 83:262-268, 1996.

162. Vos SC, Hage JJ, Woerdeman LA, et al: Acute renal failure during dextran-40 antithrombotic prophylaxis: report of two microsurgical cases, *Ann Plast Surg* 48:193-196, 2002.

163. Wass CT, Lanier WL: Glucose modulation of ischemic brain injury: review and clinical recommendations, *Mayo Clin Proc* 71:801-812, 1996.

164. Waterhouse C: Lactate metabolism in patients with cancer, *Cancer* 33:66-71, 1974.

165. Wenzel R, Osterman C, Hunting K: Hospital-acquired infections. II. Infection rates by site, service and common procedures in a university hospital, *Am J Epidemiol* 104:645-651, 1976.

166. Winkler M, Akca O, Birkenberg B, et al: Aggressive warming reduces blood loss during hip arthroplasty, *Anesth Analg* 91:978-984, 2000.

167. Wolberg AS, Meng ZH, Monroe DM 3rd, et al: A systematic evaluation of the effect of temperature on coagulation enzyme activity and platelet function, *J Trauma* 56:1221-1228, 2004.

168. Zornow MH, Prough DS: Fluid management in patients with traumatic brain injury, *New Horiz* 3:488-498, 1995.

169. Zornow MH, Scheller MS, Shackford SR: Effect of a hypertonic lactated Ringer's solution on intracranial pressure and cerebral water content in a model of traumatic brain injury, *J Trauma* 29:484-488, 1989.

170. Zunkeler B, Carson RE, Olson J, et al: Hyperosmolar blood-brain barrier disruption in baboons: an in vivo study using positron emission tomography and rubidium-82, *J Neurosurg* 84:494-502, 1996.

171. Zwaveling JH, Meulenbelt J, van Xanten NH, et al: Renal failure associated with the use of dextran-40, *Neth J Med* 35:321-326, 1989.

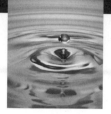

FLUID AND ELECTROLYTE DISTURBANCES IN GASTROINTESTINAL AND PANCREATIC DISEASE

Kenneth W. Simpson and Nichole Birnbaum

The gastrointestinal tract (GIT) is extremely well adapted to the task of assimilating a wide variety of nutrients and absorbs approximately 99% of the fluid presented to it (Fig. 18-1).[9] Most of the fluid absorbed in the GIT each day is derived from endogenous secretions. Exogenous fluid in the form of food and water constitutes 30 to 50 mL/kg/day, and endogenous secretions from the salivary glands, stomach, pancreas, liver, and small intestine represent two to three times this volume or 1.5 to 2 blood volumes (7% of body weight) (see Fig. 18-1). Considering this massive flux of fluid into the GIT, it is easy to see why fluid loss from or sequestration by the GIT can alter the electrolyte and acid-base status of the patient. The causes and consequences of fluid loss or sequestration are not uniform and depend on the region of the GIT involved. For example, gastric outflow obstruction is often associated with metabolic alkalosis and hypokalemia caused by loss of chloride and potassium in gastric secretions, whereas diarrhea may cause metabolic acidosis and hypokalemia because of loss of bicarbonate and potassium in the feces.

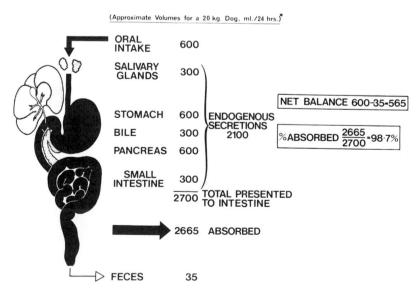

Fig. 18-1 Normal canine intestinal water balance. Of a total volume of about 3 L of fluid presented to the intestine of a 20-kg dog each day, only about 20% comes from the diet; the remainder comes from the endogenous secretions of the gastrointestinal tract. Most of this fluid is resorbed, and only a fraction of it appears in the feces. A decrease in absorption or, less commonly, an increase in secretion results in an increase in fecal water content and diarrhea. (From Burrows CF: Chronic diarrhea in the dog, *Vet Clin North Am* 13:521, 1983.)

NORMAL PHYSIOLOGY OF THE GASTROINTESTINAL TRACT

ABSORPTION AND SECRETION OF WATER AND ELECTROLYTES

Stomach

Unstimulated acid secretion by the stomach in dogs and cats is minimal (e.g., <0.04 mmol/kg$^{0.75}$/hr in the dog).[30] The "acid pump" or H$^+$,K$^+$-adenosinetriphosphatase (H$^+$,K$^+$-ATPase) is located in tubulovesicles within the cytoplasm of parietal cells.[77] In the stimulated state, H$^+$,K$^+$-ATPase and KCl transporters are incorporated in the parietal cell canalicular membrane. Hydrogen ions derived from the ionization of water within the parietal cells are transported into the gastric lumen in exchange for potassium ions. Potassium and chloride transporters in the canalicular membrane allow luminal transfer of potassium and chloride ions. Carbonic anhydrase catalyzes the combination of –OH$^-$ with CO_2 to form HCO_3^-, which diffuses into the blood (so-called alkaline tide). Acid secretion in dogs has been estimated at 30 mL/kg/day.[9] Stimulation with pentagastrin results in a rapid increase in fluid and hydrogen ion secretion, with pH rapidly decreasing to less than 1.0. Acid secretion in dogs reaches a peak of 28 mL/kg$^{0.75}$/hr or 4.1 mmol HCl/kg$^{0.75}$/hr. Potassium transport reaches a peak of 0.34 mmol/kg$^{0.75}$/hr and sodium transport a peak of 0.09 mmol/kg$^{0.75}$/hr.[30] The concentrations of K$^+$ (10 to 20 mEq/L) and Cl$^-$ (120 to 160 mEq/L) in gastric juice are higher than those of plasma (~4 mEq/L and 110 mEq/L, respectively, in the dog).

Acid secretion by parietal cells is regulated by a variety of neurochemical and neurohumoral stimuli.[49,91] Luminal peptides, digested protein, acetylcholine, and gastrin-releasing peptide stimulate gastrin secretion from G cells and cause histamine release from enterochromaffin-like cells (Fig. 18-2). Histamine is also released from mast cells. Acetylcholine and gastrin can also directly stimulate parietal cells. Somatostatin acts to decrease gastrin, histamine, and acid secretion. Acid secretion can be decreased by blocking H$_2$ (e.g., cimetidine, ranitidine, famotidine), gastrin (e.g., proglumide), and acetylcholine (e.g., atropine) receptors and by inhibiting adenyl cyclase (e.g., prostaglandin E analogues) and H$^+$,K$^+$-ATPase (e.g., omeprazole). Somatostatin directly decreases gastric acid and gastrin secretion.

Pancreas

The exocrine pancreas plays a major role in the digestion of food. It secretes enzymes that digest a wide variety of foodstuffs and bicarbonate, which serves to solubilize

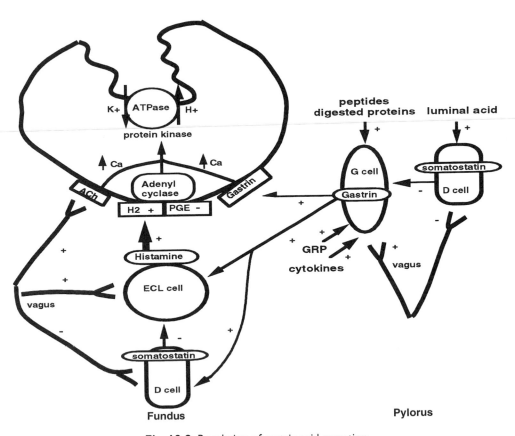

Fig. 18-2 Regulation of gastric acid secretion.

secreted enzymes and neutralize gastric acid so that optimal enzyme activity is maintained. Pancreatic secretions also play an important role in the absorption of cobalamin (vitamin B$_{12}$) and in the regulation of the bacterial flora of the small intestine, and they directly influence small intestinal function by modifying certain enzymes on the intestinal brush border and exerting trophic effects on the mucosa.

Histologically, the pancreas is composed of many secretory lobules that contain acinar cells. These secretory acini are drained by a branching ductular system that is lined by a variety of epithelial cells. A dense network of capillaries, nerves, and lymphatics surround the acini and ducts.

Pancreatic acinar cells are responsible for the synthesis of digestive enzymes, whereas the cells lining the ductular system are the major source of fluid and electrolyte secretion. The electrolyte composition of pancreatic secretion changes in response to stimulation. At low rates of secretion, the chloride concentration exceeds that of bicarbonate, whereas at higher rates, the bicarbonate concentration is higher than the chloride concentration (Fig. 18-3). In the stimulated cat pancreas, the HCO$_3^-$ concentration increases from 70 to 145 mEq/L and the Cl$^-$ concentration decreases from 100 to 30 mEq/L. Concentrations of Na$^+$ and K$^+$ in pancreatic secretions are similar to those of plasma. The concentrations of electrolytes also change within the pancreatic ductular system. A decrease in Cl$^-$ concentration from the intralobular ducts to the main ducts is thought to arise through the exchange of Cl$^-$ for HCO$_3^-$. Secretin is the principal mediator of pancreatic fluid and electrolyte secretion (Fig. 18-4) and is released in response to acidification of the proximal small intestine. Secretin and cholecystokinin have synergistic effects on fluid and elec-

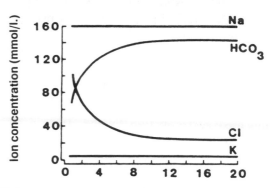

Fig. 18-3 Ionic composition of pancreatic juice secreted at different flow rates in the anesthetized cat in response to secretin. (From Argent BE, Case RM: Pancreatic ducts: cellular mechanism and control of bicarbonate. In Johnson LR, editor: *Physiology of the gastrointestinal tract,* 3rd ed, New York, 1994, Raven Press, p. 1473.)

trolyte secretion. Bicarbonate is responsible for solubilizing zymogens within the pancreatic ductular system and neutralizing gastric acid in the duodenum to provide an optimal pH for pancreatic enzyme activity. Pancreatic duct cells also produce intrinsic factor, which is a protein necessary for the absorption of cobalamin (vitamin B$_{12}$).

Classically, the pancreatic response to a meal has been divided into cephalic, gastric, and intestinal phases. During normal feeding conditions, these phases overlap and occur simultaneously, but the intestinal phase appears to be quantitatively most important. Pancreatic secretion occurs not only in response to a meal but also cyclically throughout the day. Peaks in interdigestive secretion are accompanied by an increase in biliary

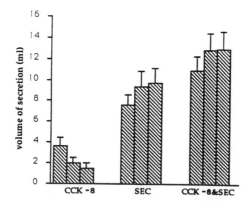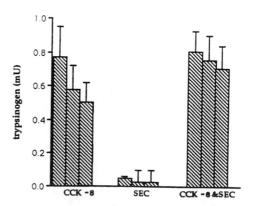

Fig. 18-4 Output of trypsinogen and fluid in pancreatic juice during intravenous infusion of cholecystokinin (CCK-8), secretin (Sec), and CCK-8 and Sec together. Data (mean ± SE) for eight dogs are expressed as total output per 15 minutes during 45-minute infusion periods. Order of secretagogues was varied, and there was a 15-minute rest period between secretagogues. (From Simpson KW, Alpers DH, DeWille J, et al: Cellular localization and hormonal regulation of pancreatic intrinsic factor secretion in dogs, *Am J Physiol* 265: G178-G188, 1993.)

secretion and intestinal motility. These cycles are thought to be mediated by motilin and may serve an intestinal housekeeping function by flushing digestive products, cell debris, and bacteria along the intestinal tract. Inhibition of exocrine pancreatic secretion has not been studied as extensively as stimulation, but glucagon and somatostatin appear to decrease pancreatic secretion.

Intestine

Net absorption of fluid and electrolytes in the intestine reflects a balance between absorption and secretion, and the final outcome in the healthy intestine represents a victory for absorption. The ability of the intestine to absorb fluid and electrolytes varies according to site. In a 20-kg dog, approximately 2.70 L of fluid (oral intake, stomach juice, saliva, pancreatic juice, and bile) is presented to the small intestine each day. Approximately 1.35 L is absorbed in the jejunum, 1 L in the ileum, and 300 mL in the colon, with 50 mL remaining in the feces.[92] From these figures, it can be calculated that the jejunum absorbs 50%, the ileum 75%, and the colon 90% of the fluid presented to the intestinal tract (Fig. 18-5). The progressive increase in absorptive efficiency along the intestinal tract is a function of enterocyte pore size, membrane potential difference, and the type of transport processes associated with each intestinal segment.[12,58,81] Whereas the jejunal epithelium is "leaky" and transfers a large amount of fluid (isotonic absorption), the tight epithelial junctions of the distal colon allow a high transepithelial voltage gradient to develop, and net solute transfer occurs against this gradient.[81]

The absorption of water is passive in the small and large intestines and follows the transport of solutes across the intestinal epithelium.[12] Passive absorption of water or electrolytes can be transcellular (i.e., through the cytoplasm of the cells) or paracellular (i.e., via the lateral intercellular spaces and tight junctions between enterocytes), and transfer occurs down a chemical or electrical gradient (e.g., passive transport of Na^+ and Cl^- in the jejunum and ileum).

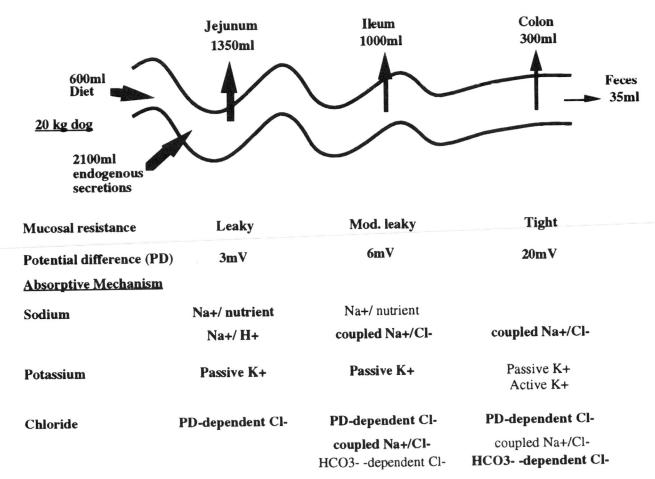

Mucosal resistance	Leaky	Mod. leaky	Tight
Potential difference (PD)	3mV	6mV	20mV
Absorptive Mechanism			
Sodium	Na+/ nutrient Na+/ H+	Na+/ nutrient coupled Na+/Cl-	coupled Na+/Cl-
Potassium	Passive K+	Passive K+	Passive K+ Active K+
Chloride	PD-dependent Cl-	PD-dependent Cl- coupled Na+/Cl- HCO3- -dependent Cl-	PD-dependent Cl- coupled Na+/Cl- HCO3- -dependent Cl-

Fig. 18-5 Fluid and electrolyte absorption in the gastrointestinal tract. (Adapted from Burrows CF: Chronic diarrhea in the dog, *Vet Clin North Am* 13:521, 1983; Chang EB, Rao MC: Intestinal water and electrolyte transport: mechanisms of physiological and adaptive responses. In Johnson LR, editor: *Physiology of the gastrointestinal tract*, ed 3, New York, 1994, Raven Press, pp. 2027-2081; and Sellin JH: Intestinal electrolyte absorption and secretion. In Sleisinger MH, Fordtran JS, Feldman M, et al, editors: *Gastrointestinal and liver disease pathophysiology, diagnosis and management*, ed 6, vol 2, Philadelphia, 1998, WB Saunders, pp. 1451-1471.)

Active transport involves transport against a concentration gradient and requires energy input (e.g., Na^+ transport driven by the Na^+,K^+ pump). The Na^+,K^+-ATPase is present in all enterocytes (Fig. 18-6, mechanism A; see also Fig. 18-5) and maintains the electrochemical Na^+ gradient required not only for net transepithelial Na^+ movement but also for the transport of many other solutes.[81] Solvent drag is the term used to describe solute movement secondary to water flow (e.g., NaCl transport in the jejunum via the paracellular route). The relative importance of each transport system is site dependent (see Figs. 18-5 and 18-6), and the location of the enterocyte in the villus or crypt is also important: villus enterocytes absorb, whereas crypt enterocytes secrete.

Jejunum

Because of the high permeability of the jejunum, passive transport processes make a major contribution to overall Na^+ and Cl^- movement in this segment of the intestinal tract. The luminal membranes of the epithelial cells in this region contain sodium-dependent transporters for hexose sugars and amino acids (see Figs. 18-5 and 18-6, mechanism B). Sodium enters the epithelial cell down its concentration gradient and is the driving force for accumulation of the nutrient intracellularly. Glucose and glutamine supply energy. Sodium is then extruded from the cell at the basolateral membrane by Na^+,K^+-ATPase while the hexose sugar or amino acid diffuses out of the cell at the basolateral membrane down a favorable concentration gradient. Therefore Na^+,K^+-ATPase drives net absorption of both Na^+ and the sugar or amino acid. Proteins that function as Na^+-H^+ exchangers are present in the luminal membranes of the enterocytes in the jejunum and allow absorbed Na^+ to be exchanged for intracellular H^+ (see Figs. 18-5 and 18-6, mechanism C). This exchange is driven by both the electrochemical gradient for Na^+ and a pH gradient that results from a moderately acidic intracellular environment.[81] As Na^+ is extruded at the basolateral membrane by Na^+,K^+-ATPase, HCO_3^- also moves out of the cell, resulting in net absorption of sodium bicarbonate. Although

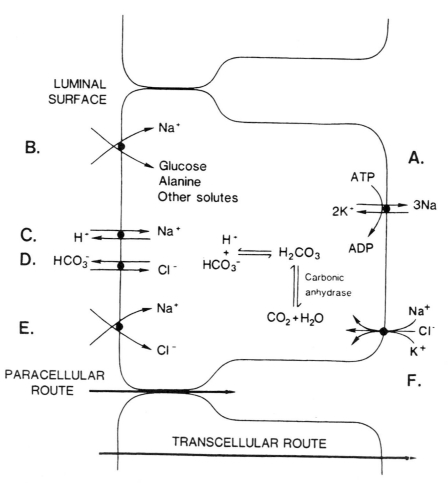

Fig. 18-6 Summary of membrane transport processes present in different regions of the small intestine. Absorptive mechanisms: all enterocytes (**A**), jejunum (**B**), and ileum (**B–E**). Secretory mechanisms (**F**). (From Moseley RH: Fluid and electrolyte disorders and gastrointestinal disease. In Kokko JP, Tannen RL: *Fluid and electrolytes*, Philadelphia, 1996, WB Saunders, p. 680.)

Na^+-nutrient absorption and Na^+-HCO_3^- absorption occur in the jejunum as already described, solvent drag–mediated Na^+ absorption secondary to monosaccharide absorption is the major mechanism for Na^+ absorption in this segment.

Movement of K^+ in the intestinal tract follows its electrochemical gradient, and secretion generally predominates.[81] In the small intestine, most K^+ secretion is passive and results from the generation of a lumen-negative potential difference across the epithelium.[81] This negative potential difference attracts K^+ into the intestinal lumen, and consequently the concentration of K^+ is always higher in intestinal contents than in plasma. In the jejunum, solvent drag created by glucose and amino acid transport causes passive absorption of Cl^- and HCO_3^-.

Ileum

The predominant form of Na^+ absorption in the ileum is neutral NaCl absorption (see Figs. 18-5 and 18-6, mechanisms C and D or E) with some contribution by Na^+-nutrient absorption (see Figs. 18-5 and 18-6, mechanism B). The contents of the ileum and colon are normally alkaline.[24,92] Solvent drag–mediated passive absorption of Cl^- and HCO_3^- does not occur in the ileum and colon, but a Cl^--HCO_3^- exchange mechanism is present. The exact mechanism of HCO_3^- secretion in duodenal, ileal, and colonic enterocytes is unknown but is thought to involve both electrogenic and electroneutral components and discrete apical and basolateral transporters.[81]

Colon

Absorption of Na^+ in the colon is achieved against a large electrochemical gradient (see Fig. 18-5) and is principally a result of active Na^+ transport.[26] Colonic Na^+ absorption is also influenced by mineralocorticoids (e.g., aldosterone). Mineralocorticoids increase the activity of Na^+ channels in the luminal membranes of colonic epithelial cells and may increase Na^+,K^+-ATPase in the basolateral membranes. The colonic epithelium contains K^+ channels and is capable of active potassium transport. Absorption of potassium is thought to be accomplished by means of a K^+-ATPase with characteristics similar to those of both basolateral membrane Na^+,K^+-ATPase and parietal cell H^+,K^+-ATPase.[7] The concentration of K^+ in colonic contents is high because of the high potential difference generated and can approach 90 mEq/L.[26] Active K^+ secretion is mediated by Na^+,K^+-ATPase or by Na^+-K^+-$2Cl^-$ cotransport. Aldosterone and cyclic adenosine monophosphate (cAMP) increase apical K^+ conductance and stimulate secretion of K^+ (see Fig. 18-5).[7] Colonic absorption is important in small-intestinal disease because the colon may compensate for fluid losses associated with small-bowel dysfunction. Alternatively, patients with small-bowel dysfunction may present with signs of large-bowel disease. This is thought to result

from impairment of colonic absorption or stimulation of colonic secretion by products of abnormal small-intestinal function, such as hydroxylated fatty acids or deconjugated bile acids.

The primary anions in the colon are short-chain fatty acids, which are generated by bacterial metabolism of carbohydrate and protein.[81] These short-chain fatty acids include acetate, propionate, and butyrate, which are the preferred metabolic substrates for colonic cells. They are known to stimulate Na^+, water, and K^+ absorption by the colon, but the exact mechanism of this process has not been defined.[76]

Intestinal secretion is a function of villus crypt cells. It is thought the electrogenic transport of Cl^- across the basolateral membrane into the enterocyte (see Fig. 18-6, mechanism F) and Cl^- efflux through Cl^- channels in the microvillus membrane into the intestinal lumen (Fig. 18-7) cause intestinal secretion.

CONTROL OF ABSORPTION AND SECRETION OF WATER AND ELECTROLYTES

Control of absorption and secretion is an autonomous process that is regulated by the neurocrine systems located in the submucosal plexus.[13,14,58,81] Acetylcholine and vasoactive intestinal polypeptide (VIP) are the major mediators of gastrointestinal secretion, whereas

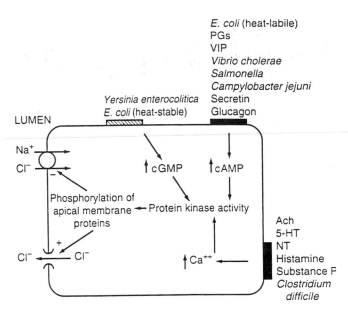

Fig. 18-7 Role of intracellular messengers cGMP, cAMP, and Ca^{2+} on NaCl absorption and Cl^- secretion by small intestine epithelium. Increases in messenger-specific protein kinase activity result in phosphorylation of specific brush border membrane phosphoproteins that alter ion movement. *PGs*, Prostaglandins; *VIP*, vasoactive intestinal polypeptide; *Ach*, acetylcholine; *5-HT*, serotonin; *NT*, neurotensin. (From Moseley RH: Fluid and electrolyte disorders and gastrointestinal disease. In Kokko JP, Tannen RL, editors: *Fluid and electrolytes*, Philadelphia, 1996, WB Saunders, p. 681.)

norepinephrine, somatostatin, and opioids are the principal regulators of absorption. At the cellular level, acetylcholine and VIP cause an increase in intracellular calcium and cAMP that inhibits neutral NaCl absorption and facilitates transcellular Cl⁻ efflux. Many bacterial agents exert their effects by increasing the intracellular concentration of cAMP in enterocytes. Norepinephrine, somatostatin, and opioids lower intracellular cAMP and calcium concentrations and stimulate neutral NaCl absorption (see Fig. 18-7).

Volume status and intestinal blood flow also influence ion transport. Systemic volume expansion results in an increase in intestinal secretion, whereas volume contraction results in adrenergic stimulation and increased absorption.[12] Osmotic forces are also important in the regulation of electrolyte and fluid transport. Luminal osmolality is normally maintained close to plasma osmolality.[12] After intake of hypertonic foods and liquids, rapid equilibration is accomplished by movement of water into the intestinal lumen. In particular, the duodenum and upper jejunum are subject to major fluid shifts. As intestinal chyme moves distally, absorptive processes steadily decrease luminal Na⁺, Cl⁻, and water. Osmotic diarrhea results if nonabsorbable solutes such as disaccharides remain in the lumen. Increased fluid absorption in the colon can compensate to some extent for fluid lost into the lumen of the small bowel, but eventually colon absorptive capacity is overwhelmed. Cations such as magnesium and anions such as sulfate are poorly absorbed and can also lead to osmotic diarrhea.

In response to inflammation, the number of immune cells in the lamina propria increases. Inflammation can lead to mucosal ulceration, exudation of protein, motility dysfunction, and loss of absorptive surface area, all of which can result in intestinal fluid loss. Many secreta-gogues associated with inflammation have been identified. Adenosine, serotonin, and histamine have both direct effects on epithelial cells and indirect effects via neural pathways. Other secretagogues include oxidants (e.g., superoxides, hydrogen peroxide, and OH⁻ released from neutrophils) that stimulate Cl⁻ secretion, cytokines (e.g., interleukin-1, interleukin-3), arachidonic acid, platelet-activating factor, substance P, kallikreins, and bradykinin.[81] *Escherichia coli* heat-labile enterotoxin and enterotoxins produced by *Vibrio cholerae, Salmonella* sp., *Campylobacter jejuni, Pseudomonas aeruginosa,* and *Shigella* sp. activate adenylate cyclase, producing cAMP and augmenting secretion in the intestine (see Fig. 18-7).[29] The eicosanoids, especially the lipoxygenase metabolites of arachidonic acid, are central to the secretory response associated with inflammation. Kinins stimulate secretion in both the small and large intestines, where they stimulate production of prostaglandin E₂.[60]

Acid-base balance may also affect intestinal electrolyte transport. In the rat, metabolic acidosis is a potent stimulus for ileal Na⁺ absorption (possibly in exchange for H⁺), whereas metabolic alkalosis decreases Na⁺ absorption but increases HCO₃⁻ secretion.[12]

PATHOPHYSIOLOGY OF THE GASTROINTESTINAL TRACT

VOMITING

Vomiting is a reflex act that is initiated by stimulation of the vomiting center in the medulla. The vomiting center can be stimulated directly or indirectly via the chemoreceptor trigger zone (CTZ), which is situated in the area postrema (Fig. 18-8). The blood-brain barrier is limited at this point, enabling blood-borne substances such as

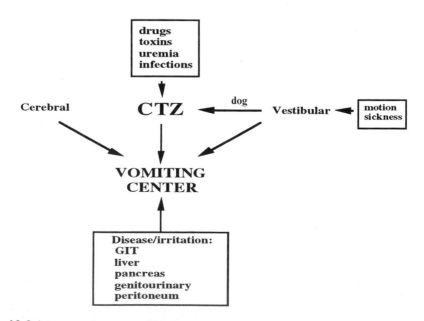

Fig. 18-8 Initiation of vomiting. *CTZ,* Chemoreceptor trigger zone; *GIT,* gastrointestinal tract.

toxins or drugs to stimulate the CTZ. Neurologic input from the vestibular nucleus can also stimulate the CTZ in the dog or the vomiting center. Disease or irritation of the GIT, abdominal organs, or peritoneum and cerebral diseases can directly stimulate the vomiting center via visceral receptors and vagal afferents.

Once the vomiting center is adequately stimulated, a series of visceral events is initiated. This sequence of events includes inhibition of proximal gastrointestinal motility, a retrograde power contraction in the small intestine, and antral relaxation, which enables transfer of intestinal contents to the stomach. These events are followed by moderate-amplitude contractions in the gastric antrum and intestine and shortening of the intraabdominal esophagus. Dilatation of the cardia and lower esophageal sphincter enables transfer of gastric contents to the esophagus during retching and vomiting. Retching often precedes vomiting and is characterized by rhythmic inspiratory movements against a closed glottis. Negative intrathoracic pressure during retching prevents expulsion of esophageal contents. During vomiting, the abdominal muscles contract and intrathoracic and intraabdominal pressures are positive, resulting in forceful expulsion of gastric contents from the mouth.

Vomiting is associated with a wide range of disease processes and, when frequent or severe, can have major effects on fluid, electrolyte, and acid-base balance. The consequences of vomiting depend to some extent on the cause. Vomiting of gastric and intestinal contents usually involves loss of fluid containing Cl^-, K^+, Na^+, and HCO_3^-, and dehydration is accompanied to a variable extent by hypochloremia, hypokalemia, and hyponatremia.[15,95] Metabolic acidosis is generally more common than metabolic alkalosis in dogs with gastrointestinal disease.[15]

With obstruction of the gastric outflow tract or proximal duodenum, loss of Cl^- can exceed that of HCO_3^-, and hypochloremia, hypokalemia, and metabolic alkalosis result.[15,72,95] Metabolic alkalosis is self-perpetuating because of increased renal reabsorption of $NaHCO_3$ in the presence of volume, chloride, and potassium depletion.[74] These metabolic disturbances arise as a result of preferential conservation of volume at the expense of extracellular pH. The renal reabsorption of almost all filtered HCO_3^- and the exchange of sodium for hydrogen ions in the distal tubule promote an acidic urine pH despite extracellular alkalemia (so-called paradoxical aciduria).[74,96]

Metabolic alkalosis in patients with gastrointestinal signs is not invariably associated with outflow obstruction and has been encountered in dogs with parvovirus enteritis and acute pancreatitis.[33] Diseases characterized by hypersecretion of acid, such as gastrinoma, may also be associated with metabolic alkalosis and aciduria. Basal gastric acid secretion in two dogs with gastrin-producing tumors (1.7 and 2.7 $mmol/hr/kg^{0.75}$ HCl) was maximal in the unstimulated state.[87] In this situation, hypochloremia, hypokalemia, metabolic alkalosis, and dehydration are probably caused by gastric hypersecretion of acid.[87]

DIARRHEA

The pathomechanisms in patients with diarrhea include increased intestinal secretion, decreased intestinal absorption, rapid transit of intestinal contents, and mesenteric, vascular, or lymphatic disease.[64]

Secretory agents include neuropeptides of the enteric system (found in neuroendocrine tumors), cholinergic agonists, gastrointestinal hormones, bacterial enterotoxins, deconjugated bile acids, and hydroxy fatty acids.[64] Secretory diarrhea results when prosecretory stimulation overwhelms absorptive forces. Secretory diarrhea is manifested by increased colonic secretion of sodium-rich fluid. Volume depletion resulting from sodium and water loss stimulates antidiuretic hormone release, which in turn stimulates water retention by the kidneys and dilutional hyponatremia.

Decreased intestinal absorption may result from decreased intestinal surface area as a consequence of damage by infectious agents (e.g., parvovirus), cellular infiltration, or surgery. Damage to the intestinal epithelial barrier may also increase intestinal permeability, disrupting paracellular and transcellular absorptive pathways. An increase in the osmolality of intestinal contents may also decrease absorption. Specific causes of osmotic diarrhea include overeating, sudden dietary change, osmotic laxative ingestion, maldigestion, or malabsorption. Absorption of water and electrolytes is retarded by accumulation of nonabsorbable solutes in the gut lumen, and there is net water movement from plasma to the gut lumen. In osmotic diarrhea, the concentration of sodium in the stool may remain below that of plasma, leading to water loss in excess of sodium, dehydration, and hypernatremia, especially when water intake is inadequate.[26] This finding has been observed in dogs and people with hepatic encephalopathy (HE) treated with lactulose.[62] Intestinal absorption may also be affected by diseases that cause increased venous pressure, lymphatic pressure, decreased interstitial osmotic pressure (hypoalbuminemia), and increased epithelial permeability. Disorders of intestinal motility result in decreased intestinal fluid absorption because of decreased contact time between luminal contents and the enterocytes.

An understanding of these pathomechanisms is useful in identifying the pathophysiology and establishing appropriate treatment of patients with diarrhea, but diarrhea caused by only one mechanism is rare in clinical practice. For example, a dog with inflammatory bowel disease may have decreased intestinal absorption caused by decreased surface area, increased mucosal permeability, increased intraluminal osmotic forces, and decreased interstitial osmotic forces coupled with rapid transit of intestinal contents and increased intestinal secretion.

Fluid and Electrolyte Abnormalities in Diarrhea

The fluid and electrolyte abnormalities associated with diarrhea include volume depletion, hyponatremia or hypernatremia, hypokalemia, and metabolic acidosis.[15,58,95] The metabolic acidosis that develops is characterized by hyperchloremia and a normal anion gap caused by loss of diarrheal fluid with relatively low chloride and high bicarbonate concentrations. Serious electrolyte and acid-base abnormalities are relatively uncommon in patients with diarrhea as a sole complaint. When diarrhea is severe and protracted or is accompanied by vomiting, acid-base and electrolyte disturbances are more likely, but it is difficult to predict which abnormalities will be present. For example, decreased total CO_2 concentrations were identified in less than 17% of 134 dogs with parvovirus enteritis in one study,[38] whereas metabolic alkalosis and hypochloremia were more common than metabolic acidosis in another study of dogs with parvovirus enteritis.[33] Another study of 22 dogs infected with parvovirus identified lower plasma concentrations of sodium, potassium, chloride, and bicarbonate than controls. Serum L-lactate concentrations were increased in some puppies with canine parvoviral enteritis, but most affected puppies developed only mild compensated metabolic acidosis.[61]

Hypoadrenocorticism should be ruled out whenever hyperkalemia and hyponatremia are present, but up to 26% of dogs with hypoadrenocorticism may have normal mineralocorticoid function and normal Na/K ratios.[48] Therefore a history of intermittent signs of gastrointestinal disease may warrant an adrenocorticotropic hormone stimulation test despite a normal Na/K ratio. Clinicopathologic findings in dogs with primary gastrointestinal disease may mimic those of hypoadrenocorticism with Na/K ratios less than 27:1 and metabolic acidosis.[21,51] Gastrointestinal diseases reported to mimic primary hypoadrenocorticism include trichuriasis, ancylostomiasis, salmonellosis, and perforated duodenal ulcer. Postulated mechanisms of these electrolyte derangements include metabolic acidosis secondary to volume depletion and fecal loss of bicarbonate with subsequent translocation of potassium from intracellular to extracellular fluid. Selective aldosterone deficiency does not appear to be responsible for hyperkalemia and hyponatremia in dogs with trichuriasis that have laboratory abnormalities that mimic those of hypoadrenocorticism.[27] Hypocalcemia and hypomagnesemia occur uncommonly in veterinary patients with diarrhea and are most often encountered in animals with protein-losing enteropathy. Ionized hypocalcemia and hypomagnesemia have been described in Yorkshire terriers with diarrhea, abdominal effusion, leukocytosis, neutrophilia,

hypoproteinemia, hypoalbuminemia, hypocholesterolemia, and increased serum activity of aspartate aminotransferase. The hypomagnesemia and hypocalcemia potentially were the result of intestinal loss, malabsorption, and abnormalities of vitamin D and parathyroid hormone metabolism.[42]

Normal stool water contains a higher concentration of potassium than sodium.[26] As stool volumes increase in human patients with diarrhea, there is a progressive increase in the sodium and chloride concentrations and a decrease in potassium concentration, and the electrolyte composition of the stool approaches that of plasma.[26] In cases of diarrhea, there is a linear relationship between fluid and sodium loss.[26] In human patients, measurements of fecal electrolyte concentrations and osmolality are used to calculate an osmolality gap, which aids in the differentiation of osmotic and secretory diarrhea. The osmolality, sodium concentration, and potassium concentration of feces from four normal cats were reported as 622 to 927 mOsm/kg, 27 to 57 mEq/L, and 19 to 46 mEq/L, respectively.[28] Stool normally contains high concentrations of potassium, and fecal potassium loss can become severe in protracted diarrheal states.[26] Stimulation of the renin-aldosterone axis as a result of volume depletion has been suggested as one potential cause of potassium loss.[58]

Dogs with gastrin-secreting tumors may be presented for evaluation of intermittent or profuse watery diarrhea, vomiting, and weight loss. In this setting, diarrhea and vomiting are probably a result of the increased volume and acidity of gastric secretions, which cause gastrointestinal ulceration and destruction of pancreatic enzymes.[87] The high concentrations of gastrin may also adversely affect intestinal function.

In humans, profuse watery intermittent or fulminant diarrhea can be caused by tumors secreting VIP (VIPomas).[46] The majority of these tumors are located in the pancreas, although the VIPoma syndrome has been associated with tumors at a number of other sites in humans. Additional findings include severe hypokalemia, metabolic acidosis, and occasionally hypochlorhydria. The profound secretory diarrhea results from the stimulatory action of VIP on intestinal secretion. The VIPoma syndrome differs from gastrinoma in that patients with VIPoma have normal serum gastrin concentrations and lack gastric acid hypersecretion and secondary upper GIT ulceration. Increased concentrations of VIP and motilin (VIP, 927 pg/mL; normal range, 0 to 84 pg/mL; motilin, 341 pg/mL; normal range, 0 to 125 pg/mL) have been documented in a dog with severe diarrhea and a heart base tumor. The dog had metabolic acidosis, hypokalemia, a normal anion gap, and no evidence of renal potassium wasting (Richter and Simpson, unpublished observations).

MANAGEMENT OF DISORDERS OF THE GASTROINTESTINAL TRACT

OVERVIEW OF FLUID THERAPY FOR VOMITING AND DIARRHEA

Correction of volume, electrolyte, and acid-base disturbances is an essential part of the management of patients with vomiting and diarrhea. The most appropriate type, route, and rate of fluid replacement are chosen based on the patient's hydration, tissue perfusion, and electrolyte and acid-base status. The presence of anemia or hypoalbuminemia and the potential for continuing fluid loss through vomiting, diarrhea, fever, and compensatory hyperventilation associated with metabolic acidosis must also be taken into account. Minimal evaluation of the patient with gastrointestinal disease should include determination of body temperature, heart rate, skin turgor, capillary refill time, packed cell volume (PCV), total protein concentration, urine specific gravity, and urine pH, as well as serum concentrations of sodium, potassium, chloride, total CO_2, and glucose. Measurement of blood gases, blood pressure (central venous and arterial), and urine output is required for optimal care of patients with severe gastrointestinal disease.

Oral fluid therapy may be useful for patients with diarrhea that can tolerate oral intake. Subcutaneous administration of an isotonic balanced electrolyte solution may be sufficient to correct mild ($\leq 5\%$) fluid deficits but is insufficient for patients with moderate (5% to 10%) or severe (>10%) dehydration. For patients with moderate to severe dehydration, inadequate oral intake, electrolyte imbalance, or signs of hypovolemic or endotoxic shock, intravenous fluid administration is necessary.

The rate of fluid administration depends on the presence or absence of shock, the extent of dehydration, and the presence of cardiac or renal disease that may predispose the patient to volume overload. Patients with a history of vomiting that are mildly dehydrated are usually responsive to crystalloids (e.g., lactated Ringer's solution or 9% NaCl) at a rate that provides maintenance needs and replaces existing deficits and ongoing losses over a 24-hour period. Patients with signs of shock require more aggressive support. The volume deficit can be replaced with crystalloids at an initial rate of 60 to 90 mL/kg/hr, which is then tailored to maintain tissue perfusion and hydration. Central venous pressure monitoring and evaluation of urine output are necessary for patients with severe gastrointestinal disease, especially those with third-space losses of fluid into the gut or peritoneum. Colloids and hypertonic solutions can also be used to reduce the amount of crystalloid required (e.g., 5 mL/kg of 7% NaCl in 6% dextran intravenously, 10 to 20 mL/kg/day of degraded gelatin [Haemaccel] intra-venously). Colloids are also useful in hypoproteinemic patients. Endotoxic shock is a common complication of severe gastrointestinal disease. Warning signs of endotoxemic shock include fever or subnormal body temperature, tachycardia, increased respiratory rate, slow capillary refill time, hyperemic or pale mucous membranes, transient leukopenia followed by leukocytosis with a left shift and toxic neutrophils, low-normal central venous pressure, and bounding pulses. Patients with endotoxic shock must be treated aggressively with fluid therapy, broad-spectrum antibiotics, glucocorticoids, oxygen, glucose, and bicarbonate as indicated.[32]

The effect of vomiting and diarrhea on acid-base balance is difficult to predict, and therapeutic intervention to correct acid-base imbalance should be based on blood gas analysis. Patients with normal acid-base status or mild metabolic acidosis may be given lactated Ringer's solution at a rate sufficient to correct fluid deficits and provide for maintenance and ongoing losses for a 24-hour period. Potassium depletion may be a consequence of prolonged diarrhea, vomiting, or anorexia, but most polyionic replacement fluids contain only small amounts of potassium. Consequently, KCl is usually added to parenteral fluids and adjusted based on serum potassium concentrations. When severe metabolic acidosis is present (pH < 7.1; $HCO_3^- < 10$ mEq/L), sodium bicarbonate (1 mEq/kg) can be given. Care should be taken to rule out respiratory acidosis before administering sodium bicarbonate and to administer it slowly and in small amounts (0.5 mEq/kg over 15 minutes) to prevent cerebrospinal fluid acidosis, aggravation of hypokalemia, or hypocalcemia. Additional bicarbonate supplementation is based on repeated blood gas analyses. Metabolic alkalosis usually responds to correction of the volume, chloride, and potassium deficits with 0.9% NaCl supplemented with KCl administered intravenously.

Diagnostic investigations should initially focus on ruling out upper gastrointestinal obstruction. Administration of antisecretory drugs (e.g., H_2 antagonists) may limit chloride efflux into gastric juice. When acid hypersecretion is present or suspected, it is best managed by administration of a proton pump inhibitor (e.g., omeprazole at 0.2 to 0.7 mg/kg every 24 hours). Somatostatin analogues may also be useful to control gastric acid hypersecretion (e.g., octreotide at 2 to 20 µg/kg subcutaneously every 8 hours).[87]

Other symptomatic treatments considered initially in patients with vomiting and diarrhea are nothing by mouth and antiemetics or antacids when vomiting persists. Prophylactic use of antibiotics (e.g., cephalosporins, ampicillin) may be warranted in animals with shock and suspected gastrointestinal barrier dysfunction. Analgesia can be provided using opioids (e.g., buprenorphine at 0.0075 to 0.01 mg/kg intramuscularly).

Oral Rehydration Solutions

The rationale for use of oral rehydration solutions (ORSs) is the coupled transport of sodium with glucose or other actively transported small organic molecules and hence the promotion of water absorption.[17,25] These cotransport processes often remain relatively unaffected in acute infectious (e.g., bacterial, viral) cases of diarrhea.[93] In secretory diarrhea, the epithelium maintains its absorptive capacity and cotransport processes that are important for the success of oral rehydration therapy.[93] With certain viral causes of diarrhea (e.g., rotaviral infection in children), patchy epithelial damage may allow oral rehydration to be of benefit.[78,79] A balanced ORS has a carbohydrate-to-sodium ratio of 1:1 to 2:1, potassium, chloride, an alkali source, and an osmolality between 250 and 310 mOsm/kg. The ideal formula still remains controversial.[89,93] Alkali sources such as bicarbonate and citrate also enhance the absorption of water and electrolytes.[90]

Clinical trials of ORSs containing complex carbohydrates or glucose polymers in place of glucose have resulted in decreased volume and duration of diarrhea. A potential explanation for the beneficial effect of such solutions is that glucose polymer molecules contain more glucose residues without delivering a high osmotic load to the intestinal lumen. Much of the breakdown of the polymer occurs at the epithelial surface, and the smaller molecules do not accumulate in the intestinal lumen. The relative hypotonicity of glucose polymer solutions may be the major contributor to their efficacy.[93]

In children, oral electrolyte solutions can be used to treat mild to severe dehydration even in the presence of vomiting as long as the patient is able to swallow small amounts frequently.[4] A volume equal to the amount that would be given intravenously is appropriate. Reports of the effectiveness of ORSs in veterinary patients are limited, but favorable results have been reported in the treatment of uncomplicated acute gastroenteritis in dogs and cats with Pedialyte (Abbott Laboratories, Abbott Park, IL) at a daily dosage of 150 mL/kg body weight until a bland diet could be reintroduced.[73] Commercial solutions such as Pedialyte are readily available but usually contain too much glucose and too little sodium and carry some risk of hypertonic diarrhea.[73] A more physiologic solution recommended by the World Health Organization contains 90 mEq/L sodium, 20 mEq/L potassium, 80 mEq/L chloride, 30 mEq/L bicarbonate, and 111 mmol/L glucose. Such a solution can be prepared by adding 3.5 g NaCl, 2.5 g $NaHCO_3$, 1.5 g KCl, and 20 g glucose to 1 L water.[73]

Nutritional Support

Growing evidence suggests that providing enteral nutrition, rather than nothing by mouth, is beneficial to patients with gastroenteritis or pancreatitis. In one study, dogs with parvovirus infection experienced increased weight gain, shorter hospital stay, decreased morbidity, and a trend toward decreased intestinal permeability (a risk factor for bacterial translocation and endotoxic shock) when fed through nasoesophageal tubes despite the presence of vomiting and diarrhea as compared with dogs in which feeding was delayed until diarrhea and vomiting had subsided.[55] Studies in dogs with experimentally induced acute pancreatitis have shown no detrimental effects of enteral feeding and better intestinal morphology and barrier function with enteral as compared with parenteral nutrition.[68,69]

Patient Monitoring

For stable patients, minimal monitoring includes regular assessment of vital signs and fluid and electrolyte balance. In patients with systemic abnormalities, monitoring should be more aggressive and should include vital signs, weight, PCV, total protein concentration, fluid intake and output, blood pressure (central venous and arterial), and determination of serum concentrations of electrolytes and glucose, acid-base status, platelets, and coagulation status.

PROTEIN-LOSING ENTEROPATHY

Hypoproteinemia characterized by a decrease in both albumin and globulin often is associated with gastrointestinal disease or blood loss. When total protein or albumin concentrations decrease to less than 4.0 g/dL or 1.5 g/dL, respectively, some type of natural or synthetic colloid replacement can be instituted to avoid interstitial fluid accumulation and pulmonary edema.[94] Benefit from colloid administration is often short lived because colloids are rapidly lost into the gut. The short duration of effect and the expense of colloids have resulted in the use of colloids for brief support, whereas long-term treatment is focused on the underlying cause of the protein loss. As described previously, ionized hypocalcemia and hypomagnesemia have been described in Yorkshire terriers with protein-losing enteropathy and may require treatment in some cases.[42] Severe hypomagnesemia (0.8 mg/dL; normal range, 1.6 to 2.3 mg/dL), hypocalcemia, and protein-losing enteropathy also have been reported in a 5-year-old castrated male shih tzu examined because of anorexia, lethargy, paresis, and abdominal distention caused by lymphangiectasia and intestinal inflammation. Treatment included administration of magnesium (0.8 mEq/kg) in a balanced electrolyte solution and resulted in normalization of serum magnesium concentration to 1.7 mg/dL, as well as resolution of lethargy, paresis, and tachycardia. Serum concentrations of ionized calcium and parathyroid hormone also increased after treatment, and findings were thought to be consistent with secondary hypoparathyroidism attributable to hypomagnesemia.[10]

GASTRIC DILATATION AND VOLVULUS

Gastric dilatation and gastric dilatation-volvulus (GDV) are life-threatening conditions that are frequently accompanied by severe hypovolemic shock. Hypovolemic shock arises as a consequence of impaired venous return caused by obstruction of the caudal vena cava by gastric distention. Devitalization of the gastric wall, splenic torsion, congestion of abdominal viscera, and endotoxic shock further exacerbate the hypovolemic crisis.

A variety of acid-base and electrolyte disturbances have been observed in dogs with GDV.[59,99] Metabolic acidosis and hypokalemia were the most common abnormalities in one study, occurring in 15 of 57 and 16 of 57 dogs, respectively.[59] Metabolic acidosis is probably caused by decreased tissue perfusion, anaerobic metabolism, and accumulation of lactic acid.[59] Metabolic alkalosis may also occur as a result of vomiting or sequestration of acid in the stomach.[59] Either respiratory acidosis or respiratory alkalosis may be observed and reflect hypoventilation or hyperventilation, respectively. The variety of acid-base and electrolyte abnormalities in dogs with GDV dictates that fluid therapy be individualized based on blood gas analysis and serum electrolyte concentrations.

Plasma lactate concentration appears to be a good predictor of gastric necrosis and survival among dogs with GDV.[20] In this study, 69 of 70 (99%) dogs with plasma lactate concentrations less than 6.0 mmol/L survived, whereas 18 of 31 (58%) dogs with plasma lactate concentrations more than 6.0 mmol/L did not. Gastric necrosis was identified in 38 (37%) dogs. The median plasma lactate concentration in dogs with gastric necrosis (6.6 mmol/L) was significantly higher than that in dogs without gastric necrosis (3.3 mmol/L). The specificity and sensitivity of plasma lactate concentration (with a cutoff of 6.0 mmol/L) for predicting which dogs had gastric necrosis were 88% and 61%, respectively. Sixty-two of 63 (98%) dogs without gastric necrosis survived compared with 25 of 38 (66%) dogs with gastric necrosis.

Gastric decompression and fluid therapy are the most important emergency treatments for dogs with GDV. Fluid therapy has traditionally consisted of shock doses (60 to 90 mL/kg/hr) of lactated Ringer's solution given via large-gauge catheters into the cephalic or jugular veins. Experimental studies that have compared crystalloids (60 mL/kg 0.9% NaCl followed by 20 mL/kg/hr) with hypertonic saline (5 mL/kg 7% NaCl in 6% dextran followed by 0.9% NaCl 20 mL/kg/hr) in dogs with GDV-induced shock indicated that hypertonic saline maintains better myocardial performance, higher heart rate, and lower systemic vascular resistance than crystalloid alone.[2] The resuscitative dose of hypertonic saline was delivered in 5 to 10 minutes as compared with 1 hour for the crystalloid. Potassium and bicarbonate are best administered based on blood gas and electrolyte measurements.

ACUTE PANCREATITIS

Acute pancreatitis is a potentially life-threatening condition affecting dogs and cats.[34,35,83,84,88] Clinical abnormalities are highly variable and in dogs range from mild dehydration and vomiting to shock, hemorrhagic diathesis, and death. Anorexia, lethargy, and weight loss are the most common clinical signs in cats with pancreatitis. The severity of clinical signs is thought to reflect the severity of pancreatitis (i.e., mild edematous versus severe necrotizing or suppurative) and the presence of systemic complications such as shock, pancreatic infection and necrosis, sepsis, and disseminated intravascular coagulation.

The cause of acute pancreatitis in dogs and cats usually remains undetermined. Regardless of the initiating cause, active pancreatic enzymes (e.g., trypsin, phospholipase, collagenase, elastase) and inflammatory mediators (e.g., kallikreins, kinins, free radicals, complement components, thromboplastins) are released in an active form into the pancreatic tissues and blood vessels. Activated factor XII (Hageman's factor) and trypsin appear to be largely responsible for activation of the coagulation, fibrinolytic, kinin, and complement cascades. Pancreatic defense mechanisms limit trypsinogen activation within the pancreas, and circulating α_1-antitrypsin and α_2-macroglobulin bind to active enzymes and prevent systemic damage.[52,63,86]

When these defense systems are overwhelmed, increased pancreatic capillary permeability leads to fluid loss into the pancreas and peritoneal cavity, a decrease in pancreatic blood flow, and further release of active pancreatic enzymes and inflammatory mediators such as tumor necrosis factor (TNF-α), interleukin-1 (IL-1), and platelet-activating factor (PAF) from the inflamed pancreas. Large numbers of leukocytes migrate to the inflamed pancreas and serve as a continued source of free radicals, inflammatory mediators, and enzymes amplifying the severity of pancreatic inflammation and precipitating thrombosis of pancreatic blood vessels, as well as contributing to pancreatic necrosis. The systemic inflammatory response contributes to widespread derangements in fluid, electrolyte, and acid-base balance and is associated with adverse effects in many organ systems, including impaired cardiovascular (e.g., hypovolemic shock, myocardial damage), hematologic (e.g., disseminated intravascular coagulation), respiratory (e.g., pleural effusion), hepatic (e.g., hepatic parenchymal damage, biliary stasis), renal (e.g., glomerular and tubular damage), and metabolic (e.g., lipemia, hypocalcemia, diabetes mellitus, hypoproteinemia) function.[8,19,53,70,75] The development of multisystemic abnormalities separates mild from severe, potentially fatal pancreatitis. Increased understanding of the systemic inflammatory response holds the promise of novel treatments for acute pancreatitis and is a focus of current research.[39,65] Bacterial translocation from the inflamed and permeable GIT may further exacerbate the disease process, causing endotoxic shock, pancreatic necrosis and infection, or pancreatic abscess formation.

Many electrolyte and acid-base disturbances have been reported in dogs and cats with acute pancreatitis. Hypokalemia, hypoglycemia, hyponatremia, hypochloremia, hypocalcemia, hypoalbuminemia, and azotemia have been reported.* Hyperkalemia, hypernatremia, and hypercalcemia have been observed less commonly. Hypokalemia, hypochloremia, and hyponatremia are probably consequences of increased loss of these electrolytes in vomitus or diarrhea, decreased oral intake, and transcellular shifts. Concomitant diabetes mellitus also contributes. Hypoproteinemia is more common in dogs with acute pancreatitis than in cats and is thought to be a consequence of intrapancreatic and peripancreatic exudation of albumin. Hypoalbuminemia also contributes to the hypocalcemia observed in dogs with pancreatitis,[54] and hypoalbuminemia and decreased total serum calcium concentration were among the few clinicopathologic changes noted in cats with experimentally induced acute pancreatitis.[44] However, hypocalcemia is not always attributable to hypoalbuminemia and did not account for the hypocalcemia observed in 30% of 40 cats with naturally occurring fatal pancreatitis.[35] The need to measure serum ionized calcium concentrations in cats with pancreatitis is highlighted by a study of 46 cats with acute pancreatitis in which low serum total calcium concentration was present in 19 of 46 (41%) cats, but plasma ionized calcium concentration was low in 28 of 46 (61%).[43] This study demonstrated that cats with pancreatitis had a significantly lower median plasma ionized calcium concentration (1.07 mmol/L) than did control cats (1.12 mmol/L). Cats with pancreatitis that died or were euthanatized had significantly lower median plasma ionized calcium concentrations (1.00 mmol/L) than did cats that survived (1.12 mmol/L). Ten of the 13 cats with pancreatitis that had plasma ionized calcium concentrations of 1.00 mmol/L or less died or were euthanatized. Additional studies of the mechanisms responsible for the changes in serum ionized calcium concentration in this setting (e.g., alteration of the parathyroid-calcium axis and sequestration of calcium in the pancreas and other tissues) clearly is needed.[5,6,37,71]

Hypercalcemia has been reported in dogs with acute pancreatitis.[34] The clinical relevance of this finding remains unclear because serum total calcium concentrations were corrected for albumin and ionized calcium concentrations were not measured.[67] Hyperglycemia and glucosuria are especially frequent in cats with pancreatitis, but ketonuria is infrequent, suggesting that stress may be a more common cause for these abnormalities than diabetes mellitus. However, mild diabetes mellitus or recrudescence of a previous diabetic state may occur in cats with acute pancreatitis. Azotemia is usually present and is often prerenal or renal in origin. Some studies report a high frequency of concurrent pancreatitis and nephritis,[23,50] whereas others[35,84] do not. Clarification of a possible relationship between pancreatitis and renal disease awaits future studies. Acid-base abnormalities in dogs and cats with acute pancreatitis usually consist of metabolic acidosis, but metabolic alkalosis may also be observed.[34]

Medical management of acute pancreatitis is usually initiated before the diagnosis is confirmed and is based on presenting clinical findings and laboratory abnormalities (e.g., PCV, urinalysis, and total protein, blood urea nitrogen, glucose, sodium, and potassium concentrations). See the information given earlier in the section on Overview of Fluid Therapy for Vomiting and Diarrhea. Hypovolemia and dehydration are evaluated and corrected by intravenous administration of fluids. The type of fluid chosen should be based on serum electrolytes (e.g., sodium, potassium, chloride, total CO_2) to restore normal electrolyte and acid-base balance. Hypocalcemia usually is not associated with tetany or seizures, and the value of supplementing calcium in patients with ionized hypocalcemia, especially cats in which hypocalcemia has been associated with prognosis, remains to be determined. If hypoglycemia is present, dextrose (2.5% to 5%) is added to the fluids. Insulin therapy is initiated if hyperglycemia, glucosuria, and ketonuria are present. Stress hyperglycemia should be ruled out when ketonuria is absent.

Other symptomatic treatments initially considered include nothing by mouth and antiemetics or antacids when vomiting is persistent. Centrally acting antiemetics such as metoclopramide or phenothiazine derivatives are indicated for patients with intractable vomiting. Prophylactic use of antibiotics (i.e., cephalosporins or ampicillin alone or in combination with enrofloxacin or amikacin) may be warranted for patients with shock, fever, diabetes mellitus, or hemorrhagic diarrhea or vomitus. Analgesia can be provided using opioids (e.g., buprenorphine at 0.0075 to 0.01 mg/kg intramuscularly).

After a diagnosis of pancreatitis is confirmed, fluid therapy is continued, and more specific therapy may be used. The majority of dogs with acute pancreatitis respond to fluid therapy and nothing by mouth for 48 hours. More specific therapy is usually reserved for dogs that do not respond to fluid therapy or that have signs of disseminated intravascular coagulation. In contrast to dogs, cats with acute pancreatitis are more commonly presented with anorexia than vomiting, but episodes of pancreatic inflammation appear to be more protracted. No treatment regimens for pancreatitis have been critically evaluated in dogs or cats with naturally occurring pancreatitis.

Specific therapy in humans consists of preventing further pancreatitis from developing and limiting the local and systemic consequences of pancreatitis. Therapy aimed at inhibiting pancreatic secretion (e.g., glucagon,

---

*References 23,34,35,66,80,84.

somatostatin) or intracellular activation of proteases (e.g., gabexate mesylate) that has been beneficial in ameliorating experimental pancreatitis has shown little benefit in the treatment of clinical patients. This lack of success may be related to the timing of therapy in relation to the development of pancreatitis. Therapy in experimental pancreatitis is usually initiated before or shortly after induction of pancreatitis, whereas most clinical patients are not presented until 24 to 48 hours after the onset of pancreatitis. These findings have led to more therapeutic emphasis on limitation of damage, including limiting the effects of inflammatory mediators or pancreatic enzymes and maintaining pancreatic perfusion.

The systemic effects of pancreatitis may be ameliorated in experimental animals by maintaining adequate pancreatic microcirculation and protease-antiprotease balance. The pancreatic microcirculation in dogs with experimental pancreatitis was maintained more effectively by use of dextran-containing solutions than by use of crystalloids.[36,45] The pancreatic microcirculation of cats with experimental pancreatitis was maintained by low-dose dopamine infusion (5 μg/kg/min).[41] Natural protease inhibitors contained in plasma help restore protease-antiprotease balance when administered in large volumes.[18] For this reason, it may be beneficial to administer fresh frozen plasma (10 to 20 mL/kg) to dogs with pancreatitis. Administration of fresh frozen plasma may also be beneficial for management of disseminated intravascular coagulation or other coagulopathies. Heparin administration (75 to 150 U/kg subcutaneously every 8 hours) may be warranted in the early stages of acute pancreatitis to delay development of disseminated intravascular coagulation. Heparin may also clear lipemia, which is a frequent finding in acute pancreatitis. Clearing of lipemia facilitates performance and interpretation of serum biochemistry tests. Oral pancreatic enzyme extracts have been reported to reduce pain in humans with chronic pancreatitis but are less likely to be effective in dogs because dogs do not appear to have a protease-mediated negative feedback system.

Emerging evidence in human patients and experimental animals supports a primary role for enteral rather than parenteral nutrition in the management of acute pancreatitis. In both humans and animals, jejunal feeding (i.e., distal to the site of pancreatic stimulation) does not exacerbate acute pancreatitis.[68,69,97] People with acute pancreatitis fed via jejunostomy tubes (including oral transpyloric tubes) experience lower morbidity, decreased systemic inflammatory response, and shorter hospital stays and incur less medical expense than those treated using total parenteral nutrition.[22,40] It now is feasible to place jejunostomy tubes nonsurgically in dogs through the nose, esophagus, or stomach, and clinical application of this feeding strategy is not restricted by requirement of a surgical procedure. However, it remains uncertain whether dogs with acute pancreatitis require jejunal delivery of nutrients. Evidence suggests that the pancreas in dogs with experimentally induced acute pancreatitis and in people with severe naturally occurring pancreatitis may not be as amenable to stimulation as the normal pancreas. Dogs recovering from naturally occurring pancreatitis also have been shown to have subnormal serum concentrations of trypsin-like immunoreactivity, suggesting that pancreatic enzyme synthesis is down-regulated. In addition, the major benefits of enteral support in human patients and experimental dogs with acute pancreatitis are caused by reductions in the systemic inflammatory response and translocation of enteric bacteria rather than by a reduction in pancreatic stimulation. Feeding a liquid diet (41% protein, 18% fat, 3% crude fiber) through a nasoesophageal tube positively impacts intestinal permeability and morbidity in dogs with parvovirus enteritis. These findings support the idea that enteral feeding in general, rather than jejunal delivery of nutrients, is the primary reason for the beneficial effects of enteral nutrition, but this hypothesis needs to be critically evaluated.[55] Parenteral nutrition should not be abandoned completely, but its use should be restricted to patients with the greatest need for it (e.g., those in which caloric intake is severely impaired by persistent vomiting). When parenteral nutrition is indicated, a choice must be made between total and partial parenteral nutrition. Partial parenteral nutrition is a more practical and manageable procedure than total parenteral nutrition in most settings and has been shown to be a safe and effective way of providing nutrition to dogs with pancreatitis and gastrointestinal disease.[11] Interestingly, dogs and cats that received a combination of enteral and partial parenteral nutrition survived more often than those receiving only partial parenteral nutrition.[11] Parenteral nutrition is discussed further in Chapter 25.

SMALL-BOWEL OBSTRUCTION

Intestinal obstruction can be classified as acute or chronic, partial or complete, and simple or strangulated. The cause of obstruction may be extraluminal compression, intramural thickening, or an intraluminal mass. The most common extraluminal cause of obstruction is intussusception.[98] Intestinal neoplasia is the most common intramural cause of obstruction in veterinary patients, but hematoma, focal granulomas related to feline infectious peritonitis, inflammatory bowel disease, stricture, and phycomycosis are also observed.[31,56,57] Foreign objects such as peach pits, toys, and fishhooks are common causes of intraluminal obstruction in dogs, whereas string linear foreign objects (frequently anchored under the tongue) are common in cats. The adverse effects of intestinal obstruction are a consequence of fluid loss into the GIT, proliferation of intestinal bacteria, and inflammation of the intestine.[16] Intestinal perforation further exacerbates the clinical situation and is common with linear foreign objects and intestinal neoplasia.

Vomiting would be expected to be a major feature of intestinal obstruction. However, complete intestinal obstruction in dogs is frequently not associated with vomiting.[47,82] Clinical signs are more often related to marked loss of fluid and electrolytes into the intestine. Bowel distention causes a steady decrease in intestinal absorptive capacity and an increase in the secretion of sodium, potassium, and albumin into the lumen.[47] With complete obstruction of the ileum, there is a gradual increase in the secretion of sodium, potassium, and water into the obstructed bowel, which can reach 13 mL/min after 60 hours of obstruction.[82] Metabolic acidosis is a consequence of bicarbonate loss, dehydration, and starvation.[47] Stagnated luminal contents and impaired motility provide a favorable environment for the proliferation of bacteria and the elaboration of bacterial toxins. Anoxia and devitalization of the bowel wall allow translocation of bacteria and toxins transmurally and then systemically. If untreated, potentially fatal endotoxemic shock can develop. Partial obstruction, especially of the distal small intestine, can be associated with chronic diarrhea and weight loss caused by intestinal stasis, and affected animals may have a history of responding to antibiotic treatment.

Physical findings range from mild dehydration to signs of septic shock and depend on the severity of fluid loss, fluid shifts, and intestinal compromise caused by obstruction. Shock and abdominal pain are often the predominant findings with strangulated obstructions such as intestinal volvulus, incarcerated obstructions, and intussusception.

Fluid therapy should be instituted based on clinical findings and initial laboratory findings. Fluid shifts can be severe, and close monitoring of central venous pressure, PCV, total protein concentration, urine output, acid-base status, and electrolyte concentrations is often initiated to detect and correct changes in fluid balance. Hypochloremia and hypokalemia are frequent in patients with intestinal obstruction. Metabolic alkalosis suggests upper duodenal obstruction. Fluid balance and electrolyte abnormalities should be corrected before surgery. In animals with experimental intestinal obstruction, administration of crystalloids caused a decrease in plasma oncotic pressure and net loss of fluid into the distended intestinal lumen, whereas colloids transiently increased plasma oncotic pressure and allowed the jejunum to maintain normal absorptive capacity.[1] Antibiotics effective against gram-negative and gram-positive aerobic and anaerobic bacteria are administered to patients with signs of sepsis or intestinal compromise and can be used prophylactically before surgery. The prognosis depends on the cause of obstruction and severity of clinical abnormalities associated with it. The prognosis ranges from very good for simple foreign bodies to grave for metastatic intestinal neoplasia. If a large portion of the intestine must be removed, the patient may be at risk for developing short-bowel syndrome.

REFERENCES

1. Allen D, Krietys PR, Grainger DN: Crystalloids versus colloids: implications in fluid therapy of dogs with intestinal obstruction, *Am J Vet Res* 47:1751-1755, 1986.
2. Allen DA, Schertel ER, Muir WW, et al: Hypertonic saline/dextran resuscitation of dogs with experimentally induced gastric dilatation-volvulus shock, *Am J Vet Res* 52:92-96, 1991.
3. Argent BE, Case RM: Pancreatic ducts: cellular mechanism and control of bicarbonate. In Johnson LR, editor: *Physiology of the gastrointestinal tract*, ed 3, New York, 1994, Raven Press, p. 1473.
4. Avery ME, Snyder JD: Oral therapy for acute diarrhea: the underused simple solution, *N Engl J Med* 323:891-894, 1990.
5. Bhattacharya SK, Crawford AJ, Pate JW, et al: Mechanism of calcium and magnesium translocation in acute pancreatitis: a temporal correlation between hypocalcemia and membrane-mediated excessive intracellular calcium accumulation in soft tissues, *Magnesium* 7:91-102, 1988.
6. Bhattacharya SK, Luther RW, Pate JW, et al: Soft tissue calcium and magnesium content in acute pancreatitis in the dog: calcium accumulation, a mechanism for hypocalcemia in acute pancreatitis, *J Lab Clin Med* 105:422-427, 1985.
7. Binder HJ, Sandle GI: Electrolyte transport in the mammalian colon. In Johnson LR, editor: *Physiology of the gastrointestinal tract*, ed 3, vol 2, New York, 1994, Raven Press, pp. 2133-2171.
8. Brady CA, Otto CM: Systemic inflammatory response syndrome, sepsis, and multiple organ dysfunction, *Vet Clin North Am Small Anim Pract* 31:1147-1162, 2001.
9. Burrows CF: Chronic diarrhea in the dog, *Vet Clin North Am* 13:521, 1983.
10. Bush WW, Kimmel SE, Wosar MA, et al: Secondary hypoparathyroidism attributed to hypomagnesemia in a dog with protein-losing enteropathy, *J Am Vet Med Assoc* 219:1732-1734, 2001.
11. Chan DL, Freeman LM, Labato MA, et al: Retrospective evaluation of partial parenteral nutrition in dogs and cats, *J Vet Intern Med* 16:440-445, 2002.
12. Chang EB, Rao MC: Intestinal water and electrolyte transport: mechanisms of physiological and adaptive responses. In Johnson LR, editor: *Physiology of the gastrointestinal tract*, ed 3, New York, 1994, Raven Press, pp. 2027-2081.
13. Cooke HJ: Role of the "little brain" in the gut in water and electrolyte homeostasis, *FASEB J* 3:127-138, 1989.
14. Cooke HJ, Reddix RA: Neural regulation of intestinal electrolyte transport. In Johnson LR, editor: *Physiology of the gastrointestinal tract*, ed 3, vol 2, New York, 1994, Raven Press, pp. 2083-2132.
15. Cornelius LM, Rawlings CA: Arterial blood gas and acid-base values in dogs with various diseases and signs of disease, *J Am Vet Med Assoc* 178:992-995, 1981.
16. Cullen JJ, Caropreso DK, Hemann LL, et al: Pathophysiology of adynamic ileus, *Dig Dis Sci* 42:731-737, 1997.
17. Curran PF: Na, Cl, and water transport by rat ileum in vitro, *J Gen Physiol* 43:1137-1148, 1960.
18. Cuschieri A, Cummings JRG, Meehan SE, et al: Treatment of acute pancreatitis with fresh frozen plasma, *Br J Surg* 70:710-712, 1983.
19. Denham W, Norman J: The potential role of therapeutic cytokine manipulation in acute pancreatitis, *Surg Clin North Am* 79:767-782, 1999.

20. de Papp E, Drobatz KJ, Hughes D: Plasma lactate concentration as a predictor of gastric necrosis and survival among dogs with gastric dilatation-volvulus: 102 cases (1995-1998), *J Am Vet Med Assoc* 215:49-52, 1999.

21. DiBartola SP, Johnson SE, Davenport DJ, et al: Clinicopathologic findings resembling hypoadrenocorticism in dogs with primary gastrointestinal disease, *J Am Vet Med Assoc* 187:60-63, 1985.

22. Duerksen DR, Bector S, Parry D, et al: A comparison of the effect of elemental and immune enhancing polymeric jejunal feeding on exocrine pancreatic function, *J Parenter Enteral Nutr* 26:205-208, 2002.

23. Duffel SJ: Some aspects of pancreatic disease in the cat, *J Small Anim Pract* 16:365-374, 1975.

24. Edmonds CJ: Salts and water. In Smyth DH, editor: *Biomembranes, Intestinal Absorption*, vol 4B, New York, 1974, Plenum, pp. 711-759.

25. Farthing MJG: History and rationale of oral rehydration and recent developments in formulating an optimal solution, *Drugs* 36(suppl 4):80-90, 1988.

26. Fordtran JS: Speculations on the pathogenesis of diarrhea, *Fed Proc* 26:1405-1414, 1967.

27. Graves TK, Schall WD, Refsal K, Nachrenier RF: Basal and ACTH-stimulated plasma aldosterone concentrations are normal or increased in dogs with trichuriasis-associated pseudohypoadrenocorticism, *J Vet Intern Med* 8:287-289, 1994.

28. Gregory CR, Guilford WG, Berry CR, et al: Enteric function in cats after subtotal colectomy for treatment of megacolon, *Vet Surg* 19:216-220, 1990.

29. Hamer DH, Gorbach SL: Intestinal diarrhea and bacterial food poisoning. In Sleisinger MH, editor: *Gastrointestinal and liver disease. Pathophysiology, diagnosis and management*, ed 6, vol 2, Philadelphia, 1998, WB Saunders, pp. 1594-1632.

30. Happe RP, DeBruijne JJ: Pentagastrin stimulated gastric secretion in the dog (orogastric aspiration technique), *Res Vet Sci* 33:232-239, 1982.

31. Harvey CJ, Lopez JW, Hendrick MJ: An uncommon intestinal manifestation of feline infectious peritonitis: 26 cases (1986-1993), *J Am Vet Med Assoc* 209:1117-1120, 1996.

32. Haskins SC: Shock. In Kirk RW, Bistner SI, Ford RB, editors: *Handbook of veterinary procedures and emergency treatment*, ed 5, Philadelphia, 1990, WB Saunders, pp. 33-52.

33. Heald RD, Jones BD, Schmidt DA: Blood gas and electrolyte concentrations in canine parvoviral enteritis, *J Am Anim Hosp Assoc* 22:745-748, 1986.

34. Hess RS, Saunders HM, Van Winkle TJ, et al: Clinical, clinicopathologic, radiographic, and ultrasonographic abnormalities in dogs with fatal acute pancreatitis: 70 cases (1986-1995), *J Am Vet Med Assoc* 213:665-670, 1998.

35. Hill RC, Van Winkle TJ: Acute necrotizing and acute suppurative pancreatitis in the cat: a retrospective study of 40 cases (1976-1989), *J Vet Intern Med* 7:25-33, 1993.

36. Horton JW, Dunn CW, Burnweit CA, et al: Hypertonic saline dextran resuscitation of acute canine bile-induced pancreatitis, *Am J Surg* 158:48-56, 1989.

37. Izquierdo R, Bermes E Jr, Sandberg L, et al: Serum calcium metabolism in acute experimental pancreatitis, *Surgery* 98:1031-1037, 1985.

38. Jacobs RM, Weiser MG, Hall RL, et al: Clinicopathologic findings of canine parvoviral enteritis, *J Am Anim Hosp Assoc* 16:809-814, 1980.

39. Johnson GB, Brunn GJ, Platt JL: Cutting edge: an endogenous pathway to systemic inflammatory response syndrome (SIRS)-like reactions through Toll-like receptor 4, *J Immunol* 172:20-24, 2004.

40. Kalfarentzos F, Kehagias J, Mead N, et al: Enteral nutrition is superior to parenteral nutrition in severe acute pancreatitis: results of a randomised prospective trial, *Br J Surg* 84:1665-1669, 1997.

41. Karanjia ND, Lutrin FJ, Chang Y-B, et al: Low dose dopamine protects against hemorrhagic pancreatitis in cats, *J Surg Res* 48:440-443, 1990.

42. Kimmel SE, Waddell LS, Michel KE: Hypomagnesemia and hypocalcemia associated with protein-losing enteropathy in Yorkshire terriers: five cases (1992-1998), *J Am Vet Med Assoc* 217:703-706, 2000.

43. Kimmel SE, Washabau RJ, Drobatz KJ: Incidence and prognostic value of low plasma ionized calcium concentration in cats with acute pancreatitis: 46 cases (1996-1998), *J Am Vet Med Assoc* 219:1105-1109, 2001.

44. Kitchell BE, Strombeck DR, Cullen J, et al: Clinical and pathologic changes in experimentally induced acute pancreatitis in cats, *Am J Vet Res* 47:1170-1173, 1986.

45. Klar E, Herfarth C, Messmer K: Therapeutic effect of isovolemic hemodilution with dextran 60 on the impairment of pancreatic microcirculation in acute biliary pancreatitis, *Ann Surg* 211:346, 1990.

46. Krejs GJ: VIPoma syndrome, *Am J Med* 82:37-47, 1987.

47. Lantz GC: The pathophysiology of acute mechanical small bowel obstruction, *Compend Contin Educ Pract Vet* 3:910-917, 1981.

48. Lifton SJ, King LG, Zerbe CA: Glucocorticoid deficient hypoadrenocorticism in dogs: 18 cases (1986-1995), *J Am Vet Med Assoc* 209:2076-2081, 1996.

49. Lloyd KKC, Debas HT: Peripheral regulation of gastric acid secretion. In Johnson LR, editor: *Physiology of the gastrointestinal tract*, ed 3, New York, 1994, Raven Press, pp. 1185-1226.

50. Macy DW: Feline pancreatitis. In Kirk RW, Bonagura JD, editors: *Current veterinary therapy X*, Philadelphia, 1989, WB Saunders, pp. 893-896.

51. Malik R, Hunt GB, Hinchlifke JM, et al: Severe whipworm infection in the dog, *J Small Anim Pract* 31:185-188, 1990.

52. Melgarejo T, Roheleder J, Williams DA, et al: Immunoelectrophoretic characterization of plasma α_1-protease inhibitor in dogs with experimental pancreatitis, *J Vet Intern Med* 10:157, A33, 1996.

53. Mentula P, Kylanpaa ML, Kemppainen E, et al: Plasma anti-inflammatory cytokines and monocyte human leucocyte antigen-DR expression in patients with acute pancreatitis, *Scand J Gastroenterol* 39:178-187, 2004.

54. Meuten DJ, Chew DJ, Capen CC, et al: Relationship of serum total calcium to albumin and total protein in dogs, *J Am Vet Med Assoc* 180:63-67, 1982.

55. Mohr AJ, Leisewitz AL, Jacobson LS, et al: Effect of early enteral nutrition on intestinal permeability, intestinal protein loss, and outcome in dogs with severe parvoviral enteritis, *J Vet Intern Med* 17:791-798, 2003.

56. Moore R, Carpenter J: Intramural hematoma causing obstruction in three dogs, *J Am Vet Med Assoc* 184:186-188, 1984.

57. Moore R, Carpenter J: Intestinal sclerosis with pseudo-obstruction in three dogs, *J Am Vet Med Assoc* 184:830-833, 1984.

58. Moseley RH: Fluid and electrolyte disorders and gastrointestinal disease. In Kokko JP, Tannen RL, editors: *Fluid and electrolytes*, Philadelphia, 1996, WB Saunders, p. 675.

59. Muir WW: Acid-base and electrolyte disturbances in dogs with gastric dilatation-volvulus, *J Am Vet Med Assoc* 181:229-231, 1982.

60. Musch MW, Miller RJ, Field M, et al: Stimulation of colonic secretion by lipoxygenase metabolites of arachidonic acid. *Science* 217:1255-1256, 1982.

61. Nappert G, Dunphy E, Ruben D, et al: Determination of serum organic acids in puppies with naturally acquired parvoviral enteritis, *Can J Vet Res* 66:15-18, 2002.

62. Nelson DC, McGrew WRG, Hoyumpa AM: Hypernatremia and lactulose therapy, *JAMA* 249:1295-1298, 1983.

63. Ohlsson K: Interactions in vitro and in vivo between dog trypsin and dog plasma protease inhibitors, *Scand J Clin Lab Invest* 28:219, 1971.

64. Ooms L, Degryse A: Pathogenesis and pharmacology of diarrhea, *Vet Res Commun* 10:355-397, 1986.

65. Oruc N, Ozutemiz AO, Yukselen V, et al: Infliximab: a new therapeutic agent in acute pancreatitis? *Pancreas* 28:E1-8, 2004.

66. Owens JM, Drazner FH, Gilbertson SR: Pancreatic disease in the cat, *J Am Anim Hosp Assoc* 11:83-89, 1975.

67. Peoples JB: The role of pH in altering serum ionized calcium concentration, *Surgery* 104:370-374, 1988.

68. Qin HL, Su ZD, Gao Q, et al: Early intrajejunal nutrition: bacterial translocation and gut barrier function of severe acute pancreatitis in dogs, *Hepatobiliary Pancreat Dis Int* 1:150-154, 2002.

69. Qin, HL, Su ZU, Hu LG, et al: Parenteral versus early intrajejunal nutrition: effect on pancreatitic natural course, entero-hormones release and its efficacy on dogs with acute pancreatitis, *World J Gastroenterol* 9:2270-2273, 2003.

70. Raraty MG, Connor S, Criddle DN, et al: Acute pancreatitis and organ failure: pathophysiology, natural history, and management strategies, *Curr Gastroenterol Rep* 6:99-103, 2004.

71. Rattner DW, Napolitano LM, Corsetti J, et al: Hypocalcemia in experimental pancreatitis occurs independently of changes in serum nonesterified fatty acid levels, *Int J Pancreatol* 6:249-262, 1990.

72. Robinson EP, Hardy RM: Clinical signs, diagnosis and treatment of alkalemia in dogs: 20 cases (1982-1984), *J Am Vet Med Assoc* 192:943-949, 1988.

73. Romatowski J: Use of oral fluids in acute gastroenteritis in small animals, *Mod Vet Pract* 66:261-263, 1985.

74. Rose BD: Metabolic alkalosis. In *Clinical physiology of acid-base and electrolyte disorders*, ed 2, New York, 1984, McGraw-Hill, pp. 374-393.

75. Ruaux CG, Pennington HL, Worrall S, et al: Tumor necrosis factor-alpha at presentation in 60 cases of spontaneous canine acute pancreatitis, *Vet Immunol Immunopathol* 72:369-376, 1999.

76. Ruppin H, Bar-Meir S, Soergel KH, et al: Absorption of short chain fatty acids by the colon, *Gastroenterology* 78:1500-1507, 1980.

77. Sachs G: The gastric H^+/K^+-ATPase. In Johnson LR, editor: *Physiology of the gastrointestinal tract*, ed 3, New York, 1994, Raven Press, p. 1119.

78. Sack DA, Chowdhury AMAK, Eusof A, et al: Oral rehydration of rotavirus diarrhea: a double blind comparison of sucrose with glucose electrolyte solution, *Lancet* 2:280-283, 1978.

79. Santosham M, Daum RS, Dillman L, et al: A controlled study of well-nourished children hospitalized in the United States and Panama, *N Engl J Med* 306:1070-1076, 1982.

80. Schaer M: A clinicopathologic survey of acute pancreatitis in 30 dogs and 5 cats, *J Am Anim Hosp Assoc* 15:681-687, 1979.

81. Sellin JH: Intestinal electrolyte absorption and secretion. In Sleisinger MH, Fordtran JS, Feldman M, et al, editors: *Gastrointestinal and liver disease pathophysiology, diagnosis and management*, ed 6, vol 2, Philadelphia, 1998, WB Saunders, pp. 1451-1471.

82. Shields R: The absorption and secretion of fluid and electrolytes by the obstructed bowel, *Br J Surg* 52:774-779, 1965.

83. Simpson KW: Current concepts of the pathogenesis and pathophysiology of acute pancreatitis in the dog and cat, *Compend Contin Educ Pract Vet* 15:247-254, 1993.

84. Simpson KW: Acute pancreatitis. In August JR, editor: *Consultations in feline internal medicine III*, Philadelphia, 1997, WB Saunders, pp. 91-98.

85. Simpson KW, Alpers DH, DeWille J, et al: Cellular localization and hormonal regulation of pancreatic intrinsic factor secretion in dogs, *Am J Physiol* 265:G178-188, 1993.

86. Simpson KW, Beechey-Newman N, Lamb CR, et al: Cholecystokinin-8 induces edematous pancreatitis in dogs which is associated with a short burst of trypsinogen activation, *Dig Dis Sci* 40:2152-2161, 1995.

87. Simpson KW, Dykes NL: Diagnosis and treatment of gastrinoma, *Semin Vet Med Surg (Small Anim)* 12:274-281, 1997.

88. Simpson KW, Shiroma JT, Biller DS, et al: Ante mortem diagnosis of pancreatitis in four cats, *J Small Anim Pract* 35:93-99, 1994.

89. Sladen GE, Dawson AM: Interrelationships between the absorptions of glucose, sodium and water by the normal human jejunum, *Clin Sci* 36:119-132, 1969.

90. Sladen GE, Parsons DS, Dupre J: Effects of bicarbonate on intestinal absorption, *Gut* 9:731, 1968.

91. Soll AH, Berglindh T: Receptors that regulate gastric acid-secretory function. In Johnson LR, editor: *Physiology of the gastrointestinal tract*, ed 3, New York, 1994, Raven Press, pp. 1139-1169.

92. Strombeck DR: Small and large intestine: normal structure and function. In Guilford WG, Center SA, Strombeck DR, et al, editors: *Strombeck's small animal gastroenterology*, ed 3, Philadelphia, 1996, WB Saunders, p. 318.

93. Thillainayagam AV, Hunt JB, Farthing MJG: Enhancing clinical efficiency of oral rehydration therapy: is low osmolality the key? *Gastroenterology* 114:197-210, 1998.

94. Tobias TA, Schertel ER: Shock: concepts and management. In DiBartola SP, editor: *Fluid therapy in small animal practice*, Philadelphia, 1992, WB Saunders, pp. 436-470.

95. Twedt DC, Grauer GF: Fluid therapy for gastrointestinal, pancreatic and hepatic disorders, *Vet Clin North Am* 12:463-485, 1982.

96. Van Slyke KK, Evans EI: The paradox of aciduria in presence of alkalosis caused by hypochloremia, *Ann Surg* 126:545-567, 1947.

97. Vu MK, van der Veek PP, Frolich M, et al: Does jejunal feeding activate exocrine pancreatic secretion? *Eur J Clin Invest* 29:1053-1059, 1999.

98. Wilson GP, Burt JK: Intussusception in the dog and cat: a review of 45 cases, *J Am Vet Med Assoc* 164:515-518, 1974.

99. Wingfield WE, Twedt DC, Moore RW, et al: Acid-base and electrolyte values in dogs with acute gastric dilatation-volvulus, *J Am Vet Med Assoc* 180:1070-1072, 1982.

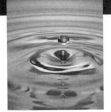

CHAPTER · 19

FLUID, ELECTROLYTE, AND ACID-BASE DISTURBANCES IN LIVER DISEASE

Sharon A. Center

Liver disease can influence many metabolic, hormonal, and hemodynamic processes. Changes in hepatic albumin synthesis affect oncotic pressure; alterations in renal function and disturbances in production and metabolism of hormones contribute to water, electrolyte, and acid-base imbalances; and stimulation of baroreceptors and osmoreceptors can evoke detrimental changes in effective circulating volume and plasma osmolality.

NORMAL PHYSIOLOGY OF THE HEPATOBILIARY SYSTEM

BILE FORMATION: COMPOSITION AND FLOW

Bile is an aqueous solution containing organic and inorganic compounds and electrolytes (Table 19-1).[134] Separate hepatic and ductular transport mechanisms allow regulation of bile composition and volume in response to changing physiological needs.[85] Bile acids are amphipathic organic anions synthesized and conjugated by the liver. The hepatocyte is a polarized secretory epithelial cell with specific transporters localized in basolateral and canalicular cell membranes.[108] The canaliculus is a confined space formed by a junction between specialized portions of cell membranes from two adjacent hepatocytes. The surfaces defining the canaliculus form a tight junction that functions as an anatomic barrier to solute diffusion. Transport processes in the basolateral hepatocellular and canalicular membranes determine bile acid uptake and biliary excretion. Active transport of osmotically active solutes into the canaliculus provides the driving force for bile flow.

Bile salts are the most concentrated organic solutes in bile and a major determinant of bile secretion. Rate-limiting secretory mechanisms involve bile acid transporters in the canalicular membranes. Bile acids impart unique properties that attenuate the osmotic forces in bile. Formation of bile acid micelles (polymolecular aggregates) protects the intestinal mucosa from highly concentrated solutes and promotes interaction between bile acids and lipids in the intestinal tract, thus facilitating digestion. Almost all bile acids are conjugated (exclusively to taurine in the cat and to taurine or glycine in the dog) and exist as organic anions rather than undissociated acids. Nonabsorbable constituents of bile (e.g., bile acids, phospholipids, cholesterol) are concentrated when water and inorganic electrolytes (e.g., sodium, chloride, bicarbonate) are absorbed from the gallbladder and biliary ducts. Stasis of bile flow or dehydration can promote a pathologic thickening of bile (inspissated or sticky consistency), whereas choleresis (increased bile flow) produces watery or dilute bile. The bicarbonate concentration of bile exceeds that of plasma and is largely under the

TABLE 19-1 Flow and Electrolyte Concentrations of Hepatic Bile

Species	Flow (μL/min/g liver)	Na$^+$ (mEq/L)	K$^+$ (mEq/L)	Cl$^-$ (mEq/L)	HCO$_3^-$ (mEq/L)	Taurocholate (Canalicular Bile) (mM/L)
Dog	0.19 (n = 24)*	171 (n = 75)	5.1 (n = 73)	66 (n = 83)	61 (n = 83)	37 (n = 80)
Cat	0.23 (n = 5)	163 (n = 16)	4.2 (n = 16)	109 (n = 16)	24 (n = 16)	26 (n = 10)

*n = Number of observations reported.

**Transcellular and Paracellular
Mechanisms Influencing Bile Flow**

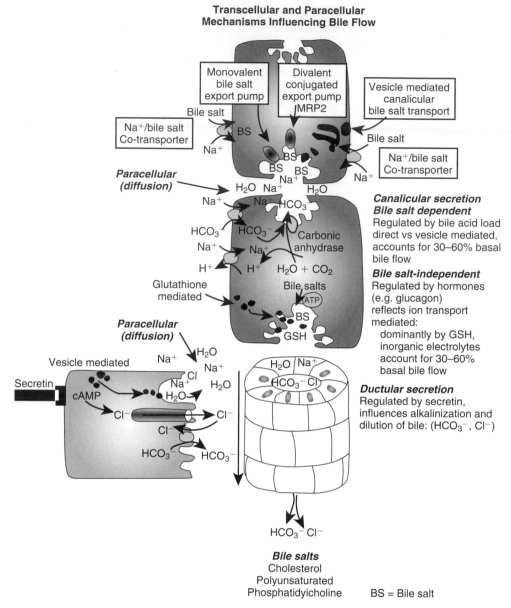

BS = Bile salt

Fig. 19-1 Transcellular (active pump-dependent) and paracellular (diffusion-dependent) mechanisms of bile formation in the hepatocyte and bile duct epithelium. Canalicular secretion depends on bile salt-dependent and -independent mechanisms. Efflux of bile acids into canaliculi involves facilitated diffusion dependent on canalicular carrier proteins, ATP-dependent mechanisms, and exocytosis of cytosolic vesicles; these involve specific monovalent bile salt, bivalent bile salt, sodium/bile salt cotransport, and vesicle-mediated bile acid transport. Bile acid-independent bile flow is mediated by a Na transport/Na$^+$, K$^+$-ATPase-linked mechanism, bicarbonate transport (associated with carbonic anhydrase and a canalicular membrane pump), and transport of organic solutes (principally glutathione [GSH]). Transcellular mechanisms in ducts primarily transport bicarbonate and chloride. Secretin initiates expression of a Cl$^-$ transmembrane channel (cystic fibrosis transmembrane regulator) and subsequent activation of the Cl$^-$/HCO$_3^-$ exchanger leading to bicarbonate secretion in ductal bile. Whereas bile formation occurs continuously, hormones (e.g., glucagon) can increase bile salt-independent mechanisms. Ductular secretions are stimulated by secretin causing bile alkalinization and dilution.

influence of secretin. Most of the bicarbonate in bile arises during bile transport through biliary ductules. Bile formation and flow are driven mainly by osmotic mechanisms. Flow is initiated by bile acid–dependent and –independent mechanisms. In the basal state, equal contributions to flow are derived from canalicular bile salt–dependent and bile salt–independent mechanisms and from ductule

processes. In the absence of bile salts, bile flow reaches only 40% to 50% of normal. Transcellular rather than paracellular mechanisms are most important in determining bile composition. Transcellular mechanisms concentrate bile acids and other solutes, whereas paracellular mechanisms permit simple diffusion (water and electrolytes) down electrochemical or osmotic gradients (Fig. 19-1).

There is a direct linear relationship between canalicular bile acid concentrations and bile flow. Non–micelleforming bile acids (e.g., dehydrocholate) have the greatest effect. Hepatocellular uptake of bile acids is an energy-dependent process linked to sodium transport. This process accounts for approximately 80% of taurocholate uptake but only 50% of unconjugated cholate uptake.[108] Protein carriers facilitate cytosolic transport of bile acids to canalicular membranes. Efflux of bile acids into canaliculi involves several mechanisms including facilitated diffusion dependent on canalicular carrier proteins, an adenosine triphosphate (ATP)-dependent mechanism, and exocytosis of cytosolic vesicles. Collectively, transcellular transport of bile acids and micelle formation maintain a marked concentration gradient between bile and blood, permitting biliary concentrations to exceed plasma bile acid concentrations by 100- to 1000-fold.

Bile acid–independent bile flow is mediated by a sodium transport Na^+,K^+-ATPase–linked mechanism, bicarbonate transport (associated with carbonic anhydrase and a canalicular membrane pump), and transport of organic solutes (e.g., glutathione [GSH]). As the most abundant organic molecule in canalicular bile (approximating 8 to 10 mM/L), GSH imposes the greatest osmotic effect even exceeding that of free bile salts. Approximately 50% of hepatic GSH, most GSSG (oxidized GSH), and all GSH-conjugates are exported into the canaliculus. Membrane pumps (canalicular multispecific organic anion transporter [cMOAT], also termed the multidrug resistance associated protein-2 [MRP2]) facilitate GSH exportation. The strong osmotic influence of GSH on bile flow derives from its hydrophilic nature, active membrane exportation, and hydrolysis by membrane affiliated γ–glutamyltransferase (γGT) into its three constituent amino acids (cysteine, glutamate, glycine) yielding three osmolar equivalents. The osmotic effect of catabolized GSH draws water and electrolyte solutes through paracellular pathways or other hepatocellular conduits.

Bile ducts contribute to bile formation and modification as well as to bile flow. Production of ductular fluid primarily is under the influence of secretin, which regulates spontaneous or basal bile flow. Gastrin (but not pentagastrin) also increases bile duct secretion in dogs, whereas somatostatin decreases ductular bile flow. Increased ductular bile flow results in bile alkalinization and dilution. Disease states causing bile ductule proliferation also increase bile flow (e.g., cirrhosis, extrahepatic bile duct occlusion, inflammatory disorders). Bile ductules and ducts can also reabsorb bile as shown in cholecystectomized dogs.[59]

HEPATIC NITROGEN METABOLISM: DETOXIFICATION, EXCRETION, AND ROLE IN ACID-BASE BALANCE
Urea Cycle and Glutamine Cycle

The liver converts waste nitrogen to an excretable form.[43] Nitrogen derived from amino acids can be converted to ammonia directly or indirectly after incorporation into glutamate or aspartate in the liver. Ammonia subsequently is detoxified by conversion to urea (Fig. 19-2). Two mechanisms exist for hepatic nitrogen detoxification. The hepatic urea cycle is best known and involves a linked series of enzymatic reactions carried out in the mitochondria and cytosol of the hepatocyte (see Fig. 19-2). The second mechanism, the glutamine cycle, involves transport of glutamine into mitochondria, where it is converted to ammonia and used as a precursor of carbamoyl phosphate (see Fig. 19-2). The urea cycle is a low-affinity system most important during alkalosis, whereas the glutamine cycle is a high-affinity system most important during acidosis. Collectively, these systems efficiently cleanse portal blood of ammonia. Approximately 25% of the ammonia for urea synthesis is derived directly from portal blood, and the remainder is derived from catabolism of proteins, peptides, and amino acids.

Urea synthesis depends on substrate supply, hormonal regulation, nutritional status, and liver cell volume. Regulation of urea cycle enzymes corresponds to the level of dietary nitrogen intake and possibly liver cell volume. The urea cycle may play an important role in acid-base homeostasis, as explained by the following reaction (using the amino acid alanine as an example of a nitrogen source)[43]:

(alanine)
$$CH_3CH(CO_2)NH_3 + 3O_2 \rightarrow 2CO_2 + HCO_3^- + NH_4^+ + H_2O$$

Generation of one positive (NH_4^+) and one negative (HCO_3^-) charge has the potential to maintain electroneutrality. However, because physiologic pH is in the range of 7.0 to 7.4, only 1% of ammonia exists as ammonia. Therefore the protons represented by the ammonium ions cannot be readily transferred to HCO_3^-, and thus catabolism of large amounts of amino acids or protein can generate high bicarbonate concentrations resulting in metabolic alkalosis. Normally, detoxification of ammonia to electroneutral urea prevents changes in systemic pH[43]:

$$2NH_4^+ + HCO_3^- \rightarrow NH_2CONH_2 \text{ (urea)} + 2H_2O + H^+$$

$$HCO_3^- + H^+ \rightarrow H_2O + CO_2$$

Net: $2NH_4^+ + 2HCO_3^- \rightarrow NH_2CONH_2$ (urea) $+ CO_2 + 3H_2O$

The preceding model probably is an oversimplification. Consumption of a diet composed of a complex mixture of amino acids (anionic, cationic, and sulfate-containing amino acids) results in a net gain of protons that must be excreted or neutralized. Urinary excretion occurs via dihydrogen phosphate (titratable acidity) and renal tubular production of ammonium from glutamine. Traditional

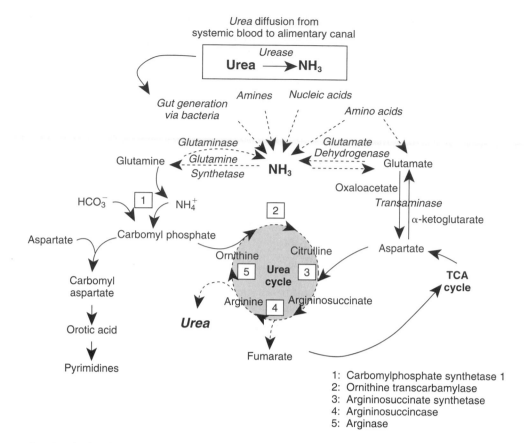

Fig. 19-2 Diagram showing the biochemical reactions involved with nitrogenous waste production, detoxification, and elimination in the liver. See text for explanations.

concepts of renal tubular acid titration consider ammonium ion formation an important mechanism of acid-base regulation. However, ammonium ions excreted in urine are incapable of titrating acid because they are already protonated.[43] An alternative view is that urinary excretion of NH_4^+ represents a mechanism by which the liver is deprived of substrates for urea synthesis, resulting in less bicarbonate neutralization and mitigation of acidosis. According to this hypothesis, the kidneys determine the route of nitrogen disposal, whereas the liver plays a more active role in systemic acid-base balance.

Serum Proteins: Albumin and Globulins
Albumin

Albumin accounts for 25% of the proteins synthesized by the liver.[114] Serum albumin concentration reflects the net result of synthesis by hepatocytes, systemic distribution, and degradation. Being relatively small in size (66,000 daltons), albumin can be lost from the circulation through pathologically altered vessels (e.g., vasculitis), gut wall (e.g., lymphangiectasia), or glomeruli (e.g., glomerulonephritis, amyloidosis) or into the peritoneal cavity as a result of hepatic sinusoidal hypertension. Impaired or down-regulated hepatic albumin synthesis or losses exceeding synthetic capability result in hypoal-buminemia of variable severity. The liver has a tremendous reserve capacity for albumin synthesis.[138] Normally, only 20% to 30% of the hepatocytes produce albumin, and synthesis can be increased as needed by a factor of 200% to 300%.[60]

Hepatic albumin production fluctuates depending on physiologic conditions and requirements (Fig. 19-3). The most important variables are nutrition and interstitial osmotic pressure as sensed by the hepatocyte.[137] The influence of nutrition on albumin production can be dramatic. Albumin synthesis decreases by 50% within 24 hours after a fast or with consumption of a protein-deficient diet. Serum albumin concentration reflects this change only after a lag period ranging from days to weeks as a new balance is achieved between exchangeable albumin pools. Feeding excessive calories in a protein-restricted ration augments development of hypoalbuminemia, as does dietary depletion of branched-chain amino acids.[88,102,138] Hypoalbuminemia, caused in part by reduced albumin synthesis, also can be a consequence of changes in serum oncotic pressure related to hyperglobulinemia and treatment with synthetic colloids (e.g., dextran).[52,137] Synthesis of albumin also decreases, sometimes dramatically, during critical illness as part of a negative acute-phase response.[23,27]

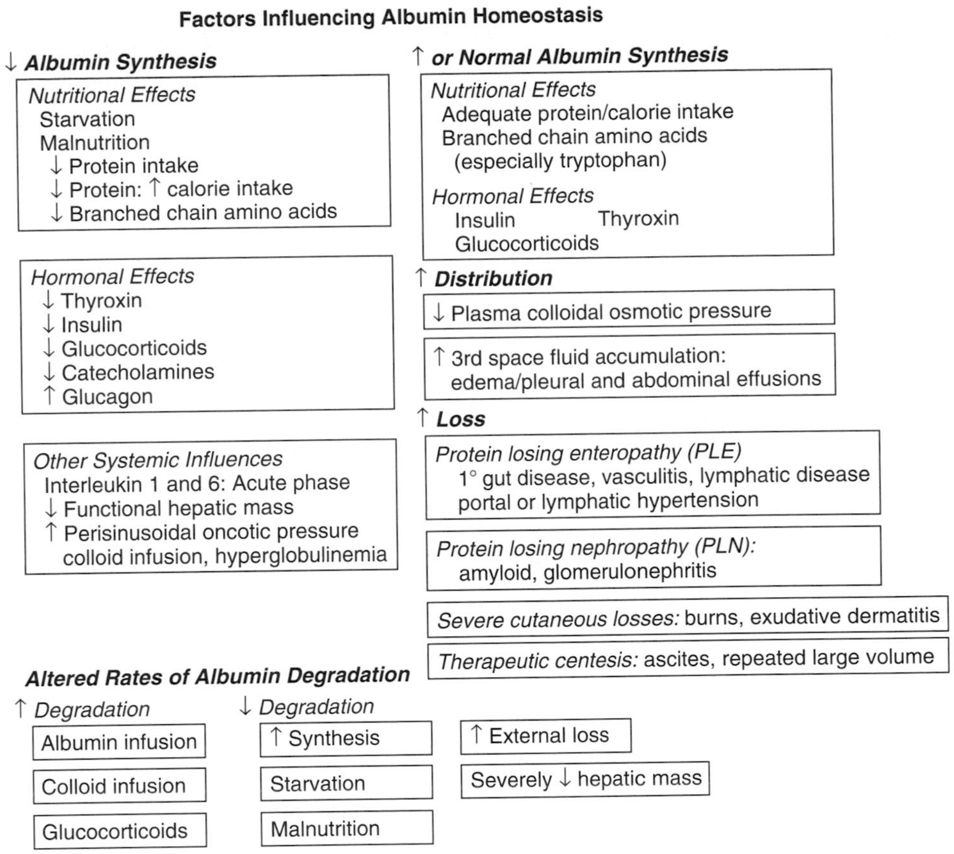

Factors Influencing Albumin Homeostasis

↓ **Albumin Synthesis**

Nutritional Effects
Starvation
Malnutrition
↓ Protein intake
↓ Protein: ↑ calorie intake
↓ Branched chain amino acids

Hormonal Effects
↓ Thyroxin
↓ Insulin
↓ Glucocorticoids
↓ Catecholamines
↑ Glucagon

Other Systemic Influences
Interleukin 1 and 6: Acute phase
↓ Functional hepatic mass
↑ Perisinusoidal oncotic pressure
colloid infusion, hyperglobulinemia

↑ **or Normal Albumin Synthesis**

Nutritional Effects
Adequate protein/calorie intake
Branched chain amino acids
(especially tryptophan)

Hormonal Effects
Insulin   Thyroxin
Glucocorticoids

↑ **Distribution**

↓ Plasma colloidal osmotic pressure

↑ 3rd space fluid accumulation:
edema/pleural and abdominal effusions

↑ **Loss**

Protein losing enteropathy (PLE)
1° gut disease, vasculitis, lymphatic disease
portal or lymphatic hypertension

Protein losing nephropathy (PLN):
amyloid, glomerulonephritis

Severe cutaneous losses: burns, exudative dermatitis

Therapeutic centesis: ascites, repeated large volume

Altered Rates of Albumin Degradation

↑ Degradation

| Albumin infusion |
| Colloid infusion |
| Glucocorticoids |

↓ Degradation

| ↑ Synthesis |
| Starvation |
| Malnutrition |

| ↑ External loss |
| Severely ↓ hepatic mass |

Fig. 19-3 Factors and conditions influencing albumin synthesis and degradation.

After synthesis in the hepatocyte, albumin is released into the space of Disse by exocytosis. It then diffuses into the hepatic sinusoids, where it mingles with the systemic circulation. It then is dispersed into the interstitial space, returning to the systemic circulation via lymphatics and the thoracic duct. In normal animals, 50% to 70% of albumin is located extravascularly, with the largest amounts in interstitial spaces in skin and muscle.[102] Normal transcapillary escape approximates 5% per hour, but inflammation may increase this several fold. This phenomenon commonly contributes to the "negative-acute-phase" effect that modestly lowers serum albumin concentrations in inflammation.

Catabolism of albumin probably occurs within or adjacent to vascular endothelium of tissues.[181] The half-life of plasma albumin in dogs is 7 to 10 days.[54,62] No half-life estimate is available for the cat. The rate of albumin catabolism is highly variable, but its fractional catabolic rate is directly proportional to the plasma albumin concentration and pool size.[81] In conditions that cause hypoalbuminemia, the fractional and absolute rate of albumin catabolism decreases. The rate of albumin catabolism increases after albumin or synthetic colloid transfusion. Thus transfusion of albumin or infusions of synthetic colloids may potentiate endogenous hypoalbu-

minemia by two separate mechanisms. As a consequence of the large space of distribution and numerous mechanisms influencing the synthesis, distribution, and catabolism of albumin, serum albumin concentration does not accurately reflect contemporary changes in total body albumin resources or its hepatic synthesis.

The strong net negative charge of albumin (−17) explains its important contribution to the strong ion difference (SID) and allows it to bind weakly and reversibly with a variety of ions. In this capacity, albumin functions as a circulating depot and transport molecule for many ions (e.g., Ca^{+2}, Mg^{+2}, Cu^{+2}) and metabolites (e.g., fatty acids, thyroxine, bilirubin, bile salts, amino acids).[104] Albumin accounts for most of the plasma thiol content (i.e., sulfhydryl bonds) and provides protection against oxidative stress.[135] Albumin also provides antioxidant activity by binding reactive transition metals (e.g., Cu^{+2}) that catalyze free radical generation.[104] Other important effects of albumin involve anticoagulant, antithrombotic, and antiinflammatory effects.

Oxidized and glycosylated forms of albumin occur in human patients with cirrhosis,[175] and these forms increase in concentration as total serum albumin concentration decreases. The increase in the oxidized form of albumin reflects its role as a scavenger of reactive oxygen species. Glycosylation of albumin influences its binding and permeability characteristics and augments platelet aggregation, which may predispose to thromboembolic complications.[175] The clinical implication of a lower reduced/oxidized albumin ratio lies in its relationship to oxidative stress imposed by low thiol substrate availability.

Numerous factors influence serum albumin concentration (see Fig. 19-3). Modest hypoalbuminemia may reflect reduced albumin synthesis or enhanced catabolism, but these usually are slow in onset. Protein catabolism caused by illness usually spares albumin and targets muscle. The acute-phase response to tissue injury enhances transcapillary escape of albumin and may reduce lymphatic clearance. The most dramatic rapid reduction in serum albumin concentration is dilutional in nature and associated with crystalloid administration (with or without synthetic colloid). Such therapeutic dilutional effects typically aggravate acute severe extracorporeal losses (e.g., hemorrhage). Albumin loss resulting from protein-losing enteropathy or nephropathy initially is compensated for by albumin flux between intravascular and interstitial pools. With chronicity, a net body albumin deficit becomes apparent, and hypoalbuminemia develops. The most severe chronic hypoalbuminemia arises from disorders that impair albumin synthesis while simultaneously increasing catabolism or extracorporeal loss (e.g., protein-losing enteropathy, protein-losing nephropathy).

Hypoalbuminemia in patients with cirrhosis is a result of many factors, including ascites associated with portal hypertension, decreased synthesis, reduced nitrogen intake, dilutional effects from expansion of splanchnic and systemic circulating volume, concurrent diseases causing extracorporeal albumin loss and an acute-phase response (e.g., decreased albumin synthesis, increased transcapillary loss).

Globulins

The plasma globulin concentration represents many different proteins, some of which are shown in Fig. 19-4. The majority of nonimmunoglobulin serum globulins are synthesized and stored in the liver. Many of these proteins function as acute-phase reactants, a group of functionally diverse proteins normally present in very small quantities. The synthesis of acute-phase proteins rapidly and markedly increases after tissue injury or inflammation under the influence of cytokines. These proteins can contribute substantially to an increased total globulin concentration. Nevertheless, determination of the total globulin concentration is not a good measure of liver synthetic function because of the contribution of immunoglobulins to the total globulin concentration.

Hyperglobulinemia is common in animals with acquired hepatic disease, and the magnitude of this response may mask hypoalbuminemia if only total serum protein concentration is determined. Along with the acute-phase response, increased globulins reflect systemic immune stimulation secondary to impaired Kupffer cell function, disturbed B- and T-cell function, and development of autoantibodies. In severe hepatic insufficiency, decreased α-globulins (e.g., haptoglobin, α_1-antitrypsin) and hypoalbuminemia portend a poor prognosis.[146]

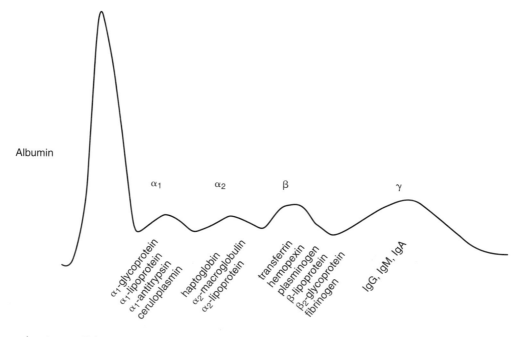

Fig. 19-4 Diagram showing a cellulose acetate electrophoretogram with representative proteins in their respective regions.

PATHOPHYSIOLOGY OF THE HEPATOBILIARY SYSTEM

INFLUENCE OF LIVER FUNCTION ON BLOOD UREA NITROGEN AND SERUM CREATININE

Urea Synthesis

The liver detoxifies waste nitrogen in two biochemical cycles, converting its primary waste product ammonia (NH_3) to an excretable form (urea). Approximately 25% of hepatic NH_3 is extracted directly from portal blood or from the kidneys, with the remainder derived from systemic and enteric metabolism of proteins, peptides, and amino acids. The *hepatic urea cycle* is the best known and dominant detoxification system for nitrogen and involves a linked series of five enzymatic reactions conducted in the mitochondria and cytosol of the hepatocyte. The second mechanism, the *hepatic glutamine cycle*, involves transport of glutamine into mitochondria, where it is converted to NH_3 and used as a precursor of carbamoyl phosphate. Hepatic NH_3 detoxification occurs in designated acinar zones, with urea synthesis dominating periportally (zone 1) and glutamine synthesis prevailing in perivenous hepatocytes (zone 3, adjacent to hepatic venules). Working cooperatively, these systems efficiently cleanse nitrogenous wastes from portal blood, thereby restricting access to the systemic circulation. Since most NH_3 produced within the liver as well as that derived from the splanchnic circulation is incorporated into urea, hepatic glutamine synthesis is considered a "backup system" scavenging residual NH_3 after splanchnic blood has traversed the hepatic sinusoid.

The hepatic urea cycle is a low affinity high capacity system that dominates in the face of alkalosis while the glutamine cycle is a high affinity low capacity system most important in the face of acidosis. Thus, during acidosis, less NH_3 is incorporated into urea partitioning relatively greater amounts for glutamine synthesis. In this way the liver vacillates between functioning as a net "importer" to a net "exporter" of glutamine effectively sparing bicarbonate utilization in urea synthesis. Detoxification of NH_3 through glutamine synthesis as occurs in muscle, is only temporary except in the kidney where glutamine is metabolized to release NH_3 into urine.

Blood urea nitrogen (BUN) concentration is directly affected by hepatic urea synthesis. Dietary protein restriction and an expanded volume of distribution for urea (e.g., hypoalbuminemia, third-space fluid accumulation, splanchnic and systemic vasodilatation) can exaggerate low BUN concentrations. Consequently, patients with acquired hepatic insufficiency and those with portosystemic shunting commonly develop abnormally low BUN concentrations. Increased water turnover associated with polydipsia and polyuria also may contribute to low BUN concentrations, whereas enteric hemorrhage in dogs with cirrhosis can increase BUN concentration into the nor-

mal range. These extrarenal factors make interpretation of BUN concentration as an indicator of renal function more difficult. BUN concentrations in dogs with cirrhosis (with and without ascites), dogs with portosystemic vascular anomaly (PSVA), and cats with hepatic lipidosis (HL) are shown in Figs. 19-5, 19-6, and 19-7.

Creatinine Synthesis

The liver also plays a major role in the biosynthesis of creatine, an organic nitrogenous compound essential for cell energy metabolism (Fig. 19-8). Creatine is derived from two amino acids (arginine and lysine), and the initial synthetic step is dependent on a rate-limiting enzyme (glycine amidinotransferase) present in a wide variety of organs. The next synthetic step occurs primarily in the liver and involves the transfer of a methyl group from *S*-adenosylmethionine (SAMe). Decreased hepatic synthesis of creatine in liver disease can result from insufficient methylation reactions and may cause subnormal serum creatinine concentrations. Approximately 98% of creatine is located in muscle tissue. Consequently, loss of muscle mass secondary to a negative nitrogen balance (or small body size in young animals with PSVA) can cause subnormal serum creatinine concentrations (see Figs. 19-5, 19-6, and 19-7). Increased water turnover associated with polydipsia and polyuria can accentuate subnormal creatinine concentrations in patients with hepatic insufficiency. In humans with hepatic cirrhosis and concurrent renal dysfunction, serum creatinine concentration fails to reflect decreased glomerular filtration rate (GFR); a similar phenomenon may occur in animals.[25,123]

HYPOALBUMINEMIA IN LIVER DISEASE

Hypoalbuminemia (serum albumin concentration, <1.5 g/dL) alters Starling's forces and favors loss of fluid from the vascular space, hypovolemia, and decreased systemic perfusion pressure. In conjunction with other disturbances in Starling's forces, a transudative effusion, edema, or both may develop. The location of third-space fluid accumulation often reflects local causal factors. With sodium retention and hepatic sinusoidal or portal hypertension, as may occur in patients with liver disease, a pure or modified transudate accumulates as ascites.

Many endogenous and exogenous compounds (including drugs) are bound to albumin, and transport of such substances is an important function of albumin. Adverse clinical consequences may arise in hypoalbuminemic patients treated with drugs that are highly protein-bound. A larger amount of unbound (free) drug may increase interactions with receptors and facilitate movement of drug across the blood-brain barrier, potentially resulting in adverse effects.

Hypoalbuminemia usually is accompanied by hypocalcemia (as reflected by measurement of serum total calcium concentration) as a result of decreased protein binding of calcium. A linear relationship between

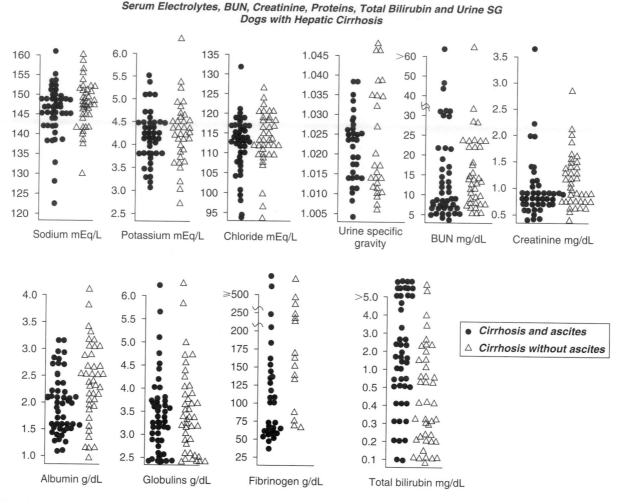

Fig. 19-5 Scattergram showing the serum electrolytes, blood urea nitrogen (BUN), creatinine, proteins, and total bilirubin and urine specific gravity in dogs with hepatic cirrhosis with and without ascites. (Data from SA Center: College of Veterinary Medicine, Cornell University, 1998).

serum protein and calcium concentrations exists in dogs and can be used to assess the clinical importance of hypocalcemia.[19,109] A reliable relationship between albumin, protein, and calcium concentrations does not occur in cats.[19,63]

Although usually attributed to synthetic failure, hypoalbuminemia in liver disease is multifactorial. In addition to decreased synthetic capacity, increased distribution into ascites, malnutrition, and a negative acute-phase response also may affect serum albumin concentration. Increased ultrafiltration into the space of Disse (caused by sinusoidal hypertension) may overwhelm the absorptive capacity of hepatic lymphatics despite a nearly tenfold increase in lymphatic flow. Hydrostatic leakage of protein-poor ultrafiltrate from the liver aggravates abdominal effusion. In such patients, newly synthesized albumin released directly into ascitic fluid may not reach the intravascular compartment and may take weeks to equilibrate with the exchangeable albumin pool.[137,183] Some human patients with severe

liver disease and hypoalbuminemia maintain normal rates of albumin synthesis. In these patients, water and sodium retention are primarily responsible for hypoalbuminemia and ascites. Serum protein concentrations in dogs with hepatic cirrhosis (with and without ascites), dogs with PSVA, and cats with HL are shown in Figs. 19-5, 19-6, and 19-7.

In patients with inflammatory liver disease, albumin synthesis may be suppressed by inflammatory mediators.[14,27,91,115] Suppression of albumin synthesis usually is inversely proportional to the rate of acute-phase protein synthesis and thus has been called a negative acute-phase response. However, the acute-phase response also increases transcapillary diffusion of albumin. Endotoxin can increase vascular permeability to albumin, and enhanced transmural passage of endotoxins during portal hypertension may contribute to splanchnic vasodilatation and transcapillary leakage of albumin.[104] Abnormal polyamine metabolism caused by altered urea cycle function and methionine metabolism also can

Serum Electrolytes, BUN, Creatinine, Proteins and Urine SG
Dogs with Portosystemic Venous Anomalies

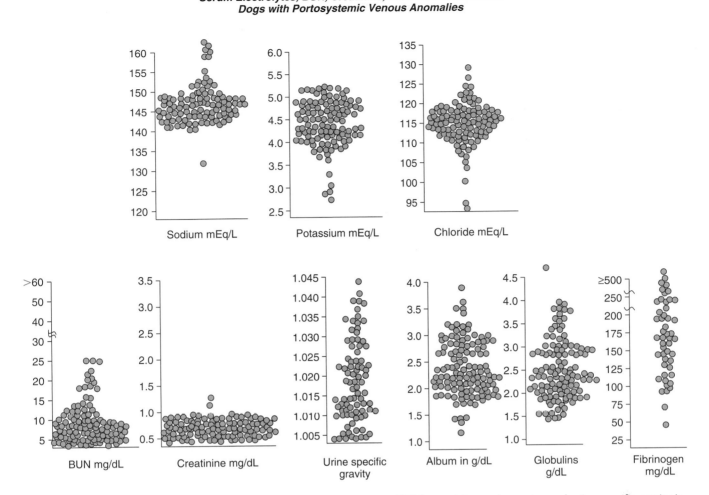

Fig. 19-6 Scattergram showing the serum electrolytes, blood urea nitrogen (BUN), creatinine, and proteins, and urine specific gravity in dogs with portosystemic vascular anomalies. (Data from SA Center: College of Veterinary Medicine, Cornell University, 1998).

impair albumin synthesis. Dietary restriction of protein is the most common correctable cause of hypoalbuminemia in liver disease patients. By increasing protein intake as tolerated and observing the response over weeks, the role of dietary protein restriction in hypoalbuminemia can be evaluated.

Hypoalbuminemia in liver disease generally is not accompanied by decreased globulin concentration (see Figs. 19-5, 19-6, and 19-7). Rather, globulin concentration is normal or increased because of a disproportionate increase in γ-globulins and acute-phase proteins. γ-Globulin concentrations increase as a result of increased systemic exposure to gut-derived antigens, microorganisms, and debris normally removed by the hepatic mononuclear phagocytes (Kupffer cells) and presence of inflammatory and immune-mediated processes associated with the underlying disease. α-Globulins (particularly haptoglobin), fibrinogen, and antithrombin III are abnormally low in dogs with end-stage cirrhosis and hepatic synthetic failure.[146]

Portosystemic shunting and severe hepatic insufficiency also decrease plasma concentration of protein C, an important anticoagulant also involved in the inflammatory response.[170] The diagnostic utility of the serum total protein concentration is complicated by the induction of haptoglobin by glucocorticoids and development of coagulopathies that can further deplete fibrinogen, antithrombin III, and protein C.[75,87]

The wide range of serum albumin concentrations in normally hydrated cirrhotic dogs with and without ascites demonstrates that hypoalbuminemia is only one factor influencing ascites formation (see Fig. 19-5). In dogs with ascites (n = 52), median serum albumin concentration was 2.0 g/dL (range, 1.2 to 3.2 g/dL), and in dogs without ascites (n = 50), median serum albumin concentration was 2.4 g/dL (range, 0.7 to 4.2 g/dL). Median serum globulin concentrations in these dogs were similar, whereas median plasma fibrinogen concentration was significantly decreased in ascitic dogs (median, 105 mg/dL; range, 30 to 780 mg/dL)

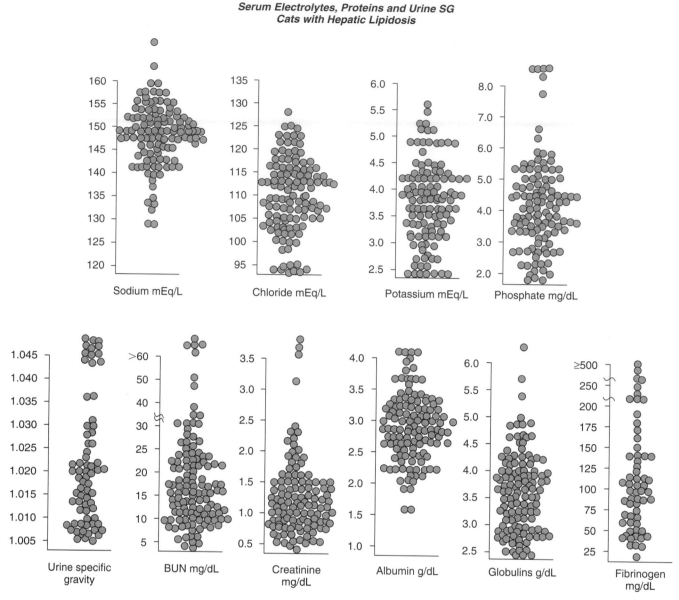

Fig. 19-7 Scattergram showing the serum electrolytes, blood urea nitrogen (BUN), creatinine, proteins, and urine specific gravity in cats with hepatic lipidosis; n = 73. (Data from SA Center: College of Veterinary Medicine, Cornell University, 1998).

compared with dogs without ascites (median, 165 mg/dL; range, 64 to 550 mg/dL).

SERUM ELECTROLYTES

Hypokalemia in Liver Disease

Hypokalemia is a serious electrolyte disturbance associated with hepatic insufficiency.[26] Contributing factors include insufficient energy intake, enteric losses (e.g., vomiting, diarrhea, nutrient malassimilation), treatment with loop diuretics, and secondary hyperaldosteronism.[164] Magnesium deficiency also can complicate hypokalemia by potentiating kaliuresis through its effects on aldosterone.[65] Hypokalemia may go unrecognized because of the transcellular shift that occurs

between potassium and hydrogen ions. Serum potassium concentrations of dogs with cirrhosis, dogs with PSVA, and cats with HL are shown in Figs. 19-5, 19-6, and 19-7. Frank hypokalemia was present in 11 of 48 cirrhotic dogs with ascites, in 10 of 42 of cirrhotic dogs without ascites, in 6 of 113 dogs with PSVA, and in 32 of 116 cats with HL. A total of 34 of 90 cirrhotic dogs (19 of 48 with ascites and 15 of 42 without ascites), 24 of 104 dogs with PSVA, and 44 of 116 cats with HL had subnormal or low normal serum potassium concentrations. Although the prognosis is worse for cats with HL and hypokalemia, the prognostic significance of hypokalemia has not been evaluated in the other disorders.[28]

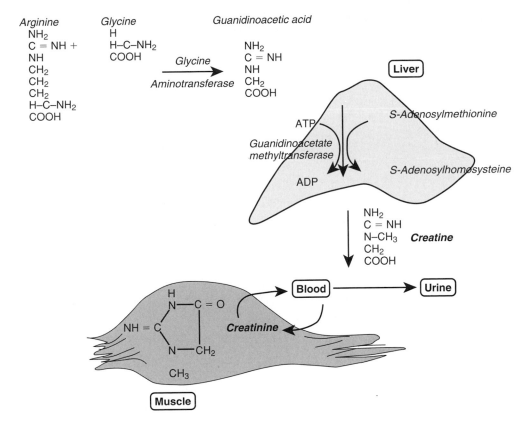

Fig. 19-8 Diagrammatic representation of hepatic contribution to creatine synthesis. (Adapted from Heymsfield SB, Arteaga C, McManus C, et al: Measurement of muscle mass in humans: validity of the 24-hour urinary creatinine method, *Am J Clin Nutr* 37:478–494, 1983. ©American Society for Clinical Nutrition.)

It is important to recognize and correct hypokalemia for several reasons. Most importantly, a reciprocal relationship exists between intracellular and extracellular potassium concentrations and renal ammoniagenesis.[71,163,164] Infusion of potassium chloride in hypokalemic patients significantly improved central nervous system (CNS) function in early hepatic encephalopathy (HE) and prolonged survival in cirrhotic humans.[182] Patients given potassium chloride to establish normokalemia experienced decreased arterial NH_3 concentration and pH, increased arterial NH_4^+/NH_3 ratio, decreased urine pH, and slightly increased 24-hour urinary ammonia excretion with a significantly increased urine NH_4^+/NH_3 ratio. Mechanistically, potassium infused into the hypokalemic patient replaces intracellular hydrogen ions. The displaced cellular hydrogen ions decrease blood pH, promoting conversion of NH_3 to the less-diffusible NH_4^+ form. This small shift in pH is not great enough to stimulate renal ammoniagenesis, but reduced urine pH leads to increased excretion of NH_4^+. This effect may be augmented by increased plasma aldosterone given its ability to increase hydrogen ion delivery into distal renal tubular fluid.[145]

Serum Potassium Concentration and Ammoniagenesis. Experimental and clinical observations of potassium depletion and loading suggest that renal NH_3 production is intimately linked with potassium homeostasis. Low serum potassium concentrations stimulate and high serum potassium concentrations suppress renal ammoniagenesis.[118,162] A closed-loop regulatory system modulates NH_3 production, hydrogen ion homeostasis, and urinary potassium excretion in response to acute and chronic changes in serum potassium concentration. Potassium deficiency stimulates H^+ secretion in the distal nephron and may stimulate HCO_3^- production by increasing collecting duct expression of an H^+-K^+-ATPase that facilitates reabsorbtion of K^+ in exchange for H^+.[92,118] Potassium deficiency also may increase luminal electronegativity in the proximal tubule, stimulating HCO_3^- secretion.[22] Hypokalemia arising from diuretics used to treat ascites can cause hyperammonemia secondary to metabolic alkalosis resulting from renal H^+ loss.

Hypophosphatemia in Liver Disease

Hypophosphatemia also may complicate hepatic insufficiency. At increased risk are cats with HL associated with diabetes mellitus or pancreatitis. Although symptomatic hypophosphatemia may develop after rehydration and insulin therapy, it is most common as a result of refeeding in cats with HL. Serum potassium, magnesium, and phosphorus concentrations in 157 cats with severe HL are shown in Fig. 19-9. In this population, only 22 of 157 (14%) HL cats had hypophosphatemia at presentation, but more than 35% of those undergoing nutritional support became hypophosphatemic with refeeding. Hypophosphatemia in patients with liver disease is thought to reflect intracellular shifts of phosphate.[64,157]

Although less common on presentation than hypokalemia, severe hypophosphatemia can produce many clinical signs including weakness (e.g., ventilatory failure severe enough to cause respiratory acidosis, neck ventroflexion in cats), vomiting, gastric atony, hemolysis, bleeding tendencies (i.e., platelet dysfunction), hemolytic anemia, and neurologic signs that can be confused with HE.[45,64] Mechanisms of hemolysis involve depletion of red cell energy related to impaired glycolysis and ATP production and diminished ability to maintain reduced GSH in erythyrocytes. Muscle weakness in

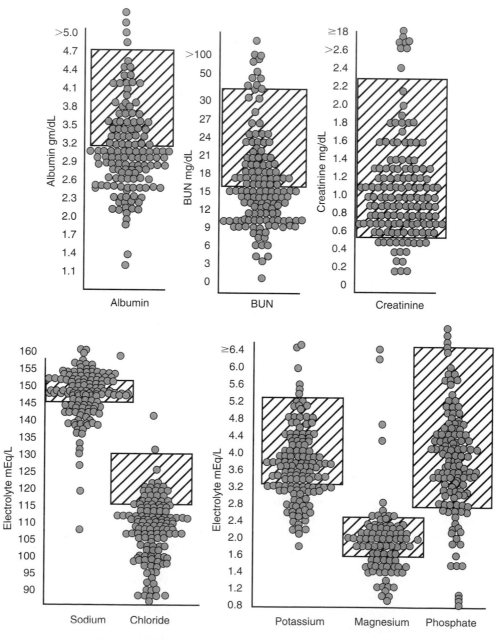

Fig. 19-9 Scattergram showing the serum potassium, magnesium, phosphate, sodium, chloride, albumin, blood urea nitrogen (BUN), and creatinine from a survey of 157 cats with severe hepatic lipidosis. Normal range indicated by slashed boxes. (Data from SA Center: College of Veterinary Medicine, Cornell University, 2004).

hypophosphatemia may be severe enough to impair ventilation, leading to ventilatory failure and respiratory acidosis. Hypophosphatemia induced by refeeding in cats with HL typically appears within the first 48 hours of alimentation, and overt clinical effects are observed with serum phosphorus concentrations less than 1.5 mg/dL.

Hypomagnesemia in Liver Disease

Symptomatic hypomagnesmia is observed infrequently in patients with liver disease. Recognition of low serum magnesium concentration is important because of the essential role of magnesium as an enzyme cofactor. The mechanisms underlying clinical signs have not been clarified but likely involve transcellular shifting of magnesium into cells with glucose. Hypomagnesemia also may be induced by citrate toxicity after large-volume transfusion with citrate-phosphate-dextrose (CPD)-anticoagulated blood in patients with limited ability for hepatic metabolism of citrate. The most important clinical manifestations of hypomagnesemia are muscle weakness, impaired contractility of the diaphragm, aggravation of preexisting cardiomyopathy, and altered sensorium that may mimic HE. These clinical signs also can be mistakenly attributed to abnormal serum potassium or phosphorus concentrations.

WATER AND SODIUM DISTURBANCES IN CHRONIC LIVER DISEASE

The most common fluid and electrolyte abnormalities in hepatic insufficiency accompanied by portal hypertension are impaired ability to excrete sodium and water and decreased GFR. Sodium retention occurs first, and water retention and impaired GFR follow. Disturbances of body water and electrolyte homeostasis become apparent with progressive liver dysfunction and precede ascites formation. When most severe, disparity between water ingestion and excretion causes dilutional hyponatremia.

Isoosmotic Renal Sodium Retention

In many patients with hepatic insufficiency prone to ascites formation, isoosmotic renal sodium retention expands extracellular volume such that total body sodium is not reflected in the serum sodium concentrations (see Fig. 19-5). In humans, the magnitude of sodium retention varies among individuals. That a similar phenomenon occurs in cirrhotic dogs is indicated by their diverse urine specific gravity (USG) values and serum sodium concentrations at presentation and their apparent resistance to diuretic therapy.

Impaired Excretion of Solute-Free Water

Up to 35% of human patients with cirrhosis develop impaired free water excretion causing dilutional hyponatremia.[124,125,148] A similar phenomenon may occur in dogs (see Fig. 19-5).[13,58,106,126,173] When dogs with cirrhosis with and without ascites were compared, the overall frequency of hyponatremia on initial presentation was approximately 25% with the lowest serum sodium concentrations found in dogs with ascites (see Fig. 19-5). As in humans, serum sodium concentration in dogs did not predict ascites formation, but marked hyponatremia was only observed in dogs with substantial free water retention and ascites.

Decreased free water excretion is linked to increased vasopression (AVP) secretion. The most plausible theories involve the sympathetic nervous system (SNS) as both a detector and effector mechanism, adjusting extracellular fluid (ECF) volume and arterial pressure. Decreased total body sodium or decreased arterial pressure reduces SNS inhibition of AVP secretion, whereas vascular distention causes inhibition of AVP secretion and adjustments in vascular tone, cardiac rate, and cardiac contractility. Endothelin may play a modulatory role in the renal AVP response.

Pathophysiology of Fluid Retention in Cirrhosis

In cirrhosis, disturbances in fluid balance precede ascites formation by several weeks. In this phase, intravascular volume expansion results from renal sodium retention.[106] Renal tubular sodium retention also precedes changes in renal blood flow, GFR, filtration fraction, and intrarenal vascular resistance associated with cirrhosis.[99] A 36% plasma volume expansion occurred in cirrhotic dogs during this active salt-retaining, preascitic phase with two thirds of the newly acquired volume distributed to the vasodilated splanchnic circulation.[98] Ascites formation is hastened by sodium ingestion or intravenous administration of sodium-containing fluids. Surgical creation of portosystemic shunting in dogs with hepatic cirrhosis abolished portal hypertension and the early tendency for renal sodium retention and ascites. In such studies, 20- to 30-lb cirrhotic dogs with shunts were able to maintain normal sodium balance with intakes as high as 85 mEq/day. Cirrhotic dogs without shunts accumulated sodium at this level of intake.[171]

Peripheral arterial and splanchnic vasodilatation initiates water and sodium conservation in cirrhosis.[69] Peripheral arterial vasodilatation ("underfilling") reenforces the signal initiating renal sodium retention (i.e., perceived reduction in circulating ECF volume). The physiologic responses observed after acute portal vein constriction (i.e., systemic arterial vasodilation and hypotension, ECF expansion, increased cardiac output) are similar to those associated with the hyperdynamic circulatory syndrome of cirrhosis.[16]

These hemodynamic maladjustments are mediated by the renin-angiotensin-aldosterone system (RAAS) and SNS in response to underfilling of the systemic arterial circulation and decreased renal perfusion. Abnormal intrarenal accumulation of angiotensin II occurs early in the disease process, even before activation of the RAAS.[97]

Renal sodium conservation may be related in part to enhanced sensitivity to aldosterone.

Effect of Portosystemic Shunting on Sodium and Water Retention

Portosystemic shunting also may affect sodium and water retention, and surgically created portosystemic shunts in experimental dogs have been used to study the effects of diverted hepatoportal perfusion on sodium and water balance. Ten weeks after end-to-side portocaval shunt formation, plasma volume, systemic blood pressure, and central venous pressures were maintained, and no changes in GFR, plasma renin activity, or aldosterone concentrations were identified.[96] Some dogs maintained normal sodium balance after ingestion of 150 mEq/day of sodium, but others developed ascites.[96] These findings indicate that in some situations portosystemic shunting alone can impair ability to adapt to increased sodium loads. This finding may explain the tendency to form ascites in some dogs with PSVA (especially those with ductus venosus) and hypoalbuminemia or after administration of sodium-rich crystalloids.

Specific Mechanisms of Water and Electrolyte Disturbances in Cirrhosis and Portosystemic Shunting

Nonosmotic Vasopressin Stimulation. Nonosmotic stimulation of AVP is a central factor mediating water retention in cirrhosis.[69] Acute changes in portal venous pressure in cirrhotic dogs initiate AVP-mediated antidiuresis. Both systemic and splanchnic arterial vasodilatation can stimulate nonosmotic AVP release and activate other antidiuretic and vasopressor systems.[69] Early in cirrhosis ("compensated cirrhosis"), transient neurohormonal responses increase plasma volume and temporarily suppress baroreceptor signaling. As the disease progresses, arterial vasodilatation worsens, and neurohormonal responses are no longer able to compensate. At this point, vasoconstrictor systems become continuously stimulated and promote the sodium and water retention that causes edema and ascites. The response is exaggerated by abnormal retention of AVP as a result of impaired metabolism. Normally, the kidney and liver metabolize AVP, but decreased AVP clearance in hepatic disease correlates with disease severity.[154]

Increased Basal Cortisol and ACTH Concentrations. Increased basal cortisol and adrenocorticotropic hormone (ACTH) concentrations complicate hepatic insufficiency associated with portosystemic shunting in dogs, but normal adrenal response to low-dose dexamethasone suppression is maintained.[139] High basal cortisol directly reflects shunting, and concentrations normalize in dogs with congenital PSVA after successful shunt ligation.[139,156] Dogs with PSVA also have high free water flux and abnormally high GFR that normalize after shunt ligation.[51] It is unknown if this

response relates to abnormal cortisol concentration or hemodynamic adjustments.

Altered Steroid Hormone Metabolism. Altered steroid hormone metabolism also may contribute to sodium retention in cirrhosis. Abnormally increased serum bile salt concentrations may inhibit 11β-hydroxysteroid dehydrogenase-2 (11β-HSD-2), the enzyme that interconverts endogenous and exogenous biologically active 11β-hydroxysteroids and their inactive 11-ketosteroid counterparts. 11β-HSD-2 selectively modulates access of aldosterone to mineralocorticoid receptors and normally is located in mineralocorticoid-responsive tissues (including the distal nephron). Absence or inhibition of 11β-HSD-2 can mimic mineralocorticoid excess by allowing inappropriate access of 11β-hydroxyglucocorticoids to mineralorcorticoid receptors.[4,132]

Abnormal Aldosterone Release and Responsiveness to Aldosterone. High (or inappropriately normal) aldosterone concentrations precede and accompany pathologic sodium retention in humans and animals with cirrhosis. Experimentally, hepatic venous congestion and acute portal hypertension stimulate aldosterone secretion.[18] The importance of aldosterone in sodium and water retention in cirrhosis in humans is demonstrated by the efficacy of spironolactone (a specific aldosterone antagonist) in mobilizing ascites and alleviating sodium retention in patients without underlying renal dysfunction. The influence of aldosterone on renal sodium retention is enhanced by increased renal sensitivity to the hormone. This phenomenon is reflected clinically by decompensation (i.e., ascites induction) of cirrhotic dogs given glucocorticoids with minimal mineralocorticoid activity (e.g., prednisone).

Splanchnic Arterial Vasodilatation. Although the cause of systemic and splanchnic arterial vasodilatation that stimulates AVP production and other antidiuretic and vasopressor mechanisms is not completely understood, nitric oxide (NO) plays an integral role. Splanchnic NO is produced by inducible NO synthetase activity in the mesenteric splanchnic endothelium. Splanchnic vasodilatation also reflects formation of arteriovenous shunts, acquired portosystemic communications, and other endothelial (e.g., prostacyclin, endothelin) and nonendothelial (e.g., glucagon, vasoactive intestinal peptide) vasodilatory mechanisms.[8] Vasodilatation of splanchnic vasculature also may reflect increased exposure to bacterial endotoxins from enhanced transmural passage of endotoxin from the gut lumen.[159]

Diminished Renal Prostaglandin Synthesis. Decreased renal prostaglandin production increases pathologic water accumulation and dilutional hyponatremia in cirrhosis and hepatorenal syndrome (HRS; see the Hepatorenal Syndrome section).[69] Endogenous renal prostaglandins normally play an important role in regulation of renal perfusion and tubular response to AVP, especially when vasoconstrictor forces predominate (as in cirrhosis). Renal synthesis of vasodilatory eicosonoids (e.g., prostaglandin [PG] I2 and PGE2) normally counterbalances vasoconstrictive stimuli (e.g., angiotensin II, AVP, increased renal sympathetic tone) and preserves renal blood flow and GFR. The protective effect of renal prostaglandins becomes apparent when cirrhotic patients with ascites are treated with nonsteroidal antiinflammatory drugs (NSAIDs). These patients may experience decreased renal blood flow and GFR, activation of vasoconstrictor systems, and sodium and fluid retention that can cause acute renal failure and HRS.

Water and Sodium Disturbances in Cats with Liver Disease

Cats with HL do not have consistent changes in serum electrolyte concentrations (see Fig. 19-7). This finding is not unexpected because many conditions that cause anorexia and rapid weight loss lead to HL. In a survey of cats with severe HL, 14 of 72 had USG values less than 1.010, 29 of 114 were hyponatremic, and only 1 was hypernatremic. Cats with chronic cholangitis or cholangiohepatitis also do not have consistent changes in serum sodium concentration or USG.

Summary of Effects of Cirrhosis on Total Body Sodium and Water and Ascites Formation

In cirrhotic patients, there is a relative inability to adjust water excretion to the amount of water ingested and decreased ability to eliminate sodium in the urine. Impaired water and sodium elimination arises from several factors: (1) enhanced sodium reabsorption in the proximal nephron and decreased delivery of glomerular filtrate to the distal nephron; (2) decreased GFR caused by splanchnic vasodilatation, low systemic blood pressure, altered cardiac output, and inappropriate vasoconstriction of the glomerular efferent arterioles; (3) decreased renal prostaglandin synthesis (PGE2) and impaired autoregulation of renal blood flow; (4) pathologic redistribution of renal blood flow away from the cortex; (5) increased response to or activity of aldosterone; and (6) nonosmotic stimulation of AVP release. The most important factors favoring dilutional hyponatremia are disturbed hemodynamics involving the splanchnic and systemic circulation and nonosmotic AVP release. Medical treatment of impaired water and sodium is difficult and may be facilitated by aquaretic agents and vasopressors specific for the splanchnic circulation.[68,89,178] The importance of sodium retention in ECF volume expansion associated with portal hypertension is evidenced by patient response to dietary sodium restriction and diuretic stimulation of natriuresis. The severity of sodium retention relative to water retention varies among individuals, and serum sodium concentration does not predict ascites formation (see Fig. 19-5). Some patients produce urine that is virtually free of sodium, whereas others produce inappropriately concentrated urine because of excessive AVP release and are at high risk for dilutional hyponatremia.

ASCITES RESULTING FROM LIVER DISEASE

Pathophysiologic mechanisms underlying ascites formation are complex, and no specific clinical features clearly identify patients prone to ascites formation. Serum electrolyte, BUN, creatinine, protein, and total bilirubin concentrations for 109 cirrhotic dogs with and without ascites are shown in Fig. 19-5. Better understanding of the pathophysiology of ascites formation has led to a shift from the classical underfilling and overflow hypotheses to the forward theory (Fig. 19-10). Currently, splanchnic arterial vasodilatation and associated systemic and renal counter-regulatory responses are thought to be the main pathophysiologic events underlying ascites formation. Decreased systemic vascular resistance initially arises as a consequence of marked splanchnic arterial vasodilatation. The mechanisms underlying splanchnic vasodilatation are poorly understood but likely involve enhanced availability, synthesis, or activity of vasodilatory factors such as NO, glucagon, vasoactive intestinal peptide, endotoxin, bile acids, prostaglandins, and increased local autonomic tone. Splanchnic vasodilatation promotes abnormal distribution of circulating blood volume away from the systemic circulation. The resulting systemic hypoperfusion is sensed by arterial baroreceptors, which signal a need for vasoconstriction and sodium and water retention by the kidneys (e.g., activation of the RAAS and SNS, release of AVP). These events establish a hyperdynamic state characterized by increased cardiac output, decreased systemic vascular resistance, and arterial vasodilatation affecting both the splanchnic and systemic circulation.

Increased splanchnic capillary hydrostatic pressure arises from increased splanchnic blood flow and portal hypertension, which are caused by increased hepatic sinusoidal resistance resulting from hepatic fibrosis. Increased intrasinusoidal pressure combined with high splanchnic capillary pressure and decreased oncotic pressure can cause an up to twentyfold increase in hepatic lymph formation, exceeding the drainage capacity of the thoracic and hepatic lymphatics. Lymph subsequently weeps from the surface of the liver or splanchnic vasculature into the peritoneal space, causing ascites. Hypoalbuminemia is notably absent early in this syndrome. Formation of ascites continues in response to the ongoing systemic counter-regulatory response (e.g., RAAS-mediated renal sodium retention, nonosmotic stimulation of AVP release). In some patients, these

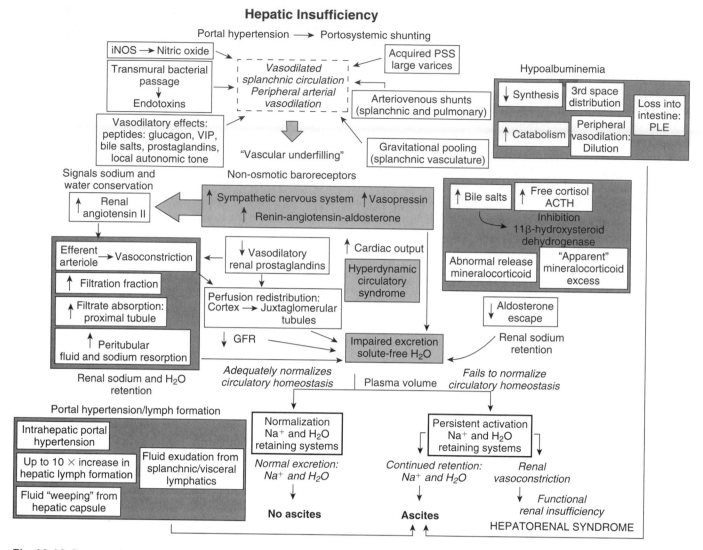

Fig. 19-10 Diagram showing the pathophysiologic mechanisms associated with ascites formation in patients with chronic hepatic insufficiency.

compensatory responses can culminate in development of HRS and acute renal failure.

Albumin infusions do not consistently improve circulatory and renal function in cirrhotic patients with ascites because of enhanced movement of albumin from vessels into the interstitium and severe vasodilatation of the splanchnic circulation. Although acute volume expansion in cirrhotic human patients increases peripheral blood volume, limited improvement occurs in central blood volume (i.e., splanchnic, hepatic, and cardiopulmonary circulation). However, infusion of albumin in combination with administration of a long-acting synthetic AVP analogue terlipressin can cause splanchnic vasoconstriction and improved systemic perfusion.

Assessment of Ascites

A sample of the abdominal effusion should be evaluated biochemically, cytologically, and by culture if cytology suggests infection. Ascites arising from liver disease typically is a pure transudate with a total protein concentration of less than 2.5 g/dL and specific gravity between 1.010 and 1.015. Cytologically, the fluid has low cellularity with only a few mesothelial cells and neutrophils present. In the jaundiced patient, the fluid is yellow and bilirubin crystals may be observed, but the bilirubin concentration of the effusion is less than that of serum. A serum-to-effusion albumin gradient greater than 1.1 suggests portal hypertension as a causative mechanism.[131] Body weight and abdominal girth measurements should be taken as a reference for evaluating changes in fluid accumulation. Girth measurements are meaningful only if a consistent method is used. A mark is made on the abdomen with a permanent ink pen, and the owner is taught to monitor ascites accumulation by measuring girth circumference using a consistent technique.

ABNORMAL RENAL FUNCTION IN LIVER DISEASE

As liver function deteriorates and portal hypertension worsens, several maladaptive responses threaten renal function. Decreased GFR reduces delivery of glomerular filtrate to the distal diluting segments of the nephron. Coupled with increased resorption in the proximal tubule, this increases renal sodium and water reabsorption, impairs renal escape from abnormally increased aldosterone, and favors resistance to atrial natriuretic peptides.[57] Systemic counter-regulatory responses that normally preserve filtration fraction increase production of angiotensin II and further provoke vasoconstriction of the efferent arterioles. Although these events maintain glomerular capillary pressure, increase filtration fraction, and alter peritubular Starling's forces favoring fluid reabsorption, they do so at the expense of decreased renal blood flow.[69] Functional disruption of solute conservation in the loop of Henle by loop diuretics (e.g., furosemide) may further impair the ability of the nephron to dilute or concentrate urine.

Increased Water Turnover and Glomerular Filtration Rate

The influence of hepatic insufficiency on BUN and serum creatinine concentrations is aggravated by increased water turnover and development of a supranormal GFR as observed in dogs with PSVA.[51] Primary polydipsia associated with HE, stimulation of hepatoportal osmoreceptors, and an impaired renal medullary concentration gradient (e.g., chronic hypokalemia, decreased urea synthesis) may contribute to abnormal water balance in these animals.[72,93,162]

Polyuria and Polydipsia

Polydipsia, polyuria, and renal dysfunction may be associated with liver disease in both dogs and cats. Dogs with PSVA may be presented primarily for evaluation of polyuria and polydipsia.[29,72] Mechanisms may include psychogenic polydipsia associated with HE; sensory input signaling splanchnic vasodilatation, decreased hepatic portal perfusion, or altered osmolality; renal medullary washout caused by low urea concentration; renal tubular dysfunction associated with potassium depletion; or increased concentrations of endogenous steroids.[93]

Evaluation of USG before fluid therapy in dogs with PSVA showed that 47 of 87 had a USG less than 1.020, and 12 of 87 were hyposthenuric (see Fig. 19-6). Serum electrolyte concentrations were not significantly correlated with USG, but subnormal BUN concentrations occurred in 58 of 123 dogs, and low normal or subnormal creatinine concentrations were found in 83 of 123. These findings suggest that diuresis contributes to low USG in these patients, as supported by presence of supranormal GFR in dogs with PSVA.[51] Subnormal

BUN concentrations in dogs with PSVA could impair maintenance of the renal medullary solute gradient necessary for water reabsorption in response to AVP. Low serum creatinine concentration probably reflects reduced muscle mass associated with the young age and small size of many affected dogs, hepatic insufficiency, and increased water turnover.[25,51,79,123]

Similar mechanisms are likely to be operative in dogs with acquired hepatic insufficiency. Of cirrhotic dogs with ascites, 15 of 26 with urinalysis performed before treatment had USG less than 1.020 (see Fig. 19-5). Of these, only 3 of 26 were hyposthenuric. In the same group, 11 of 42 had low BUN concentrations, and 21 of 42 had low or subnormal serum creatinine concentrations. In cirrhotic dogs without ascites, 16 of 34 with urinalysis performed before treatment had a specific gravity less than 1.020, and only 1 of 34 was hyposthenuric. In the same group, 20 of 47 had low BUN concentrations, and 36 of 47 had low normal or subnormal serum creatinine concentrations.

Altered Intrarenal Hemodynamics

Subtle changes in intrarenal hemodynamics contribute to deranged renal function in cirrhosis. Normally, renal blood flow is predominantly distributed to cortex (90%) with less blood flow to the outer (9%) and inner medulla (1%). Autoregulation of renal blood flow maintains proper balance between afferent and efferent arteriolar tone to regulate GFR and filtration fraction. Redistribution of blood flow from outer cortical to juxtamedullary nephrons occurs in approximately 60% of human patients with ascites. Redistribution of renal blood flow and increased intrarenal arterial resistance are correlated with increased plasma renin activity.[16,90] Changes in systemic and splanchnic hemodynamics (e.g., low systemic arterial blood pressure, decreased systemic vascular resistance, splanchnic vasodilatation) associated with the hyperdynamic circulatory state of cirrhosis initiate renal vasoconstrictor responses that further compromise renal perfusion. Arterial vasodilatation expands vascular capacity and makes effective circulating blood volume difficult or impossible to maintain. High SNS activity further reduces renal cortical blood flow, whereas low systemic pressure and increased renal interstitial pressure compromise renal blood flow, GFR, sodium excretion, and water diuresis.

Hepatorenal Syndrome

HRS is a state of functional renal failure associated with low GFR, preserved tubular function, and normal renal histology that occurs in some human patients with cirrhosis and ascites.[111] A similar syndrome rarely may occur in veterinary patients. Reduced renal cortical perfusion resulting from increased renal vascular resistance precedes renal failure in this syndrome. The cause of intrarenal vasoconstriction is complex and poorly understood

(Fig. 19-11). Factors associated with development of HRS in humans are listed in Box 19-1. Essential diagnostic criteria for HRS in humans include a spontaneously acquired acute decline in GFR, impaired urinary sodium excretion (<10 mEq/day), urine osmolality greater than plasma osmolality, and absence of other causes of renal failure.

Prevention of HRS requires early intervention to minimize circulatory instability and renal hypoperfusion. Treatment in human patients has included plasma expanders (e.g., albumin, colloids), the long-acting α-adrenergic agonist midodrine to improve systemic blood pressure and renal perfusion, and the somatostatin analogue octreotide and the AVP analogue terlipressin to attenuate splanchnic vasodilatation.[3,10,89,142,172]

ACID-BASE DISTURBANCES IN LIVER DISEASE

Although experimental studies support a role for hepatic urea and glutamine cycles in regulation of systemic pH by their effects on renal ammoniagenesis, there is no consistent pattern of acid-base disturbances in patients with liver disease.[117,147] The most common disturbance

in humans with hepatic insufficiency and coma is respiratory alkalosis, but metabolic acid-base disturbances may also occur.[117,133,147] Patients with stable cirrhosis and those with portal hypertension attenuated by surgically created portosystemic shunts commonly develop compensated respiratory or metabolic alkalosis. Respiratory alkalosis is closely associated with the extent of functional liver impairment rather than the presence of portosystemic shunting and nearly always is compensated.[133]

Mechanism of Respiratory Alkalosis

Respiratory alkalosis in cirrhosis may evolve subsequent to reduced arterial oxygen saturation secondary to acquired venoarterial shunting, ventilation-perfusion mismatch (derived from ascites-induced restriction of ventilatory efforts or changes in pulmonary capillaries), a shift to the right in the oxyhemoglobin dissociation curve, direct stimulation of the respiratory center by encephalopathic toxins (e.g., NH_3), or development of CNS acidosis.[78] Respiratory alkalosis may also develop as compensation for metabolic acidemia (e.g., lactic acido-

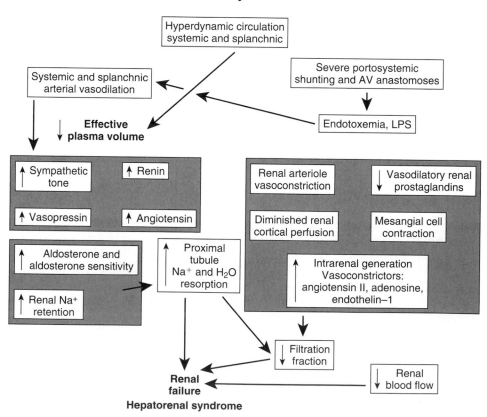

Fig. 19-11 Pathophysiologic mechanisms of the hepatorenal syndrome based on human clinical studies and experimental animal modeling of cirrhosis. (From Guzman JA, Rosado AE, Kruse JA: Vasopressin vs norepinephrine in endotoxic shock: systemic, renal, and splanchnic hemodynamic and oxygen transport effects, *J Appl Physiol* 95:803–809, 2003.)

<table>
<tr><td>Box 19-1</td><td>Health Factors Associated with Development of the Hepatorenal Syndrome in Humans</td></tr>
</table>

Constant associations
  Ascites
  Intravascular volume disturbances

Variable associations
  Gastrointestinal bleeding
  Large-volume paracentesis
  Overzealous use of diuretics
  Progressive jaundice
  Sepsis
  Nephrotoxic drugs
  Nonsteroidal antiinflammatory drugs
  Radiographic contrast media

sis, increased concentrations of free fatty acids, impaired renal tubular acid excretion, or renal hypoperfusion).[7,136]

Mechanism of Metabolic Alkalosis

Hypoalbuminemia produces an apparent metabolic alkalosis even in the presence of a normal serum bicarbonate concentration because of loss of the buffering capacity of the negative charges on the albumin molecule.[105] A decrease of 1 g/dL of plasma albumin results in a calculated base excess of +3.7 mEq/L. Hypoalbuminemia appears to be the dominant alkalinizing influence in cirrhotic dogs, whereas hypochloremia appears to be more influential in cats with severe HL.

Metabolic alkalosis in some patients is caused by excessive diuretic therapy, repeated vomiting of gastric secretions, or alkali loading arising from transfusion of citrate-anticoagulated blood. Immediately after blood collection, CPD-preserved blood has low bicarbonate and high citrate concentrations.[56] During storage, red cell metabolism consumes bicarbonate as a result of gly-colysis and lactic acid production. After infusion, citrate-preserved blood products favor development of metabolic alkalosis because both lactate and citrate can be metabolized to HCO_3^-. The total potential bicarbonate concentration in 450 mL of CPD-preserved human blood is approximately 58 mEq/L (i.e., the initial 24 mEq/L in the plasma itself and an additional 34 mEq/L as citrate).[56] Although transfused blood is transiently acidifying because of free citric acid, this effect is quickly counteracted by the metabolism of citrate to CO_2 and water.

Persistent secondary hyperaldosteronism, as occurs in some patients prone to ascites formation, also contributes to metabolic alkalosis. This effect is augmented when administered diuretics increase distal renal tubular delivery of sodium and water. Metabolic alkalosis also is favored by loss of effective extracellular volume (i.e., concentration alkalosis).[56]

Mechanisms of Metabolic Acidosis

Metabolic acidosis is more common in patients in the terminal stages of cirrhosis complicated by hypoxia, systemic hypotension, lactic acidosis, and renal dysfunction. Patients that develop lactic acidosis have severely compromised hepatic function and cardiovascular stability. Both dogs and cats with severe liver disease accumulate unidentified anions, presumably lactate. As compared with cirrhotic dogs, cats with severe HL appear to be at greater risk for acidemia, metabolic acidosis, accumulation of unmeasured anions, and dilutional acidosis.

Lactate Metabolism in Liver Disease

All cells can produce lactate and can add it to the systemic circulation, and all cells (with the exception of red blood cells [RBCs]) also can extract lactate from the blood for metabolism. Estimates of the lactate flux (production and utilization under basal conditions) indicate production primarily in the skin, RBCs, brain, and skeletal muscle (Table 19-2).[128] Skeletal muscle contributes considerably more lactate to the systemic circulation after strenuous exercise or generalized seizure activity (as may occur in

TABLE 19-2 Rates of Basal Lactate Production and Utilization (mmol/day/kg) in Humans

Tissue	Basal Lactate Production	Tissue	Basal Lactate Utilization
Skin	5.0	Liver	10.3
Red blood cells	4.3	Kidney	5.5
Brain	3.4	Heart	1.1
Muscle	3.1	Other	1.5
Intestinal mucosa	1.6		
White blood cells, platelets	1.0		
Total	18.4	Total	18.4

From Park R, Arieff AI: Lactic acidosis, Adv Intern Med 25:33-68, 1980.

patients with HE). The liver and kidneys are the primary sites of lactate removal, with the liver predominating at rest (see Table 19-2). The normal dog liver can extract at least 19% of a physiologic lactate load per hour.[127] Lactate utilization is governed by conversion to pyruvate via lactate dehydrogenase (LDH), and the pyruvate formed is either metabolized to glucose or oxidized in the tricarboxylic acid (Krebs) cycle to carbon dioxide and water (Fig. 19-12). Lactate generation by RBCs, brain, and skin with subsequent gluconeogenesis by liver and kidneys is known as the Cori cycle, an important mechanism of energy provision during starvation.

Pyruvate, an intermediate common to several metabolic pathways, is the immediate precursor of lactic acid. Glucose and alanine are the physiologically important pyruvate precursors. Pathologic conditions stimulating conversion of glucose or alanine to pyruvate predispose to lactic acidosis. The enzyme pyruvate dehydrogenase (PDH) plays an integral role in lactate metabolism, catalyzing the intramitochondrial conversion of pyruvate to acetyl coenzyme A (acetyl CoA), which enters the Krebs cycle (see Fig. 19-12).

Removal of lactic acid normally occurs through three pathways: two depend on hepatic function, and the third on renal excretion.[94] At rest, the liver metabolizes 40% to 60% of endogenously produced lactate by oxidation in the mitochondrial tricarboxylic acid cycle or by conversion of lactate to glucose in the cytosolic Cori cycle (see Fig. 19-12). Each mechanism of lactate metabolism regenerates bicarbonate. Hepatic utilization of lactate depends on substrate uptake, hepatic gluconeogenic capacity, and hepatic blood flow. In the absence of metabolic acidosis or tissue perfusion deficits, hyperlactatemia usually is associated with conditions that favor glycolysis (e.g., high catecholamine concentrations, alkalosis) and increase conversion of pyruvate to lactate.[50] Respiratory alkalosis, common in cirrhotic patients, is thought to increase lactate production by enhancing phosphofructokinase (PFK) activity.[66] Lactate accumulation also is favored when symptomatic hypoglycemia increases catecholamine release, when high blood ammonia concentrations inhibit PDH and cause preferential conversion of pyruvate to lactate, and when acidosis inhibits pyruvate carboxylase and impairs hepatic gluconeogenesis from lactate (see Fig. 19-12). Reduction in systemic pH compromises hepatic uptake of lactate, and decreased hepatic pH arising from lactic acidosis directly disables hepatic lactate metabolism in dogs.[11,41]

Lactic acidosis results in a high anion gap metabolic acidosis caused by excessive production or decreased

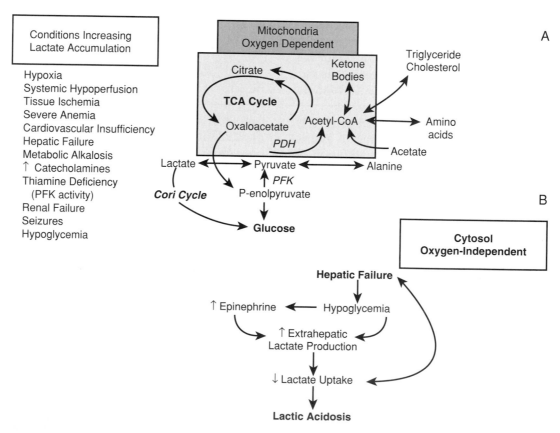

Fig. 19-12 Metabolic generation and interactions of lactate **(A)** and the mechanisms leading to lactic acidosis in liver failure **(B)**. *PFK*, Phosphofructokinase; *PDH*, pyruvate dehydrogenase.

utilization of lactic acid. It is most commonly associated with tissue hypoxia, hypoperfusion, or fulminant hepatic failure. Lactate production is a late sign of inadequate oxygen supply and therefore is neither a sensitive nor early indicator of impending hepatic insufficiency.[20,21] Lactic acidemia also may develop in some conditions without perfusion deficits or hypoxic injury (e.g., diabetes mellitus, renal failure, fulminant hepatic failure, sepsis).[50,66,101]

Hypoperfusion, hypoxia, and ischemic damage of the liver convert it from a lactate-consuming to a lactate-producing organ.[50] Intraoperative hypotension, hepatic ischemia, vascular thrombosis, and fulminant hepatic failure each can lead to lactic acidemia. In fulminant hepatic failure, lactic acidemia indicates severe circulatory insufficiency, anaerobic metabolism, and diffuse panlobular parenchymal damage.[20] The direct relationship between plasma lactate concentrations and the severity of parenchymal damage permits prognostic use of systemic lactate concentrations in human hepatic transplant patients.[50]

Serum lactate concentrations have not been commonly measured in veterinary patients, and the prevalence of lactic acidemia is unknown in dogs and cats with most forms of liver disease. However, cats with severe HL have been shown to develop hyperlactatemia.[35] The tendency for affected cats to develop lactate intolerance may be related to impaired mitochondrial function, thiamine deficiency (thiamine is a cofactor for PDH activity), impaired sinusoidal blood flow resulting from hepatocellular cytosolic expansion with triglyceride causing sinusoidal compression, or other underlying disorders causing hypoxia or a predilection for lactic acidosis (e.g., diabetes mellitus, pancreatitis). Dogs with experimentally induced acute hepatic failure developed mild increases in plasma lactate concentrations despite markedly increased concentrations in the brain (Fig. 19-13).[121] High brain lactate concentrations are associated with cerebral edema, increased intracranial pressure (>50 mm Hg), decreased cerebral perfusion pressure (<40 mm Hg), and death within 2 days.[121]

Transfusion of stored blood also can cause lactic acidosis. Immediately after collection into CPD solution, human blood has reduced bicarbonate concentration, increased PCO_2 (CO_2 slowly diffuses through the plastic), and high citrate concentration.[56] Glycolysis in RBC generates lactic acid during storage, and concentrations of approximately 12 mEq/L can be achieved in anticoagulated blood within 14 days. Comparable studies have not been performed using canine or feline blood.

Citrate Metabolism in Liver Disease

Citrate-rich blood products can lead to symptomatic hypercitratemia in patients with hepatic insufficiency caused by impaired metabolism of citrate. This effect is most common in very small animals (<5 kg) when large amounts of blood components are transfused. Owing to the chelating capacity of citrate, hypercitratemia can provoke symptomatic ionized hypocalcemia and more rarely hypomagnesemia. Clinical effects include coagulopathy, cardiac arrhythmias, and neuromuscular signs. Large citrate loads also can cause metabolic alkalosis as a result of hepatic metabolism of citrate to bicarbonate. The CPD solution used as an anticoagulant and preservative for blood components is a mixture of sodium citrate, citric acid, sodium phosphate, and dextrose. A 450-mL unit of blood mixed with 63 mL of CPD solution has a final sodium citrate concentration of 34 mEq/L.[56] Hemorrhagic tendencies initiated or aggravated by transfusion of large amounts of citrate-containing blood products should prompt measurement of serum ionized calcium concentration. Symptomatic ionized hypocalcemia requires treatment with intravenously administered calcium gluconate or calcium chloride (see Chapter 6).

Acid-Base Disturbances in Dogs with Cirrhosis

Evaluation of clinical data from dogs with cirrhosis indicates that conventional interpretation can cause unmeasured anions to be overlooked and result in underestimation of the complexity of the acid-base disturbance (Fig. 19-14). Mixed acid-base disturbances in these dogs may include metabolic alkalosis associated with hypoalbuminemia (83%) and hypochloremia (13%) and metabolic acidosis associated with unmeasured anions (67%). Overall, alkalemia was detected in 30% (25% of these animals had clinical signs and laboratory data consistent with emerging HRS), and acidemia was found in 17%. Conventional calculation of anion gap resulted in an abnormal value in 10%, but after correction of serum sodium concentration for water excess or deficit, 30% had abnormal anion gap values. Low serum sodium concentration (water excess) was found in 17% of dogs with cirrhosis.

Acid-Base Disturbances in Cats with Severe Hepatic Lipidosis

Clinical data from cats with severe HL also support the idea that conventional interpretation may underestimate the complexity of acid-base disturbances in patients with liver disease (Fig. 19-15). Mixed acid-base disturbances in these cats may include metabolic alkalosis associated with hypochloremia (74%) and hypoalbuminemia (48%), and metabolic acidosis associated with unmeasured anions (96%). Alkalemia was detected in 17% and acidemia was found in 26% of these cats. Conventionally calculated anion gap was abnormal in 39%, but abnormal values increased to 52% after correction of serum sodium concentration for water excess or deficit. Low serum sodium concentration (water excess) was found in 57% of cats with severe HL.

A.

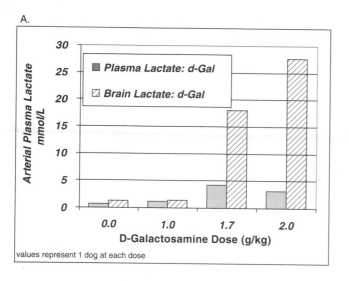

B.

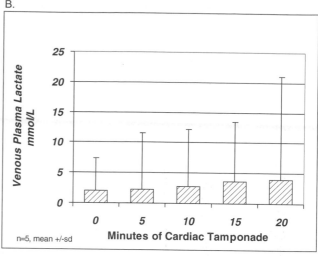

C.

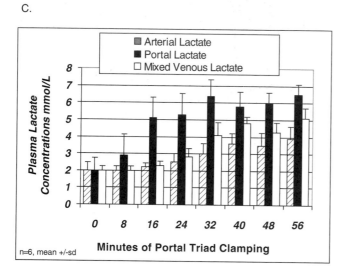

D.

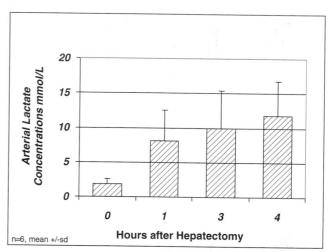

Fig. 19-13 Graphic display of plasma and brain lactate concentrations in dogs with fulminant hepatic failure (n = 4) and plasma lactate concentrations in dogs with induced cardiac tamponade (n = 5), dogs with portal triad clamping (n = 6), and in hepatectomized dogs (n = 6). Plasma concentrations of lactate in dogs with fulminant hepatic failure were significantly lower than lactate values achieved within the central nervous systems. Plasma lactate concentrations in dogs with fulminant hepatic failure were similar to those associated with systemic hypotension induced by pericardial tamponade and portal triad clamping. Data adapted from **(A)** Nyberg SL, Cerra FB, Gruetter R: Brain lactate by magnetic resonance spectroscopy during fulminant hepatic failure in the dog, *Liver Transpl Surg* 4:158–165, 1998; **(B)** Mathias DW, Clifford PS, Klopfenstein HS: Mixed venous blood gases are superior to arterial blood gases in assessing acid-base status and oxygenation during acute cardiac tamponade in dogs, *J Clin Invest* 82:833–838, 1988;. **(C)** Nemec A, Pecar J, Seliskar A, et al: Assessment of acid-base status and plasma lactate concentrations in arterial, mixed venous, and portal blood from dogs during experimental hepatic blood inflow occlusion, *Am J Vet Res* 64:599–608, 2003; **(D)** Park R, Arieff AI, Leach W, et al: Treatment of lactic acidosis with dichloroacetate in dogs, *J Clin Invest* 70:853–862, 1982.

HEPATIC ENCEPHALOPATHY

HE is a complex neurophysiologic syndrome involving the CNS that implies a critical loss of functional hepatic mass (65% to 70%) or extensive hepatofugal circulation (portosystemic shunting). The pathogenesis of HE is multifactorial. The most highly suspected contributing factors and their mechanisms are summarized in Box 19-2, Table 19-3, and Fig. 19-16.[38] Abnormal cerebral function may arise from a variety of neuroactive toxins, as well as functional and structural alterations affecting neurotransmission and energy metabolism. Most changes are reversible with recovery of hepatic function and appropriate management of the acute metabolic crisis.

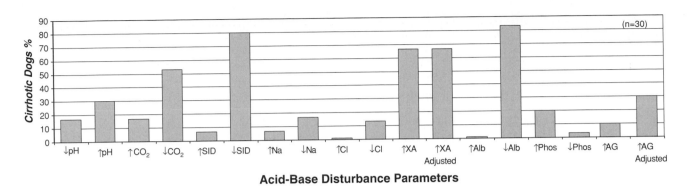

Fig. 19-14 Graphic representation of parameters and calculated values used to identify acid-base derangements (number of patients with abnormal values) derived from dogs with hepatic cirrhosis (n = 30). *Alb*, Albumin; *AG*, anion gap; *Cl*, chloride; *Phos*, phosphorus; *SID*, strong ion difference; *XA*, unmeasured anions; *Adjusted*, value adjusted for change in free water as represented by serum sodium concentration. Values used to determine SID were calculated using conventional formulas as described in Chapter 13. (Data from SA Center: College of Veterinary Medicine, Cornell University, 2004).

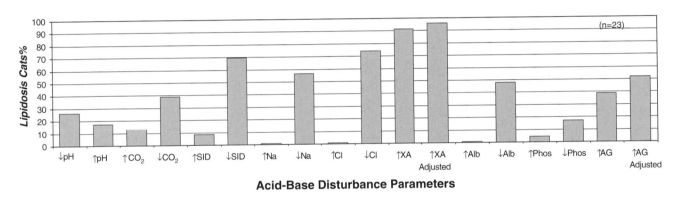

Fig. 19-15 Graphic representation of parameters and calculated values used to identify acid-base derangements (number of patients with abnormal values) derived from cats with severe HL (n = 23). *Alb*, Albumin; *AG*, anion gap; *Cl*, chloride; *Phos*, phosphorus; *SID*, strong ion difference; *XA*, unmeasured anions; *Adjusted*, value adjusted for change in free water as represented by serum sodium concentration. Values used to determine SID were calculated using conventional formulas as described in Chapter 13. (Data from SA Center: College of Veterinary Medicine, Cornell University, 2004).

Diagnosis of HE is based on clinical signs and clinicopathologic features in the setting of confirmed severe liver disease or portosystemic shunting. In companion animals, HE is rarely associated with acute hepatic failure. The onset of clinical signs can be acute or chronic and episodic or progressive. Progressive HE is characterized by widely variable signs that include decreased level of consciousness progressing to lethargy, somnolence, stupor, and coma.

CLINICAL MANAGEMENT OF PATIENTS WITH LIVER DISEASE

Important therapeutic considerations in the patient with liver disease include provision of appropriate nutrition for the stage of disease including assessment of protein and sodium tolerance, as well as maintenance of euglycemia, hydration, and electrolyte balance. Circumstances that promote development of HE should be avoided, and HE should be treated aggressively if it does develop. Therapy to eliminate or ameliorate ascites should be carried out as necessary, and coagulation abnormalities should be identified and managed.

NUTRITIONAL CONSIDERATIONS IN LIVER DISEASE

The primary goal of nutritional support is to achieve positive (or at least neutral) nitrogen balance and to provide adequate energy, vitamin, and micronutrient intake.

Protein and Sodium Intake

Protein intake should be restricted only in the presence of hyperammonemia, ammonium biurate crystalluria, or

TABLE 19-3   Conditions Associated with Development of Hepatic Encephalopathy

Condition	Mechanism
Dehydration	Prerenal azotemia
	Renal azotemia
Azotemia	$\uparrow$ NH$_3$
Alkalemia	$\uparrow$ NH$_3$, $\uparrow$diffusion across BBB into CNS
Hypokalemia	$\uparrow$ NH$_3$, $\uparrow$renal ammoniagenesis
	Promotes alkalemia
	Polyuria and anorexia
Hypoglycemia	Neuroglycopenia: augments NH$_3$ toxicity
Catabolism	$\uparrow$ Protein turnover: $\uparrow$ NH$_3$
	$\downarrow$ Muscle NH$_3$ detoxication
Infection	$\uparrow$ Protein turnover: $\uparrow$ NH$_3$
	Urease producers $\rightarrow$ urea $\rightarrow$ $\uparrow$ NH$_3$
Polydipsia/polyuria	$\downarrow$ K$^+$ $\rightarrow$ alkalosis, $\uparrow$ NH$_3$
	Provokes: inappetence, weakness
Anorexia	Catabolism
	$\downarrow$ K$^+$: promotes alkalemia $\rightarrow$ augments NH$_3$ toxicity
	$\downarrow$ Zinc: impairs urea cycle NH$_3$ detoxification
	Dehydration
	Hypoglycemia
Constipation	$\uparrow$ Toxin production
	$\uparrow$ Toxin absorption
Hemolysis	$\uparrow$ RBC breakdown $\rightarrow$ $\uparrow$Protein
Blood transfusion	$\uparrow$ RBC breakdown $\rightarrow$ $\uparrow$ Protein: $\uparrow$ NH$_3$
	$\uparrow$ NH$_3$ content in stored blood, endotoxins
GI hemorrhage	
RBC digestion	$\uparrow$ Protein: $\uparrow$ NH$_3$
Inflammation	$\uparrow$ Protein: $\uparrow$ NH$_3$
Parasitism	$\uparrow$ Protein: $\uparrow$ NH$_3$
High dietary protein (animal, fish, eggs)	$\uparrow$ Protein load: $\uparrow$ NH$_3$,
	Aromatic amino acids
	$\uparrow$ Many other toxins
Drugs: (examples)	
Benzodiazepines	Tetracyclines
Antihistamines	Methionine
Barbiturates	Organophosphates
Phenothiazines	Diuretic overdosage
Metronidazole	Certain anesthetics

BBB, Blood-brain barrier; CNS, central nervous system; RBC, red blood cell.

clinically apparent HE or as a therapeutic trial when subtle clinical signs suggest occult HE. In the latter situation, protein intake should be increased cautiously according to individual patient tolerance so as to avoid inadequate nutrition. Nitrogen tolerance is estimated based on response to initial protein intake and sequential assessments of clinical status. Dogs experiencing nitrogen intolerance require dietary modification of both protein quantity and quality along with treatments targeting enteric toxin production (see the section on Acute and Chronic Hepatic Encephalopathy).

Sodium intake should be limited to 100 mg/100 kcal energy requirement in hypoalbuminemic dogs and cats and in those with ascites. A diet that is less than 0.1% sodium on a dry matter basis is considered very low in sodium for dogs.

Vitamin Supplementation

Water-soluble vitamins should be given to all patients with liver disease. Intravenous fluids should be supplemented with a water-soluble B complex vitamin preparation. Anorectic cats seem to be predisposed to B-vitamin depletion.

Signs of vitamin B$_1$ deficiency (i.e., hypothiaminosis or Wernecke's encephalopathy) are easily confused with those of HE but can be rapidly corrected with 50 to 100 mg of thiamine given parenterally or orally

Hepatic Encephalopathy

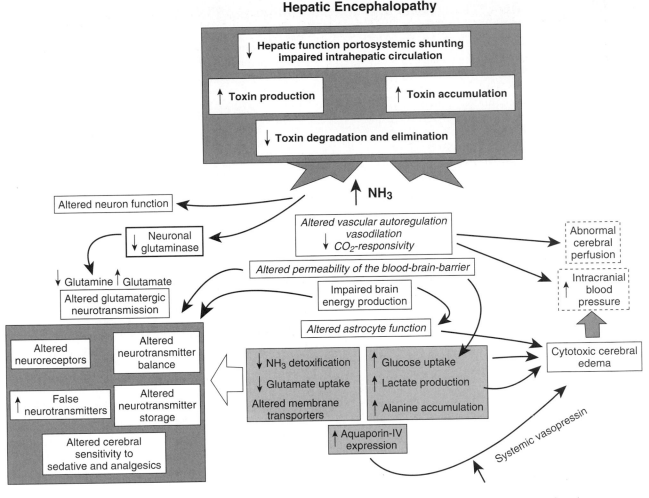

Fig. 19-16 Diagram demonstrating pathomechanisms contributing to hepatic encephalopathy, as discussed in the text.

every 12 hours followed by every 24 hours for 3 days. Thereafter, thiamine can be adequately provided using a B-vitamin preparation added to intravenous fluids. Oral administration of thiamine is preferred to parenteral administration to avoid the rare but severe vasovagal or anaphylactic reactions to injectable thiamine observed in some animals.

Cats with intestinal malassimilation or pancreatic dysfunction are at increased risk for vitamin B_{12} deficiency because of inadequate intrinsic factor or impaired cobalamin uptake in the small intestine,[149] and a link between cobalamin insufficiency and HL is suspected.[34] Parenteral treatment with vitamin B_{12} is begun after a sample for measurement of baseline serum B_{12} concentration has been obtained. Pretreatment determination of serum B_{12} concentration is mandatory because it is on this basis that chronic repletion therapy is prescribed. Initially, parenteral cobalamin treatment should provide 0.5 to 1.0 mg of B_{12} intramuscularly or subcutaneously

every 7 days to every 21 days. Chronic supplementation is based on sequential weekly measurements of the serum cobalamin concentration. Patients receiving cobalamin also should be treated with a thiol compound (GSH donor) such as *N*-acetylcysteine or *S*-adenosylmethionine to facilitate detoxification and removal of cyanide from cyanocobalamin (the usual therapeutic form of cobalamin) and α-tocopherol (vitamin E). Experimental evidence suggests that α-tocopherol may increase formation of active cobalamin from the therapeutically administered synthetic form of vitamin B_{12}.

Hepatic (and possibly systemic) depletion of fat-soluble vitamin E (α-tocopherol) may complicate inflammatory and cholestatic liver disease. Specific deficiencies have not been quantified in companion animals with spontaneous liver disease, but experimental evidence, information from human medicine, and evidence of deficient hepatic thiol antioxidant status in companion animals argue that α-tocopherol supplementation is

Box 19-2	Putative Hepatoencephalopathic Toxins and Their Mechanisms

Ammonia
↓ Microsomal Na^+, K^+-ATPase in the brain
↓ ATP availability (ATP consumed in glutamine production)
↑ Excitability (if mild ↑ NH_3)
Disturbed malate-aspartate shuttle: ↓ energy
↓ Glycolysis
Brain edema (acute liver failure)
↓ Glutamate, altered glutamate receptors
↑ BBB transport: glutamate, tryptophan, octopamine

Bile Acids
Membranocytolytic effects alter cell or membrane permeability
BBB more permeable to other HE toxins
Impaired cellular metabolism because of cytotoxicity

Endogenous Benzodiazepines
Neural inhibition: hyperpolarize neuronal membrane
Induction of peripheral (mitochondrial) benzodiazepine receptors

GABA
Neural inhibition: hyperpolarize neuronal membrane
↑ BBB permeability to GABA in HE
↓ α-Ketoglutarate: impairs energy metabolism, NH_3 detoxification
Diversion from TCA cycle for NH_3 detoxification
↓ ATP availability

Aromatic Amino Acids
↓ Neurotransmitter synthesis: ↓dopa
↓ Gluconeogenesis: compete with BCAA for CNS transporter
Accumulation of octopamine, phenylethanolamine, serotonin
Octopamine and phenylethanolamine compete with dopa, norepinephrine

Altered Neuroreceptors
Abnormal mediators and response
↑ Production false neurotransmitters

Methionine → Toxic Metabolites: Mercaptans
(Methanethiol and dimethyldisulfide)
Synergistic with other toxins: NH_3, SCFA
Gut derived → fetor hepaticus (distinct breath odor in HE)
↓ NH_3 detoxification in brain
↓ Microsomal Na^+, K^+-ATPase

Tryptophan
Directly neurotoxic
↑ Serotonin: neuroinhibition

Glutamine
Alters BBB amino acid transport
NH_3 transfer

SCFA
↓Microsomal Na^+, K^+-ATPase in brain
Uncouples oxidative phosphorylation
Impairs oxygen utilization
Displaces tryptophan from albumin → ↑ free tryptophan

Phenol (Derived from Phenylalanine and Tyrosine)
Synergistic with other toxins
↓A multitude of cellular enzymes
Neurotoxic and hepatotoxic

False Neurotransmitters (Tyrosine → Octopamine, Phenylalanine → Phenylethylamines)
Impair norepinephrine action

ATP, Adenosine triphosphate; *BBB*, blood-brain barrier; *HE*, hepatic encephalopathy; *GABA*, γ-aminobutyric acid; *TCA*, tricarboxylic acid; *BCAA*, branched chain amino acids; *CNS*, central nervous system; *SCFA*, short chain fatty acids.

appropriate. Vitamin E can protect both lipid-soluble and water-soluble cell constituents from oxidative damage, and experimentally provides antioxidant protection in various types of liver injury, including those associated with cholestasis.[151,152] The amount of vitamin E needed to protect membrane polyunsaturated fatty acids (PUFAs) from oxidative damage ranges from 0.4 to 0.8 mg of vitamin E/g of dietary PUFA.[176] However, patients on diets rich in long-chain PUFA may require more than 1.5 mg of vitamin E/g of dietary PUFA. The complex relationship between vitamin E status and dietary PUFA intake makes definitive recommendations difficult.[107] Vitamin E uptake by enterocytes is dependent on the presence of enteric bile acids, and cholestasis may increase vitamin E requirement because of impaired enterohepatic bile acid circulation.[46] Using a water-soluble form of α-tocopheral can circumvent problems created by impaired enteric bile acid circulation (e.g., α-tocopherol formulated with polyethylene glycol-1000 succinate, Eastman Chemical Company, Kingsport, TN).

A dosage of at least 10 U/kg body weight/day is recommended but has not been critically evaluated for efficacy in dogs and cats with spontaneous liver disorders.

Vitamin K_1 is given to all jaundiced patients during the first 12 hours of hospitalization to prevent coagulopathies associated with its deficiency. Since vitamin K is a fat-soluble vitamin, its enteric availability may be substantially reduced by impaired enterohepatic bile acid circulation. Consequently intramuscular or subcutaneous administration of vitamin K is recommended. A vitamin K_1 dosage of 0.5 to 1.5 mg/kg, repeated three times at 12-hour intervals, has been clinically shown to ameliorate coagulation abnormalities in most cats and many dogs with liver disease.[32] The dose of vitamin K should be calculated carefully because excessive amounts can cause oxidant damage to the liver, erythrocytes, and other organs (especially in sick cats).

Maintenance of Euglycemia

Patients with hepatic dysfunction may have insufficient liver and muscle glycogen reserves to maintain glycogenolysis. If hepatic gluconeogenesis also is impaired, these patients are prone to symptomatic hypoglycemia. Animals with portosystemic shunting and those with fulminant hepatic failure are at greatest risk. Neuroglycopenia must be avoided in animals with PSVA during surgical and anesthetic procedures because neurologic recovery can be permanently impaired. In HE, hypoglycemia can intensify neurologic signs by augmenting ammonia-associated brain energy deficits. Intravenous fluids initially should be supplemented with 2.5% dextrose with sequential determinations of blood glucose concentration guiding maintenance treatment. Symptomatic hypoglycemia is managed by administration of 0.5 to 1.0 mL/kg of a 50% dextrose solution given by bolus intravenous injection (diluted 1:2 to 1:8 in saline). Thereafter, glucose supplementation is sustained by adding glucose to fluids to effect using a continuous 24-hour infusion.

TREATMENT OF HEPATIC ENCEPHALOPATHY
General Considerations

Treatment of HE is based on clinical signs and a comprehensive understanding of the underlying pathophysiologic mechanisms. Syndrome severity is difficult to quantify with biochemical tests and does not correlate with hepatic histologic lesions. The degree of HE reflects circulatory complications, portosystemic shunting, fluid and electrolyte disturbances, hypoglycemia, accumulation of toxins associated with HE (especially ammonia), systemic complications caused by liver dysfunction, and concurrent disease processes. Stratification of patients into two major categories facilitates therapeutic decisions. The first category consists of patients with episodic HE that are relatively normal between episodes and

likely have a resolvable precipitating circumstance (see Table 19-3). The second category consists of patients with spontaneous acute encephalopathy in which an underlying cause cannot be found. Management of HE involves detection and treatment of precipitating events, modulation of causative mechanisms, and treatment of the underlying liver disease.

Major treatment strategies for HE include (1) reducing systemic and cerebral NH_3 concentrations by therapeutically targeting the gastrointestinal tract (the primary source of NH_3 production); (2) maintaining stable systemic blood pressure; (3) ensuring euhydration (i.e., avoiding dehydration or overhydration); (4) correcting or avoiding detrimental electrolyte disturbances (e.g., hypokalemia, hypophosphatemia); (5) maintaining euglycemia; (6) controlling hemorrhage (especially enteric bleeding); (7) avoiding catabolic events and maintaining body condition and muscle mass by feeding a diet tailored to the patient's nitrogen tolerance and energy requirements; (8) providing supplemental vitamins and micronutrients in the event that increased requirements may be present in hepatic insufficiency (i.e., reduced hepatic storage or activation); (9) identifying and eliminating infectious complications including enteric parasites that may provoke catabolism and nitrogenous waste production; and (10) using metabolic strategies to improve NH_3 metabolism or ameliorate NH_3 toxicity (e.g., supplementing L-carnitine [L-CN], L-ornithine, L-aspartate, and possibly branched-chain amino acids).

Adjusting the enteric bacterial flora, providing fermentable carbohydrates, and avoiding constipation are common strategies used to modify enteric factors contributing to HE. Constipation is detrimental because many encephalopathic toxins are produced and absorbed in the large intestine. Excessively aggressive nitrogen restriction and failure to provide enough energy for maintenance requirements encourages a catabolic state and muscle wasting, which impair protein and NH_3 tolerance. Cachexia, starvation, and glucocorticoid administration increase nitrogenous waste production from muscle catabolism, including NH_3 and other toxic metabolites.

Antianabolic effects of certain drugs (e.g., tetracyclines) may promote release of nitrogenous waste products, exceeding hepatic capacity for detoxification. Avoiding hypokalemia and metabolic alkalosis are crucial because these disturbances favor high blood NH_3 concentrations. Metabolic alkalosis facilitates brain uptake and intracerebral trapping of NH_3. Hypokalemia promotes renal ammoniagenesis and H^+ loss, promoting metabolic alkalosis and increasing renal tubular NH_3 reabsorption. Severe hypokalemia also may impair urinary concentrating ability, leading to diuresis and dehydration. Persistence of either hypokalemia or hypophosphatemia can lead to weakness and anorexia, compromising adequate nutritional support and fluid balance. In some animals, hypoglycemia precipitates encephalopathic signs. While hypoglycemia can directly or indirectly provoke neurologic and systemic signs (e.g., weakness, lethargy, confusion) and increased neuronal susceptibility to cerebral neurotoxins, hyperglycemia can contribute to an increase in astrocyte osmolal load thereby provoking cerebral edema. A number of neuroactive drugs (e.g., sedatives, analgesics, anesthetics) can directly interact with dysfunctional neuroreceptors causing encephalopathic signs. Maintaining adequate hydration is important in avoiding prerenal azotemia, which can increase enteric NH_3 production and hyperammonemia. Volume expansion can attenuate hyperammonemia caused by enteric hemorrhage when NH_3 arises largely from enhanced renal ammoniagenesis. However, avoiding overhydration also is important because it can promote ascites, cerebral edema, or pulmonary edema associated with occult cardiopulmonary complications of hepatic insufficiency. Fluid volumes and drug dosages must be calculated based on estimated lean body mass in patients with ascites. Failure to do so can lead to fluid overload or life-threatening drug toxicities. Administration of a highly protein-bound drug to a patient with hypoalbuminemia without dosage adjustment potentially can lead to an inadvertent drug overdose that could be lethal.

Acute Severe Hepatic Encephalopathy or Liver Injury

Treatments should be targeted at controlling hyperammonemia and cerebral edema. Critical supportive care should address circumstances that increase cerebral blood flow and compromise cerebral or hepatic metabolism. Effort should be made to attenuate systemic inflammatory responses and provoking causative factors. Although acute hepatic failure usually is associated with high blood NH_3 concentrations, strategies targeting enteric NH_3 production generally are less effective in patients with acute HE than in those with episodic HE caused by chronic liver disease or portosystemic shunting.

Careful management of systemic blood pressure is important; both hypotension and hypertension must be avoided. Analogues of AVP used to counteract splanchnic hypoperfusion and enteric bleeding in severe hepatic insufficiency are contraindicated in patients with signs of cerebral edema based on experimental studies and observations in human patients.[39] Body temperature should be monitored, and hyperthermia should be avoided. Hyperthermia increases metabolic rate and cerebral blood flow, which can increase intracranial pressure. Modest hypothermia may prevent emerging cerebral edema in acute HE but cannot be maintained long term. Glucose infusion may ensure euglycemia, but hyperglycemia and hyponatremia may provoke cerebral edema in acute hepatic failure. Hypercapnia must be avoided because it may increase cerebral blood flow and intracranial pressure. However, hyperventilation must also be avoided because severe hypocapnia may decrease cerebral perfusion. Monitoring blood pH to avoid alkalemia or acidemia is essential. Alkalemia can facilitate diffusion of NH_3 across the blood-brain barrier, and acidemia may indicate the presence of unmeasured anions, especially lactate. Hyperlactatemia should be avoided because it contributes to cerebral edema, increased cerebral blood flow, and increased intracranial pressure. Infusion of branched-chain amino acids and supplemental L-CN may be appropriate in patients with acute severe HE and suspected cerebral edema, but these treatments remain controversial. Supplemental vitamin K and water-soluble vitamins should be given, and fluids containing lactate should be avoided. Antimicrobials should be administered to prevent enteric organisms from gaining access to the systemic circulation.

Chronic Hepatic Encephalopathy

Dietary Management. The mainstay of nutritional support is judicious protein restriction taking care to avoid a catabolic state.[37] Nitrogen allowances should be tailored individually for each patient. Excessively severe protein restriction can contribute to the malnutrition of chronic liver disease, increasing catabolic loss of muscle. Positive nitrogen balance should be maintained and catabolism should be avoided because muscle is an important site for transient NH_3 detoxification. Vegetable and dairy sources of protein are superior to meat, fish, or egg sources in dogs. Cats are strict carnivores and require meat-derived protein as part of their restricted protein allowance. Energy requirements may be increased in hepatic insufficiency, and the patient's body condition and behavior at home should be evaluated sequentially to assess the adequacy of nutritional support.

Conventional recommendations for chronic management of hyperammonemia and HE in dogs include limiting dietary protein intake to between 14% and 16% of energy intake with a minimum of 2.5 g protein/kg body weight/day. Recommendations for cats include limiting dietary protein to 25% to 30% of energy intake with a minimum of 4.5 g protein/kg body weight/day. In cats, insufficient arginine or citrulline may increase susceptibility to hyperammonemia. Titration of individual protein tolerance from an initial severely restricted allocation is done by adding 0.25 to 0.5 g protein/kg body weight/day and evaluating clinical response over time (e.g., sequential body weight, body condition scores, serum albumin and creatinine concentrations, and patient cognition and behavior). Use of L-CN (parenteral administration) may avert NH_3 toxicity, but this approach has not yet been widely applied clinically. Conventional total parenteral nutrition solutions have been used safely in dogs and cats with HE with formula modification to achieve protein restriction on an individual basis. In the author's hospital, supplemental L-CN

(25 to 50 mg/kg body weight/day) also is provided in such solutions.

Modification of the Enteric Environment: Ammonia Detoxification. Many factors contribute to HE, and no single treatment is appropriate and effective for all patients in all circumstances. A common approach incorporates strategies that reduce enteric and extraintestinal NH_3 production and increase enteric NH_3 detoxification (Table 19-4). The kidneys may be a major source of NH_3 production in patients with enteric hemorrhage, and volume expansion may facilitate renal NH_3 elimination.[122]

Orally administered disaccharides that are fermented in the gut (e.g., lactulose, lactitol, or lactose in lactase-deficient patients) commonly are combined with parenterally administered antimicrobial agents to modify enteric flora and suppress urease-producing bacteria. Transient repopulation of the gut with beneficial (i.e., non–urease-producing) microorganisms (e.g., lactobacilli) may provide short-term benefits. Collectively, these efforts often ameliorate clinical signs of HE. In neurologically impaired patients that cannot tolerate oral medications, cleansing enemas are used to rid the colon of retained toxins and debris and are followed by retention enemas (see Table 19-4). Retention enemas contain enteric-modulating medications with effects similar to those described for oral administration. Simultaneous oral and per-rectal dosing should be avoided to prevent diarrhea, cramping, and potential drug overdose.

Fermentable Carbohydrates Dietary management of HE optimally is combined with oral administration of a fermentable carbohydrate such as lactulose (β-galactosidofructose, most commonly used), lactitol (β-galactosidosorbitol), or lactose (in lactase-deficient patients) because this strategy increases patient nitrogen tolerance. Lactulose and lactitol are synthetic disaccharides not digested by mammalian enzymes. Lactose may achieve a similar effect in lactase-deficient patients and is much cheaper. These compounds undergo bacterial fermentation in the intestinal tract, yielding lactic, acetic, and formic acids, which acidify the enteric lumen (pH < 5.0). These organic acids constitute an osmolal load provoking a cathartic influence (softening feces and increasing

TABLE 19-4 Methods Used to Modify Enteric Production and Absorption of Toxins

Dietary modifications
↓ Protein quantity
Altered protein quality: dairy and vegetable preferred
↑ Dietary soluble fiber

Modification of enteric microbial population

Alter enteric pH:	Lactose, lactulose, lactitol, fiber		
Antimicrobials:			
Neomycin	22 mg/kg	PO	BID-TID
Metronidazole	7.5 mg/kg	PO	BID-TID
Amoxicillin	11 g mg/kg	PO	BID

Administration of lactobacilli: live yogurt cultures
Modify enteric substrates: dietary, nonabsorbable disaccharides fiber

Lactulose	0.25-0.5 mL/kg	PO	BID-TID

(This is a STARTING dose. Start low and gradually work dose up to required amount based on stool consistency and frequency: aim for 2-3 soft pudding-like stools per day.)

Lactitol	0.5-0.75 g/kg	PO	BID
Lactose	Slightly sweet solution		BID
Fiber	Metamucil, psyllium		

(Each of the above are used to effect, attaining several soft stools per day.)

Direct elimination of enteric microorganisms, substrates, and products

Cleansing enemas	5-10 mL/kg, repeat until clear: use warm polyionic fluids	
Retention enemas	As necessary, respect total systemic drug dose	
Neomycin	15-20 mL 1% solution	TID
	(No > 22 mg/kg body weight up to TID)	
Lactulose	5-15 mL diluted 1:3 with water	TID
Lactitol	0.5-0.75 g/kg	BID
Metronidazole	7.5 mg/kg (systemic dose) with water	BID
Betadine	Dilute 1:10 with water, flush out within 10 min	
Dilute vinegar	Dilute 1:10 with water, alters pH	BID-TID
Activated charcoal	Administered and retained in crisis situation	

PO, *Orally;* BID, *twice daily;* TID, *thrice daily.*

the frequency of defecation). This cathartic effect increases the gastrointestinal transit rate, which commonly is slow in patients with HE and portal hypertension. The acidic luminal pH suppresses bacterial urease activity, renders the enteric environment inhospitable for many ammonia-generating organisms, and traps NH_3 as the NH_4^+, thereby increasing its elimination in feces. Carbohydrate fermentation also increases microbial incorporation of nitrogen, thereby decreasing the nitrogen available for systemic absorption. Fecal nitrogen excretion increases up to fourfold because of increased fecal volume and nitrogen trapping. Carbohydrate fermentation also decreases formation of potentially toxic short-chain fatty acids (e.g., propionate, butyrate, valerate) thought to contribute to HE. The dose of fermentable carbohydrate administered must be individually titrated to achieve several soft stools each day. Too much lactulose induces abdominal cramping (because of fermentation and gas production), stimulates peristalsis (causing borborygmus), and causes watery diarrhea. Generation of organic acids from lactulose rarely can result in metabolic acidosis, dehydration, and hypernatremia.[119]

Given together, lactulose and an enteric antimicrobial synergistically improve nitrogen tolerance in most animals. Lactulose (0.25 to 1 mL/kg orally every 12 hours to every 8 hours) commonly is combined with metronidazole (7.5 mg/kg orally every 12 hours to every 8 hours), amoxicillin (22 mg/kg orally every 12 hours), or neomycin (22 mg/kg orally every 12 hours) to decrease enteric production of NH_3 from urea and other nitrogenous substrates. Caution should be exercised when using neomycin because it potentially can be absorbed from the intestinal tract to an extent sufficient to result in ototoxicity or nephrotoxicity, especially if coexisting inflammatory bowel disease increases its absorption. Rarely, concurrent administration of an antimicrobial may reduce the efficacy of lactulose by decreasing its bacterial fermentation. This effect can be detected by checking fecal pH, which should be less than 6.0 if effective lactulose fermentation has occurred. Transient repopulation of the intestine with non–urease-producing microorganisms (e.g., lactobacilli) may provide only short-term benefit but carries little risk. Products that deliver lactobacilli or similar probiotic organisms also provide fermentable carbohydrate substrates, which may explain their benefits. Rarely, hepatic or systemic infections with the probiotic organism have been encountered.

Cleansing and Retention Enemas Conventional measures that decrease systemic NH_3 concentrations are directed at cleansing and removing noxious substrates from the colon and modifying the enteric environment. Initially, this approach involves cleansing rectal lavage using warm isotonic fluids and removal of residual ingesta, nitrogen-containing compounds, urease-producing microorganisms, and encephalopathic toxins. Next, a retention enema containing an antimicrobial, a fermentable carbohydrate, an acidifying solution, or activated charcoal is instilled. Use of a fermentable carbohydrate is preferred because it reduces enteric pH and traps NH_3 and eliminates it as NH_4^+.

FLUID THERAPY IN LIVER DISEASE
General Considerations

Selection of the most appropriate fluid for patients with hepatobiliary disease must take into consideration their propensity for third-space fluid accumulation (e.g., edema, ascites), hypoalbuminemia, hyponatremia, hypokalemia, coagulopathies, and hyperlactatemia and whether preexisting acid-base disturbances put them at risk for HE. In patients without evidence of synthetic failure or HE, balanced polyionic solutions are appropriate and should be supplemented with KCl as routinely recommended for maintenance needs.

When ascites or edema precedes fluid administration or develops after infusion of polyionic solutions, fluid support must be modified to reduce the administered load of sodium. Ascites has been experimentally induced in medium-sized dogs with cirrhosis by ingestion of only 85 mEq of sodium per day. Considering that a 15-kg dog has a maintenance volume requirement of approximately 1 L/day, the sodium content of commonly used polyionic crystalloid solutions may promote ascites formation when maintenance volumes are administered. Selection of commercially available solutions with restricted sodium content or mixing of commercially available solutions to achieve restricted sodium content is necessary for these patients. Slow infusion of both a crystalloid and a colloid is a useful approach for many of these patients because it expands intravascular volume, limits the requirement for crystalloids, and reduces the tendency for third-space fluid sequestration. Crystalloid administration is reduced to 33% of normal maintenance requirement when administered with 20 mL/kg/day of synthetic colloid. The potential bleeding complications associated with synthetic colloid use and their cost must be carefully considered. See Chapter 27 for more information on colloid therapy.

Hypoalbuminemic patients with tense ascites require individually tailored fluid therapy combined with a synthetic colloid or plasma, large-volume paracentesis, and diuretics (furosemide and spironolactone). Simply adjusting fluid sodium intake or restricting water intake is not efficacious. Water restriction is hazardous because of inadequate home monitoring. Although providing a synthetic colloid may seem reasonable, this approach alone will not interrupt the complex physiologic signals impairing renal water excretion. Low plasma oncotic pressure is not the sole driving force of ascites in these patients.

Hyponatremia presents a therapeutic challenge in patients with liver disease because the underlying physiology is complex and involves increased secretion of AVP (see Fig. 19-10). Availability of aquaretic agents (AVP receptor antagonists) may facilitate management of water retention in the future.[68,178]

Influence of Diuresis, Fluid Expansion, and Diuretics on Ammonia Concentration

Hyperammonemia in patients with hepatic insufficiency can be attenuated by systemic volume expansion because volume expansion reduces renal and hepatic ammoniagenesis. Renal ammoniagenesis is curtailed by increased renal plasma flow and GFR, which increases fractional NH_3 excretion. Enhanced renal NH_3 elimination occurs secondary to increased glutamine delivery to the proximal tubules, increased urine flow rate (i.e., decreased NH_3 reabsorption), and suppression of antidiuretic hormone secretion. Total body NH_3 load is decreased by redirection of ammonia into urine rather than into the renal vein. Volume expansion in well-compensated human patients with cirrhosis also decreases plasma renin activity and angiotensin II production. The latter effect may be important because angiotensin II enhances ammoniagenesis in the proximal tubules.[83] Improved systemic perfusion increases uptake of NH_3 by liver, skeletal muscle, and brain where it can be detoxified.

Enhanced sodium reabsorption in the ascending limb of Henle's loop and distal tubule is a disturbance associated with cirrhosis that may cause resistance to conventional doses of furosemide. Decreased response to furosemide also may reflect impaired drug access to the tubular lumen where it achieves its pharmacologic effect. When very large doses of furosemide are administered to initiate diuresis, the risk of hypovolemia and excessive loss of Cl^- (in excess of Na^+) is increased. Although retention of HCO_3^- maintains electroneutrality, it contributes to metabolic alkalosis that can increase NH_3 flux through an impaired urea cycle. Collectively, these effects promote persistent hyperammonemia in the patient with hepatic insufficiency. Dopamine may act synergistically with furosemide in this setting because dopamine inhibits proximal renal tubular Na^+/HCO_3^- cotransport.[95]

Administration of a carbonic anhydrase inhibitor (e.g., acetazolamide) or a thiazide (e.g., chlorothiazide) diuretic can indirectly augment hyperammonemia by inhibiting HCO_3^- generation in the renal tubular epithelium. Bicarbonate is necessary for mitochondrial synthesis of carbomyl phosphate (an essential urea cycle substrate), and urea cycle function may be impaired (see Fig. 19-2).[77]

Fluid Therapy Aggravating Electrolyte Depletions and Transcellular Shifts

Hyperglycemia caused by oral carbohydrate loading, diabetes mellitus, or glucose-supplemented fluids aggravates electrolyte depletion by osmotic diuresis. During the initial stages of refeeding in cats with HL, hyperglycemia also may provoke symptomatic hypothiaminosis (in patients with marginal thiamine reserves) because thiamine is a cofactor for several enzymatic reactions involving glucose utilization. Provision of thiamine is mandatory during refeeding of cats with HL and is accomplished using a water-soluble B-complex vitamin supplement. Glucose supplementation is contraindicated in cats with HL because it favors metabolic adaptations that precipitate refeeding syndrome, compromises adaptation to fatty acid oxidation, and may potentiate hepatic triglyceride accumulation via enhanced lipogenesis. Carbohydrates should not be used to increase the energy density of diets fed to cats with HL. However, carbohydrate supplementation of parenteral fluids may be necessary in very small or young dogs with PSVA because they may have inadequate gluconeogenic and glycolytic enzyme activity and insufficient muscle and liver glycogen stores to maintain euglycemia during anorexia or recovery from anesthesia and surgery.

TREATMENT OF ACID-BASE DISTURBANCES IN LIVER DISEASE

Respiratory and Metabolic Alkalosis

Respiratory alkalosis usually does not cause clinical complications or require intervention. Amelioration of HE often attenuates hyperventilation. If loss of acid-rich gastric juice underlies development of metabolic alkalosis, treatment with an H_2 blocker or acid pump inhibitor (e.g., omeprazole) may allow normalization of systemic pH. In patients with hypokalemia, KCl supplementation of fluids is required for recovery from alkalosis. In the absence of impending ascites or edema, 0.9% NaCl may be administered to replace the chloride deficit. In the presence of ascites or edema, infusion of 0.45% NaCl in 2.5% dextrose is preferable. Induction of a bicarbonate diuresis by administration of the carbonic anhydrase inhibitor acetazolamide can also be effective if conventional therapy fails.[53]

Metabolic Acidosis

If alkalinization is necessary, a bicarbonate- or acetate-containing polyionic solution (e.g., Normosol-R, Plasma-Lyte) can be used for patients with hepatic insufficiency. Consideration of the patient's sodium tolerance is essential because sodium bicarbonate delivers a sodium load that may increase ascites formation. In general, treatment with alkalinizing solutions or medications should be avoided in patients with signs of HE because alkalosis worsens hyperammonemia and increases NH_3 delivery to the CNS. Lactate-containing solutions should be avoided in cats with severe HL. If lactic acidemia is suspected, identification and correction of systemic hypoperfusion are warranted. An important potential cause of metabolic acidosis in animals with severe liver disease is renal dysfunction, which may develop as a result of hemodynamic disruptions associated with portal hypertension and systemic hypoperfusion or the underlying cause of liver injury (e.g., copper toxicosis, immune-mediated injury, infectious disease), chronic interstitial nephritis, or glomerulonephropathy. Renal tubular acidosis also has been recognized in dogs with copper-associated hepatotoxicity, drug-induced fulminant hepatic failure (e.g., carprofen or other NSAIDs), and in cats with HL.[24,33]

Lactic Acidosis

With the exception of cats with HL and animals in fulminant hepatic failure, the importance of lactic acidosis in patients with spontaneous liver disease remains unclear. High anion gap metabolic acidosis, in the absence of renal failure or administration of unusual drugs, suggests lactic acidemia. In this circumstance, lactate-containing fluids should be avoided. Marked lactic acidosis in a patient with liver disease suggests the presence of some other complicating condition (i.e., endotoxemia, severe infection, disorders causing hypoperfusion) or acute fulminant hepatic failure. At a normal rate of lactate production, abrupt cessation of hepatic lactate metabolism does not result in clinically significant lactate accumulation because of a compensatory increase in lactate extraction by extrahepatic tissues.[179] As a result of lack of correlation between systemic and CNS lactate concentrations, however, it is difficult to determine which patients may suffer from lactate administration (see Fig. 19-13).[121] Therefore acetated Ringer's solution (or a comparable crystalloid solution) has been recommended as an alternative alkalinizing solution for patients with serious hepatic dysfunction.[9,161] As a bicarbonate precursor, acetate is more readily metabolized by peripheral tissues than is lactate (acetate combines with CoA, forming acetyl CoA). This process consumes one hydrogen ion from carbonic acid and yields one bicarbonate ion for each millimole of acetate metabolized. Although acetate usually is considered nontoxic, excessive administration of acetate may impair myocardial contraction and induce vasodilatation.[6,174]

It is unclear whether treatment with bicarbonate or a bicarbonate precursor is beneficial in patients with liver disease and lactic acidosis.[5,73] Administration of bicarbonate to dogs with hypoxic lactic acidosis does not facilitate recovery but rather increases blood lactate concentrations. Administered bicarbonate may have detrimental effects on hepatic and splanchnic circulation, increasing CO_2 delivery to the liver and decreasing hepatic intracellular pH.[73,129]

Respiratory Acidosis

Respiratory acidosis is a grave prognostic finding in patients with liver disease and requires diagnostic investigation. Ventilatory support should be provided if hypoventilation is present, but caution should be exercised to avoid hyperventilation and hypocapnia, which can decrease cerebral blood flow and metabolic rate. Calculation of the PA-PaO$_2$ gradient identifies impaired gas diffusion and ventilation-perfusion mismatch in patients with normal arterial PO$_2$ values. A PA-PaO$_2$ gradient greater than 15 mm Hg warrants consideration of oxygen therapy. Respiratory acidosis and increased PA-PaO$_2$ gradient justify a grave prognosis in animals with hepatic disease.

MANAGEMENT OF ASCITES IN PATIENTS WITH LIVER DISEASE

Increased abdominal pressure caused by tense ascites can increase portal venous pressure. This effect can potentiate gastrointestinal hemorrhage from newly expanded varices, ectatic vessels, or ulcerative lesions, as well as protein loss from the intestines. Tense ascites also has negative hemodynamic effects on cardiac output. Studies of patients before and after fluid removal have shown a progressive increase in cardiac output, stroke volume, and ventricular ejection rate. Tense ascites also can impair ventilation by restricting diaphragmatic movement and chest expansion and also can impair appetite by imposing gastric compression.

Management of factors contributing to ascites formation is essential. Treatment must be carefully supervised because iatrogenic problems related to ascites mobilization (e.g., sodium restriction, paracentesis, diuretic administration) can lead to complications (e.g., abnormalities of hydration, electrolytes, and acid-base balance).

Before treatment, the patient's body condition score, body weight, and abdominal girth are recorded, and serum sodium, potassium, BUN, and creatinine concentrations and USG are determined to provide baseline information.

Sodium Restriction

Sodium restriction as proposed for dogs with cardiac or renal disease is instituted. A positive response to dietary management alone is rare. Low sodium intake for dogs and cats is less than 100 mg/100 kcal energy requirement or less than 0.1% to 0.2% sodium on a dry matter basis. By calculating daily sodium intake and measuring 24-hour urinary excretion of sodium, 24-hour sodium balance can be estimated in patients refractory to dietary sodium restriction. If negative sodium balance has not been achieved, additional sodium restriction can be recommended.

Diuretics

Combined use of a loop diuretic (furosemide, 1 to 2 mg/kg orally every 12 hours) and an aldosterone antagonist (spironolactone, loading dosage of 2 to 4 mg/kg followed by 1 to 2 mg/kg orally every 12 hours) is recommended initially. The goal of diuretic therapy is to achieve a net negative sodium balance such that ascites can be resolved and avoided in the future. Combined use of furosemide and spironolactone produces greater effect in humans than either drug used alone and usually does not result in iatrogenic hypokalemia. A similar strategy has been used in dogs, but at least one study failed to identify a diuretic response to spironolactone even at high dosages in healthy dogs.[84] If sequential evaluation of the patient every 5 to 7 days fails to identify sufficient mobilization of ascites but serum electrolyte concentrations and renal function remain normal and the owner has consistently fed a sodium-restricted diet, the dosage of each diuretic may be doubled. The rate of weight loss should not exceed 1% of body weight per day.[112] If treatment still fails to mobilize ascites after an additional 7 to 14 days, large-volume paracentesis is recommended. In some patients with tense ascites, large volume paracentesis is used initially to improve patient comfort and well being, as other strategies for ascites management are employed.

Complications of diuretic therapy include development or worsening of hyponatremia, decreased GFR, hypokalemia or hyperkalemia, metabolic acidosis, and induction of HE. Diuretics are contraindicated in patients with preexisting hyponatremia (i.e., serum sodium concentration < 130 mEq/L), known renal dysfunction, or active bacterial infection because these factors may predispose the patient to development of HRS. Although water restriction is used to manage hyponatremia in human patients, this approach is discouraged in veterinary medicine because it is difficult to closely monitor water intake in dogs and cats, and dehydration predisposes these animals to acute renal failure.

Albumin

Although administration of colloids may expand the intravascular compartment and facilitate mobilization of edema and ascites, these effects are short-lived because of transcapillary escape of albumin. Despite this limitation, hypoalbuminemic patients with liver disease and ascites may benefit from administration of albumin or synthetic colloids during large-volume paracentesis. Colloid infusion also may counter hypovolemia and hypotension during anesthesia and surgical procedures, in sepsis, and at the onset of HRS. Selection of the most appropriate colloid for a given situation depends on the required duration of effect, whether abnormalities of hemostasis are present, and whether other disease processes are aggravating hypoproteinemia. In patients with severe ongoing extracorporeal protein loss (e.g., intestinal loss, urinary loss), administered colloids may have very short retention time in plasma. If hypoalbuminemia is only the result of hepatobiliary disease, colloids have a longer plasma retention time.

Hypoalbuminemia does not appear to be a dominant factor in the pathophysiology of ascites formation in patients with liver disease. In fact, the presence of albumin in the effusion actually aggravates fluid accumulation. Studies in human patients with cirrhosis indicate that large-volume paracentesis of ascites should be coupled with intravascular colloid replacement using autologous albumin or plasma or synthetic colloids.

Blood component products are used to supply albumin in small patients because concentrated species-specific albumin is not available for veterinary use. Albumin concentrations range from 3.5 to 4.5 g/dL in whole blood or fresh frozen plasma and from 1.5 to 1.9 g/dL in packed RBCs, making it difficult and expensive to adequately correct albumin deficits. An infusion rate of 10 mL/kg/hr typically is used in dogs and cats with liver disease and hypoalbuminemia that require treatment with colloid. This approach provides important coagulation and transport proteins in addition to albumin. Plasma infusion also may decrease tendencies for adverse drug effects with medications that are highly protein-bound. In the absence of extrahepatic routes of protein loss, albumin has a longer retention time than synthetic colloids.[140] The patient's size determines whether plasma administration can reasonably be expected to achieve adequate colloid repletion. Unfortunately, plasma administration can lead to complications associated with hypercitratemia such as symptomatic hypocalcemia and hypomagnesemia caused by chelation of these cations by citrate. Stored blood products also may be a source of additional NH_3 and may introduce endotoxins, pyrogens, or bacteria if contaminated products are administered.[53]

Benefits and Hazards of Using Human Albumin in Animals. Some clinicians advocate administration of commercially available human albumin to veterinary patients. In particular, this practice has been recommended in patients presented for acute critical care. Veterinary clinicians should carefully consider the benefits and risks of this therapy. Use of albumin for similar purposes in human patients remains controversial.[40,167,177] Meta-analysis of autologous albumin compared with crystalloids or synthetic colloids in human patients failed to demonstrate advantage for albumin administration in several diseases. Opponents of its use emphasize the risks of infusing albumin in patients with disorders associated with increased vascular permeability.

Maintaining serum albumin concentration within a defined range theoretically may have clinical benefit, but limited clinical evidence supports this view with a few notable exceptions (e.g., emergency resuscitation, impending HRS, colloid replacement during large-volume paracentesis). The relatively mild clinical signs observed in genetically analbuminemic humans (with serum albumin concentrations < 1 g/L) suggest that albumin is far from essential. These patients have other plasma constituents (e.g., globulins, lipids) that compensate for the absence of albumin's colloidal effects.

Potential complications associated with albumin infusion include fluid overload (especially pulmonary edema) when infused too rapidly, decreased GFR caused by presence of microaggregates that impede glomerular filtration and impaired renal sodium and water excretion. These renal effects may predispose to acute renal failure and are thought to result from increased peritubular oncotic pressure. Infused albumin also may impede the renal response to furosemide by limiting luminal delivery to the ascending loop of Henle. Endogenous albumin may have antiinflammatory effects such as binding NO, oxidants, cytokines, and other inflammatory mediators, whereas manufactured albumin appears to permissively foster inflammation. Administered albumin also can have anticoagulant effects, exerting heparin-like activity on antithrombin III and inhibiting platelet aggregation.

Infusing albumin specifically to improve the oncotic pressure gradient and control interstitial fluid accumulation provides only a temporary benefit. Infused albumin initially may draw some fluid from the interstitium into the intravascular compartment, but later, when infused albumin escapes into the interstitium, it favors third-space accumulation of fluid. In septic patients, up to two thirds of administered albumin moves to the interstitial space within 4 hours and thereafter promotes interstitial fluid accumulation. Thus the colloidal benefit of albumin is transient at best, and it may worsen third-space fluid accumulation in the presence of vasculitis or impaired lymphatic function. In cirrhotic patients with ascites, extravasation of albumin into the peritoneal effusion has the potential to aggravate fluid retention. Use of human albumin products derived from pooled donor plasma also has the risk of infectious agent transmission. Consideration must be given to the potential for exposing clinicians and technicians to potentially infectious agents that are transmissible to human beings (e.g., prions).

Synthetic Colloids

Dextran and hydroxyethyl starch (HES, hetastarch) are macromolecular colloids developed for use as acute volume expanders. Dextrans are linear polymers of glucose produced by bacterial enzyme systems. The preferred dextran for oncotic effect is dextran 70, which has an effective half-life of 24 hours in normal dogs. HES, a highly branched polymer of glucose (synthetic hydroxyethyl substitute of amylopectin), also has a plasma half-life of 24 hours in normal dogs.[180] The pharmacokinetics of HES are complex owing to the molecular size and heterogeneity of component polymers. Elimination of HES occurs by glomerular filtration of small polymers, hydrolysis of larger polymers by α-amylase, or reticuloendothelial phagocytosis and metabolism in the liver, spleen, and lymph nodes.[110] The HES that is retained in reticuloendothelial cells does not appear to have a detrimental effect on organ function in normal dogs, but its

effects have not been evaluated in dogs with liver disease or portosystemic shunting where it may impede macrophage surveillance.[110,116,130,168] Although HES expands plasma in humans for 12 to 48 hours, it increased oncotic pressure for less than 12 hours in hypoalbuminemic dogs.[76,82,113] When used for oncotic support, synthetic colloids usually are given at a dosage of 20 mL/kg/day and can be administered by slow infusion over many hours.

Adverse Effects of Synthetic Colloids in Patients with Liver Disease. Synthetic volume expanders have predictable effects on hemostasis. The risk of bleeding with dextran is related to the dosage and type of dextran used. Hemostatic abnormalities may be related to dilutional effects on one or more coagulation factors, interference with platelet activity, decreased activity of von Willebrand factor, or increased fibrinolytic activity.* Regardless of cause, hemostatic abnormalities are notable in animals with hepatobiliary disease given dextran 70.[33] Intraoperative use of dextran 70 in dogs with PSVA has resulted in bleeding tendencies in patients assessed presurgically as having normal hemostasis (i.e., normal results for mucosal bleeding time, prothrombin time, activated partial thromboplastin time, activated coagulation time, and proteins induced by vitamin K absence or antagonism [PIVKA]). In addition to rapid hemodilution causing moderate to severe reduction in hematocrit, some patients with liver disease treated with synthetic colloids also have developed transient pulmonary edema.

In normal dogs and humans, the influence of HES on coagulation is dose-dependent and negligible when small doses are administered. However, normal dogs do develop a dose-dependent increase in bleeding time after blood replacement with HES. Induced hemostatic abnormalities in humans have involved von Willebrand factor and factor VIII coagulation activity, and cumulative dosages greater than 30 mL/kg have induced von Willebrand's disease or hemophilia-like syndromes. Little information is available regarding HES use in veterinary patients, and no reports describe its effects on coagulation tests in patients with spontaneous hepatobiliary disease. Although HES is contraindicated in the presence of severe coagulopathies, its use in dogs with low serum albumin concentration not attributable to liver disease but with preexisting coagulation abnormalities resulted in normalization of coagulation in five of seven dogs.[150]

Acute allergic reactions are possible with use of dextrans and HES. Adverse effects associated with nonalbumin plasma extenders have been well studied only in healthy dogs. Isovolemic hemodilution with HES and

---

References 1,2,15,42,47,48,67,70,86,100,103,143,158,160,169.

polymerized bovine collagen did not have adverse effects on hepatic histology,[155] but normal dogs receiving hypertonic saline (6%) and dextran 70 at a maximally tolerated dosage (20 mL/kg) experienced increases in alanine aminotransferase, aspartate aminotransferase, and alkaline phosphatase during the first 72 hours.[55]

Therapeutic or Large-Volume Paracentesis

Therapeutic or large-volume paracentesis usually is safe. However, severe consequences (including death) have been reported in patients with hepatic cirrhosis. Characteristic hemodynamic maladaptations in these patients include increased plasma renin activity, increased norepinephrine concentrations, decreased systemic vascular resistance, and an increased hepatic venous pressure gradient.[141] The most common complications of therapeutic abdominocentesis in humans include HE, decreased renal function, and hyponatremia.[12] The influence of rapid abdominocentesis on portal pressure and vena caval pressure has been evaluated in humans and dogs. These studies have not identified deleterious effects on portal or systemic venous pressure. The effect of large-volume paracentesis on reformation of ascites in cirrhotic dogs treated by sodium restriction or high sodium intake is shown in Fig. 19-17.[98] These data explain why sodium restriction is so important in overall management of patients with ascites and must be established before or concurrent with therapeutic paracentesis.

Use of Colloids and Large-Volume Paracentesis

Intravenous colloid administration can facilitate mobilization of ascites in the hypoalbuminemic patient when salt restriction and diuretics are ineffective. In these patients, large-volume paracentesis is coupled with intravenous colloid administration. Without colloids, therapeutic or large-volume paracentesis can lead to contraction of effective circulating blood volume, renal dysfunction, and dilutional hyponatremia.

Large-volume paracentesis coupled with albumin administration is safe and useful for management of

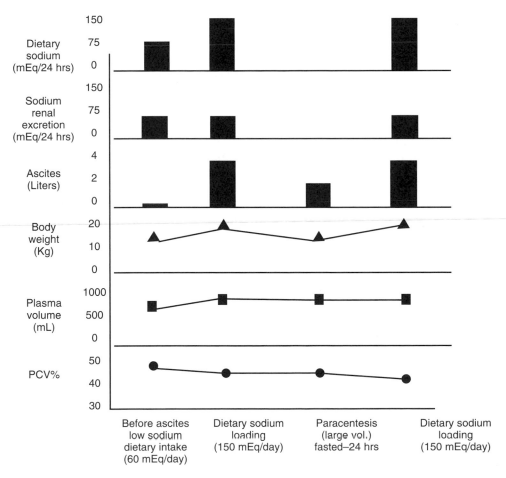

Dogs (n=5) with dimethylnitrosamine induced cirrhosis

Fig. 19-17 Experimental data showing the response of cirrhotic dogs to different levels of sodium ingestion, ascites formation, and response to paracentesis. Data derived from five dogs with cirrhosis induced with dimethylnitrosamine. (Adapted from Levy M: Sodium retention and ascites formation in dogs with experimental portal cirrhosis, *Am J Physiol* 233:F572–F585, 1977.)

intractable ascites. Alternative colloids have been investigated because of the high cost of homologous albumin. In comparative studies, postparacentesis circulatory dysfunction occurred twice as frequently in patients receiving synthetic colloids as in those receiving homologous albumin.[69] Humans given dextran 70 at 12 hours after paracentesis experienced resolution of their hemodynamic abnormalities and became normovolemic (84 ± 14 mL of dextran 70 for each 1000 mL of ascites removed).[165] Patients receiving dextran 70 concurrently with paracentesis did not develop significant hemodynamic changes in the first 24 hours after paracentesis.[165] Unfortunately, gastrointestinal bleeding as a complication of dextran infusion precipitated HE in some patients. As a result of the short plasma retention time of dextran 70, some of these patients developed hypovolemia 24 hours after paracentesis.[166] An alternative approach with a more reliable outcome was accomplished by combining smaller volume daily paracentesis with dextran 70 (6 g for each 1000 mL of ascites removed).[61] Compared with single diuretic therapy, large-volume paracentesis combined with intravenous dextran 70 and diuretics resulted in a better outcome and fewer adverse effects in cirrhotic patients (i.e., a high frequency of HE occurred when diuretics alone were used to mobilize ascites).[44,153]

The use of large-volume paracentesis in dogs and cats is complicated by lack of available autologous albumin and the necessity to use human albumin, species-specific plasma, or synthetic colloids. Plasma is preferred in small patients, and HES can be used in larger patients (more hemorrhagic complications result from use of dextran 70 than HES in the author's experience). Fluid removal is completed aseptically using a 14-gauge Teflon catheter. A sterile closed-end polypropylene tomcat catheter can be used to maintain patency of the Teflon catheter. For large-volume paracentesis, fluid is removed over 30 to 45 minutes. After paracentesis, the patient rests quietly with the puncture site positioned uppermost to avoid formation of a subcutaneous seroma; if possible, a pressure bandage is applied to the puncture site. Avoiding the midline as the site of abdominal puncture prevents gravitational pooling of subcutaneous fluid (a ventrolateral flank approach is preferred). Ventral midline puncture also increases the risk of visceral laceration (due to ovariohysterectomy adhesions). Confirming that the urinary bladder is empty, reviewing abdominal radiographs for abnormally positioned organs, and ballotting the puncture site immediately before needle insertion help avoid visceral laceration.

MANAGEMENT OF BLEEDING TENDENCIES IN PATIENTS WITH LIVER DISEASE

Blood Transfusion and Vitamin K_1 Administration

Whole-blood transfusions are indicated for patients with symptomatic anemia or coagulopathy. Anemia usually becomes symptomatic in dogs when the packed cell volume (PCV) is 18% or less and in cats when the PCV is 15% or less. Cats with liver disease seem predisposed to hemolysis associated with formation of Heinz bodies. Sometimes hemolysis occurs after treatment with certain drugs or products that provoke oxidative damage (e.g., excessive vitamin K_1, propofol, propylene glycol-containing drugs, onion powder used to enhance food palatability) or as a result of hypophosphatemia. Coagulation abnormalities in liver disease result from several different deficiencies or abnormalities. The most commonly considered cause of bleeding is factor deficiency arising from hepatic synthetic failure. However, clinical evidence suggests that these patients more often develop a vitamin K–responsive coagulopathy. This observation may be related to intestinal malabsorption (e.g., secondary to abnormal enterohepatic bile acid turnover), insufficient dietary intake, or impaired enteric synthesis of vitamin K secondary to prophylactic antimicrobial therapy. Vitamin K deficiency is avoided or corrected by administration of vitamin K_1 at a dosage of 0.5 to 1.5 mg/kg for two or three treatments at 12-hour intervals initially and then once weekly as required. Sequential PIVKA clotting tests can determine the relationship of a coagulopathy to vitamin K deficiency and the need for weekly vitamin K_1 injections. Other conditions that may contribute to bleeding tendencies in patients with liver disease include increased factor consumption or utilization as occurs with extensive gastrointestinal bleeding and disseminated intravascular coagulation.

If a blood transfusion is required, fresh whole blood is most helpful. Stored blood products may contain lactate, can deliver substantial amounts of NH_3 that may exacerbate HE, and also may introduce pyrogens or endotoxins that are poorly tolerated in patients with liver disease.[144] The rate of blood administration depends on the circumstances and urgency imposed by bleeding tendencies. Usually, an infusion rate of 5 to 10 mL/kg/hr is safe and effective.

DDAVP Administration

In addition to blood component therapy, coagulopathies may be ameliorated by administration of 1-deamino-8-D-arginine AVP (DDAVP, desmopressin) at a dosage of 0.5 to 5.0 μg/kg subcutaneously or diluted in 10 to 20 mL of saline and given intravenously slowly over 10 minutes during the perioperative period (e.g., before liver biopsy) or during a bleeding crisis. Administration usually is coupled with transfusion of fresh frozen plasma. Although DDAVP can mitigate bleeding in humans and animals with hepatobiliary disease, its mechanism of action in this circumstance remains uncertain. Hemostatic responses to DDAVP administration to dogs include liberation of preformed endothelial von Willebrand factor monomers and increased factor VIII activity (Fig. 19-18).[17] The benefits in patients with liver

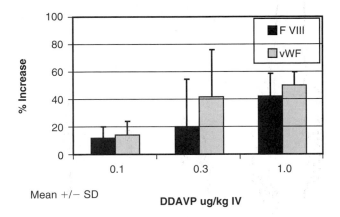

Fig. 19-18 Graphic depiction of the influence of desmopressin (DDAVP) on von Willebrand factor and factor VIII activity in healthy dogs. (Adapted from Bernat A, Hoffmann P, Dumas A, et al: V2 receptor antagonism of DDAVP-induced release of hemostasis factors in conscious dogs, *J Pharmacol Exp Ther* 282:597–602, 1997.)

disease seem too great to be explained based on these mechanisms because neither of these factors is notably deficient in hepatic insufficiency. DDAVP may have hemodynamic or vasoactive actions that have a salutary effect on microvasculature in areas of active hemorrhage. DDAVP has a narrow (4 to 6 hours) therapeutic window of effectiveness, and administration must be planned for optimal response (e.g., immediately before an invasive procedure). Administration of additional doses does not offer therapeutic benefit in terms of von Willebrand factor and may aggravate edema or ascites by increasing water retention.

Hemorrhage Caused by Citrate Loading

In very small patients (<10 kg) receiving large quantities of blood or blood components preserved with CPD, acquired hemorrhagic tendency is treated with 0.1 mL/kg of 10% $CaCl_2$ suspended in 10 to 20 mL of 0.9% saline and given over 10 to 20 minutes. Treatment is repeated until ionized hypocalcemia has been corrected.

REFERENCES

1. Aberg M, Hedner V, Bergentz S: Effect of dextran on factor VIII and platelet function, *Ann Surg* 189:243-247, 1979.
2. Aberg M, Bergentz S, Hedner U: Effect of dextran and induced thrombocytopenia on the lysability of ex vivo thrombi in dogs, *Acta Chir Scand* 143:91-94, 1977.
3. Abraldes JG, Bosch J: Somatostatin and analogues in portal hypertension, *Hepatology* 35:1305-1311, 2002.
4. Ackermann D, Vogt B, Escher G, et al: Inhibition of 11β-hydroxysteroid dehydrogenase by bile acids in rats with cirrhosis, *Hepatology* 30:623-629, 1999.
5. Adrogue HJ, Tannen RL: Ketoacidosis, hyperosmolar states, and lactic acidosis. In Kokko JP, Tannen RL, editors: Fluids and Electrolytes, ed 3, Philadelphia, 1996, WB Saunders, pp. 643-674.
6. Aizawa Y, Ohmori T, Imai K, et al: Depressant action of acetate upon the human cardiovascular system, *Clin Nephrol* 8:477-480, 1977.
7. Amatuzio DS, Nesbitt S: A study of pyruvic acid in the blood, spinal fluid and urine of patients with liver disease with and without hepatic coma, *Clin Invest* 29: 1486-1490, 1950.
8. Angeli P, Volpin R, Gerunda G, et al: Reversal of type 1 hepatorenal syndrome with administration of midodrine and octreotide, *Hepatology* 29:1690-1697, 1999.
9. Arai K, Kawamoto M, Yuge O, et al: A comparative study of lactated Ringer and acetated Ringer solution as intraoperative fluids in patients with liver dysfunction, *Masui* 35:793-799, 1986.
10. Angeli P: Prognosis of hepatorenal syndrome: has it changed with current practice? *Aliment Pharmacol Ther* 20:(suppl 3):44-48, 2004.
11. Arieff AI, Park R, Leach J, et al: Pathophysiology of experimental lactic acidosis in dogs, *Am J Physiol* 239: F135-F142, 1980.
12. Arroyo V, Gines P, Planas R: Treatment of ascites in cirrhosis. Diuretics, peritoneovenous shunt, and large-volume paracentesis, *Gastroenterol Clin North Am* 21: 237-256, 1992.
13. Arroyo V, Rodes J, Gutierrez-Lizarraga MA, et al: Prognostic value of spontaneous hyponatremia in cirrhosis with ascites, *Am J Dig Dis* 21:249-256, 1976.
14. Baumann H, Gauldie J: The acute phase response, *Immunol Today* 15:74-80, 1994.
15. Bergqvist D: Dextrans and haemostasis: a review, *Acta Chir Scand* 31:320-324, 1982.
16. Bernardi M: Renal sodium retention in preascitic cirrhosis: expanding knowledge, enduring uncertainties, *Hepatology* 35:1544-1547, 2002.
17. Bernat A, Hoffmann P, Dumas A, et al: V2 receptor antagonism of DDAVP-induced release of hemostasis factors in conscious dogs, *J Pharmacol Exp Ther* 282:597-602, 1997.
18. Better OS, Schrier RW: Disturbed volume homeostasis in patients with cirrhosis of the liver, *Kidney Int* 23:303-309, 1983.
19. Bienzle D, Jacobs RM, Lumsden JH: Relationship of serum total calcium to serum albumin in dogs, cats, horses and cattle, *Can Vet J* 34:360-364, 1993.
20. Bihari D, Gimson AE, Waterson M, et al: Tissue hypoxia during fulminant hepatic failure, *Crit Care Med* 13:1034-1039, 1985.
21. Bihari D, Smithies M, Gimson A, et al: The effects of vasodilation with prostacyclin on oxygen delivery and uptake in critically ill patients, *N Engl J Med* 317:397-403, 1987.
22. Boron VF, Hediger MA, Boulpaep EL, et al: The renal electrogenic Na+:HCO3-cotransporter, *J Exp Biol* 200: 263-268, 1997.
23. Brenner DA, Buck M, Feitelberg SP, et al: Tumor necrosis factor-alpha inhibits albumin gene expression in a murine model of cachexia, *J Clin Invest* 85:248-255, 1990.
24. Brown SA, Spyridakis LK, Crowell WA: Distal renal tubular acidosis and hepatic lipidosis in a cat, *J Am Vet Med Assoc* 189:1350-1352, 1986.
25. Caregaro L, Menon F, Angeli P, et al: Limitations of serum creatinine level and creatinine clearance as filtration markers in cirrhosis, *Arch Intern Med* 154:201-205, 1994.

26. Casey TH, Summerskill WHJ, Bickford RG, et al: Body and serum potassium in liver disease: II. Relationships to arterial ammonia, blood pH, and hepatic coma, *Gastroenterology* 48:208-215, 1965.

27. Castell JV, Gomez-Lechon MJ, David M, et al: Acutephase protein synthesis by interleukin-6, *Hepatology* 12:1179-1186, 1990.

28. Center SA, Crawford MA, Guida L, et al: A retrospective study of cats (n=77) with severe hepatic lipidosis: (1975-1990), *J Vet Intern Med* 7:349-359, 1993.

29. Center SA, Magne M: Historical, physical examination, and clinicopathologic features of portosystemic vascular anomalies in the dog and cat, *Sem Vet Med Surg Small Anim* 5:83-93, 1990.

30. Center SA, Harte J, Watrous D, et al: The clinical and metabolic effects of rapid weight loss in obese pet cats and the influence of supplemental oral l-carnitine, *J Vet Intern Med* 14:598-608, 2000.

31. Center SA, Sunvold GD: Investigations of the effect of l-carnitine on weight reduction, body condition, and metabolism in obese dogs and cats. In Reinhart GA, Carey DP, editors: *Recent advances in canine and feline nutrition,* vol III, Iams Nutrition Symposium Proceedings, Orange Frazer Press, 2000, Wilmington, OH, pp. 113-122.

32. Center SA, Warner K, Corbett J, et al: Proteins invoked by vitamin K absence and clotting times in clinically ill cats, *J Vet Intern Med* 14:292-297, 2000.

33. Center SA: Unpublished observations, College of Veterinary Medicine, Cornell University, 2005.

34. Center SA: Feline hepatic lipidosis, *Vet Clin North Am Small Anim Pract* 35:225-269, 2005.

35. Center SA, Thompson M, Wood PA, et al: Hepatic ultrastructural and metabolic derangements in cats with severe hepatic lipidosis. Proceedings of the 9th ACVIM Forum, 1991, pp. 193-196.

36. Center SA, Warner KL, Erb HN: Liver glutathione concentrations in dogs and cats with naturally occurring liver disease, *Am J Vet Res* 63:1187-1197, 2002.

37. Center, SA: Nutritional support for dogs and cats with hepatobiliary disease, *J Nutr* 128:2733S-2746S, 1998.

38. Center SA: Pathophysiology of liver disease: normal and abnormal function. In Guilford GA, Center SA, Strombeck DR, et al, editors: *Strombeck's small animal gastroenterology,* ed 3, Philadelphia, 1996, WB Saunders, pp. 553-632.

39. Chung C, Vaquero J, Gottstein J, et al: Vasopressin accelerates experimental ammonia-induced brain edema in rats after portocaval anastomosis, *J Hepatol* 39:193-199, 2003.

40. Cochrane Injuries Group Albumin Reviewers: Human albumin administration in critically ill patients: systematic review of randomized controlled trials, *BMJ* 317: 235-239, 1998.

41. Cohen RD, Iles RA, Barnett D, et al: The effect of changes in lactate uptake on the intracellular pH of the perfused rat liver, *Clin Sci* 41:159-170, 1971.

42. Concannon KT, Haskins S, Feldman BF: Hemostatic defects associated with two infusion rates of dextran 70 in dogs, *Am J Vet Res* 53:1369-1375, 1992.

43. Cooper AJL: Role of the liver in amino acid metabolism. In Zakim D, Boyer TD, editors: *Hepatology: a textbook of liver disease,* ed 3, Philadelphia, 1996, WB Saunders, pp. 563-604.

44. Cotrim HP, Garrido V, Parana R, et al: Paracentesis associated with dextran-70 in the treatment of ascites in patients with chronic liver diseases: a randomized therapeutic study, *Arq Gastroenterol* 31:125-129, 1994.

45. Craddock PR, Yawata Y, VanSanten L, et al: Acquired phagocyte dysfunction: a complication of hypophosphatemia of parenteral hyperalimentation, *N Engl J Med* 290:1403-1407, 1974.

46. Davit-Spraul A, Cosson C, Couturier M, et al: Standard treatment of alpha-tocopherol in Alagille patients with severe cholestasis is insufficient, *Pediatr Res* 49:232-236, 2001.

47. Damon L, Adams M, Stricker R, et al: Intracranial bleeding during treatment with hydroxyethyl starch, *N Engl J Med* 317:964-965, 1987.

48. Dalrymple-Hay M, Aitchison R, Collins P, et al: Hydroxyethyl starch induced acquired von Willebrand's disease, *Clin Lab Haematol* 14:209-211, 1992.

49. Dawson DJ, Babbs C, Warnes TW, et al: Hypophosphataemia in acute liver failure, *BMJ* 295:1312-1313, 1987.

50. DeGasperi A, Mazz E, Corti A, et al: Lactate blood levels in the perioperative period of orthotopic liver transplantation, *Int J Clin Lab Res* 27:123-128, 1997.

51. Deppe TA, Center SA, Simpson KW, et al: Glomerular filtration rate and renal volume in dogs with congenital portosystemic vascular anomalies before and after surgical ligation, *J Vet Intern Med* 13:465-471, 1999.

52. Dich J, Hansen SE, Thieden HID: Effect of albumin concentration and colloid osmotic pressure on albumin synthesis in perfused rat liver, *Acta Physiol Scand* 89:352-358, 1973.

53. Dillingham MA, Anderson RJ: Electrolyte, water, mineral, and acid base disorders in liver disease. In Maxwell MH, Kleeman CR, Narins RG, editors: *Clinical disorders of fluid and electrolyte metabolism,* ed 4, New York, 1987, McGraw-Hill, New York, pp. 879-896.

54. Dixon FJ, Maurer PH, Deichmiller MP: Half-lives of homologous serum albumins in several species, *Soc Exp Bio Med* 83:287-288, 1953.

55. Dubick MA, Zaucha GM, Korte DW Jr, et al: Acute and subacute toxicity of 7.5% hypertonic saline-6% dextran-70 (HSD) in dogs. 2. Biochemical and behavioral responses, *J Appl Toxicol* 13:49-55, 1993.

56. Emmitt M, Narins RG: Mixed acid-base disorders. In Maxwell MH, Kleeman CR, Narins RG, editors: *Clinical disorders of fluid and electrolyte metabolism,* ed 4, New York, 1987, McGraw-Hill, pp. 743-788.

57. Epstein M: Atrial natriuretic factor and liver disease. In Epstein M, editor: *The kidney in liver disease,* ed 4, Philadelphia, 1996, Hanley & Belfus Inc., pp. 339-358.

58. Epstein M: Derangements of renal water handling in liver disease, *Gastroenterology* 89:1415-1425, 1985.

59. Erlinger S: Physiology of bile secretion and enterohepatic circulation. In Johnson LR, editor: *Physiology of the gastrointestinal tract,* ed 2, New York, 1987, Raven Press, pp. 1557-1580.

60. Evans TW: Review article: albumin as a drug—biological effects of albumin unrelated to oncotic pressure, *Aliment Pharmacol Ther* 16(suppl 5):6-11, 2002.

61. Fassio E, Terg R, Landeira G, et al: Paracentesis with Dextran 70 vs paracentesis with albumin in cirrhosis with tense ascites. Results of a randomized study, *J Hepatol* 14:310-316, 1992.

62. Fink RM, Enns R, Kimball CP, et al: Plasma protein metabolism: observations using heavy nitrogen in lysine, *J Exp Med* 80:455-475, 1944.

63. Flanders JA, Scarlett JM, Blue JT, et al: Adjustment of total serum calcium concentration for binding to albumin

and protein in cats: 291 cases (1986-1987), *J Am Vet Med Assoc* 194:1609-1611, 1989.

64. Forrester SD, Moreland KJ: Hypophosphatemia: causes and clinical consequences, *J Vet Intern Med* 3:149-159, 1989.

65. Francisco LL, Sawin LL, Dibona GF: Mechanism of negative potassium balance in the magnesium-deficient rat, *Proc Soc Exp Biol Med* 168:382-388, 1981.

66. Frommer JP: Lactic acidosis, *Med Clin North Am* 67:815-829, 1983.

67. Garzon AA, Cheng C, Lerner B, et al: Hydroxyethyl starch (HES) and bleeding: an experimental investigation of its effect on hemostasis, *J Trauma* 7:757-766, 1967.

68. Gerbes AL, Gulberg V, Gines P, et al: Therapy of hyponatremia in cirrhosis with a vasopressin receptor antagonist: a randomized double-blind multicenter trial, *Gastroenterology* 124:933-939, 2003.

69. Gines P, Berl T, Bernardi M, et al: Hyponatremia in cirrhosis: from pathogenesis to treatment, *Hepatology* 28:851-864, 1998.

70. Gollub S, Schaefer C, Squitieri A: The bleeding tendency associated with plasma expanders, *Surg Gynecol Obstet* 124:1203-1211, 1967.

71. Good DW: Effects of potassium on ammonia transport by medullary thick ascending limbs of the rat, *J Clin Invest* 80:1358-1365, 1987.

72. Grauer GF, Pitts RP: Primary polydipsia in three dogs with portosystemic shunts, *J Am Anim Hosp Assoc* 23:197-200, 1987.

73. Graf H, Leach W, Arieff AI: Metabolic effects of sodium bicarbonate in hypoxic lactic acidosis in dogs, *Am J Physiol* 249:F630-F635, 1985.

74. Guzman JA, Rosado AE, Kruse JA: Vasopressin vs norepinephrine in endotoxic shock: systemic, renal, and splanchnic hemodynamic and oxygen transport effects, *J Appl Physiol* 95:803-809, 2003.

75. Harvey JW, West CL: Prednisone-induced increases in serum alpha-2-globulin and haptoglobin concentrations in dogs, *Vet Pathol* 24:90-92, 1987.

76. Haupt MT, Rackow EC: Colloid osmotic pressure and fluid resuscitation with hetastarch, albumin, and saline solutions, *Crit Care Med* 10:159-162, 1982.

77. Haussinger D, Kaiser S, Stehle T, et al: Liver carbonic anhydrase and urea synthesis. The effect of diuretics, *Biochem Pharmacol* 35:3317-3322, 1986.

78. Heinemann HO, Emirgil C, Mijnssen JP: Hyperventilation and arterial hypoxemia in cirrhosis of the liver, *Am J Med* 28:239-246, 1960.

79. Heymsfield SB, Waki M, Reinus J: Are patients with chronic liver disease hypermetabolic? *Hepatology* 11:502-504, 1990.

80. Heymsfield SB, Arteaga C, McManus C, et al: Measurement of muscle mass in humans: validity of the 24-hour urinary creatinine method, *Am J Clin Nutr* 37:478-494, 1983.

81. Hoffenberg R: Control of albumin degradation in vivo and in the perfused liver. In Rothschild MA, Waldmann T, editors: *Plasma protein metabolism: regulation of synthesis, distribution and degradation*, New York, 1970, Academic Press, pp. 239-255.

82. Hulse J, Yacobi A: Hetastarch: an overview of the colloid and its metabolism, *Drug Intel Clin Pharmacol* 17:334-341, 1983.

83. Jalan R, Kapoor D: Enhanced renal ammonia excretion following volume expansion in patients with well compensated cirrhosis of the liver, *Gut* 52:1041-1045, 2003.

84. Jeunesse E, Woehrle F, Schneider M, et al: Spironolactone as a diuretic agent in the dog: is the water becoming muddy (abstract), *J Vet Intern Med* 18:448, 2004.

85. Kanno N, LeSage G, Glaser S, et al: Regulation of cholangiocyte bicarbonate secretion, *Am J Physiol* 281:G612-G625, 2001.

86. Karlson KE, Garzon AA, Shaftan GW, et al: Increased blood loss associated with administration of certain plasma expanders: Dextran 75, Dextran 40, and hydroxyethyl starch, *Surgery* 62:670-678, 1967.

87. Kelly DA, Summerfield JA: Hemostasis in liver disease, *Semin Liver Dis* 7:182-191, 1987.

88. Kirsch RF, Saunders SJ, Frith L, et al: Plasma amino acid-regulation of albumin synthesis, *J Nutr* 98:395-403, 1969.

89. Kiszka-Kanowitz M, Henriksen JH, Hansen EF, et al: Effect of terlipressin on blood volume distribution in patients with cirrhosis, *Scand J Gastroenterol* 5:486-492, 2004.

90. Knepper MA: Molecular physiology of urinary concentrating mechanism: regulation of aquaporin water channels by vasopressin, *Am J Physiol* 272:F3-F12, 1997.

91. Koj A, Gauldie J, Regoeezi E, et al: The acute-phase response of cultured rat hepatocytes, *Biochem J* 224:505-514, 1984.

92. Kone BC, Higham SC: A novel N-terminal splice variant of the rate H+-K+-ATPase α2 subunit, *J Biol Chem* 273:3543-3552, 1998.

93. Kozlowski S, Krzysztof D: The role of osmoreception in portal circulation in control of water intake in dogs, *Acta Physiol Pol* 24:325-330, 1973.

94. Kreisberg RA: Lactate homeostasis and lactic acidosis, *Ann Intern Med* 92:227-237, 1980.

95. Kunimi M, Seki G, Hara C, et al: Dopamine inhibits renal $Na^+:HCO_3^-$ cotransporter in rabbits and normotensive rats but not in spontaneously hypertensive rats, *Kidney Int* 57:534-543, 2000.

96. Levy M, Wexler MJ: Renal sodium retention and ascites formation in dogs with experimental cirrhosis but without portal hypertension or increased splanchnic vascular capacity, *J Lab Clin Med* 91;520-536, 1978.

97. Levy M: Pathogenesis of sodium retention in early cirrhosis of the liver: evidence for vascular overfilling, *Semin Liver Dis* 14:4-13, 1994.

98. Levy M: Sodium retention and ascites formation in dogs with experimental portal cirrhosis, *Am J Physiol* 233:F572-F585, 1977.

99. Levy M: Sodium retention in dogs with cirrhosis and ascites: efferent mechanisms, *Am J Physiol* 233:F586-F592, 1977.

100. Lewis JH, Szeto IL, Bayer WL: Severe hemodilution with hydroxyethyl starch and dextrans, *Arch Surg* 93:941-950, 1966.

101. Luft FC: Lactic acidosis update for critical care clinicians, *J Am Soc Nephrol* 12:S15-S19, 2001.

102. Lunn PC, Austin S: Excess energy intake promotes the development of hypoalbuminemia in rats fed on low-protein diets, *Br J Nutr* 49:9-16, 1983.

103. Macintyre E, Mackie IJ, Ho D, et al: The haemostatic effects of hydroxyethyl starch (HES) used as a volume expander, *Intensive Care Med* 11:300-303, 1985.

104. Margarson MP, Soni N: Serum albumin: touchstone or totem? *Anaesthesia* 53:789-803, 1998.

105. McAuliffe JJ, Lind LJ, Leith DE, et al: Hypoproteinemic alkalosis, *Am J Med* 81:86-90, 1986.

106. McCullough AJ, Mullen KD, Kalhan SC: Measurements of total body and extracellular water in cirrhotic patients

with and without ascites, *Hepatology* 14:1102-1111, 1991.

107. McGuire SO, Alexander DW, Fritsche KL: Fish oil source differentially affects rat immune cell alpha-tocopherol concentration, *J Nutr* 127:1388-1394, 1997.

108. Meier PJ: Molecular mechanisms of hepatic bile salt transport from sinusoidal blood into bile, *Am J Physiol* 269:G801-G812, 1995.

109. Meuten DJ, Chew DJ, Capen CC, et al: Relationship of serum total calcium to albumin and total protein in dogs, *J Am Vet Med Assoc* 180:63-67, 1982.

110. Mishler JM: *Pharmacology of hydroxyethyl starch. Use in therapy and blood banking*, Oxford, 1982, Oxford University Press, pp. 1-118.

111. Moller S, Henriksen JH: Pathogenesis and pathophysiology of hepatorenal syndrome—is there scope for prevention? *Aliment Pharmacol Ther* 20(suppl 3):31-41, 2004.

112. Moore KP, Wong F, Gines P, et al: The management of ascites in cirrhosis: report on the consensus conference of the international ascites club, *Hepatology* 38:258-266, 2003.

113. Moore LE, Garvey MS: The effect of hetastarch on serum colloid oncotic pressure in hypoalbuminemic dogs, *J Vet Intern Med* 10:300-303, 1996.

114. Morgan EH, Peters T: The biosynthesis of rat serum albumin: V. Effect of protein depletion and refeeding on albumin and transferrin synthesis, *J Biol Chem* 246:3500-3507, 1971.

115. Moshage H: Cytokines and the hepatic acute phase response, *J Pathol* 181:257-266, 1997.

116. Murphy GP, Demaree DE, Gagnon JA: The renal and systemic effects of hydroxyethyl starch solution infusions, *J Urol* 93:534-539, 1965.

117. Moreau R, Hadengue A, Soupison T, et al: Arterial and mixed venous acid-base status in patients with cirrhosis. Influence of liver failure, *Liver* 13:20-24, 1993.

118. Nagami GT: Effect of bath and luminal potassium concentration on ammonia production and secretion by mouse proximal tubules perfused in vitro, *J Clin Invest* 86:32-39, 1990.

119. Nelson DC, McGrew WRG, Hoyumpa AM: Hypernatremia and lactulose therapy, *JAMA* 249:1295-1298, 1983.

120. Nemec A, Pecar J, Seliskar A, et al: Assessment of acid-base status and plasma lactate concentrations in arterial, mixed venous, and portal blood from dogs during experimental hepatic blood inflow occlusion, *Am J Vet Res* 64:599-608, 2003.

121. Nyberg SL, Cerra FB, Gruetter R: Brain lactate by magnetic resonance spectroscopy during fulminant hepatic failure in the dog, *Liver Transpl Surg* 4:158-165, 1998.

122. Olde Damink SWM, Jalan R, Deutz NE, et al: The kidney plays a major role in the hyperammonemia seen after simulated or actual GI bleeding in patients with cirrhosis, *Hepatology* 37:1277-1285, 2003.

123. Papadakis MA, Arieff AI: Unpredictability of clinical evaluation of renal function in cirrhosis. Prospective study, *Am J Med* 82:945-953, 1987.

124. Papper S: The role of the kidney in Laennec's cirrhosis of the liver, *Medicine (Baltimore)* 37:299-309, 1958.

125. Papper S, Belsky JL, Bleifer KH: Renal failure in Laennec's cirrhosis of the liver. I. Description of the clinical and laboratory features, *Ann Intern Med* 51:759-765, 1959.

126. Papper S, Saxon L: The diuretic response to administered water in patients with liver disease. II. Laennec's cirrhosis of the liver, *Arch Intern Med* 103:750-757, 1959.

127. Park R, Leach WJ, Arieff AI: Determination of the liver intracellular pH in vivo and its homeostasis in acute acidosis and alkalosis, *Am J Physiol* 236:F240-F245, 1979.

128. Park R, Arieff AI: Lactic acidosis, *Adv Int Med* 25:33-68, 1980.

129. Park R, Arieff AI, Leach W, et al: Treatment of lactic acidosis with dichloroacetate in dogs, *J Clin Invest* 70:853-862, 1982.

130. Parth E, Jurecka W, Szepfalusi Z: Histological and immunohistochemical investigations of hydroxyethyl starch deposits in rat tissues, *Eur Surg Res* 24:13-21, 1992.

131. Pembleton-Corbett JR, Center SA, Schermerhorn T, et al: Serum-effusion albumin gradient in dogs with transudative abdominal effusion, *J Vet Intern Med* 14:613-618, 2000.

132. Perschel FH, Buhler H, Hierholzer K: Bile acids and their amidates inhibit 11 beta-hydroxysteroid dehydrogenase obtained from rat kidney, *Pflugers Arch* 418:538-543, 1991.

133. Prytz H, Thomsen AC: Acid-base status in liver cirrhosis. Disturbances in stable, terminal and porta-caval shunted patients, *Scand J Gastroenterol* 11:249-256, 1976.

134. Pugh P, Stone SL: The ionic composition of bile, *J Physiol* 201:50P-51P, 1969.

135. Quinlan GJ, Margarson MP, Mumby S, et al: Administration of albumin to patients with sepsis syndrome: a possible beneficial role in plasma thiol repletion, *Clin Sci (Lond)* 95:459-465, 1998.

136. Record CO, Iles RA, Cohen RD, et al: Acid-base and metabolic disturbances in fulminant hepatic failure, *Gut* 16:144-149, 1975.

137. Rothschild MA, Oratz M, Dessler R, et al: Albumin synthesis in cirrhotic subjects with ascites studied with carbonate 14, *J Clin Invest* 48:344-350, 1969.

138. Rothschild MA, Oratz M, Schreiber SS: Serum albumin, *Hepatology* 8:385-401, 1988.

139. Rothuizen J, Biewenga WJ, Mol JA: Chronic glucocorticoid excess and impaired osmoregulation of vasopressin release in dogs with hepatic encephalopathy, *Domest Anim Endocrinol* 12:13-24, 1995.

140. Rudloff E, Kirby R: The critical need for colloids: selecting the right colloid, *Compend Contin Educ* 19:811-825, 1997.

141. Ruiz-del-Arbol L, Monescillo A, Jimenez W, et al: Paracentesis-induced circulatory dysfunction: mechanisms and effect on hepatic hemodynamics in cirrhosis, *Gastroenterology* 113:579-586, 1997.

142. Saner FH, Fruhauf NR, Schafers RF, et al: Terlipressin plus hydroxyethyl starch infusion: an effective treatment for hepatorenal syndrome, *Eur J Gastroenterol Hepatol* 15:925-927, 2003.

143. Sanfilippo MJ, Suberviola PD, Geimer NF: Development of a von Willebrand-like syndrome after prolonged use of hydroxyethyl starch, *Am J Clin Pathol* 88:653-655, 1987.

144. Schenker S, Breen KJ, Hoyumpa AM: Hepatic encephalopathy: current status, *Gastroenterology* 66:121-151, 1974.

145. Sebastian A, Sutton JM, Hulter HM, et al: Effect of mineralocorticoid replacement therapy on renal acid-base homeostasis in adrenalectomized patients, *Kidney Int* 18:762-763, 1980.

146. Sevelius E, Andersson M: Serum protein electrophoresis as a prognostic marker of chronic liver disease in dogs, *Vet Rec* 137:663-667, 1995.

147. Shangraw RE, Jahoor F: Effect of liver disease and transplantation on urea synthesis in humans: relationship to acid-base status, *Am J Physiol* 276:G1145-G1152, 1999.

148. Shear L, Kleinerman J, Gabuzda GJ: Renal failure in patients with cirrhosis of the liver. I. Clinical and pathologic characteristics, *Am J Med* 39:184-189, 1965.

149. Simpson KW, Fyfe J, Cornetta A, et al: Subnormal concentrations of serum cobalamin (vitamin B_{12}) in cats with gastrointestinal disease, *J Vet Intern Med* 15:26-32, 2001.

150. Smiley LE, Garvey MS: The use of hetastarch as adjunct therapy in 26 dogs with hypoalbuminemia: a phase two clinical trial, *J Vet Intern Med* 8:195-202, 1994.

151. Sokol RJ, Devereaux M, Khandwala RA: Effect of dietary lipid and vitamin E on mitochondrial lipid peroxidation and hepatic injury in the bile duct-ligated rat, *J Lipid Res* 32:1349-1357, 1991.

152. Sokol RJ, McKim JM, Goff MC, et al: Vitamin E reduces oxidant injury to mitochondria and the hepatotoxicity of taurochenodeoxycholic acid in the rat, *Gastroenterology* 114:164-174, 1998.

153. Sola R, Vila MC, Andreu M, et al: Total paracentesis with dextran 40 vs diuretics in the treatment of ascites in cirrhosis: a randomized controlled study, *J Hepatol* 282-288, 1994.

154. Solis-Hernuzo JA, Gonzalez-Gamarra A, Castellano G, et al: Metabolic clearance rate of arginine vasopressin in patients with cirrhosis, *Hepatology* 16:974-979, 1992.

155. Standl T, Lipfert B, Reeker W, et al: Acute effects of complete blood exchanges with ultra-purified hemoglobin solution or hydroxyethyl starch on liver and kidney in the animal model, *Anasthesiol Intensivemed Notfallmed Schmerzther* 31:354-361, 1996.

156. Sterczer A, Meyer HP, Van Sluijs FJ, et al: Fast resolution of hypercortisolism in dogs with portosystemic encephalopathy after surgical shunt closure, *Res Vet Sci* 66:63-67, 1999.

157. Stoff JS: Phosphate homeostasis and hypophosphatemia, *Am J Med* 72:489-495, 1982.

158. Stump DC, Strauss RG, Henriksen RA, et al: Effects of hydroxyethyl starch on blood coagulation, particularly factor VIII, *Transfusion* 25:230-234, 1985.

159. Such J, Frances R, Munoz C, et al: Detection and identification of bacterial DNA in patients with cirrhosis and culture-negative, nonneutrocytic ascites, *Hepatology* 36:135-141, 2002.

160. Symington BE: Hetastarch and bleeding complications, *Ann Intern Med* 105:627-628, 1986.

161. Tanifuji Y, Kamide M, Shudo Y, et al: Clinical evaluation of acetated ringer as intraoperative fluids for patients with liver cirrhosis, *Masui* 32:1347-1352, 1983.

162. Tannen RL: Relationship of renal ammonia production and potassium homeostasis, *Kidney Int* 11:453-465, 1977.

163. Tannen RL, Kunin AS: Effect of pH on ammonia production by renal mitochondria, *Am J Physiol* 231:1631-1637, 1976.

164. Tannen RL: Ammonia and acid base homeostasis, *Med Clin North Am* 67:781-798, 1983.

165. Terg R, Berreta J, Abecasis R, et al: Dextran administration avoids hemodynamic changes following paracentesis in cirrhotic patients. A safe and inexpensive option, *Dig Dis Sci* 37:79-83, 1992.

166. Terg R, Miguez CD, Castro L, et al: Pharmacokinetics of Dextran-70 in patients with cirrhosis and ascites undergoing therapeutic paracentesis, *J Hepatol* 25:329-333, 1996.

167. The SAFE Study Investigators: A comparison of albumin and saline for fluid resuscitation in the intensive care unit, *N Engl J Med* 350:2247-2256, 2004.

168. Thompson WL, Fukushima T, Rutherford RB, et al: Intravascular persistence, tissue storage, and excretion of hydroxyethyl starch, *Surg Gynecol Obstet* 131:965-972, 1970.

169. Thompson WL, Gadsden RH: Prolonged bleeding times and hypofibrinogenemia in dogs after infusion of hydroxyethyl starch and dextran, *Transfusion* 5:440-446, 1965.

170. Toulza O, Center SA, Brooks MB, et al: Protein C deficiency in dogs with liver disease, *J Vet Int Med* 18:445, 2004 (abstract).

171. Unikowsky B, Wexler MJ, Levy M: Dogs with experimental cirrhosis of the liver but without intrahepatic hypertension do not retain sodium or form ascites, *J Clin Invest* 72:1594-1604, 1983.

172. Uriz J, Gines P, Cardenas A, et al: Terlipressin plus albumin infusion: an effective and safe therapy of hepatorenal syndrome, *J Hepatol* 33:43-48, 2000.

173. Vaamonde CA: Renal water handling in liver disease. In Epstein M, editor: *The kidney in liver disease*, ed 3, Baltimore, 1988, Williams & Wilkins, pp. 31-72.

174. Vinay P, Cardoso M, Tejedor A, et al: Acetate metabolism during hemodialysis: metabolic considerations, *Am J Nephrol* 7:337-354, 1987.

175. Watanabe A, Matsuzaki S, Moriwaki H, et al: Problems in serum albumin measurement and clinical significance of albumin microheterogeneity in cirrhotics, *Nutrition* 20:351-357, 2004.

176. Weber P, Bendich A, Machlin LJ: Vitamin E and human health: rationale for determining recommended intake levels, *Nutrition* 13:450-460, 1997.

177. Wilkes MM, Navickis RJ: Patient survival after human albumin administration: a meta-analysis of randomized, controlled trials, *Ann Intern Med* 135:149-164, 2001.

178. Wong F, Blei AT, Blendis LM, et al: A vasopressin receptor antagonist (VPA-985) improves serum sodium concentration in patients with hyponatremia: a multicenter, randomized, placebo-controlled trial, *Hepatology* 37:182-191, 2003.

179. Woods HF, Connor H, Tucker GT: The role of altered lactate kinetics in the pathogenesis of type B lactic acidosis. In Porter R, editor: *Metabolic acidosis*, CIBA Found Symp 87:307-323, 1982.

180. Yacobi A, Gibson TP, McEntegart CM, et al: Pharmacokinetics of high molecular weight hydroxyethyl starch in dogs, *Res Comm Chem Pathol Pharmacol* 36:199-204, 1982.

181. Yedgar S, Carew RE, Pittman RC, et al: Tissue sites of catabolism of albumin in rabbits, *Am J Physiol* 244:E101-E107, 1983.

182. Zavagli G, Ricci G, Bader G, et al: The importance of the highest normokalemia in the treatment of early hepatic encephalopathy, *Miner Electrolyte Metab* 19:362-367, 1993.

183. Zimmon DS, Oratz M, Kessler R, et al: Albumin to ascites. Demonstration of a direct pathway bypassing the systemic circulation, *J Clin Invest* 48:2074-2078, 1969.

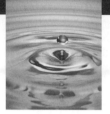

FLUID THERAPY IN ENDOCRINE AND METABOLIC DISORDERS

David L. Panciera

Metabolic disorders such as complicated diabetes mellitus, hypoadrenocorticism, and heatstroke are associated with marked disturbances in fluid homeostasis, electrolyte balance, and acid-base status. Prompt recognition of the complications associated with these and other metabolic disorders is essential for effective management. The dynamic nature of these illnesses during treatment requires the attending clinician to be vigilant in monitoring and to recognize when therapy needs to be altered. An understanding of the pathophysiology of the metabolic abnormalities encountered in each disorder is necessary for proper management.

DIABETIC KETOACIDOSIS

Diabetic ketoacidosis (DKA) is a life-threatening complication of diabetes mellitus that results from a combination of factors, including insulin resistance (counter-regulatory hormones), fasting, a lack of insulin, and dehydration in an animal with diabetes mellitus. Dehydration, electrolyte disturbances, and metabolic acidosis are consistent findings in affected patients that must be addressed during treatment. Most animals with DKA have concurrent diseases including pancreatitis, urinary tract infection, hyperadrenocorticism, neoplasia, hepatic disease, and renal failure. In addition to clinical signs typical of diabetes mellitus, dogs and cats with ketoacidosis frequently exhibit lethargy, anorexia, vomiting, weakness, depression, dehydration, tachypnea, and weight loss. Other clinical signs may be present depending on the underlying illness. A tentative diagnosis is made by documenting ketonuria in a diabetic animal with clinical signs of systemic illness and diabetes mellitus. The prognosis more often is determined by the nature and severity of the concurrent disease than by the ketoacidotic state.

PATHOPHYSIOLOGY

A combination of events must take place for ketoacidosis to occur. Insulin deficiency, presence of counter-regulatory hormones, fasting, and dehydration combine to create the metabolic aberrations that result in the syndrome of DKA.[29] The insulin deficiency may be relative or absolute. The diagnosis of diabetes mellitus is most often made at the time of presentation for DKA, but a minority of dogs and cats are receiving insulin at the time of diagnosis. The concurrent illness present in the majority of cases of DKA is the cause of insulin resistance and contributes to the increase in counter-regulatory hormones.

Carbohydrate Metabolism

Hyperglycemia occurs as a result of insulin deficiency, increases in counter-regulatory hormones, and dehydration. Increased hepatic glucose output primarily caused by increased gluconeogenesis appears to be the primary factor causing hyperglycemia.[9,29] Gluconeogenic substrates include amino acids derived from proteolysis and decreased protein synthesis, lactate from glycolysis, and glycerol from lipolysis. Increased glucagon and β-adrenergic activation by catecholamines in the face of inadequate insulin stimulate glycolysis and gluconeogenesis. The osmotic diuresis induced by glycosuria contributes to dehydration and subsequent hyperglycemia.[9,29] Dehydration also may cause decreased insulin delivery to sensitive tissues such as skeletal muscle and therefore may reduce insulin action. In addition, antagonism of the cellular actions of insulin by growth hormone and cortisol contribute to insulin resistance.

Lipid Metabolism

Ketoacids are derived from the increased free fatty acids that are present as a consequence of increased lipolysis. An increase in catecholamines results in activation of hormone-sensitive lipase in adipose tissue, liberating free fatty acids and glycerol.[9,29] In the liver, the large quantity of free fatty acids is oxidized to ketone bodies under the influence of glucagon, although cortisol, epinephrine, and growth hormone also play a role in stimulating ketogenesis. Anorexia that is usually present in patients with DKA contributes to the hormonal changes mentioned above and lack of substrate for anabolic functions. Utilization of ketones is impaired in DKA as well, contributing to their increased concentration.

Fluid and Electrolyte Metabolism

Dehydration is a consistent finding in dogs and cats with DKA.[6,8,11,37] It occurs because of osmotic diuresis secondary to glycosuria and ketonuria, and as a result of gastrointestinal losses associated with vomiting and diarrhea. Electrolyte loss also occurs in these patients because of the diuresis and the cation excretion that accompanies ketoacid excretion.[29] Insulin deficiency also results in loss of electrolytes because insulin is required for normal sodium, chloride, potassium, and phosphorus reabsorption in tubular epithelial cells. Loss of sodium, potassium, chloride, magnesium, phosphorus, and calcium occur to a substantial degree in DKA. However, the resulting electrolyte abnormalities are reflected variably in plasma concentrations.[6,8,11,37]

Acid-Base Changes

Loss of ketoacids in the urine results in buffering by plasma bicarbonate. Urinary bicarbonate excretion contributes to the metabolic acidosis induced by accumulation of ketoacids.[29] Retention of these unmeasured anions results in an increased anion gap.

TREATMENT

Fluid Therapy

The goals of fluid therapy in DKA are to restore circulating volume, replace water and sodium deficits, correct electrolyte imbalances, improve tissue delivery of nutrients, and decrease the blood glucose concentration. Initial fluid therapy should improve intravascular volume, reduce secretion of counter-regulatory hormones, and enhance tissue delivery of insulin. It generally is recommended that insulin administration be delayed for 1 to 2 hours after fluid therapy is instituted when hyperglycemia is severe, hypotension is present, or clinically relevant hypokalemia exists. Reduction of blood glucose concentration before replacement of intravascular volume could result in loss of water from the intravascular space along with glucose and worsening of hypotension. Severe hyperglycemia and hypotension are likely. A substantial reduction of blood glucose will occur despite a delay in insulin administration because fluid therapy alone reduces insulin resistance, increases insulin availability at peripheral tissues such as skeletal muscle, dilutes the blood glucose, and enhances urinary loss subsequent to an increase in glomerular filtration rate (GFR).[51] After initial rehydration, consideration should be given to the decrease in the plasma effective osmolality and thus plasma volume that occurs after reduction of the blood glucose concentration, necessitating administration of fluids at a higher rate than would be needed in a euglycemic patient. After hydration status has been normalized and blood glucose concentration reduced, additional fluid administration should be based on calculation of maintenance needs plus ongoing losses from the gastrointestinal tract (e.g., vomiting, diarrhea) and in the urine (i.e., polyuria caused by continued glycosuria). Aggressive treatment is not necessary in dogs or cats with ketonuria if signs of systemic illness are not present. The presence of a concurrent disease, present in most dogs and cats with DKA, may necessitate modification of the fluid therapy plan.

Fluid Composition

Because of the marked deficits of water and sodium present in animals with DKA, 0.9% saline is the fluid of choice for initial management. Administration of an isotonic solution allows for rapid expansion of intravascular volume in patients with severe dehydration or hypovolemic shock.

Serum osmolality usually is high in animals with DKA, often moderately to markedly so. The median measured osmolality in 23 cats with DKA was 353 mOsm/kg (reference range, 280 to 300 mOsm/Kg), and the median calculated osmolality in 19 other cats was 333 mOsm/kg.[6] The hyperosmolality is attributable primarily to hyperglycemia, azotemia, and ketone bodies. Because treatment rapidly resolves these abnormalities, the osmolality decreases predictably without the use of hypotonic solutions. Cerebral edema has been documented in humans, particularly children during treatment of DKA. Clinical signs of cerebral edema are rare despite its common occurrence.[31] Rapid reduction in plasma osmolality is a major factor in development of cerebral edema. Cerebral edema is caused in part by the accumulation of idiogenic osmoles in the central nervous system (CNS) secondary to chronic hyperosmolality.[13] Idiogenic osmoles are produced in response to plasma hyperosmolality, and they increase the osmolality of the brain to prevent cerebral dehydration. If the plasma osmolality decreases quickly, the idiogenic osmoles will persist and cause water accumulation in the cerebrum because of the difference in osmolality between the brain and plasma. Because of this, administration of hypotonic fluids such as 0.45% saline is discouraged by some endocrinologists, particularly during initial treatment.[9,29] The importance of this pathophysiology in dogs and cats is unknown, but it seems prudent to avoid rapid reduction in plasma osmolality during treatment of DKA. Although 0.45% saline approximates the composition of electrolytes lost as a result of osmotic diuresis and has been recommended for administration after rehydration, the author rarely uses it for treatment of DKA.

Once the blood glucose concentration decreases to less than 250 mg/dL, 50% dextrose should be added to the 0.9% saline to make a 2.5% to 5% dextrose solution.[8,36,37] Adjustments in the dextrose content of the fluids should be made based on Table 20-1. The addition of dextrose will prevent hypoglycemia and allow for continued insulin administration to stop ketoacid formation.

Rate and Volume of Fluid Administration

The primary goal of initial fluid therapy is to restore intravascular fluid volume to improve tissue perfusion, including GFR. Fluids should be administered at a rate sufficient to replace volume deficits in 12 to 24 hours, with 50% of the estimated deficit replaced in the first 4 to 6 hours. An estimated volume of fluid to account for ongoing losses should be added to the maintenance and replacement fluid volume, with special consideration of urine output in the presence of polyuria. Fluids should be administered cautiously to animals with impaired cardiac function or the potential for oliguric renal failure. Monitoring should consist of estimates or quantitation of urine output, serial body weights, packed cell volume, total solids, and serum concentrations of creatinine, electrolytes, and glucose. Urine output should be evident within 2 to 4 hours of initiating fluid therapy unless oliguric renal failure is present.

Insulin Therapy

Intravenous fluid therapy will decrease the blood glucose concentration and reduce lactic acidosis, but insulin administration is required to halt ketogenesis, increase ketone body utilization, decrease gluconeogenesis, promote glucose utilization, and decrease proteolysis.[9,29] Ketogenesis will be decreased by an insulin concentration 50% less than that required for promotion of peripheral utilization of glucose, and consequently ketoacid formation is decreased rapidly after insulin administration. For insulin to be most effective, tissue perfusion must be restored, and intravenous fluid therapy should be instituted first or at least concurrently. Insulin sensitivity is increased by reduction in hyperosmolality and decreased concentrations of counter-regulatory hormones. An additional important effect of insulin is its action on electrolyte transport and resolution of acidosis that cause a transcellular shift of potassium into cells causing hypokalemia. In patients with serum potassium concentrations less than 3.5 mEq/L, insulin administration should be delayed until potassium supplementation has successfully increased the serum potassium concentration above this limit to avoid worsening of hypokalemia. In addition, hypotensive animals should receive fluid therapy sufficient to stabilize circulatory status before insulin administration to avoid the decrease in plasma volume that occurs when glucose and water are translocated into cells in response to insulin.

Administration of small doses of regular insulin has a clear advantage over large doses because the smaller doses are less likely to cause severe hypokalemia or hypoglycemia.[28] In addition, if the reduction in the blood glucose concentration is too rapid, the associated decrease in osmolality may promote development of cerebral edema. Two methods of delivering low-dose insulin therapy to dogs have been described: the low-dose intramuscular technique and the continuous low-dose intravenous infusion.[8,37] With either technique, regular insulin is administered with a desired effect of decreasing the blood glucose by not more than 50 to 75 mg/dL/hr. Similar treatment has been used in cats with DKA.[36]

The low-dose intramuscular insulin protocol is an effective and straightforward, but somewhat time-consuming, method for insulin administration in DKA.[8] Intramuscular administration is recommended because absorption from subcutaneous sites may be reduced or inconsistent in the presence of dehydration. However, absorption is similar from the two administration sites in humans with DKA.[18] The initial dose of regular insulin is

TABLE 20-1 Adjustment in Insulin and Dextrose Administration Using the Continuous Low-Dose Intravenous Insulin Infusion Protocol

Blood Glucose Concentration (mg/dL)	Intravenous Fluid Solution	Rate of Intravenous Insulin Solution (mL/hr)*
>250	0.9% saline	10
200–250	0.9% saline, 2.5% dextrose	7
150–200	0.9% saline, 2.5% dextrose	5
100–150	0.9% saline, 5% dextrose	5
<100	0.9% saline, 5% dextrose	Stop insulin infusion

*Intravenous insulin solution contains 2.2 U/kg (dog) or 1.1 U/kg (cat) of regular insulin in 250 mL of 0.9% saline.
Adapted from Macintire DK: Treatment of diabetic ketoacidosis in dogs by continuous low-dose intravenous infusion of insulin, J Am Vet Med Assoc 202:1266–1272, 1993.

0.2 U/kg intramuscularly, followed by hourly measurement of blood glucose concentrations.[8] Subsequent insulin administration continues hourly at 0.1 U/kg intramuscularly until the blood glucose concentration is 250 mg/dL or less. Dogs weighing less than 10 kg are given 2 U and cats are given 1 U initially, followed by 1 U every hour unless diluted insulin is available.[8] If the blood glucose concentration decreases by more than 100 mg/dL, the dosage is decreased. Once the blood glucose concentration is less than 250 mg/dL, the hourly insulin injections are stopped, and 50% dextrose is added to the intravenous fluid solution in a quantity sufficient to make a 5% dextrose solution. Additional doses of regular insulin are administered every 4 to 6 hours at 0.1 to 0.4 U/kg subcutaneously with the dosage and dosing interval determined by measurement of blood glucose concentration every 1 to 2 hours to maintain blood glucose concentration between 200 and 300 mg/dL. The primary disadvantage of the low-dose intramuscular protocol is that it requires considerable technical effort to accomplish hourly injections and blood glucose measurements. In addition, the decrease in blood glucose concentration seems to occur more rapidly and less predictably than with the continuous intravenous infusion method.

The continuous low-dose intravenous infusion protocol involves administration of regular insulin diluted in normal saline using an intravenous infusion pump.[37] It is the author's preferred technique of insulin administration to dogs with DKA because of the predictable and consistent response, the gradual decrease in blood glucose concentration (mean of 28 mg/dL/hr in dogs), and the ease of use.[37] Unlike the low-dose intramuscular protocol, treatment is not dependent on hourly injections, and the decrease in blood glucose concentration is more gradual using the intravenous protocol. An insulin solution is made by adding regular insulin at 2.2 U/kg for dogs and 1.1 U/kg for cats to 250 mL 0.9% saline.[36,37] This solution is administered as a constant-rate infusion at 10 mL/hr to deliver a dosage of 0.09 U/kg/hr in dogs and 0.045 U/kg/hr in cats. Because insulin may adhere to plastic in the administration set, it is recommended that 50 mL of the insulin solution be allowed to flow through the administration set before use. During insulin administration, intravenous fluid therapy with 0.9% saline is continued through a separate line as indicated for rehydration and maintenance needs. Blood glucose concentration is measured every 60 to 90 minutes. When the blood glucose is less than 250 mg/dL, the infusion rate is decreased according to Table 20-1, and dextrose is added to the hydration fluids to a final concentration of 2.5% to 5% (see Table 20-1).[37] The primary disadvantage of the continuous low-dose intravenous infusion protocol is the need for an infusion pump and the time required to monitor blood glucose serially.

The high-dose intramuscular or subcutaneous insulin protocol is the simplest for management of DKA, requiring the least amount of monitoring and equipment.[5] However, it has some shortcomings, including a rapid decrease in blood glucose concentration that predisposes to hypoglycemia, a greater magnitude of hypokalemia, and a substantial decrease in osmolality over a short period. It is for these reasons that this technique is no longer used in humans and is considered less desirable for use in dogs and cats. Regular insulin is administered at 0.25 U/kg every 4 hours intramuscularly until the patient is rehydrated, followed by subcutaneous administration every 6 to 8 hours.[5] The dosage and frequency of insulin administration are based on monitoring blood glucose concentration hourly, with a goal of decreasing the glucose concentration by approximately 50 mg/dL/hr. Once the glucose concentration is near 250 mg/dL, dextrose is added to the intravenous saline solution to a final concentration of 5%, and the subsequent insulin dosage is decreased by 25% to 50%.

Regardless of the initial insulin administration protocol used, intermediate or long-acting insulin treatment can be instituted when the animal is eating normally.

Potassium Supplementation

Regardless of the serum potassium concentration, almost all patients with DKA have a deficit of total body potassium.[9,29] Before treatment, hypokalemia is found in approximately 30% to 43% of dogs and 55% to 67% of cats, whereas hyperkalemia is found in less than 10% of cases.[6,8,11,14,37] Hypokalemia occurs because of urinary potassium losses caused by osmotic diuresis, deficient renal tubular potassium absorption caused by insulin deficiency, and excretion with ketoacids, as well as through gastrointestinal losses from vomiting and diarrhea. Treatment of DKA rapidly lowers plasma potassium concentration because correction of acidosis causes a transcellular shift of potassium into cells, insulin enhances transport of potassium into cells, and intravenous fluid administration causes diuresis and dilution of plasma potassium. Hypokalemia can cause muscle weakness, arrhythmias, and impaired renal function.

Potassium should be supplemented in virtually all animals with DKA, but the initial dose rate is dependent on the pretreatment serum potassium concentration. If the serum potassium concentration is above the reference range, intravenous fluids should be administered without addition of potassium for 2 hours at which time serum potassium concentration should be rechecked if possible. If the serum potassium concentration has decreased into the normal range, supplementation is given according to Table 20-2. The dose rate of KCl should not exceed 0.5 mEq/kg/hr because of the risk of cardiac arrhythmia. If a serum potassium measurement is not available after initial treatment and urine output appears adequate, 30 to 40 mEq KCl should be added to each liter of fluids. Urine production should be monitored closely to ensure that oliguric renal failure is not present. In humans with hypokalemia before treatment, it is recommended that insulin administration be delayed until the serum potassium concentration can be increased into the normal range because the potassium concentration will decrease during insulin administration.[29] A similar recommendation is made for veterinary patients with substantial hypokalemia (<3.5 mEq/L). Serum potassium concentration should be monitored 4 hours after initiating potassium supplementation and at least every 8 to 12 hours thereafter, with dosage adjustments to maintain normokalemia (see Table 20-2).

Phosphorus Supplementation

Similar to potassium, phosphate is deficient in animals with DKA regardless of the serum phosphorus concentration. Phosphorus is lost in patients with DKA because of a shift from the intracellular to the extracellular compartment secondary to hyperosmolality that is followed by urinary loss, decreased cellular uptake caused by insulin deficiency, inhibition of renal tubular phosphate absorption caused by acidosis, and osmotic diuresis.[21,29] During treatment of DKA, the reduction in osmolality and insulin administration result in translocation of phosphate into the cell from the extracellular compartment. This translocation frequently causes a marked decrease in the plasma phosphorus concentration. However, clinically important consequences of hypophosphatemia are noted only when the serum phosphorus concentration is less than 1.0 to 1.5 mg/dL, and these signs are observed inconsistently. Hemolysis, muscle weakness, seizures, depression, and decreased leukocyte and platelet function leading to infection and bleeding can result from hypophosphatemia. The only abnormalities documented as caused by hypophosphatemia in veterinary DKA patients are hemolytic anemia in cats and possibly stupor and seizures in a dog.[1,6,53] Hemolysis can occur despite phosphate supplementation and may have causes other than hypophosphatemia including oxidative injury.[6,10] Hypophosphatemia is present at initial evaluation in 13% to 48% of cats with DKA; the prevalence in dogs is unknown.[6,11]

Treatment of hypophosphatemia is indicated when the serum phosphorus concentration before treatment is less than 1.5 mg/dL or if the serum phosphorus concentration is less than 1.0 mg/dL in the dog and less than 1.5 mg/dL in the cat at any time. Potassium phosphate typically is the treatment of choice because potassium supplementation is also necessary in most cases, but sodium phosphate is also available for use. Potassium phosphate is available as a solution containing 3 mmol/mL of phosphorus (99 mg/dL) and 4.36 mEq/mL of potassium. Excessive phosphate supplementation can cause hypocalcemia, hyperphosphatemia, tetany, soft tissue mineralization, and renal failure.[21,52] Because phosphate deficits vary widely and are not necessarily reflected by serum phosphorus concentrations, phosphate administration should be guided by repeated serum phosphate measurements during treatment. Potassium phosphate should be administered by constant-rate infusion at an initial dosage of 0.01 to 0.06 mmol/kg/hr.[52] Higher infusion rates can be administered as necessary. Monitoring should consist of measurement of serum potassium, phosphate, and calcium concentrations every 8 to 12 hours during phosphate administration. Hyperphosphatemia, clinically relevant hypocalcemia, and hyperkalemia are indications to discontinue phosphate administration. Treatment also should be discontinued when the serum phosphorus concentration is normal and the animal is eating. Some have suggested that potassium phosphate be routinely administered to animals with DKA regardless of the initial serum phosphorus concentration, but there is no evidence in veterinary or human medicine that such treatment is beneficial.[17]

Magnesium Supplementation

Magnesium deficiency is present in some cats with DKA as reflected by measurement of ionized magnesium concentrations.[41] However, total magnesium concentrations were high in many of the same cats, and the widely available total magnesium concentration is unlikely to reflect active plasma magnesium status.[41] Because clinical signs such as arrhythmia, weakness, seizures, and refractory hypocalcemia and hypokalemia have not been documented to result from hypomagnesemia in dogs or cats with DKA, magnesium supplementation is not recommended.

Bicarbonate Administration

The acidosis of DKA typically is a high anion gap acidosis, although hyperchloremic acidosis also can be present at presentation. The unmeasured anions are ketoacids that act as precursors of bicarbonate during treatment with insulin because insulin enhances utilization of ketones and inhibits further production of ketoacids by decreasing lipolysis.[9,29] Because of this, the acidosis asso-

TABLE 20-2 Potassium Supplementation in Intravenous Fluids

Serum Potassium Concentration (mEq/L)	Potassium Supplement (mEq) in 1 L Intravenous Fluids
>3.5	20
3.0–3.5	30
2.5–3.0	40
2.0–2.5	60
<2.0	80

ciated with DKA does not usually need to be treated with bicarbonate, although animals with severe acidosis may benefit from treatment. Studies in humans have not shown a beneficial effect of bicarbonate administration in DKA.[23,39] However, few patients with severe acidosis have been studied, and it is currently recommended to administer bicarbonate to individuals with a blood pH less than 7.0, particularly if the pH does not improve after the first hour of intravenous fluid administration.[29] Humans with hyperchloremic metabolic acidosis have a slower recovery from acidosis compared with those with high anion gap, probably because they have relatively less ketoacid to convert to bicarbonate. Therefore patients that present with hyperchloremic metabolic acidosis may benefit from bicarbonate administration.[2] Potential complications of bicarbonate administration in animals with ketoacidosis include impaired ketone utilization, paradoxical intracellular or CNS acidosis, and contribution to cerebral edema. The most common detrimental effect of bicarbonate is likely to be worsening of hypokalemia because concurrent intravenous fluid therapy and insulin administration cause a decrease in serum potassium concentration.

Recommendations for bicarbonate therapy are to administer a conservative dose when acidosis is severe. If the blood pH is less than 7.0 or the plasma bicarbonate concentration is less than 8 mEq/L, bicarbonate treatment should be instituted. The bicarbonate deficit in milliequivalents can be estimated by the following formula: $0.3 \times$ body weight (kg) $\times (24 -$ patient bicarbonate). One fourth to one half of this dose is administered over 2 to 4 hours. Blood gases should be measured after completion of bicarbonate administration with additional bicarbonate administered if the blood pH remains less than 7.2 or the plasma bicarbonate concentration is less than 12 mEq/L. If blood gases are not available, bicarbonate should not be administered.

HYPERGLYCEMIC HYPEROSMOLAR STATE

Formerly named hyperglycemic hyperosmolar nonketotic coma, hyperglycemic hyperosmolar state (HHS) is defined as diabetes mellitus with a blood glucose concentration greater than 600 mg/dL and serum osmolality more than 350 mOsm/kg in the absence of ketonuria.[14,30] In humans, acidosis is mild if present, but acidosis may be more common in dogs and cats with HHS.[29,30] The pathogenesis of this syndrome is similar to that of ketoacidosis, but it is thought that plasma insulin concentrations are higher in HHS than in DKA.[29] This difference results in insulin activity sufficient to prevent ketosis but inadequate to prevent hyperglycemia. Reductions in secretion or activity of growth hormone, glucagon, or both also may play a role in development of HHS. Loss of water in urine and decreased water intake cause dehydration with subsequent decreased renal perfusion and resultant retention of glucose. The stress of concurrent illness that usually is present results in increased counter-regulatory hormones, which contribute to further increases in blood glucose concentration.

Clinical signs are related to diabetes mellitus, concurrent disease, and hyperosmolality. Dehydration, hypothermia, and abnormalities of mentation ranging from depression to stupor or coma are common.[30] Other neurologic signs include weakness, abnormal pupillary light reflexes, cranial nerve deficits, and seizures. Neurologic signs likely result from intracellular dehydration of the brain secondary to hyperosmolality. Typical laboratory abnormalities include severe hyperglycemia, azotemia, hyperphosphatemia, and hypochloremia.[30] Concurrent diseases, including renal failure, congestive heart failure, and various infections, are common in cats with HHS.[30]

TREATMENT

Management of HHS is similar to management of DKA. Osmolality should be reduced gradually to avoid cerebral edema. Because volume depletion is integral to the pathology of HHS, restoration of circulating volume is critical to early, successful management. The goals of fluid therapy initially are to restore circulating volume and then to completely replace the estimated fluid deficits plus maintenance requirements over 36 to 48 hours. Blood glucose concentration is expected to decrease as a result of increased renal perfusion and increased urine glucose excretion, as well as increased perfusion of other tissues causing enhanced cellular glucose uptake. Administration of 0.9% NaCl is indicated for the initial 4 to 6 hours of treatment. Subsequent intravenous fluids should be either 0.9% or 0.45% saline. The composition of urine electrolyte losses closely resembles 0.45% saline, but sodium deficits typically are present in these patients. Because renal function often is impaired in patients with HHS, caution should be used when considering the appropriate potassium and phosphate supplementation, and supplementation should be based on serial measurements of serum electrolyte concentrations.

It is recommended that insulin administration be withheld until intravascular volume has been restored because intracellular movement of glucose and water from the extracellular space could cause a further decrease in intravascular volume resulting in shock. Therefore insulin administration should be delayed until fluid therapy has successfully replenished vascular volume. Insulin should be administered in a manner similar to that recommended for DKA, but additional caution is warranted to ensure that a rapid decrease in blood glucose concentration does not occur. Frequent monitoring of electrolytes and appropriate supplementation is necessary, as is the case for patients with DKA.

HYPOADRENOCORTICISM

Hypoadrenocorticism (Addison's disease) usually is the result of destruction of the adrenal cortex, resulting in deficiencies of both glucocorticoids and mineralocorticoids. Rarely, glucocorticoid deficiency occurs alone, resulting in a more vague presentation without the typical electrolyte abnormalities. Clinical signs vary considerably, and dogs with chronic illness have nonspecific clinical signs, whereas those with acute manifestations may have a life-threatening hypotensive crisis and severe hyperkalemia.[15,38,43] Prompt, appropriate treatment of this life-threatening illness should include correction of the volume depletion, hyperkalemia, hyponatremia, and glucocorticoid deficiency.

PATHOPHYSIOLOGY

Hypoadrenocorticism typically results in combined mineralocorticoid and glucocorticoid deficiency. Aldosterone, the primary mineralocorticoid secreted by the adrenal cortex, enhances reabsorption of sodium and water and excretion of potassium and hydrogen ions by the connecting segment and cortical collecting ducts of the kidneys. Aldosterone deficiency causes loss of sodium and water in the urine, resulting in hyponatremia and dehydration, as well as retention of potassium and hydrogen ions, resulting in hyperkalemia and metabolic acidosis. Gastrointestinal losses caused by vomiting and diarrhea may contribute to worsening dehydration, hyponatremia, and hypochloremia. Glucocorticoids are necessary for normal vascular tone, endothelial function, vascular permeability, water distribution, and the vasoconstrictive response to catecholamines.[33] Decreased cardiac contractility and vascular tone secondary to glucocorticoid deficiency can result in hypotension. In addition, cortisol enhances gluconeogenesis and glycogenolysis and modulates cytokine production and leukocyte response during inflammation. Cortisol deficiency is associated with hypotension, gastrointestinal signs (vomiting, diarrhea, melena), hypoglycemia, and an impaired response to stress.

Primary hypoadrenocorticism accounts for the majority of cases, with the cause presumed to be immune-mediated in most instances. The resultant mineralocorticoid and glucocorticoid deficiency results in the typical clinicopathologic picture. Glucocorticoid deficiency alone occurs infrequently and may be primary in origin (caused by loss of the zona fasciculata and zona reticularis) or secondary to adrenocorticotropic hormone (ACTH) deficiency. Primary and secondary "atypical" hypoadrenocorticism can be distinguished by measurement of plasma ACTH concentration, which is high in primary hypoadrenocorticism and low to undetectable in secondary hypoadrenocorticism.

CLINICAL FINDINGS

Dogs with chronic hypoadrenocorticism or atypical disease usually are evaluated because of lethargy, anorexia or inappetence, weight loss, weakness, polyuria, polydipsia, vomiting, and regurgitation, sometimes with a waxing and waning course.[15,38,43] Findings on physical examination are nonspecific and include lethargy, generalized weakness, dehydration, poor body condition, and melena. Dogs with an Addisonian crisis have a shorter history of weakness, lethargy, collapse, and gastrointestinal signs such as vomiting and melena.[15,38,43] Physical examination abnormalities include dehydration, weakness, hypothermia, weak pulses, bradycardia, prolonged capillary refill time, and melena. Bradycardia or low-normal heart rate in an animal with evidence of dehydration or shock should prompt the veterinarian to consider hypoadrenocorticism and other diseases causing hyperkalemia. An electrocardiogram often is the most expedient method for confirming the presence of hyperkalemia. Severe hypotension and shock are caused by volume depletion, decreased vascular tone, and decreased cardiac output secondary to the inappropriately slow heart rate.

Laboratory tests provide important information that will lead the clinician to test specifically for hypoadrenocorticism. A mild to moderate nonregenerative anemia is common but frequently is masked by dehydration. Lack of a stress leukogram in an ill dog with normal numbers of lymphocytes and eosinophils is consistent with an absence of glucocorticoid activity and provides evidence for hypoadrenocorticism.[15,38,43] The majority of dogs with hypoadrenocorticism have hyperkalemia, hyponatremia, and hypochloremia.[15,38,43] However, other causes of low sodium/potassium ratios exist, including oliguric renal failure, urinary tract obstruction, uroabdomen, severe gastrointestinal diseases including trichuriasis, pancreatitis, DKA, pleural effusion, and congestive heart failure.[22,48] Moderate to severe increases in BUN, creatinine, and phosphorus concentrations are common and usually are the result of decreased renal blood flow caused by hypovolemia and hypotension. Urine specific gravity usually is less than 1.030 because hyponatremia results in loss of the renal medullary concentration gradient. Hypoglycemia occurs in approximately 33% of cases and may be of sufficient severity to result in clinical signs including weakness, ataxia, and seizures.[15,38,43] Hypercalcemia also occurs in about 30% of cases.[15,38,43] Hypoalbuminemia, mild increases in liver enzymes, and hypocholesterolemia are present in some cases. Dogs with isolated glucocorticoid deficiency have similar hematologic changes and normal serum electrolyte concentrations, and azotemia is mild and less frequent than in dogs with concurrent mineralocorticoid deficiency.[34,49] Dogs with atypical hypoadrenocorticism frequently have hypocholesterolemia, hypoalbuminemia, and hypoglycemia.[34,49]

DIAGNOSIS

Only by demonstration of subnormal concentrations of plasma cortisol after ACTH administration can diagnosis of hypoadrenocorticism be made. The test should be performed before administration of a glucocorticoid or dexamethasone should be used because most other corticosteroids will be detected by the cortisol assay. Blood samples are collected before and 1 hour after intravenous administration of cosyntropin (5 µg/kg; 250 µg maximum) or before and 2 hours after intramuscular administration of ACTH gel (2.2 U/kg; 40 U maximum).[15] Cortisol concentrations are very low in dogs with primary hypoadrenocorticism, with the post-ACTH cortisol concentration typically below the normal resting range.[15,38,43] Recent administration of a glucocorticoid can suppress the pituitary-adrenal axis and decrease the post-ACTH cortisol concentration; therefore a careful history about systemic or topical corticosteroid use should be obtained. Serum aldosterone concentration can be measured during the ACTH response test if recent corticosteroid administration is likely to suppress the cortisol response.

TREATMENT

The goals of initial treatment of hypoadrenocorticism are to resolve hypotension, replace the volume deficit, decrease the plasma potassium concentration, correct other electrolyte abnormalities, and resolve the metabolic acidosis. These goals are most rapidly and effectively achieved by appropriate intravenous fluid therapy. Correction of hypoglycemia and replacement of glucocorticoids and mineralocorticoids also are important considerations during the initial management of hypoadrenocorticism.

Fluid Therapy

Fluid therapy should rapidly increase intravascular fluid volume, replace fluid deficits, and decrease the serum potassium concentration. Deficits of water, sodium, and chloride in the animal with an Addisonian crisis are large, and the magnitude of volume depletion usually is greater than estimated on physical examination. Many dogs present in hypovolemic shock and require immediate resuscitation.

Fluid Composition

Because of the deficits of sodium and chloride, as well as the hyperkalemia that is found in hypoadrenocorticism, 0.9% NaCl is the most appropriate fluid for initial treatment. If normal saline is not available, lactated Ringer's or similar replacement solutions can be used despite the presence of 4 mEq/L of potassium.

Rate and Volume of Fluid Administration

Administration of a bolus of NaCl will not only be effective for treatment of hypovolemia but also will reduce hyperkalemia and metabolic acidosis and subsequently increase heart rate, cardiac output, and blood pressure. Initially, fluids should be given at a rate of 40 to 80 mL/kg/hr for the first 1 to 2 hours depending on the severity of hypotension and hyperkalemia.[15] Once an adequate response to the initial fluid therapy is observed, the fluid rate can be decreased to two to three times maintenance, based on the estimated fluid deficit and ongoing losses. It is crucial to note urine output to ensure that oliguric renal failure is not present as a primary condition (rather than hypoadrenocorticism) or has occurred because of inadequate renal perfusion secondary to hypoadrenocorticism. Inadequate urine output may be the result of continued volume depletion caused by inadequate fluid therapy or ongoing losses, or as the result of oliguric renal failure. If urine output appears inadequate, placement of a urinary catheter is indicated to document oliguria and institute treatment for acute renal failure if present.

A rapid increase in serum sodium concentration and osmolality in the patient with hyponatremia and hypoosmolality may be associated with dehydration of the brain and neurologic signs caused by myelinolysis. This complication is more likely to occur with chronic hyponatremia than with that of 24 hours' duration or less. Myelinolysis appears to be rare during treatment of dogs with hypoadrenocorticism.[4]

Hypoglycemia should be treated with an initial bolus of 0.5 to 1 mL/kg 50% dextrose if clinical signs are present. If signs are not present and hypoglycemia is mild to moderate, sufficient 50% dextrose to make a 5% solution should be added to the normal saline.

Glucocorticoid Replacement

Glucocorticoids should be administered after fluid therapy has corrected the severe hypovolemia. Because appropriate intravenous fluid administration alone is very effective in resolving the most serious manifestations of the hypoadrenocortical crisis, glucocorticoid treatment can be delayed for several hours if necessary. Unless dexamethasone is administered, glucocorticoid treatment should be delayed until the ACTH response test is completed because other glucocorticoids will interfere with the cortisol assay. A rapid-acting glucocorticoid should be administered intravenously. Hydrocortisone sodium succinate or phosphate (cortisol) probably is the best initial glucocorticoid treatment, primarily because it has mineralocorticoid activity as well. Hydrocortisone should be administered as a constant-rate infusion of 0.3 mg/kg/hr or as an initial intravenous bolus (given over 5 minutes) of 5 mg/kg followed by 1 mg/kg every 6 hours.[15,32] Alternatively, dexamethasone sodium phosphate (0.1 to 0.2 mg/kg intravenously) or prednisolone sodium succinate (1 to 2 mg/kg intravenously) can be administered if hydrocortisone is not available.[45,46] Subsequent treatment should consist of subcutaneous administration of dexamethasone every 12 hours or prednisolone every 6 hours until oral treatment with prednisone (0.4 to 0.6 mg/kg daily) can be tolerated. The oral prednisone dosage should be reduced over 7 to 10 days to a maintenance dose of approximately 0.2 mg/kg daily and then adjusted as necessary to control clinical signs. The glucocorticoid dosage should be increased if stress or illness occurs in a dog with hypoadrenocorticism.

Mineralocorticoid Replacement

Because electrolyte abnormalities are rapidly corrected with intravenous administration of normal saline, and a short-acting injectable mineralocorticoid preparation is not available, specific mineralocorticoid treatment generally is delayed until oral fludrocortisone (0.01 mg/kg twice daily) can be administered.[15,27,45] Hydrocortisone has some mineralocorticoid activity and for this reason is the preferred glucocorticoid replacement. Administration of the long-acting injectable mineralocorticoid desoxycorticosterone pivalate (DOCP) should be reserved for use when a definitive diagnosis has been made, although it reportedly can be safely administered to dogs with normal adrenocortical function.[15] Serum electrolyte concentrations should be monitored and dosage adjustments of mineralocorticoids made as appropriate.[27,35]

Management of Hyperkalemia

Rarely is specific treatment of hyperkalemia indicated because appropriate fluid therapy rapidly corrects this electrolyte abnormality by dilution of plasma, increasing urine output, and shift of potassium into cells during correction of acidosis. Indications for more aggressive treatment of hyperkalemia are severe bradyarrhythmia or failure to respond to initial appropriate fluid therapy. Sodium bicarbonate administration will correct acidosis and decrease serum potassium concentration. The bicarbonate deficit can be calculated as described in the section on DKA, and 25% of the deficit should be administered.[45] Alternatively, 1 to 2 mEq/kg of sodium bicarbonate can be administered slowly intravenously. Another effective method to rapidly decrease the plasma potassium concentration is administration of regular insulin (0.2 U/kg intravenously) with concurrent administration of 1 g dextrose per unit of insulin as an intravenous bolus and 1 to 2 g dextrose per unit of insulin added to the volume of intravenous fluids to be administered during a 6-hour period.[42] The most rapid protection against the cardiac effects of hyperkalemia is accomplished by administration of calcium gluconate (2 to 10 mL intravenously over 10 minutes with electrocardiographic monitoring).[45] Calcium does not alter serum potassium concentration; rather, it temporarily counteracts the impairment of myocardial membrane excitability induced by hyperkalemia, allowing time for other treatments to decrease the serum potassium concentration.

Management of Metabolic Acidosis

Metabolic acidosis associated with hypoadrenocorticism usually is mild to moderate, with the total CO_2 14 mEq/L or more in at least 75% of cases.[43] The acidosis usually is corrected by fluid therapy alone. If acidosis is severe (pH < 7.1 or bicarbonate < 10 mEq/L), sodium bicarbonate may be provided by administering 50% of the calculated bicarbonate deficit over 2 to 4 hours. The need for additional bicarbonate treatment is determined by repeated blood gas analysis, with a bicarbonate less than 12 and pH less than 7.2 being indications for further therapy. If acidosis is persistent, concurrent disorders such as renal failure should be considered.

HYPOGLYCEMIA

Hypoglycemia is a common metabolic abnormality with a variety of causes, including neonatal hypoglycemia, juvenile hypoglycemia, starvation, hepatic insufficiency, hypoadrenocorticism, insulin overdose, sepsis, insulinoma, non–islet cell tumors, glycogen storage disease, pregnancy, hunting dog hypoglycemia, and an error in sample handling or analysis.[42] When severe, clinical signs including weakness, seizures, ataxia, collapse, stupor, and muscle tremors commonly are observed.

Animals in the home environment with mild clinical signs can be fed a normal meal if willing to eat or can be administered a sugar solution orally. During a hypoglycemic crisis in the hospital, intravenous administration of 0.5 to 1 mL/kg of 50% dextrose given to effect is recommended.[42] It is preferable to dilute the dextrose to a 25% or less concentrated solution to avoid phlebitis that may occur with 50% dextrose. This dose can be repeated if hypoglycemia does not resolve. Blood glucose concentration initially should be monitored after dextrose administration and then hourly with a goal of maintaining blood glucose concentration between 60 and 150 mg/dL. After administration of the intravenous dextrose bolus and resolution of signs of hypoglycemia, intravenous fluids with 2.5% to 5% dextrose are administered. In some cases, a 10% dextrose solution must be administered to maintain euglycemia. If a balanced electrolyte solution is indicated, dextrose can be added to the appropriate crystalloid solution. Hypertonic solutions should be administered through a central vein if possible. If hypoglycemia persists despite appropriate intravenous dextrose administration, glucagon can be administered as a constant-rate infusion.[16,50] The initial dosage is 5 ng/kg/min, which can be increased in 5-ng/kg/min increments up to 20 ng/kg/min or higher as necessary to maintain the blood glucose concentration greater than 60 mg/dL.[50] The neurologic signs caused by hypoglycemia should resolve within several minutes of dextrose administration. If they do not and if the blood glucose concentration is normal, neuroglycopenic brain injury may be present. It can result in temporary or permanent neurologic deficits including coma, blindness, ataxia, and behavioral changes. A glucocorticoid (dexamethasone sodium phosphate, 1 to 2 mg/kg intravenously), mannitol (0.5 to 1.0 g/kg intravenously over 20 minutes), and furosemide (1 to 2 mg/kg intravenously) can be administered, but the efficacy of this treatment is questionable.

MYXEDEMA STUPOR AND COMA

Myxedema coma is a rare, life-threatening complication of hypothyroidism. In addition to typical clinical signs of hypothyroidism, impaired mental status ranging from obtundation to coma, hypothermia without shivering, bradycardia, cold extremities, poor pulse quality, and myxedema usually are present.[7,24,26] Common laboratory findings consist of nonregenerative anemia, hyponatremia, hypercholesterolemia, lipemia, hypercapnia, and hypoxemia.[7,24,26] Pleural effusion and pulmonary edema have been reported, but idiopathic dilated cardiomyopathy could have been present in some of these dogs based on the case descriptions.[24,26] Concurrent disease almost always is present in humans with myxedema coma but occurred in only one of the five dogs reported with this disease.[7,24,26,40] A high index of suspicion is necessary to make the diagnosis of myxedema stupor because the syndrome is rare and many of the clinical signs are similar to those of other disorders.

Fluid therapy with 0.9% NaCl should be administered judiciously because although blood volume is decreased, cardiac function often is decreased. In addition, water excretion is impaired secondary to inappropriate secretion of arginine vasopressin and reduced renal perfusion.[40] Alternatively, water restriction is effective in correcting hyponatremia if the patient is well hydrated. Initial treatment in humans consists of intravenous administration of levothyroxine, but the initial dosage is controversial.[25,40,47,54] A loading dose of levothyroxine three to five times the standard daily dose (0.066 to 0.11 mg/kg in the dog) generally is recommended, but a lower dose approximating the standard replacement levothyroxine dose in uncomplicated hypothyroidism (0.022 mg/kg in the dog) also has been used. After the initial loading dose, intravenous treatment is continued at 0.022 mg/kg daily until oral treatment can be administered at 0.022 mg/kg every 12 hours. Supportive treatment is critical to successful management and consists of resolution of hypothermia, treatment of dehydration and hypotension, correction of hypoglycemia, and resolution of glucocorticoid deficiency.[24,25,40] Passive warming to relieve the hypothermia is recommended unless hypothermia is severe because active warming by applying an external heat source may cause vasodilatation of cutaneous vessels, leading to worsening of hypotension and circulatory collapse. If present, hypoglycemia should be managed by dextrose administration and ventilatory support given if indicated. Glucocorticoid supplementation is recommended in humans because plasma cortisol concentrations may be inappropriately low for the degree of illness, but this phenomenon has not been documented to occur in critically ill dogs.[44] If evidence of infection is present, broad-spectrum antibiotic treatment should be instituted.

HEATSTROKE

Heatstroke is a progressive and life-threatening illness caused by severe hyperthermia. In dogs and cats, hyperthermia usually is induced by increased environmental temperature or excessive exercise or muscle activity. Thermal injury extends to all tissues, and multiple organ failure, intravascular coagulation, and CNS dysfunction ensue. Prompt and aggressive treatment and monitoring are necessary to avoid or treat irreversible and fatal organ damage.

PATHOPHYSIOLOGY

The normal response to hyperthermia is increased cardiac output as a result of increased heart rate and decreased peripheral vascular resistance.[3,20] A shift of blood flow from the central to peripheral circulation increases delivery of blood to the muscles and skin to dissipate heat. If dehydration, impaired cardiac function, or prolonged hyperthermia occurs, decreased splanchnic blood flow will result in hypoxic injury to the intestinal tract and liver, causing cytokine production, endothelial dysfunction, bacterial translocation, endotoxemia, and hepatocellular dysfunction.[3,20] These abnormalities cause splanchnic vasodilatation and hypotension that will contribute to continued hyperthermia. Myocardial injury caused by direct heat injury, hypoxia, acidosis, and thromboembolic events decreases cardiac contractility and causes cardiac arrhythmias. Thus shock associated with heatstroke is a combination of hypovolemic, cardiogenic, and endotoxic shock. Pulmonary endothelial damage causes increased pulmonary vascular resistance and permeability that contribute to pulmonary edema and hemorrhage, as well as acute respiratory distress syndrome.[20] Endothelial and platelet damage secondary to hyperthermia and release of cytokines lead to disseminated intravascular coagulation (DIC) that is common in heatstroke. Platelet, megakaryocyte, and hepatocellular injury, as well as DIC, can lead to hemorrhage that frequently is evident on presentation and can worsen during management. A combination of factors, including hyperthermic injury, ischemia caused by endothelial swelling and intravascular coagulation, and edema can cause severe and irreversible brain injury, resulting in stupor, coma, blindness, seizures, and other signs of CNS injury.[3,20] Acute renal failure can result from impaired renal perfusion, myoglobinemia or hemoglobinemia, or thermal injury. A mixed metabolic acidosis and respiratory acidosis also is common.

TREATMENT

The goals of treatment of heatstroke are to decrease the core body temperature, support cardiovascular function, correct fluid and electrolyte abnormalities, and address other complications as they arise. Correction of hyperthermia is the priority. Owners should initiate this treatment before transporting the animal if possible because it appears to improve survival in dogs.[12] Cooling can be accomplished by spraying with or immersing the animal in cool water, followed by placing it in the airflow of a fan.[19] Ice water should be avoided because it may cause cutaneous vasoconstriction and impair heat dissipation. Massaging the skin can help increase blood flow and speed cooling. The target temperature should be 103° F to prevent hypothermia as the body temperature continues to decrease.[19]

Isotonic fluids (0.9% NaCl or lactated Ringer's solution) should be administered initially at a rapid rate (up to 90 mL/kg/hr) to restore intravascular volume and reduce core body temperature.[19] The volume and rate of fluid administration should be determined by severity of signs and response to the therapy. Hypokalemia can occur in some animals with heatstroke, and it may be necessary to add potassium chloride to intravenous fluids after initial resuscitation. If hypoalbuminemia is present, a colloid (hetastarch at 10 mL/kg) may be combined with the crystalloid treatment.[19] Monitoring should be performed frequently during initial treatment, consisting of pulse rate and quality, capillary refill time, blood pressure, respiratory rate, urine output, and central venous pressure when necessary. A coagulopathy usually is present. Therefore plasma transfusion and, if indicated, treatment for DIC should be considered early in therapy. Gastrointestinal hemorrhage is common and may be of sufficient severity to result in anemia necessitating transfusion with packed red blood cells or whole blood. Because of compromise of the gastrointestinal tract and bacterial translocation, intravenous administration of a broad-spectrum antibacterial drug is indicated. Gastroprotectant treatment can be administered but is likely to be of limited efficacy. Acid-base disturbances should be managed when present, but the acidosis associated with heatstroke often responds to intravenous fluid therapy alone. If cerebral edema is suspected, administration of mannitol, furosemide, and dexamethasone should be considered. Corticosteroids have not been shown to be beneficial for treatment of heatstroke and should be avoided unless indicated for a specific complication.

After an adequate response to initial fluid therapy, subsequent rates of administration and composition of fluids should be determined by estimating fluid deficits, noting urine output, and monitoring serum electrolyte concentrations. Recognition of complications including DIC, coagulation factor deficiency, severe thrombocytopenia, hepatic failure, renal failure, pulmonary edema, cardiac arrhythmias, seizures, and sepsis requires careful monitoring. Many of these complications may not develop until 48 to 72 hours after presentation.

REFERENCES

1. Adams LG, Hardy RM, Weiss DJ, et al: Hypophosphatemia and hemolytic anemia associated with diabetes mellitus and hepatic lipidosis in cats, *J Vet Intern Med* 7:266-271, 1993.
2. Androgue JC, Wilson H, Boyd AE, et al: Plasma acid-base patterns in diabetic ketoacidosis, *N Engl J Med* 301: 1603-1610, 1982.
3. Bouchama A, Knochel JP: Heat stroke, *N Engl J Med* 346:1978-1988, 2002.
4. Brady CA, Vite CH, Drobatz KJ: Severe neurologic sequelae in a dog after treatment of hypoadrenal crisis, *J Am Vet Med Assoc* 215:222-225, 1999.
5. Broussard JD, Wallace MS: Insulin treatment of diabetes mellitus in the dog and cat. In Bonagura JD, editor: *Kirks current veterinary therapy XII*, Philadelphia, 1995, WB Saunders, pp. 393-398.
6. Bruskiewicz KA, Nelson RW, Feldman ED, et al: Diabetic ketosis and ketoacidosis in cats: 42 cases (1980-1995), *J Am Vet Med Assoc* 211:188-192, 1997.
7. Chastain CB, Graham CL, Riley MG: Myxedema coma in two dogs, *Canine Pract* 9:20-34, 1982.
8. Chastain CB, Nichols CE: Low-dose intramuscular insulin therapy for diabetic ketoacidosis in dogs, *J Am Vet Med Assoc* 178:561-564, 1981.
9. Chiasson JL, Aris-Jilwan N, Belanger R, et al: Diagnosis and treatment of diabetic ketoacidosis and the hyperglycemic hyperosmolar state, *CMAJ* 168:859-866, 2003.
10. Christopher MM, Broussard JD, Peterson ME: Heinz body formation associated with ketoacidosis in diabetic cats, *J Vet Intern Med* 9:24-31, 1995.
11. Crenshaw KL, Peterson ME: Pretreatment clinical and laboratory evaluation of cats with diabetes mellitus: 104 cases (1992-1994), *J Am Vet Med Assoc* 209:943-949, 1996.
12. Drobatz KJ, Macintire DK: Heat-induced illness in dogs: 42 cases (1976-1993), *J Am Vet Med Assoc* 209:1894-1899, 1996.
13. Edge JA: Cerebral oedema during treatment of diabetic ketoacidosis: are we any nearer finding a cause? *Diabetes Metab Res Rev* 16:316-324, 2000.
14. Feldman EC, Nelson RW: Diabetic ketoacidosis. In *Canine and feline endocrinology and reproduction*, ed 3, Philadelphia, 2004, WB Saunders, pp. 580-615.
15. Feldman EC, Nelson RW: Hypoadrenocorticism (Addison's disease). In *Canine and feline endocrinology and reproduction*, ed 3, Philadelphia, 2004, WB Saunders, pp. 394-439.
16. Fischer JR, Smith SA, Harkin KR: Glucagon constant-rate infusion: a novel strategy for the management of hyperinsulinemic-hypoglycemic crisis in the dog, *J Am Anim Hosp Assoc* 36:27-32, 2000.
17. Fisher JN, Kitabchi AE: A randomized study of phosphate therapy in the treatment of diabetic ketoacidosis, *J Clin Endocrinol Metab* 57:177-180, 1983.
18. Fisher JN, Shahshahani MN, Kitabchi AE: Diabetic ketoacidosis: low-dose insulin therapy by various routes, *N Engl J Med* 297:238-241, 1977.

19. Flournoy WS, Macintire DK, Wohl JS: Heatstroke in dogs: clinical signs, treatment prognosis, and prevention, *Compend Cont Educ Pract Vet* 25:422-431, 2003.

20. Flournoy WS, Wohl JS, Macintire DK: Heatstroke in dogs: pathophysiology and predisposing factors, *Compend Cont Educ Pract Vet* 25:410-418, 2003.

21. Forrester SD, Moreland KJ: Hypophosphatemia: causes and consequences, *J Vet Intern Med* 3:149-159, 1989.

22. Graves TK, Schall WD, Refsal K, et al: Basal and ACTH-stimulated plasma aldosterone concentrations are normal or increased in dogs with trichuriasis-associated pseudohypoadrenocorticism, *J Vet Intern Med* 8:287-289, 1994.

23. Green SM, Rothrock SG, Ho JD, et al: Failure of adjunctive bicarbonate to improve outcome in severe pediatric diabetic ketoacidosis, *Ann Emerg Med* 31:41-48, 1998.

24. Henik RA, Dixon RM: Intravenous administration of levothyroxine for treatment of suspected myxedema coma complicated by severe hypothermia in a dog, *J Am Vet Med Assoc* 216:713-717, 2000.

25. Jordan RM: Myxedema coma: pathophysiology, therapy, and factors affecting prognosis, *Med Clin North Am* 79:185-194, 1995.

26. Kelly MJ, Hill JR: Canine myxedema stupor and coma, *Compend Cont Educ Pract Vet* 6:1049-1055, 1984.

27. Kintzer PP, Peterson ME: Treatment and long-term follow-up of 205 dogs with hypoadrenocorticism, *J Vet Intern Med* 11:43-49, 1997.

28. Kitabchi AE, Ayyagari V, Guerra SMO: The efficacy of low-dose versus conventional therapy of insulin for treatment of diabetic ketoacidosis, *Ann Intern Med* 84:633-638, 1976.

29. Kitabchi AE, Umpierrez GE, Murphy MB, et al: Management of hyperglycemic crises in patients with diabetes, *Diabetes Care* 24:131-153, 2001.

30. Koenig A, Drobatz KJ, Beal AB, et al: Hyperglycemic, hyperosmolar syndrome in feline diabetics: 17 cases (1995-2001), *J Vet Emerg Crit Care* 14:30-40, 2004.

31. Krane EJ, Rockoff MA, Wallman JK, et al: Subclinical brain swelling in children during treatment of diabetic ketoacidosis, *N Engl J Med* 312:1147-1151, 1985.

32. Lamb WA, Church DB, Emslie DR: Effect of chronic hypocortisolaemia on plasma cortisol concentrations during intravenous infusions of hydrocortisone sodium succinate in dogs, *Res Vet Sci* 57:349-352, 1994.

33. Lamberts SWJ, Bruining HA, de Jong FH: Corticosteroid therapy in severe illness, *N Engl J Med* 337:1285-1292, 1997.

34. Lifton SJ, King LG, Zerbe CA: Glucocorticoid deficient hypoadrenocorticism in dogs: 18 cases (1986-1995), *J Am Vet Med Assoc* 209:2076-2081, 1996.

35. Lynn RC, Feldman EC, Nelson RW: Efficacy of microcrystalline desoxycorticosterone pivalate for treatment of hypoadrenocorticism in dogs. DOCP Clinical Study Group, *J Am Vet Med Assoc* 202:392-396, 1993.

36. Macintire DK: Emergency therapy of diabetic crises: insulin overdose, diabetic ketoacidosis, and hyperosmolar coma, *Vet Clin North Am Small Anim Pract* 25:639-650, 1995.

37. Macintire DK: Treatment of diabetic ketoacidosis in dogs by continuous low-dose intravenous infusion of insulin, *J Am Vet Med Assoc* 202:1266-1272, 1993.

38. Melian C, Peterson ME: Diagnosis and treatment of naturally occurring hypoadrenocorticism in 42 dogs, *J Small Anim Pract* 37:268-275, 1996.

39. Morris LR, Murphy MB, Kitabchi AE: Bicarbonate therapy in severe diabetic ketoacidosis, *Ann Intern Med* 105:836-840, 1986.

40. Nicoloff JT, LoPresti JS: Myxedema coma: a form of decompensated hypothyroidism, *Endocrinol Metab Clin North Am* 22:279-290, 1993.

41. Norris CR, Nelson RW, Christopher MM: Serum total and ionized magnesium concentrations and urinary fractional excretion of magnesium in cats with diabetes mellitus and diabetic ketoacidosis, *J Am Vet Med Assoc* 215:1455-1459, 1999.

42. Peterson ME: Endocrine emergencies. In Torrance AG, Mooney CT, editors: *Manual of small animal endocrinology*, ed 2, Shurdington, 1996, British Small Animal Veterinary Association, pp. 163-171.

43. Peterson ME, Kintzer PP, Kass PH: Pretreatment clinical and laboratory findings in dogs with hypoadrenocorticism: 225 cases (1979-1993), *J Am Vet Med Assoc* 208:85-91, 1996.

44. Prittie JE, Barton LJ, Peterson ME, et al: Pituitary ACTH and adrenocortical secretion in critically ill dogs, *J Am Vet Med Assoc* 220:615-619, 2002.

45. Reusch CE: Hypoadrenocorticism. In Ettinger SJ, Feldman EC, editors: *Textbook of veterinary internal medicine*, ed 5, Philadelphia, 2000, WB Saunders, pp. 1488-1499.

46. Rijnberk A: Adrenals. In *Clinical endocrinology of dogs and cats: an illustrated text*, Dordrecht, The Netherlands, 1996, Kluwer Academic Publishers, pp. 61-93.

47. Rodriguez I, Fluiters E, Perez-Mendez LF, et al: Factors associated with mortality of patients with myxoedema coma: prospective study in 11 cases treated in a single institution, *J Endocrinol* 180:347-350, 2004.

48. Roth L, Tyler RD: Evaluation of low sodium:potassium ratios in dogs, *J Vet Diagn Invest* 11:60-64, 1999.

49. Sadek D, Schaer M: Atypical Addison's disease in the dog: a retrospective survey of 14 cases, *J Am Anim Hosp Assoc* 32:159-163, 1996.

50. Smith SA, Harkin KR, Fischer JR: Glucagon constant rate infusion for hyperinsulinemic hypoglycemic crisis with neuroglycopenia in 6 dogs, *J Vet Intern Med* 14:344, 2000.

51. Waldhausl W, Keinberger G, Korn A, et al: Severe hyperglycemia: effects of rehydration on endocrine derangements and blood glucose concentration, *Diabetes* 28:577-584, 1979.

52. Willard MD, DiBartola SP: Disorders of phosphorus. In DiBartola SP, editor: *Fluid therapy in small animal practice*, ed 2, Philadelphia, 2000, WB Saunders, pp. 163-174.

53. Willard MD, Zerbe CA, Schall WD, et al: Severe hypophosphatemia associated with diabetes mellitus in six dogs and one cat, *J Am Vet Med Assoc* 190:1007-1010, 1987.

54. Yamamoto T, Fukuyama J, Fujiyoshi A: Factors associated with mortality of myxedema coma: report of eight cases and literature survey, *Thyroid* 9:1167-1174, 1999.

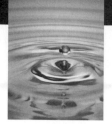

CHAPTER · 21

FLUID AND DIURETIC THERAPY IN HEART FAILURE

John D. Bonagura, Linda B. Lehmkuhl, and Helio Autran de Morais

Congestive heart failure (CHF) is a clinical syndrome characterized by cardiac dysfunction, abnormal hemodynamics, neurohormonal activation, release of cytokines, and renal retention of sodium and water. A cardiac or vascular lesion that limits cardiac output and decreases arterial blood pressure (ABP) triggers heart failure. The stereotypical compensatory response to heart failure supports ABP but also promotes a maladaptive state that leads to substantial morbidity and mortality.

Advanced CHF, as well as the therapy of this syndrome, often is associated with alterations in renal function and a variety of fluid, electrolyte, and serum biochemical abnormalities. Some of these disturbances are mild and seemingly well tolerated, but others, such as hyponatremia and acute renal failure, indicate severe circulatory dysfunction and a need for urgent therapy.[69] There are circumstances in which cardiac patients actually require fluid therapy to maintain optimal ventricular filling and prevent deterioration of renal function. However, it is more common for fluid therapy to produce edema or effusions in a previously compensated cardiac patient. Safe restoration of fluid and electrolyte balance in the patient with cardiovascular disease is challenging. To orchestrate such treatment, the clinician must appreciate the pathophysiology of heart failure and the compensatory changes that develop. This chapter addresses some of the clinically relevant pathophysiologic and therapeutic aspects of heart failure.

Much of our understanding of hemodynamics, renal function, and neurohumoral activity in heart failure stems from many experimental studies in dogs and from a limited number of clinical investigations of dogs and cats with spontaneous heart disease. However, studies of fluid therapy in spontaneous CHF in dogs and cats are largely unavailable. Accordingly, the recommendations offered here represent our interpretation of relevant animal studies and personal experience with the treatment of dogs and cats with CHF.

THE NORMAL CIRCULATION

The central circulation is regulated largely by a need to maintain plasma volume, mean ABP, and tissue perfusion. Of prime importance is the maintenance of normal effective plasma volume and ABP in the central circulation.[133,141] These two variables depend on cardiac output, systemic vascular impedance, and renal regulation of sodium and water excretion. The reflexes that control the circulation have evolved so that blood pressure and plasma volume are maintained within a narrow range even in the presence of sudden physiologic stresses, such as exercise, hypotension, or hemorrhage. Blood pressure and plasma volume are monitored by different mechanoreceptors and osmoreceptors located in the arteries, veins, heart, kidney, and central nervous system. Ultimately, two factors—cardiac output and systemic vascular resistance (more precisely, vascular impedance)—determine ABP (Fig. 21-1). A change in either one of these two variables causes a parallel change in blood pressure. Numerous physiologic variables can affect cardiac output and vascular impedance (Box 21-1), and many of these factors are perturbed in CHF. Of particular relevance in this chapter are determinants of plasma volume in health and disease (Box 21-2). Plasma volume is a major contributor to venous pressure and cardiac filling. The serum sodium concentration, as described more fully in Chapter 3, plays a central role in determining plasma volume. Renal tubular activity, vascular dynamics, hormones, and other vasoactive factors regulate sodium balance. Abnormalities of sodium excretion are pivotal to the development of CHF.

Attention also must be directed to the microcirculation and factors controlling fluid movement across capillaries. Tissue perfusion is crucial for organ functions such as the formation of urine, muscle contraction, and exchange of oxygen and carbon dioxide. Assuming the maintenance of adequate mean ABP, vascular resistance largely governs tissue perfusion across the arterial side of the microcirculation. Vascular

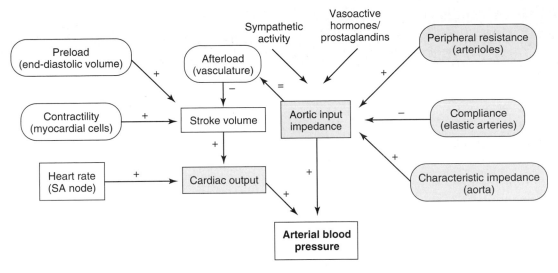

Fig. 21-1 Control of arterial blood pressure. Arterial blood pressure is a function of the cardiac output and the arterial impedance. Contractility, preload, and afterload determine the stroke volume, which, multiplied by the heart rate, yields the cardiac output. Changes in arterioles, elastic arteries, and the aorta all influence the aortic input impedance (afterload). *(+)*, Increases in the parameter increase aortic input impedance, stroke volume, cardiac output, or arterial blood pressure; *(–)*, increases in the parameter decrease aortic input impedance or stroke volume. (Modified from de Morais HSA: Pathophysiology of heart failure and clinical evaluation of heart function. In Ettinger SJ, Feldman EC, editors: *Textbook of veterinary internal medicine*, ed 5, Philadelphia, 2000, WB Saunders.

Box 21-1	**Factors Controlling Arterial Blood Pressure**

Variables Affecting Cardiac Output
Venous pressure and venous return
   Plasma volume
   Renal regulation of sodium and water
   Serum albumin
   Venous tone
      Sympathetic activity
      Local factors (e.g., kinins)
Ventricular diastolic function
   Venous pressure and venous return
   Myocardial relaxation
   Ventricular chamber compliance
   Pericardial restraint
   Ventricular filling
Ventricular systolic function
   Myocardial contractility
   Preload (ventricular end-diastolic volume)
   Afterload (arterial impedance)
   Valvular function
Electrical activity of the heart
   Heart rate
   Cardiac rhythm and conduction

Variables Affecting Systemic Vascular Impedance
Vasoconstriction
   Sympathetic nervous system
   Angiotensin II
   Arginine vasopressin (ADH)
   Endothelin
   Some prostaglandins

Vasodilatation
   Atrial natriuretic peptide (ANP)
   Brain natriuretic peptide (BNP, ventricular origin)
   Some prostaglandins (e.g., prostacyclin)
   Endothelium-derived relaxation factor (nitric oxide)
Aortic dynamic compliance

Arterial and Cardiac Baroreceptor (Mechanoreceptor) Reflexes

resistance for any regional circulation is the sum of structural, autonomic, hormonal, and local vasoactive factors (see Box 21-1). Conversely, plasma volume and venous pressure exert the greatest effect at the venous end of the capillary. The interplay of hydrostatic pressures, oncotic pressures, capillary permeability, and lymphatic function determines whether the interstitium and serous body cavities accumulate or remain free of excess solute and water.[69,147,156] The effect of these so-called Starling's forces on fluid dynamics is summarized in Fig. 21-2.

THE CIRCULATION IN HEART FAILURE

Heart failure is characterized clinically by hemodynamic abnormalities triggered by cardiac dysfunction.[75] The causes of heart failure include numerous structural and functional disorders of the cardiac valves, myocardium,

---

Box 21-2 Factors Regulating Plasma Volume in Heart Failure

Controlled Variables

Arterial blood pressure (arterial and ventricular mechanoreceptors)

Plasma osmolality (central nervous system)

Serum sodium concentration (juxtaglomerular apparatus)

Renal perfusion pressure (kidney)

Atrial volume and pressure (left atrium)

Effectors Modifying Renal Glomerular and Tubular Function

Norepinephrine (sympathetic activity)

Renin-angiotensin

Arginine vasopressin (ADH)

Aldosterone

Renal blood flow (and distribution)

Natriuretic peptides (ANP, BNP)

Plasma Protein (albumin)

Drug Therapy

Diuretics

Loop diuretics (furosemide, bumetanide, torsemide)

Thiazide diuretics (hydrochlorothiazide)

Potassium-sparing diuretics (triamterene, amiloride)

Spironolactone (blocks renal effects of aldosterone)

Carbonic anhydrase inhibitors (acetazolamide)

Angiotensin-converting enzyme inhibitors (captopril, enalapril, benazepril, lisinopril, ramapril)

Digitalis glycosides, pimobendan, and other cardiotonic drugs

Vasodilator drugs (hydralazine, nitrates, angiotensin-converting enzyme inhibitors)

Fluid Balance

Fluid therapy (volume and type)

Dietary sodium intake

Voluntary water intake

Gastrointestinal function

---

pericardium, and blood vessels, as well as sustained cardiac arrhythmias (Box 21-3). In response to impaired cardiac output, potent homeostatic mechanisms are activated that preserve perfusion of the brain and heart but at the expense of less vital regional circulations. Preservation of blood pressure mandates dramatic alterations in neural, hormonal, and cardiovascular function and structure. These adaptations (summarized in Box 21-4) include (1) activation of the sympathetic nervous system[45,169] and release of hormones,[42,114] (2) increased systemic vascular resistance[43,44] and impedance,[35] (3) reduction of autonomic reflex activity,[75,176] and (4) cardiac dilatation and hypertrophy that together with myocardial tissue changes are collectively referred to as "cardiac remodel-

ing."[50,70,106] Heart failure also alters renal function[115,176] and enhances reabsorption of sodium and water.[14,170] In combination, these potent control systems are capable of maintaining normal ABP in all but the most severe cases of cardiac failure.

Hemodynamic abnormalities in the central circulation and microcirculation in CHF (Box 21-5) can be traced to both decreased cardiac performance and renal retention of sodium and water.[115,133,143] Decreased cardiac output, valvular insufficiency, or diminished ventricular compliance increases ventricular end-diastolic pressure, which is transmitted back to the venous and capillary beds ("backward" failure). Higher venous and capillary pressures are augmented by renal fluid retention and expansion of the plasma volume. Renal sodium and water retention as a consequence of reduced cardiac output often is described in the medical literature as "forward" heart failure.[133] Forward failure, in this regard, does not refer to clinical signs of low cardiac output but instead describes the renal responses triggered by low cardiac output. Forward failure is a critical factor in the development of edema and effusions in right-sided and biventricular heart failure. These concepts and some of the factors responsible for increased venous and capillary pressures are shown in Fig. 21-3. The important role of the kidney in the pathogenesis of edema and effusions is discussed in the section on Renal Function in Heart Failure.

High venous pressures and increased ventricular end-diastolic pressure enhance cardiac filling and allow the ventricle to generate a greater contractile response. As shown in Fig. 21-4, ventricular stroke volume is directly related to ventricular filling pressure.[41,154] High venous pressure also maintains cardiac filling when ventricular compliance is decreased, as in hypertrophic cardiomyopathy, pericardial disease, or severe ventricular dilatation[50] (see Fig. 21-4, bottom). The clinical relevance of this relationship becomes obvious when the edematous patient is treated with diuretics and venous pressures, ventricular filling, and cardiac output decline, causing systemic hypotension or prerenal azotemia.

The term **congestive heart failure** implies a situation of increased venous and capillary hydrostatic pressures, increased transudation of fluid across capillary walls, and net accumulation of fluid in the interstitial compartment (i.e., edema) or serous body cavities (i.e., effusion). A safety margin normally prevents this accumulation of fluid, and venous pressures must increase substantially (usually to two or three times above the normal upper limit) before edema develops.[56,148,156,171] Development of pulmonary edema in the dog usually requires left atrial pressure to increase acutely to more than 20 mm Hg.[56] Substantial increases in lymphatic drainage permit much higher pressure to be tolerated chronically.[14,30] In addition to increased venous pressures, hypoalbuminemia

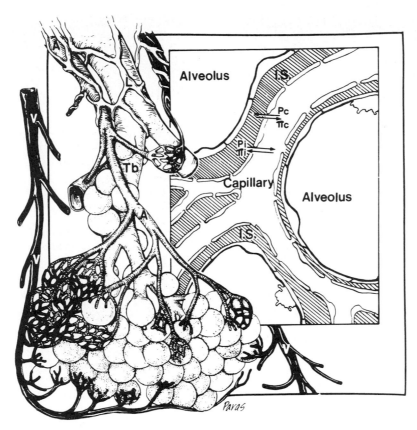

Fig. 21-2 Microcirculation of the respiratory unit. The arteriole branches into the capillary plexus surrounding alveoli. Starling's forces controlling fluid movement into or out of the capillary or interstitial space (IS) are indicated. Capillary hydrostatic pressure in the lung must generally exceed 20 to 25 mm Hg before edema develops. Chronically, even higher hydrostatic pressures can be tolerated before edema develops. This is explained by the increased lymphatic drainage of the interstitium that develops in chronic edematous states. P_c, Capillary hydrostatic pressure, which forces fluid into the interstitium; π_c, capillary colloid osmotic pressure principally because of albumin, which causes fluid to be retained within the capillary; P_i, interstitial hydrostatic pressure, which is negative in the lung; π_i, interstitial colloid osmotic pressure, which is controlled by pulmonary lymphatics and maintains the interstitium relatively free of albumin; A, arteriole; V, venule; L, lymphatic vessel; Tb, terminal bronchiole. (From Ware WW, Bonagura JD: Pulmonary edema. In Fox PR, editor: *Canine and feline cardiology*, Philadelphia, 1999, WB Saunders, p. 252. Medical illustration by Felicia Paras.)

can contribute to edema formation.[56,174] As a consequence of variable lymphatic drainage and other factors such as capillary permeability and compartment compliance, edema is not uniformly distributed in the tissues.[171] This nonuniform distribution is evident clinically inasmuch as acute cardiogenic pulmonary edema in the dog is most prominent in perihilar and in right-sided lung lobes.

The edema of CHF develops predominantly in the capillary beds drained by the failing side of the heart. This finding is pertinent because CHF is classified clinically as left-sided, right-sided, or biventricular. Increased pulmonary venous and capillary hydrostatic pressures cause pulmonary edema (see Fig. 21-2), the cardinal finding of left-sided CHF. Right-sided heart failure increases systemic venous pressures leading to jugular venous distention or pulsation, hepatic congestion, ascites, or (infrequently in small animals) subcutaneous

edema. Increased systemic venous pressure even may contribute to pulmonary edema formation.[96]

Pleural effusions develop as a result of left-sided, right-sided, or, most often, biventricular failure. This finding can be explained by the dual venous drainage of the pleural surfaces (i.e., parietal drainage is systemic, whereas visceral drainage is pulmonary). Although veterinary textbooks usually attribute pleural effusion to isolated right-sided CHF, this is not common in human patients. Pleural effusion correlates better with pulmonary capillary wedge pressure than with right atrial pressure.[174] Similarly, pleural effusions in small animals most often indicate biventricular CHF. Although pleural effusion does occur in some dogs and cats with predominantly right-sided cardiac disease (e.g., pulmonic stenosis, tricuspid malformation), ascites is more common in dogs. Clinically significant pleural effusions are rare in animals with isolated right ventricular failure caused by

Box 21-3 Causes of Heart Failure

Valvular Heart Disease
Congenital malformations
    Aortic stenosis
    Mitral valve malformation
    Pulmonic stenosis
    Tricuspid valve malformation
Acquired diseases
    Degenerative, myxomatous atrioventricular valvular
      disease
    Ruptured chordae tendineae
    Bacterial endocarditis

Myocardial Diseases
Malformations: defects of the atrial and ventricular septum
Dilated cardiomyopathy
Hypertrophic cardiomyopathy
Restrictive cardiomyopathy (endomyocardial fibrosis)
Undefined feline cardiomyopathies
Atrial muscle degeneration
Right ventricular cardiomyopathy
Myocarditis
Secondary myocardial diseases (hyperthyroidism,
    acromegaly, hypertension)

Pericardial Diseases
Idiopathic pericardial hemorrhage/pericarditis
Cardiac neoplasia leading to pericardial effusion
Infective pericarditis
Constrictive pericardial disease

Vascular Diseases
Malformation: patent ductus arteriosus
Arteriovenous fistula
Heartworm disease

High-Output States
Anemia
Thyrotoxicosis

Cardiac Arrhythmia
Chronic bradyarrhythmia
Chronic tachyarrhythmia

Box 21-4 Neurohormonal, Renal, and Cardiovascular Activities in Congestive Heart Failure

Autonomic
Heightened sympathetic nervous system activity
    Increase heart rate
    Augmentation of myocardial contractility
    Vasoconstriction
    Release of renin
Blunting of arterial blood pressure reflexes

Hormonal or Autocrine
Vasoconstricting or sodium-retaining systems
    Activation of the renin-angiotensin-aldosterone system
    Release of arginine vasopressin (antidiuretic hormone)
    Release of vasoactive prostaglandins and local
      vasoconstricting factors
      Endothelin-1
      Thromboxane
      Neuropeptide Y
Vasodilating or natriuretic systems
    Release of natriuretic peptides (impaired responsiveness
      of end organ)
    Increased basal nitric oxide (reduced release after
      receptor stimulation)
    Increased release of prostaglandins (E_2, I_2)
    Decrease in kallikreins
    Increased dopamine
    Decreased calcitonin gene-related peptide
Increased release of tumor necrosis factor and other
    cytokines

Renal
Efferent arteriolar constriction (via angiotensin II)
Increased filtration fraction (ratio of glomerular filtration
    rate to renal plasma flow)
Redistribution of renal blood flow
Increased sodium and water reabsorption

Cardiovascular
Cardiac adaptations
    Ventricular dilatation
    Ventricular hypertrophy
    Tissue changes (e.g., fibrosis, hypertrophy, altered
      collagen matrix)
    Cardiomyocyte death including apoptosis
    Intrinsic changes in cardiac isoenzymes
    Down-regulation of cardiac β receptors
Vascular adaptations
    Vasoconstriction
    Increased systemic vascular resistance and arterial
      impedance
    Redistribution of blood flow
    Vascular remodeling

heartworm-induced pulmonary hypertension.[13,160] Conversely, pleural effusions are common when end-stage CHF develops in dogs with severe mitral regurgitation, pulmonary hypertension, and secondary right ventricular dysfunction or in cats with severe cardiomyopathy. Pleural effusion may become chylous in nature in those with advanced CHF.

The relative contribution of renal sodium retention in CHF probably depends on the type and acuteness of heart failure. The development of ascites, pleural effusion, or subcutaneous edema in right-sided or biventricular cardiac failure is accompanied by avid renal sodium retention (see section on Renal Function in Heart Failure). Dramatic weight loss, sometimes exceeding

5 kg in giant-breed dogs, may be observed after successful diuresis. This degree of weight loss after diuretic

Box 21-5	Hemodynamic Consequences of Congestive Heart Failure

Reduced cardiac output
Increased systemic vascular resistance and arterial impedance
Increased pulmonary vascular resistance
Increased plasma volume
Increased ventricular end-diastolic pressure
Increased venous pressure
   Systemic (central) venous pressure
   Pulmonary venous pressure
Increased capillary hydrostatic pressure
   Edema
   Serous cavity effusion

therapy is uncommon in isolated left-sided failure. Thus successful therapy of right-sided CHF depends in the short term on initiation of a brisk diuresis or paracentesis. Long-term management hinges on improving cardiac function, reducing neurohormonal activation, and overcoming the potent sodium-retaining effects of forward cardiac failure.

In contrast to right-sided or biventricular CHF, severe left-sided heart failure can develop without substantial sodium retention or weight gain.[64] Two common examples in veterinary medicine can be cited. The first example is rupture of a mitral chorda tendinea in an older dog with previously stable mitral regurgitation. The sudden increase in mitral regurgitant volume increases mean left atrial and pulmonary capillary pressures, leading to peracute pulmonary edema. The second example is a cat with hypertrophic cardiomyopathy and a noncompliant left ventricle (see Fig. 21-4, bottom left curve). It is not uncommon for severe pulmonary edema to follow a bout of protracted tachycardia (e.g., stress). Development of pulmonary edema in these situations can be explained by acute deterioration of left ventricular systolic or diastolic performance that rapidly increases left atrial and pulmonary venous pressures. Although diuresis is a critical treatment in this situation, short-term success may hinge on therapy that reduces mitral regurgitant fraction (i.e., afterload reduction) or enhances filling of the stiff left ventricle.

Another issue of relevance to CHF and fluid therapy of the cardiac patient is the relative size of the vascular compartments. The vascular compliance of the pulmonary circulation is much smaller than that of the systemic circulation, and sudden expansion of the plasma volume usually increases pulmonary venous pressure more than systemic venous pressure. This is particularly true in the patient with left-sided heart disease and explains why some dogs and cats develop pulmonary edema after intravenous administration of a so-called maintenance volume of crystalloid solution. Furthermore, central venous pressure (CVP) cannot be used to

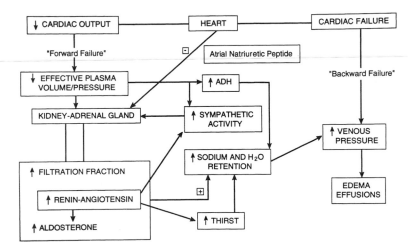

Fig. 21-3 Prominent mechanisms responsible for fluid accumulation in heart failure. The combined effects of abnormally high venous pressure and renal retention of sodium and water can explain the development of pulmonary edema, subcutaneous edema, or the transudative effusions in body cavities. Ventricular systolic or diastolic failure increases venous pressure behind the failing ventricle ("backward" failure). This may be the predominant mechanism of edema formation in acute left-sided heart failure. In contrast, chronic heart failure, especially when right-sided or biventricular in nature, is characterized by avid sodium retention. Although atrial distention causes the release of atrial natriuretic peptide (ANP), the effects of sympathetic activity, angiotensin II, aldosterone, vasopressin (ADH), and local vasoconstrictor factors dominate, leading to vasoconstriction in systemic vessels and increased sodium and water reabsorption in the renal tubules. This is a simplified view because other local and systemic factors can be involved. (Modified from Bonagura JD: Fluid management of the cardiac patient, *Vet Clin North Am Small Anim Pract* 12:503, 1982.)

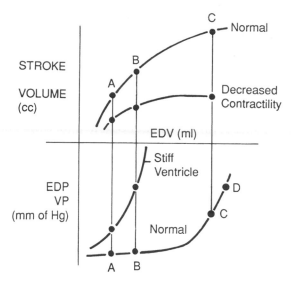

Fig. 21-4 Ventricular function curves in heart failure. Ventricular function curves demonstrate the potential relationships between venous pressure (a determinant of ventricular filling and end-diastolic volume), ventricular compliance or distensibility (which determines the venous and atrial pressures required to fill the ventricle), and stroke volume (determined by ventricular end-diastolic volume, ventricular afterload, and myocardial contractility). The top of the graph demonstrates ventricular systolic function, and the lower curves demonstrate ventricular filling dynamics.

Top, When inotropic ("contractile") state and afterload are held constant, the ventricular stroke volume depends on cardiac filling (preload), although this relationship is depressed in patients with myocardial failure. Patients treated with excessive dosages of diuretics may develop inadequate ventricular filling, leading to decreased stroke volume and cardiac output and causing prerenal azotemia. Reduction of diuretic dosage or fluid therapy is generally required to reestablish cardiac output.

Bottom, Ventricular distensibility—the tangent of any point on the diastolic pressure-volume curve—depends on the amount of ventricular hypertrophy, myocardial fibrosis, and the volume of the ventricle. Animals with stiff ventricles resulting from ventricular hypertrophy or myocardial fibrosis require high ventricular filling pressures and are poorly tolerant of fluid infusions. Note that increased cardiac filling can progress only at disproportionately higher venous pressures, a situation that predisposes to pulmonary edema. Recognize that even dilated ventricles can develop diastolic dysfunction (*bottom right*). Once the grossly dilated ventricle reaches a certain point, distensibility decreases. Compare the slope at the extreme right of this diastolic filling curve with that of the smaller, hypertrophied ventricle. The benefit of diuretic therapy in this setting can be appreciated because even small reductions in plasma volume and preload may permit the ventricle to fill at substantially lower venous pressures.

gauge the effect of intravenous fluid therapy on left-sided cardiac filling pressures, especially in the setting of isolated left-sided CHF.[133] Owing to differences in vascular compliance and cardiac function, left-sided filling pressures may increase much more rapidly than CVP.

RENAL FUNCTION IN HEART FAILURE

Remarkably, the kidney often is able to maintain glomerular filtration in the setting of decreased blood pressure or cardiac output. Decreases in renal perfusion are countered by dilatation of the afferent arteriole mediated by the release of prostaglandin E_2, and constriction of the efferent arteriole primarily by angiotensin II. Efferent arteriolar constriction also is augmented by arginine vasopressin (antidiuretic hormone [ADH]) and norepinephrine.[115] These microvascular responses increase glomerular filtration pressure, increase filtration fraction, and maintain glomerular filtration in the setting of reduced renal blood flow (see Chapter 2).[109,130,150] However, progressive renal failure is not uncommon in dogs and cats with CHF, and treatment of patients with both intrinsic renal disease and heart failure is difficult. This situation also occurs in human patients in whom worsening of renal function is associated with a poorer prognosis and higher mortality.[53] Neurohormones and cytokines, angiotensin in particular, are considered central to the progression of renal disease in heart failure.[74] Aggressive therapy of heart failure may slow progression of renal disease in humans.[83]

The renal response to decreased cardiac output is central to the pathogenesis of edema and effusions in heart failure. Studies of induced right-sided heart failure and spontaneous CHF in dogs have demonstrated avid retention of administered salt loads.[7,78] Numerous mechanisms have been identified for persistent sodium retention in CHF (see Fig. 21-3). These alterations include redistribution of renal blood flow,[7,124] enhanced tubular sodium reabsorption,[6,85,95] release of prostaglandins,[32,34,104] greater renal sympathetic nerve activity,* increased renal interstitial pressure,[54,94] and increased hormonal activity. The last includes increases in vasopressin (ADH),[14,128] angiotensin II, and aldosterone† (see Box 21-4). Presumably, these mechanisms also operate in animals with spontaneous heart failure.[126]

Particular emphasis has been placed on the increased concentrations of renin, angiotensin II, and aldosterone found in patients with CHF.[114] There are a number of triggers for the release of renin in the cardiac patient.[106] One mechanism is the stimulation of renal β-adrenergic receptors by sympathetic efferent traffic activated in response to hypotension. Renin also is released in response to reduced renal blood flow related to heart failure or volume depletion caused by diuretic therapy of CHF.[173] Severe sodium restriction, especially in dogs with signs of heart disease but without overt CHF, can

*References 21,61,84,107,142,159.
†References 20,24,33,47,52,58,63,65,71,80,82,109,111,129,130,150.

lead to renin release.[120] Clinically, the effects of angiotensin II and aldosterone can be mitigated in part by drugs that inhibit formation of angiotensin II (angiotensin-converting enzyme [ACE] inhibitors such as enalapril) or drugs that block the AT-1 receptor of angiotensin II such as losartan and candesartan.

Other factors promote renal fluid retention in CHF. Changes in intrarenal blood flow can lead to redistribution of flow to the salt-conserving juxtamedullary nephrons.[14,85,87] Increased filtration fraction maintains the glomerular filtration rate (GFR) but predisposes to renal tubular reabsorption of water (see Chapter 2). Arginine vasopressin (ADH) also plays a role. In CHF, increases in plasma ADH concentration probably represent nonosmotic release in response to low ABP.[115] Increased thirst (mediated by angiotensin II), when combined with increases in ADH, can contribute to free-water retention and hyponatremia.[31,92,113] Endothelin is another hormone released from endothelial cells in CHF.[125,167] This hormone reduces renal blood flow, GFR, and urinary sodium excretion.[91,115] The sequence in which these mechanisms are activated varies with the type and severity of heart failure.[42,133] However, it is clear that with deterioration in cardiac function, sodium- and water-retaining mechanisms are exacerbated, and further expansion of the plasma volume occurs. Blunting the renal response generally requires appropriate medical treatment of CHF, progressive restriction of dietary sodium, and administration of diuretics.

In CHF, the vasoconstrictive and sodium-retaining mechanisms overwhelm local and systemic vasodilator and natriuretic systems. Distention of the atria and ventricles signals release of atrial natriuretic peptide (ANP) and brain natriuretic peptide (BNP). These peptides of cardiac origin stimulate formation of cyclic GMP, leading to diuresis, vasodilatation, and improved ventricular relaxation.[100,106] Although increased circulating concentrations of ANP and BNP can be measured in dogs with experimentally induced and spontaneous CHF,[4,55,90,166] it also has been shown that the renal response to these hormones is blunted or antagonized.[19,97,127] If dogs or people with CHF are treated with pharmacologic doses of ANP, however, or if the degradation of ANP is reduced by administration of a neutral endopeptidase inhibitor, diuresis may follow.[97,103] Other vascular-modulating factors, such as the vasodilator nitric oxide, are more difficult to assess in CHF, but metabolites of this endothelial-derived substance reportedly are decreased in some dogs with mitral regurgitation.[119]

CARDIOVASCULAR DRUGS AND RENAL FUNCTION

EFFECTS OF DIURETICS ON RENAL FUNCTION

Diuretics used in management of CHF prevent reabsorption of solute and water, leading to increased urine flow. Diuretics are essential to both the short- and long-term management of CHF. The clinical pharmacology of these drugs and effects on renal function (Tables 21-1 and 21-2) are relevant to understanding their effectiveness and limitations.

All of the commonly used diuretics, except spironolactone, are delivered by renal blood flow and secreted in the proximal tubule. Circulatory failure, reduced renal blood flow, or primary renal failure may reduce the renal delivery of a diuretic. In the case of renal failure, endogenous organic acids can compete with furosemide for transport across the proximal nephron. Once secreted into the filtrate, a diuretic inhibits salt and water transport via a specific mechanism and at relatively specific sites along the nephron.[67,105,134]

Fig. 21-5 demonstrates the general sites of action of the commonly used diuretics. The importance of understanding these details can be illustrated by two examples. First, the effectiveness of a diuretic depends on the ability of cells distal to the site of diuretic action to reabsorb sodium and water. Initially in CHF, loop diuretics, which act on the thick portion of Henle's loop, are highly effective. However, in severe chronic CHF, the more distal tubular cells can increase their reabsorption of sodium and water and overcome the effects of the diuretic.[133] This problem can be counteracted with additional treatment such as the combination of hydrochlorothiazide and spironolactone, which act more in the distal nephron. This type of sequential nephron blockade can induce a marked diuresis in some dogs but not without risk of volume depletion. A second example pertains to the adverse effects of diuretics. Loop diuretics increase the delivery of sodium to cells of the late distal convoluted tubules and collecting ducts. At those sites, sodium is reabsorbed in exchange for potassium (under the influence of aldosterone) or hydrogen ions that are secreted.[67] These ion exchange mechanisms have the potential to cause hypokalemia or metabolic alkalosis, especially with high doses or chronic therapy.

The carbonic anhydrase inhibitors, such as acetazolamide, act on the proximal tubule by inhibiting bicarbonate reabsorption. These diuretics are limited in effectiveness because they induce metabolic acidosis, and the loop of Henle and distal nephron can reabsorb much of the increased salt and water that is delivered to these segments. Carbonic anhydrase inhibitors are rarely, if ever, used in CHF.

Furosemide, ethacrynic acid, bumetanide, and torsemide exert their effects on the ascending limb of Henle's loop.[105,134,161] These so-called loop diuretics block the Na^+-K^+-$2Cl^-$ cotransporter (symport) and prevent the active transport across the tubular lumen of two chloride ions, one sodium ion, and one potassium ion. Loop diuretics are potent with a good dose response ("high ceiling"). This is related to the high capacity for reabsorbing filtrate at this site (normally ~25% of the

TABLE 21-1 Effects of Cardiovascular Drugs on Renal Function

Pharmacologic Class	Examples	Mechanism of Action	Effects on Renal Function
Angiotensin-converting enzyme inhibitors	Captopril, benazepril, enalapril, lisinopril, ramipril	Inhibit converting enzyme, preventing conversion of AT-1 to AT-2; also reduce degradation of vasodilator kinins	Reduce the activity of the renin-angiotensin-aldosterone system; can reduce intra-glomerular filtration pressure by blocking angiotensin II-mediated vasoconstriction of the efferent arteriole
Angiotensin receptor blockers	Losartan, candesartan	Block AT-1 receptors of angiotensin II	As described for angiotensin-converting enzyme inhibitors; may also affect tissue renin-angiotensin-aldosterone systems
Catecholamines	Dobutamine, dopamine	Stimulate beta and alpha receptors to increase cardiac output and blood pressure; low doses of dopamine stimulate dopaminergic receptors in renal arterioles	Increase renal perfusion pressure; dilate renal blood vessels (dopamine)
β-Adrenergic blockers	Metoprolol Carvedilol	Block β-adrenoceptor Block α-adrenoceptor	Decrease renin Vasodilator effect May reduce renal blood flow (dose related)
Digitalis glycosides	Digoxin	Sensitize baroreceptors	Reduce sympathetic nerve activity; may reduce activation of the renin-angiotensin system
Diuretics*	Loop diuretics (furosemide) Thiazide diuretics Potassium-sparing diuretics (amiloride, spironolactone)	Prevent reabsorption of electrolytes and water at various sites along the renal tubules Furosemide (administered IV) can release atrial natriuretic peptide and prostaglandins	Increase urine volume and urinary electrolyte loss; high dose can precipitate volume depletion and acute renal failure; IV furosemide may cause dilation of renal arterioles
Human brain natriuretic peptide	Nesiritide	Increase cycle GMP Probable dilation of afferent arteriole	Increase GFR, decreases RPF Increase sodium excretion and urine volume
Neutral endopeptidase inhibitors	Sinorphan, ecadotril	Prevent degradation of atrial natriuretic peptide	Renal vasodilatation, increase urinary loss of sodium and water
Vasodilators	Hydralazine, sodium nitroprusside, prazosin	Dilate systemic arterioles by diverse mechanisms (e.g., generation of nitric oxide; α-adrenergic blockade)	May increase renal perfusion; if hypotension develops renal blood flow can decrease

*Also see Table 21-2.

filtrate is reabsorbed at this site). Urinary concentration is impaired because blocking the Na^+-K^+-$2Cl^-$ carrier impedes development of a hypertonic renal interstitium. Urinary dilution also is impaired because dilution of the filtrate is a normal function of this segment. After administration of a loop diuretic, there are substantial losses of chloride, sodium, water, and other electrolytes (including potassium, magnesium, and calcium) in the urine. Some hemodynamic and renal effects of loop diuretics may arise from direct vascular effects that cause vasodilatation or increased venous capacitance.[28] Intravenous administration of furosemide releases vasodilator prostaglandins that increase renal blood flow.[11,102,110,117]

The thiazide and thiazide-like diuretics act on the cortical distal convoluted tubule by competing with the

TABLE 21-2 Diuretics

Diuretic Class	Examples	Primary Site of Action	Mechanisms of Action	Adverse Effects in Dogs and Cats
Carbonic anhydrase inhibitors	Acetazolamide	Proximal tubules	Inhibit membrane and cytoplasmic carbonic anhydrase	Metabolic acidosis
Loop diuretics	Furosemide Bumetanide Torsemide Ethacrynic acid	Thick ascending loop of Henle	Block Na^+-K^+-$2Cl^-$ cotransporter (symport)	Volume depletion, azotemia, hypokalemia, hypomagnesemia, hyponatremia, ototoxicity
Thiazides	Hydrochlorothiazide	Distal convoluted tubules	Block the Na^+-Cl^- cotransporter (symport)	As described for loop diuretics
Thiazide-like diuretics	Chlorthalidone			Potential for hyponatremia
	Metolazone			Ventricular arrhythmias (from hypokalemia)
Potassium-sparing diuretics	Triamterene Amiloride	Late distal tubules	Inhibit renal epithelial sodium channels (triamterene, amiloride)	Hyperkalemia
Aldosterone antagonists	Spironolactone Eplerenone	Collecting ducts	Inhibit mineralocorticoid receptors (spironolactone, eplerenone)	

DIURETIC SITES OF ACTION

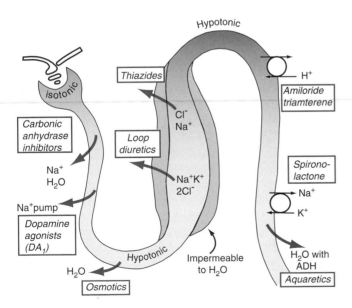

Fig. 21-5 Renal effects of diuretics. Loop diuretics such as furosemide are most commonly used in treatment of congestive heart failure (CHF). Spironolactone works in the distal nephron and is therefore a relatively weak diuretic; however, it also demonstrates cardiac-protecting properties. In the concept of "sequential nephron blockade," a loop diuretic would be combined with a thiazide and spironolactone or eplerenone to prevent solute and water reabsorption at multiple levels. (From Opie LH, Gersch BJ: *Drugs for the heart*, ed 6, Philadelphia, 2005, WB Saunders.)

luminal Na-Cl cotransporter and preventing movement of NaCl into the distal tubular cells. This effect impairs the ability to dilute urine (and excrete solute-free water) but does not necessarily affect urine concentration, which is a medullary function. Accordingly, in hyponatremia, when there is impaired free-water clearance, the thiazide diuretics are relatively contraindicated.[69,134] The overall potency of thiazide diuretics is limited, in part because about 90% of the filtrate already has been reabsorbed before the distal nephron has been reached. Nevertheless, when combined with furosemide, dangerous volume depletion can result.

The late distal tubules and collecting ducts are sites of sodium reabsorption, aldosterone-controlled secretion of potassium ions, ADH-mediated water reabsorption, and urine concentration. Diuretics acting at these sites initiate diuresis by preventing movement of sodium through luminal channels, either by directly blocking the channels (e.g., amiloride, triamterene) or by antagonizing the effect of aldosterone (e.g., spironolactone, eplerenone). These drugs also exert a potassium-sparing effect and often are classified by that description. They act very distally in the nephron, and their quantitative potential to inhibit sodium reabsorption is low, resulting in a weak diuretic effect. The diuretic effect of spironolactone depends on prevailing aldosterone concentrations (which are low in animals with mild CHF or in those receiving appropriate dosages of ACE inhibitors). The main value of these drugs is for maintenance of normal serum potassium concentration or antagonism of aldosterone-induced cardiac injury.[122,151,152,172]

There are a number of clinically relevant issues regarding the dosage and administration of diuretics.[26,134,144,149] Many of the commonly used diuretics are organic anions at physiologic pH and are highly bound to serum proteins. To be effective, the diuretic must be delivered to the urinary space by glomerular filtration or active secretion in the proximal renal tubule. Active secretion is the more important mechanism because the drug is concentrated in tubular fluid. Reduced renal perfusion associated with heart failure, as well as primary renal disease, may limit the effectiveness of a diuretic unless a high dosage is used and the drug is sufficiently concentrated in renal tubular fluid. The concern about renal perfusion is one rationale for initial high-dose, intravenous administration of furosemide in patients with severe CHF. Gastrointestinal absorption of diuretics such as furosemide may be impaired in CHF, especially with right-sided failure and intestinal edema. Temporarily switching from oral to parenteral administration of furosemide can have a dramatic diuretic benefit in some patients. Pain, administration of opiates (which stimulate ADH release), high sodium intake, and acute worsening of heart failure all represent clinical situations in which diuretics may fail, and the dosage required to establish diuresis successfully may be substantially higher or an alternative route of administration may be required.

Diuretic therapy triggers neurohormonal responses,[42,173] and diuretic monotherapy is no longer considered an appropriate management strategy for long-term treatment of CHF. Diuretic-induced volume depletion leads to a rebound in renal retention of salt and water. This effect is mediated by decreased tubular flow rate, salt retention in segments of the nephron unaffected by the diuretic used, increased sympathetic activity, and activation of the renin-angiotensin-aldosterone system (RAAS).[105,133] Consequently, most patients with CHF should be treated with an ACE inhibitor and a diuretic. If diuretic monotherapy is prescribed, administration of the drug two or three times daily may become necessary, and even at this frequency, the diuretic may become less effective ("braking" effect).

The dosage of diuretics used must be effective but should be carefully controlled to prevent the common complications of dehydration, azotemia, and electrolyte imbalance. The initial dosage of furosemide chosen for a patient with life-threatening pulmonary edema often is high (2 to 5 mg/kg, intravenously every 1 to 3 hours) to ensure diuresis. Symptomatic improvement, brisk diuresis, and decrease in pulmonary capillary wedge pressure often develop within 1 to 2 hours of administration of furosemide,[66] but a lag period (24 to 48 hours) may be noted between obvious clinical improvement and clearing of radiographic pulmonary densities. Owing to the potential for overzealous diuresis and iatrogenic renal failure and electrolyte disturbances, the clinician should evaluate serum biochemistry every 24 to 48 hours until the patient is eating and drinking satisfactorily. After a stable diuretic course of 2 to 3 weeks, most dogs maintain relatively normal renal function and serum potassium concentration unless a decompensating factor (e.g., vomiting, anorexia) intervenes. This is especially true when ACE inhibitors are prescribed concurrently because they reduce aldosterone concentration and decrease potassium loss. Thus stable serum creatinine and potassium concentrations over two or three reevaluation periods are likely to be maintained for some time.[133] The overall dosage of diuretics should be limited by using combination therapy for CHF, including progressive sodium restriction, ACE inhibitors, and digoxin or pimobendan if there are no contraindications.[72,89,116] Cats receiving furosemide are more prone to develop mild to moderate azotemia and hypokalemia than are dogs, even at dosages that are 50% lower than daily dosages typically used for dogs.

EFFECTS OF OTHER CARDIOVASCULAR DRUGS ON RENAL FUNCTION

Angiotensin II is one of the factors responsible for efferent arteriolar vasoconstriction and increased filtration fraction in CHF. The ACE inhibitors, such as enalapril, may antagonize efferent arteriolar constriction sufficiently in some patients to cause an abrupt decrease in glomerular perfusion pressure. This effect is especially likely in volume-depleted patients. The result is acute renal failure, with serum creatinine concentration often exceeding 5 mg/dL. Renal failure in this setting generally can be reversed by reducing diuretic dosage, decreasing the dosage of the ACE inhibitor, and providing judicious fluid therapy (see the section on Therapy of Fluid and Electrolyte Imbalances in Congestive Heart Failure). After volume repletion, the dosage of the ACE inhibitor is increased over 2 to 4 weeks, and the drug combination is adjusted while monitoring body weight, clinical signs of CHF, ABP, and serum creatinine concentration.

Normal autonomic responses to changes in blood pressure and normal heart rate variability are blunted in CHF.[61,88] This allows sympathetic activity to dominate in cardiac failure. Sympathetic nerve activity can increase renin release and affect renal blood flow.[115] Digitalis glycosides such as digoxin appear to exert a neurotropic effect and restore baroreceptor sensitivity and parasympathetic tone, and this effect is independent of the inotropic action of the drug.[75,157] By this or some other effect, digoxin also can blunt the RAAS in CHF.

Cardiac patients sometimes are treated with aspirin and other antiprostaglandin drugs to prevent blood clots (cats) or to alleviate signs of osteoarthritis (dogs). Nonsteroidal antiinflammatory drugs (NSAIDs) may be deleterious when used in CHF patients. By preventing prostaglandin-induced dilatation of the afferent arteriole, NSAIDs may decrease glomerular filtration pressure. They may be especially hazardous when used in combination with furosemide and ACE inhibitors. Other drugs including β-adrenergic blockers, human BNP, neutral endopeptidase inhibitors, and direct vasodilators also may affect renal function. Some of the major effects of these drugs are summarized in Table 21-1. The effects of BNP on renal hemodynamics are still under investigation, and these effects may differ in normal subjects from those in patients with CHF or systemic hypertension.[68,163]

SERUM BIOCHEMICAL ABNORMALITIES IN CONGESTIVE HEART FAILURE

The majority of serum biochemical abnormalities in heart failure can be attributed to alterations in renal function, changes in dietary intake of water and electrolytes, diuretic and other drug therapy, and drug toxicosis. Most alterations are mild, and two surveys of serum biochemical concentrations of patients at our hospitals have failed to demonstrate severe changes in the majority of cardiac patients.[8,10] Nevertheless, some animals with CHF develop substantial disorders of fluid and electrolyte balance that may require fluid therapy and adjustment of cardiac medications.

SODIUM

Serum sodium concentration usually is normal in heart failure, but total body sodium and total body water are likely to be increased. Severe right-sided or biventricular CHF can be associated with hyponatremia. Salt wasting secondary to concurrent diuretic use may contribute to hyponatremia, but it is uncommon for low serum sodium concentration in an edematous patient to be caused solely by salt depletion. Multiple factors are probably involved.[31,39,48,92,113] One likely cause of hyponatremia in CHF is dilution resulting from markedly reduced renal free-water clearance (see Chapter 3). This effect probably is mediated by the nonosmotic release of arginine vasopressin (ADH) and indicates insufficient cardiac output. Continued release of ADH and polydipsia are important factors to be considered in the pathogenesis of hyponatremia in the patient with CHF. In one study of dogs with CHF, dogs with severe heart failure caused by dilated cardiomyopathy were more likely to develop hyponatremia.[169] Activation of the RAAS is predictable in the setting of severe CHF, and glomerular filtration pressure may depend largely on efferent arteriolar constriction mediated in part by angiotensin II.[109,130] Consequently, ACE inhibitors must be used very carefully in such patients. However, such treatment often is effective in improving CHF and, despite a reduction in serum aldosterone concentration, increasing serum sodium concentration (see the section on Therapy of Fluid and Electrolyte Imbalances). Another reason for profound hyponatremia is concurrent use of several diuretics with sequential nephron blockade. In particular, the addition of a thiazide diuretic to furosemide and spironolactone may provoke marked hyponatremia, hypokalemia, and hypochloremia, often in a matter of 1 or 2 days. Thiazides are more commonly associated with hyponatremia than are loop diuretics because they induce loss of effective solutes (sodium and potassium) in excess of water and do not interfere with the renal effects of ADH.[132]

POTASSIUM

Serum potassium concentration may be normal, increased, or decreased in patients with heart failure. Mild hyperkalemia may be observed in acute low-output heart failure because of an abrupt reduction in GFR. Overzealous administration of potassium salts and potassium supplementation in the presence of potassium-sparing diuretics, beta-blockers, or ACE inhibitors are causes of iatrogenic hyperkalemia.[135] Profound hyperkalemia can occur in cats with CHF and concurrent aortic thromboembolism. This probably is related to multiple factors, such as muscle necrosis, reperfusion of infarcted tissues,[119] metabolic acidosis, and renal failure with inadequate urinary excretion of potassium. Management of life-threatening hyperkalemia may be required as discussed in Chapter 5.

Hypokalemia is particularly injurious because it predisposes to digitalis intoxication and muscular weakness and may induce cardiac arrhythmias. Hypokalemia in the cat has been linked to abnormal taurine metabolism and taurine deficiency–associated myocardial failure.[29] Numerous factors predispose to hypokalemia in the cardiac patient.[133] Anorexia resulting from chronic disease or digitalis intoxication can lead to inadequate potassium intake. Cardiac cachexia and tissue wasting also lead to increased potassium loss. Activation of the RAAS may be important because potassium excretion is enhanced by aldosterone. Fortunately, aldosterone concentrations are readily reduced by administration of an ACE inhibitor. Reduced renal perfusion may influence potassium handling because inadequate delivery of sodium to the distal tubule causes potassium to be secreted with organic acids.[69,134] Kaliuresis of variable magnitude occurs with diuretic therapy unless a potassium-sparing diuretic, such as spironolactone or triamterene, or an ACE inhibitor is prescribed. We have observed hypokalemia even when potassium-sparing diuretics have been administered. Cats seem particularly prone to diuretic-induced hypokalemia. The potent loop diuretics, such as furosemide, also promote kaliuresis by accelerating delivery of sodium to the distal nephron, leading to an overall increase in the rate of sodium-potassium exchange.[18,69,134] Combination diuretic therapy is especially likely to lead to hypokalemia, even in the presence of ACE inhibitors or spironolactone. Lastly, metabolic alkalosis is a frequent complication of volume contraction, vomiting, or diuretic-induced chloriuresis.[133,134] Alkalosis increases the concentration of potassium in the renal tubular cell and promotes its secretion into the tubular fluid.

OTHER ELECTROLYTES

Serum chloride concentration usually is normal in heart failure. However, it is common for an animal to develop mild hypochloremia after diuretic therapy. Mild hypochloremia is the most commonly observed diuretic-induced electrolyte disturbance in our practice. This observation probably is the result of the inhibitory effect of furosemide and other loop diuretics on chloride transport and may be associated with a small but commensurate increase in serum bicarbonate concentration as estimated by the total CO_2. Serum calcium and phosphorus concentrations are normal in CHF unless renal failure or another unrelated disorder is present. **Hypomagnesemia** has received little attention in veterinary medicine, but it is common in human patients undergoing diuresis induced by loop diuretics.[25,138,153] In one survey of hypomagnesemia in a veterinary hospital, cardiovascular disease was a prominent risk factor for development of hypomagnesemia.[73] The potential importance of magnesium is emphasized by the association of hypomagnesemia with cardiac arrhythmias and the use of magnesium infusions to treat digitalis-induced cardiac arrhythmias in human patients. Serum magnesium concentration in dogs with CHF did not decrease significantly after furosemide therapy in one study of dogs[36] but was 20% lower than that of a control population in another study of dogs.[18] Digitalis also has been shown to increase urinary magnesium excretion.

ACID-BASE DISTURBANCES

Blood pH in heart failure is the product of competing factors that alter acid-base balance. Complex acid-base disorders are common because of disturbances in tissue oxygenation and in pulmonary and renal function. As a result, simple determination of total CO_2 without direct measurement of blood pH and calculation of bicarbonate may lead to erroneous conclusions (see Chapters 9 through 13). In our experience, respiratory alkalosis and metabolic acidosis are the most commonly encountered acid-base disorders in acute heart failure. Mild metabolic alkalosis is not uncommon in patients receiving chronic diuretic therapy.

Metabolic acidosis may be caused by a stagnant circulation with hypoxia and lactic acidemia,[49] by prerenal azotemia, or by tissue ischemia as may occur with aortic thromboembolism. In uncomplicated cases, the venous pH and bicarbonate concentrations are mildly decreased and arteriovenous oxygen difference is increased. In severe CHF, with avid vasoconstriction, mixed venous Po_2 often is less than 30 mm Hg. **Respiratory acidosis** is a less common but more serious complication and indicates the presence of severe respiratory failure, pulmonary edema, compression atelectasis (from pleural effusion), or respiratory muscle fatigue. Respiratory acidosis is characterized by the development of arterial hypoxemia and hypercapnia and a decrease in blood pH unless a mixed disorder is present (see Chapter 12). **Metabolic alkalosis**, with increased bicarbonate concentration and blood pH, is common and often is a complication of diuretic therapy with resultant volume contraction (contraction alkalosis) and renal loss of chloride and potassium.[69,134] Vomiting, a common complication of digitalis intoxication, also leads to chloride loss and metabolic alkalosis. **Respiratory alkalosis** with a low Pco_2 may be detected in some patients because animals with moderate pulmonary edema tend to hyperventilate as a result of stimulation of stretch and nociceptive receptors in the lungs.[133] Patients with low cardiac output without pulmonary edema have increased muscle fatigability that may be manifested as dyspnea and subsequent hypocapnia. Dyspnea in this subset of patients may be related to skeletal muscle changes that occur during CHF. Abnormal muscle function during CHF has been linked to the decrease in muscle bulk, increased reliance on anaerobic metabolism, decreased muscle blood flow, and metaboreceptor activation.[17]

SERUM PROTEINS

Serum protein concentration frequently is decreased in severe heart failure, especially in dogs with right-sided or biventricular failure. In a survey of dogs with CHF and atrial fibrillation, about one fourth had low serum protein concentrations.[10] Concurrent disorders (e.g., liver disease, renal disease, gastrointestinal disease) also may influence serum protein concentration.

The mechanisms responsible for decreased serum protein concentration in CHF are undetermined. Possible explanations include lymphatic loss of protein through a congested intestine, decreased hepatic synthesis, cardiac cachexia, and enhanced endothelial permeability caused by increased capillary pressure and hypoxia. Ascitic fluid is higher in protein concentration than is a transudate collecting in the pleural space because the hepatic sinusoid is more leaky than other capillary beds. Consequently, considerable protein can pool in the peritoneal cavity of a cardiac patient with ascites, and the protein concentration in ascitic fluid can exceed 3.5 g/dL. Repeated abdominal paracentesis also can contribute to total body depletion of protein. Plasma volume contraction after diuretic therapy usually increases serum protein concentration, but total serum protein concentration may remain subnormal or in the low-normal range. Hypoproteinemia in dogs with CHF caused by heartworm disease may be related to glomerular injury and renal protein loss. Dramatic proteinuria has been observed in heartworm-infected dogs with concurrent renal amyloidosis.

There are a number of clinical consequences of hypoproteinemia in CHF. Effective plasma volume is decreased further when moderate to severe hypoalbuminemia develops. As demonstrated in experimental studies of dogs with left atrial hypertension, edema is more likely to occur at lower venous pressures when there is hypoalbuminemia.[56] Marked protein loss through the gut may indicate a need for additional nutritional support. Hypoalbuminemia also predisposes to metabolic alkalosis (see Chapter 10). Infusions of plasma may be required in the patient with severe hypoalbuminemia and may promote a substantial diuresis.

RENAL FUNCTION TESTS

The blood urea nitrogen (BUN) and serum creatinine concentrations may increase in CHF, indicating reduced glomerular filtration. There are several reasons for development of azotemia in heart failure, but the most common are preexisting renal disease, reduced cardiac output, and iatrogenic problems (i.e., overzealous use of diuretics and ACE inhibitors). Common causes of azotemia in dogs or cats with CHF are listed in Box 21-6.

Approximately 25% of dogs with CHF are azotemic at the time of admission.[10] The magnitude of azotemia generally is mild to moderate. Renal function should be assessed both before and after initiation of therapy. Azotemia is common in patients with dilated cardiomyopathy and cardiogenic shock and may improve only after aggressive therapy with inotropic agents and

Box 21-6	Causes of Azotemia in Heart Failure

Renal Disease
Preexisting renal disease
Renal thromboembolism (feline cardiomyopathy, bacterial endocarditis)
Heartworm disease (glomerulonephritis, amyloidosis)

Inadequate Renal Blood Flow
Dehydration
  Anorexia and hypodipsia
  Vomiting
  Water restriction (by the client or veterinarian)
Severe heart failure (low cardiac output, hypotension)

Drug Related
Volume contraction resulting from diuretics
Angiotensin-converting enzyme inhibitors (hypotension, efferent arteriolar vasodilatation)
Vasodilator therapy (hypotension)
Digitalis intoxication (secondary to anorexia or vomiting)

reestablishment of hydration (see the section on Therapy of Heart Failure). The development of azotemia in a patient with previously normal renal function suggests overzealous diuresis, an adverse reaction to an ACE inhibitor, inappropriate water restriction, or a worsening of heart failure. Return of serum creatinine concentration to normal after intravenous or subcutaneous administration of a crystalloid solution or after reduction of drug dosage indicates a prerenal or drug-induced cause of azotemia. Acute renal failure that responds promptly to intravenous administration of a crystalloid solution has been observed in some dogs treated with ACE inhibitors.

THERAPY OF HEART FAILURE

The initial goals of therapy in CHF include increasing arterial PO_2, reducing oxygen demand, establishing a diuresis, and unloading the ventricles while supporting ABP, tissue perfusion, and renal function. Long-term treatments are aimed at preventing fluid retention, load reduction, maintaining cardiac output to support exercise and organ perfusion, and blunting progressive neurohormonal injury to cardiac and vascular tissues.

HOSPITAL THERAPY

The first goals are attained with supplemental oxygen therapy and sedation as needed to reduce distress or air hunger. Traditionally, dogs in heart failure have been sedated with morphine (initial dosage of 0.05 to 0.1 mg/kg intramuscularly), but vomiting after morphine injection occasionally precipitates cardiac arrest. For this reason, we prefer butorphanol (0.2 to 0.3 mg/kg, intramuscularly) as an effective and safer sedative for dogs in CHF. Stress in cats can be alleviated with an acepromazine-butorphanol combination (0.05 to 0.1 mg/kg acepromazine and 0.25 mg/kg butorphanol intramuscularly). In the presence of moderate to severe pleural effusion, thoracocentesis is performed to decrease pulmonary atelectasis. Tense ascites, sufficient to impair ventilation, is reduced by abdominocentesis. About one third to one half of the total ascitic volume is drained. The high protein content of hepatic lymph and the dynamic equilibrium between the third-space and plasma compartments argue against complete drainage of the peritoneal space.[133] Pulmonary edema sufficient to cause respiratory failure and respiratory muscle fatigue is an indication for artificial ventilation.

Diuresis is initiated and maintained with parenterally administered furosemide. An initial intravenous bolus of 2 to 5 mg/kg can be followed by serial intravenous or intramuscular boluses of 1 to 4 mg/kg every 6 to 8 hours or more frequently when necessitated by insufficient clinical response. The use of constant rate infusion (CRI) of furosemide also may be used to treat dogs and cats with life-threatening pulmonary edema. In healthy dogs and in human patients with CHF, furosemide CRI increases urine output and minimizes electrolyte disturbances when compared with repeated bolus injections.[2,27] Our approach is to initially administer an intravenous bolus of furosemide, estimate the furosemide dosage required for the next 24 hours, and then infuse this volume by syringe pump. Supplemental boluses also can be given if required during the CRI. A novel approach for treatment of severe CHF in human patients has been advocated by Licata et al.[86] They administered small-volume, hypertonic saline combined with furosemide and demonstrated enhanced diuresis in refractory CHF. This therapy has not been studied in animals with spontaneous disease but deserves consideration, especially in hyponatremic patients. Another approach that may be adopted in veterinary practice involves addition of intravenous synthetic human brain natriuretic factor (h-BNP) or nesiritide to the hospital treatment protocol.[100] Although expensive, nesiritide is labeled for human use and appears to be effective in dogs. The h-BNP increases urine output and decreases the effects of aldosterone in furosemide-treated dogs,[15] increases urine volume in normal dogs and those with experimental CHF,[16,158] and has limited electrophysiological effects on the canine heart.[37]

Both preload reduction and afterload reduction are beneficial to the failing left ventricle. Nitrates such as nitroglycerin ointment and sodium nitroprusside increase concentrations of the vasodilator nitric oxide in vascular smooth muscle, leading to relaxation of arterioles and systemic veins.[106] Two percent nitroglycerin ointment ($\frac{1}{4}$ to 1 inch of the 2% ointment, topically every 12 hours) acts primarily as a systemic venodilator, and this treatment is well tolerated by both dogs and cats. Although some question exists about the efficacy of topically administered nitroglycerin, the anticipated venodilation should work in concert with furosemide to decrease venous and capillary hydrostatic pressures. The need for arteriolar dilators in the hospital setting depends on the cause and severity of CHF. Although vasodilator therapy has the potential to induce systemic hypotension, such treatment generally is safe in dogs when baseline ABP is greater than 95 mm Hg. For dogs with severe CHF, sodium nitroprusside (1 to 5 µg/kg/min intravenously by CRI), enalapril (0.5 mg/kg orally every 12 hours), and hydralazine (1 to 2 mg/kg orally every 12 hours) are effective vasodilators in the hospital setting. Each drug can increase stroke volume and reduce pulmonary edema. Afterload reduction is particularly useful in the treatment of severe mitral regurgitation arising from canine endocardiosis or when left ventricular dysfunction is evident, as in dogs with dilated cardiomyopathy.[9] The choice of vasodilator in dogs depends on the urgency of the situation. In florid pulmonary edema, nitroprusside can be infused to a specific endpoint, such as a systolic ABP of 85 to 90 mm Hg.

In less urgent cases, or when intravenous therapy is impractical, enalapril or hydralazine can be administered orally to provide afterload reduction. After stabilization, enalapril or another ACE inhibitor is initiated (or continued) as part of the home treatment plan. Nitroprusside and hydralazine rarely are used in cats, and most cats with CHF are treated with furosemide, nitroglycerin, and eventually an ACE inhibitor.

Cardiac output, ABP, and tissue perfusion are supported when necessary by providing inotropic support. In dogs or cats with severe systemic hypotension (ABP < 80 mm Hg), inotropic support with dobutamine (2.5 to 10 µg/kg/min) or dopamine (2 to 10 µg/kg/min) is indicated. Catecholamines most often are administered to dogs with CHF caused by dilated cardiomyopathy. Occasionally, this approach is used in patients with severe mitral regurgitation or pulmonary embolism. Cats with any form of cardiomyopathy may develop cardiogenic shock characterized by bradycardia, hypothermia, and hypotension. Treatment with dobutamine can be life saving in affected cats. Infusions should be titrated to a systolic ABP of 90 to 120 mm Hg and can be combined with slow external warming in an oxygen incubator. When treatment with catecholamines is impractical, oral administration of the calcium sensitizer pimobendan should be considered once this drug is available for general use. Intravenous administration of a related compound, levosimendan, may become a treatment of choice in the future. Both pimobendan and levosimendan exert potent positive inotropic effects combined with vasodilatation, which unloads the left ventricle.[89,155]

HOME THERAPY

Chronic therapy of CHF targets the kidney, heart, and vascular tree, while attempting to minimize neurohormonal injury to cardiac and vascular tissues. By combining diuretics (usually furosemide and spironolactone) with an ACE inhibitor and dietary sodium restriction, fluid retention is prevented. In dogs, cardiac performance is enhanced by administration of digoxin or, where available, by orally administered pimobendan. Further cardiac protection is achieved by gradual up-titration of a β-adrenergic blocker such as carvedilol. Specific heart rhythm disturbances such as atrial fibrillation or ventricular tachycardia require additional antiarrhythmic drug treatments. Many of these treatments impact renal function and fluid and electrolyte balance in the cardiac patient. The rationale for medical therapy is considered below.

A fundamental feature of CHF is dominance of vasoconstrictive-sodium–retaining mechanisms over competing vasodilator-natriuretic systems.[42,129,131] Chronic activation of the sympathetic nervous system, increased formation of endothelin, and progressive stimulation of the RAAS injures the myocardium, blood vessels, and the kidney.[62,151] Neurohormonal activation clearly occurs in many dogs with spontaneous heart disease, especially those with advanced heart failure.[79,118,146,169] Many laboratory and clinical investigations in humans have emphasized the beneficial effect that pharmacologic blockade of the RAAS has in limiting the progression of myocardial disease and reducing morbidity and mortality in CHF.[23,106,145] Another therapeutic advance is aldosterone blockade at the tissue level by administration of an aldosterone antagonist (spironolactone or eplerenone).[122,172] A tissue RAAS is present in the canine heart, and the local chymases that convert angiotensin to its active form may not be inhibited by ACE inhibitors. Aldosterone antagonism produces measurable survival benefits in human patients with CHF and has been shown to reduce left ventricular remodeling in dogs with experimentally induced heart failure.[152] Aldosterone also blunts baroreceptor reflexes in dogs, an effect that can be partially reversed by administration of digitalis glycosides.[168] As with the ACE inhibitors, β-adrenergic blockers also improve left ventricular ejection fraction and inhibit myocardial remodeling and fibrosis in humans and in animal models of myocardial failure.[1,12,38,139,140] Beta-blockers are now standard therapy for human heart failure and increasingly are considered for treatment of dogs and cats with heart disease.

These data along with results of clinical trials in veterinary medicine have impacted modern therapy of CHF in dogs and, to a lesser extent, cats. Increasingly, treatment is directed beyond diuretics and inotropes to drugs that reduce the deleterious effects of neurohormones on cardiac and vascular tissues. A prominent example is the adoption of ACE inhibitors and spironolactone in the treatment of spontaneous CHF in dogs and cats. Two prospective North American studies of dogs with CHF have demonstrated the efficacy of enalapril at 0.5 mg/kg orally every 24 hours or every 12 hours,[22,66] and another investigation demonstrated the relative renal safety of monotherapy with enalapril.[5] Other studies have shown efficacy for benazepril,[76] including the relatively large BENCH study of dogs with CHF caused by mitral regurgitation or dilated cardiomyopathy.[123] In the latter trial, benazepril dosages of 0.5 mg/kg every 24 hours or every 12 hours both were effective and well tolerated in terms of renal function. Alternatively, lisinopril (0.25 to 0.5 mg/kg every 24 hours or every 12 hours) or another ACE inhibitor such as ramipril can be prescribed because all ACE inhibitors should be beneficial in CHF. Based on clinical observations,[3,137] cats with chronic CHF also can benefit from ACE inhibition, but a blinded, controlled, prospective study has not yet been published. Although the initial dosage of ACE inhibitors in cats is relatively low (0.25 to 0.5 mg/kg every 24 to 48 hours orally), higher dosages (0.25 to 0.5 mg/kg every 12 hours orally) may be well tolerated or result in only mild azotemia. Spironolactone frequently is prescribed for dogs and cats with chronic heart failure because ACE

inhibition does not fully inhibit aldosterone formation in advanced CHF. Thus in most dogs and cats, CHF is managed by a combination of furosemide, ACE inhibitor, and spironolactone.

The use of beta-blockers as a treatment for the failing heart has lagged somewhat in veterinary clinical practice, probably as a consequence of the advanced state of CHF observed in so many affected dogs and cats. Nevertheless, β-blockade can be achieved in many patients with heart failure. Although metoprolol has been most widely studied in canine models of heart failure,[98,139,140] ample evidence exists in humans and other species that carvedilol is at least equally cardioprotective.[1,38] Carvedilol is our beta-blocker of choice in dogs because the available dosage forms (3.125 mg, 6.25 mg, and 12.5 mg) provide more dosing flexibility. Unfortunately, drug interventions that alter neurohormonal activation and renal sodium retention have some limitations depending on the drug and stage of heart failure. Although both ACE inhibition and β-adrenergic blockade retard progression of cardiomyopathy in experimental canine models, early treatment with enalapril in small-breed dogs with mitral regurgitation does not delay onset of CHF.[81] Another limitation occurs with the use of natriuretic hormones such as BNP and neutral endopeptidase inhibitors such as ecadotril, which prevents the breakdown of natriuretic peptides. CHF improves when these drugs are administered acutely to humans or dogs,[16] and in those with very early heart failure, chronic therapy with ecadotril produces favorable results. However, in a pivotal clinical trial of dogs with advanced CHF, chronic ecadotril therapy was ineffective and no better than placebo in improving CHF. Similarly, initial trials with inhibitors of endothelin have been disappointing in human patients.[112] Treatments that should be beneficial based on theoretical considerations may not in fact have clear benefit in controlled clinical trials.

Thus the typical home therapy of CHF in dogs includes administration of an ACE inhibitor as described above (0.5 mg/kg orally every 24 hours to every 12 hours), furosemide (2 to 4 mg/kg orally every 12 to 8 hours), and either digoxin (0.005 to 0.0075 mg/kg orally every 12 hours) or pimobendan (0.2 to 0.3 mg/kg orally every 12 hours). Spironolactone (0.5 to 1 mg/kg/day orally) also is prescribed. Once CHF is well controlled, an up-titration of carvedilol can be initiated. The daily dosage is critical, and it takes months to achieve target daily dosages of about 0.5 mg/kg/day in dogs with cardiomyopathy. The negative inotropic effects of carvedilol can worsen CHF, and consequently we start with a very low dosage. Initial dosages of 0.05 to 0.1 mg/kg PO twice daily can be started once the patient is completely free of edema. Gradual up-titration every 2 to 4 weeks to a target dosage of 0.2 to 0.25 mg/kg orally twice daily can be achieved in many dogs. A beta-blocker should not be given to "wet" patients, and the dosage may need to be reduced by 50% if fluid retention worsens despite diuretic and inotropic therapy. When CHF is complicated by atrial fibrillation, digoxin should be given, and either diltiazem (starting at 0.5 mg/kg orally every 8 hours and increasing the dosage by 0.5 mg/kg every day to a maximum of 2 mg/kg orally every 8 hours) or a beta-blocker should be prescribed to gain better control of ventricular rate response. Both diltiazem and beta-blockers are negative inotropes and must be used carefully in CHF. Our current approach is to control heart rate (100 to 150 beats/min) with digoxin and diltiazem and then to add carvedilol. Should the heart rate decrease to less than 100 beats/min, serum digoxin concentration is measured (trough target concentration of 0.9 to 1.2 ng/mL), and the dosage of diltiazem is reduced. Low sodium diets also may be beneficial in dogs with CHF.[136] Other dietary measures may be considered. The addition of omega-3 fatty acids found in fish oil may inhibit proinflammatory cytokines and reduce cardiac cachexia.[46] Typical dosages are 30 to 40 mg/kg orally daily for eicosapentaenoic acid (EPA) and 20 to 25 mg/kg orally daily for docosahexaenoic acid (DHA). Nutriceuticals, such as taurine or L-carnitine, may be indicated for some patients.[77] Amlodipine may be used for treatment of concurrent hypertension that is unresponsive to the above-mentioned measures, but direct vasodilator drugs, particularly hydralazine, may activate the RAAS[57] and can lead to additional fluid retention.

Home management of cats with progressive CHF or recurrent pulmonary edema or pleural effusion secondary to cardiomyopathy often includes furosemide (1 to 2 mg/kg orally every 24 hours or every 12 hours) and enalapril or benazepril (0.25 to 0.5 mg/kg every 24 hours to every 12 hours orally). Spironolactone (6.25 mg orally every 24 hours) also can be added to the treatment plan. Digoxin (one fourth of a 0.125-mg tablet orally every 48 hours) rarely is used in cats today, unless dilated cardiomyopathy has been identified by echocardiography. Diltiazem (30 mg of a sustained release product orally initially every 24 hours) or atenolol (6.25 to 12.5 mg per cat orally every 12 hours) often is recommended for long-term management of cats with hypertrophic cardiomyopathy, but based on a multicenter clinical trial, neither of these drugs was beneficial in short-term treatment of cats with CHF (Fox PR, personal communication). Once the cat with CHF is stabilized, a cardiologist should be consulted regarding other drug options, including inodilators such as pimobendan.

REFRACTORY EDEMA AND EFFUSIONS

Some patients become refractory to diuretic therapy and continue to develop edema or effusions.[134] Three commonly encountered examples of this problem are (1) progressive ascites and pleural effusion in dogs with biventricular heart failure, (2) progressive pleural effu-

sion in cats with cardiomyopathy, and (3) recurrent pulmonary edema in dogs with left-sided heart failure. Successful therapy of some of these patients may be attained by skillful use of cardiac medications[103] and by addressing the following points:

- Ensure medication compliance, and educate the client about medications, dosages, and methods of administration.
- Consistently enforce a low-sodium diet.
- Enforce rest.
- Optimize current medication dosages, especially the daily dosage of an ACE inhibitor.
- Improve left-sided heart function with an inodilator or load reducer.
- Reduce the dosage of any negative inotropic drugs.
- Adjust the dosage or route of administration of furosemide.
- Consider using combination diuretic therapy.
- Identify and treat extracardiac complications such as hyperthyroidism, anemia, and hypertension.

The first three points are straightforward but by no means easy to achieve. With progressive CHF, the sodium intake should be progressively limited unless the patient is hyponatremic. Periods of enforced rest are useful in mobilizing edema and decreasing cardiac work. Rest alone can lead to considerable diuresis in patients with right-sided CHF. The remaining guidelines require some explanation.

Current medication dosages should be optimal for the stage of CHF with furosemide given at least twice daily and spironolactone part of the daily treatment plan (once or twice daily). The effect of an ACE inhibitor in CHF may be dose dependent.[164] Frequently, veterinarians prescribe ACE inhibitors but do not always maximize the dosage for fear of precipitating hypotension or renal failure. For both enalapril and benazepril, the daily dosage should be increased to at least 0.5 mg/kg orally every 12 hours when tolerated. In addition, the inodilator pimobendan should be prescribed or the dosage optimized (to 0.3 mg/kg orally every 12 hours) in dogs. Pimobendan is not available in all countries but often can be obtained under compassionate protocols. If pulmonary edema persists, and especially if the systolic ABP exceeds 150 mm Hg, another vasodilator can be prescribed such as amlodipine (0.05 to 0.1 mg/kg orally every 24 hours to every 12 hours). Unless digitalization is contraindicated (e.g., complex ventricular ectopia, atrioventricular block, sinus node disease, moderate to severe renal failure), digoxin should be prescribed. The dosage should produce a trough serum digoxin concentration of 0.9 to 1.2 ng/mL, but trough concentrations as high as 1.5 ng/mL may be acceptable in dogs with atrial fibrillation and rapid ventricular response rate.

Modifying the diuretic dosage may be necessary, especially in dogs with chronic renal failure, in those that develop severe polydipsia, and in those with apparent intestinal malabsorption of furosemide. Low dosages of furosemide (e.g., 1 to 2 mg/kg every 12 hours or every 24 hours), in combination with an ACE inhibitor, are quite effective in patients with mild heart failure. However, patients with renal failure or low cardiac output may require higher dosages to deliver sufficient active drug to the renal tubules.[51] In the case of furosemide, gradually increasing the dosage and frequency from 2 mg/kg every 12 hours to 6 mg/kg every 8 hours may be sufficient to maximally inhibit renal tubular chloride and sodium reabsorption. Once this "ceiling" effect is achieved, no further diuresis develops with increasing dosage.[134] This "ceiling" effect is especially apparent with loop diuretics (e.g., furosemide, bumetanide, torsemide), which typically have a short duration of action (see previous section on Diuretics). Furosemide may be poorly absorbed by a congested intestine,[165] and subcutaneous administration of furosemide in patients with refractory ascites and pleural effusion should be considered. Frequently, the same daily dosage, given subcutaneously instead of orally, leads to substantial diuresis. We have taught clients to administer one of the daily doses of furosemide subcutaneously to their animals every other day, and such therapy can be beneficial when used chronically. Combination diuretic therapy with sequential nephron blockade represents another option for the patient with refractory edema or effusion.[60,105,108,134] The combination of three diuretics (furosemide, hydrochlorothiazide, and spironolactone) acting on different segments of the nephron (see Fig. 21-5) may be effective in treating dogs with progressive ascites or pleural effusion. However, hyponatremia (<130 mEq/L) and hypokalemia are contraindications to thiazide diuretics, and thiazide diuretics often induce profound hyponatremia. When hydrochlorothiazide is prescribed, the initial dosage should be low, approximately 1 to 2 mg/kg orally every 48 hours. Renal function and serum electrolyte concentrations should be evaluated within 1 week of treatment before the dosage is increased.

THERAPY OF FLUID AND ELECTROLYTE IMBALANCES IN CONGESTIVE HEART FAILURE

INDICATIONS

The cardiac patient, in contrast to many other sick animals, is not an ideal candidate for parenteral fluid therapy. Volume expansion poses substantial risks in terms of increasing venous pressures, sodium retention, and edema. In managing cardiac patients, we prefer to offer water (of low sodium content) ad libitum, provide a sodium-restricted but palatable diet, treat CHF medically, and allow the patient's kidneys to correct any fluid and electrolyte disturbances. This approach may lack technical sophistication, but it often works well in the clinical setting. Dogs are especially resilient to the complications of diuretic therapy provided their intake of water and food is adequate. In fact, it is common to observe a dog or cat begin drinking shortly after receiving successful therapy for life-threatening pulmonary edema or pleural effusion.

Some patients with heart failure do develop problems that require fluid and electrolyte supplementation. Indications for fluid therapy in the patient with CHF include persistent anorexia, dehydration, renal failure, moderate to severe hypokalemia, digitalis intoxication, drug-induced hypotension, gastroenteritis, anemia, and serious metabolic (e.g., diabetes mellitus), neoplastic, or infectious diseases. Another indication is the need for intravenous infusion to deliver drugs such as dobutamine, sodium nitroprusside, or lidocaine. When animals with heart disease undergo general anesthesia, a catheter should be placed and intravenous fluids administered. Ventricular filling is impaired in pericardial disease, and this abnormality may demand volume expansion with parenteral fluid therapy. Hypertrophied ventricles may be more difficult to distend unless CVP is maintained at a normal to slightly increased level. However, overinfusion of fluids can lead to peracute pulmonary edema in dogs and in cats with marked left ventricular hypertrophy, and care must be taken.

Thus a number of situations may necessitate fluid therapy in the cardiac patient. What fluid should be infused? The following recommendations are based on our clinical experience and theoretical considerations for fluid, electrolyte, and diuretic therapy in patients with CHF. Controlled, prospective evaluations of such therapy in dogs and cats are unavailable. The following discussion considers basic principles of therapy; selection of fluids, additives, and rates of administration; monitoring of the patient (including Swan-Ganz catheterization); and our approach to some specific problems related to fluid therapy in the cardiac patient.

PARENTERAL SOLUTIONS

Fluid Volume

The daily fluid volume is guided by the current state of edema, estimated maintenance needs (40 to 60 mL/kg/day), hydration status, body weight, oral fluid intake, estimated urine output, total serum protein concentration, serum sodium concentration, serum creatinine concentration, and, when available, CVP and pulmonary capillary wedge pressure. It is prudent to consider a minimal fluid infusion initially (e.g., no more than 30 to 40 mL/kg/day) and to assess the effect of fluid therapy on the patient. The daily volume should be infused slowly and distributed evenly over 24 hours to reduce the risk of pulmonary edema and pleural effusion. The choice of fluid depends largely on concerns about sodium retention. The intravenous route of administration is preferred, but either 0.45% NaCl in 2.5% dextrose or lactated Ringer's solution can be given subcutaneously if necessary. When the patient can drink, fluid therapy is tapered, low-sodium fresh water is supplied ad libitum, and dietary sodium intake is regulated while ensuring a palatable diet.

The CHF patient continues to retain sodium, and diuretics must be given concurrently to prevent untoward retention of sodium derived from the diet or crystalloid therapy. Although it may seem paradoxical to administer diuretics to a patient receiving fluid therapy, these drugs are important adjuncts to the overall fluid and electrolyte management in treatment of the edematous cardiac patient.[59,69,134] Diuretic therapy also promotes redistribution of extracellular water from edematous sites to the venous system. Furosemide also acts initially to increase GFR (possibly by releasing vasodilating prostaglandins). After diuresis and contraction of the plasma volume, however, cardiac filling and GFR decrease unless the patient drinks adequately or receives supplemental fluid therapy. A fine balance is required, and the clinician must learn to control the risk of edema while preventing an increase in BUN or serum creatinine concentration. Human BNP (nesiritide) may represent another option for preventing fluid retention in cardiac patients receiving fluid therapy; however, this drug also increases the serum creatinine in some human patients.

Sodium

Dogs with cardiac failure do not respond normally to a sodium load, and after saline infusion, marked retention of sodium and water can occur.[7] Healthy dogs can maintain normal serum sodium concentration with a diet containing sodium at only 0.5 mEq/kg/day (11.5 mg/kg/day).[93,99] This amount is equivalent to approximately 175 mg of sodium or 435 mg of sodium chloride per day for a 15-kg dog. In Canine Prescription Diet H/d (Hill's Pet Nutrition, Topeka, KS) there are approximately 23 mg of sodium and 542 kcal in a 418-gram serving of canned food. The H/d dry product contains about 15 mg sodium and 407 kcal in a 99-gram serving. Another highly sodium-restricted diet, CV-Formula (Nestlé Purina PetCare Company, St. Louis, MO), contains about 20 mg of sodium and 638 kcal in a 354-gram serving. Early Cardiac Support Diet (Royal Canin/Waltham) delivers 61 mg of sodium and 300 kcal in a 73-gram, dry food serving. A 2.5-oz jar of chicken baby food contains approximately 40 to 60 mg of sodium. A number of over-the-counter dog foods also are relatively restricted in sodium (e.g., Cycle Senior [Del Monte, San Francisco, CA], Alpo Senior [Nestlé Purina PetCare Company]). The extent of dietary sodium

restriction required in animals with CHF has not been determined, but it seems prudent to limit daily sodium intake to less than 12 mg/kg/day in dogs with advanced cardiac failure. The average sodium content of Feline Prescription Diet H/d (Hill's Pet Nutrition) is about 354 mg per 14.25-oz can (70 mg/100 kcal; 506 kcal/can), and a 5.5-oz can of CV-Formula (Nestlé Purina PetCare Company) contains about 112 mg of sodium (50 mg/100 kcal; 223 kcal/can). Dietary sodium requirements for cats with CHF are not available.

The clinician also must be mindful of the sodium content of crystalloid solutions. Normal saline solution (0.9% NaCl) contains 154 mEq of sodium per liter. Therefore 500 mL of 0.45% NaCl in 2.5% dextrose contains 37.5 mEq (862 mg) of sodium, an amount that conceivably represents the minimal daily requirement for a normal 75-kg dog. If severe metabolic acidosis in a cardiac patient must be treated with sodium bicarbonate, an additional sodium load is imposed because there are 23 mg of sodium per milliequivalent of sodium bicarbonate. Metabolic acidosis in those with CHF often is caused by lactic acidosis, a condition that may not be responsive to bicarbonate treatment, and is best treated by improving cardiac output (see Chapter 10).

Based on these concepts, either 5% dextrose or 0.45% NaCl in 2.5% dextrose, supplemented with potassium chloride, is recommended when routine fluid therapy is required for rehydration, maintenance of hydration, or drug infusions in patients with CHF. Unfortunately, therapy with 5% dextrose or 0.45% NaCl in 2.5% dextrose is sometimes associated with inadequate free-water excretion, weight gain, hyponatremia, and hypokalemia. These electrolyte disturbances are similar to those observed when some dogs and cats with severe CHF are treated with diuretics and given free access to water. Development of hyponatremia in this clinical setting is especially common in cats. Because of the potential for hyponatremia, balanced crystalloid such as lactated Ringer's solution or Plasma-Lyte is preferable as a replacement fluid for cardiac patients with dehydration. The short-term use (<12 hours) of such sodium-replete fluids usually is well tolerated, provided the volume is small and the rate of infusion is slow (e.g., 2.5 to 5 mL/kg/hr). Therapy of hyponatremia is discussed later and in Chapter 3.

Potassium Supplementation

Potassium (as the chloride salt) is administered routinely to cardiac patients receiving fluid therapy. Administration of glucose-containing, salt-poor solutions, especially during diuretic therapy of anorexic patients, tends to decrease serum potassium concentration. Typical intravenous potassium dosages of 0.5 to 2.0 mEq/kg/day are given using accepted guidelines for intravenous administration of potassium (see Chapter 5). For hypokalemic animals, higher dosages of potassium chloride are used up to a rate not to exceed 0.5 mEq/ kg/hr intravenously. Oliguria, hyperkalemia, and concurrent administration of potassium-sparing diuretics, beta-blockers, or ACE inhibitors are relative contraindications for parenteral potassium therapy, unless serum potassium concentration is known to be low. When providing the patient with oral potassium chloride supplementation, the clinician should consider that there is 1 mEq of potassium in each 89 mg of potassium chloride salt (or in 234 mg of potassium gluconate).

Blood Products

Moderate to severe anemia increases the demand for cardiac output and can precipitate CHF. In most cases, the packed cell volume must decrease to less than 22% or it must decrease rapidly for cardiac complications to occur. Although anemia alone can cause high-output heart failure, the development of pulmonary edema or pleural effusion is even more common in the setting of a preexisting heart disease such as cardiomyopathy or chronic valvular heart disease. Anemic patients often receive fluid therapy to maintain blood pressure and organ perfusion, and this poses another risk for the dog or cat with underlying cardiac dysfunction. Similarly, the hemoglobin solution Oxyglobin (Biopure Corporation, Cambridge, MA) expands plasma volume and can cause CHF in susceptible patients (this product currently is unavailable). Management of these animals involves medical therapy of CHF, treatment of the underlying cause of anemia, and often a slow infusion of packed cells to reduce the demand for cardiac output.

MANAGING ELECTROLYTE DISORDERS IN CHF

Electrolyte disturbances, notably hypokalemia, hypochloremia, and metabolic alkalosis, are common complications of diuretic therapy. Digitalis intoxication with anorexia and vomiting can have similar effects. Mild reductions in serum chloride concentration are of limited concern, but hypokalemia should be avoided in cardiac patients because it predisposes to cardiac arrhythmias, digitalis intoxication, muscle weakness (and necrosis), and renal fibrosis and may decrease serum taurine concentration in cats.[29] Fortunately, most dogs do not develop marked hypokalemia during the initial hospital therapy of CHF.[8] With the widespread use of ACE inhibitors and spironolactone (which spare potassium loss), hypokalemia also is relatively uncommon during chronic management of CHF, except in the settings of digitalis intoxication, vomiting, or prolonged anorexia or when combination diuretic therapy is prescribed. Cats are more prone to hypokalemia. Even a 1-day course of parenteral furosemide can decrease the serum potassium concentration in cats. Hypokalemia is common with chronic furosemide administration in cats unless prevented by an ACE inhibitor or potassium supplementation.

Hypokalemia can be prevented in the hospital setting by encouraging food intake and supplementing parenteral fluids with KCl. Constant-rate infusion of furosemide also may be associated with less severe urinary potassium loss. Routine oral potassium supplementation is needed only when diuretics are administered chronically, but neither an ACE inhibitor nor potassium-sparing diuretic is part of the treatment plan. In such cases, a KCl "salt substitute" can be sprinkled on the food, or the client can administer a prescription formulation of potassium gluconate or potassium chloride daily. As a rule, potassium supplementation should not be given to patients receiving an ACE inhibitor because hyperkalemia may develop.[135] In practice, mild hyperkalemia is not uncommon in patients receiving both an ACE inhibitor and spironolactone, but it usually is ignored. Use of oral potassium supplements and the hospital management of severe hypokalemia are described in detail in Chapter 5.

Serum sodium concentration generally is normal in cardiac patients, and the finding of hyponatremia is a serious sign. Low serum sodium concentration in the setting of excess extracellular fluid volume suggests decreased effective arterial blood volume with impaired renal water excretion related to persistent release of ADH. Diuretics also may contribute to hyponatremia (and hypochloremia) by causing hypokalemia, inducing plasma volume depletion and release of ADH, and impairing function in the diluting segments of the nephron.[39,48,69] Thiazide diuretics are especially likely to cause hyponatremia because they favor excretion of relatively concentrated urine. These abnormalities are exacerbated by increased water intake associated with polydipsia, which can be prominent in dogs with CHF, or by infusion of a sodium-poor crystalloid. The general causes of and approach to hyponatremia are described in Chapter 3.

Therapy of hyponatremia in CHF is difficult. Mild hyponatremia (130 to 145 mEq/L in dogs) simply is an indication to adjust cardiac therapy. Moderate hyponatremia (<130 mEq/L), especially when associated with prerenal azotemia, is an indication for cage rest, mild water restriction, frequent determination of body weight and serum biochemistry, and vigorous therapy of CHF. Furosemide is continued because studies in human patients suggest that furosemide may promote the formation of more dilute urine, thereby increasing free-water clearance, whereas thiazides do not.[134] Thiazide diuretics should be discontinued. If the patient is receiving fluids, either lactated Ringer's solution or 0.9% NaCl, supplemented with KCl, should be used initially at conservative infusion rates (e.g., 20 to 30 mL/kg per 24 hours). Infusion for 48 to 72 hours of a catecholamine (dobutamine or dopamine) or addition of an inodilator such as milrinone, pimobendan (if available), or levosimendan should be considered to increase cardiac output.

Box 21-7 | Evaluation of the Cardiac Patient

Inspection and Examination
Body weight
Estimated hydration
Jugular venous pressure
Arterial blood pressure (indirect or direct)
Body temperature
Pulse rate and quality
Respiratory rate
Pattern of ventilation
Cardiac auscultation
Pulmonary auscultation and percussion
Level of consciousness
Muscle strength
Mucous membrane color and capillary refill time
Evaluation for ascites (measurement of girth)

Laboratory Evaluation
Blood urea nitrogen and serum creatinine
Serum electrolytes (sodium, potassium, chloride)
Blood gas tensions (P_{O_2}, P_{CO_2})
Blood pH and bicarbonate

Chest Radiograph
Evaluation of heart size
Pulmonary vascularity
Pulmonary infiltrates or edema
Pleural effusion

Electrocardiogram
Heart rate and rhythm
ST segment (myocardial perfusion or ischemia)
T wave

Echocardiography and Doppler Studies
Morphologic diagnosis
Ventricular systolic function (ejection fraction)
Ventricular diastolic function (Doppler studies)
Estimation of right atrial and ventricular filling (preload)
Hemodynamic estimates of left atrial pressure (Doppler studies)

Determination or Calculation of:
Intravenous fluid requirements
Oral water intake
Urinary output
Total daily sodium intake (intravenous and dietary)
Total daily potassium intake (intravenous and dietary)
Total daily caloric intake
Environmental temperature and humidity

Hemodynamic Measurements
Central venous pressure (right-sided filling pressures)
Pulmonary capillary wedge pressure (left-sided filling pressures)
Cardiac output
Pulmonary vascular resistance
Systemic vascular resistance (if arterial line in place)

Current Therapy
Diuretic drugs
Crystalloid and additives
Cardiotonic agents, including digitalis
Vasodilators and angiotensin-converting enzyme inhibitors
Additional measures: paracentesis, oxygen, antiarrhythmic drugs, bronchodilator, omega-3 fatty acids

---

Gradually increasing the dosage of ACE inhibitor up to the maximal dosage tolerated (at least 0.5 mg/kg of enalapril or benazepril every 12 hours) is important to antagonize the RAAS.[31,113] Despite the theoretical concern that an ACE inhibitor may reduce serum sodium concentration, clinical experience in this setting is just the opposite. Severe hyponatremia (<120 mEq/L) requires water restriction and cautious infusion of 0.9% saline or low-volume hypertonic saline to prevent the neurologic consequences of hyponatremia (see Chapter 3). Mannitol or low-volume hypertonic saline may increase delivery of filtrate to the distal diluting segments of the nephron and may increase free-water clearance. With few exceptions, patients with CHF and severe hyponatremia have been unresponsive to therapy. Therapy with ADH (vasopressin) receptor antagonists that block the effects of ADH on the distal nephron may become available in the future, and these antagonists have been effective in treatment of experimental canine CHF.[101,141,175]

MONITORING OF PATIENTS

Cardiac patients require careful monitoring of clinical, hematologic, cardiac, and hemodynamic variables. It is important to tabulate and establish the trend of important clinical signs: body temperature, respiratory rate and depth, breath sounds, heart rate, heart rhythm, mucous membrane color and refill time, pulse strength, attitude, noninvasively determined arterial blood pressure, and pulse oximetry if available (Box 21-7). Frequent determination of such simple variables as water and food intake, estimated urine output, body weight, infused fluid volume, and diuretic dosage provides the clinician with useful information about fluid dynamics and the need for fluid therapy. Serial determination of serum creatinine, BUN, sodium, and potassium concentrations is useful for adjusting fluid, diuretic, and cardiac therapy. Physical and radiographic signs of fluid accumulation may indicate a need to reduce fluid volume and increase diuretic dosage or to consider additional treatments, such as vasodilator drugs. More accurate hemodynamic information can be obtained using a percutaneously placed pulmonary arterial catheter, as described in the following section. The effect of fluid therapy on CVP and pulmonary venous pressure is a prime concern in patients with heart failure and can be a major determinant of the rate of fluid administration. Insufficient venous pressure reduces cardiac output, whereas very high pressures promote formation of edema. In heart failure, an optimal venous pressure is necessary to maintain cardiac output, but pulmonary venous pressures greater than 20 mm Hg and CVPs greater than 10 to 12 cm H_2O may be associated with formation of edema.

The CVP is simple to measure using an indwelling jugular venous catheter, and its determination quantifies and indicates the directional changes of right heart filling pressures. Inspection and estimation of jugular venous pressure provide similar qualitative information. A CVP line is useful in guiding fluid management of seriously ill patients without heart disease, but CVP is **not** an accurate reflection of pulmonary venous pressure in those with CHF. The ability of the left and right ventricles to accept and pump blood may be different in CHF. Accordingly, the effects of a volume infusion on the left ventricle and pulmonary circulation may not be accurately gauged by measuring the filling pressures of the right ventricle.[40,41,154] It is common to observe animals with high pulmonary venous pressure but relatively low CVP. This is especially true after diuretic therapy. Even in animals with right-sided CHF, ascites may continue to develop despite a relatively low CVP, possibly as a result of avid sodium retention, hypoproteinemia, or the devel-

opment of cardiac cirrhosis and portal hypertension secondary to chronic hepatic congestion. In the future, noninvasive estimation of CVP can be accomplished by 2D echocardiography and Doppler techniques, but such use awaits further verification.

To obtain measurements of pulmonary venous and left-sided cardiac filling pressures, a catheter must be advanced into a lobar pulmonary artery under fluoroscopic or pressure-monitored guidance (Fig. 21-6). Special end-hole, balloon-tipped catheters (Swan-Ganz) can be used to occlude pulmonary arterial flow temporarily, permitting measurement of the damped left atrial pressure waveform, which is transmitted through the valveless pulmonary venous and capillary beds.[40,41,72,154] The mean value of such a determination is called the **pulmonary capillary wedge pressure** and is equivalent to the mean left ventricular filling pressure (but not equivalent to the end-diastolic pressure in some patients) (Fig. 21-7). Pulmonary edema generally is associated with pulmonary capillary wedge pressures greater than 20 to 25 mm Hg. These values are guidelines, and even higher values may not be associated with edema in chronic left-sided heart failure. The clinician can measure the pressure filling the left ventricle and estimate the tendency to form pulmonary edema by determining whether low (<7 mm Hg), optimal (12 to 18 mm Hg), or high (>20 mm Hg) venous pressures are present in the cardiac patient (see Figs. 21-6 and 21-7).[41]

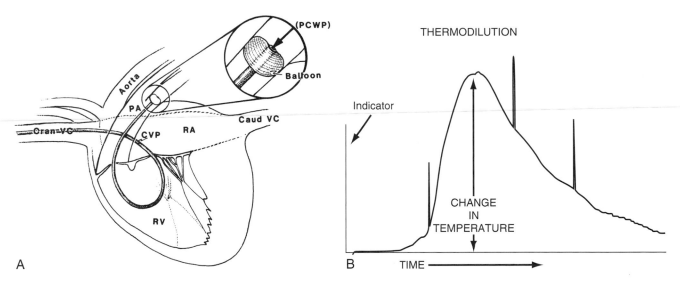

Fig. 21-6 Swan-Ganz pulmonary catheterization. **A,** Determination of central venous pressure (CVP) and pulmonary capillary wedge pressure. Determination of right and left ventricular filling pressures (*left lateral view*). A balloon-tipped, flow-directed catheter (Swan-Ganz) is inserted into the jugular vein and passed through the cranial vena cava (Cran VC), right atrium (RA), right ventricle (RV), and pulmonary artery (PA). Two independent catheter lumina permit pressure determinations in both the right atrium and the pulmonary artery. The proximal lumen in the RA measures the CVP, and the distal tip measures the PA pressure. When the balloon is inflated, blood flow is temporarily occluded, and the pulmonary capillary wedge pressure (PCWP) is measured (*inset*). *Caud VC,* Caudal vena cava. **B,** Cardiac output curve of a 21-kg dog in heart failure. The curve was obtained using a Swan-Ganz catheter equipped with a distal thermistor tip for measuring blood temperature. The recording demonstrates the change in blood temperature that developed after 3 mL of iced 5% dextrose was injected into the right atrial port of the catheter. Cardiac output is inversely related to the area under the curve. The calculated cardiac output in this case was 2.3 L/min. (A from Bonagura JD: Fluid management of the cardiac patient, *Vet Clin North Am Small Anim Pract* 12:509, 1982.)

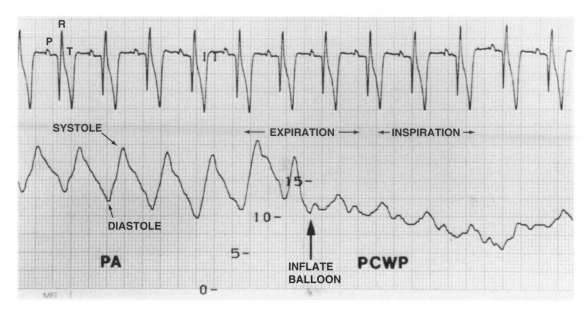

Fig. 21-7 Pressure tracing recorded from the pulmonary artery of a dog undergoing diuretic treatment of congestive heart failure. The pulmonary artery pulsatile pressure and occlusion (wedge) pressure are indicated. Balloon inflation is complete at the arrow. Notice that the pulmonary artery diastolic pressure is closely related to the wedge pressure. The pulmonary artery diastolic pressure is often used to track changes in the wedge pressure (provided there is no pulmonary vascular disease). Variations in the pressure recording baseline are related to ventilation. Measurements are generally made during expiration to avoid the "dips" associated with negative intrapulmonary pressures.

The rate of fluid administration, diuretic dosage, and cardiac therapy are guided by these measurements. Marked reductions in pulmonary capillary wedge pressure can be observed in some patients after administration of furosemide, hydralazine, or sodium nitroprusside. Noninvasive estimation of left atrial pressure may be possible in the future by application of advanced Doppler echocardiographic methods, in particular, the ratio of early ventricular filling velocity (E-wave) to the tissue Doppler velocity (Ea-wave).

Cardiac output also can be measured when the catheter is equipped with a thermistor near the catheter tip and a cardiac output computer is available (see Fig. 21-6, *B*). With this information, four potential **hemodynamic subsets** may be encountered[40]:

- Normal cardiac output and normal pulmonary capillary wedge pressure (the normal situation)
- Normal cardiac output with high pulmonary capillary wedge pressure predisposing to edema (left-sided CHF with volume expansion)
- Low cardiac output and low pulmonary capillary wedge pressure (volume depletion, as with excessive diuresis)
- Low cardiac output and high pulmonary capillary wedge pressure (severe left-sided heart failure, cardiogenic shock)

The CVP also can be measured through dual-port Swan-Ganz catheters (see Fig. 21-6, *A*). In biventricular CHF, both the wedge pressure and CVP are abnormally high (see Figs. 21-7 and 21-8). With excessive diuresis of the patient, both pressures are reduced. A relatively common situation after diuresis in those with primary left-sided heart failure is persistently high wedge pressure with relatively low (<5 mm Hg) CVP. This situation can lead to reduced right-sided filling and prerenal azotemia. Reducing the diuretic dosage improves cardiac output but may exacerbate pulmonary edema. Noninvasive determination of cardiac output is feasible with Doppler echocardiography. The greatest value of this technique is found in the following of trends, as the aortic velocity-time integral increases or decreases with changes in ventricular stroke volume.

REFERENCES

1. Abbott JA: Beta-blockade in the management of systolic dysfunction, *Vet Clin North Am Small Anim Pract* 34:1157-1170, 2004.
2. Adin DB, Taylor AW, Hill RC, et al: Intermittent bolus injection versus continuous infusion of furosemide in normal adult greyhound dogs, *J Vet Intern Med* 17:632-636, 2003.
3. Amberger CN, Glardon O, Glaus T, et al: Effects of benazepril in the treatment of feline hypertrophic cardiomyopathy: results of a prospective, open-label, multicenter clinical trial, *J Vet Cardiol* 1:19-26, 1999.
4. Asano K, Masuda K, Okumura M, et al: Plasma atrial and brain natriuretic peptide levels in dogs with congestive heart failure, *J Vet Med Sci* 61:523-529, 1999.
5. Atkins CE, Brown WA, Coats JR, et al: Effects of long-term administration of enalapril on clinical indicators of renal function in dogs with compensated mitral regurgitation,

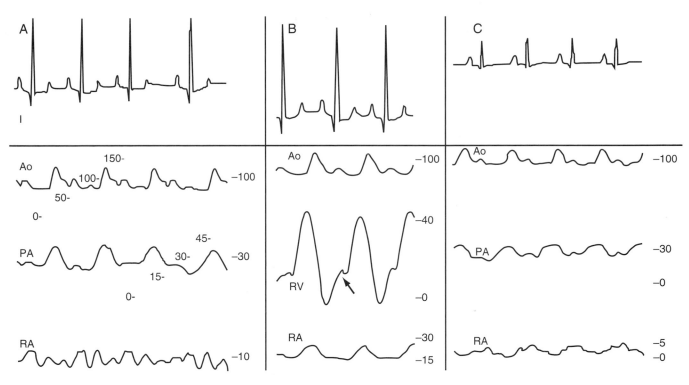

Fig. 21-8 A, Electrocardiogram and pressure recordings from a standing dog with dilated cardiomyopathy and biventricular cardiac dysfunction. There is pulmonary hypertension secondary to abnormally high wedge pressure (not shown) and left-sided cardiac dysfunction. The pulmonary artery pressures are approximately 39/23 (systolic/diastolic) mm Hg. The right atrial pressure (central venous pressure) is also abnormally high, with a mean value of approximately 9 mm Hg. Scales indicate millimeters of mercury for the adjacent curves. *Ao,* Pressure in the descending aorta; *PA,* pressure in the pulmonary artery; *RA,* pressure in the right atrium. **B,** Electrocardiograph (ECG) and pressure recordings from a standing dog with dilated cardiomyopathy and mitral and tricuspid regurgitation during infusion of 0.9% saline solution. Volume expansion has led to a marked increase in the right atrial pressure (mean, 16 mm Hg). The right ventricular pressure (RV) tracing also indicates an increase in the end-diastolic ventricular pressure (*arrow*). Pulmonary hypertension from left-sided heart failure accounts for the increase in systolic RV pressure (42 mm Hg, normal is <25 mm Hg). Scales on the right indicate millimeters of mercury for the preceding curves. **C,** ECG and pressure recordings from a standing dog with mitral regurgitation and mild left-sided heart failure. Pulmonary hypertension secondary to abnormally high wedge pressure (not shown) and left-sided cardiac dysfunction are present. The pulmonary artery pressures are approximately 34/25 (systolic/diastolic) mm Hg. The wedge pressure in this case was approximately 23 mm Hg. Despite the high left-sided filling pressures, note that right atrial pressure is normal, with a mean (central venous pressure) value of approximately 3 mm Hg. Scales on the right indicate millimeters of mercury for the preceding curves.

J Am Vet Med Assoc 221:654-658, 2003. (Erratum in *J Am Vet Med Assoc* 15:221:1149, 2002).

6. Auld RB, Alexander EA, Levinsky NG: Proximal tubular function in dogs with thoracic caval constriction, *J Clin Invest* 50:2150-2158, 1971.

7. Barger AC, Yates FE, Rudolph AM: Renal hemodynamics and sodium excretion in dogs with graded valvular damage, and in congestive failure, *Am J Physiol* 200:601-608, 1961.

8. Bonagura JD, Lehmkuhl LB: Fluid therapy in heart failure. In DiBartola SJ, editor: *Fluid therapy in small animal practice,* ed 1, Philadelphia, 1992, WB Saunders, pp. 529-553.

9. Bonagura JD, Rush J: Heart failure. In Birchard SJ, Sherding RG, editors: *Saunders manual of small animal practice,* ed 2, Philadelphia, 2000, WB Saunders.

10. Bonagura JD, Ware WA: Atrial fibrillation in the dog: clinical findings in 81 cases, *J Am Anim Hosp Assoc* 22: 111-120, 1986.

11. Bourland WA, Day DK, Williams HE: The role of the kidney in the early nondiuretic action of furosemide to reduce elevated left atrial pressure in the hypervolemic dog, *J Pharmacol Exp Ther* 202:221-229, 1977.

12. Bristow MR: Mechanism of action of beta-blocking agents in heart failure, *Am J Cardiol* 80:26L-40L, 1997.

13. Calvert CA, Rawlings CA: Canine heartworm disease. In Fox PR, editor: *Canine and feline cardiology,* New York, 1988, Churchill Livingstone, pp. 519-549.

14. Cannon PJ: The kidney in heart failure, *N Engl J Med* 296:26-32, 1977.

15. Cataliotti A, Boerrigter G, Costello-Boerrigter LC, et al: Brain natriuretic peptide enhances renal actions of furosemide and suppresses furosemide-induced aldosterone activation in experimental heart failure, *Circulation* 109:1680-1685, 2004.

16. Chen HH, Grantham JA, Schirger JA, et al: Subcutaneous administration of brain natriuretic peptide in experimental heart failure, *J Am Coll Cardiol* 36:1706-1712, 2000.

17. Clark AL, Poole-Wilson PA, Coats AJ: Exercise limitation in chronic heart failure: central role of the periphery, *J Am Coll Cardiol* 28:1092-1102, 1996.

18. Cobb M, Michell AR: Plasma electrolyte concentrations in dogs receiving diuretic therapy for cardiac failure, *J Small Anim Pract* 33:526-529, 1992.

19. Cogan MG: Atrial natriuretic peptide, *Kidney Int* 37:1148:1160, 1990.

20. Cohn JN, Levine TB: Angiotensin-converting enzyme inhibition in congestive heart failure: the concept, *Am J Cardiol* 49:1480-1483, 1982.

21. Cohn JN, Levine TB, Olivar MT, et al: Plasma norepinephrine as a guide to prognosis in patients with chronic congestive heart failure, *N Engl J Med* 311:819-823, 1984.

22. Co-operative Veterinary Enalapril (COVE) Study Group: Controlled clinical evaluation of enalapril in dogs with heart failure—results of the Cooperative Veterinary Enalapril Study Group, *J Vet Intern Med* 9:243-252, 1995.

23. Creager MA, Cusco JA: Treatment of congestive heart failure with angiotensin-converting enzyme inhibitors. In McCall D, Rahimtoola SH, editors: *Heart failure,* New York, 1995, Chapman & Hall, pp. 316-344.

24. Creager MA, Halperin JL, Bernard DB, et al: Acute regional circulatory and renal hemodynamic effects of converting-enzyme inhibition in patients with congestive heart failure, *Circulation* 64:483-489, 1981.

25. Decarli C, Spouse G, Larosa JL: Serum magnesium levels in symptomatic atrial fibrillation and their relation to rhythm control by intravenous digoxin, *Am J Cardiol* 57:956-959, 1986.

26. Dirks JH, Cirksena WJ, Berliner RW: Micropuncture study of the effect of various diuretics on sodium reabsorption by the proximal tubules of the dog, *J Clin Invest* 45:1875-1885, 1966.

27. Dormans TP, Pickkers P, Russel FG, et al: Vascular effects of loop diuretics, *Cardiovasc Res* 32:988-997, 1996.

28. Dormans TP, van Meyel JJ, Gerlag PG, et al: Diuretic efficacy of high dose furosemide in severe heart failure: bolus injection versus continuous infusion, *J Am Coll Cardiol* 28:376-382, 1996.

29. Dow SJ, Fettman MJ, Smith KR, et al: Taurine depletion and cardiovascular disease in adult cats fed a potassium-depleted acidified diet, *Am J Vet Res* 53:402-405, 1992.

30. Dumont AE, Clauss RH, Reed GE, et al: Lymph drainage in patients with congestive heart failure: comparison with findings in hepatic cirrhosis, *N Engl J Med* 269:949-952, 1963.

31. Dzau VJ, Hollenberg NK: Renal response to captopril in severe heart failure: role of furosemide in natriuresis and reversal of hyponatremia, *Ann Intern Med* 100:777-781, 1984.

32. Dzau VJ, Swartz SL: Dissociation of the prostaglandin and renin-angiotensin systems during captopril therapy for chronic congestive heart failure secondary to coronary artery disease, *Am J Cardiol* 60:1101-1105, 1987.

33. Dzau VJ, Colucci WS, Hollenberg NK, et al: Relation of the renin-angiotensin-aldosterone system to clinical state in congestive heart failure, *Circulation* 63:645-651, 1981.

34. Dzau VJ, Packer M, Lilly LS, et al: Prostaglandins in severe congestive heart failure: relation to activation of the renin-angiotensin system and hyponatremia, *N Engl J Med* 310:347-352, 1984.

35. Eaton GE, Cody RJ, Brinkley PF: Increase in aortic impedance precedes peripheral vasoconstriction at the early stage of ventricular failure in the paced canine model, *Circulation* 88:2714-2721, 1993.

36. Edwards JN: Magnesium and congestive heart failure. *Proceedings of the American College of Veterinary Internal Medicine,* New Orleans, 1991, pp. 679-680.

37. Fenelon G, Protter AA, Stambler BS: Examination of the in vivo cardiac electrophysiological effects of nesiritide (human brain natriuretic peptide) in conscious dogs, *J Card Fail* 8:320-325, 2002.

38. Feuerstein GZ, Yue TL, Cheng HY, et al: Myocardial protection by the novel vasodilating beta-blocker, carvedilol: potential relevance of anti-oxidant activity, *J Hypertens Suppl* 11:S41-48, 1993.

39. Fichman MP, Vorherr H, Kleeman CR, et al: Diuretic-induced hyponatremia, *Ann Intern Med* 75:853-863, 1971.

40. Forrester JS, Diamond G, Chatterjee K, et al: Medical therapy of acute myocardial infarction by application of hemodynamic subsets, *N Engl J Med* 295:1404-1413, 1976.

41. Franciosa JA, Dunkman WB, Wilen M, et al: "Optimal" left ventricular filling pressure during nitroprusside infusion for congestive heart failure, *Am J Med* 74:457-464, 1983.

42. Francis GS, McDonald KM: Neurohumoral mechanisms in heart failure. In McCall D, Rahimtoola SH, editors: *Heart failure,* New York, 1995, Chapman & Hall, pp. 90-116.

43. Francis GS, Goldsmith SR, Levine TB, et al: The neurohumoral axis in congestive heart failure, *Ann Intern Med* 101:370-377, 1984.

44. Francis GS, Siegel RM, Goldsmith SR, et al: Acute vasoconstrictor response to intravenous furosemide in patients with chronic congestive heart failure. Activation of the neurohumoral axis, *Ann Intern Med* 103:1-6, 1985.

45. Francis GS: Neurohumoral mechanisms involved in congestive heart failure, *Am J Cardiol* 55:15A-21A, 1985.

46. Freeman LM, Rush JE, Kehayias JJ, et al: Nutritional alterations and the effect of fish oil supplementation in dogs with heart failure, *J Vet Intern Med* 12:440-448, 1998.

47. Freeman RH, Davis JD, Williams GM, et al: Effects of the oral angiotensin converting enzyme inhibitor, SQ 14225 in a model of low cardiac output in dogs, *Circ Res* 45:540-545, 1979.

48. Friedman E, Shadel M, Halkin H, et al: Thiazide-induced hyponatremia, *Ann Intern Med* 110:24-30, 1989.

49. Fulop M, Horowitz M, Aberman A, et al: Lactic acidosis in pulmonary edema due to left ventricular failure, *Ann Intern Med* 79:180-186, 1973.

50. Gaasch WH, Freeman GL: Functional properties of normal and failing hearts. In McCall D, Rahimtoola SH, editors: *Heart failure,* New York, 1995, Chapman & Hall, pp. 14-29.

51. Gerlag PGG, van Meijel JJM: High-dose furosemide in the treatment of refractory congestive heart failure, *Arch Intern Med* 148:286-291, 1988.

52. Gottlieb SS, Weir MR: Renal effects of angiotensin-converting enzyme inhibition in congestive heart failure, *Am J Cardiol* 66:14D-21D, 1990.

53. Gottlieb SS, Abraham W, Butler J, et al: The prognostic importance of different definitions of worsening renal

function in congestive heart failure, *J Card Fail* 8: 136-141, 2002.

54. Granger JP: Regulation of sodium excretion by renal interstitial hydrostatic pressure, *Fed Proc* 45:2892-2896, 1986.

55. Greco DS, Biller B, Van Liew CH: Measurement of plasma atrial natriuretic peptide as an indicator of prognosis in dogs with cardiac disease, *Can Vet J* 44:293-297, 2003.

56. Guyton AC, Lindsey AW: Effect of elevated left atrial pressure and decreased plasma protein concentration on the development of pulmonary edema, *Circ Res* 7:649-657, 1959.

57. Haggstrom J, Hansson K, Karlberg BE, et al: Effects of long-term treatment with enalapril or hydralazine on the renin-angiotensin-aldosterone system and fluid balance in dogs with naturally acquired mitral valve regurgitation, *Am J Vet Res* 57:1645-1652, 1996.

58. Hall JE, Guyton AC, Jackson TE, et al: Control of glomerular filtration rate by the renin-angiotensin system, *Am J Physiol* 233:F366-F372, 1977.

59. Hamlin RL, Smith RC, Powere TE, et al: Efficacy of various diuretics in normal dogs, *J Am Vet Med Assoc* 146:1417-1420, 1965.

60. Heinemann HO: Right-sided heart failure and the use of diuretics, *Am J Med* 64:367-369, 1978.

61. Higgins CB, Vatner SF, Eckberg DL, et al: Alterations in the baroreceptor reflex in conscious dogs with heart failure, *J Clin Invest* 51715-51724, 1972.

62. Hirsch AT, Muellerleile M, Dzau VJ: Cardiovascular tissue angiotensin systems: activation and actions in heart failure. In McCall D, Rahimtoola SH, editors: *Heart failure,* New York, 1995, Chapman & Hall, pp. 117-134.

63. Hirsch AT, Pinto YM, Schunkert H, et al: Potential role of the tissue renin-angiotensin system in the pathophysiology of congestive heart failure, *Am J Cardiol* 66:22D-32D, 1990.

64. Hollander W, Judson WE: The relationship of cardiovascular and renal hemodynamic function to sodium excretion in patients with severe heart disease but without edema, *J Clin Invest* 35:970-979, 1956.

65. Ichikawa I, Pfeffer JM, Pfeffer MA, et al: Role of angiotensin II in the altered renal function of congestive heart failure, *Circ Res* 55:669-675, 1984.

66. IMPROVE Study Group: Acute and short-term hemodynamic, echocardiographic, and clinical effects of enalapril maleate in dogs with naturally acquired heart failure: results of the Invasive Multicenter Prospective Veterinary Evaluation of Enalapril study, *J Vet Intern Med* 9:234-242, 1995.

67. Jackson EK: Diuretics. In Hardman JG, Limbird LE, Molinoff PB, et al: *Goodman & Gilman's the pharmacological basis of therapeutics,* ed 9, New York, 1996, McGraw-Hill, pp. 685-714.

68. Jensen KT, Carstens J, Pedersen EB: Effect of BNP on renal hemodynamics, tubular function and vasoactive hormones in humans, *Am J Physiol* 274:F63-72, 1998.

69. Kaloyanides GJ: Pathogenesis and treatment of edema with special reference to the use of diuretics. In Maxwell MH, Kleeman CR, editors: *Clinical disorders of fluid and electrolyte metabolism,* New York, 1980, McGraw-Hill, pp. 647-701.

70. Katz AM: Cardiomyopathy of overload: a major determinant of prognosis in congestive heart failure, *N Engl J Med* 322:100-110, 1990.

71. Keane WR, Shapiro BE: Renal protective effects of angiotensin-converting enzyme inhibition, *Am J Cardiol* 65:491-531, 1990.

72. Keene BW, Rush JE: Therapy of heart failure. In Ettinger SJ, editor: *Textbook of veterinary internal medicine,* ed 3, Philadelphia, 1989, WB Saunders, pp. 939-975.

73. Khanna C, Lund EM, Raffe M, et al: Hypomagnesemia in 188 dogs: a hospital population-based prevalence study, *J Vet Intern Med* 12:304-309, 1998.

74. Kim S, Iwao H: Molecular and cellular mechanisms of angiotensin II-mediated cardiovascular and renal diseases, *Pharmacol Rev* 52:11-34, 2001.

75. Kinugawa T, Thames MC: Baroreflexes in heart failure. In McCall D, Rahimtoola SH, editors: *Heart failure,* New York, 1995, Chapman & Hall, pp. 30-45.

76. Kitagawa H, Wakamiya H, Kitoh K, et al: Efficacy of monotherapy with benazepril, an angiotensin converting enzyme inhibitor, in dogs with naturally acquired chronic mitral insufficiency, *J Vet Med Sci* 59:513-520, 1997.

77. Kittleson M, Keene B, Pion PD, et al: Results of the Multicenter Spaniel Trial (MUST): taurine and carnitine responsive dilated cardiomyopathy in American cocker spaniels with decreased plasma taurine concentration, *J Vet Intern Med* 11:204-211, 1997.

78. Knowlen GG, Kittleson MD, Nachreiner RF, et al: Comparison of plasma aldosterone concentration among clinical status groups of dogs with chronic heart failure, *J Am Vet Med Assoc* 183:991-996, 1983.

79. Koch J, Pedersen HD, Jensen AL, et al: Activation of the renin-angiotensin system in dogs with asymptomatic and symptomatic dilated cardiomyopathy, *Res Vet Sci* 59:172-175, 1995.

80. Kubo SH: Neurohormonal activation and the response to converting enzyme inhibitors in congestive heart failure, *Circulation* 81(suppl III):107-114, 1990.

81. Kvart C, Haggstrom J, Pedersen HD, et al: Efficacy of enalapril for prevention of congestive heart failure in dogs with myxomatous valve disease and asymptomatic mitral regurgitation, *J Vet Intern Med* 16:80-88, 2002.

82. Levens NR: Control of renal function by intrarenal angiotensin II in the dog, *J Cardiovasc Pharmacol* 16(suppl 4):565-569, 1990.

83. Levin A, Djurdjev O, Barret B, et al: Cardiovascular disease in patients with chronic kidney disease: getting to the heart of the matter, *Am J Kidney Dis* 38:1398-1407, 2001.

84. Levine TB, Francis GS, Goldsmith SR, et al: Activity of the sympathetic nervous system and renin-angiotensin system assessed by plasma hormone levels and their relation to hemodynamic abnormalities in congestive heart failure, *Am J Cardiol* 49:1659-1666, 1982.

85. Levy M: Effects of acute volume expansion and altered hemodynamics on renal tubular function in chronic caval dogs, *J Clin Invest* 51:922-938, 1972.

86. Licata G, Di Pasquale P, Parrinello G, et al: Effects of high-dose furosemide and small-volume hypertonic saline solution infusion in comparison with a high dose of furosemide as bolus in refractory congestive heart failure: long-term effects, *Am Heart J* 145:459-466, 2003.

87. Lifschitz MD, Schrier RW: Alterations in cardiac output with chronic constriction of thoracic inferior vena cava, *Am J Physiol* 225:1364-1370, 1973.

88. Little CJ, Julu PO, Hansen S, et al: Non-invasive real-time measurements of cardiac vagal tone in dogs with cardiac disease, *Vet Rec* 156:101-105, 2005.

89. Luis Fuentes V: Use of pimobendan in the management of heart failure, *Vet Clin North Am Small Anim Pract* 34:1145-1155, 2004.

90. MacDonald KA, Kittleson MD, Munro C, et al: Brain natriuretic peptide concentration in dogs with heart disease and congestive heart failure, *J Vet Intern Med* 17:172-177, 2003.

91. Margulies KG, Hilderbrand FL, Lerman A, et al: Increased endothelin in experimental heart failure, *Circulation* 82:2226-2232, 1990.

92. Mettauer B, Roulearu J-L, Bichet D, et al: Sodium and water excretion abnormalities in congestive heart failure, *Ann Intern Med* 105:161-167, 1986.

93. Michell AR: Physiological aspects of the requirement for sodium in mammals, *Nutr Res Rev* 2:149-160, 1989.

94. Migdal S, Alexander EA, Levinsky NG: Evidence that decreased cardiac output is not the stimulus to sodium retention during acute constriction of the vena cava, *J Lab Clin Med* 89:809-816, 1977.

95. Millard RW, Higgins CB, Franklin D, et al: Regulation of the renal circulation during severe exercise in normal dogs and dogs with experimental heart failure, *Circ Res* 31:881-888, 1972.

96. Miller WC, Simi WW, Rice DL: Contribution of systemic venous hypertension to the development of pulmonary edema in dogs, *Circ Res* 43:598-600, 1978.

97. Molina CR, Fowler MB, McCrory S, et al: Hemodynamic, renal, and endocrine effects of atrial natriuretic peptide infusion in severe heart failure, *J Am Coll Cardiol* 12:175-186, 1988.

98. Morita H, Suzuki G, Mishima T, et al: Effects of long-term monotherapy with metoprolol CR/XL on the progression of left ventricular dysfunction and remodeling in dogs with chronic heart failure, *Cardiovasc Drugs Ther* 16:443-449, 2002.

99. Morris ML, Patton RL, Teeter SM: Low sodium diet in heart disease: how low is low? *Vet Med Small Anim Clin* 9:1225-1227, 1976.

100. Munagala VK, Burnett JC Jr, Redfield MM: The natriuretic peptides in cardiovascular medicine, *Curr Probl Cardiol* 29:707-769, 2004.

101. Naitoh M, Suzuki H, Murakami M, et al: Effects of oral AVP receptor antagonists OPC-21268 and OPC-31260 on congestive heart failure in conscious dogs, *Am J Physiol* 267:H2245-2254, 1994.

102. Nomura A, Yasuda H, Minami M, et al: Effect of furosemide in congestive heart failure, *Clin Pharmacol Ther* 30:177-182, 1981.

103. O'Connor CM, Gattis WA, Swedberg K: Current and novel pharmacologic approaches in advanced heart failure, *Am Heart J* 135:S249-S263, 1998.

104. Oliver JA, Sciacca RR, Pinto J, et al: Participation of the prostaglandins in the control of renal blood flow during acute reduction of cardiac output in the dog, *J Clin Invest* 67:229-237, 1981.

105. Opie LH, Kaplan NM: Diuretics. In Opie LH, Gersh BJ, editors: *Drugs for the Heart*, ed 6, Philadelphia, 2005, Elsevier/WB Saunders, pp. 80-103.

106. Opie LH: *Heart physiology: from cell to circulation*, ed 4, Baltimore, 2003, Lippincott Williams & Wilkins.

107. Osborn JL, Holdaas H, Thames MD, et al: Renal adrenoreceptor mediation of antinatriuretic and renin secretion responses to low frequency renal nerve stimulation in the dog, *Circ Res* 53:298-305, 1983.

108. Oster JR, Epstein M, Smoller S: Combination therapy with thiazide-type and loop diuretic agents for resistant sodium retention, *Ann Intern Med* 99:405-406, 1983.

109. Packer M, Lee WH, Kessler PD: Preservation of glomerular filtration rate in human heart failure by activation of the renin-angiotensin system, *Circulation* 74:766-774, 1986.

110. Packer M, Lee WH, Medina N, et al: Functional renal insufficiency during long-term therapy with captopril and enalapril in severe chronic heart failure, *Ann Intern Med* 106:346-354, 1987.

111. Packer M, Lee WH, Medina N, et al: Influence of renal function on the hemodynamic and clinical responses to long-term captopril therapy in severe chronic heart failure, *Ann Intern Med* 104:147-154, 1986.

112. Packer M, McMurray J, Massie BM, et al: Clinical effects of endothelin receptor antagonism with bosentan in patients with severe chronic heart failure: results of a pilot study, *J Card Fail* 11:12-20, 2005.

113. Packer M, Medina N, Yshak M: Correction of dilutional hyponatremia in severe chronic heart failure by converting-enzyme inhibition, *Ann Intern Med* 100:782-789, 1984.

114. Packer M: Neurohumoral interactions and adaptations in congestive heart failure, *Am J Cardiol* 55:1A-10A, 1985.

115. Paradiso G, Bakris GL, Stein JH: The kidney and heart failure. In McCall D, Rahimtoola SH, editors: *Heart failure*, New York, 1995, Chapman & Hall, pp. 135-158.

116. Parmley WW: Pathophysiology of congestive heart failure, *Am J Cardiol* 55:9A-14A, 1985.

117. Patak RV, Fadem SZ, Rosenblatt SG, et al: Diuretic-induced changes in renal blood flow and prostaglandin E excretion in the dog, *Am J Physiol* 236:F494-F500, 1979.

118. Pedersen HD, Koch J, Poulsen K, et al: Activation of the renin-angiotensin system in dogs with asymptomatic and mildly symptomatic mitral valvular insufficiency, *J Vet Intern Med* 9:328-331, 1995.

119. Pedersen HD, Schutt T, Sondergaard R, et al: Decreased plasma concentration of nitric oxide metabolites in dogs with untreated mitral regurgitation, *J Vet Intern Med* 17:178-184, 2003.

120. Pedersen HD: Effects of mild mitral-valve insufficiency, sodium-intake, and place of blood-sampling on the renin-angiotensin system in dogs, *Acta Vet Scand* 37:109-118, 1996.

121. Pion PD, Kittleson MD: Therapy for feline aortic thromboembolism. In Kirk RW, editor: *Current veterinary therapy X*, Philadelphia, 1989, WB Saunders, pp. 295-301.

122. Pitt B, Zannad F, Remme WJ, et al: The Randomized Aldactone Evaluation Study Investigators: the effect of spironolactone on morbidity and mortality in patients with severe heart failure, *N Engl J Med* 341:709-717, 1999.

123. Pouchelon JL (for the Benazepril in Canine Heart Disease Study Group (BENCH): The effect of benazepril on survival times and clinical signs of dogs with congestive heart failure: results of the multicenter, prospective, randomized, double-blind, placebo-controlled, long term clinical trial, *J Vet Cardiol* 1:7-18, 1999.

124. Priebe H, Heimann JC, Hedley-Whyte J: Effects of renal and hepatic venous congestion on renal function in the presence of low and normal cardiac output in dogs, *Circ Res* 47:883-890, 1980.

125. Prosek R, Sisson DD, Oyama MA, et al: Plasma endothelin-1 immunoreactivity in normal dogs and dogs with acquired heart disease, *J Vet Intern Med* 18:840-844, 2004.

126. Reinhardt HW, Kaczmarczy KG, Eisele R, et al: Left atrial pressure and sodium balance in conscious dogs on a low sodium intake, *Pflugers Arch* 370:59-66, 1977.

127. Riegger GA, Elsner D, Kroner EP, et al: Atrial natriuretic peptide in congestive heart failure in the dog: plasma

levels, cyclic guanidine monophosphate, ultrastructure of atrial myoendocrine cells, and hemodynamic, hormonal, and renal effects, *Circulation* 77:398-406, 1988.

128. Riegger GA, Liebau G, Kochsiek K: Antidiuretic hormone in congestive heart failure, *Am J Med* 72:49-52, 1982.

129. Riegger GA, Liebau G, Holzschuh M, et al: Role of the renin-angiotensin system in the development of congestive heart failure in the dog as assessed by chronic converting-enzyme blockade, *Am J Cardiol* 53:614-618, 1984.

130. Ritz E, Nowack R: Detrimental and beneficial effects of converting enzyme inhibitors on the kidney, *J Cardiol Pharmacol* 16(suppl 4):570-575, 1990.

131. Roche BM, Schwartz D, Lehnhard RA, et al: Changes in concentrations of neuroendocrine hormones and catecholamines in dogs with myocardial failure induced by rapid ventricular pacing, *Am J Vet Res* 63:1413-1417, 2003.

132. Rose BD, Post TW: *Clinical physiology of acid base and electrolyte disorders,* ed 5, New York, 2001, McGraw Hill, p. 702.

133. Rose BD, Post TW: *Clinical physiology of acid base and electrolyte disorders,* ed 5, New York, 2001, McGraw Hill, p. 677.

134. Rose BD: Diuretics, *Kidney Int* 39:336-352, 1991.

135. Roudebush P, Allen TA, Kuehn NF, et al: The effect of combined therapy with captopril, furosemide, and a sodium-restricted diet on serum electrolyte concentrations and renal function in normal dogs and dogs with congestive heart failure, *J Vet Intern Med* 8:337-342, 1994.

136. Rush JE, Freeman LM, Brown DJ, et al: Clinical, echocardiographic, and neurohormonal effects of a sodium-restricted diet in dogs with heart failure, *J Vet Intern Med* 14:513-520, 2000.

137. Rush JE, Freeman LM, Brown DJ, et al: The use of enalapril in the treatment of feline hypertrophic cardiomyopathy, *J Am Anim Hosp Assoc* 34:38-41, 1998.

138. Ryan MP: Diuretics and potassium/magnesium depletion: directions for treatment, *Am J Med* 82(suppl 3A):38-47, 1987.

139. Sabbah HN, Sharov VG, Gupta RC, et al: Chronic therapy with metoprolol attenuates cardiomyocyte apoptosis in dogs with heart failure, *J Am Coll Cardiol* 36:1698-1705, 2000.

140. Sabbah HN, Shimoyama H, Kono T, et al: Effects of long-term monotherapy with enalapril, metoprolol, and digoxin on the progression of left ventricular dysfunction and dilation in dogs with reduced ejection fraction, *Circulation* 89:2852-2859, 1994.

141. Schrier RW, Abraham WT: Hormones and hemodynamics in heart failure, *N Engl J Med* 341:577-585, 1999.

142. Schrier RW, Humphreys MH, Ufferman RC: Role of cardiac output and the autonomic nervous system in the antinatriuretic response to acute constriction of the thoracic superior vena cava, *Circ Res* 29:490-498, 1971.

143. Schrier RW: Pathogenesis of sodium and water retention in high output and low output cardiac failure, nephrotic syndrome, cirrhosis and pregnancy, *N Engl J Med* 319:1065-1072; 1127-1134, 1988.

144. Seely JF, Dirks JH: Site of action of diuretic drugs, *Kidney Int* 11:1-8, 1977.

145. Shimoyama H, Sabbah HN, Rosman H, et al: Effects of long-term therapy with enalapril on severity of functional mitral regurgitation in dogs with moderate heart failure, *J Am Coll Cardiol* 25:768-772, 1995.

146. Sisson DD: Neuroendocrine evaluation of cardiac disease, *Vet Clin North Am Small Anim Pract* 34:1105-1126, 2004.

147. Starling EH: The influence of mechanized factors on lymph production, *J Physiol (Lond)* 10:14-155, 1894.

148. Staub NC: Pathophysiology of pulmonary edema. In Staub NC, Taylor AE, editors: *Edema,* New York, 1984, Raven Press, pp. 719-746.

149. Suki WN, Rector FC Jr, Seldin DW: The site of action of furosemide and other sulfonamide diuretics in the dog, *J Clin Invest* 44:1458-1469, 1965.

150. Suki WN: Renal hemodynamic consequences of angiotensin-converting enzyme inhibition in congestive heart failure, *Arch Intern Med* 149:669-673, 1989.

151. Sun Y, Weber KT: Cardiac remodelling by fibrous tissue—Role of local factors and circulating hormones, *Ann Med* 30(suppl 1):S3-S8, 1998.

152. Suzuki G, Morita H, Mishima T, et al: Effects of long-term monotherapy with eplerenone, a novel aldosterone blocker, on progression of left ventricular dysfunction and remodeling in dogs with heart failure, *Circulation* 106:2967-2972, 2002.

153. Swales JD: Magnesium deficiency and diuretics, *BMJ* 285:1377-1378, 1982.

154. Swan HJC, Ganz W, Forrester J, et al: Catheterization of the heart in man with use of a flow-directed balloon-tipped catheter, *N Engl J Med* 283:447-451, 1970.

155. Tachibana H, Cheng HJ, Ukai T, et al: Levosimendan improves LV systolic and diastolic performance at rest and during exercise after heart failure, *Am J Physiol (Heart Circ Physiol)* 288:H914-922, 2005.

156. Taylor AE: Capillary fluid filtration: Starling forces and lymph flow, *Circ Res* 49:557-575, 1982.

157. Thames MD: Acetylstrophanthidin-induced reflex inhibition of canine renal sympathetic nerve activity mediated by cardiac receptors with vagal afferents, *Circ Res* 44:8-15, 1979.

158. Thomas CJ, Woods RL: Haemodynamic action of B-type natriuretic peptide substantially outlasts its plasma half-life in conscious dogs, *Clin Exp Pharmacol Physiol* 30:369-375, 2003.

159. Thomas JA, Marks BH: Plasma norepinephrine in congestive heart failure, *Am J Cardiol* 41:233-243, 1978.

160. Thrall DE, Calvert CA: Radiographic evaluation of canine heartworm disease coexisting with right heart failure, *Vet Radiol* 24:124-126, 1983.

161. Uechi M, Matsuoka M, Kuwajima E, et al: The effects of the loop diuretics furosemide and torsemide on diuresis in dogs and cats, *J Vet Med Sci* 65:1057-1061, 2003.

162. Uechi M, Sasaki T, Ueno K, et al: Cardiovascular and renal effects of carvedilol in dogs with heart failure, *J Vet Med Sci* 64:469-475, 2002.

163. van der Zander K, Houben AJ, Kroon AA, et al: Does brain natriuretic peptide have a direct renal effect in human hypertensives? *Hypertension* 41:119-123, 2003.

164. Van Veldhuisen DJ, Genth-Zoth S, Brouwer J, et al: High-versus low-dose ACE inhibition in chronic heart failure: a double-blind, placebo-controlled study of imidapril, *J Am Coll Cardiol* 32:1811-1818, 1998.

165. Vasko MR, Brown-Cartwright D, Knochel JP, et al: Furosemide absorption altered in decompensated congestive heart failure, *Ann Intern Med* 102:314-318, 1985.

166. Vollmar AM, Montag C, Preusser U, et al: Atrial natriuretic peptide and plasma volume of dogs suffering from heart failure or dehydration, *Zentralbl Veterinarmed A* 41:548-557, 1994.

167. Vollmar AM, Preusser U, Gerbes AL, et al: Endothelin concentration in plasma of healthy dogs and dogs with congestive heart failure, renal failure, diabetes mellitus, and hyperadrenocorticism, *J Vet Intern Med* 9:105-111, 1995.

168. Wang W: Chronic administration of aldosterone depresses baroreceptor reflex function in the dog, *Hypertension* 24:571-575, 1994.

169. Ware WA, Lund DD, Subieta AR, et al: Sympathetic activation in dogs with congestive heart failure caused by chronic mitral valve disease and dilated cardiomyopathy, *J Am Vet Med Assoc* 197:1475-1481, 1990.

170. Watkins L Jr, Burton JA, Haber E, et al: The renin-angiotensin-aldosterone system in congestive failure in conscious dogs, *J Clin Invest* 57:1606-1617, 1976.

171. Weaver LJ, Carrico CJ: Congestive heart failure and edema. In Staub NC, Taylor AE, editors: *Edema*, New York, 1984, Raven Press, pp. 543-562.

172. Weber KT: Aldosterone and spironolactone in heart failure [editorial], *N Engl J Med* 341:709-717, 1999.

173. Weber KT: Furosemide in the long-term management of heart failure: the good, the bad, and the uncertain, *J Am Coll Cardiol* 44:1308-1310, 2004.

174. Wiener-Kronish JP, Goldstein R, Matthay RA, et al: Lack of association of pleural effusion with chronic pulmonary arterial and right atrial hypertension, *Chest* 92:967-970, 1987.

175. Yatsu T, Tomura Y, Tahara A, et al: Pharmacological profile of YM087, a novel nonpeptide dual vasopressin V1A and V2 receptor antagonist, in dogs, *Eur J Pharmacol* 321:225-230, 1997.

176. Zucker IH, Share L, Gilmore JP: Renal effects of left atrial distension in dogs with chronic congestive heart failure, *Am J Physiol* 236:H554-H560, 1979.

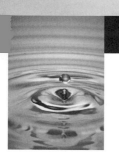

CHAPTER · 22

FLUID THERAPY DURING INTRINSIC RENAL FAILURE

Dennis J. Chew and Jennifer A. Gieg

Normal renal function, including maintenance of extracellular fluid (ECF) volume and osmolality, normal electrolyte concentrations, and acid-base balance, is essential for stability of the internal milieu. Excretion of metabolic waste products, biosynthesis of hormones, and degradation of reabsorbed peptides are additional essential renal functions. The amount of water and electrolytes presented to and processed by the kidneys on a daily basis is enormous. Consequently, it is not surprising that failure of normal renal function is associated with failure to regulate the volume and composition of the ECF. An overview of normal renal function is presented in Chapter 2.

Intrinsic (primary) renal failure is present whenever functional and histopathologic lesions in the kidneys result in accumulation of nitrogenous waste products (e.g., urea, creatinine) in the blood. Loss of at least 75% of renal excretory function (reversible or irreversible) must occur before blood urea nitrogen (BUN) or serum creatinine concentrations become increased (i.e., before azotemia is detected). Serum phosphorus concentration becomes increased with further loss (≥85%) of excretory renal function.

Intrinsic renal failure may be divided further into failure with acute or chronic causes.[26,106] The approach to fluid therapy in the patient with renal failure is similar regardless of the specific histologic diagnosis. Although a specific diagnosis is important in establishing a prognosis and making adjustments in therapy, it is not necessary for the initial treatment of the patient with intrinsic renal failure.

Chronic renal failure (CRF) may occur with greater frequency in older cats than in older dogs.[92] A survey found renal disease to be more prevalent in cats than dogs receiving care at veterinary clinics.[93] CRF is much more common than acute renal failure (ARF) in both species. ARF was diagnosed in approximately 30% of dogs with renal disease in one series[129] but in only 5% in another study.[5] Isolated ischemic events accounted for 33% of the cases in dogs, followed by 22% in which no underlying cause could be found, 21% with isolated exposure to a nephrotoxicant, 18% with multiple disorders, and 5% with isolated miscellaneous disorders (e.g., leptospirosis, pyelonephritis, renal lymphoma).[129] In a series of dogs with hospital-acquired ARF, 72% had been exposed recently to a nephrotoxicant and 14% had undergone anesthesia within the previous 2 weeks; chronic heart disease, neoplasia, and fever were conditions commonly associated with ARF.[5]

Both CRF and ARF may be subdivided into oliguric or nonoliguric forms (Box 22-1). CRF usually is characterized by polyuria, but affected animals may be transiently oliguric when dehydrated, and permanent oliguria develops during terminal decompensation. Patients with ARF can be either oliguric or nonoliguric. Animals with ARF often are clinically more ill (based on history, clinical signs, and laboratory evaluation) than are those with compensated CRF. However, decompensated CRF patients may be as sick as those with ARF. "Acute-on-chronic" renal failure is a common situation in which acute prerenal azotemia caused by vomiting, anorexia, and hypodipsia aggravates preexisting azotemia. The CRF patient also is at greater risk for developing acute tubular necrosis resulting from ischemia caused by dehydration. Thirty-five percent of dogs with hospital-acquired renal failure had preexisting renal disease.[5] Severe anemia may necessitate blood transfusion in CRF patients and occasionally in ARF patients. Hypoproteinemia arising from chronic glomerular disease may require infusion of plasma, hetastarch, or human albumin, but this aspect of therapy is not addressed in this chapter. See Box 22-2 for a list of the clinical abnormalities that may require fluid therapy in patients with renal failure.

Parenteral fluid therapy is the most important treatment consideration for patients in uremic crisis whether because of ARF or CRF. Fluid therapy goals include ECF volume expansion, correction of serious electrolyte and acid-base disturbances, reduction of the magnitude of azotemia, and provision of red blood cells when needed. Nutritional support during early stabilization has not received much emphasis in veterinary literature but is important. Fluid therapy must be integrated with other treatments in the uremic patient. In those with oliguric intrinsic renal failure, the patient must be monitored for retention of water and electrolytes, whereas losses of water and electrolytes must be replaced in patients with polyuric intrinsic renal failure.

GENERAL PRINCIPLES AND GOALS

Rarely is the exact nature of the underlying disease process responsible for intrinsic renal failure known at the time therapy must be instituted. Consequently, treatment and further diagnostic testing must be carried out simultaneously. Box 22-3 presents an overview of the goals of fluid therapy in the patient with renal failure, and Box 22-4 presents a recommended diagnostic and therapeutic approach.

Box 22-2	Uremic Signs and Problems That May Require Fluid Therapy Support

Gastrointestinal
Anorexia
Vomiting
Diarrhea
Hypodipsia

Altered Urine Production
Polydipsia
Polyuria
Oliguria
Anuria

Blood
Anemia
Lack of production
Blood loss
Decreased red cell life span

Hypoproteinemia
Blood loss
Increased glomerular permeability

Box 22-1	Renal Failure Syndromes Requiring Fluid Therapy

Common
Polyuric chronic renal failure
Oligoanuric acute renal failure
Nonoliguric acute renal failure

Uncommon
Oliguric chronic renal failure
Nephrotic syndrome

The primary aim of therapy during severe uremia is to correct alterations in the patient's internal milieu. Ideally, treatment allows the patient to live long enough to allow repair of renal damage in acute injury and hypertrophy of viable remnant nephrons in chronic injury, resulting in improved renal function and ability to sustain life without extensive medical support. Existing renal lesions are not directly amenable to therapy. Adequate ECF volume must be maintained to maximize renal perfusion and facilitate excretory function. Fluid therapy during uremic crises usually is successful at least until a definitive diagnosis and prognosis can be made.

Intravenous fluid therapy also provides an avenue for intensive diuresis so that azotemia is reduced. A combination of fluid administration for rehydration, maintenance, and mild volume expansion and diuretic administration can be used in an attempt to increase glomerular filtration rate (GFR), renal blood flow (RBF), and renal tubular fluid flow rate in animals with apparent primary (intrinsic) renal failure. BUN, serum creatinine, and serum phosphorus concentrations decrease if therapy successfully increases GFR. BUN concentration can decrease without a change in GFR because increased renal tubular fluid flow rate reduces passive tubular reabsorption of urea, but creatinine is not affected by changes in tubular flow rate.[53,56] For these reasons, BUN often decreases out of

---

Box 22-3 | **General Goals of Parenteral Fluid Therapy for Uremic Patients**

Survival
Temporary
Awaiting a specific diagnosis
Formulating a prognosis
Awaiting results of a renal biopsy
Awaiting implementation of dialysis

Long-Standing
Recompensation in chronic renal failure
Reclamation of renal function and histology in acute renal failure

Reduction in Magnitude of Azotemia
Improvement in Renal Function or Resolution of Renal Lesions
Maximization of Endogenous Renal Excretory Function
Correct prerenal component
Increase glomerular filtration rate (GFR)
Increase tubular flow rate (with or without an increase in GFR)
Preferential decrease in blood urea nitrogen versus serum creatinine

Improved Quality of Life

Box 22-4 | **Initial Diagnostic and Therapeutic Sequence for the Uremic Patient**

Obtain Baseline Data (Before Any Treatment)
Body weight, skin turgor, vital signs
Packed cell volume and total protein, urinalysis
Blood urea nitrogen, serum creatinine, serum phosphorus
Sodium, potassium, chloride
Total CO_2 or blood gases

Rule Out Prerenal and Postrenal Azotemia Immediately

Start Fluid Treatments

Fluid Challenge Response

Rule Out Other Potentially Reversible Causes for Decreased Glomerular Filtration Rate
Urinary tract infection
Hypercalcemia
Hypokalemia and potassium depletion
Leptospirosis

Determine the Cause of the Intrinsic Renal Failure
Complete urinalysis
Urine specific gravity before fluids
Urine dipstrip
Fresh urine sediment
Urine protein-to-creatinine ratio
Urine culture
Renal imaging
    Radiography
    Ultrasonography
    Excretory urography
Renal biopsy

Repeat Baseline Data During Fluid Treatments

---

proportion to serum creatinine concentration when diuresis ensues.

Initial therapy for uremic animals is directed at correction of all potential prerenal factors that may be contributing to the azotemia. The intravenous route is used for fluid administration to ensure rapid access to the circulation and maximize renal perfusion. The volume of fluid administered must be chosen and monitored carefully. Animals that remain oligoanuric may become overhydrated by excessive fluid infusion, whereas it may be difficult to administer sufficient fluid volume to correct dehydration in animals with severe polyuria. Overhydration also may occur in animals without oliguria if their ability to excrete a water load is severely impaired.

The most life-threatening fluid, electrolyte, and acid-base disturbances should be corrected first while searching for potential causes of intrinsic renal failure. Drugs capable of causing ARF (e.g., aminoglycosides) should be discontinued. Hypovolemia should be corrected during a 4- to 6-hour period to enhance renal perfusion rapidly. Loss of renal autoregulatory function may prevent kidneys damaged by ischemia, nephrotoxins, or chronic disease from protecting themselves against ongoing or future episodes of reduced renal perfusion. Further renal injury is sustained in these instances if renal hypotension develops or persists. Fluid therapy regimens for treatment of uremic patients have not been standardized in veterinary medicine, and what follows is based largely on empirical experience.

INITIAL STABILIZATION

ROUTE OF FLUID ADMINISTRATION

The oral and subcutaneous routes of fluid administration are not satisfactory for the initial phase of treatment of severely uremic patients. The azotemic patient may be vomiting and have unreliable gastrointestinal absorption of water and electrolytes. Subcutaneous absorption of fluid also may be unreliable, especially if moderate or severe dehydration is present. Also, it is difficult to administer large volumes of fluid by the subcutaneous route. Consequently, the intravenous route is essential during the initial treatment of uremic patients with substantial dehydration, severe ongoing fluid losses (e.g., vomiting, diarrhea, polyuria), or serious disturbances of electrolyte and acid-base balance.

Placement of a sterile indwelling jugular venous catheter is preferred for the initial management of severe uremia so that central venous pressure (CVP) can be monitored during aggressive fluid administration. Fluid administration should be discontinued temporarily or markedly curtailed if CVP exceeds 13 cm H_2O or if it increases acutely by 2 cm H_2O or more during any 10-minute period. A fluid challenge with 20 mL/kg administered over 10 minutes can be used to assess the likelihood of subsequent volume overload. The CVP should not increase more than 2 cm H_2O if cardiovascular function is normal.[25] If available, measurement of pulmonary capillary wedge pressure can provide an earlier warning about impending volume overload.

REHYDRATION

Fluid needs for rehydration can be calculated (estimated percentage of dehydration × body weight in kilograms = liters required) or administered as two to three times the required maintenance fluid (i.e., 120 to 180 mL/kg/day). Hypovolemic shock, if present, should be treated with fluids administered at a rate of 90 mL/kg/hr with or without CVP monitoring until cardiovascular status has been stabilized. Additional fluids are administered to match sensible (urinary volume), insensible (respiratory and gastrointestinal losses of ~20 mL/kg/day), and contemporary (estimated volume from vomiting and diarrhea) fluid losses. Urine output is variable in patients with intrinsic renal failure, and it is advisable to place an indwelling urinary catheter to monitor urine output and facilitate fluid therapy for the initial 24 to 48 hours. Alternatively, urine can be collected in a metabolic cage. For cats, the weight of the litter pan or saturated cage pads can be determined sequentially, provided that a starting dry weight is known. Visualization of urinations and serial palpation of bladder filling during fluid therapy are the least reliable methods for determining urine production.

URINE OUTPUT

Recognition of Oliguria

Prompt recognition of oliguria is important because it dictates the volume of fluid that can be safely administered. Oliguria at presentation may result from hypovolemia (caused by hypodipsia, anorexia, vomiting, and diarrhea), severe intrarenal damage, or both. Although not present initially, oliguria may develop later during treatment of patients with ARF and CRF. Development of oliguria at any point during the course of treatment mandates meticulous attention to further fluid infusion to avoid overhydration.

Oliguria has been defined variably as less than 0.27 mL/kg/hr,[48] less than 0.48 mL/kg/hr,[41,106] and less than 1.0 to 2.0 mL/kg/hr.[76] Normal dogs and cats produce a minimal urine volume of approximately 1.0 mL/kg/hr if not under the stress of acute study,[6,71,121] whereas dogs suddenly caged without food produced approximately half this volume.[41] Liberal criteria should be used to document oliguria in uremic patients. Urine production of less than 1.0 mL/kg/hr (24 mL/kg/day) is considered absolute oliguria, whereas urine production of 1.0 to 2.0 mL/kg/hr during intravenous fluid infusion is considered relative oliguria. Healthy kidneys are expected to produce a brisk diuresis (urine output ranging from 2.0 to 5.0 mL/kg/hr) after intravenous administration of fluids for correction of dehydration and expansion of the ECF volume.[111] A prompt and brisk diuresis during intravenous fluid infusion suggests that initial oliguria probably was physiologic (prerenal) in nature.

Anuria (0 mL/kg/hr in 18%) and oliguria (0.1 to 1.0 mL/kg/hr in 43%) were documented in more than 60% of 44 dogs with ARF whose urine output was measured. Normal urine output (1 to 2 mL/kg/hr in 25%) and polyuria (>2 mL/kg/hr in 14%) were found in the remaining dogs.[129] Dogs that were oliguric (<0.25 mL/kg/hr) at the time of diagnosis of hospital-acquired ARF and that remained oliguric after at least 6 hours of fluid therapy were 20 times more likely to die or be euthanized than were dogs with greater urine production.[5]

"Ins and Outs"

Direct measurement of urine output allows the clinician to match fluid therapy to the needs of the dehydrated animal with either severe oliguria or diuresis. When this approach is not used, fluid requirements in an oliguric animal may be overestimated (resulting in overhydration), and requirements in an animal undergoing extensive diuresis may be underestimated (resulting in failure to correct dehydration). Using this technique, the day is divided into six 4-hour intervals. Other intervals (e.g., every hour, every 6 hours, every 8 hours) may be chosen based on the animal's condition. The fluid requirement for this interval is determined using both insensible (20 mL/kg divided by 6 for a 4-hour interval) and measured sensible (urine volume) losses during the same period. The measured volume of sensible (urinary) losses from the previous 4-hour period is given back to the patient in the next 4-hour period along with the calculated insensible requirement. Previously calculated dehydration needs are replaced first, and then the "ins and outs" method just described is carried out. This close attention to fluid volume is of benefit in the initial treatment of critically ill animals, especially when cardiovascular and renal status is uncertain.

FLUID QUALITY

Normal saline (0.9% NaCl) often is the initial fluid of choice for intravascular rehydration because it contains abundant sodium (154 mEq/L) and is devoid of potassium. The type of fluid chosen for correction of dehydration should be based on the patient's serum sodium concentration. Lactated Ringers and Plasmalyte-148 both contain slightly lower sodium at 130 mEq/L and 140 mEq/L respectively. If hypernatremia is persistent despite use of low sodium crystalloids, 0.45% NaCl may be needed (77 mEq/L). When rehydration has been accomplished, hypotonic fluids (0.45% NaCl in 2.5% dextrose) may be used for maintenance needs to prevent development of hypernatremia. Hypernatremia commonly develops in patients with primary renal failure that continue to receive fluids high in sodium relative to sodium maintenance needs (e.g., lactated Ringer's solution, 0.9% NaCl) after initial rehydration.

Potassium supplementation of fluids must be monitored carefully by measurement of serum potassium concentration. Serum potassium concentration is affected by urine output, renal excretory function, metabolic acidosis, oral intake, and rate of parenteral fluid administration (see Chapter 5). In general, potassium supplementation is not recommended during the initial hours of stabilization until renal excretory function has been maximized and serum potassium concentration measured, especially if the patient is oliguric. Supplementation of fluids with potassium often is needed during polyuric renal failure, but the magnitude of potassium supplementation should be less than that used in patients with normal renal function. Rather than the usual 20 to 30 mEq/L of KCl per liter of fluids, 10 to 20 mEq/L may be more appropriate in patients with renal failure.

METABOLIC ABNORMALITIES

Dogs and cats with compensated CRF generally have normal serum sodium, potassium, and chloride concentrations. However, electrolyte and acid-base disorders commonly develop in patients with decompensated CRF and ARF with severe reductions in GFR.[5,16,42,127,129] Hyperkalemia, hypokalemia, hypernatremia, hyponatremia, hyperphosphatemia, hypocalcemia, and metabolic acidosis may be encountered. Depending on the severity of these metabolic abnormalities, specific treatment may be required.

Sodium

Serum sodium concentration often is normal in dehydrated uremic patients as a consequence of isonatremic fluid loss (e.g., polyuria, diarrhea). However, hypernatremia may develop when losses of free water exceed sodium losses. Hypernatremia commonly develops after uremic patients are treated for several days with replacement solutions containing large amounts of sodium. Hypernatremia also may develop after several doses of sodium bicarbonate have been administered for treatment of metabolic acidosis. Less commonly, patients with renal failure have dehydration and hyponatremia because of continued water consumption and dilution of ECF sodium concentration after isonatremic sodium losses. In addition, a hypercatabolic state results in increased endogenous water production that can contribute to overhydration and hyponatremia if additional water cannot be excreted by the kidneys.[50]

Isotonic isonatremic fluids (Normosol, Plasma-Lyte 148, lactated Ringer's solution, 0.9% NaCl) are indicated for the initial correction of dehydration in patients with normal serum sodium concentrations. After hypovolemic shock has been corrected with isotonic fluids, hypotonic solutions (0.45% NaCl or 5% dextrose in water) are indicated for patients with initially high serum sodium concentrations. Usually, isotonic solutions are administered to patients with hyponatremia in an effort to provide sodium and water with the expectation that the kidneys will excrete excess water and the serum sodium concentration will return to normal. Rarely, hypertonic sodium chloride solutions (3% NaCl) may be needed for treatment of severe and symptomatic hyponatremia (see Chapter 3).

Chloride

Serum chloride concentration usually parallels serum sodium concentration during free water loss. Proportionally more chloride may be lost during vomiting of gastric fluid, and hypochloremia may develop in some uremic patients. The fluid of choice in this instance is 0.9% NaCl (see Chapter 4).

Potassium

Hyperkalemia. Life-threatening hyperkalemia is most likely to be encountered in severely oliguric patients, especially when metabolic acidosis is severe. Mild to moderate hyperkalemia can develop in patients with poor renal function receiving intravenous fluids supplemented with potassium. Hyperkalemia usually docs not occur in CRF unless severe oliguria or metabolic acidosis develops. Hyperkalemia was uncommon in dogs with intrinsic ARF in one study. Serum potassium concentration was less than 5.0 mEq/L in 75% of affected dogs despite the presence of oligoanuria in more than 60% of the dogs.[129] Severe hyperkalemia is more likely in azotemic dogs and cats with urethral obstruction, uroabdomen, or hypoadrenocorticism. Serum potassium concentration was above the reference range in more than 50% of male cats with urethral obstruction in one study.[47] Serial or continuous electrocardiographic (ECG) monitoring is recommended in these instances because severe hyperkalemia can lead to life-threatening cardiac arrhythmias.

Hyperkalemia can be managed temporarily by volume expansion with 0.9% NaCl and sodium bicarbonate infusion (1 to 4 mEq/kg, intravenously). Any ECG changes compatible with hyperkalemia should be managed to stabilize the cardiac rhythm. These measures are discussed in Chapter 5 and include administration of sodium bicarbonate, hypertonic glucose, or calcium gluconate. Glucose infusion may be preferred over sodium bicarbonate when total calcium or ionized calcium concentrations are precariously low because an infusion of alkali may further decrease ionized and total calcium concentrations. Glucose infusions also are preferred over bicarbonate if seizures already are a problem or if metabolic alkalosis exists. Calcium gluconate directly counteracts the effect of potassium on the heart but does not decrease serum potassium concentration. Calcium salts may have an additional benefit in patients with hypocalcemia but may promote deleterious soft tissue mineralization if hyperphosphatemia is present.

The ECG should revert to normal within minutes of these treatments, but they provide only temporary relief from the effects of hyperkalemia. Maximizing renal excretory function and maintaining blood pH and bicarbonate within the normal range help to decrease serum potassium concentration more permanently. Chronic hyperkalemia may be treated with an ion exchange resin (sodium polystyrene sulfonate) or may require dialysis. Peritoneal dialysis is discussed in Chapter 28; and hemodialysis is discussed in Chapter 29.

Hypokalemia. Hypokalemia is most likely to occur at presentation in patients with polyuric renal failure, especially when anorexia is present. Hypokalemia is much more common than hyperkalemia in animals with CRF, and it occurs more commonly in cats than in dogs. Hypokalemia also may develop after rehydration with potassium-deficient fluids, during periods of spontaneous diuresis, and during periods of intensive therapeutic diuresis. Chronic hypokalemia can cause functional renal lesions (e.g., defective urinary concentrating ability, decreased GFR), structural renal lesions, and CRF. Chronic metabolic acidosis and potassium depletion in cats apparently can result in CRF, but the exact mechanisms remain unknown. Cats with marked potassium depletion and hypokalemia may demonstrate truncal weakness manifested by ventroflexion of the head and inability to move.

Potassium should be added cautiously to daily fluids (see Table 5-2 in Chapter 5) in animals with primary renal failure. Serum potassium concentration should be measured serially to ensure that hyperkalemia does not develop because excretion of an acute potassium load is delayed in patients with renal failure. Severe hypokalemia usually is defined as a potassium concentration of 2.5 mEq/L or less and often is associated with clinical signs. Serum potassium concentrations of 2.0 mEq/L or less are life threatening.

If possible, intravenous fluids should be avoided during initial treatment of cats with primary renal failure and severe hypokalemia. This recommendation was based on the observation of paradoxical decreasing of serum potassium concentration or failure of serum potassium concentration to increase after potassium supplementation of intravenous fluids in cats with chronic potassium depletion.[44-46] This may be a result of ECF volume expansion and has been observed despite maximal rates of potassium supplementation with fluids containing up to 80 mEq/L potassium. Instead of supplementing intravenous fluids with potassium, oral supplementation with potassium gluconate is recommended for the correction of severe hypokalemia during the first 12 to 24 hours. After this time, aggressive fluid therapy with potassium supplementation can be instituted. An initial daily dosage of 5 to 10 mEq of potassium gluconate is recommended until serum potassium concentration approaches the normal range.[45,46] Afterward, 3 to 8 mEq/day is given orally for maintenance of serum potassium concentration, and this dosage is tapered to 2 to 4 mEq/day for chronic maintenance.[45,46] Alternatively, subcutaneous fluids containing up to 35 mEq/L potassium chloride can be given at the time of initial oral supplementation. In this case, volume expansion and concomitant diuresis are not as great as observed with intravenous fluids, resulting in less dilution of ECF potassium concentration and less renal excretion of administered potassium.

Potassium depletion and hypokalemia at concentrations of 2.0 mEq/L or less may result in paralysis of respiratory muscles and require ventilatory support. In these instances, infusion of intravenous fluids containing 80 to 150 mEq/L potassium may be justified at the maximal rate of 0.5 mEq/kg/hr. Dopamine infusion at 0.5 µg/kg/min has been suggested for severe hypokalemia to allow translocation of intracellular potassium to ECF.[44-46] The action of dopamine on adrenocortical receptors also selectively inhibits angiotensin II–induced aldosterone secretion,[23] which could be helpful in minimizing kaliuresis.

Phosphorus

Hyperphosphatemia. Hyperphosphatemia is a frequent finding in patients with ARF and CRF, and it may be severe (>10 mg/dL). Hyperphosphatemia may be severe relative to increases in BUN or serum creatinine concentrations in patients with ARF. Acute hyperphosphatemia in the absence of primary renal injury is not deleterious to renal excretory function or renal histology but may be of consequence in the development of additional primary renal injury during acute and chronic intrinsic renal failure. During ARF, hyperphosphatemia may contribute to worsening of histologic lesions and excretory function by several mechanisms, including renal mineralization, direct nephrotoxicity, and renal vasoconstriction.[138]

Hyperphosphatemia also can adversely influence the progression of CRF in dogs and cats and contribute to the development of hypocalcemia during CRF and ARF. At present, it is not known whether rigorous control of serum phosphorus concentration during the uremic crises of patients with ARF or CRF will improve recovery of renal excretory function or enhance healing of renal lesions. Regardless, it seems clinically prudent to make an effort to reduce serum phosphorus concentration to some degree, preferably to within the normal range. Less severe hyperphosphatemia was associated with improved survival in a group of dogs with hospital-acquired ARF.[5]

No specific fluid therapy counteracts increased serum phosphorus concentration. However, therapeutic efforts to increase GFR also tend to decrease serum phosphorus concentration. If the patient is not vomiting, intestinal phosphorus-binding agents (e.g., aluminum hydroxide, calcium carbonate, calcium acetate) may be administered in an attempt to maintain serum phosphorus concentration below 6.0 mg/dL. Phosphorus binders are much more effective when given with meals but may decrease serum phosphorus concentration in anorexic patients, presumably by binding phosphorus in gastrointestinal secretions.[113] See Chapter 7 for more information on the use of phosphate binders.

Hypophosphatemia. Hypophosphatemia is an unlikely occurrence in patients with primary renal failure. Rarely, excessive treatment with intestinal phosphorus

binders and intensive diuresis results in transient hypophosphatemia.

Calcium

Approximately 50% to 75% of dogs with CRF had normal serum calcium concentrations in one report,[28] depending on whether the serum total or ionized calcium concentration was measured (see Chapter 6). Similarly, 10% to 40% of these patients had hypocalcemia, and 6% to 14% were hypercalcemic. Approximately 75% of cats with CRF had normal serum total calcium concentrations, whereas 15% had hypocalcemia and 12% had hypercalcemia.[42] Mean serum calcium concentration was normal in dogs with ARF, but 25% of affected dogs had concentrations less than the reference range.[129]

Serum total calcium concentration can markedly underestimate the severity of ionized hypocalcemia, especially in azotemic patients. Seventy-five percent of cats with urethral obstruction and azotemia had low ionized calcium concentrations, but serum total calcium concentrations were simultaneously low in only 27% of patients. Low total calcium concentrations predicted low ionized calcium concentrations in these cats, but normal total calcium concentrations did not accurately predict low ionized calcium concentrations.[47]

Symptomatic hypocalcemia (i.e., tremors, seizures, muscular weakness, muscular rigidity) is not common in patients with renal failure but may require intravenous administration of calcium salts when it does occur (see Chapter 6). However, administered calcium may interact with an increased serum phosphorus concentration, resulting in metastatic mineralization of soft tissues, including the heart and kidneys. Hypocalcemia has been attributed to mass law interactions between calcium and phosphorus when serum phosphorus concentration is very high and also to deficits of calcitriol (e.g., reduced intestinal absorption of calcium, increased skeletal resistance to parathyroid hormone). Measures to decrease serum phosphorus concentration may increase serum calcium concentration through more favorable mass law ionic interactions between phosphorus and calcium. Symptomatic hypocalcemia appears to be more common in dogs with ethylene glycol poisoning and ARF, but it also can be seen after $NaHCO_3$ therapy and reductions in serum ionized calcium concentration.

Hypercalcemia occasionally is encountered in dogs and cats with CRF.[28,42,57] Hypercalcemia in these instances usually is mild, but some dogs with renal failure have been observed to have serum total calcium concentrations as high as 14 mg/dL.[111] In most instances, dogs with CRF and hypercalcemia have an associated ionized calcium concentration that either is normal or low.[28,99,109] Accordingly, these patients do not require specific therapy for hypercalcemia. When serum ionized calcium concentration is increased, specific therapy to decrease the ionized calcium concentration is warranted (see

Chapter 6). Lactated Ringer's solution contains supplemental calcium (3 mEq/L) and should be avoided in hypercalcemic patients.

Magnesium

Serum magnesium concentration may be increased in patients with severe renal failure.[28] Ionized and total magnesium concentrations occasionally are increased in dogs and cats with renal failure.[123] Total serum magnesium concentrations were increased in 11 of 14 cats with urethral obstruction.[47] Magnesium-containing drugs, such as antacids, should be avoided because any absorbed magnesium may not be readily excreted by the kidneys and could exacerbate hypermagnesemia. Hypomagnesemia has been associated with peritoneal dialysis using dialysate that did not contain magnesium.[37] See Chapter 8 for more information on magnesium.

Metabolic Acidosis

Metabolic acidosis commonly is associated with severe reductions in renal mass and GFR. In CRF, progressive inability to excrete hydrogen ions develops because total urinary ammonia excretion declines with reduction in renal mass. Increased serum phosphorus concentration also contributes to the degree of metabolic acidosis in both ARF and CRF (see Chapter 10). Metabolic acidosis often is well compensated in patients with stable CRF owing to renal tubular adaptation and hyperventilation. However, patients with decompensated CRF or ARF often have severe metabolic acidosis. Ethylene glycol frequently is associated with severe metabolic acidosis in the early phases after its ingestion and metabolism to organic acids.[64,127]

Metabolic acidosis may be severe (blood pH, <7.2) and require treatment. In the absence of blood gas analysis, a total CO_2 concentration less than 15 mEq/L in a patient with primary renal failure usually indicates the presence of metabolic acidosis severe enough to require alkali supplementation. More aggressive correction of metabolic acidosis is indicated if hyperkalemia also is present. To correct metabolic acidosis, sodium bicarbonate is added to calcium-free maintenance fluids at a dosage of 1 to 5 mEq/kg, depending on the severity of the acidosis. Alternatively, the bicarbonate deficit of the extracellular space can be calculated from blood gas data using the formula 0.3 × body weight (kg) × (target bicarbonate − current bicarbonate) = milliequivalents of bicarbonate to be given over several hours, or one fourth to one half given as a slow bolus with the remainder given in maintenance fluids. Partial correction of the bicarbonate deficit is preferable to attempts to fully correct the deficit. When calculating the amount of bicarbonate to be given, the target bicarbonate chosen should be in the low normal range (e.g., 16 mEq/L).

This method requires use of serial blood gas analysis and adjustment of therapy based on the results. Hypernatremia, hyperosmolality, metabolic alkalosis, decreasing of serum ionized calcium concentration with resultant seizures, and paradoxical cerebrospinal fluid acidosis are all potential complications during alkali therapy (see Chapter 10).[27]

INTENSIVE DIURESIS

The goal of intensive diuresis is to increase the turnover of body water, electrolyte, and metabolic waste products. Diuresis hopefully will result in loss of some substances that have accumulated in the uremic environment and have caused many of the clinical signs. Increases in GFR, RBF, and urine flow may be independent of one another. In certain instances, GFR actually increases during diuresis, but in other cases increased urine production is not accompanied by increased GFR. Increased urine volume should not be equated with improved renal excretory function. In some cases, it is not possible to increase urine flow.

Most studies in humans have failed to show any benefit of mannitol or furosemide either prophylactically or as treatment for established nephrotoxic or ischemic ARF.[32,116,126] One study of the potential renoprotective effects of furosemide against ischemic injury before cardiac surgery suggested a detrimental effect.[87] The use of diuretics is justified to increase urine output and facilitate fluid therapy, but no data suggest that diuretics improve clinical outcome. The ability of diuretics to alter favorably the course of a uremic crisis is not established in veterinary medicine, but most clinicians administer them anyway. Success with these agents includes reduced azotemia and conversion from oligoanuria to increased urine flow. Diuretics most commonly are used in states of oliguria, usually associated with ARF. Osmotic diuretics and furosemide have been used to augment urinary flow in animals with polyuric CRF, but their superiority over rehydration and mild ECF volume expansion has not been established. The use of diuretics in patients with polyuric renal failure sometimes is not advocated on the grounds that urine production may become excessive and result in dehydration. These patients may benefit from diuretics that cause vasodilatation, increased GFR, increased RBF, and natriuresis, but this has not been studied. In all instances, rehydration should be completed before administration of diuretics.[28,29,83,89]

CONVERSION FROM OLIGURIA TO NONOLIGURIA

Oliguria and persistence of azotemia during initial fluid therapy may result from inadequate correction of renal perfusion, intrarenal vasoconstriction, or underlying renal damage. To distinguish among these possibilities, a fluid "push" often is advocated to ensure that clinically undetectable dehydration or hypovolemia is not the cause of the oliguria. ECF volume expansion may override some forms of intrarenal vasoconstriction. A fluid volume of approximately 3% to 5% (30 to 50 mL/kg) of the animal's body weight has been recommended after correction of apparent dehydration.[53] The rationale for this additional fluid load is that dehydration of 3% to 5% of body weight may be clinically undetectable, and renal function may improve when additional fluid is administered. Slight overhydration is preferable to ongoing dehydration and possible additional renal damage.[106] If oliguria persists after this maneuver, it is likely to be pathologic. Fluid administration must be closely monitored because an animal with severely diseased kidneys may not be able to tolerate volume expansion, and overhydration may result. Performing a fluid push with CVP monitoring may be safer, but even this approach does not guarantee avoidance of overhydration.

The use of diuretics to convert oliguria to nonoliguria should be considered after rehydration has been accomplished.[25,29,83,89] Rehydration allows greater delivery of the diuretic to the kidney, and beneficial effects are more likely to occur. If diuresis is initiated before rehydration, dehydration could result in additional renal injury. It is easier to manage nonoliguric animals because hyperkalemia and overhydration are less likely to occur, and the severity of nitrogenous waste product retention may be less. It is not certain whether conversion from oliguria to nonoliguria after diuretic administration changes the natural course of the disease or merely identifies animals with less severe underlying renal lesions.[89] Animals that remain oliguric despite diuretic administration have a poor prognosis because of the relative impracticality of dialysis.

Dextrose, mannitol, furosemide, and dopamine (or combinations of these) are the diuretics most often used in an attempt to convert oliguria to nonoliguria. Administration of diuretics to normal animals can increase GFR, RBF, tubular fluid flow rate, and osmolar clearance. Decreased release of renin and inhibition of tubuloglomerular feedback are features of some diuretics that are theoretically attractive in the treatment of ARF.[29,89] Reduced transport of sodium by damaged tubules after use of diuretics has the potential advantage of limiting further injury in acute but sublethally injured tubular cells, especially those located in areas of relative hypoxia (outer medulla and the pars recta and thick ascending limb of the loop of Henle).[9,114]

The phase of ARF during which diuretics are given dramatically influences their ability to improve renal function. In some experimental models, diuretics given prophylactically can preserve renal excretory function, but the extent of tubular necrosis may not be limited. In experimental animals and some clinical trials in humans, diuretics were most effective when given prophylactically, somewhat effective if given during the induction phase, and least effective when given during the maintenance phase of ARF. Mannitol or furosemide given prophylactically to human patients with CRF who were about to undergo radiocontrast agent infusion were less renoprotective than 0.45% sodium chloride infusion alone.[122] Radiocontrast-induced vasoconstriction was overcome in human patients by the infusion of mannitol or atrial natriuretic peptide (ANP), but both infusion groups experienced a similar extent of ARF.[84]

Diuretic administration may not result in immediate improvement of renal excretory function, but conversion from oliguria to nonoliguria represents some measure of success. In the authors' experience, oliguric animals in the maintenance phase of ARF usually can be converted to nonoliguria by administration of diuretics, with the notable exception of patients with oligoanuria caused by ethylene glycol poisoning.[127] Usually, conversion to nonoliguria occurs without a detectable increase in GFR and is characterized by an increase in urine volume without reduction in the magnitude of azotemia. Increased tubular flow rate has the potential to relieve obstruction of tubular lumina and, secondarily, to improve GFR. Adequate intravenous fluid administration should be maintained to prevent dehydration and additional renal injury in patients that experience a marked increase in urine volume after diuretic administration.

During attempts to initiate diuresis, careful attention must be given to body weight, urine output, and changes in BUN or serum creatinine concentration. After the hydrated body weight of the patient has been established as a baseline, attempts should be made to maintain body weight while administering diuretics. Progressive weight loss during attempts to maintain diuresis indicates dehydration, whereas progressive weight gain indicates overhydration. Meticulous attention to fluid therapy is required after diuresis has been established by administration of diuretics or spontaneous renal repair because a tendency toward dehydration, hyponatremia, and hypokalemia may persist for weeks.

Hypertonic Dextrose

Osmotic diuresis using 20% dextrose in water has been used at a total daily dosage of 22 to 66 mL/kg. Solutions containing 2.5% or 5% dextrose do not provide sufficient dextrose to initiate diuresis. To create hyperglycemia, a 20% dextrose solution is administered at a rate of 2 to 10 mL/min for the first 10 to 15 minutes, followed by a rate of 1 to 5 mL/min. Alternatively, the dextrose dosage can be calculated as 0.5 to 1.0 g/kg infused during 15 to 20 minutes.[111] Development of glucosuria indicates that sufficient hyperglycemia has been achieved to saturate renal tubular transport of glucose. Urine output should approach 1 to 4 mL/min if treatment has been successful. After dextrose has been given, a polyionic solution (e.g., lactated Ringer's solution) is administered intravenously to prevent dehydration and electrolyte depletion. Treatment is repeated two to three times daily as needed. If adequate urine volume is not achieved, further attempts at osmotic diuresis using hypertonic dextrose are not warranted.

Some believe hypertonic dextrose to be as effective as mannitol in promoting diuresis, and dextrose is less expensive and easily detected in the urine. In addition, hypertonic dextrose solutions provide calories and increased urine flow. However, the salutary effects of dextrose solutions on renal function and urine flow have not been compared with those of other diuretics. It is the authors' opinion that other diuretics are more potent in conversion of oliguria to nonoliguria.

Mannitol

Mannitol may be used as an alternative to dextrose in promoting osmotic diuresis. No controlled studies support the use of mannitol prophylactically or during established ARF in human patients.[32] Mannitol administration results in ECF volume expansion, which favors increased GFR and reduced tubular sodium reabsorption. However, the beneficial effects of mannitol are not simply the result of volume expansion because the same effect is not observed after volume expansion with 0.9% NaCl.[89] After filtration, mannitol exerts a hyperosmotic effect along the entire nephron and also inhibits renin release,[89] which may be important in forms of ARF that are dependent on the renin-angiotensin-aldosterone system. Mannitol may induce release of ANP, which may produce salutary effects on renal function.[84] After renal ischemia, mannitol attenuates a deleterious increase in intramitochondrial calcium concentration and also acts as a free-radical scavenger.[116]

A combination of bicarbonate, mannitol, and diuresis has been used in people for treatment and prevention of renal failure caused by pigmenturia (e.g., hemoglobinuria, myoglobinuria). One study of human patients with high creatine kinase activity consistent with crush injury found no benefit of a mannitol and bicarbonate combination in prevention of renal failure, dialysis, or death.[15] In this study, however, 85% of the patients had increased serum creatinine concentration at presentation, consistent with the possibility that renal damage had already taken place. Another study evaluating this treatment approach in earthquake crush victims began therapy in the field with the intent of beginning treatment before the onset of renal failure. In this study, time between trauma and initiation of fluid therapy was longer in patients who ultimately required dialysis than in those who did not. In addition to mannitol and bicarbonate, these patients received aggressive fluid therapy with isotonic saline, and it is difficult to differentiate the beneficial effects of mannitol and bicarbonate from those of fluid therapy alone.[66]

Mannitol may be superior to dextrose in promoting diuresis in animals with ARF when cellular swelling is important in the maintenance of oliguria or reduced GFR. Dextrose equilibrates with intracellular fluid and ECF spaces, but mannitol remains in the extracellular space and consequently may be more effective in reversing cellular swelling. Mannitol also may be superior to furosemide in the treatment of ARF in patients that are not yet overhydrated.

Mannitol may be infused at an initial dosage of 0.25 to 0.50 g/kg body weight given intravenously over 3 to 5 minutes to initiate diuresis. Diuresis is expected within 20 to 30 minutes after infusion. The concerns about dextrose also apply to mannitol, but there is no practical way to monitor the appearance of mannitol in the urine. If increased urine flow rate or decreased azotemia occurs, intermittent bolus injections or constant infusion as a 5% to 10% solution may be necessary to maintain this salutary effect. To maintain diuresis, a 5% to 10% mannitol solution may be administered intravenously at 2 to 5 mL/min. Mannitol may be diluted in lactated Ringer's solution to provide fluid needs. The total daily dosage of mannitol should not exceed 2 g/kg[102] because high-dose mannitol therapy has been reported to cause ARF in some human patients,[9] and it has been associated with nervous system toxicity in functionally anephric dogs.[118]

If a beneficial effect (urine production of 1 to 3 mL/min)[102] is not seen within 1 hour, mannitol infusion is discontinued because additional doses may not be excreted and may result in severe hyperosmolality, hyponatremia, hypervolemia, pulmonary edema, and congestive heart failure. Animals that are already overhydrated should not be given mannitol.

Furosemide

Furosemide may be given as the initial therapy, after mannitol has failed to have a salutary effect, or in combination with dopamine (see the section on Dopamine). Furosemide may promote diuresis when dextrose and mannitol have failed to do so. This loop diuretic acts by inhibiting the reabsorption of chloride in the thick ascending limb of the loop of Henle after secretion by the proximal tubule. A small amount of the administered dose is filtered.[29] Furosemide also may impair tubuloglomerular feedback.[9] A dosage of 2 to 4 mg/kg is administered intravenously, and this dosage may be doubled or even tripled if no beneficial effect is seen within 30 to 60 minutes. When successful, diuresis may last as long as 2 hours, and furosemide may be given every 8 hours to maintain diuresis.

Furosemide can cause permanent or reversible ototoxicity and deafness in human patients, usually when given at high dosages or to patients with renal failure.[131] Hearing impairment in dogs and cats receiving furosemide for primary renal failure has not been investigated. High dosages (e.g., 50 mg/kg) of furosemide administered to normal dogs may cause hypotension, apathy, and staggering, and a dosage of 10 mg/kg administered to normal cats caused apathy and anorexia.[106] Furosemide potentiates tubular injury in some types of experimental ARF, including aminoglycoside nephrotoxicity, but the mechanism of such injury is unclear.[1,89] Based on these studies, furosemide should not be given to patients as treatment for ARF caused by aminoglycosides. Furosemide exacerbated renal injury in experimental dogs when given at the same time as the nephrotoxin, but furosemide has not been studied as a treatment for ARF caused by aminoglycoside administration in hydrated dogs. In one study of hospital-acquired ARF, all three dogs that received a combination of gentamicin and furosemide therapy did not survive.[5]

Dopamine and Other Dopaminergic Agents

Dopamine is a catecholamine capable of interacting with two subtypes of dopamine receptors (DA-1 and DA-2), as well as with α- and β-adrenergic receptors.[13,120] In both human and veterinary medicine, low-dose ("renal dose") dopamine (<5 μg/kg/min) has been advocated as a potential means of increasing RBF and urine output either for prevention of oliguria or transition from oliguria to nonoliguria. At this low infusion rate, the potentially beneficial dopaminergic and β-adrenergic effects of dopamine predominate.[78,94] However, interaction with adrenergic receptors can limit its usefulness because of the tachycardia and increased systemic and renal vascular resistance that follow vasoconstriction at higher dosages.

Dopamine receptors have been identified at both vascular and tubular sites. Dopamine receptors that regulate renal vasodilatation have been demonstrated in the kidney of the dog, rat, and rabbit.[31] Until recently, it was thought that feline kidneys did not contain dopamine receptors and thus could not respond to dopamine. A DA-1 or DA-1–like receptor has been identified in feline kidney using anti–DA-1 receptor antibodies.[59] Proximal renal tubules of rats, rabbits, and humans contain specific dopamine receptors that inhibit sodium and water reabsorption when stimulated, but detailed characteristics of these receptors are not yet available.[31]

Postsynaptic DA-1 receptors cause vasodilatation of renal, mesenteric, coronary, and cerebral vascular beds.[63] The second type of dopamine receptor (DA-2) is located on postganglionic sympathetic nerve endings and ganglia, and activation of these receptors inhibits release of norepinephrine. These receptors also are located in the emetic center of the brain.[63]

The first type of dopamine receptor has not been identified in glomeruli but is found in nonglomerular renal vessels.[72] Stimulation of DA-1 receptors results in direct vasodilatation, whereas DA-2 receptor activation indirectly results in vasodilatation by inhibiting release of norepinephrine from postganglionic sympathetic nerve endings with subsequent reduction of tonic sympathetic vasoconstriction.[4,62,72,120] Stimulation of DA-2 receptors also can result in nausea and vomiting.[120] These receptors have been identified in the glomeruli and tubules of the rat kidney.[62] The first type of receptor also has been identified in the juxtaglomerular cells of the rat kidney. When stimulated, some studies report that it increases

renin secretion,[91] but inhibition of renin release has been noted by others.[39]

After dopamine administration, RBF usually is increased to a greater degree than is GFR.[62,72] When they occur, increases in GFR may be a consequence of increased cardiac output rather than a direct renal effect. In some species, however, GFR is highly dependent on RBF, and increased RBF could contribute to increased GFR. Increased RBF and decreased renal vascular resistance occurred in a dose-dependent manner in anesthetized dogs receiving dopamine at rates of 1 to 48 μg/kg/min.[69] In dogs, the effects of dopamine on RBF and electrolyte excretion are mediated by activation of DA-1 receptors, and these effects are abolished by administration of the DA-1-specific receptor antagonist SCH 23390.[62] Renal vasodilatation mediated via DA-2 vascular receptor activation is considered important by some investigators.[72] Dopamine causes natriuresis largely by inhibition of sodium, potassium-adenosinetriphosphatase (Na^+,K^+-ATPase) in the proximal tubule, medullary thick ascending limb of Henle's loop, and cortical collecting duct via DA-1 and DA-2 receptor interaction. Inhibition of aldosterone release also may play a role in sodium loss and subsequent diuresis after dopamine infusion.[81] Dopamine's ability to limit oxygen consumption in high-risk tubules could limit tubular injury and accelerate renal repair in ARF.[39] However, in rats treated with higher dosages of dopamine (10 μg/kg/min), measurements of medullary and cortical blood flow and medullary Po_2 indicated an increase in medullary blood flow without a corresponding increase in medullary Po_2. This finding suggests that, at some doses, dopamine may cause an increase in workload and oxygen demand without allowing for an increase in oxygen supplied to the tissue. This may upset the already fragile oxygen balance within the renal medulla and worsen hypoxic injury.[77,81] Free-water excretion also is enhanced because dopamine inhibits central release of antidiuretic hormone (ADH) and antagonizes the action of ADH at the collecting tubule.[39]

The renal response to dopamine infusion varies by species, dosage, and degree of renal impairment. Pronounced differences in the response to dopamine exist between dogs and cats. "Renal-dose" dopamine (0.2 to 2.0 μg/kg/min) activates both dopamine DA-1 and DA-2 receptors, whereas β-adrenergic receptors are activated at higher dosages (2 to 5 μg/kg/min), and α-adrenergic receptors become increasingly activated at even higher dosages (>5 μg/kg/min).[23,75] An ideal dosage of dopamine for beneficial renal effects is one at which dopaminergic and β-adrenergic effects exceed vasoconstrictive α-adrenergic effects (<5 μg/kg/min).[23] Increased RBF, increased urine volume, decreased urine osmolality, and increased urinary fractional excretions of electrolytes typically occur during dopamine infusion in dogs.[62,69] In dogs, GFR is either increased or unchanged during dopamine infusion.[62] Low-dose dopamine infusion (<10 µg/kg/min) increases RBF largely as a consequence of efferent arteriolar dilatation.[72] High-dose dopamine infusion (≥10 µg/kg/min) predominantly activates α-adrenergic receptors. Renal α-adrenergic receptor activation results in renal vasoconstriction. Renal α-adrenergic receptors are located on renal tubular cells and produce antidiuretic and antinatriuretic effects when stimulated.[72] Activation of β-adrenergic receptors in the kidney may enhance renin release.[72]

In the normal cat, diuresis occurs during dopamine infusion, but increases in GFR and RBF are not observed. A combination of fluid therapy, dopamine, and furosemide resulted in lower GFR as compared with fluids alone in normal cats.[96] Similarly, fenoldopam does not cause any renal effects in anesthetized cats.[31] This lack of response was thought to reflect a lack of specific dopamine receptors in the cat's renal vasculature or tubules.[31,130] Although DA-1 receptors are now known to be present in the feline kidney, the response to dopaminergic agonists remains poor in this species. Regardless, diuresis and natriuresis ensue during dopamine infusion in cats. This effect probably is caused by stimulation of α-adrenergic receptors that increase blood pressure and decrease sodium reabsorption in the late distal tubule and collecting tubule.[31] This diuretic response can be abolished by nonselective α-adrenergic antagonists but not by selective dopamine receptor antagonists.[31] Pressure diuresis may partially explain the diuresis during dopamine infusion at dosages of approximately 10 µg/kg/min because systemic arterial blood pressure is increased at this dosage in cats.[31]

So-called "renal dose" dopamine (i.e., a dosage less than the vasopressor dosage, often 2 to 5 µg/kg/min) has surprisingly little documentation to support its use in clinical patients in either human[39,116,126] or veterinary medicine. Efficacy studies of dopamine in clinically uremic dogs or cats with or without oliguria are not available. Based on results for experimental dogs and cats and clinical trials in human patients, dopamine infusion for the conversion of oliguria to nonoliguria seems reasonable. In oliguric human patients, dopamine infusion can result in diuresis and natriuresis after high-dose furosemide therapy has failed to establish diuresis.[72] Low-dose dopamine infusion (4 µg/kg/min) attenuated the adverse effects of ibuprofen on RBF in a canine model of endotoxic shock and counteracted the vasoconstrictive effects of systemically administered norepinephrine.[58] Despite increases in RBF documented in humans receiving "renal dose" dopamine, there does not appear to be any lasting benefit or protection provided by dopamine infusion. No difference in mortality rate, need for renal replacement therapy, or prevention of renal failure in high-risk groups has been documented.[3,81] With evidence accumulating that dopamine is not efficacious in treatment of ARF in people, many investigators are suggesting it no longer has a place in renal critical care medicine.

Fenoldopam, a specific DA-1 receptor agonist, is more specific and potent than dopamine in causing renal vasodilatation in dogs.[10,30,69] Fenoldopam and derivatives that maintain increased RBF are well absorbed from the intestinal tract of the dog.[11] Fenoldopam maintained or increased RBF despite systemic arterial hypotension in anesthetized dogs in one study.[4] Increased systemic arterial pressure and tachycardia do not occur with fenoldopam because, unlike dopamine, it does not stimulate adrenergic receptors. Renal perfusion is maintained at higher dosages of fenoldopam despite induction of systemic hypotension. Fenoldopam stimulated release of renin in anesthetized dogs, an effect that opposes fenoldopam's inhibition of tubular function and its vasodepressor actions.[30] Oral and intravenous fenoldopam given to a small number of dogs with spontaneous chronic renal insufficiency increased RBF nearly 100% over baseline, whereas GFR as estimated by creatinine clearance increased by 25% to 50%.[13] Fenoldopam ameliorated cyclosporine-induced nephrotoxicity in rats[12] and provided renal protection during subacute amphotericin nephrotoxicity in dogs. Some enhanced recovery of renal function was seen during acute amphotericin nephrotoxicity.[100] Fenoldopam increased renal reserve for RBF but not for GFR in dogs in which amino acids were simultaneously infused.[10] Patients undergoing liver transplantation and receiving fenoldopam had lower BUN and serum creatinine concentrations and required fewer doses of furosemide to maintain urine output than did patients receiving an infusion of low-dose dopamine.[38] After transplantation, significantly better creatinine clearance was seen in patients receiving fenoldopam as compared with those receiving dopamine or placebo.[7] Although fenoldopam may be of benefit to patients at risk for development of ARF, no benefit was found for veterinary patients with normal renal function undergoing nephrotomy.[139] Of concern is a recent study evaluating the effect of fenoldopam in a canine model of renal injury secondary to rhabdomyolysis. Not only was no renoprotective effect of fenoldopam observed but also administration of the drug appeared to worsen renal function in the hours after renal injury. Although renal function was only followed for 3 hours after injury, the possible negative effects of dopamine agonists in ARF warrant further investigation.[98]

Zelandopam (formerly YM435) is a potent and selective dopamine DA-1 receptor agonist with no α- or β-adrenoreceptor agonist activity. Infusion of zelandopam in anesthetized dogs caused RBF to increase more than 10 times as much as with dopamine infusion. RBF also was slightly increased over that achieved with fenoldopam infusion.[137] Zelandopam can overcome renal vasoconstriction of afferent and efferent arterioles induced by angiotensin II and endothelin in rats[125] and angiotensin II or norepinephrine in dogs.[136] Increased RBF, GFR, urinary flow rate, and urinary sodium excretion followed infusion of zelandopam in anesthetized dogs in a dose-dependent manner without effect on heart rate.[134] Zelandopam reversed angiotensin II–induced decreases in RBF, GFR, and urine flow rate in the same study of dogs and prevented decreases induced by renal nerve stimulation or platelet-activating factor. Infusion of zelandopam reversed decreases in GFR, urinary flow rate, and urinary sodium excretion that occurred after 1 hour of renal ischemia in experimental dogs but not when the infusion was stopped. Beneficial effects were not observed during infusion of 0.9% saline.[135] Zelandopam given before administration of cisplatin in rats prevented increases in BUN and serum creatinine concentration that typically are seen with cisplatin-induced renal failure.[133] Although the efficacy of zelandopam in established renal failure is not known, it may be of benefit in animals receiving known nephrotoxins.

The potentially beneficial effects of dopaminergic compounds have been studied in human patients with CRF. In these patients, dopamine infusion increased GFR and RBF.[72] In another study of human patients with advanced CRF, GFR did not increase, but RBF, urine flow, and sodium excretion were increased after dopamine infusion.[72] Oral ibopamine has been given to human patients with CRF in an attempt to retard progressive deterioration of excretory renal function, and increased creatinine clearance, diuresis, and natriuresis were observed.[24]

In human patients, there is marked individual variation in the rate of dopamine infusion required to achieve activation of various receptors. Consequently, patients must be carefully monitored to achieve the desired effect.[63] Variation in the response to dopamine may be because of differences in the number or sensitivity of dopamine receptors among different species and among individuals in a given species.[128] The adverse effects of dopamine may be severe and counterproductive to renal excretory function. Therefore dopamine must be infused accurately at a low dosage, usually 1 to 5 μg/kg/min. Such precise infusion is best achieved with an infusion pump. A large vein should be chosen for infusion of dopamine to avoid vasoconstriction that may be associated with a relatively high concentration of dopamine locally. Otherwise, ischemia and necrosis can occur, and extravasation of dopamine-containing fluids warrants the same concern.[79]

Dopamine should not be administered in fluids containing sodium bicarbonate or in other alkaline fluids because the drug is inactivated in an alkaline environment.[9,72] Metoclopramide is a DA-2 receptor antagonist.[120] Consequently, intermittent injection or constant infusion of metoclopramide to control vomiting should be avoided or discontinued during dopamine infusion.

Dopamine hydrochloride is most appropriate for small animal patients, but must always be diluted before administration. It can be added safely to most commercially available saline or dextrose-containing solutions and is stable in fluids at room temperature for at least 24 hours. A separate intravenous line is recommended for infusion of dopamine to ensure accuracy of dose administration. Alternatively, two intravenous lines can be connected by a Y-piece administration set to one intravenous catheter. Dopamine is administered via one intravenous line, and the other intravenous line is used to administer fluids for maintenance and rehydration. First, the total number of micrograms per minute to be infused is calculated, and then the number of drops per minute required to achieve this dose is calculated. An infusion pump is set at this number of drops per minute. In the absence of an infusion pump, an administration set that delivers 60 drops/mL (pediatric drip chamber) is used. Each drop contains 1 μg of dopamine. For example, to infuse dopamine at 2 μg/kg/min to a 10-kg dog, 20 μg/min is required. This can be accomplished using a 60-drops/mL drip chamber at 20 drops/min or 1 drop/3 sec. Alternatively, 50 mg (1.25 mL of a 40-mg/mL solution) of dopamine may be added to 500 mL of fluids, resulting in a dopamine concentration of 100 μg/mL, and the drip rate is adjusted accordingly.[33]

ECG monitoring is recommended during dopamine infusion to ensure rapid detection of arrhythmias. The resting heart rate should be determined and recorded after hydration but before starting the dopamine infusion. The heart rate should be determined every 15 minutes for the first hour and hourly thereafter if no problems have been encountered. A sudden increase in heart rate (>180 beats/min in dogs or >200 beats/min in cats) indicates the need to reduce the rate of dopamine infusion. Emergence of a serious cardiac arrhythmia (e.g., ventricular tachycardia) during dopamine infusion may preclude further administration of the drug. Promptly discontinuing dopamine infusion usually results in cessation of cardiac arrhythmias. Animals with underlying cardiac disease may be more susceptible to arrhythmias during dopamine infusion, but this usually is not a problem at the low dosage of dopamine used for renal effects. Serial blood pressure measurements may be helpful in detection of adrenergic receptor activation when higher dosages of dopamine (≥5 μg/kg/min) are used in attempt to convert oliguria to nonoliguria. The infusion rate should be decreased if systemic arterial blood pressure continuously increases during dopamine infusion.

It is the authors' impression that oliguric renal failure that has failed to respond to mannitol or furosemide may be converted to nonoliguria after combined infusion of dopamine and furosemide. Experimental studies in dogs showed this combination to be superior to either dopamine or furosemide alone in maintaining GFR, RBF, osmolar clearance, and urine flow during a model of nephrotoxic ARF.[90] A synergistic effect of dopamine in combination with furosemide has been found for the conversion of oliguria to nonoliguria in human patients with ARF. A salutary response necessitates previous volume repletion and institution of combination therapy diuretics within 24 hours of the onset of oliguria.[72] Dopamine-induced renal vasodilatation may increase the delivery of furosemide to its site of action in the ascending limb of Henle's loop.[115]

Most of the authors' experience with combined use of dopamine and furosemide has been in dogs, but this regimen has been used safely in cats. Dopamine is continuously infused at a rate of 2 to 5 µg/kg/min in combination with furosemide at 1 mg/kg/hr given by intravenous bolus injections. If no improvement occurs within 6 hours, additional efforts to convert oliguria to nonoliguria with dopamine are unlikely to be successful, and the infusion should be discontinued. Clinicians often select this combination regimen as a last resort, but it may be more beneficially used in the initial management of oliguric ARF. As noted earlier, decreased BUN and serum creatinine concentrations do not necessarily accompany an increase in urine production. Studies of the more potent and specific dopaminergic renal vasodilators and natriuretics should be undertaken in the future to determine their ability to alter the course of uremic crises in dogs and cats. It may prove valuable to study higher dosages of dopamine after α- and β-adrenergic blockade.

Calcium Channel Blockers

Felodipine is a calcium channel blocker with renal vasodilatory and natriuretic properties that also warrants further study in the treatment of uremic crises.[43,104] Recovery of GFR is more rapid in human patients with intrinsic ARF when they are treated with the calcium channel blocking agent verapamil or gallopamil.[32] Calcium channel blockers also may provide a protective effect if given before or at the time of ischemic insult. Calcium channel blockers have been shown to improve outcome in postischemic myocardial injury and may have similar potential in renal transplantation. Verapamil may protect the kidney against ischemic and reperfusion injury if given at the time of transplantation.[37a] A lower incidence of acute tubular necrosis is seen in patients treated with a calcium channel blocker at the time of transplantation.[117]

Atrial Natriuretic Peptide

ANP causes diuresis, natriuresis, increased GFR, and maintenance of RBF during periods of increased vasoconstriction.[84] ANP promotes both vasodilatation of the afferent arteriole and vasoconstriction of the efferent arteriole, which selectively increases GFR independently of RBF.[80] ANP also may provide renoprotection independently of its hemodynamic effects in that renal tubular cell exfoliation, necrosis, and cast formation are reduced and ATP regeneration is enhanced. ANP exerts beneficial effects immediately after ischemia and also during established postischemic ARF in which sustained increases in GFR and tubular function may occur.[80,116] ANP prevented radiocontrast-induced renal vasoconstriction in a study of dogs and proved beneficial in models of ischemic and nephrotoxic ARF.[84] Results from a multicenter study of human patients with ARF suggest that ANP may be beneficial in patients with oliguria.[84] ANP was most beneficial when started early in the course of ARF in human patients.[32] In a double-blinded placebo-controlled study in people undergoing cardiac surgery, patients receiving ANP had decreased need for dialysis and maintained higher creatinine clearance than those in the placebo group.[124] ANP also has been shown to ameliorate the effects of ischemic injury in dogs. Control subjects and those receiving ANP were subjected to aortic cross-clamping for 90 minutes. Renal function was better in those dogs receiving ANP than in control dogs receiving a saline placebo.[97] High doses of ANP cause peripheral vasodilatation that can result in systemic hypotension as a limiting factor. A combination of ANP and dopamine may provide the beneficial effects of ANP without the hypotension.[116]

Emerging Treatments

N-acetylcysteine. *N*-acetylcysteine (NAC), an amino acid analogue, is used most often in veterinary medicine as a mucolytic agent in patients with respiratory disease and as an antioxidant in treatment of acetaminophen toxicity. Its antioxidant properties arise from its role as a glutathione precursor. This potential benefit has been explored for treatment and prevention of renal failure secondary to oxidative damage, most notably radiocontrast-induced renal failure. Despite several studies, the benefit of NAC in prevention of contrast-induced nephropathy remains controversial. One recent randomized study suggested that baseline serum creatinine concentration affected the risk of nephropathy after intravenous contrast administration, and administration of NAC, regardless of the magnitude of azotemia, did not provide any benefit.[108] Similarly, a study examining the potential benefit of NAC in prevention of the oxidative damage in pigmenturia showed an increase in antioxidant activity in vitro with NAC administration but no clear benefit in renal function.[105] An experimental model of amphotericin B–induced nephrotoxicity indicated that NAC given before and during amphotericin B administration resulted in increased GFR and decreased renal tubular necrosis compared with rats that received amphotericin B alone.[51] Although no clear benefit has been shown in treatment of ARF with NAC, there may be a role for NAC in the prevention of nephrotoxicity.

Growth Factors. Growth factors including epidermal growth factor (EGF), insulin-like growth factor 1 (IGF-1), and hepatocyte growth factor (HGF) are some of the newer drugs being investigated for the treatment of ARF. Growth factors may play a role as mitogens in the recovery of renal tubules after severe injury.[115a] Prepro-EGF is produced primarily in the renal distal convoluted tubule.[107] Up-regulation of EGF receptors and high concentrations of EGF have been documented in the proximal renal tubule in experimental ARF.[115a] Preliminary evidence suggests that administration of EGF may hasten renal recovery in experimental ARF. HGF and IGF-1 have been identified in the kidney and are thought to have similar mitogenic potential as EGF. One study comparing the effects of these growth factors in cells exposed to hypoxic and hypoglycemic injury showed that only HGF resulted in a decrease in apoptosis and an increase in cell viability.[40]

FAILURE TO CONVERT OLIGURIA TO NONOLIGURIA

When oliguria persists, the daily volume of intravenous fluids administered must be curtailed to avoid overhydration. Fluids should not be discontinued unless the animal is already obviously overhydrated (e.g., inappropriate weight gain, subcutaneous edema, pulmonary edema, distended jugular veins). Fluid administration should be adjusted in patients with persistent oliguria to replace insensible losses (respiratory and normal gastrointestinal losses are ~20 mL/kg/day) and contemporary fluid losses from vomiting or diarrhea (this volume must be estimated).

Providing insensible fluid needs may allow the animal to survive long enough for spontaneous diuresis to occur. Dialysis may be required to maintain life if the animal is severely uremic, has severe hyperkalemia and metabolic acidosis, or is markedly overhydrated. Therapeutic phlebotomy may be a lifesaving maneuver in a critically overhydrated patient. Acute removal of approximately 25% of the patient's blood volume (~20 mL/kg) may be useful in this setting. Peritoneal dialysis is discussed in Chapter 28, and hemodialysis is discussed in Chapter 29.

BLOOD

Transfusion with whole blood or packed red cells is indicated if the packed cell volume (PCV) is less than 20% and the patient is showing clinical signs related to anemia. It may be of benefit in some patients with PCV values of 20% to 25% (see Chapter 24). Packed red blood cells are preferable in overhydrated patients. Transfusion with whole blood is satisfactory if overhydration is not present or if total plasma protein concentration is less than 5.0 g/dL.

Severe anemia may be apparent at presentation in animals with advanced CRF or may develop later in those with ARF. Anemia may become apparent after correction of dehydration or may develop suddenly after gastrointestinal blood loss in both ARF and CRF patients.

Anemia usually is not apparent in the early phases of ARF, but it frequently becomes apparent during a protracted maintenance phase, especially when the magnitude of azotemia is severe.

Blood loss through gastrointestinal ulceration can be severe yet may go undetected until melena is observed later. Blood loss may be aggravated by poor platelet function and capillary fragility in uremia at a time when replacement with new red blood cells (reticulocytes and nucleated red blood cells) is inefficient because of reduced renal erythropoietin production by the diseased kidneys. Shortened red blood cell life span and suppression of bone marrow as a consequence of uremia also may contribute to anemia.[26,106] Lastly, repeated blood sampling for diagnostic testing and ongoing crystalloid fluid therapy contribute to the observed anemia. Concomitant management of gastrointestinal ulcers with proton-pump inhibitors (e.g., omeprazole, pantoprazole) and sucralfate, as well as reduction in the magnitude of azotemia, aids in reduction of blood loss. If proton-pump inhibitors are unavailable or cost-prohibitive, an H2 receptor antagonist (e.g., famotidine, cimetidine) may be used intravenously in patients unable to tolerate oral gastroprotectants. Even in vomiting patients, sucralfate may be of benefit if mixed with water and given as a slurry, allowing it to coat the gastric and esophageal mucosa as it is ingested.

NUTRITIONAL ASPECTS OF MANAGEMENT

Treatment of human patients with ARF with parenteral alimentation solutions containing amino acids and glucose resulted in a more rapid decrease in serum creatinine concentration and lower mortality.[32] Primary renal failure is a catabolic state[9,106] in which breakdown of body proteins potentiates the observed increases in BUN, serum phosphorus, serum potassium, and hydrogen ion concentrations. Most animals with severe uremia are anorexic and consequently suffer protein-calorie malnutrition, which may become life threatening. Spontaneous intake of nutrients is unlikely in animals that remain severely azotemic (BUN, >100 mg/dL) during initial medical management of a uremic crisis. Some animals resume nutrient intake after medical therapy has reduced the severity of gastrointestinal ulceration, central stimuli for vomiting have been blunted, and the magnitude of azotemia has been reduced. Animals undergoing successful dialysis often eat on their own.

Some form of nutritional support usually is prescribed for anorexic uremic animals with decompensated CRF or protracted ARF. The aim of nutritional therapy is to promote anabolism and reduce endogenous protein catabolism, which serves as a source of nitrogenous solutes, phosphorus, potassium, and hydrogen ions. Forced feeding can be attempted but often is not successful in providing enough nutritional support. Nutrient intake should consist of a reduced quantity of high-quality protein. Sufficient nonprotein calories must be supplied to prevent the dietary protein source from being catabolized for energy.

Some sparing of body protein can be accomplished by hypertonic glucose infusion, particularly when administered in conjunction with amino acids during total parenteral nutrition.[9,26,106] The BUN is reduced in these instances as a consequence of reduced catabolism and enhanced anabolism, and this may improve the animal's quality of life. In addition, provision of nutrients during renal healing may facilitate the recovery process, but the proper nutrient composition in this setting is not known. Care must be taken to prevent overhydration when administering hypertonic alimentation solutions to patients with oliguria. Infusion of 20% to 25% dextrose to supply caloric needs and a balanced amino acid solution at 0.3 g/kg/day via a jugular catheter has been recommended for parenteral nutritional support.[55] One liter of 5% dextrose solution provides only 170 kcal. Thus standard glucose supplementation of intravenous fluids at 2.5% or 5% dextrose does not provide sufficient nonprotein calories to prevent catabolism of endogenous proteins. Parenteral nutrition is discussed in Chapter 25.

Enteral alimentation using nasogastric tube feedings can be attempted after initial reduction of azotemia by fluid therapy and medical management of the gastrointestinal manifestations of uremia using H2 receptor blocking drugs, metoclopramide, and sucralfate. Nasogastric tube feedings are relatively easy to maintain and are well tolerated by cats and most dogs. In the absence of more specific information regarding nutritional requirements during uremic episodes in dogs or cats, commercially available liquid diets for human and veterinary patients have been used for nasogastric tube feedings at the Ohio State University Veterinary Teaching Hospital. Some severely azotemic animals are able to tolerate nasogastric tube feedings well. Pulse feedings four to six times per day through the nasogastric tube often are tolerated without vomiting. Continuous pump infusion of liquid nutrition frequently is tolerated when previous pulse feedings resulted in vomiting. Pureed veterinary foods designed to reduce waste retention during renal failure do not flow through small-diameter nasogastric tubes well but can be administered readily through a gastrostomy tube. If long-term nutritional support is necessary during support of renal healing, placement of a gastrostomy or esophagostomy tube facilitates this therapy.

MONITORING THE EFFECTS OF FLUID THERAPY

Frequent monitoring of the patient in uremic crisis is essential, especially during the first 3 days, when these patients are likely to be most unstable and rapid changes are most likely.

Serial body weight measurements using the same scale facilitate proper fluid therapy during initial management. Weight gain sufficient to account for rehydration should occur during the initial 24 hours of intravenous fluid therapy. Failure to gain weight during attempts at rehydration may indicate that an inadequate volume of fluid has been administered, possibly because of underestimation of ongoing losses through vomiting or diarrhea. Precise body weight should be determined three to four times during the first 24 hours of hospitalization to help determine whether rehydration is being accomplished. Mild progressive weight loss should occur thereafter in the absence of caloric intake. Failure to lose some weight during this period can be a clue that inappropriate fluid retention has occurred. It is easy to overlook gradual fluid accumulation that ultimately may lead to clinical signs related to overhydration. Anticipated daily weight loss for anorexic animals has been estimated as 0.1 to 0.3 kg body weight per 1000 kcal of daily caloric need[53] or 0.5% to 1.0% of body weight per day.[48] Body weight should be determined twice daily for the duration of hospitalization to ensure that a sudden inappropriate increase in body weight does not occur. Conversely, sudden excessive loss of body weight may indicate episodes of unappreciated fluid loss and dehydration that could threaten ongoing renal healing.

Measurement of urine output via an indwelling urethral catheter facilitates fluid therapy decisions in conjunction with serial body weight as described previously. Animals that have questionable urine output after the administration of fluids for rehydration should have a urinary catheter placed at this time. The hour-to-hour decision-making process during fluid challenges and diuretic treatments is facilitated by precise quantitative information about urine output.

PCV and total plasma protein (TPP) concentration should be determined twice daily for the first 48 hours and daily thereafter while the patient is receiving parenteral fluids. This can be helpful in documenting intravascular rehydration (decreasing PCV and TPP), overhydration (progressively decreasing PCV and TPP), dehydration (increasing PCV and TPP), or blood loss (decreasing PCV and TPP). The amount of blood withdrawn for each PCV and TPP determination should be minimized by using a 25-gauge needle and filling the microhematocrit tube directly from the hub of the needle when a drop of blood first appears or by using an insulin syringe.

Although body weight and PCV or TPP measurements are recommended for monitoring patients on intravenous fluid therapy, they are better used as general rather than absolute indicators of hydration status. In the first 24 to 48 hours of fluid therapy, little correlation between fluid administered and PCV, TPP, and body weight changes was found.[73] Thus these measurements should always be used along with serial physical examinations to determine the success of fluid therapy. Serial physical examination is focused on evaluation of hydration because overhydration can result in the death of the animal and dehydration can lead to further renal injury. The subcutaneous tissues may feel gelatinous ("slippery") during overhydration before development of overt peripheral edema. Increased lung sounds and respiratory rate may indicate early overhydration and pneumonia or compensatory hyperventilation in response to metabolic acidosis. Jugular venous distention suggests hypervolemia or overt congestive heart failure. Ongoing hemorrhage (e.g., gastrointestinal blood loss) should be suspected when mucous membranes suddenly become pale.

Serial measurements of serum biochemistry are necessary to determine whether the animal's azotemia is responding to treatment. Frequent serum biochemical evaluation is indicated for patients with progressive or rapid changes in BUN and creatinine concentrations, those with persistent oliguria, and those that suddenly develop polyuria. Patients with severe electrolyte or acid-base disturbances should be followed more frequently than those with relatively stable biochemistry. Adjustment of the dosage of oral phosphorus-binding agents is based on serial measurement of serum phosphorus concentration. Chest radiographs, urine culture, and blood culture should be considered for patients that develop fever, cough, or leukocytosis with a left shift during hospitalization. Intravenous catheter sites should be inspected. The intravenous catheter should be removed and its tip cultured when catheter sepsis is suspected. Maintenance of intravenous catheters is discussed further in Chapter 15.

Blood pressure monitoring is an important component of treatment of the ARF patient. Hypertension is defined as systolic blood pressure greater than 150 to 160 mm Hg, diastolic blood pressure greater than 80 to 90 mm Hg, or both.[35,61] CRF has long been considered a risk factor for development of hypertension.[19] Hypertension also occurs in the majority of dogs with ARF with systolic hypertension occurring in 78% and diastolic hypertension occurring in 84% of dogs with ARF at presentation.[61] The presence of hypertension did not vary significantly with etiology, hydration status, or degree of urine production.[61] These findings suggest that physical examination and clinical monitoring cannot be substituted for direct or indirect blood pressure determination. Direct blood pressure monitoring is not practical in most clinical settings, but indirect measurements can be made using Doppler or oscillometric techniques. Some animals with ARF may have normal systolic blood pressure at presentation, but progressive increases in blood pressure may occur during intravenous fluid therapy.

Renal biopsy should be performed if it is not clear whether the intrinsic renal disease is chronic or acute. The finding of acute lesions on renal biopsy may justify further expense and effort, whereas severe chronic lesions associated with nonresponsive uremia may warrant euthanasia.

OUTCOME DURING FLUID TREATMENTS OF UREMIC CRISES

Ideally, fluid therapy provides sufficient time for adequate renal healing, improved renal excretory function, and at least partial resolution of azotemia and the clinical signs of uremia. The magnitude of residual azotemia and loss of other renal functions (e.g., concentrating ability, acidifying ability) after withdrawal of aggressive fluid therapy determine whether an animal can eventually be treated without administration of parenteral fluids.

Fluid therapy may not be sufficient for patients with renal failure and advanced irreversible loss of excretory function. In these cases, the serum concentrations of urea nitrogen, creatinine, phosphorus, and other unmeasured uremic solutes do not decrease sufficiently to allow adaptation to the uremic environment. The nature of the underlying renal disease, the extent of systemic uremic signs, and the presence of concomitant abnormalities in other organ systems interact to determine whether survival is possible. Many animals with severe uremia are euthanized because of severe clinical signs that do not improve rapidly during initial treatment. Electrolyte imbalances, acid-base disturbances, uremic solute retention, hormonal dysfunction, hematologic abnormalities, and malnutrition can be extensive and difficult to manage effectively.

In the absence of dialysis, persistence of oliguria or development of oliguria during fluid and diuretic treatment of dogs with ARF is associated with a poor prognosis.[5,16,129] Nonoliguric renal failure was common in one study of aminoglycoside nephrotoxicity,[16] but 50% of affected patients were oliguric in a later report.[5] The prognosis is worse for dogs with oliguric forms of aminoglycoside nephrotoxity, but the absence of oliguria does not guarantee survival. The prognosis is grave for dogs or cats that develop anuric ARF, a situation most likely to develop in ethylene glycol intoxication.[64,82,101,112,127] Anuric ARF also may be encountered in cats after ingestion of Easter or day lilies.[70] The prognosis in cats with lily ingestion depends on the presence of ARF at the time of diagnosis. Of 11 cats with known lily ingestion, 7 of 11 cats had ARF at the time of presentation. Of the five for which follow-up data were available, none survived despite the use of peritoneal dialysis in one cat. By contrast, all of the cats presented with gastrointestinal signs alone survived after gastrointestinal decontamination and diuresis.[68] Another case series suggests that some cats with ARF at presentation can survive. Of six cats with ARF at the time of presentation, 50% survived with aggressive supportive care, but CRF developed in all of the survivors. Degree of azotemia did not appear to predict outcome, but urine production did appear to be a factor. Two of the surviving cats were reported to be polyuric at the time of presentation, whereas all of the cats that died or were euthanized were oligoanuric at the time of presentation.[85] Some dogs and cats with severe oliguric ARF have been shown to survive with return of renal function and urine production after several months of hemodialysis.[34,36,86]

Since 2001, reports have emerged of ARF in dogs after ingestion of grapes or raisins.[22,67,95,119] In a study of 43 affected dogs with azotemia at the time of presentation, only 53% survived with 12% of dogs dying and 35% being euthanized.[49] Dogs that did survive had complete clinical recovery and resolution of azotemia. Oligoanuria, ataxia, and weakness were negative prognostic indicators, and dogs that did not survive had higher serum total calcium and potassium concentrations and calcium-phosphorus products at presentation than did dogs that survived. Many toxic principles have been proposed for grape- or raisin-induced ARF, but thus far none has been identified. The dosages of grapes and raisins known to have caused renal failure range from 3 to 36 g/kg of raisins and from as few as four or five grapes per dog to 148 g/kg.[49,95] In a recent study, there was no association between survival and ingested dose (g/kg) of fruit.[49] Because of the unpredictability and severity of this toxicity, decontamination and aggressive treatment are recommended for any dog with known exposure. Grape and raisin toxicity has not yet been reported in cats.

Many animals with acute decompensation of CRF can be successfully treated if a substantial proportion of their azotemia is prerenal in nature. In these cases, the goal is to return the animal to its previous level of azotemia by careful rehydration.

The outlook is less optimistic for animals with intrinsic ARF. In a series of dogs with intrinsic ARF, more than 50% died or were euthanized, whereas 24% survived with CRF and 19% returned to normal as evaluated by serum creatinine concentration.[129] Survival in another retrospective study was only 20% with 69% of dogs dying and 11% being euthanized.[60] Of these dogs, those with ethylene glycol toxicity and multiple disorders had the highest mortality rates (100% and 75%, respectively). Leptospirosis, documented in 8 of the 80 dogs, carried a better prognosis with only 33% mortality. Another series of 15 dogs with leptospirosis had a similar mortality rate of 27%.[8] Somewhat better survival (83%) was reported in a series of 36 cases, and survival was similar for dogs treated by hemodialysis (86%) and conventional medical therapy (82%).

In a series of dogs with hospital-acquired ARF of various causes, 38% survived, 24% died, and 38% were euthanized.[5] In another study of dogs with ARF, severe azotemia (serum creatinine concentration, >10 mg/dL), hypocalcemia (<8.6 mg/dL), anemia (PCV, <33%), proteinuria, ethylene glycol ingestion, and disseminated intravascular coagulation were associated with failure to survive, but advanced age was not a factor.[129] Odds ratios for failure to survive were lowest for dogs with presenting serum creatinine concentrations of 1.8 to 5.0 mg/dL, intermediate for those serum creatinine concentrations of 5.1 to 10.0, and very high for dogs with serum creatinine concentrations in excess of 10.0 mg/dL. Dogs that did not survive hospital-acquired ARF in another study had higher serum phosphorus and anion gap concentrations than dogs that survived.[5] In that study, dogs older than 7 years or those that had oliguria at presentation were at increased risk for failure to survive, but magnitude of azotemia at the time of diagnosis did not predict survival. In a retrospective study of cats with ARF, mortality was 56%. In this study, nephrotoxicity was the most common cause of ARF (12 of 25 cats). Azotemia did not affect outcome, but urine production was crucial. All nonoliguric cats survived, whereas none of the oliguric or anuric cats survived.[132] When intrinsic ARF in dogs is caused by leptospirosis, aggressive fluid therapy and administration of antibiotics often lead to resolution of nephritis and survival.[14,74,110] In the unusual circumstance in which hospital-acquired ARF follows use of nafcillin, the prognosis for recovery of normal renal function is fair. Four of seven dogs regained normal renal function, two had persistent isosthenuria with normal BUN and creatinine concentrations, and one was euthanized because of failure to respond to treatment.[103]

Early identification of the cause of ARF allows aggressive targeted therapy. This is most crucial in cases of toxicity (e.g., ethylene glycol, ibuprofen, lilies) in which a narrow window of time is available for induction of emesis and administration of antidotes. A high index of suspicion is necessary. Suspicion of leptospirosis traditionally has been based on laboratory findings and risk of exposure, whereas definitive diagnosis relied on seroconversion or, rarely, identification of leptospires on biopsy or in urine. A real-time quantitative PCR has recently been reported for use in humans and has been shown to identify pathogenic serovars of leptospirosis without cross-reacting with nonpathogenic serovars or other bacterial organisms.[88] This technique holds promise for early and definitive identification of this disease.

Prognosis for survival and recovery of adequate renal function after episodes of intrinsic ARF requires clinical consideration and integration of the cause of renal failure, severity of histopathologic renal injury, severity of laboratory abnormalities, other organ system dysfunction, response time after initial therapy, adequacy of response to therapy, and access to dialysis. In the future, targeted therapy to augment renal hemodynamics with atrial natriuretic peptide, assisted recovery of denuded tubular basement membranes with growth factors, and resolution of intratubular obstruction with disintegrins and fluid therapy may improve prognosis for recovery from intrinsic ARF.[80,126]

How long should one wait for the return of adequate renal function? There is no well-defined period in patients with renal failure over which the magnitude of azotemia substantially diminishes as renal lesions heal and renal function improves, if this occurs at all. Consequently, the duration of treatment is determined individually for each patient. Fluid therapy is continued as long as the BUN, serum creatinine, and serum phosphorus concentrations are progressively decreasing to a level tolerated by the patient.

Long-term supportive care may be required for animals in which the magnitude of severe azotemia either does not decrease or actually increases during initial aggressive fluid therapy. Some animals tolerate severe azotemia during ARF or CRF better than others. In these patients, meticulous attention to fluid therapy is indicated for 2 to 4 weeks during ARF, for 5 to 7 days during uncomplicated decompensated CRF, and for 2 to 4 weeks during ARF-on-CRF. This usually provides adequate time for the diseased kidneys to undergo healing of acute lesions or recompensation in chronic renal disease. The time required for renal compensation and improved clinical condition is variable and depends on the extent of renal injury.

In the absence of dialysis, euthanasia should be considered for animals with severe azotemia and clinical signs of uremia if clinical and laboratory improvement is not seen after 5 to 7 days of intensive treatment. Dialysis may substantially lessen the patient's discomfort by reducing the magnitude of azotemia. Early and aggressive hemodialysis has been shown to improve the prognosis for survival of ARF in dogs and cats (see Chapter 29). Animals that remain severely oliguric, develop progressive oliguria, or develop overhydration during aggressive fluid therapy probably should be euthanized if dialysis is not an option. Likewise, euthanasia should be considered for animals with intractable hyperkalemia or severe metabolic acidosis.

Bacterial infections are important complications during the management of uremic crises and may result in death. Uremic patients have diminished host defenses at a time when indwelling urinary catheterization is necessary to monitor urine output and placement of an intravenous catheter is required to administer fluids. Urinary tract infection is a common cause of bacterial sepsis in dogs.[21] Recumbency may favor the development of pneumonia in the septic animal and increases the risk of aspiration pneumonia after episodes of vomiting.

Severe encephalopathy and uremic pneumonitis may be manifestations of advanced renal failure that are not readily treated. Blood loss into the gastrointestinal tract can be severe. Gastrointestinal ulcers that contribute to hemorrhage, diarrhea, and vomiting may continue to develop despite conventional medical management of uremia. Malnutrition can become severe when nutrient intake is absent or poor and when catabolism is increased. Such malnutrition results in severe loss of lean body mass.

TAPERING PARENTERAL FLUID THERAPY

If oliguria persists despite attempts at intensive diuresis, the volume of administered fluid is immediately reduced until diuresis ensues. Replacement of insensible fluid losses is continued at approximately 20 mL/kg/day, and contemporary losses from vomiting or diarrhea are replaced.

In nonoliguric patients, the volume of fluid administered is reduced gradually after BUN and serum creatinine concentrations have decreased substantially. Alternatively, fluids are tapered if BUN and serum creatinine concentrations remain increased but are stable for three consecutive days after an initial reduction in the magnitude of azotemia and improved clinical status. It has been the authors' experience that animals with BUN concentrations greater than 100 mg/dL and serum creatinine concentrations greater than 8 mg/dL after aggressive fluid therapy are not likely to be managed adequately with fluids, and certainly not when fluid therapy is withdrawn.

Patients with polyuric renal failure have an obligatory diuresis, and successful tapering of intravenous fluids depends on increased spontaneous fluid intake by the animal (drinking and eating) and reduced fluid losses through vomiting or diarrhea. Fluid therapy should not be abruptly discontinued during the treatment of uremic patients to avoid development of dehydration and a subsequent sudden increase in the magnitude of azotemia. In general, parenteral fluid volume is reduced by approximately 25% daily for each of two to three consecutive days before discontinuing fluid therapy. It is important to monitor the patient closely during this time to ensure that the animal remains well hydrated (as determined by skin turgor and stable body weight) and that the magnitude of azotemia either stabilizes or decreases. A substantial increase in BUN and serum creatinine concentrations in conjunction with deterioration of the animal's clinical condition necessitates resumption of fluid therapy. During more rapid tapering of intravenous fluids, it is advisable to provide supplemental fluids subcutaneously.

Some animals with worsening azotemia after initial tapering of fluid volume can successfully undergo a later reduction of fluid volume after an additional few days of full fluid support. At that time, the tapering of fluid therapy should be more gradual. Some uremic patients develop a worsening degree of azotemia after each tapering of intravenous fluids and cannot be successfully treated. In some instances, chronic fluid loading by the subcutaneous route (administered by the owners at home) can alleviate the degree of azotemia to an extent that the animal remains functional.

REFERENCES

1. Adelman AD, Spangler WL, Beasom F, et al: Furosemide enhancement of experimental gentamicin nephrotoxicity, *J Infect Dis* 140:342-352, 1979.

2. Adin CA, Cowgill LD: Treatment and outcome of dogs with leptospirosis: 36 cases (1990-1998), *J Am Vet Med Assoc* 216:371-375, 2000.

3. ANZICS Clinical Trials Group: Low-dose dopamine in patients with early renal dysfunction: a placebo-controlled randomized trial, *Lancet* 356:2139-2143, 2000.

4. Aronson S, Goldberg LI, Roth S, et al: Preservation of renal blood flow during hypotension induced with fenoldopam in dogs, *Can J Anaesth* 37:380-384, 1990.

5. Behrend EN, Grauer GF, Mani I, et al: Hospital-acquired acute renal failure in dogs: 29 cases (1983-1992), *J Am Vet Med Assoc* 208:537-541, 1996.

6. Bentinck-Smith J, French TW: A roster of normal values for dogs and cats. In Kirk RW, editor: *Current veterinary therapy X,* Philadelphia, 1989, WB Saunders, pp. 1335-1345.

7. Biancofiore G, Della Rocca G, Bindi L, et al: Use of fenoldopam to control renal dysfunction early after liver transplantation, *Liver Transpl* 10:986-992, 2004.

8. Boutilier P, Carr A, Schulman RL: Leptospirosis in dogs: a serologic survey and case series 1996 to 2001, *Vet Ther* 4:178-187, 2003.

9. Brezis M, Rosen S, Epstein FH: Acute renal failure. In Brenner BM, Rector FC, editors: *The kidney,* Philadelphia, 1991, WB Saunders, pp. 993-1061.

10. Brooks DP, DePalma D: The dopamine DA-1 receptor agonist fenoldopam enhances amino-acid-induced hyperemia in dogs, *Pharmacology* 47:43-49, 1993.

11. Brooks DP, DePalma PD, Cyronak MJ, et al: Identification of fenoldopam prodrugs with prolonged renal vasodilator activity, *J Pharmacol Exp Ther* 254:1084-1089, 1990.

12. Brooks DP, Goldstein R, Koster PF, et al: Effect of fenoldopam in dogs with spontaneous renal insufficiency, *Eur J Pharmacol* 184:195-199, 1990.

13. Brooks DP, Drutz DJ, Ruffolo RR Jr: Prevention and complete reversal of cyclosporine A-induced renal vasoconstriction and nephrotoxicity in the rat by fenoldopam, *J Pharmacol Exp Ther* 254:375-379, 1990.

14. Brown CA, Roberts AW, Miller MA, et al.: *Leptospira interrogans* serovar *grippotyphosa* infection in dogs, *J Am Vet Med Assoc* 209:1265-1267, 1996.

15. Brown CV, Rhee P, Chan L, et al: Preventing renal failure in patients with rhabdomyolysis: do bicarbonate and mannitol make a difference? *J Trauma* 56:1191-1196, 2004.

16. Brown SA, Barsanti JA, Crowell WA: Gentamicin-associated acute renal failure, *J Am Vet Med Assoc* 186:686-690, 1985.

17. Brown SA, Henik RA: Diagnosis and treatment of systemic hypertension, *Vet Clin North Am Small Anim Pract* 28:1481-1494, 1998.

18. Brown SA, Brown CA, Crowell WA, et al: Effects of dietary polyunsaturated fatty acid supplementation in early renal insufficiency in dogs, *J Lab Clin Med* 135:275-286, 2000.

19. Brown SA, Henik RA, Finco DR: Diagnosis of systemic hypertension in dogs and cats. In Bonagura JD, editor: *Current veterinary therapy XIII,* Philadelphia, 2000, WB Saunders, pp. 835-838.

20. Buffington CA, DiBartola SP, Chew DJ: Effect of low potassium commercial nonpurified diet on renal function of adult cats, *J Nutr* 121:S91-S92, 1991.

21. Calvert CA, Dow SW: Cardiovascular infections. In Greene CE, editor: *Infectious diseases of the dog and cat,* ed 2, Philadelphia, 1990, WB Saunders, pp. 97-113.

22. Campbell A, Bates N: Raisin poisoning in dogs, *Vet Rec* 152:376, 2003.

23. Carcoana OV, Hines RL: Is renal dose dopamine protective or therapeutic? Yes. *Crit Care Clin* 12:677-685, 1996.

24. Casagrande C, Merlo L, Ferrini R, et al: Cardiovascular and renal action of dopaminergic prodrugs, *J Cardiovasc Pharmacol* 14(suppl 8):540-559, 1989.

25. Chew DJ: Acute intrinsic renal failure, 14th Kal Kan Symposium, Columbus, OH, 1991, pp. 69-92.

26. Chew DJ, DiBartola SP: Diagnosis and pathophysiology of renal disease. In Ettinger SJ, editor: *Textbook of veterinary internal medicine,* ed 3, vol 2, Philadelphia, 1989, WB Saunders, pp. 1893-1961.

27. Chew DJ, Leonard M, Muir W: Effect of sodium bicarbonate infusions on ionized calcium and total calcium concentrations in serum of clinically normal cats, *Am J Vet Res* 50:145-150, 1989.

28. Chew DJ, Nagode LN: Renal secondary hyperparathyroidism, Fourth Annual Meeting of the Society for Comparative Endocrinology, Washington, DC, 1990, pp. 17-26.

29. Chonko AM, Grantham JJ: Treatment of edema states. In Maxwell MH, Kleeman CR, Narins RG, editors: *Clinical disorders of fluid and electrolyte metabolism,* ed 4, New York, 1987, McGraw-Hill, pp. 429-460.

30. Clark KL, Hilditch A, Robertson MJ, et al: Effects of dopamine DA1-receptor blockade and angiotensin converting enzyme inhibition on the renal actions of fenoldopam in the anaesthetized dog, *J Hypertens* 9:1143-1150, 1991.

31. Clark KL, Robertson MJ, Drew GM: Do renal tubular dopamine receptors mediate dopamine-induced diuresis in the anesthetized cat? *J Cardiovasc Pharmacol* 17:267-276, 1991.

32. Conger JD: Interventions in clinical acute renal failure: what are the data? *Am J Kidney Dis* 26:565-576, 1995.

33. Cornelius LM: Fluid therapy in the uremic patient. In Kirk RW, editor: *Current veterinary therapy VIII,* Philadelphia, 1983, WB Saunders, pp. 989-994.

34. Cowgill LD: Application of peritoneal and hemodialysis in the management of renal failure. In Osborne CA, Finco DR, editors: *Canine and feline nephrology and urology,* Baltimore, 1995, Williams & Wilkins, pp. 335-367.

35. Cowgill LD, Langston CE: Role of hemodialysis in the management of dogs and cats with renal failure, *Vet Clin North Am Small Anim Pract* 26:1347-1378, 1996.

36. Cowgill LD: Hypertension and the kidney, Proceedings of the American College of Veterinary Internal Medicine, 22nd Annual Forum, Minneapolis, MN, 2004.

37. Crisp MS, Chew DJ, DiBartola SP, et al: Peritoneal dialysis in dogs and cats: 27 cases (1976-1987), *J Am Vet Med Assoc* 195:1262-1266, 1989.

37a. Dawidson et al: 1992. Verapamil (VP) improves the outcome after renal transplantation (CRT), *Transpl Int* 5 Suppl 1:S60-S62, 1992.

38. Della Rocca G, Pompei L, Costa MG, et al: Fenoldopam mesylate and renal function in patients undergoing liver transplantation: a randomized, controlled pilot study, *Anesth Analg* 99:1604-1609, 2004.

39. Denton MD, Chertow GM, Brady HR: "Renal-dose" dopamine for the treatment of acute renal failure: scientific rationale, experimental studies and clinical trials, *Kidney Int* 50:4-14, 1996.

40. De Souza Durao M, Razvickas CV, Goncalves EA, et al: The role of growth factors on renal tubular cells submitted to hypoxia and deprived of glucose, *Ren Fail* 25:341-353, 2003.

41. DiBartola SP, Chew DJ, Jacobs G: Quantitative urinalysis including 24 hour protein excretion in the dog, *J Am Anim Hosp Assoc* 16:537-546, 1980.

42. DiBartola SP, Rutgers HC, Zack PM, et al: Clinico-pathologic findings associated with chronic renal disease in cats: 74 cases (1973-1984), *J Am Vet Med Assoc* 190:1196-1202, 1987.

43. DiBona GF: Effects of felodipine on renal function in animals, *Drugs* 29(suppl 2):168-175, 1985.

44. Dow SW: Studies of potassium depletion in cats, 12th Annual Kal Kan Symposium, Columbus, OH, 1989, pp. 61-64.

45. Dow SW, Fettman MJ, Curtis CR, et al: Hypokalemia in cats: 186 cases (1984-1987), *J Am Vet Med Assoc* 194:1604-1608, 1989.

46. Dow SW, LeCouteur RA, Fettman MJ, et al: Potassium depletion in cats: hypokalemic polymyopathy, *J Am Vet Med Assoc* 191:1563-1568, 1987.

47. Drobatz KJ, Hughes D: Concentration of ionized calcium in plasma from cats with urethral obstruction, *J Am Vet Med Assoc* 211:1392-1395, 1997.

48. English PB: Acute renal failure in the dog and cat, *Aust Vet J* 50:384-392, 1974.

49. Eubig PA, Brady MS, Gwaltney-Brant SM, et al: Acute renal failure in dogs subsequent to the ingestion of grapes or raisins: a retrospective evaluation of 43 dogs (1992-2002), *J Vet Intern Med* 19(5):663-674, 2005.

50. Feld LG, Cachero S, Springate JE: Fluid needs in acute renal failure, *Pediatr Clin North Am* 37:337-350, 1990.

51. Feldman L, Efrati S, Dishy V, et al: N-acetylcysteine ameliorates amphotericin-induced nephropathy in rats, *Nephron Physiol* 99:23-27, 2005.

52. Fettman MJ: Feline kaliopenic polymyopathy/nephropathy syndrome, *Vet Clin North Am Small Anim Pract* 19:415-432, 1989.

53. Finco DR: Fluid therapy. In Kirk RW, editor: *Current veterinary therapy VI*, Philadelphia, 1977, WB Saunders, pp. 3-12.

54. Finco DR: Kidney function. In Kaneko JJ, Harvey JW, Burss ML, editors: *Clinical biochemistry of domestic animals*, ed 5, San Diego, 1997, Academic Press, pp. 441-484.

55. Finco DR, Barsanti JA: Parenteral nutrition during a uremic crisis. In Kirk RW, editor: *Current veterinary therapy VIII*, Philadelphia, 1983, WB Saunders, pp. 994-996.

56. Finco DR, Duncan JR: Evaluation of blood urea nitrogen and serum creatinine concentrations as indicators of renal dysfunction: a study of 111 cases and review of related literature, *J Am Vet Med Assoc* 168:593-601, 1976.

57. Finco DR, Rowland GN: Hypercalcemia secondary to chronic renal failure in the dog: a report of four cases, *J Am Vet Med Assoc* 173:990-994, 1978.

58. Fink M, Nelson R, Roethal R: Low-dose dopamine preserves renal blood flow in endotoxin shocked dogs treated with ibuprofen, *J Surg Res* 38:582-591, 1985.

59. Fluornoy WS, Wohl JS, Albrecht-Schmitt TJ, et al: Pharmacologic identification of putative D_1 dopamine receptors in feline kidneys, *J Vet Pharmacol Ther* 26:283-290, 2003.

60. Forrester SD, McMillan NS, Ward DL: Retrospective evaluation of acute renal failure in dogs, Proceedings of the American College of Veterinary Internal Medicine, 20th Annual Forum, Dallas, TX, 2002.

61. Francey T, Cowgill LD: Hypertension in dogs with severe acute renal failure, Proceedings of the American College of Veterinary Internal Medicine, 22nd Annual Forum, Minneapolis, MN, 2004.

62. Fredrickson ED, Bradley T, Goldberg L: Blockade of renal effects of dopamine in the dog by the DA1 antagonist SCH 23390, *Am J Physiol* 249:F236-F240, 1985.

63. Goldberg LI, Rajfer SI: Dopamine receptors: applications in clinical cardiology, *Circulation* 72:245-248, 1985.

64. Grauer GF, Thrall MA, Henre BA, et al: Early clinicopathologic findings in dogs ingesting ethylene glycol, *Am J Vet Res* 45:2299-2303, 1984.

65. Green J, Abassi Z, Winaver J, et al: Acute renal failure: clinical and pathophysiologic aspects. In Seldin DW, Giebisch G, editors: *The kidney: physiology and pathophysiology*, ed 3, vol 2, Philadelphia, 2000, Lippincott, Williams, and Wilkins, pp. 2329-2373.

66. Gunal AI, Celiker H, Dogukan A, et al: Early and vigorous fluid resuscitation prevents acute renal failure in the crush victims of catastrophic earthquakes, *J Am Soc Nephrol* 15:1862-1867, 2004.

67. Gwaltney-Brant S, Holding JK, Donaldson CW, et al: Renal failure associated with ingestion of grapes or raisins in dogs, *J Am Vet Med Assoc* 218:1555-1556, 2001.

68. Hadley RM, Richardson JA, Gwaltney-Brant SM: A retrospective study of day lily toxicosis in cats, *Vet Hum Toxicol* 45:38-39, 2003.

69. Hahn RA, Wardell JR, Sarau HM, et al: Characterization of the peripheral and central effects of SK&F 82526, a novel dopamine receptor agonist, *J Pharmacol Exp Ther* 223:305-313, 1982.

70. Hall JO: Lily nephrotoxicity. In August JR: *Consultations in feline internal medicine*, ed 4, Philadelphia, 2001, WB Saunders, pp. 309-310.

71. Hamlin RL, Rasjian RJ: Water intake and output and quantity of feces in healthy cats, *Vet Med* 59:746-747, 1964.

72. Hammond PG, Cutler RE: Dopamine, dopaminergic agents, and the kidney. Part 1: Pharmacology, vascular and tubular effects, *Dial Transplant* 18:36-37, 1989.

73. Hansen B, DeFrancesco T: Relationship between hydration estimate and body weight change after fluid therapy in critically ill dogs and cats, *J Vet Emerg Crit Care* 12:235-243, 2002.

74. Harkin KR, Gartrell CL: Canine leptospirosis in New Jersey and Michigan: 17 cases (1990-1995), *J Am Anim Hosp Assoc* 32:495-501, 1996.

75. Harper L, Savage CO: The use of dopamine in acute renal failure (letter), *Clin Nephrol* 47:347-349, 1997.

76. Haskins SC: Anesthetic management of the end-stage renal failure patient, *Calif Vet* 33:13-15, 1979.

77. Heyman SN, Kaminski N, Brezis M: Dopamine increases renal medullary blood flow without improving regional hypoxia, *Exp Nephrol* 3:331-337, 1995.

78. Holmes CL, KR Walley: Bad medicine: low-dose dopamine in the ICU, *Chest* 123:1266-1275, 2003.

79. Hosgood G: Pharmacologic features and physiologic effects of dopamine, *J Am Vet Med Assoc* 197:1209-1211, 1990.

80. Humes hd: Acute renal failure: prevailing challenges and prospects for the future, *Kidney Int Suppl* 50:S26-S32, 1995.

81. Kellum JA, JM Decker: Use of dopamine in acute renal failure: a meta-analysis, *Crit Care Med* 29:1526-1531, 1996.

82. Kersting EJ, Nielsen SW: Experimental ethylene glycol poisoning in the dog, *Am J Vet Res* 27:574-582, 1966.

83. Kirby R: Acute renal failure as a complication in the critically ill animal, *Vet Clin North Am Small Animal Pract* 19:1189-1208, 1989.

84. Kurnik BR, Weisberg LS, Cuttler IM, et al: Effects of atrial natriuretic peptide versus mannitol on renal blood flow during radiocontrast infusion in chronic renal failure, *J Lab Clin Med* 116:27-36, 1990.

85. Langston CE, Cowgill LD, Spano JA: Applications and outcome of hemodialysis in cats: a review of 29 cases, *J Vet Intern Med* 11:348-355, 1997.

86. Langston CE: Acute renal failure caused by lily ingestion in six cats, *J Am Vet Med Assoc* 220:49-52, 2002.

87. Lassnigg A, Donner E, Grubhofer G, et al: Lack of renoprotective effects of dopamine and furosemide during cardiac surgery, *J Am Soc Nephrol* 11:97-104, 2000.

88. Levett PN, Morey RE, Galloway RL, et al: Detection of pathogenic leptospires by real-time quantitative PCR, *J Med Microbiol* 54:45-49, 2005.

89. Levinsky NG, Bernard DB, Johnston PA: Mannitol and loop diuretics in acute renal failure. In Brenner BM, Lazarus JM, editors: *Acute renal failure,* Philadelphia, 1983, WB Saunders, pp. 712-722.

90. Lindner A, Cutler RE, Goodman WG: Synergism of dopamine plus furosemide in preventing acute renal failure in the dog, *Kidney Int* 16:158-166, 1979.

91. Lokhandwala MF, Hegde SS: Cardiovascular dopamine receptors: role of renal dopamine and dopamine receptors in sodium excretion, *Pharmacol Toxicol* 66:237-243, 1990.

92. Lulich JP, Osborne CA, O'Brien TD, et al: Feline renal failure: questions, answers, questions, *Compend Cont Ed Pract Vet* 14:127-151, 1992.

93. Lund EM, Armstrong PJ, Kirk CA, et al: Health status and population characteristics of dogs and cats examined at private veterinary practices in the United States, *J Am Vet Med Assoc* 214:1336-1341, 1999.

94. Marik PE: Low-dose dopamine: a systematic review, *Intensive Care Med* 28:877-883, 2002.

95. Mazzaferro EM, Eubig PA, Hackett TB, et al: Acute renal failure associated with raisin or grape ingestion in 4 dogs, *J Vet Emerg Crit Care* 14:203-212, 2004.

96. McCabe J, Goldstein R, Cowgill L, et al: The effects of fluids and diuretic therapies on glomerular filtration rate, renal blood flow and urine output in healthy cats, 22nd Annual Forum, American College of Veterinary Internal Medicine, Minneapolis, MN, 2004.

97. Mitaka C, Hirata Y, Habuka K, et al: Atrial natriuretic peptide infusion improves ischemic renal failure after suprarenal abdominal aortic cross-clamping in dogs, *Crit Care Med.* 31:2205-2210, 2003.

98. Murray C, Markos F, Snow HM: Effects of fenoldopam on renal blood flow and its function in a canine model of rhabdomyolysis, *Eur J Anaesthesiol* 20:711-718, 2003.

99. Nachreiner RF, Refsal KR: The use of parathormone, ionized calcium and 25-hydroxyvitamin D assays to diagnose calcium disorders in dogs, 8th Annual Forum, American College of Veterinary Internal Medicine, Washington, DC, 1990, pp. 251-254.

100. Nichols AJ, Koster PF, Brooks DP, et al: Effect of fenoldopam on the acute and subacute nephrotoxicity produced by amphotericin B in the dog, *J Pharmacol Exp Ther* 260:269-274, 1992.

101. Nunamaker DM, Medway W, Berg P: Treatment of ethylene glycol poisoning in the dog, *J Am Vet Med Assoc* 159:310-314, 1971.

102. Osborne CA, Low DG, Finco DR: Fluid therapy in renal failure. In Osborne CA, Low DG, Finco DR, editors: *Canine and feline urology,* Philadelphia, 1972, WB Saunders, pp. 291-309.

103. Pacoe PJ, Ilkiw JE, Kass PH, et al: Case-control study of the association between intraoperative administration of nafcillin and acute postoperative development of azotemia, *J Am Vet Med Assoc* 208:1043-1047, 1996.

104. Pettersson K, Noble MIM, Bjorkman J-A, et al: The positive inotropic effect of felodipine in isovolumically beating dog heart, *J Cardiovasc Pharmacol* 10(suppl 1): S112-S118, 1987.

105. Polo-Romero FJ, Fernandez-Funez A, Broseta Viana L, et al: Effect of N-acetylcysteine on oxidative status in glycerol-induced acute renal failure in rats, *Ren Fail* 26:613-618, 2004.

106. Polzin D, Osborn C, O'Brien T: Diseases of the kidneys and ureters. In Ettinger SJ, editor: *Textbook of veterinary internal medicine,* ed 3, vol 2, Philadelphia, 1989, WB Saunders, pp. 1962-2046.

107. Rall LB, Scott J, Bell GI, et al: Mouse prepro-epidermal growth factor synthesis by the kidney and other tissues, *Nature* 313:228-331, 1985.

108. Rashid ST, Salman M, Myint F, et al: Prevention of contrast-induced nephropathy in vascular patients undergoing angiography: a randomized controlled trial of intravenous N-acetylcysteine, *J Vasc Surg* 40:1136-1141, 2004.

109. Refsal KR, Nachreiner RF, Graham PA: Laboratory assessment of hypercalcemia, 16th Annual American College of Veterinary Internal Medicine Forum, San Diego, 1998, pp. 646-647.

110. Rentko VT, Clark N, Ross LA, et al: Canine leptospirosis. A retrospective study of 17 cases, *J Vet Intern Med* 6:235-244, 1992.

111. Ross LA: Fluid therapy for acute and chronic renal failure, *Vet Clin North Am Small Anim Pract* 19:343-359, 1989.

112. Rowland J: Incidence of ethylene glycol intoxication in dogs and cats seen at Colorado State University Veterinary Teaching Hospital, *Vet Hum Toxicol* 29:41-44, 1987.

113. Schiller LR, Santa Ana CA, Sheikh MS, et al: Effect of the time of administration of calcium acetate on phosphorus binding, *N Engl J Med* 320:1110-1113, 1989.

114. Schrier RW, Arnold PE, van Putten VJ, et al: Cellular calcium in ischemic acute renal failure, *Kidney Int* 32:313, 1987.

115. Schwartz LB, Gewertz BL: The renal response to low dose dopamine, *J Surg Res* 45:574-588, 1988.

115a. Green J, Abassi Z, Winaver J, et al: Acute renal failure: clinical and pathophysiologic aspects. In Seldin DW, Giebisch G: *The kidney: physiology and pathophysiology,* ed 3, Philadelphia, 2000, Lippincott Williams and Wilkins, pp. 2329-2372.

116. Shilliday I, Allison ME: Diuretics in acute renal failure, *Ren Fail* 16:3-17, 1994.

117. Shilliday IR, Sherif M: Calcium channel blockers for preventing acute tubular necrosis in kidney transplant recipients, *Cochrane Database Syst Rev* CD003421, 2004.

118. Silber SJ, Thompson N: Mannitol induced central nervous system toxicity in renal failure, *Invest Urol* 9:310, 1972.

119. Singleton VL: More information on grape or raisin toxicosis, *J Am Vet Med Assoc* 219:434, 436, 2001.

120. Smith GW, Farmer JB, Ince F, et al: FPL 63012AR: a potent D1-receptor agonist, *Br J Pharmacol* 100:295-300, 1990.

121. Smith RC, Haschen T, Hamlin RL, et al: Water and electrolyte intake and output and quantity of feces in the healthy dog, *Vet Med* 59:743-746, 1964.

122. Solomon R, Werner C, Mann D, et al: Effects of saline, mannitol, and furosemide to prevent acute decreases in renal function induced by radiocontrast agents, *N Engl J Med* 331:1416-1420, 1994.

123. Summers A, Chew DJ, Buffington CAT: Serum ionized magnesium and calcium concentrations in a population of sick dogs and cats, *Compend Cont Ed Pract Vet Suppl*, in press.

124. Sward K, Valsson F, Odencrants P, et al: Recombinant human atrial natriuretic peptide in ischemic acute renal failure: a randomized placebo-controlled trial, *Crit Care Med* 32:1310-1315, 2004.

125. Takenaka T, Forster H, Epstein M: Characterization of the renal microvascular actions of a new dopaminergic (DA1) agonist, YM435, *J Pharmacol Exp Ther* 264:1154-1159, 1993.

126. Thadhani R, Pascual M, Bonventre JV: Acute renal failure, *N Engl J Med* 334:1448-1460, 1996.

127. Thrall MA, Grauer GF, Mero KN: Clinicopathologic findings in dogs and cats with ethylene glycol intoxication, *J Am Vet Med Assoc* 184:37-41, 1984.

128. Trim CM, Moore JN, Clark ES: Renal effects of dopamine infusion in conscious horses, *Equine Vet J Suppl* 7:124-128, 1989.

129. Vaden SL, Levin J, Breitschwerdt EB: A retrospective case-control of acute renal failure in 99 dogs, *J Vet Intern Med* 11:58-64, 1997.

130. Wasserman K, Huss R, Kullman R: Dopamine-induced diuresis in the cat without changes in renal hemodynamics, *Arch Pharm* 312:77-83, 1980.

131. Weiner IM, Mudge GH: Diuretics and other agents employed in the mobilization of edema fluid. In Gilman AG, Goodman LS, Rall TW, et al, editors: *The pharmacologic basis of therapeutics,* New York, 1985, Macmillan Publishing, pp. 887-907.

132. Worwag S, Langston CE: Acute renal failure in cats: 25 cases (1997-2002), Proceedings of the American College of Veterinary Internal Medicine, 22nd Annual Forum, Minneapolis, MN, 2004.

133. Yatsu T, Arai Y, Takizawa K, et al: Renal effect of YM435, a new dopamine D1 receptor agonist, in anesthetized dogs, *Eur J Pharmacol* 322:45-53, 1997.

134. Yatsu T, Takizawa K, Kasia-Nakagawa C, et al: Hemodynamic characterization of YM435, a novel dopamine DA1 receptor agonist, in anesthetized dogs, *J Cardiovasc Pharmacol* 29:382-388, 1997.

135. Yatsu T, Uchida W, Inagaki O, et al: Dopamine DA1 receptor agonist activity of YM435 in the canine renal vasculature, *Gen Pharmacol* 29:229-232, 1997.

136. Yatsu T, Arai Y, Takizawa K, et al: Effect of YM435, a dopamine DA1 receptor agonist, in a canine model of ischemic acute renal failure, *Gen Pharmacol* 31:803-807, 1998.

137. Yatsu T, Aoki M, Inagaki O: Preventive effect of zelandopam, a dopamine D1 receptor agonist, on cisplatin-induced acute renal failure in rats, *Eur J Pharmacol* 461:191-195, 2003.

138. Zager RA: Hyperphosphatemia: a factor that provokes severe experimental acute renal failure, *J Lab Clin Med* 100:230-239, 1982.

139. Zimmerman-Pope N, Waldron DR, Barber DL, et al: Effect of fenoldopam on renal function after nephrotomy in normal dogs, *Vet Surg* 32:566-573, 2003.

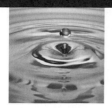

CHAPTER • 23

SHOCK SYNDROMES

Thomas K. Day and Shane Bateman

Shock is a complex and fascinating condition. Although often thought of as a disease of the cardiovascular system, the consequences of shock are cellular in nature and result from inadequate delivery of oxygen and nutrients to tissues by an impaired cardiovascular system. Shock represents the final common pathway to death in many critical care patients in veterinary and human medicine. Veterinary patients can be presented with shock, develop shock during the diagnosis and treatment of a wide variety of medical and surgical diseases, or develop shock during the postoperative period. All of the shock syndromes in veterinary medicine can result in high morbidity and mortality if not recognized and treated immediately. Advances in our knowledge of the pathophysiology of shock and shock syndromes and advances in noninvasive and invasive monitoring techniques have resulted in the ability to anticipate, recognize, and treat shock syndromes more effectively. Although we have learned a great deal about the pathophysiology of this devastating condition, much work remains to be completed. The future for shock researchers and clinicians alike holds considerable promise.

DEFINITION OF SHOCK

A true understanding of the shock syndromes must begin with the definition of shock. Shock is not defined by tachycardia, hypotension, circulatory collapse, stupor, coma, pale mucous membranes, or dehydration. These clinical signs may be associated with shock and are easily recognized, but they are common to many other conditions. The underlying problem or inciting event for all causes of shock is a decrease in effective blood flow and oxygen delivery to tissues that results in failure to meet the demands of the tissues.[43] Stated differently, shock is "the state in which profound and widespread reduction of *effective* tissue perfusion leads first to reversible and then, if prolonged, to irreversible cellular injury."[35] The decrease in effective perfusion can occur by many mechanisms, either cardiac or vascular in nature. Poor tissue perfusion initiates a complex series of events that eventually result in altered cellular metabolism, cellular death, organ failure, and ultimately the death of the animal.

PATHOPHYSIOLOGY

The delivery of oxygen to the tissues must meet their oxygen consumption demands. In the normal animal, oxygen consumption by the tissues is relatively constant. Clinical syndromes that can result in increased tissue oxygen consumption include status epilepticus, tremoro-genic toxins (e.g., strychnine, mold), heatstroke, and malignant hyperthermia. An examination of the oxygen delivery variables and formulas may be beneficial in evaluating all of the potential mechanisms by which oxygen delivery can be altered to produce shock (Table 23-1). The delivery of oxygen is dependent on cardiac output and the content of oxygen in arterial blood. Cardiac output is the product of heart rate and stroke volume, which consists of preload, afterload, myocardial contractility, and myocardial synchrony (cardiac rhythm). The content of oxygen in arterial blood consists of the amount of hemoglobin and the saturation of the existing hemoglobin with oxygen. Alteration of any of the components of oxygen delivery can result in inadequate oxygen delivery to the tissues. Many of these variables are difficult to measure and require the use of a pulmonary artery catheter or measurement of blood gases. An alternative way of considering oxygen delivery to tissues is to consider all the components of the cardiovascular system that must be functioning effectively. The heart must be pumping effectively, adequate intravascular blood volume (and hemoglobin) must be present, and the vascular tree must be responding normally to local blood flow requirements for effective tissue perfusion to take place. Therefore defects or dysfunction in any component or aspect of the cardiovascular system could lead to ineffective tissue perfusion or shock.

Blood pressure is the product of cardiac output and systemic vascular resistance. By definition, it is the lateral force that the blood exerts on the blood vessel wall at any given portion of the vascular system. Blood pressure is not synonymous with blood flow, perfusion, or cardiac output. These variables have complex influences on one another but cannot be used interchangeably. Therefore blood pressure is not a primary determinant of oxygen delivery but may be affected when cardiac output or vascular resistance is pathologically altered. Clinical assessment of patients with shock includes assessment of blood pressure, but it must be interpreted in conjunction with the patient's history, other clinical signs, and measured variables.

TABLE 23-1 Oxygen Delivery Variables, Equations, and Normal Values

Term and Abbreviation	Formula	Normal Value
Oxygen delivery (Do_2)	$Do_2 = CO \times Cao_2$	500-800 mL/min/m²
O_2 content in arterial blood (Cao_2)	$Cao_2 = (Hb \times 1.34 \times Sao_2) + (Pao_2 \times 0.003)$	16-22 mL O_2/dL
O_2 content in mixed venous blood (Cvo_2)	$Cvo_2 = (Hb \times 1.34 \times Svo_2) + (Pvo_2 \times 0.003)$	12-17 mL O_2/dL
Arterial-venous O_2 content difference (oxygen extraction)	$Ca\text{-}vo_2 = Cao_2 - Cvo_2$	3-5 mL O_2/dL
Oxygen consumption (Vo_2)	$Vo_2 = (Cao_2 - Cvo_2) \times CO$	100-150 mL/min/m²
Cardiac output (CO)	$CO = SV \times HR$	150-200 mL/kg/min

Sao₂, Saturation of oxygen in arterial blood; Svo₂, saturation of oxygen in venous blood; MAP, mean arterial blood pressure; SVR, systemic vascular resistance.

Alteration of tissue perfusion resulting from dysfunction within the cardiovascular system is detected by numerous triggers or sensors located throughout the organism. Detection of inadequate perfusion in this way initiates a neurohormonal compensatory response intended to counterbalance the failure within the cardiovascular delivery system (Fig. 23-1).[28] Examples of this compensatory response include specialized stretch receptors located in the aorta and carotid arteries that detect a decrease in cardiac output. Detection of a decrease in cardiac output prompts signal transmission to the vasomotor center of the medulla oblongata and results in release of the inhibition of the sympathetic center and activation of inhibition of the parasympathetic center. The adrenal medulla (activated by increased sympathetic tone) plays a large role in the neurohormonal response by releasing epinephrine and norepinephrine. The direct effects of increased sympathetic activity and higher circulating catecholamine concentrations from the adrenal gland are an increase in heart rate, increased cardiac contractility, and vasoconstriction (arterial and venous). Perfusion to individual tissue beds becomes dependent on their metabolic activity and importance. The brain and heart are able to autoregulate relatively effectively in the face of systemic vasoconstriction to maintain effective perfusion and oxygen and nutrient delivery. Most other tissue beds, including the skin, muscles, splanchnic beds, and the kidneys, possess much less effective autoregulatory mechanisms and fall victim to decreased perfusion as shock progresses.

Decreased glomerular filtration rate (GFR) in the kidneys is a direct effect of decreased cardiac output and initiates a potent series of compensatory responses. Activation of the renin-angiotensin-aldosterone axis assists in the maintenance of effective GFR, but production of angiotensin II has a potent systemic vasoconstrictive effect in addition to serving as a potent stimulus for aldosterone release from the adrenal glands. Aldosterone acts on the renal tubules to promote retention of sodium and water and thus increase intravascular volume. The release of adrenocorticotropic hormone (ACTH) and vasopressin (antidiuretic hormone [ADH]) from the pituitary gland also serves important compensatory roles. The combination of catecholamine stimulation and ACTH release increases circulating cortisol, which

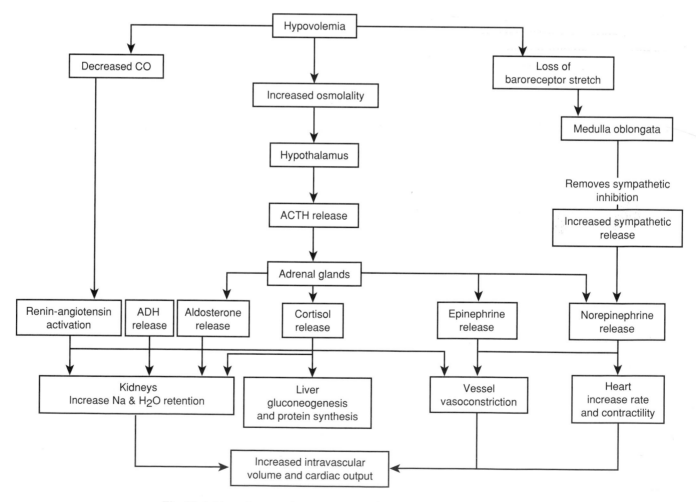

Fig. 23-1 Neurohormonal responses to a decrease in intravascular volume.

mobilizes substrates necessary for energy production. The renal tubules under the influence of ADH retain additional water to increase intravascular volume. Vasopressin, like angiotensin II, is a potent vasoconstrictive hormone.

The vasoconstriction that occurs in major arteries and veins as a result of the neurohormonal response to shock also occurs at the capillary level. Both precapillary and postcapillary vessels constrict. Precapillary constriction results in decreased perfusion to tissues. As shock progresses and oxygen supply decreases, anaerobic metabolism ensues. The combination of decreased oxygen supply and anaerobic metabolism alters the reaction of the terminal vessels in response to continual sympathetic stimulation. In this situation, the precapillary vessels dilate while the postcapillary vessels remain constricted. The results are increased blood flow to the capillary system, pooling of blood in the capillaries, and maldistribution of blood volume. This loss of additional blood volume exacerbates hypovolemia in the macrocirculation. In addition to the macrocirculation effects, the increased hydrostatic filtration pressure in the capillaries causes fluid loss in the tissues. The changes in the microcirculation have been termed the circulus vitiosus of shock (Fig. 23-2).[45] The changes at the capillary level also are responsible for what is termed maldistribution of blood flow. This alteration in microvascular function has been shown to persist past the point of successful restoration of adequate cardiac output and blood pressure and is thought to play a significant role in the development of multiple organ failure and death in shock patients.[24,25]

Although failure of the delivery system to the cell is vital to understanding shock, so too are the intracellular consequences of inadequate oxygen and nutrient delivery. Cell injury can occur via several important pathways. Initial deprivation of oxygen results in mitochondrial dysfunction and increasing dependence on anaerobic glycolysis and thus lactate production. As a result of decreased intracellular pH, enzymatic function is depressed, making the cell more susceptible to other injury. Ultimately, the need for adenosine triphosphate (ATP) to maintain cellular ionic and osmotic gradients exceeds the ATP production capacity of the cell, and

bioenergetic failure occurs. Loss of osmotic gradients can produce damaging intracellular swelling and potential cell rupture. The loss of calcium from endoplasmic reticulum reserves (Ca-ATPase failure) is a potent trigger for arachidonic acid breakdown and the production of inflammatory mediators such as prostaglandins and leukotrienes. Free radical damage also can occur in cells as a result of lysosomal membrane degradation or during reperfusion. Free radicals can propagate extensive cell membrane injury through lipid peroxidation, damage to cell DNA, and triggering of apoptosis pathways. Numerous cytokine mediators produced during cellular injury may play a crucial role in vascular endothelial injury resulting in white blood cell, platelet, or hemostatic plugging of the microvasculature and produce a no-reflow phenomenon. In fact, more than 150 locally produced mediators have been implicated in shock.[8,31,45,47,50] The mononuclear phagocytes are the most critical cells in initiating the release of cytokines.

CLASSIFICATION OF SHOCK SYNDROMES

Historically, shock has been classified into various categories and etiologies to assist in understanding this complex disorder. Numerous classification schemes have been presented to assist in understanding the clinical syndromes of shock. Many classification schemes are aimed at simplifying a complex disorder of the cardiovascular system into isolated components either on an anatomic basis or functional basis. Anatomic classification schemes typically are devised from the important components of the system: the heart, blood, and vessels. These categorizations isolate and attempt to explain dysfunction into cardiogenic, hypovolemic, and vascular (obstructive and distributive) types of shock.[35,43] Hypovolemic shock can occur by loss of intravascular volume of any etiology, including dehydration, blood loss, and third-space loss of fluids. Cardiogenic shock can occur as a result of any cardiac abnormality that causes pump failure such as heart disease, myocardial injury, or arrhythmia. Inappropriate vasodilatation is the hallmark of distributive shock and can occur through loss of neurological input (e.g., sympathetic trunk transection) or inflammatory mediators.

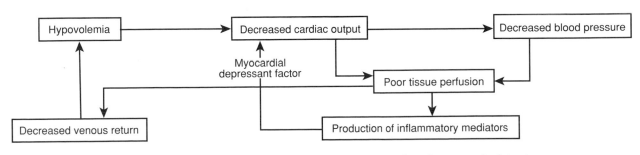

Fig. 23-2 Circulatory events that lead to the vicious circle (circulus vitiosus) of shock.

Sepsis, endotoxemia, and anaphylaxis all are common causes of distributive shock. Obstructive shock occurs as a result of any obstruction of blood flow out of or into the heart. Pericardial effusion and cardiac tamponade, pulmonary thromboembolism, caval syndrome, gastric dilatation-volvulus (GDV) syndrome, acute portal hypertension, and intracardiac tumors are clinical examples of shock that could be considered primarily obstructive. Physiologic classification schemes tend to categorize shock syndromes according to the attendant oxygen delivery variables: cardiac output, oxygen content of the blood, and cellular utilization of oxygen.[58] Shock also has been categorized based on normal or abnormal circulatory mechanisms.[68] The emphasis of this classification scheme is on the dynamics of precapillary and postcapillary vascular changes that occur and the resultant redistribution and pooling of blood.

Although such categorical organization of shock syndromes is helpful to understand the complex nature of shock, it is crucial to recognize that most clinical forms of shock affect multiple components simultaneously. The utility of anatomic or functional categories of shock is questionable when viewed from a clinical perspective, and some have argued that such a classification is misleading because clinicians may approach a one-dimensional easy-to-understand representation of shock with a simplistic one-dimensional approach to therapy.[58] Unfortunately, shock is complex—it does not begin with a common pathophysiologic event and does not necessarily end with survival after a simple universal initial treatment. Each etiology of shock sets in motion a complex series of events that include neural and hormonal responses, as well as numerous inflammatory cascades.

Perhaps the most useful feature of these schemes is to force the clinician to consider potential dysfunction of multiple components of the cardiovascular system and thus consider therapies that support each component of dysfunction.

Additional disagreement also centers on the use of the term distributive shock. The term distributive has been used to describe various types of high-flow shock under the assumption that blood flow is not normally distributed to tissue beds. Used in this context, "distributive shock" is a theoretical designation of a type of shock syndrome that is not defined by criteria that can be easily measured in a clinical setting. Maldistribution of blood flow has been documented in people in clinically accessible microscopic vascular beds (e.g., sclera, liver, nail bed). Direct observations have documented the phenomenon of maldistribution of blood flow, but such measurements are not necessarily representative of all areas and are not quantitative measures of the extent of maldistribution throughout the body. Therefore maldistribution of blood flow is a physiologic concept that may be relevant to all shock states.[58] Clinically measurable,

quantitative criteria are required for distributive shock to qualify as a specific type of shock.

The various classifications of shock syndromes in veterinary and human medicine have been created in an attempt to simplify a complex series of physiologic events. Unfortunately, laboratory research and clinical experience have not supported any one classification of the shock syndromes as being the easiest to understand or teach. The specific details surrounding the presentation of the patient with shock should rank as most important, and valuable time should not be wasted deciding which classification scheme best describes the patient. This chapter emphasizes the concepts that (1) important initial decisions based on physical examination determine the clinical stage of shock, (2) initial therapy should be based on the clinical stage of the specific shock syndrome, and (3) classification of the etiology of shock, response to initial therapy, and laboratory and other diagnostic evaluations all determine additional therapeutic interventions.

HYPOVOLEMIC SHOCK

Hypovolemia can be either absolute or relative in nature and is a common presentation of shock. Hemorrhagic shock is considered an absolute cause of hypovolemia because an actual loss of intravascular blood volume has occurred. Common clinical presentations include hemoperitoneum secondary to hemorrhage from splenic or hepatic neoplasia, coagulopathies (e.g., anticoagulant rodenticide toxicity, thrombocytopathia, thrombocytopenia), gastrointestinal hemorrhage, epistaxis, and traumatic lacerations of arteries or other major blood vessels.[14,41] Nonhemorrhagic shock is associated with relative hypovolemia despite no direct loss of whole blood from the intravascular space. The primary physiologic event is loss of plasma volume. Examples of loss of plasma volume include severe dehydration and third-space loss (e.g., peritoneum, intestinal tract). Anaphylactic shock is a clinical form of shock that has important hypovolemic and distributive components. It occurs as a result of immunoglobulin E–mediated release of vasoactive substances that produce massive vasodilatation and pooling of as much as 60% to 80% of the circulating blood volume (i.e., distributive), as well as endothelial injury and the leak of large volumes of fluid and plasma proteins from the intravascular to interstitial spaces (i.e., hypovolemic).[42]

CARDIOGENIC SHOCK

Cardiogenic shock can be associated with cardiac disease of any cause, acquired or congenital. It most commonly occurs in veterinary patients with cardiomyopathy, rupture of the chordae tendinae, or other conditions that adversely affect myocardial contractility.[12] It rarely occurs with the absence of congestive heart failure. It is a very common finding in human patients who have experienced myocardial infarction or during the postoperative period after coronary artery bypass graft surgery or other cardiac surgery requiring cardiopulmonary bypass. The clinical signs of cardiogenic shock are similar to those of other types of shock with notable exceptions. Respiratory distress and exercise intolerance or collapse are prominent features of cardiogenic shock, and bilateral crackles caused by pulmonary edema may be heard on thoracic auscultation. Cardiac murmurs also may be heard. Jugular distention may be present (jugular veins are collapsed in other types of shock), and mucous membranes may have a greater tendency to become cyanotic. Arrhythmias also are common at presentation in patients with cardiogenic shock and can be a primary cause of decreased cardiac output and decreased oxygen delivery.

OBSTRUCTIVE SHOCK

Obstructions of blood flow from the heart or returning to the heart can contribute to obstructive shock. Examples of obstructive shock include pericardial tamponade caused by pericardial effusion, caval syndrome of heartworm disease, pulmonary thromboembolism, aortic thromboembolism, and intracardiac neoplasia. The dilated stomach in patients with GDV can decrease ventricular filling as a result of obstruction of the caudal vena cava. Acute portal hypertension after surgical ligation of portosystemic shunts also was a common cause of obstructive shock in the past, but increased usage of ameroid constrictors (i.e., gradual attenuation of the shunt) has decreased the frequency of this form of obstructive shock. Clinical signs associated with this form of shock are variable and dependent on the location of obstruction.

DISTRIBUTIVE SHOCK

For the reasons discussed previously, distributive shock probably is the most controversial category in this classification scheme. The most common examples of this form of shock are systemic inflammatory response syndrome (SIRS) or sepsis, anaphylactic shock, and spinal shock. The unifying feature of these clinical syndromes is dysfunction of the microcirculation that causes inappropriate and widespread vasodilatation. Most often, vasodilatation results from inflammatory mediators that have induced nitric oxide synthetase enzymes to produce large quantities of nitric oxide, a potent vasodilating cytokine.[8,47] This form of shock differs substantially from most other forms of shock because it generally results in warm and well-perfused extremities in the early stages of the disorder.

COMMON CLINICAL FORMS OF SHOCK IN SMALL ANIMAL MEDICINE

Traumatic Shock

Traumatic shock is perhaps the most common form of shock in small animal veterinary medicine. Traumatic shock most often occurs as a result of accidental blunt trauma but can also be seen in the perioperative period of extensive soft tissue or orthopedic surgery. The surgical operation can be viewed as controlled trauma, allowing us to know the time and type of event that has induced shock.[5] Cardiovascular dysfunction in the early stages arises from the abnormalities of normal blood volume that occur as a consequence of hemorrhage or unreplaced evaporative fluid loss during long surgical procedures. Uncontrolled pain also may trigger substantial sympathetic outflow that can have profound vasoconstrictive effects on many tissue beds, resulting in decreased blood flow, altered perfusion, and meeting the criteria for the definition of shock. Traumatized patients with severe pain presented with signs of shock may not have significant blood loss, and their clinical signs may in fact be caused by severe pain. Such patients do not have clinical signs consistent with external or internal hemorrhage and typically have very high blood pressure. Treatment in such cases should consist of cautious initial fluid resuscitation and appropriate pain management. Tissue damage and ischemia in some patients also can trigger SIRS. Typically, the inflammatory response requires many hours to manifest fully, and this manifestation of traumatic injury may not be apparent until well after initial fluid resuscitation and pain management have successfully restored normal cardiovascular activity. Thus adequate and aggressive monitoring of the patient for signs consistent with SIRS allows early intervention.

Systemic Inflammatory Response Syndrome and Septic Shock

SIRS is a term applied to the widespread inflammatory and immune activity mounted by an organism against several kinds of microbial infections or in response to severe tissue trauma, injury, or necrosis.[31,50,59,60] The inflammatory response to both infectious and noninfectious triggers is nearly identical. It is composed of multiple intersecting and connected pathways of inflammation, endothelial dysfunction, and hemostatic abnormalities. Although the inflammatory response theoretically protects the organism by eliminating the microbial invader and repairing damaged tissues, the inflammatory response itself is damaging to multiple organs in many cases. The detrimental consequences of this response are referred to as multiple organ dysfunction syndrome (MODS). A consensus strategy for diagnosis of SIRS has been developed for both humans and veterinary patients. Physical examination findings and routine laboratory diagnostic tests are used to determine whether a patient fulfills appropriate criteria to diagnose SIRS (Table 23-2). Sepsis is a term used solely for patients meeting criteria for SIRS but with a proven microbial cause. Septic shock is a term reserved for septic patients displaying signs of cardiovascular dysfunction and altered tissue perfusion.

TABLE 23-2 Criteria for Systemic Inflammatory Response Syndrome*

Rectal temperature	>103.5° F, <100° F
Heart rate	>160 beats/min (dog)
	>250 beats/min (cat)
Respiratory rate	>20 breaths/min
$PaCO_2$	<32 mm Hg
White blood cell count	>12,000, <1000, or >10% bands

A patient is considered to have systemic inflammatory response syndrome if two or more of the criteria are fulfilled.

The primary effects of the inflammatory mediators on the cardiovascular system are vasodilatation, endothelial cell injury, and myocardial dysfunction. Dysfunction of the cardiovascular system as a result of these injuries can produce hypovolemia because of increased vascular permeability, dysfunction caused by decreased cardiac contractility, arrhythmias caused by circulating inflammatory mediators such as myocardial depressant factor, or some combination of these.[59,60] Clinically, high-output and low-output states of septic shock have been observed. In the high-output state, mild vasodilatation produced by the effects of cytokines on the vasculature results in an increase in cardiac output. Mucous membranes are bright red; capillary refill time is shortened; core body temperature usually is increased; and peripheral pulses are bounding. In the low-output state, peripheral vasodilatation overwhelms the cardiovascular system and, combined with poor ventricular performance in the latter stages of sepsis, cardiac output decreases. Mucous membranes are pale; capillary refill time is prolonged; core body temperature is decreased; pulses are weak; and blood pressure is low.

Successful management frequently relies on rapid and early identification and treatment of the primary cause of the inflammatory response. Despite extensive research into effective clinical therapies to modulate the inflamma-tory response, little has been achieved.[15] Only one therapy has shown promise in randomized clinical trials in human patients with severe sepsis and MODS. Recombinant activated human protein C, an important antithrombotic and antiinflammatory protein, is the only therapy that has reduced mortality in human patients with this devastating condition.[3,4] In veterinary patients, supportive care of organ injury and optimization of cardiovascular function and oxygen delivery are the mainstays of therapy.[8,47] Vasodilatation and increased vascular permeability dominate the cardiovascular effects of SIRS and septic shock, and aggressive, appropriate fluid therapy and cardiovascular support are crucial in successful treatment. The combination of cardiovascular effects results in a maldistribution of blood flow to tissues, at times in the presence of normal or increased cardiac output. Common causes of SIRS in small animal medicine include pancreatitis, heatstroke, pyometra, septic peritonitis, GDV, snake envenomation, neoplasia, and multiple trauma.

CLINICAL STAGES OF SHOCK

Three clinical stages of shock depict the progression of shock: compensatory stage, early decompensatory stage, and decompensatory (terminal) stage (Table 23-3).[54] As described above, the initiating event is an acute decrease in tissue perfusion. Shock develops when the normal compensatory neurohormonal response to restore blood volume and maintain the metabolic needs of the tissues is unsuccessful in restoring perfusion. When cardiac output decreases and autoregulation is lost, shock progresses from the compensatory stage to early decompensatory to terminal decompensatory stages.

COMPENSATORY STAGE

The compensatory stage of shock occurs as a result of baroreceptor-mediated release of catecholamines. Systemic vascular resistance (arteries and veins), heart rate, and contractility increase to produce an increase in

TABLE 23-3 Clinical Stages and Signs of Shock

Clinical Stage of Shock	Characteristics	Clinical Signs
Compensatory stage	Increases in CO, HR, and SVR Neurohormonal response Hypermetabolic, hyperdynamic state	Mild increases in HR, RR Normal mentation and blood pressure "Brick" red MM, CRT < 1 sec
Early decompensatory stage	Redistribution of blood flow to heart and brain Consumption of oxygen dependent on oxygen delivery Development of lactic acidosis	Tachycardia, tachypnea, pale MM, poor CRT, weak pulse, poor mentation, usually hypothermic, hypotension
Decompensatory (terminal) stage	Autoregulatory escape, sympathetic center lost, chronotropic and inotropic response lost	Low heart rate despite low CO, absent CRT, severe hypotension

CO, *Cardiac output;* HR, *heart rate;* SVR, *systemic vascular resistance;* RR, *respiratory rate;* CRT, *capillary refill time;* MM, *mucous membranes.*

cardiac output. The neurohormonal response described earlier also increases venous return via water retention by the kidneys and movement of interstitial fluid to the intravascular space. These compensatory mechanisms require a large amount of energy, resulting in a hypermetabolic state at the cellular level. The increased metabolic rate produced in the compensatory stage of shock requires an above-normal amount of oxygen to be delivered. Additional substrates required to produce energy are provided by the actions of glucagon, corticotrophin (ACTH), cortisol, and growth hormone. The compensatory stage of shock can maintain adequate cardiac output during mild to moderate acute loss of intravascular volume. The hypermetabolic state cannot be maintained indefinitely. If intravascular volume remains inadequate, systemic vascular resistance begins to decrease, cardiac dysfunction occurs, and decompensation begins.

Veterinarians commonly overlook the clinical signs of compensatory shock. The hyperdynamic cardiovascular system can easily be mistaken as normal. Although heart rate and respiratory rate usually are increased (in some cases, heart rate is only mildly increased), mucous membranes are injected (bright pink to reddish in color), capillary refill is more rapid than normal (usually <1 second), mentation is normal, blood pressure is normal to increased, and pulse pressure is normal to increased (bounding pulses). Adequate volume resuscitation is warranted immediately to remove the stimulus for the hypermetabolic state and prevent the decompensatory stage of shock. Injected mucous membranes may not be as consistent a clinical entity in cats as compared with dogs.

EARLY DECOMPENSATORY STAGE

The early decompensatory stage of shock is marked by redistribution of blood flow to preferred organs (heart and brain) with further decreases in oxygen delivery to all other organs. Oxygen consumption in tissues becomes dependent on oxygen delivery, and anaerobic metabolism, lactic acidosis, and tissue hypoxia result. Organ response to the redistribution of blood flow during early decompensatory shock varies. Intestinal integrity may be compromised, resulting in microulceration. Normal intestinal flora can translocate to the bloodstream through the compromised mucosa. The pancreas responds to hypoxia by releasing myocardial depressant factor, which decreases myocardial contractility, predisposes the heart to cardiac arrhythmias, and decreases the activity of the reticuloendothelial system. Vasoconstriction of the pulmonary vasculature results in microvascular shunting and impairment of oxygen transport. Blood is shunted from renal cortical to juxtamedullary nephrons, and constriction of the afferent glomerular arterioles can reduce renal blood flow enough to produce oliguria and potentially induce tubular necrosis.

Veterinary patients commonly are presented with the early decompensated stages of shock. Tachycardia, normal to decreased pulse pressure, hypotension, pale mucous membranes, prolonged capillary refill time, decreased mentation, and decreased body temperature are all signs of early decompensatory shock. Aggressive fluid resuscitation is required to stop the pathologic process, reduce morbidity, and prevent mortality. Cats with shock may not develop tachycardia as frequently as do affected dogs. Cats that have all of the other signs of shock except tachycardia should be considered in a state of shock and treated appropriately.

DECOMPENSATORY (TERMINAL) STAGE

Prolonged tissue hypoxia can result in a phenomenon termed autoregulatory escape. The local responses override sympathetic-mediated vasoconstriction, and massive vasodilatation occurs in all organs, including the heart and brain. Complete circulatory collapse is the endpoint of autoregulatory escape. The sympathetic center of the brain no longer functions, and chronotropic and inotropic responses are lost. This outcome is the culmination of all types of shock and is termed decompensatory (terminal) shock.

Clinical signs of decompensatory (terminal) shock include low heart rate despite low cardiac output and severe hypotension, pale or cyanotic mucous membranes, absent capillary refill, weak or absent pulses, decreased heart sounds, low body temperature, no urine production, and stupor or coma. Cardiopulmonary arrest is imminent without very aggressive resuscitation and organ support. The decompensatory stage of shock commonly is not responsive to aggressive fluid resuscitation alone and requires intensive monitoring and support of multiple organ systems simultaneously.

TREATMENT

The most successful approach to therapy of shock syndromes commences with anticipation of events that could lead to inadequate perfusion. Under most circumstances, however, the clinician cannot anticipate events that will lead to a state of shock except during the perioperative period. Early recognition and intervention also are important in the successful treatment of shock. A quotation from Shoemaker and Kram[61] provides an effective philosophy of shock therapy: "The single most important factor in successful resuscitation from shock is time...rapid expeditious therapy in early stages may lead to good results, but adequate therapy that is delayed may be ineffective." Advances in fluid types and monitoring techniques are not an excuse for delays in therapy but have increased the likelihood of successful initial therapy.

STANDARD ABCs OF RESUSCITATION

The standard ABCs of resuscitation (**airway, breathing, bleeding, circulation**) should form the initial consideration for therapy for all shock patients. A patent airway should be established and maintained at all times. Abnormal breathing patterns should be recognized. Supplemental oxygen should be delivered at a high flow rate by facemask or by the "blow by" technique if the animal resists a facemask. In most intraoperative and postoperative patients, an endotracheal tube is in place. If not, the clinician must be certain the patient is able to breathe adequately and should provide supplemental oxygen. For patients in the perioperative period, rapid evaluation of the anesthetic drug record should occur. All anesthetic drugs that may have deleterious effects on the cardiovascular system should be antagonized or discontinued. All α_2 agonists should be antagonized because their expected cardiovascular responses include decreased cardiac output.

Controversy exists whether to antagonize opioid agonists. Bradycardia is not typically an adverse effect of opioids during shock. In most instances, the sympathetic response overrides the parasympathomimetic effects of opioid agonists. Analgesia is an important component in the treatment of shock syndromes, and consequently most opioids should not be antagonized. The most important reason to antagonize an opioid is respiratory depression. Pure agonists are most likely to produce deleterious respiratory depression. Therefore the opioid agonist-antagonists should receive stronger consideration as analgesics for mild to moderate pain during shock.

The phenothiazines cannot be antagonized, but knowledge of their previous use aids in therapy. The benzodiazepines have minimal effects on the cardiovascular system and do not require antagonists. The inhalation anesthetics are eliminated primarily by respiration. Both halothane and isoflurane can have deleterious effects on the cardiovascular system, including decreased cardiac output (halothane) and decreased systemic vascular resistance (isoflurane). Isoflurane also is a potent respiratory depressant.

Circulatory support begins by control of internal and external bleeding. The primary method of circulatory support is fluid therapy in all of the shock syndromes, with the exception of cardiogenic shock (Table 23-4). Hypovolemic and distributive forms of shock will be the most fluid-responsive kinds of shock, depending on the clinical stage of shock. Obstructive forms of shock vary in their responsiveness to volume resuscitation, depending on the location of the obstruction. At the very least, partial shock dosages should be administered to such patients to determine responsiveness. Volume resuscitation with any type of fluid typically is contraindicated in patients with cardiogenic shock.

VOLUME RESUSCITATION

Vascular access must be obtained to begin adequate volume resuscitation. Fluids administered subcutaneously or into the peritoneal cavity are not considered adequate for shock therapy. The neurohormonal response to low cardiac output results in peripheral vasoconstriction and poor absorption of fluids administered subcutaneously or intraperitoneally. In addition, crystalloid fluids require administration as rapidly as possible to expand the intravascular space effectively.

Central veins (e.g., jugular vein) allow larger volumes of crystalloids to be administered faster, but jugular vein catheterization requires more time. Catheterization of a peripheral vein should be completed before placing a catheter in the jugular vein, and the decision to place an indwelling catheter in the jugular vein should be made based on the initial response to fluid therapy and the underlying cause of shock. Peripheral venous catheterization is simpler, and a patent catheter can be established

TABLE 23-4 Fluid Choices for Patients with Shock

Fluid Type	Dosage	Indications for Use
Crystalloids (lactated Ringer's solution, 0.9% NaCl, Normosol, Plasma-Lyte)	90 mL/kg as fast as possible (dog) 55 mL/kg as fast as possible (cat)	Acute volume resuscitation, interstitial fluid replacement (dehydration)
Hypertonic solutions (7% NaCl, 23.4% NaCl)	4 mL/kg over 5 min for a 7% solution; see Table 23-5 for dilution of 23.4% NaCl with colloid	Acute volume resuscitation in normally hydrated animals
Colloids		
Whole blood	22 mL/kg/hr maximum	>30% loss of blood
Plasma	10-20 mL/kg	Loss of oncotic pressure, secondary hemostatic disorders
Packed red blood cells	Based on PCV	Hemolytic anemia, oxygen-carrying source
Hemoglobin-based oxygen carriers (Oxyglobin)	15-30 mL/kg	Hemolytic anemia, acute loss of intravascular volume
Hetastarch, pentastarch	10-20 mL/kg initial bolus (dog) 20 mL/kg/day infusion	Acute volume resuscitation, source of oncotic pressure

in a fraction of the time required for jugular venous catheterization. Appropriate peripheral veins readily available include the cephalic and lateral saphenous veins in dogs and the cephalic and medial saphenous veins in cats. Catheter placement in the lateral saphenous vein is contraindicated in GDV in dogs unless the stomach has been adequately decompressed to allow fluids given at the site to return unhindered to the heart. Catheterization of more than one peripheral vein may be necessary to administer adequate volumes of fluids in very large dogs or to administer two or more different types of fluids. Venous cutdown procedures may become necessary in patients with no visible veins as a result of severe hypotension and poor peripheral circulation.

The type of catheter used also can be an important factor in the speed of fluid administration. A large-gauge, short, over-the-needle catheter placed in a peripheral vein allows administration of larger volumes of fluid more rapidly than a smaller gauge, long, through-the-needle catheter placed in a central (e.g., jugular) vein.

The intraosseous route of administration may be of value in patients weighing less than 2 kg, especially puppies and kittens. Intraosseous placement of large-gauge needles in the trochanteric fossa, tibial crest, iliac wing, or proximal humerus can allow rapid administration of any type of fluid (see Chapter 15).

Crystalloids

Isotonic crystalloid fluids historically have been the most common type of fluid recommended initially for the shock patient, but the basis for the popularity of crystalloids is unclear.[37] Two experiments were performed in the 1960s that may have popularized crystalloid fluid therapy for animals and people with hemorrhagic shock.[40,62] One experiment showed that the physiologic response to mild hemorrhage is a shift of fluid from the interstitial space to the intravascular space.[40] The second experiment indicated that survival was improved in an animal model of hemorrhagic shock when crystalloids were administered simultaneously with reinfusion of the blood that was removed.[62] The conclusions from these two experiments, which have endured over the years, are that an interstitial fluid deficit is a major consequence of hemorrhage and that crystalloid fluid replacement is important for survival. Changes in interstitial fluid occur only when blood loss is less than 15% of total blood volume. When blood volume loss exceeds 15%, a fluid type that will not move into the interstitial space must support intravascular volume.

Crystalloids effectively replenish the interstitial space. Dehydration is defined as loss of water in the extravascular tissue (interstitial and intracellular). Tonicity of the interstitial compartment increases as fluid is lost, which promotes movement of fluid out of the intravascular space. Severe dehydration can result in poor tissue perfusion, but the terms dehydration and perfusion should

not be used interchangeably. Crystalloids contribute to effective fluid resuscitation when used with colloids if dehydration also is present. Another consequence of large volumes of crystalloid fluids is decreased intravascular oncotic pressure caused by dilution of impermeant protein anions.[37] Decreased oncotic pressure impairs maintenance of intravascular volume and promotes extravasation of fluids into the interstitial space.

Approximately 75% to 85% of isotonic crystalloids move to the interstitial space within the first hour after intravenous administration.[26] For example, if an animal loses 300 mL of intravascular volume, approximately 1200 mL of isotonic crystalloid must be administered to support the circulation. Therefore crystalloid fluids do not maintain intravascular volume or tissue perfusion for extended periods and should not be considered the sole source of intravascular fluid support for shock patients. Massive crystalloid administration can produce body compositional changes similar to those of the late stages of shock: expanded total body water and interstitial water with contracted plasma volume and intracellular fluid.[58] Increased interstitial water and excessive total body water do not necessarily contribute to correction of intravascular volume deficits. Hypovolemia can occur in the presence of interstitial edema. Increased amounts of interstitial fluid do not play a role in circulatory function and may impair oxygen transport by impairing diffusion of oxygen from the intravascular space to the cells.

Examples of isotonic crystalloids include lactated Ringer's solution, physiologic saline, Plasma-Lyte 148 (Baxter, Deerfield, IL), and Normosol-R (Abbott Laboratories, Abbott Park, IL). Hyperchloremic metabolic acidosis has been reported after administration of large doses of physiologic saline. Plasma-Lyte 148 and Normosol-R contain approximately twice the amount of bicarbonate precursors (as acetate and gluconate) compared with lactated Ringer's solution and thus may be more efficient alkalinizing fluids for shock patients with clinically relevant metabolic acidosis. The rate of administration of isotonic crystalloids in dogs and cats traditionally has been considered to be 90 mL/kg/hr and 55 mL/kg/hr, respectively. However, because of the rapid extravasation of crystalloids to the interstitial space, the recommended rate of administration to dogs and cats has been revised to 90 and 55 mL/kg, respectively, **as rapidly as possible**. The entire shock dose can be administered within as short a time as 10 to 15 minutes if necessary. Many clinicians divide this shock dose into several smaller aliquots and reassess the patient before administering the next aliquot. Not all patients have a similar volume deficit, and thus shock fluid therapy should be titrated to effect. Administration can be hastened by utilizing pressurized fluid infusion systems, large-gauge short catheters, and more than one catheter.

Most normal healthy animals can tolerate additional interstitial volume for short periods. Most of the interstitial fluid either is returned to the intravascular space via lymphatics or excreted by the kidneys. Although crystalloids historically have been recommended for initial fluid therapy in those with shock (except for cardiogenic shock), the veterinarian should consider the clinical stage of shock and the possible detrimental effects of large volumes of crystalloid solutions.

During the postoperative period, most anesthetized patients have received large volumes of crystalloid fluids, effectively diluting intravascular proteins and the interstitial space and predisposing the patient to interstitial edema. Therefore crystalloid solutions are contraindicated, and other types of intravascular volume support (e.g., colloids, hypertonic fluids) are more beneficial if inadequate perfusion states develop during the postoperative period.

The patient with SIRS or anaphylactic shock also benefits from other types of intravascular volume expansion in addition to crystalloids because an important component of these syndromes is increased capillary membrane permeability. The goal with SIRS patients is to maintain intravascular volume with colloids and to attempt to avoid interstitial edema that may occur with very large doses of crystalloids.

Colloids

Colloid oncotic pressure (COP) is important in maintaining fluid balance between the intravascular and interstitial compartments.[11,32] The primary source of oncotic pressure within the intravascular compartment is albumin (69,000 daltons), and normal COP in most veterinary species is approximately 20 to 25 mm Hg. Synthetic colloids were produced with molecular weights similar to or greater than that of albumin.

Colloid solutions are divided into biologic (e.g., whole blood, albumin, plasma) and synthetic (hetastarch, pentastarch, dextrans, gelatins, hemoglobin-based oxygen carriers [HBOCs]; see Chapters 24 and 27). Biologic colloids are indicated in specific conditions but rarely are used alone in shock therapy. Most biologic colloids are used in addition to other types of fluid therapy (e.g., crystalloids, hypertonic solutions, synthetic colloids). Whole-blood transfusions may be warranted as a primary fluid choice during hemorrhagic shock, but caution must be taken to avoid potential complications, including transfusion reaction, hemolysis of red blood cells, citrate toxicity, and hypocalcemia. The recommended rate of whole-blood transfusion has been reported not to exceed 22 mL/kg/hr, but some clinical situations require administration as quickly as possible.[14] Whole blood is not a practical primary source of intravascular volume support because of a lack of readily available blood donors and the large volumes required for larger dogs.

Hemorrhagic shock caused by traumatic hemoperitoneum can be treated using the technique of autotransfusion in addition to synthetic colloid and crystalloid fluid therapy.[9,13,38] In most instances, autotransfusion of blood from the peritoneal cavity does not supply active platelets or clotting factors. Potential complications include dyspnea, respiratory insufficiency, and disseminated intravascular coagulation caused by red blood cell fragments or other microaggregates. Administering blood collected from the peritoneal space that has been passed through a commercial blood filter minimizes the number of microaggregates. Blood that has remained in the peritoneal cavity for several days or hemorrhages as a result of suspected splenic or hepatic neoplasia should not be used for autotransfusion.

The primary determinant of the oncotic activity of plasma is albumin, which supplies about 75% to 80% of the total COP of plasma. The COP of albumin is nearly identical to that of plasma (20 to 25 mm Hg).[32,51] Intuitively, albumin could be considered the ideal colloid. However, it is incorrect to assume that albumin distributes only to the intravascular space. Albumin distributes throughout the extracellular space, and the amount of time it spends in the intravascular space is longer than that of a crystalloid but shorter than that of hetastarch. The plasma half-life of albumin is 16 hours, and more than 90% of infused albumin remains in the intravascular space.

Rarely is there a need for plasma transfusion as the sole fluid therapy for shock in veterinary patients, with the rare exception of severe burn injury in which a massive loss of protein has occurred and hypovolemia has developed. Human albumin is packaged as either a 5% or 25% solution. A 5% solution can be administered at a dosage of 10 to 20 mL/kg as rapidly as necessary during shock.[54] Many institutions and clinics may be severely limited in their in-house supply of fresh, frozen, or fresh-frozen plasma.

Packed red blood cells (PRBCs) have been considered colloids, but the red blood cell itself does not exert COP. Red blood cells alone expand the intravascular space by the volume they occupy, but unlike other fluids they cannot expand intravascular volume to a volume larger than the volume that is administered. The greatest advantage of administration of PRBCs is the increased oxygen-carrying capacity they provide. There are valid clinical situations in which PRBCs are indicated for shock patients to increase the oxygen-carrying capacity of the blood, but PRBCs should not be considered a type of fluid for volume expansion.

Synthetic colloids are high molecular weight substances that remain in the vascular space. Hydroxyethyl starch (hetastarch) is the most commonly used synthetic colloid.[32,37] The use of dextran 70 has decreased because of complications, whereas hetastarch administration has few known clinical complications. Pentastarch is a low molecular weight derivative of hetastarch that currently is not approved for use in the United States.

The primary purpose of colloid solutions is to provide volume expansion and oncotic pressure by remaining in the intravascular space and attracting sodium and water from the interstitial space. Colloids are used primarily as initial therapy for early decompensatory and decompensatory (terminal) shock and are valuable in the treatment of shock during the postoperative period when large amounts of crystalloids have been administered, saturating the interstitial space. Colloid solutions should be considered the primary method of initial and continued volume expansion in patients with SIRS or in other patients with severe capillary leak syndrome or severe protein depletion.[32] Colloids replace intravascular deficits only, and crystalloids also should be administered to replace interstitial deficits that may be present or that may be created by administration of colloids and hypertonic solutions.

The molecular weight of each colloid determines its oncotic pressure.[11] Most synthetic colloid solutions have a wide range of molecule sizes. Two terms are used to measure the size of colloid molecules: weight average molecular weight (M_w) and number average molecular weight (M_n). The M_w is determined by light scattering and is not as accurate a measure of the size of the colloid as M_n, which is the arithmetic mean of the range of molecular weights in the solution. The M_w is larger than the M_n, and as the molecular weight distribution of the colloid becomes narrower, M_w approaches and eventually equals M_n. Albumin (69,000 daltons) is used as a reference to compare oncotic activity.

Dextran 70 is synthesized from sucrose by the bacterium *Leuconostoc mesenteroides* and is processed to a clinically useful size. The M_w of dextran 70 is approximately 70,000 (hence the name dextran 70), and 80% of the molecules have molecular weights between 20,000 and 200,000 daltons. The size of dextran 70 is similar to that of albumin, and it would appear that dextran 70 is the ideal colloid solution. However, the M_n of dextran 70 may be as low as 39,000. Administration of dextran 70 results in an 80% to 100% expansion of plasma volume. Its plasma half-life is approximately 25.5 hours with a 24-hour duration of clinical effect. Coagulopathy is the main adverse effect and is dose related. The bleeding tendencies have been attributed to coating of platelets, precipitation and dilution of clotting factors, increased thrombolysis, and decreases in von Willebrand's factor and factor VIII activity. Dextran 70 should not be administered to animals with coagulation disorders or thrombocytopenia. Administration of dextran 70 at 20 mL/kg over 20 to 30 minutes to dogs resulted in decreased von Willebrand's factor antigen concentration and factor VIII activity, and buccal mucosal bleeding time and partial thromboplastin time were increased. Dextrans are adsorbed onto the red blood cell membranes and can interfere with crossmatching of blood products for transfusion. The dosage of dextran should not exceed 20 mL/kg/day as a combination of bolus and constant-rate infusion. This dosage has been exceeded without apparent adverse effects.

Hydroxyethyl starch (hetastarch) is produced by a chemical modification of amylopectin, which is a complex carbohydrate molecule similar to glycogen. Hetastarch also has a wide range of M_w in solution (M_w = 480,000), but 80% of the molecules have molecular weights between 30,000 and 2 million daltons. The M_n of hetastarch is 69,000. Administration of hetastarch at a dosage of 20 mL/kg results in a 70% to 200% (average, 141%) increase in plasma volume because of a COP of 32 mm Hg, which exceeds the COP of plasma (20 to 25 mm Hg). The plasma half-life of hetastarch is 25.5 hours, and the duration of volume expansion is 12 to 48 hours, with longer retention time with higher doses. Hetastarch prolongs partial thromboplastin time, but clinical episodes of bleeding have not been reported in human or veterinary patients when daily administration does not exceed currently recommended guidelines. Hetastarch does not interfere with platelet function, but hetastarch administration for several days can result in interference with crossmatching.

The dosage of hetastarch used clinically is 10 to 20 mL/kg in the dog and 10 to 15 mL/kg in the cat.[54] This initial dosage is administered as a rapid bolus in dogs and over 10 to 15 minutes in cats because rapid administration has been reported to cause nausea in cats. This initial dosage has been exceeded without adverse effects. A constant-rate infusion of 20 mL/kg/day can be administered after the initial bolus if the animal's disease process and cardiovascular status require continued COP support. Hetastarch has been a useful, lifesaving colloid solution, especially in patients with SIRS.

Pentastarch is an analogue of hetastarch and has a lower M_w than hetastarch (264,000 versus 480,000). Pentastarch originally was used for leukophoresis in people and currently is being investigated as a colloidal plasma expander.[52] Pentastarch has clinical qualities similar to those of hetastarch with fewer potential adverse effects. The COP of pentastarch is approximately 40 mm Hg, which should result in volume expansion 1.5 times greater than that achieved with plasma.

The metabolism of synthetic colloids depends primarily on the size of the molecule. Dextran molecules smaller than 20,000 daltons and hetastarch molecules smaller than 72,000 daltons are rapidly excreted by renal glomerular filtration. Hetastarch is hydrolyzed in the plasma by α-amylase, resulting in hyperamylasemia. The larger molecules of dextran and hetastarch are degraded by the reticuloendothelial system. Other molecules are absorbed into the interstitial space and recirculated through the lymphatic system.

HBOCs have been studied as a replacement for whole blood or PRBCs and as an ideal fluid for resuscitation during shock. The two acellular oxygen carriers that have been evaluated are hemoglobin solutions (e.g., stroma-free hemoglobin, pyridoxylated hemoglobin, polymerized hemoglobin) and perfluorocarbon emulsions.

HBOCs must effectively transport oxygen and support circulatory hemodynamics. The most useful features of HBOCs include lack of a need to do crossmatching, ready availability, stability at room temperature, long storage time, prolonged residence and activity in the vascular space, and effective oxygen transport without supplemental oxygen.

The HBOC Oxyglobin (Biopure Corporation, Cambridge, MA), which is a polymerized hemoglobin of bovine origin, has been released to the veterinary market. Oxyglobin is a universally compatible fluid that immediately enhances oxygen-carrying capacity by providing a hemoglobin source to plasma. In addition to oxygen-carrying capacity, Oxyglobin exerts a colloid effect in blood, potentially making it the ideal fluid for resuscitation. Its shelf life is approximately 2 years at room temperature, and supplemental oxygen is not required for the positive effects on oxygen-carrying capacity. Compared with whole blood, Oxyglobin has a higher P_{50} (partial pressure of O_2 at which hemoglobin is 50% saturated), which allows oxygen to be delivered to the tissues more readily. The oxygen affinity of Oxyglobin is dependent on chloride and not 2,3-diphosphoglycerate, as occurs with hemoglobin in red blood cells. The half-life of Oxyglobin is dose dependent and generally is 24 hours at clinically useful dosages. The COP of Oxyglobin is approximately 43 mm Hg.[51]

The most common adverse effects of Oxyglobin administration are transient and include discoloration of the mucous membranes, sclera, and urine; mild gastrointestinal effects (vomiting, diarrhea); and the potential for volume overloading in euvolemic anemic patients because of the high COP and subsequent volume expansion.

The primary use of Oxyglobin in most veterinary patients is to treat anemia, whether it is the result of hemolysis, blood loss, or ineffective erythropoiesis. There also is great interest in the use of Oxyglobin for patients with hypovolemic or hemorrhagic shock and especially SIRS because of the colloidal effects of Oxyglobin in addition to its ability to increase oxygen delivery. Oxyglobin will probably play a crucial role in the management of shock syndromes in veterinary medicine in the near future.

Crystalloids or Colloids?

Neither crystalloids nor colloids administered alone have resulted in an increase in survival in human patients with hypovolemic shock.[6,10,61,71] Colloids provide superior intravascular volume support based on physiology and clinical experience. One analogy, called the "hole in the bucket," has been presented in the medical literature to help resolve the argument over whether crystalloids or colloids should be used for intravascular volume expansion.[37] The goal of therapy is to expand intravascular volume by filling a bucket. The volume of crystalloid required to expand intravascular volume (i.e., fill the bucket) is approximately three times the volume of colloid required. Assuming that the bucket filled with colloid is full, it will be necessary to punch holes in the bucket filled with crystalloid to allow excess fluid to escape and prevent overflow. The question is if the goal is to fill the bucket with fluid, do you want to punch holes in the bucket and make the bucket more difficult to fill? It would certainly be more efficient to fill the bucket without having to punch holes in it to deliver a volume of crystalloid equivalent to the volume of colloid. Controversy will continue to keep this debate alive. Ultimately, however, both types of fluids have advantages in certain instances and should be thought of as partners in resuscitation. Clinicians must understand the basic biologic behavior of both types of fluids to capitalize on the advantages of each fluid.

Hypertonic Solutions

Hypertonic crystalloid solutions (7% and 23.4% NaCl) became popular in veterinary medicine in the 1980s and were described as small-volume resuscitation.[55] A single bolus of 7% NaCl (4 mL/kg) provides plasma volume expansion comparable with that of colloids at one fourth of the volume. The primary mechanism of action is provision of an immediate and large osmotic gradient to allow movement of water from the interstitial space to the intravascular space. Hypertonic saline also has been reported to increase myocardial contractility and dilate precapillary blood vessels that may play a role in the maldistribution of blood flow.

The duration of effects is similar to that of isotonic crystalloids, and additional intravascular support with colloids is required to maintain effective volume expansion. A convenient method for administering hypertonic saline with a colloid is to dilute 23.4% NaCl with 6% hetastarch (preferred) or 6% dextran 70 to make a 7.5% solution and infuse at a dosage of 4 mL/kg. The rate of administration of all hypertonic saline solutions should not exceed 1 mL/kg/min, and therefore solutions should be administered during a 5-minute period in dogs and cats.

Complications of hypertonic saline administration may occur when solutions are infused too rapidly and include bradycardia, hypotension, bronchoconstriction, and rapid, shallow breathing. The mechanism of the cardiopulmonary effects may involve a reflex mediated by the vagus nerve and the lungs, but atropine does not blunt the response.[57] Slow administration is highly recommended and does not induce this reflex. Cellular dehydration is another potential complication of administering hypertonic solutions, an effect that is more likely when multiple doses are used or when hypertonic saline is used in dehydrated patients. Hypernatremia can occur when more than two doses are administered in close succession. Serum sodium concentration should be monitored if more than two doses are required.

Hypertonic solutions, either alone or in combination with colloids, are useful alternatives for fluid resuscitation in postoperative patients requiring intravascular volume support and large volumes of crystalloid fluids. Hypertonic saline and colloids do not place more burden on an already saturated interstitial space and may be beneficial in partially correcting some interstitial edema states. Hypertonic solutions are contraindicated for patients with hypernatremia and in severely dehydrated patients. Some evidence in the literature suggests that hypertonic saline/colloid combination fluids carry a clinical benefit when used to resuscitate humans with head trauma.[2,34] A trial comparing the use of hypertonic saline/dextran combination and traditional fluid resuscitation strategies in dogs with GDV did not show significant differences in measured outcomes.[56]

Combination Fluid Therapy

Combinations of fluids are the most effective method of fluid therapy, especially for early decompensatory shock, decompensatory (terminal) shock states, and shock secondary to dehydration and third-space loss of fluids. Isotonic and hypertonic crystalloid fluids can be combined with hetastarch to produce effective intravascular volume expansion at lower total volumes than for isotonic crystalloid solutions alone in patients with compensatory shock. Isotonic crystalloids may not be as effective in early decompensatory shock and SIRS and are not effective in decompensatory (terminal) shock. Hetastarch decreases the total amount of isotonic crystalloids required by 40% to 60%, which can be useful for volume resuscitation in very large dogs. A combination of 23.4% NaCl and hetastarch (Table 23-5), followed by smaller volumes of crystalloids, is useful. Intravascular volume expansion is rapid and sustained, and the dose of crystalloids required to maintain the interstitial space is reduced. Another important reason to administer crystalloids in most types of shock is that both hypertonic solutions and colloids can produce a state of relative dehydration in the interstitial space.

In summary, if the goal of immediate fluid resuscitation is to expand the intravascular space, colloids should be used. If the goal of immediate fluid resuscitation is to expand the entire extracellular space, crystalloids should be used. If the goal is to expand both the intravascular and extracellular spaces, both colloids with or without hypertonic solutions and crystalloids should be used.

Cardiogenic Shock

Adequate volume resuscitation is the most important treatment for all types of shock with the notable exception of cardiogenic shock. Fluid redistribution from the lungs to the circulation, inotropic support, and antiarrhythmic therapy are the primary goals of therapy for patients with cardiogenic shock. An animal that has received therapy to reduce or redistribute intravascular

TABLE 23-5 Quick Reference for the Combination of 23.4% NaCl and 6% Hetastarch (4 mL/kg)*

Weight (lb)	Weight (kg)	mL 23.4% NaCl	mL Hetastarch
2	1	1.3	2.7
5	2	2.6	5.4
10	4.5	6	12
15	7	9	18
20	9	12	24
25	11	15	30
30	14	19	38
35	16	21	42
40	18	24	48
45	20.5	27	54
50	23	31	62
55	25	33	66
60	27	36	72
65	29.5	39	78
70	32	43	86
75	34	45	90
80	36	48	96
85	38.5	51	102
90	41	55	110
95	43	57	114
100	45.5	61	122
125	57	76	152
150	68	91	182

Administer no faster than 1 mL/kg/min.

volume may become dehydrated and volume depleted. Fluid therapy is warranted for these patients, and appropriate monitoring should determine both the type and rate of fluid therapy in patients treated for cardiogenic shock. Current investigations have provided evidence that low dosages and slow administration of colloids may provide the necessary volume to maximize cardiac output in some patients with heart failure.

ANCILLARY SUPPORTIVE THERAPY

Other treatment regimens should be used after volume replacement, especially when the patient is not responsive to initial therapy. Shock should be treated based on knowledge of pathophysiology and not necessarily initial clinical observations.[58] In most instances, for example, if the animal is hypotensive, vasopressors should not be administered immediately. Likewise, diuretics should not be administered immediately to treat oliguria in the shock patient. Further treatment should be based on monitoring the effectiveness of initial fluid therapy (see section on Monitoring).

SUPPORT OF THE CARDIOVASCULAR SYSTEM

Evidence of poor perfusion (e.g., hypotension, increased central venous pressure [CVP], oliguria) after initial resuscitation with appropriate fluid therapy is an indication for the use of drugs to support cardiac output and blood pressure. Clinicians can anticipate the probable need for continued pharmacologic cardiovascular support from the cause of shock. Animals that have evidence of prolonged shock, decompensatory shock, and SIRS are likely to require drugs that act on the cardiovascular system to support blood flow and blood pressure. Inotropes are the drugs most useful in these situations. Inotropes require adequate intravascular volume to be effective and are ineffective in states of uncorrected hypovolemia. Examples of inotropes that can be used in patients with continued evidence of poor output despite adequate volume expansion include the sympathomimetic agents dobutamine and dopamine.

Dobutamine is a synthetic sympathomimetic agent that exerts effects on the β_1-adrenoceptors of the myocardium to increase the force of contraction. Dobutamine exerts weak effects on β_2-adrenoceptors located on blood vessels to produce mild vasodilatation. The combination of mild arterial vasodilatation and increased force of myocardial contraction results in increased cardiac output without a dramatic increase in arterial blood pressure. The dosage range of dobutamine is wide (2 to 15 μg/kg/min), but most clinicians begin with continuous-rate infusion of 2 to 5 μg/kg/min and increase the dosage as needed based on hemodynamic monitoring. Adequate intravascular volume is required for dobutamine to exert positive inotropic effects.[33] The most common adverse effect of dobutamine infusion is development of ventricular arrhythmias. Dobutamine infusion should be temporarily discontinued if ventricular arrhythmias occur and can be safely restarted at a lower infusion rate on resolution of the arrhythmias. Dobutamine has minimal effects on the heart rate.

Dopamine is a precursor of norepinephrine and exerts dose-dependent effects. Low infusion rates (1 to 5 μg/kg/min) stimulate dopaminergic receptors in renal, coronary, and cerebral arteries, resulting in arterial dilatation. Somewhat higher infusion rates (5 to 10 μg/kg/min) produce a sympathomimetic effect by stimulating β_1-adrenergic receptors in the sinus node and myocardium, resulting in positive chronotropic and inotropic effects. Cardiac output is increased as a result of increased heart rate and force of myocardial contraction. Blood pressure is increased to a greater extent than occurs with dobutamine. High infusion rates (>10 μg/kg/min) stimulate α_1-adrenergic receptors located in arterial blood vessels and result in vasoconstriction and increased blood pressure. The most common adverse effect of dopamine is development of ventricular arrhythmias. Heart rate should increase with a moderate infusion rate of dopamine.

Vasopressors such as epinephrine (0.1 to 0.3 μg/kg/min) can be used during life-threatening states of hypotension that are refractory to initial fluid resuscitation. The goal of vasopressors is to increase blood pressure sufficiently to maintain blood flow to the heart and brain. Use of vasopressors should be considered temporary because vasoconstriction occurs in other tissues and decreases blood flow and organ function. The most common adverse effects of epinephrine are ventricular arrhythmias, including ventricular fibrillation. Other vasopressors that can be administered include the α_1-adrenoceptor agonist methoxamine (0.05 to 0.2 mg/kg intravenously), norepinephrine (0.1 to 10 μg/kg/min), and dopamine in a high-dose infusion (>10 μg/kg/min).

ANTIARRHYTHMIC THERAPY

Any type of arrhythmia can occur during shock, but ventricular arrhythmias (e.g., ventricular premature complexes, paroxysmal ventricular tachycardia, ventricular tachycardia) are most common. Arrhythmias that occur during shock before initial volume resuscitation are most likely the result of inadequate myocardial perfusion and may respond to volume expansion alone. Cardiogenic shock is a notable exception because arrhythmias may be the primary cause of decreased cardiac output and corresponding shock. Other causes of ventricular arrhythmias, depending on the cause of shock, include trauma, electrolyte imbalances, SIRS, hypoxemia, anemia, pain, and underlying cardiac disease.

The decision to treat ventricular arrhythmias should be based on several factors in addition to the number of premature ventricular complexes (PVCs) that occur during 1 minute. There is little debate that isolated PVCs rarely require antiarrhythmic therapy and that rapid ventricular tachycardia (>200 PVCs/min) almost always requires treatment. However, there is considerable debate whether to administer antiarrhythmic drugs in many other clinical settings, especially considering the arrhythmogenic effects of many of these drugs. A common guideline states that when more than 20 PVCs occur per minute, antiarrhythmic therapy should be instituted. However, if the patient's blood pressure is not affected and there is no evidence of a serious arrhythmia (e.g., R-on-T phenomenon), there is little reason to administer drugs. PVCs that occur in the following patterns should be treated: bigeminy, trigeminy, paroxysmal and sustained ventricular tachycardia, and multiform PVCs. Ventricular arrhythmias that affect hemodynamics (e.g., blood flow, blood pressure) should always be treated. Close coupling of the QRS and T wave (R-on-T phenomenon) should always be treated because this presentation predisposes to ventricular tachycardia and ventricular fibrillation. Antiarrhythmic drugs are indicated for arrhythmias that persist after initial fluid resuscitation, administration of analgesic agents (see section on Analgesia), and correction of electrolyte disturbances.

Intravenous bolus and continuous-rate infusions are the preferred methods of administration. The antiarrhythmic agents most commonly used during shock include lidocaine and procainamide.

Lidocaine usually is considered the first choice for ventricular arrhythmias. It is administered as an intravenous bolus (2 mg/kg) followed by a continuous-rate infusion (40 to 80 µg/kg/min) if needed. Lidocaine has a very short half-life and a very large volume of distribution and usually warrants continuous-rate infusion to maintain adequate plasma concentrations. Common adverse effects include vomiting and seizures. Hypotension can occur at very high dosages. Procainamide may be administered intravenously (3 to 6 mg/kg) as a bolus followed by a continuous-rate infusion (10 to 40 µg/kg/min) if lidocaine is ineffective. Procainamide impairs contractility to a greater extent than lidocaine.

Ventricular arrhythmias that do not respond to initial administration of antiarrhythmic drugs should be considered refractory arrhythmias. A logical approach should be used to determine the reason for ineffective antiarrhythmic therapy. Electrolytes should be evaluated because adequate amounts of potassium are required for lidocaine and procainamide to be effective. Intravascular volume should be adequate as determined by monitoring cardiovascular variables such as CVP. Appropriate analgesia should be administered, and adequate oxygenation of arterial blood should be maintained based on blood gas analysis. Serum magnesium concentration should be determined if refractory ventricular arrhythmias are present after all of the preceding variables have been determined to be adequate, especially in patients that may have chronic underlying disease.

Antiarrhythmic therapy should be discontinued slowly to determine whether additional therapy is warranted. No specific guidelines are available on the rate at which lidocaine or procainamide infusions should be decreased. Patients without underlying cardiac disease should have complete resolution of ventricular arrhythmias.

ANALGESIA

Pain and the physiologic response to pain can be detrimental to the shock patient. The primary physiologic effects of pain are manifested by the cardiovascular system and include increased heart rate, vasoconstriction, and arrhythmias. Vasoconstriction secondary to unrelieved pain, inadequate intravascular volume, and poor myocardial function can dramatically decrease cardiac output. Adequate and safe analgesia should be provided for shock patients that have concurrent pain.

Opioid analgesics are preferred for patients with shock (Table 23-6). The opioid agonist-antagonist butorphanol (0.2 to 0.6 mg/kg intravenously) is a safe and effective analgesic agent for mild to moderate pain. Butorphanol produces little effect on cardiovascular and pulmonary function. The approximate duration of action is reported to range from 20 minutes to 4 hours. Other alternatives include the opioid partial agonist buprenorphine (0.005 to 0.02 mg/kg intravenously). Although pure agonists such as oxymorphone have been reported to suppress pulmonary function in a dose-dependent manner, they are very unlikely to produce important clinical effects except in the unstable patient. A viable alternative for continuous analgesia is a constant-rate intravenous infusion of morphine (0.1 to 0.2 mg/kg/hr) or fentanyl (1 to 5 µg/kg/hr). Although morphine can

TABLE 23-6 Useful Intravenous or Intramuscular Analgesics for Dogs and Cats with Shock

Agent	Dose and Route	Approximate Duration	Comments
Butorphanol	0.2-0.6 mg/kg, IV or IM	20 min-4 hr	Rarely causes bradycardia, minimal respiratory depression
Buprenorphine	0.005-0.02 mg/kg, IV or IM	2-6 hr	Rarely causes bradycardia, minimal respiratory depression
Oxymorphone/hydromorphone	0.025-0.1 mg/kg, IV or IM 2-4 hr		Dose-dependent bradycardia and respiratory depression
Fentanyl	1-5 µg/kg or 1-5 µg/kg/hr infusion IV	20–30 min Continuous	Rarely causes bradycardia, minimal sedation
Morphine	0.1-0.2 mg/kg/hr infusion (dogs only)	Continuous	Minimal respiratory and cardiovascular (heart rate) depression

decrease heart rate and impair pulmonary function at higher dosages, administration as an intravenous infusion at the recommended dosage has little effect on cardiopulmonary function. Morphine is relatively inexpensive and, when used appropriately, provides adequate analgesia and produces few adverse effects.

Analgesic therapy should be discontinued when the initiating cause of pain has been resolved. An animal that has sustained a fracture should have analgesia administered continuously or on a predetermined schedule until the fracture can be repaired. An animal with SIRS caused by peritonitis also should have continuous administration of analgesia. Analgesic agents can be decreased and discontinued when the clinician is confident that the patient is no longer showing signs of pain.

ANTIBIOTIC THERAPY

The decision whether to administer antibiotics should be based on several factors including the stage of shock and the underlying problem. Antibiotics are not indicated for patients with the compensatory stage of shock unless contaminated skin wounds or other justifiable reasons to consider antibiotic therapy are present. In the absence of other justifiable reasons to initiate and continue antibiotic therapy, broad-spectrum antibiotics should be administered to patients with decompensatory shock for at least 24 hours because of the potential for bacterial translocation. If antibiotics are justified because of the potential for infection and provided it is relevant to do so, cultures of blood, urine, peritoneal or pleural fluid, and any discharges should be submitted whenever possible before antibiotic administration. Patients with septic shock require intravenous administration of broad-spectrum bactericidal antibiotics. Choice of antibiotic should be based on the pathogens suspected, the penetration of the antibiotic into the infected tissue, and knowledge of local or hospital bacterial resistance patterns.

CONTROVERSY ON GLUCOCORTICOID USE IN SHOCK SYNDROMES

Historically in veterinary medicine, glucocorticoid administration as an initial therapy was suggested for many, if not all, shock patients.[68] Today only a few clinical uses of glucocorticoids in shock patients seem justified. However, considerable controversy still exists, and clinicians must use a common sense approach to the administration of any therapy for the treatment of shock, including corticosteroids, and not utilize any therapy reflexively.

The primary benefit and strongest argument for the use of glucocorticoids is their strong antiinflammatory effect.[54] The prevention of cytokine production by macrophages is of particular interest. Potent inflammatory mediators of SIRS, such as tumor necrosis factor, interleukin-1, interleukin-6, and platelet-activating factor are inhibited by glucocorticoids. Glucocorticoids inhibit cyclooxygenase and lipoxygenase activity that is stimulated by cytokines and inhibit production of eicosanoids (e.g., prostaglandins, thromboxanes, leukotrienes). The earlier glucocorticoids are administered in the inflammatory response, the more effective is their inhibition of cytokines and eicosanoid production. In addition to their potent antiinflammatory effects, glucocorticoids reduce reperfusion injury. The effects of reperfusion injury are best prevented if glucocorticoids are present at the time of reperfusion of tissues. This effect is difficult to achieve in the clinical setting. The two most commonly administered glucocorticoids are dexamethasone sodium phosphate (0.25 to 1 mg/kg intravenously) and prednisolone sodium succinate (10 to 20 mg/kg intravenously). There are two types of clinical shock in veterinary patients in which it is appropriate to administer glucocorticoids. Patients presenting with shock related to hypoadrenocortical crisis have substantial cardiovascular dysfunction because of the role glucocorticoids play in maintaining adrenoreceptor density and function in the heart and blood vessels. These patients benefit from the positive effect these drugs play in restoring more normal adrenoreceptor density and function, and thus corticosteroids should be administered early, soon after initial fluid resuscitation. Patients with anaphylactic shock also benefit from the antiinflammatory effects of corticosteroids and should receive glucocorticoids soon after fluid resuscitation has been initiated.

The potential deleterious effects of glucocorticoids are numerous. Glucocorticoids relax arterioles and venules and can improve microcirculation. Although this is a positive cardiovascular effect, glucocorticoid administration is not recommended in the presence of hypovolemia without adequate fluid resuscitation because relaxation of peripheral vessels can produce hypotension. Sudden death has been reported in people after rapid administration of glucocorticoids. Gastrointestinal effects include development of ulcers that are attributed to antiprostaglandin activity and decreased mucosal blood flow. Arguments exist against the use of glucocorticoids in advanced stages of shock when the integrity of the intestinal mucosa may be compromised, resulting in microulceration. Glucocorticoids impair the cellular immune response and can predispose to bacterial infection. The beneficial effects of glucocorticoids have been reported by some investigators as being useful only with concurrent administration of antibiotics to counteract suppression of the immune system.[45]

Because of the negative effects of glucocorticoids on the cellular immune response, glucocorticoids generally are contraindicated in patients that have signs of SIRS or are considered to have septic shock.[45,54,60] Glucocorticoids may have beneficial effects in septic shock if administered before or shortly after shock ensues by decreasing production of metabolites of the inflammatory cascade.[45] However, administration before shock is impossible in nonhospitalized patients. Two large, multicenter, clinical trials in people provided evidence that glucocorticoids have negative effects on patients with septic shock.[7,70] These two studies have resulted in the recommendation not to administer glucocorticoids to patients with septic shock.

BICARBONATE THERAPY

Recommendations on the use of sodium bicarbonate in patients with shock have changed in the literature. Bicarbonate is no longer routinely recommended for shock patients.[45,58] Animals with shock usually have metabolic acidosis because of decreased tissue perfusion, and it previously was recommended that the acidosis be treated with sodium bicarbonate. However, increasing tissue perfusion should treat metabolic acidosis related to poor tissue perfusion. In most instances, improving tissue perfusion reverses metabolic acidosis. Animals with underlying diseases that predispose to metabolic acidosis (e.g., bicarbonate loss related to diarrhea or renal disease) usually require additional intervention.

The degree of metabolic acidosis in shock depends on the severity and duration of poor tissue perfusion. Mild metabolic acidosis (pH 7.2 to 7.4) has few metabolic consequences. Animals with compensatory or early decompensatory shock of short duration usually have mild metabolic acidosis. Animals with prolonged early decompensatory shock or decompensatory (terminal) shock may have severe metabolic acidosis (pH < 7.2). Severe metabolic acidosis (pH < 7.2) decreases cardiac performance and can predispose the heart to ventricular arrhythmias. Acute metabolic acidosis also can result in a transient hyperkalemia related to transcellular shifting of potassium from the intracellular to extracellular space.

Current recommendations for administration of bicarbonate begin with documentation of metabolic acidosis by blood gas analysis.[18] Bicarbonate should be administered only when the pH is less than 7.2 and only in amounts necessary to increase the pH to 7.2. An 8.4% sodium bicarbonate solution is high in sodium and can result in volume overload, decreased serum ionized calcium concentration, "overshoot" metabolic alkalosis, paradoxical central nervous system acidosis, and hypokalemia caused by a transcellular shift of potassium from the extracellular to intracellular space. Current recommended dosages range from 0.25 to 1.0 mEq/kg intravenously administered as a bolus over 10 to 15 minutes. Alternatively, a calculated dose of bicarbonate can be determined using a formula: mEq $NaHCO_3$ = 0.3 × body weight (kg) × desired change in serum $[HCO_3^-]$. Repeated blood gas analysis is used to assess the effect of the initial dose.

BLOOD PRODUCTS

Some clinical situations require administration of blood or blood products. Hemorrhagic shock from excessive blood loss usually requires administration of whole blood (preferred), PRBCs, or an HBOC (Oxyglobin). The extent of acute blood loss cannot be determined reliably by monitoring the packed cell volume (PCV) alone because the PCV is unlikely to decrease for several hours after acute blood loss. Monitoring clinical signs or quantitating the amount of blood loss should facilitate the decision of whether to administer blood or blood products. In most instances, crystalloid, colloid, or hypertonic fluid therapy should be instituted first because whole blood or blood products may not be immediately available. In addition, external or internal blood loss must be controlled for administration of blood or blood products to be effective.

The amount of blood administered usually is based on a mathematical formula, but such formulas are based on the animal's current PCV and the desired increase in PCV. As mentioned previously, however, the PCV may not change acutely, although the animal's vital signs may indicate the need for blood. The amount of blood to administer can be estimated without using the PCV as a guide. Most animals can tolerate a 10% to 15% loss of blood acutely without requiring blood transfusion. Acute blood loss of more than 20% usually requires blood transfusion in addition to initial fluid therapy. Most animals that lose more than 50% of their blood acutely do not survive for an extended period. Therefore estimating an approximate percentage blood loss and multiplying by blood volume (90 mL/kg in dogs or 70 mL/kg in cats) can provide an initial volume of blood to administer. One should be cautious when using this approach to calculate the volume of blood to be transfused because it represents a very crude estimate. The animal should be monitored closely for its response to blood administration and for potential complications, including volume overload, transfusion reactions, and metabolic acidosis or hypocalcemia caused by massive doses of anticoagulant (e.g., anticoagulant citrate dextrose solutions).

HBOCs (e.g., Oxyglobin) have been developed to provide a readily available source of oxygen-carrying fluid. Advantages include no transfusion reactions, ready availability off of the shelf at room temperature, and colloidal effects. The effects can last more than 24 hours, depending on the dose administered. Internal or external hemorrhage must be controlled for this approach to be effective. The colloidal effects associated with Oxyglobin in addition to its oxygen-carrying capability make it an attractive fluid for maximal volume resuscitation and oxygen delivery. For example, synthetic colloids (e.g., hetastarch) provide colloidal effects and support cardiac output but do not have oxygen-carrying capacity.

FUTURE CONSIDERATIONS

Several novel approaches to therapy currently are on the verge of clinical relevance. Ethyl pyruvate is a novel molecule that has potent oxygen free radical scavenging effects and an important impact on intracellular viability in a number of animal models of shock and SIRS. The use of ethyl pyruvate in a resuscitation crystalloid solution has shown remarkable improvement in survival and outcome in a number of animal models.[20,21,23,66,69] Rapid induction of hypothermia has also been shown to significantly alter outcome in a number of animal models of hemorrhagic or traumatic shock.* Currently, the optimal method of inducing hypothermia has yet to be established, and clinical devices to achieve this goal currently are being evaluated.

MONITORING

Many variables can be monitored in the shock patient, including physical findings (e.g., mucous membrane color, capillary refill time, pulse rate and quality, heart rate, respiratory rate), arterial blood pressure (by invasive or noninvasive means), PCV, urine output, CVP, cardiac output, and blood gases (arterial and venous). Which of these is the most important variable to monitor? Which variable gives the clinician the most valuable information? The answers to these questions depend on the pathophysiology of shock in the patient in question. Oxygen transport variables (e.g., cardiac output, content of oxygen in arterial and venous blood, oxygen consumption, and oxygen delivery) provide the most important and most accurate information.[39] Unfortunately, most veterinary practices do not have the capability to monitor oxygen transport variables. Many of the easily measured variables may be normal, and the animal still can progress to end-stage organ failure and death. Therefore the information that can be obtained by the clinician must be used carefully to make decisions about further therapeutic intervention.

Another common question is how often to monitor the patient with shock. The answer depends on the clinical status of the patient. The most critically ill patients require continuous, even minute-by-minute monitoring, whereas more stable patients require less frequent monitoring. Clinical judgment must be used to determine the interval of monitoring.

PHYSICAL FINDINGS

Physical findings are important and simple to monitor for trends that may be early indications of deterioration or improvement in cardiovascular status. The interpretation of these findings is subjective, and final decisions should be made using more objective monitoring techniques. Peripheral pulse rate and rhythm; respiratory rate, rhythm, and effort; mucous membrane color; and capillary refill time provide subjective information on the status of the

cardiopulmonary system. Other physical findings that are important include the animal's mentation, character of peripheral pulses, and assessment of the jugular veins.

PACKED CELL VOLUME AND TOTAL PLASMA PROTEINS

Measurements of PCV and total plasma proteins provide essential information. The PCV provides information on the oxygen-carrying potential of the blood because hemoglobin is the major contributor to the oxygen content of arterial blood. Acute changes in blood volume may not be reflected in the PCV due to fluid shifting and potential for splenic contraction in dogs. The PCV should be maintained between 25% and 35% in all critically ill animals. Blood or blood products should be considered when the PCV is less than 20% acutely and the animal is showing signs of decreased oxygen delivery (e.g., tachypnea, exercise intolerance, decreased mentation). Patients with a chronic decrease in PCV may not require blood products until the PCV is less than 15%.

Measurement of total plasma proteins provides much useful information. The color of the plasma can identify hemolysis or icterus. The refractometer reading of the total plasma protein concentration can provide subjective information on COP in patients that have not received synthetic colloids. Proteins are large molecules that are confined to the intravascular space. The presence of these large, nondiffusible molecules creates a force that draws water into the vascular space. Decreased concentration of proteins related to blood loss or extravasation from the intravascular space because of defects in the endothelium (as in SIRS) results in decreased COP. A decrease in COP can cause loss of intravascular water to the interstitial space and predispose to interstitial edema. The total plasma protein concentration should remain greater than 3.5 g/dL to maintain adequate COP. Colloid therapy should be strongly considered when the total plasma protein concentration is less than 3.5 g/dL. Colloid oncotic pressure also can be measured directly with an oncometer or colloid osmometer. The COP of plasma in normal patients is approximately 20 to 25 mm Hg, and values less than 15 mm Hg often are found in critically ill patients. Patients with COP less than 15 mm Hg will benefit from supplemental synthetic colloid administration.

CENTRAL VENOUS PRESSURE

Measurement of CVP can provide valuable information about right ventricular function and intravascular volume status and is relatively easy to monitor in most veterinary practices.[16] Monitoring CVP involves placement of an indwelling jugular catheter with the tip of the catheter in the thoracic cranial vena cava. If the animal has appropriate right-sided heart function, CVP provides information on filling pressures of the heart (i.e., preload). The CVP should range between 10 and 15 cm H_2O in the

---

*References 27,46,49,64,65,67,72–74.

shock patient, although normal CVP values range from 0 to 2 cm H_2O. Other determinants of CVP also must be considered when interpreting values, including intrathoracic pressure and venous distensibility.

Appropriate fluid resuscitation should result in an increase in CVP. However, the nature of crystalloid therapy is such that intravascular volume expansion is temporary because of normal movement of the crystalloid into the interstitial space. A general rule is that if the CVP increases to an acceptable value after initial fluid resuscitation with crystalloids but then decreases to less than 3 cm H_2O and physical parameters also deteriorate, further therapy is warranted. A rapid decrease in CVP also may indicate acute blood loss.

ARTERIAL BLOOD PRESSURE

Arterial blood pressure is defined as the force that is exerted by the blood on the arterial wall. Arterial blood pressure is not cardiac output, and it should not be assumed that adequate blood pressure is synonymous with adequate cardiac output. In fact, cardiac output is a determinant of mean arterial blood pressure (i.e., mean arterial pressure = cardiac output × systemic vascular resistance). If systemic vascular resistance is increased secondary to vasoconstriction, the result is increased blood pressure. However, cardiac output can decrease during hypertension. An animal in pain can have hypertension yet have lower than normal cardiac output. The animal with poor myocardial performance because of SIRS and vasoconstriction caused by pain or hypothermia can have very poor cardiac output. Therefore blood pressure monitoring should be used in addition to other monitoring techniques to provide the most accurate assessment of cardiovascular status.

Arterial blood pressure can be measured by direct or indirect methods. Direct measurement of arterial blood pressure requires a catheter placed in a peripheral artery (usually dorsal pedal or femoral), a pressure transducer, and a monitor. Accurate measurement of systolic, diastolic, and mean arterial pressures can be obtained with proper positioning of the transducer (i.e., at the level of the heart) and adequate calibration of equipment. The arterial waveform also can be monitored for early deterioration of the cardiovascular system (i.e., flattening of the waveform). Placement of an arterial catheter is a challenge, especially in patients weighing less than 10 kg, and the equipment is expensive, which may deter many clinicians from measuring arterial blood pressure directly.

Indirect measurement of arterial blood pressure is most feasible for the practicing veterinarian. The most important factor to remember with indirect methods is that the values obtained are not necessarily accurate, especially in smaller animals (<10 kg). However, the trend of values obtained is extremely important and should be considered more important than the actual values.

The two available methods of indirect arterial blood pressure monitoring are oscillometric and Doppler ultrasonic. The oscillometric method (e.g., Dinamap, GE Healthcare Systems, Waukesha, WI; Cardell, CAS Medical Systems Inc., Branford, CT) involves placement of an appropriate-sized blood pressure cuff over a peripheral artery. The mechanism of blood pressure measurement is to determine the oscillation of the artery at systolic and mean arterial pressures and convert this measurement to a numerical blood pressure. The diastolic pressure is the pressure at which the maximal oscillation has decreased by 80%. Therefore diastolic pressure measurements are least accurate. The most common artery used is the dorsal pedal artery, but the coccygeal and metacarpal arteries have been used with less success. The area over the artery should be clipped, and the animal should be placed in lateral recumbency to ensure that the limb is near the level of the heart. Appropriate cuff size is critical to obtain adequate readings. The width of the cuff should be approximately 40% of the circumference of the limb. A cuff that is too large results in falsely decreased values, and a cuff that is too small results in falsely increased values. The oscillometric method provides systolic, diastolic, and mean arterial pressures, as well as heart rate. The primary disadvantages of the oscillometric method include the cost of the equipment and inaccurate or unobtainable readings in animals weighing 5 to 10 kg.

The Doppler ultrasonic method uses the Doppler effect to detect movement of red blood cells past a crystal that emits Doppler waves. Each pulse of blood is converted to a sound that can easily be heard. The crystal is placed over the metacarpal artery with an appropriate-sized cuff placed proximal to the crystal. A sphygmomanometer is attached to the cuff and inflated until no sound is detected. The pressure is slowly reduced until the first audible pulse is detected. Only systolic blood pressure is measured on a reliable basis, but diastolic pressure also can be obtained. The first audible pulse is the systolic blood pressure as indicated on the sphygmomanometer. The pressure continues to be slowly removed from the cuff until the audible signal changes tone. The change in tone occurs at the diastolic blood pressure. Advantages of the Doppler method include detection of an audible pulse, reasonable cost, and reliable use in very small patients.

OXYGEN TRANSPORT VARIABLES

Oxygen transport variables (e.g., cardiac output, content of oxygen in arterial and venous blood, oxygen consumption, oxygen delivery) provide the most valuable information on cardiovascular function, but the cost of instrumentation and need to place specialized catheters tend to limit the use of these parameters.

Cardiac Output

Cardiac output is defined as the total output of blood from the heart and is synonymous with blood flow.

Cardiac output measurement requires thermodilution catheters to be placed in the pulmonary artery and a cardiac output computer.[39] Although the cost of Doppler ultrasound equipment is high, the technique to determine blood flow with an ultrasound probe is less difficult than placement of a thermodilution catheter but requires experience to produce accurate and reliable estimates.

Urine Output

Urine output can be used as an indirect measurement of renal blood flow and therefore as an indirect measurement of cardiac output. If urine production decreases to less than 1 mL/kg/hr in an animal without previously detected renal disease, low cardiac output should be suspected. Urine production is relatively easy to monitor by placement of a urethral catheter and hourly recording of urine production.

Oxygen Content

Determination of oxygen content variables requires arterial and mixed venous blood gas determination. Most of the variables in Table 23-1 are calculated. The assessment of adequate cardiopulmonary function ultimately is determined by oxygen delivery variables.

Blood Gas Analysis

Arterial and venous blood gas analysis can provide valuable information about cardiopulmonary function. The production of portable "point of care" blood gas analyzers has greatly increased the clinician's ability to monitor blood gases. Laboratory blood gas analyzers are prohibitively expensive unless high caseload allows nearly constant usage, whereas portable blood gas analyzers can easily pay for themselves in several years. One disadvantage of blood gas analysis (arterial or venous) is that the results obtained represent a single moment in time. The status of the patient may change minute by minute, which may limit the value of intermittent blood gas analysis. The partial pressure of oxygen also reflects the amount of oxygen dissolved in plasma. Saturation of hemoglobin with oxygen is much more important because oxygen is delivered by hemoglobin in the red blood cell. The saturation of hemoglobin can be determined from the oxyhemoglobin dissociation curve.

Arterial blood gas analysis provides information about gas exchange in the lung and arterial acid-base balance. Arterial blood samples are collected from the femoral or dorsal pedal artery in a heparinized syringe. The partial pressure of oxygen in arterial blood (PaO_2) is correlated with oxygen exchange in the lung. Acid-base balance is discussed in Chapters 9 to 13.

A true mixed venous blood gas sample must be obtained from the pulmonary artery, which requires placement of specialized catheter. The partial pressure of oxygen in mixed venous blood (PvO_2) represents information about perfusion of tissues on a global basis. Normal PvO_2 values range from 35 to 45 mm Hg. Values less than 30 mm Hg indicate poor perfusion of the peripheral tissues. If a thermodilution catheter is not placed in the pulmonary artery to collect blood for PvO_2 determination, a jugular catheter placed to monitor CVP can be used to collect a venous blood sample that may approximate a true mixed venous sample.

Pulse Oximetry

Pulse oximetry allows continuous monitoring of the saturation of hemoglobin with oxygen (SaO_2). The PaO_2 provides information about oxygen dissolved in plasma, whereas SaO_2 provides information about the ability of the red blood cell to carry oxygen. To be of value, pulse oximetry requires pulsatile flow of blood to the periphery. Many patients with shock have decreased blood flow to the periphery, which limits the effectiveness of pulse oximetry. In addition, the device is applied to the tongue for the most accurate readings, a technique that is difficult in the conscious patient. Other areas where the probe may be placed include the ear, axilla, vulva, and prepuce. A rectal probe may be of value in the conscious patient.

Lactate

The clinical use of lactate measurement has gained acceptance and popularity in veterinary practice during the past several years because of the ready accessibility and the reasonable cost of portable lactate analyzers. Increased lactate concentrations have been correlated with inadequate tissue oxygenation in many clinical shock syndromes, and lactate measurement has found an important place in the evaluation and monitoring of shock syndromes.[30] Normal reference intervals vary with the equipment used, but changes in lactate concentration in the presence of other clinical indicators of shock are useful for monitoring the success of therapy. In some cases, lactate concentration can increase transiently after initiation of therapy as improved perfusion results in collection of waste products that did not previously have access to the vascular system. Lactate concentration should decrease over time if successful cardiovascular resuscitation from shock has occurred. Lactate measurement has been shown to be an effective predictor of gastric necrosis in dogs with GDV and thus serves as a useful predictor of prognosis and survival.[17]

OTHER CONCERNS

The following aspects of fluid resuscitation are beyond the scope of this chapter but are of great importance when treating patients with severe shock and shock secondary to trauma. They are mentioned briefly here.

RESUSCITATION-INDUCED HEMORRHAGE AND HYPOTENSIVE RESUSCITATION

The hypotensive patient with uncontrolled internal hemorrhage is a challenge. Fluid resuscitation should begin before surgical intervention, but aggressive fluid resuscitation may increase blood pressure and cardiac output sufficiently to exacerbate hemorrhage.[13] Dilution of existing hemostatic factors also can occur, which may weaken forming clots and also may contribute to further hemorrhage.[36] Hypotensive resuscitation is defined as fluid therapy administered at rates and volumes below current recommendations with an endpoint below normal values of blood pressure.[38] The optimal endpoint of this type of resuscitation has not been determined.[19,53,63] Blood pressures higher than presentation but lower than normal have been suggested. More clinical information on hypotensive resuscitation is necessary before precise recommendations can be made.

POSTRESUSCITATION INJURY

Most clinicians have witnessed deterioration of patients that seemingly have been resuscitated successfully from advanced stages of shock. The development of SIRS and MODS is likely to play an important role in this deterioration. Two processes have been implicated in injury after successful resuscitation: the no-reflow phenomenon and reperfusion injury.[38]

No-Reflow Phenomenon

Perfusion can be decreased even after seemingly adequate fluid resuscitation. Several mechanisms have been proposed to explain this phenomenon, including calcium-induced vasoconstriction, leukocyte, platelet or hemostatic plugging of the microvasculature, and vascular compromise caused by edema of surrounding tissues. Lack of flow to the intestinal tract can result in translocation of intestinal pathogens and lead to postresuscitation septicemia, SIRS, and septic shock. The occurrence and severity of the no-reflow phenomenon seem to be related to the duration of poor perfusion during shock. At present, there is no therapy that can prevent the no-reflow phenomenon.

Reperfusion Injury

The phenomenon of reperfusion injury has been well established and can occur in any organ after adequate resuscitation. Toxic oxygen metabolites are produced by a cascade of events that result in the production of superoxide and hydroxyl radicals.[22] As with the no-reflow phenomenon, reperfusion injury can occur in any organ, but its effects on the brain are most detrimental to the survival of the patient. Antioxidants, corticosteroids, calcium channel blockers, free radical scavengers, and iron chelators have been studied as potential treatments, but no single approach has been determined to be most effective. The most effective therapy is likely to be one

that can be administered before resuscitation, which is nearly impossible in the clinical setting.

FLUID THERAPY FOR SHOCK WITH CONCURRENT HEAD TRAUMA AND PULMONARY CONTUSIONS

Patients with shock with concurrent head trauma and pulmonary contusions present special challenges to fluid therapy. Head trauma patients with cerebral edema are probably not able to handle large volumes of crystalloid fluids because most of the crystalloid extravasates into the interstitium within 1 hour of administration. Many patients with head trauma deteriorate soon after crystalloid administration. Hypertonic saline and synthetic colloids, either alone or in combination, are the fluids of choice for patients with head trauma (see Table 23-5).[1,44,48] Crystalloid therapy should be administered cautiously.

Fluid therapy in patients with pulmonary contusions is controversial.[29] In this clinical setting, the alveolar-capillary membranes have sustained damage, and the alveoli have been flooded with blood. Administration of large volumes of crystalloids potentially may worsen the clinical signs associated with pulmonary contusions. Although controversial, no definitive recommendations can be made until further research has been completed to determine the effectiveness of different fluid resuscitation strategies. Clinically, the current recommendation is similar to that for patients with cerebral edema. Consequently, hypertonic solutions and colloids, or a combination of the two, are the treatment of choice, with judicious administration of crystalloids.

CLINICAL EXAMPLES OF FLUID THERAPY FOR THE THREE STAGES OF SHOCK

Compensatory Shock

A 2-year-old male mixed-breed dog weighing 20 kg is presented after being hit by a car 20 minutes earlier. The dog walks into the clinic and seems normal. Physical examination shows hydration, normal; heart rate, 150 beats/min; respiratory rate, 90 breaths/min; mucous membranes, bright red; capillary refill time, less than 1 second; strong femoral pulses; and normal blood pressure. The dog has compensatory shock and requires fluid therapy. Alternatively, the dog may have severe pain, and the perfusion parameters identified previously have resulted from pain-induced sympathetic stimulation. An 18-gauge catheter is placed in a cephalic vein. Shock dose choices of fluids include 1.8 L of lactated Ringer's solution or 80 mL of 7% NaCl plus 500 mL of lactated Ringer's solution. Fluid should be administered in divided aliquots until the patient has achieved targeted endpoints for physical variables after therapy that include heart rate, 80 beats/min; respiratory rate, 30 breaths/min; mucous membranes, pink; and capillary refill time, 2 seconds. Measurement of systemic blood pressure and administering pain medications after the initial aliquot of fluids has been administered may be useful ways of differentiating the source of the sympathetic output in this dog.

Early Decompensatory Shock

A 5-year-old female mixed-breed dog weighing 25 kg is presented after being hit by a car 2 to 4 hours earlier. The dog also has a luxation of the coxofemoral joint. The dog is in lateral recumbency with a decreased level of consciousness. Physical examination shows normal hydration; heart rate, 180 beats/min; respiratory rate, 90 breaths/min; mucous membranes, pale; capillary refill time, difficult to elicit; weak femoral pulses; hypotension (70 mm Hg systolic blood pressure); and mild abdominal distention. Abdominocentesis shows hemoabdomen. This dog has early decompensatory shock (hemorrhagic and/or traumatic) and requires aggressive fluid therapy and monitoring. An oxygen mask is placed, and oxygen is delivered at 5 L/min. An 18-gauge catheter is placed in the cephalic vein, and therapy begins as another catheter is placed in the jugular vein. Fluid options include 125 mL of 7% NaCl alone or with 1 L of lactated Ringer's solution, 500 mL of 6% of hetastarch, or 125 mL of 7% NaCl plus 500 mL of 6% hetastarch. CVP, arterial blood pressure (Doppler), and physical findings are monitored continuously as fluid resuscitation occurs and for several hours to determine whether further fluid resuscitation is required. Analgesia is administered in the form of a parenteral opioid (butorphanol or oxymorphone). The coxofemoral luxation should not be addressed until the animal is adequately stabilized. Two hours later, the abdominal hemorrhage is not progressing, arterial blood pressure now is 150 mm Hg, mucous membranes are pink, capillary refill time is 2 seconds, and CVP has remained between 8 and 12 cm H_2O.

Decompensatory (Terminal) Shock and SIRS

A 10-year-old 10-kg male schnauzer is presented after 24 hours of intractable vomiting and diarrhea. The dog had eaten garbage 2 days previously. The dog is in lateral recumbency with severe abdominal pain and a decreased level of consciousness. Physical examination shows hydration, 10% dehydrated; heart rate, 70 beats/min; respiratory rate, 60 breaths/min; mucous membrane, pale; capillary refill time, cannot be elicited; rectal temperature, 37° C; no palpable femoral pulses; barely audible heart sounds; severe hypotension (50 mm Hg systolic blood pressure). The dog has decompensatory (terminal) shock and requires aggressive fluid therapy and cardiovascular support. An oxygen mask is placed, and oxygen is delivered at 5 L/min. Twenty-gauge catheters are placed in both cephalic veins, and therapy begins as a catheter is placed in the jugular vein. Fluid therapy includes 1 L of lactated Ringer's solution as fast as can be administered via one cephalic catheter

and then at twice the maintenance rate and 200 mL of 6% hetastarch via the other cephalic catheter. Antibiotics and analgesia (morphine infusion) are administered. The CVP is monitored by means of the jugular catheter, and arterial blood pressure is continuously monitored or repeatedly assessed. The dog does not produce urine after initial fluid therapy; blood pressure decreases; and CVP increases. The dog may be in cardiac failure or unresponsive to fluid therapy because of decreased oncotic pressure secondary to SIRS and increased vascular permeability. Venous blood gas analysis shows a Pvo_2 of 30 mm Hg. Fluid therapy is continued; 6% hetastarch (50 mL) is repeated; another hetastarch infusion (20 mL/kg/day) is begun for oncotic support; and dobutamine infusion (5 µg/kg/min) is started. One hour later, the dog begins to show a response: urine production is 3 mL/kg/hr, CVP decreases, blood pressure increases, and the dog begins to respond to verbal commands.

REFERENCES

1. Bayir H, Clark RS, Kochanek PM: Promising strategies to minimize secondary brain injury after head trauma, *Crit Care Med* 31:S112, 2003.
2. Bentsen G, Breivik H, Lundar T, et al: Predictable reduction of intracranial hypertension with hypertonic saline hydroxyethyl starch: a prospective clinical trial in critically ill patients with subarachnoid haemorrhage, *Acta Anaesthesiol Scand* 48:1089, 2004.
3. Bernard GR, Ely EW, Wright TJ, et al: Safety and dose relationship of recombinant human activated protein C for coagulopathy in severe sepsis, *Crit Care Med* 29:2051, 2001.
4. Bernard GR, Vincent JL, Laterre P, et al: Efficacy and safety of recombinant human activated protein C for severe sepsis, *N Engl J Med* 344:699, 2001.
5. Bishop MH, Shoemaker WC, Appel PL, et al: Influence of time and optimal circulatory resuscitation in high-risk trauma, *Crit Care Med* 21:56, 1993.
6. Bisonni RS, Holtgrave DR, Lawler F, et al: Colloids versus crystalloids in fluid resuscitation—an analysis of randomized controlled trials, *J Fam Pract* 32:387, 1991.
7. Bone RC, Fisher CJ, Clemmer TP, et al: A controlled clinical-trial of high-dose methylprednisolone in the treatment of severe sepsis and septic shock, *N Engl J Med* 317:653, 1987.
8. Brady CA, Otto CM: Systemic inflammatory response syndrome, sepsis, and multiple organ dysfunction, *Vet Clin North Am Small Anim Pract* 31:1147, 2001.
9. Brooks M: Transfusion medicine. In Murtaugh RJ, Kaplan PM, editor: *Veterinary emergency and critical care medicine*, St. Louis, 1992, Mosby Yearbook.
10. Choi PTL, Yip G, Quinonez LG, et al: Crystalloids vs. colloids in fluid resuscitation: a systematic review, *Crit Care Med* 27:200, 1999.
11. Concannon KT: Colloid oncotic pressure and the clinical use of colloidal solutions, *J Vet Emerg Crit Care* 3:49, 1993.
12. Cote E: Cardiogenic shock and cardiac arrest, *Vet Clin North Am Small Anim Pract* 31:1129, 2001.

13. Crowe DT, Devey JJ: Assessment and management of the hemorrhaging patient, *Vet Clin North Am Small Anim Pract* 24:1095, 1994.

14. Crystal MA, Cotter SM: Acute hemorrhage: a hemotologic emergency in dogs, *Compend Cont Educ Prac Vet* 14:1, 1992.

15. Deitch EA: Animal models of sepsis and shock: a review and lessons learned, *Shock* 9:1, 1998.

16. de Laforcade AM, Rozanski EA: Central venous pressure and arterial blood pressure measurements, *Vet Clin North Am Small Anim Pract* 31:1163, 2001.

17. de Papp E, Drobatz KJ, Hughes D: Plasma lactate concentration as a predictor of gastric necrosis and survival among dogs with gastric dilatation-volvulus: 102 cases (1995-1998), *J Am Vet Med Assoc* 215:49, 1999.

18. DiBartola SP: Metabolic acidosis. In Dibartola SP, editor: *Fluid therapy in small animal practice*, ed 1, Philadelphia, 1992, WB Saunders.

19. Dries DJ: Hypotensive resuscitation, *Shock* 6:311, 1996.

20. Fink MP: Ethyl pyruvate: a novel anti-inflammatory agent, *Crit Care Med* 31:S51, 2003.

21. Fink MP: Ethyl pyruvate: a novel treatment for sepsis and shock, *Minerva Anestesiol* 70:365, 2004.

22. Fink MP: Reactive oxygen species as mediators of organ dysfunction caused by sepsis, acute respiratory distress syndrome, or hemorrhagic shock: potential benefits of resuscitation with Ringer's ethyl pyruvate solution, *Curr Opin Clin Nutr Metab Care* 5:167, 2002.

23. Fink MP: Ringer's ethyl pyruvate solution: a novel resuscitation fluid for the treatment of hemorrhagic shock and sepsis, *J Trauma* 54:S141, 2003.

24. Garrison RN, Cryer HM: Role of the microcirculation to skeletal muscle during shock, *Prog Clin Biol Res* 299:43, 1989.

25. Garrison RN, Spain DA, Wilson MA, et al: Microvascular changes explain the "two-hit" theory of multiple organ failure, *Ann Surg* 227:851, 1998.

26. Griffel MI, Kaufman BS: Pharmacology of colloids and crystalloids, *Crit Care Clin* 8:235, 1992.

27. Guven H, Amanvermez R, Malazgirt Z, et al: Moderate hypothermia prevents brain stem oxidative stress injury after hemorrhagic shock, *J Trauma* 53:66, 2002.

28. Guyton AC: Transport of oxygen and carbon dioxide in the blood and body fluids. In Guyton AC, editor: *Textbook of medical physiology*, ed 8, Philadelphia, 1991, WB Saunders.

29. Hackner SG: Emergency management of traumatic pulmonary contusions, *Compend Cont Educ Prac Vet* 17:677, 1995.

30. Hughes D: Lactate measurement: diagnostic, therapeutic and prognostic implications. In Bonagura JD, editor: *Current veterinary therapy XIII*, Philadelphia, 2000, WB Saunders.

31. Kirby R: Septic shock. In Bonagura JD, editor: *Current veterinary therapy XII*, Philadelphia, 1995, WB Saunders.

32. Kirby R, Rudloff E: The critical need for colloids: maintaining fluid balance, *Compend Cont Educ Prac Vet* 19: 705, 1997.

33. Klein LW: Cardiovascular therapeutics. In Parillo JE, editor: *Current therapy in critical care medicine*, ed 3, St. Louis, 1977, CV Mosby.

34. Kramer GC: Hypertonic resuscitation: physiologic mechanisms and recommendations for trauma care, *J Trauma* 54:S89, 2003.

35. Kumar A, Parillo JE: Shock: classification, pathophysiology, and approach to management. In Parillo JE, Dellinger RP, editors: *Critical care medicine: principles of diagnosis and management in the adult*, ed 2, Philadelphia, 2001, Mosby.

36. Ledgerwood AM, Lucas CE: A review of studies on the effects of hemorrhagic shock and resuscitation on the coagulation profile, *J Trauma* 54:S68, 2003.

37. Marino PL: Colloid and crystalloid resuscitation. In Marino PL, editor: *The ICU book*, ed 2, Baltimore, 1998, Williams & Wilkins.

38. Marino PL: Hemorrhage and hypovolemia. In Marino PL, editor: *The ICU book*, ed 2, Baltimore, 1998, Williams & Wilkins.

39. Mellema M: Cardiac output, wedge pressure, and oxygen delivery, *Vet Clin North Am Small Anim Pract* 31:1175, 2001.

40. Moore FD: The effects of hemorrhage on body composition, *N Engl J Med* 273:567, 1965.

41. Moore KE, Murtaugh RJ: Pathophysiologic characteristics of hypovolemic shock, *Vet Clin North Am Small Anim Pract* 31:1115, 2001.

42. Mueller DL, Noxon JO: Anaphylaxis: pathophysiology and treatment, *Compend Cont Educ Prac Vet* 12:2, 1990.

43. Muir WW: Overview of shock. In *Proceedings of the 14th Annual Kal Kan Symposium Emergency/Critical Care*, Columbus, OH, 1990, p. 7.

44. Munar F, Ferrer AM, de Nadal M, et al: Cerebral hemodynamic effects of 7.2% hypertonic saline in patients with head injury and raised intracranial pressure, *J Neurotrauma* 17:41, 2000.

45. Neugebauer E, Lechleuthner A, Rixen D: Pharmacotherapy of shock. In Chernow B, editor: *The pharmacologic approach to the critically ill patient*, ed 3, Baltimore, 1994, Williams & Wilkins.

46. Norio H, Takasu A, Kawakami M, et al: Rapid body cooling by cold fluid infusion prolongs survival time during uncontrolled hemorrhagic shock in pigs, *J Trauma* 52:1056, 2002.

47. Otto CM: Sepsis. In Raffe MR, Wingfield WE, editors: *The veterinary ICU book*, Jackson, WY, 2002, Teton NewMedia.

48. Pfenninger J, Wagner BP: Hypertonic saline in severe pediatric head injury, *Crit Care Med* 29:1489, 2001.

49. Prueckner S, Safar P, Kentner R, et al: Mild hypothermia increases survival from severe pressure-controlled hemorrhagic shock in rats, *J Trauma* 50:253, 2001.

50. Purvis D, Kirby R: Systemic inflammatory response syndrome: septic shock, *Vet Clin North Am Small Anim Pract* 24:1225, 1994.

51. Raffe MR, Wingfield WE: Hemorrhage and hypovolemia. In Raffe MR, Wingfield WE, editors: *The veterinary ICU book*, Jackson, WY, 2002, Teton NewMedia.

52. Rainey TG, Read CA: Pharmacology of colloids and crystalloids. In Chernow B, editor: *The pharmacologic approach to the critically ill patient*, ed 3, Baltimore, 1994, Williams & Wilkins.

53. Revell M, Greaves I, Porter K: Endpoints for fluid resuscitation in hemorrhagic shock, *J Trauma* 54:S63, 2003.

54. Rudloff E, Kirby R: Hypovolemic shock and resuscitation, *Vet Clin North Am Small Anim Pract* 1015, 1994.

55. Schertel ER: Hypertonic fluid therapy. In DiBartola SP, editor: *Fluid therapy in small animal practice*, ed 1, Philadelphia, 1992, WB Saunders.

56. Schertel ER, Allen DA, Muir WW, et al: Evaluation of a hypertonic saline-dextran solution for treatment of dogs with shock induced by gastric dilatation-volvulus, *J Am Vet Med Assoc* 210:226, 1997.

57. Schertel ER, Schneider DA, Zissimos AG: Cardiopulmonary reflexes induced by osmolality changes in the airways and pulmonary vasculature, *Fed Proc* 44:835, 1985.

58. Shoemaker WC: Diagnosis and treatment of shock syndromes. In Shoemaker WC, Ayers S, Genvick A, editors: *Textbook of critical care*, ed 3, Philadelphia, 1995, WB Saunders.

59. Shoemaker WC, Appel PL, Kram HB: Sequence of physiologic patterns in surgical septic shock, *Crit Care Med* 21:1876, 1993.

60. Shoemaker WC, Appel PL, Kram HB: Temporal hemodynamics and oxygen transport patterns in medical patients with sepsis and septic shock, *Chest* 104:1529, 1993.

61. Shoemaker WC, Kram HB: Comparison of the effects of crystalloids and colloids on hemodynamic oxygen transport, mortality and morbidity. In Simmon RS, Udeko AJ, editors: *Debates in general surgery*, Chicago, 1991, Year Book Medical Publishers.

62. Shores T, Carrico J, Lightfoot S: Fluid therapy in hemorrhagic shock, *Arch Surg* 88:688, 1964.

63. Stern SA: Low-volume fluid resuscitation for presumed hemorrhagic shock: helpful or harmful? *Curr Opin Crit Care* 7:422, 2001.

64. Takasu A, Norio H, Gotoh Y, et al: Effect of induced-hypothermia on short-term survival after volume-controlled hemorrhage in pigs, *Resuscitation* 56:319, 2003.

65. Takasu A, Norio H, Sakamoto T, et al: Mild hypothermia prolongs the survival time during uncontrolled hemorrhagic shock in rats, *Resuscitation* 54:303, 2002.

66. Tawadrous ZS, Delude RL, Fink MP: Resuscitation from hemorrhagic shock with Ringer's ethyl pyruvate solution improves survival and ameliorates intestinal mucosal hyperpermeability in rats, *Shock* 17:473, 2002.

67. Tisherman SA: Suspended animation for resuscitation from exsanguinating hemorrhage, *Crit Care Med* 32:S46, 2004.

68. Tobias TA, Schertel ER: Shock. In Dibartola SP, editor: *Fluid therapy in small animal practice*, ed 1, Philadelphia, 1992, WB Saunders.

69. Venkataraman R, Kellum JA, Song M, et al: Resuscitation with Ringer's ethyl pyruvate solution prolongs survival and modulates plasma cytokine and nitrite/nitrate concentrations in a rat model of lipopolysaccharide-induced shock, *Shock* 18:507, 2002.

70. Veterans Administration Systemic Sepsis Cooperative Group: Effect of high dose glucocorticoid therapy on mortality in patients with clinical signs of systemic sepsis, *N Engl J Med* 317:659, 1987.

71. Webb AR: The appropriate role of colloids in managing fluid imbalance: a critical review of resent meta-analytic findings, *Crit Care* 4:S26, 2000.

72. Wu X, Stezoski J, Safar P, et al: After spontaneous hypothermia during hemorrhagic shock, continuing mild hypothermia (34 degrees C) improves early but not late survival in rats, *J Trauma* 55:308, 2003.

73. Wu X, Stezoski J, Safar P, et al: Mild hypothermia during hemorrhagic shock in rats improves survival without significant effects on inflammatory responses, *Crit Care Med* 31:195, 2003.

74. Wu X, Stezoski J, Safar P, et al: Systemic hypothermia, but not regional gut hypothermia, improves survival from prolonged hemorrhagic shock in rats, *J Trauma* 53:654, 2002.

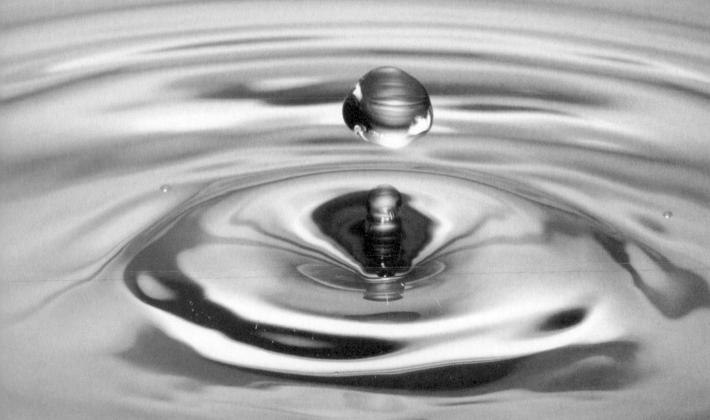

SPECIAL THERAPY

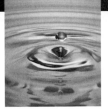

CHAPTER · 24

BLOOD TRANSFUSION AND BLOOD SUBSTITUTES

Ann E. Hohenhaus

Blood transfusions have many things in common with fluid therapy. Like crystalloid and colloid solutions, blood products are not used to treat disease; they are supportive therapies given to correct deficiencies in the patient until the underlying disease process can be treated. For example, a red blood cell transfusion is given to replace red blood cells lost as a result of a traumatic laceration. The transfusion of red blood cells increases the oxygen-carrying capacity of the blood, allowing for surgical repair of the laceration; it is not the primary treatment for hemorrhage. Likewise, sodium chloride is used to replace sodium, chloride, and water in a dehydrated patient with hypoadrenocorticism until adrenal hormones can be replaced.

The use of both blood transfusions and fluid therapy must be carefully assessed before inclusion in a patient's treatment plan, and the veterinarian should evaluate the risk/benefit ratio for each patient. Volume overload, electrolyte disturbances, and transmission of infection can occur from administration of pathogen-contaminated blood products or fluids.[18,46,91] Despite the potential negative effects of transfusion, most veterinarians view it as lifesaving therapy allowing the transfusion recipient to receive other necessary treatments such as surgery, chemotherapy, or medical care.[38]

Three major differences exist between the more commonly used fluids and blood products. The differences between crystalloid or colloid solutions and blood products are their immunogenicity, availability, and cost. The immunogenicity of blood products stems from the proteins and cellular material in the blood. Because crystalloid solutions lack proteins and cellular material, they are not considered immunogenic; however, certain colloid solutions such as hydroxyethyl starch have been reported to cause acute anaphylaxis in rare instances in humans.[70] The mechanism of this reaction is unknown.

Crystalloid and colloid solutions are readily available because they can be manufactured according to market demand. Only a living animal can produce blood, and production is limited to the donor's physi-

ologic capability. The small number of commercial canine and feline blood banks that provide a convenient source of blood for the veterinary practitioner further limits availability of blood for transfusion (Box 24-1). Furthermore, blood products require a more regulated storage environment and have a significantly shorter shelf life than crystalloid or colloid solutions, making blood a less convenient product to stock and use in a veterinary hospital.

The actual costs associated with canine blood transfusions are not known, but in 1992, veterinarians estimated the cost of a 500-mL whole blood transfusion to range from $25 to more than $300.[38] The cost of 500 mL of lactated Ringer's solution is less than $1.

Despite the fact that the first documented transfusion was given to a dog in 1665 by Richard Lower at Oxford University, veterinary transfusion medicine scientifically and technologically lags behind its counterpart in human medicine.[54] Information in this chapter is based on animal studies whenever possible. When none is available, currently accepted guidelines from human medicine will be applied to the veterinary patient. The purpose of this chapter is to provide the reader with the following:

1. A basic understanding of the theory of blood component therapy
2. Information on the technical aspects of obtaining blood for transfusion
3. Suggestions for the administration and monitoring of transfusions
4. A description of the clinical applications of a veterinary blood substitute

BASICS OF BLOOD COMPONENTS

Blood, as it is collected from the donor, contains all the elements of blood: red blood cells, white blood cells, platelets, coagulation factors, immunoglobulins, and albumin. Whole blood can be transfused into the recipient as

Box 24-1 **Veterinary Blood Banks**

Animal Blood Bank
800-243-5759
www.animalbloodbank.com

"Buddies for Life"
248-334-6877
www.ovrs.com

Eastern Veterinary Blood Bank
800-949-3822
www.evbb.com

Hemopet
310-828-4804
www.hemopet.com

Midwest Animal Blood Services
517-851-8244
www.midwestabs.com

Penn Animal Blood Bank
215-573-PABB
http://www.vet.upenn.edu/research/centers/penngen/
services/transfusionlab/pabb.html

Sun States Blood Bank
954-639-2231
www.ssabb.org

The Pet Blood Bank
800-906-7059
www.petshelpingpets.com

and coordinating the equipment and donors for successful blood collection. Preparation of blood components from whole blood requires that the blood from the donor be collected into the anticoagulant-containing bag of a multibag plastic blood collection system. The whole blood then is separated into packed red blood cells (PRBCs) and plasma by differential centrifugation, and the plasma is transferred into one or more of the satellite bags via the sterile tubing linking the bags. The bags are separated, and PRBCs are stored in a refrigerator while plasma is frozen. Blood collected into glass bottles is not amenable to centrifugation and cannot be processed into components. Additionally, storage of canine blood in a glass bottle results in lower levels of 2,3-diphosphoglycerate and adenosine triphosphate (ATP) than blood stored in plastic bags; consequently, plastic bags are the preferred storage container for blood.[16] Most general practitioners do not have access to the type of centrifuge required to properly separate blood into components. It is possible to acquire a used centrifuge or request the local blood bank to process the blood collected by the veterinarian. However, production of components is not feasible for most veterinarians, and the technical aspects of component production are not included in this chapter but can be found elsewhere.[60,72]

The most commonly used blood products, their indications, and suggested dosages are described below. The dosage of a blood product depends on the physical state of the patient and the response of the patient to the treatment: in essence, the treatment is "to effect."

WHOLE BLOOD

Whole blood is the blood collected from the donor plus the anticoagulant. In veterinary medicine, no standards have been established for the volume of blood that constitutes 1 unit. When a human blood collection system is used for dogs, 450 ± 45 mL of blood is collected in 63 mL of anticoagulant and often is designated as 1 unit. Whole blood contains red blood cells, clotting factors, proteins, and platelets and is the product most commonly transfused into dogs and cats.[38] Once whole blood is refrigerated, the white blood cells and platelets become nonfunctional. As a starting point, the dosage for whole blood is 10 to 22 mL/kg.

PACKED RED BLOOD CELLS

PRBCs are the cells and the small amount of plasma and anticoagulant that remains after the plasma is removed from 1 unit of whole blood. If 450 mL of blood is collected, the volume of PRBCs obtained is approximately 200 mL. Because the plasma has been removed, the total volume transfused is less than 1 unit of whole blood but contains the same oxygen-carrying capacity as 450 mL of whole blood. In cats, the increase in packed

it is collected from the donor, but it is neither a specific therapy nor economical use of blood. The optimal method of preservation of blood for transfusion is to separate whole blood into its component parts. Appropriate use of blood components not only conserves the products but also allows the most specific and safe product to be used for each animal. When blood components are used instead of whole blood for transfusion, two dogs can benefit from 1 unit of whole blood. A plasma transfusion counteracts the anticoagulant effects of rodenticide intoxication in one dog, and red blood cells from the same donor can provide enhanced oxygen-carrying capacity in a second, anemic dog. Component transfusions also have been used in cats, but preparation of components is more difficult because of the small volume of blood collected from donor cats.[35,48,72]

Veterinarians need to become familiar with the use of blood components because blood components are the predominant products available through commercial blood banks. Component therapy requires planning to maintain an adequate blood inventory either through ordering blood from a blood bank or through acquiring cell volume (PCV) after transfusion of 1 unit of PRBCs has been shown to be equivalent to the increase after transfusion of 1 unit of whole blood.[48] PRBCs are used only to treat clinically symptomatic anemia because they do not contain platelets or clotting factors. Red blood cell transfusions are administered to cats for a variety of reasons. Data on 126 cats administered whole blood or PRBCs indicated 52% were transfused for blood loss anemia, 38% for erythropoietic failure, and 10% for hemolytic anemia.[48] Similar reasons for transfusion of cats have been reported in Germany.[90] Dogs more commonly are transfused for blood loss anemia (70%) with 14% to 22% being transfused for hemolytic anemia and 8% to 14% for erythropoietic failure.[8,45] The initial dosage of PRBCs is 6 to 10 mL/kg, and transfusion is continued until the clinical signs of anemia are improved.

FRESH FROZEN PLASMA

Fresh frozen plasma is the plasma obtained from whole blood plus the anticoagulant, frozen within 8 hours of collection. When whole blood is centrifuged to produce plasma and PRBCs, the anticoagulant is collected in the plasma fraction. Fresh frozen plasma contains all clotting factors, which, if frozen at $-30°$ C in a blood bank freezer, maintain activity for 12 months.[85] Fresh frozen plasma maintained in an upright freezer at $-20°$ C maintains clotting factor activity for 6 months. When frozen, the plastic storage bag becomes brittle and if not carefully handled can crack, rendering the plasma unusable. For this reason, plasma is stored in special boxes to protect the plastic bag and must be handled carefully before transfusion. Fresh frozen plasma has been used to treat a wide variety of clinical patients. A retrospective analysis of fresh frozen plasma usage in dogs identified multiple indications for administration of fresh frozen plasma, including replacement of coagulation factors, albumin, α2-macroglobulin, and immunoglobulin despite the recommendation that fresh frozen plasma should not be used as a source of albumin, for volume expansion, or nutritional support.[53,62] Calculations suggest that 45 mL/kg of plasma would need to be given to increase albumin serum concentration by 1 g/dL.[84] In cases of coagulation factor deficiencies, plasma should be given to effect (i.e., until active bleeding ceases).[50] For the treatment of coagulation disorders, 6 to 10 mL/kg is the recommended starting dosage. Multiple doses may be required to control bleeding because of the short half-life of clotting factors, especially in patients with disseminated intravascular coagulation. Normalization of previously abnormal coagulation tests can be used as a guide for discontinuation of plasma therapy.

CRYOPRECIPITATE

Cryoprecipitate is prepared by thawing fresh frozen plasma at 0 to 6° C. A white precipitate forms, the plasma is removed after centrifugation, and both aliquots are refrozen. The cryoprecipitate is a concentrated source of von Willebrand's factor, fibrinogen, and factors XIII and VIII (antihemophilia factor). It is useful in the treatment of deficiencies of these clotting factors and is handled in the same manner as fresh frozen plasma. Two studies have shown cryoprecipitate to be the blood product of choice for the treatment of von Willebrand's disease because it concentrates the larger, more hemostatically active von Willebrand's multimers into a smaller volume than fresh frozen plasma.[12,78] Cryoprecipitate is equivalent to fresh frozen plasma for the treatment of hemophilia A. The dosage is 1 unit per 10 kg body weight.[59]

CRYO-POOR PLASMA

Cryo-poor plasma is the plasma remaining after the cryoprecipitate is removed. Cryo-poor plasma contains factors II, VII, IX, and X, which make it useful for the treatment of rodenticide intoxication. Storage and handling of cryo-poor plasma is similar to fresh frozen plasma. The initial dosage is 1 unit per 10 kg of body weight.

PLATELET-RICH PLASMA

Platelet-containing components are prepared from fresh whole blood by centrifugation at a slower rate than is used for production of PRBCs and plasma.[60] The platelets are suspended in a small amount of plasma to facilitate transfusion. Storage of fresh platelets is impractical outside a blood bank, because it requires a temperature of 20 to 24° C in special plastic bags under continuous agitation.[1] It has been shown that transfused platelets are rapidly destroyed in human patients with immune-mediated thrombocytopenia, and because immune-mediated thrombocytopenia is a common cause of profound thrombocytopenia in dogs, most cases of thrombocytopenia-mediated hemorrhage may not be amenable to successful platelet transfusion. If a platelet transfusion is given, the dosage is the platelets collected from 1 unit of whole blood per 10 kg body weight.

FROZEN PLATELET CONCENTRATE

Frozen platelets are collected from a single donor via plateletpheresis, and one bag contains 1×10^{11} platelets preserved in dimethyl sulfoxide (DMSO).[39] The bag also contains a small amount of fresh frozen plasma. Efficacy data on this product have not been published, but the manufacturer recommends this product be used for the treatment of immune-mediated thrombocytopenia. Because the product contains DMSO, it must be infused slowly, or bradycardia will result. The dosage is 1 unit of frozen platelets per 10 kg of body weight. This dosage should increase the platelet count 20,000/µL when a platelet count is obtained 1 to 2 hours posttransfusion.

SERUM

The use of serum has been recommended for the treatment of kittens and puppies with failure of passive transfer.

Kittens treated with 5 mL subcutaneously or intraperitoneally three times in 24 hours achieved immunoglobulin G (IgG) concentrations comparable to kittens receiving colostrum.[52] Treatment of puppies with 22 mL/kg of serum given orally or subcutaneously at birth did not result in equivalent IgG and IgA concentrations when nursing puppies were compared with serum-treated puppies.[65] IgM was higher in the puppies treated with serum administered subcutaneously.

SOURCES OF BLOOD AND BLOOD PRODUCTS FOR TRANSFUSION

The most convenient source of blood for a veterinary clinic is a commercial blood bank. Currently, there are only a few commercial veterinary blood banks in the United States, and they cannot adequately supply all the small animal practices in the country with blood (see Box 24-1). Veterinary school blood donor programs may serve as an additional source of blood for the practitioner.[38]

Most small animal practitioners borrow a donor from an employee or maintain a blood donor on the premises.[38] Borrowing a donor from either an employee or a client is a frequently used, if less convenient, option and is less expensive than maintaining an in-hospital donor. Maintaining a donor on the premises is advantageous because they are readily available for donation and their health status and disease exposure can be controlled, but the expense associated with feeding, housing, and caring for a blood donor is significant.[36] Some institutions have instituted volunteer blood donor programs.[6,40] Donors are recruited from clients, employees, or the general public. Collecting blood from stray animals is unsafe because infectious disease exposure and health status are unknown.

BLOOD DONOR SELECTION

Identification of donor dogs and cats before blood is needed is essential to allow blood type to be determined and the health status of the donor to be assessed before blood collection, thus ensuring the safety of the blood being transfused. Recommendations on infectious disease screening for canine and feline blood donors recently have been published as a consensus statement. The recommendations are included in the sections below.[88]

Dogs

More than 50 years ago, the best blood donor was believed to be a large, quiet dog not requiring anesthesia during blood collection.[56] The current recommendation is unchanged. A canine blood donor weighing more than 27 kg can safely donate 450 mL of blood in one donation, allowing collection of blood into commercially manufactured blood collection bags designed to facilitate sterile processing of components. Dogs weighing 27 kg or more have been shown to consistently donate 1 unit of blood for 2 years at 3-week intervals.[67] Bags for collecting 225 mL of blood (Terumo Medical Corporation, Somerset, NJ) have successfully been used in dogs weighing 16 to 27 kg.[72] Dogs selected as donors also should have an easily accessible jugular vein to facilitate venipuncture.

Greyhounds have been promoted as ideal blood donors because of their gentle disposition, high hematocrits, and lean body type, which simplifies blood collection.[30] Many greyhounds are euthanized because of poor racing performance, and these dogs are available from racetracks, breeders, and rescue organizations.[22]

Veterinarians choosing greyhounds as blood donors should be aware of certain breed idiosyncrasies that will impact on the management of a greyhound donor. The greyhound idiosyncrasy most important in transfusion medicine is the high red blood cell count, PCV and hemoglobin concentration, and low white blood cell counts and platelet count compared with mixed breed dogs.[66,79] Greyhounds in Florida have a seroprevalence of babesiosis of 46%.[81] Because the geographic origin of greyhounds serving as blood donors cannot always be determined, all greyhounds being screened as donors should have serologic testing for *Babesia canis* performed, and dogs with positive titers should be excluded as donors. Greyhounds with negative titers against *B. canis* should have *B. canis* polymerase chain reaction (PCR) performed, and if the test is positive, the dog should be excluded as a donor.

In addition to the tendency of greyhounds to be asymptomatic carriers of *B. canis*, some other breeds of dogs should be used cautiously as blood donors because they are known to be asymptomatic carriers of infectious organisms transmitted by transfusion. American pit bull terriers and Staffordshire bull terriers recently have been recognized as carriers of *Babesia gibsoni*.[4,55] Use of these dogs as blood donors should be restricted to those dogs seronegative and PCR-negative for *B. gibsoni*. Leishmaniasis has been identified in American foxhounds.[32] Transfusion of *Leishmania infantum*-infected blood from American foxhounds resulted in clinical leishmaniasis in transfusion recipients.[64] All potential foxhound donors should be screened for *Leishmania* sp.

Although seven canine blood groups or blood type systems have received international standardization, typing sera are available for only five types (Box 24-2). Red blood cells can be negative or positive for a given blood type, except for the dog erythrocyte antigen (DEA) 1 system which has three subtypes, DEA 1.1, 1.2, and 1.3. Canine red blood cells can be negative for all three subtypes (a DEA 1-negative blood type) or positive for

Box 24-2	Blood Types in Dogs and Cats for Which Typing Antisera Currently Exist	
Dogs		
Dog erythrocyte antigen (DEA)	1.1, 1.2	
	3	
	4	
	5	
	7	
Cats		
Type	A	
	B	
	AB	

any one of the three subtypes. Alloantibodies, occurring naturally and without previous sensitization from transfusion, do not appear to cause transfusion incompatibility in the dog.

The blood type of the ideal canine blood donor is not uniformly agreed on among transfusion experts. Of the five blood groups for which typing sera are available, a transfusion reaction has been attributed to antibody against DEA 1.1 induced by a DEA 1.1-positive transfusion in a DEA 1.1-negative recipient and to an antibody induced by a DEA 4-positive transfusion in a DEA 4-negative dog.[26,58] In theory, red blood cells expressing DEA 1.2 can sensitize a DEA 1.2-negative transfusion recipient, resulting in an acute hemolytic transfusion reaction if a second transfusion of DEA 1.2-positive blood is given. In a laboratory setting, antibodies against DEA 1.2 have been reported to cause transfusion reactions, but clinical reports of hemolytic transfusion reactions mediated by anti-DEA 1.2 antibodies are lacking. Approximately 45% of dog red blood cells are positive for DEA 7. It is believed DEA 7 is structurally related to an antigen found in common bacteria. A naturally occurring antibody against DEA 7 has been described in 20% to 50% of DEA 7-negative dogs and may result in accelerated removal of DEA 7-positive cells from a DEA-negative donor with anti-DEA 7 antibodies.[73] Based on this information, the recommendation has been made to select donors that are negative for DEA 1.1, 1.2, and 7. Others suggest the donor dog should also have red blood cells positive for DEA 4 to be designated as a universal donor.[33] Ninety-eight percent of dogs are DEA 4-positive, making it easy to find donors of this blood type. The importance of DEA 3 and 5 in blood donor selection remains to be determined.

One other feature that should be considered before selection as a blood donor is the dog's plasma von Willebrand factor concentration. Von Willebrand's disease is the most common inherited coagulopathy in dogs

and has been reported in many breeds of dogs and in dogs of mixed breeding as well. Because of the high frequency of this disease in the canine population, plasma from a canine blood donor is likely to be used to transfuse a dog with von Willebrand's disease-induced hemorrhage, and a donor with a normal concentration of von Willebrand's factor is essential to replace the deficient coagulation factor.

CATS

The physical requirements for a feline blood donor are similar to those for a canine donor. The ideal feline donor is a large cat, more than 5 kg body weight, with a pleasant disposition. Easily accessible jugular veins facilitate collection of blood, and choosing a shorthair cat decreases the clipping required before phlebotomy.

It is essential to determine the blood type of potential donors. Only one feline blood group system has been identified with three blood types: A, B, and AB (see Box 24-2).[3] Unlike dogs, cats have naturally occurring alloantibodies against type A or type B cells.[24] Cats of blood type B have strong hemagglutinating antibodies of the IgM type against type A cells, and cats of blood type A have weak hemolysin and hemagglutinating antibodies of the IgM and IgG type against type B cells. The clinical significance of these alloantibodies is threefold in transfusion medicine. First and most importantly, a cat may have a transfusion reaction without sensitization from a previous transfusion; second, type A kittens born to a type B queen are at risk for neonatal isoerythrolysis[11]; and third, the antibodies are useful in determining the blood type of a cat.

Donors of both type A and type B blood must be available because there is no universal donor in cats. Incompatible transfusions result in shortened red blood cell survival in the transfusion recipient and potentially death; therefore the serologic compatibility between recipient and donor must be determined before every transfusion in cats.[24] Donors of type A blood are easy to find because more than 99% of the domestic cats in the United States are type A.[28] The prevalence of domestic cats with type B blood varies geographically. In the United States, the western states have the highest percentage of type B cats, 4% to 6%.[28] Australia has the highest reported percentage of type B cats in their domestic cat population, 73%.[3] In Europe, the frequency of blood type B in domestic cats varies from 0% in Finland to 14.9% in France.[27] Some purebred cats have a higher frequency of type B in their population.[25] The British shorthair and the Devon rex have been reported to have the highest proportion of type B individuals, approximately 50%. The Siamese, Oriental shorthair, Burmese, Tonkinese, American shorthair, and Norwegian forest cat breeds have not been reported to have any members with type B blood. Blood type AB is extremely rare, occurring in 0.14% of cats in the United States and Canada.[31] Fortunately, a type AB donor is not required to successfully transfuse a type AB cat. Blood from a type A cat is adequate.

BLOOD DONOR SCREENING

Screening blood donors for infectious diseases transmitted by blood transfusion is an integral step in maintaining a safe blood supply. Infectious disease screening of canine and feline blood donors varies within the different geographic regions of the United States and with the breed of the blood donor. A consensus statement developed by a committee consisting of members of the Infectious Disease Study Group and the Association of Veterinary Hematology and Transfusion Medicine should serve as the guideline for donor screening.[88]

Infectious organisms known to be transmitted by blood transfusion include *B. canis*, *B. gibsoni*, *Haemobartonella canis*, and *Leishmania* sp.[18,51,64,76] All canine blood donors should be screened for *Ehrlichia canis* and *Brucella canis*, and if they test positive, they should be eliminated from the donor pool. Titers against *E. canis* less than 1:80 may be false positives and should be repeated in 2 to 3 weeks. Dogs with initially negative titers to *E. canis* can receive additional screening with a PCR test. Splenectomy of donor dogs to facilitate identification of *B. canis* and *H. canis* carriers is not recommended. In neutered dogs, a single negative test for *Brucella canis* is adequate. Based on travel history and breed, additional screening for *Trypanosoma cruzi*, *Bartonella vinsonii*, *B. canis*, *B. gibsoni*, *L. donovani*, and organisms previously classified as *Ehrlichia* spp. (*Anaplasma phagocytophilum* and *Anaplasma platys*) may be indicated.[88] Dogs should not donate if they are ill or have fever, vomiting, or diarrhea; using donors with these clinical signs has resulted in *Yersinia entercolitica* contamination of human units of blood.[19]

Outdoor cats should not be used as blood donors because restricting access to other cats can prevent most infectious diseases potentially transmitted to cats by transfusion. Potential donor cats should be screened for feline leukemia virus (FeLV) and feline immunodeficiency virus (FIV). Because FeLV infection can take up to 3 months to become patent, cats being considered as donors should be screened monthly for FeLV for 3 consecutive months. Testing for FIV antibodies can be performed simultaneously. *Bartonella henselae* is an emerging feline infectious disease and has been transmitted to cats by infected blood.[49] The use of cats with positive serology or cultures for *B. henselae* as blood donors is controversial. Because fleas are the vectors of agents potentially transmitted by transfusion, flea control is essential in donor cats. Cats that are infected with organisms formerly classified as *Haemobartonella* sp. (*Mycoplasma haemofelis* and *Mycoplasma haemonominutum*) also should be eliminated from the donor pool. Testing

should include both light microscopy and PCR for *Mycoplasma* sp. Screening of donor cats for feline infectious peritonitis (FIP) is problematic because there is no reliable test to identify the FIP-causing coronavirus. Feline blood donors should be screened for infection with *Cytauxzoon felis* and the agents causing feline ehrlichiosis if they are known to have traveled to endemic locations.

BLOOD DONOR HEALTH MAINTENANCE

A safe blood supply begins with healthy blood donors. All blood donors should undergo a complete physical examination each time they donate blood. Complete and differential blood counts, biochemical profile, and fecal examination should be performed annually. Blood donors should be vaccinated on a schedule appropriate to the donor's geographic location and risk factors for contracting infectious diseases. Because the ideal feline blood donor lives in an indoor environment and is not exposed to other cats, the author believes vaccinations against FeLV, FIV, and FIP are unnecessary in donor cats. Heartworm testing should be performed and prophylaxis should be administered to donor dogs and cats on the schedule recommended for pets in the geographic region of the blood bank. Because many infectious diseases potentially transmitted by transfusion are vector-borne, control of ectoparasites in blood donors is critical to providing the safest blood possible.

EQUIPMENT AND SUPPLIES FOR COLLECTION OF BLOOD

SKIN PREPARATION

Strict aseptic technique must be used during the blood collection process to prevent contamination. Whenever possible, solutions and equipment used for the collection process should be single-use products to prevent inadvertent contamination of blood.[37] After clipping the hair over the venipuncture site, the skin is surgically scrubbed. The ideal skin preparation regimen is yet to be determined in animals; however, in human blood donors, a 30-second, 70% isopropyl scrub followed by a 2% iodine tincture resulted in better skin surface disinfection than alcohol followed by chlorhexidine or green soap.[29] Venipuncture is accomplished while wearing sterile gloves and without touching the scrubbed area.

ANTICOAGULANT SOLUTIONS

Several different solutions are available to anticoagulate and preserve blood for transfusion (Table 24-1). Anticoagulants provide no nutrients to preserve red cell

TABLE 24-1 Anticoagulants and Preservatives for Blood

Canine Blood	Ratio with Blood	Storage Time @ 0-6°C
Anticoagulant		
Heparin	625 U/50 mL blood	For immediate transfusion
3.8% sodium citrate	1 mL/9 mL blood	For immediate transfusion
Anticoagulant-preservative		
CPDA-1	1 mL/7 mL blood	20 days
ACD "B"	1 mL/7-9 mL blood	21 days
Additive solutions	100 mL/250 mL packed red blood cells	37-42 days
Feline Blood		
Anticoagulant		
Heparin	625 U/50 mL blood	For immediate transfusion
3.8% sodium citrate	1 mL/9 mL blood	For immediate transfusion
Anticoagulant-preservative		
ACD "B"	1 mL/7-9 mL blood	30 days
Additive solutions		Not evaluated

metabolism during storage. Blood collected in anticoagulants should be transfused immediately. Anticoagulant-preservative solutions have been designed to provide nutrients to maintain red blood cell function during storage.

CPDA-1

One common anticoagulant solution for preservation of canine red blood cells, citrate phosphate dextrose adenine (CPDA-1), is found in commercially prepared, multiple-bag systems. Maximal storage time for feline blood in CPDA-1 has yet to be determined but may be as long as 35 days.[7]

ACD

Acid citrate dextrose or anticoagulant citrate dextrose (ACD) formula B can be used to store either canine or feline blood.[17,57] It can be purchased in 500-mL bags and placed in syringes for collection of blood.

Additive Solutions

Additive solutions are contained in a multibag system containing citrate phosphate dextrose (CPD) or citrate phosphate dextrose 2 (CPD-2) as the anticoagulant. The additive solution is contained in a bag separate from the main bag and is added to PRBCs after the plasma is removed. Additive solutions that have been evaluated in

dogs are Adsol (Fenwal Laboratories, Baxter Health Care Corporation, Deerfield, IL) and Nutricel (Miles Pharmaceutical Division, West Haven, CT).[87,89] Storage time of canine red blood cells with these solutions is approximately equal (5 weeks). Additive solutions have not been evaluated for storage of feline blood.

LEUKOREDUCTION FILTERS

White blood cells are responsible for some adverse effects of transfusion and do not contribute to transfusion efficacy (see "Adverse Effects of Transfusion"). An integral filter to remove white blood cells from whole blood is incorporated into some blood bag systems. One system has been evaluated using canine blood and effectively removed white blood cells without affecting red blood cell viability.[5]

COLLECTION OF BLOOD

DOGS

Dogs that have not previously donated blood may require sedation, whereas dogs that have previously donated often do not. If sedation is necessary, the author prefers butorphanol (0.1 mg/kg intravenously, 10 to 15 minutes before donation). This calms the donor but does not induce lateral recumbency. Some prefer to collect blood from dogs in lateral recumbency, especially if the femoral artery is used.[71] The choice is strictly a matter of personal preference and skill. Acepromazine is not recommended because it causes hypotension and platelet dysfunction.

The flow of blood into the bag can occur by gravity or suction. Blood collected by suction does not have a greater rate of hemolysis than that collected by gravity flow, and it can be collected more rapidly.[15] Suction collection of blood is facilitated using a device (Vacuum Chamber) manufactured by the Animal Blood Bank (Dixon, CA). This device requires an external vacuum source during collection of blood.

CATS

It is unusual to find a feline blood donor that does not require sedation during blood donation. The author prefers a combination of ketamine (10 mg) and diazepam (0.5 mg) intravenously for cats. Other protocols using midazolam and isoflurane have been described.[71] If the sedative agent is to be given intravenously, a peripheral vein (cephalic or medial saphenous) should be used to preserve the jugular veins for blood collection.

No commercially available system is manufactured for the collection of blood from cats because of the small volume of blood that can safely be withdrawn from a cat. Typically, anticoagulant can be withdrawn from a blood bag port using a syringe. It is placed in one or two large syringes (25 to 60 mL) depending on the volume of blood to be collected (see Table 24-1). A large (19-gauge) butterfly needle is used for jugular venipuncture so that if a second syringe of blood is to be collected, the full syringe can be removed and the second syringe connected without a second venipuncture. By the definition of the American Association of Blood Banks, this is an "open" system, and blood collected in this manner should not be transfused more than 24 hours after collection.[83] Alternatively, the excess CPDA-1 can be expelled from the bag and cat blood collected directly into the bag.[68] A commercially available vacuum system can be used for collecting blood from cats, but some authors find this system less satisfactory than the syringe method.[44,71]

PRETRANSFUSION COMPATIBILITY TESTING

Selection and transfusion of compatible blood is one component of the process to provide a safe and efficacious red cell transfusion. The current recommendations are different for cats and dogs at the time of the first red cell transfusion. The recommendation for subsequent transfusions is the same in both species. Because each unit of red blood cells is antigenically distinct, the recipient may form antibodies after transfusion of any unit of blood. The immune system will take a minimum of 5 days to make antibodies against transfused red blood cells; consequently, a crossmatch should be performed if more than 4 days elapse between transfusions. Performing a crossmatch will not prevent an immune reaction to subsequent transfusions; it can only identify those units of blood with potential to cause acute hemolytic transfusion reactions.

Dogs

Because of the lack of clinically significant preformed alloantibodies in the dog, blood typing and crossmatching are not routinely performed before the first transfusion of DEA 1.1-negative donor blood. If DEA 1.1-positive blood were being transfused, it would ideally be given to a DEA 1.1-positive recipient. DEA 1.1 status can be determined by using the card typing system available from DMS Laboratories (Flemington, NJ). The typing kit contains all necessary equipment and reagents to determine DEA 1.1 blood type in minutes. Blood typing or crossmatching is not required before transfusion of canine plasma.

Cats

At the time of the first red blood cell transfusion, blood type should be performed on all cats because any breed of cat can be blood type B and transfusion of type A blood to a type B cat will result in an acute hemolytic

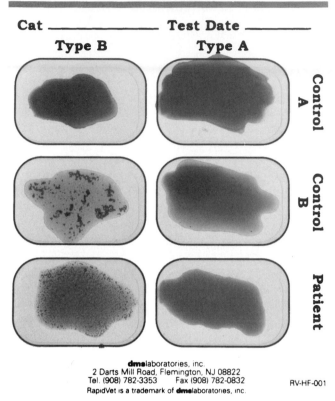

Fig. 24-1 A feline blood typing card. The patient is blood type B. (Courtesy of DMS Laboratories, Inc., Flemington, NJ.)

transfusion reaction. Blood typing in the cat has been simplified by the availability of typing cards (DMS Laboratories; Fig. 24-1). A special situation with regard to blood typing and crossmatching exists in cats. When blood typing is unavailable, crossmatching will prevent an A-B mismatch transfusion in a cat. In cats, an incompatible major crossmatch, when crossmatching is performed with a known type A donor, strongly suggests the potential recipient is a type B cat because of the preformed alloantibodies that exist in all type B cat plasma regardless of transfusion status. If cat plasma is administered, it should be the same blood type as the recipient. If blood typing is not available, crossmatching the donor to the recipient cat will prevent a reaction because of A-B incompatibility.

ADMINISTRATION OF BLOOD AND PLASMA

The person administering the blood should pay careful attention to the blood bag label before transfusion. The most common reason for an acute hemolytic transfusion reaction in human patients is clerical error—the wrong unit of blood is released from the blood bank or a unit of blood is given to a patient who was not intended to receive a transfusion.[80] In veterinary medicine, it is crucial to confirm that the blood comes from the correct species of blood donor in addition to being typed and matched to the patient requiring a transfusion. The contents of the bag also should be examined for normal color and consistency. Bacterially contaminated blood often appears brown or purple because of deoxygenation, hemolysis, and formation of methemoglobin.[37]

Blood and plasma can be administered using several routes. Most commonly, blood is given intravenously. The diameter of the catheter used for transfusion is important in determining the rate of blood flow because blood flows more slowly through a small catheter; however, small diameter catheters have not been associated with increased risk of hemolysis during transfusion.[83]

The intraosseous route can be used successfully for administration of blood and plasma.[63] In normal dogs, 93% to 98% of red blood cells administered through an intraosseous catheter are found in the peripheral circulation within 5 minutes.[13] This rapid and simple method is especially useful in animals with vascular collapse and in extremely young puppies and kittens. Special intraosseous catheters are available, but a spinal needle, bone marrow aspiration needle, over-the-needle catheter, or even an ordinary hypodermic needle can be used. Sites for the placement of the intraosseous catheter include the trochanteric fossa of the femur, the medial tibia, and the iliac crest. Blood flows very rapidly through an intraosseous catheter, and rate of administration should be monitored closely. Plasma can be administered intraperitoneally in emergency situations, but red blood cells are slowly and poorly absorbed by this route, and it is not recommended for red blood cell transfusions.

A blood transfusion administration set should be used for any transfusion of blood or component because the incorporated filter removes blood clots and debris that could cause embolism. The filter typically used in veterinary medicine is 170 μm in size. For small-volume transfusions, an 18-μm filter that can be attached to intravenous tubing is useful. An 18-μm filter does not work well for large-volume transfusions because it rapidly becomes obstructed with debris, and flow slows. A blood administration set does not remove air from stored blood. Although glass bottles are convenient blood collection systems because they do not require an extrinsic vacuum source, the risk of an air embolism is increased when blood is collected into glass bottles. Glass bottles are not recommended for collection and storage of blood.

The American Association of Blood Banks explicitly states that medications should not be added to blood or components.[83] In addition, no fluid should be added to blood except 0.9% sodium chloride when it is necessary

to decrease the viscosity of PRBCs. Fluids containing calcium such as lactated Ringer's solution may overcome the anticoagulant properties of citrate, resulting in coagulation of the blood. Solutions such as 5% dextrose in water are hypotonic and may induce hemolysis.

The recommended rate of transfusion of red blood cells depends on the status of the recipient. In massive hemorrhage, the transfusion should be given as rapidly as possible. In a normovolemic, stable transfusion recipient, some clinicians recommend a rate of 0.25 mL/kg for the first 30 minutes, after which the rate is increased if no reaction is seen.[82] In patients with heart disease, a rate of 4 mL/kg/hr should not be exceeded.[30] Plasma can be given more rapidly (4 to 6 mL/min).[47] Whatever the rate chosen, it should be rapid enough to complete the transfusion within 4 hours of initiation because of the risk of bacterial growth in blood maintained at room temperature for a prolonged period.

Control of delivery rate can be accomplished by use of infusion pumps to deliver a preset volume over a specific period. The use of infusion pumps must be limited to devices approved for use with blood because some infusion pumps can result in hemolysis of red blood cells as a result of excessive pressure.[77]

Because blood does not contain any antibacterial agents, it must be refrigerated until used to retard bacterial growth and maintain red blood cell viability. If the clinical status of the animal requires that the transfusion be given more slowly than over 4 hours, the blood can be split into smaller units with a transfer bag. One portion of the blood is transfused while the other is returned to the refrigerator until the first half of the transfusion is completed. In patients with cardiac disease at risk for volume overload, the risk can be minimized by use of PRBCs, which require infusion of a lower volume than whole blood. Diuretics can be administered before transfusion to decrease intravascular volume in cardiac patients.

Warming of blood before transfusion has been recommended to prevent hypothermia in the transfusion recipient. Warming of blood probably is only necessary if a large volume of blood is to be given or if the recipient is a neonate. For adult animals receiving a single unit of blood, the blood can be administered at refrigerator temperature. Warming blood has the potential for excessive heating, causing red blood cell membrane damage and hemolysis or bacterial growth if contamination is present. Blood warming devices that use dry heat, radio waves, microwaves, or electromagnetic energy are available, but cost often is prohibitive. Refrigerated human blood can be warmed quickly by admixing it with warm (45 to 60° C) 0.9% saline in a ratio of 1:1 without damage to red blood cells.[42] This method has not been tested for dogs or cats. Once blood is warmed to 37° C, it deteriorates rapidly and, if not used, should be discarded. Fresh frozen plasma must be thawed before transfusion. A method for thawing canine fresh frozen plasma in a microwave oven has been described, but the author has found this unsatisfactory because of uneven heating by household microwave ovens.[41] Plasma can be thawed at room temperature, and if the thawing time needs to be shortened, the plasma can be placed into a plastic bag and thawed in a 37° C water bath. The plastic bag is necessary to prevent contamination of the infusion ports in the water bath. Plasma should be used within 4 hours of thawing.

Transfusion recipients should be monitored during transfusion to allow early detection of a transfusion reaction. Rectal temperature, heart rate, and respiratory rate should be recorded every 10 minutes during the first 30 minutes and then every 30 minutes thereafter. The patient should be monitored for vomiting, diarrhea, urticaria, and hemoglobinuria or hemoglobinemia. Changes in vital signs or clinical status may indicate a transfusion reaction. Patients developing volume overload will become tachypneic or dyspneic, and tachycardic.

Patients receiving large transfusions (≥1 blood volume in 24 hours) of stored blood may develop specific abnormalities. Consequently, patients receiving large transfusions should be monitored for changes in serum potassium, ionized calcium, and ionized magnesium concentrations, as well as hypothermia and coagulation abnormalities.[43]

ADVERSE EFFECTS OF TRANSFUSION

DEFINITION

An adverse effect of transfusion or transfusion reaction consists of the range of immunologic and metabolic changes that occur during or after administration of a blood product. Four classes of adverse effects of transfusion have been described (Box 24-3). Acute transfusion reactions occur during or within a few hours after a transfusion, and delayed transfusion reactions occur after the completion of the transfusion. The delay may be months to years. Reports describing adverse effects of transfusion in dogs and cats are limited to case reports and retrospective series.*

ACUTE IMMUNOLOGIC TRANSFUSION REACTIONS

Acute immunologic transfusion reactions occur because antibodies that elicit an immune response are present in the plasma of either the donor or recipient. The sequelae of an acute immunologic transfusion reaction are rapid, often irreversible, and sometimes fatal. Current theories on the pathogenesis of acute hemolytic transfu-

---

*References 2,18,23,24,26,35,45,48,51,64,76,84,86,92.

| Box 24-3 | Classification of Transfusion Reactions |

Acute Immunologic
Acute hemolytic reaction
Febrile nonhemolytic reaction
Urticaria

Acute Nonimmunologic
Electrolyte disturbances
   Hypocalcemia
   Hyperkalemia
   Hypomagnesemia
Embolism (air or clotted blood)
Endotoxic shock
Circulatory overload
Contamination of blood
   Bacteria
   Spirochetes
   Protozoa
Physical damage
   Freezing
   Overheating
Hypothermia
Dilutional coagulopathy

Delayed Immunologic
Delayed hemolytic
Posttransfusion purpura

Delayed Nonimmunologic
Infectious disease transmission
   Feline leukemia virus
   Feline infectious peritonitis
   Feline immunodeficiency virus
   Bartonellosis
   Babesiosis
   Hemotrophic mycoplasma
   Ehrlichiosis
   Leishmaniasis
   Brucellosis
Hemochromatosis

---

sion reaction in humans propose that hemolysis induces the release of cytokines such as tumor necrosis factor, interleukin-1 (IL-1), IL-6, and IL-8, complement, endothelium-derived relaxing factor (nitric oxide), and endothelin, resulting in the clinical syndrome of disseminated intravascular coagulation, shock, and acute renal failure.[10] The pathophysiology of acute hemolytic transfusion reaction in dogs and cats must differ in some manner from that described in humans because acute renal failure is not reported to be a feature in dogs and cats.[2,23,26,92]

The best example of an acute hemolytic transfusion reaction in veterinary medicine is the administration of type A red blood cells to a type B cat. In the recipient cat, naturally occurring alloantibodies and complement bind to the transfused red blood cells and cause hemolysis. Clinical signs described in cats having an acute hemolytic transfusion reaction include fever, vomiting, lethargy, icterus, and death.[2] Results of laboratory testing often show a positive Coombs test, rapidly declining PCV, and increasing serum bilirubin concentration.

Dogs experiencing an acute hemolytic transfusion reaction show clinical signs similar but not identical to those observed in cats. Most affected dogs exhibit fever, restlessness, salivation, incontinence, and vomiting. Some dogs develop shock, and an occasional dog experiences acute death. Plasma and urine hemoglobin concentrations increase within minutes of transfusion. Incompatible cells are cleared from circulation in less than 2 hours. Dogs whose red blood cells lack the DEA 1.1 antigen that have previously been sensitized by transfusion of DEA 1.1-positive cells are at the greatest risk for an acute hemolytic transfusion reaction.[26]

Other acute immunologic transfusion reactions reported in dogs and cats include nonhemolytic fever and urticaria.[8,35,45,84] In humans, nonhemolytic fever is a result of antibodies against donor white blood cells, and urticaria occurs as a result of antibodies-against donor plasma proteins. Nonhemolytic febrile transfusion reactions do not require treatment, but antipyretics may be used if the patient is uncomfortable (Table 24-2). Urticaria is the most common reaction to plasma transfusion in dogs.[84] If urticaria caused by plasma administration is diagnosed, it should be treated with short-acting corticosteroids and antihistamines. The plasma transfusion then may be restarted at a slower rate and the recipient observed carefully.

DELAYED IMMUNOLOGIC TRANSFUSION REACTIONS

Delayed immunologic transfusion reactions are classified as delayed hemolytic, transfusion-induced immunosuppression, posttransfusion purpura, and graft-versus-host disease. These reactions are not preventable by crossmatching or blood typing. Delayed hemolytic transfusion reactions invariably occur in persons who have been previously sensitized to allogenic red blood cell antigens by transfusion or pregnancy. Even though compatible blood is given to a patient, the recipient may develop antibodies against any one of the hundreds of red blood cell antigens present on the transfused cells. An anamnestic response to the antigens on the transfused red blood cells results in a delayed hemolytic transfusion reaction that occurs 7 to 10 days after a transfusion and is a well-described complication of red cell transfusion in humans. It has not been reported in dogs, but there is

TABLE 24-2 Drug Dosages and Route of Administration for Use in Acute Transfusion Reactions

Type of Reaction	Drugs to Consider
Acute hemolytic	Methylprednisolone succinate 30 mg/kg, IV, once
	Dexamethasone sodium phosphate 4-6 mg/kg, IV, once
Febrile nonhemolytic	Aspirin 10 mg/kg, PO once
Urticaria	Diphenhydramine 2 mg/kg, IV, prn
	Prednisone 0.5-1 mg/kg every 12-24 hr PO
Hypocalcemia	Calcium gluconate (10% solution)
	50-150 mg/kg, IV over 20-30 min
	Discontinue if bradycardia occurs.
	Repeat if hypocalcemia persists.
	Calcium chloride (10% solution)
	50-150 mg/kg, IV over 20-30 min
	Discontinue if bradycardia occurs.
	Repeat if hypocalcemia persists.
Hypomagnesemia	Magnesium sulfate 0.75-1 mEq Mg^{2+}/kg IV over 24 hr
	Magnesium sulfate 0.15-0.30 mEq/kg IV over 5-15 min
Hyperkalemia	Regular insulin
	0.5 U/kg, IV given with 50% dextrose 2 g/U of insulin prn
	Infuse 0.9% saline
Circulatory overload	Nitroglycerine paste (2%) $\frac{1}{4}$ to 1 inch applied to skin, once (monitor blood pressure, may cause hypotension)
	Furosemide 2-4 mg/kg, IV once
	Oxygen therapy
Dilution coagulopathy	Fresh frozen plasma 3-5 mL/kg until coagulation tests normalize.

IV, Intravenous; PO, *orally;* prn, *as needed.*

no reason it could not occur. Fever is the most common sign of a delayed hemolytic transfusion reaction in humans. Icterus also may be noticed 4 to 7 days after a transfusion.

The only delayed immunologic transfusion reaction that has been reported in veterinary medicine is post-transfusion purpura.[86] It occurred in a dog with hemophilia A that had previously received a transfusion. Five to 8 days after subsequent transfusions, thrombocytopenia and petechiation were evident. Blood collected during a thrombocytopenic episode was positive for platelet-bound IgG, indicating an immune mechanism for platelet destruction.

ACUTE NONIMMUNOLOGIC TRANSFUSION REACTIONS

Acute nonimmunologic transfusion reactions are caused by physical changes in the red blood cells during collection, storage, or administration.

Collection-associated Changes in Blood

Improper collection of blood can result in an adverse reaction to transfusion. Introduction of air when collecting blood into glass bottles increases the likelihood of venous air embolism. Venous air embolism causes sudden onset pulmonary vascular obstruction, a precordial murmur, hypotension, and death as a result of respiratory failure. Collection of blood from an inadequately screened donor can result in transmission of bacteria, spirochetes, or protozoa and eventually clinical signs of the associated disease in the recipient. Transfusion of blood contaminated by bacteria can cause shock, which is managed with volume expansion and pressor agents, as well as empirical antibiotic administration based on results of a Gram stain. Endotoxic shock results from transfusion of blood heavily contaminated with endotoxin-producing bacteria. Clinical signs in cats transfused with blood contaminated by bacteria include collapse, vomiting, diarrhea, and acute death, but most cats did not exhibit clinical signs after receiving bacterially contaminated blood.[37] Hypotensive shock developed in a dog that received a *B. canis*–infected transfusion.[18]

Storage-associated Changes in Blood

During storage, the ATP content of red blood cells decreases, and some cells undergo hemolysis resulting in leakage of potassium out of the cells into the storage medium. The increase in potassium in the storage medium is a contributing factor in the development of hyperkalemia in patients receiving large volume transfusions of stored blood. A large-volume transfusion of stored blood can cause hyperkalemia, but this is rare unless the patient has renal failure or preexisting hyperkalemia.[43] Hyperkalemia in a transfusion recipient is as it would be in any patient with hyperkalemia. The transfusion should be discontinued and 0.9% NaCl administered because

0.9% NaCl does not contain added potassium and will facilitate renal excretion of potassium. Intravenous administration of insulin, followed by administration of 50% dextrose and frequent monitoring of blood glucose and potassium concentrations until serum potassium concentration normalizes, is all that is necessary. Routine empirical administration of calcium to transfusion recipients cannot be recommended because of the risk of hypercalcemia and increased myocardial irritability, but animals with ionized hypocalcemia resulting from large transfusion should be treated with calcium gluconate or calcium chloride to effect.[14] Physical damage (such as freezing or overheating) to red blood cells during storage causes hemolysis. While being transfused, the patient exhibits hemoglobinuria and hemoglobinemia without evidence of other signs of an acute hemolytic transfusion reaction, such as fever, vomiting, or collapse. During storage of blood, formation of clots and other debris may occur and can result in embolism during transfusion.

Administration-associated Changes in Blood

In instances of large-volume transfusion, ionized hypocalcemia or ionized hypomagnesemia can result from the citrate used as an anticoagulant complexing with calcium or magnesium and lead to myocardial dysfunction and potential cardiac arrest and tetany.[46] Hypothermia is common after large-volume transfusion in veterinary patients, and use of warming blankets should be instituted whenever possible. Dilution of coagulation factors by large-volume transfusion of coagulation factor-depleted stored blood results in prolongation of coagulation times. In dogs receiving large-volume transfusions, prolongation of coagulation times is associated with a poor prognosis.[43] Administration of fresh frozen plasma is indicated to correct the coagulation abnormalities. Dogs and cats with chronic severe anemia or compromised cardiac and pulmonary systems are at greater risk for circulatory overload and pulmonary edema than are those without cardiopulmonary disease. Dogs and cats developing volume overload from transfusion are treated with oxygen supplementation, diuretics, and vasodilators. Improvement should be seen within 1 to 2 hours.

DELAYED NONIMMUNOLOGIC TRANSFUSION REACTIONS

In humans, human immunodeficiency virus, hepatitis virus, and cytomegalovirus infections are documented as late effects of transfusion. The transmission of infection to a recipient cat from a donor cat infected with FeLV or FIV would be a veterinary example of a delayed nonimmunologic transfusion reaction. A recently described late complication of transfusion is hemochromatosis in a miniature schnauzer.[75] The dog received blood transfusions every 6 to 8 weeks for 3 years to treat chronic anemia. It was euthanized because of progressive liver disease, and the diagnosis of hemochromatosis was confirmed by necropsy.

EVALUATION OF A PATIENT WITH A SUSPECTED TRANSFUSION REACTION

Immediate intervention is critical because of the life-threatening nature of acute hemolytic transfusion reactions. In all animals suspected of having some form of acute transfusion reaction, the transfusion should be stopped and samples of patient blood and urine obtained for baseline evaluation of biochemical, hematologic, and coagulation values. The unit of blood should be inspected to ensure it is from the appropriate species and is the intended unit based on the crossmatch or blood type. Urine can be visually inspected to determine the presence or absence of hemoglobin. A Gram stain and bacterial culture of the blood remaining in the blood bag should be done. Rectal temperature of the recipient should be compared with the pretransfusion value. A transfusion-associated fever is defined as an increase in 1° F over the pretransfusion temperature.[83] The cardiovascular system should be monitored by electrocardiogram and blood pressure measurement. Immediate evaluation of serum ionized calcium and potassium concentrations would be useful, but certain electrocardiographic changes suggest hypocalcemia (long QT interval with a normal heart rate) or hyperkalemia (decreased height of P waves, loss of P waves, or widening of the QRS complex with large T waves) if rapid measurement of serum electrolyte concentrations cannot be obtained. Venous access and blood pressure should be maintained by an infusion of a crystalloid solution such as lactated Ringer's solution or 0.9% NaCl. Intravenous administration of short-acting glucocorticoids may suppress some of the mediators of acute hemolytic transfusion reactions and lessen the clinical progression, but their efficacy in transfusion reactions has not been evaluated in veterinary patients. When the evaluation of a patient with a suspected transfusion reaction suggests that an acute hemolytic transfusion reaction is occurring, the blood typing and crossmatching must be repeated to determine whether a laboratory error is responsible for the reaction. When fever occurs without evidence of hemolysis and the Gram stain is negative for bacterial contamination, the transfusion may be restarted.

It is important to recognize the late effects of transfusion and not mistake them for another disease process. Delayed transfusion reactions usually are managed with supportive care. The only specific treatment for a delayed transfusion reaction consists of treating a transfusion-acquired infection appropriately.

PREVENTION STRATEGIES

A special effort is not necessary to prevent transfusion reactions. Simply by following the transfusion guidelines discussed here with reference to donor selection, blood typing, blood storage, and administration, most transfusion reactions can be prevented. Crossmatching detects antibodies in the plasma of the recipient or donor that may cause an acute hemolytic transfusion reaction. A transfusion reaction may still occur despite a compatible crossmatch. Crossmatching does not prevent sensitization to red blood cell antigens, which may result in a hemolytic reaction during future transfusions, because it detects only antibodies that are currently present in the donor or recipient. Crossmatching is a specific procedure designed to minimize acute transfusion reactions. It should be performed routinely in veterinary clinics.

Crossmatch Procedure

Performing a crossmatch is an intimidating but simple procedure, once all the equipment is assembled (Box 24-4). Several descriptions of the procedure have been published, all of which describe the same basic procedure with minor variations.[6,21,74] Not all protocols recommend the use of phosphate-buffered saline; others have an additional step at the end using species-specific Coombs reagent to increase test sensitivity, and some recommend that tubes be incubated at 4° C, 37° C, and 42° C. The following is the protocol the author uses:

1. Obtain EDTA-anticoagulated blood from the recipient and the potential donor or the tube segments of blood from the units being considered for transfusion.
2. Centrifuge both donor and recipient blood for 5 minutes at 1000 g.
3. Using pipettes, remove the plasma, and save in separate labeled tubes.
4. Wash the red blood cells by adding phosphate-buffered saline to the red cells to fill the tube. Resuspend the red cells in the saline by tapping the bottom of the tube with a finger.
5. Centrifuge the red cells and saline for 5 minutes at 1000 g. Pipette off saline, and discard.
6. Repeat steps 4 and 5 twice.
7. After third washing of the red cells in saline, resuspend the red cells to a 3% to 5% solution. It will appear bright cherry red.
8. For each potential donor, mix two drops of recipient plasma and one drop of donor red cell suspension for the major crossmatch. Mix gently.
9. For each potential donor, mix two drops of donor plasma and one drop of recipient red cell suspension for the minor crossmatch. Mix gently.
10. For the recipient control, mix two drops of recipient plasma and one drop of recipient red cell suspension. Mix gently.
11. Incubate the tubes at room temperature for 15 minutes.
12. Centrifuge the tubes for 15 seconds at 1000 g.
13. Observe the plasma for hemolysis.
14. Resuspend the centrifuged cells by shaking gently.
15. Observe the red blood cells for agglutination.

Interpretation. Hemolysis or agglutination in a crossmatch indicates transfusion incompatibility. The degree of agglutination is graded 0 to 4+ (Box 24-5 and Fig. 24-2). Units of blood that are incompatible should not be used. If all available units are incompatible, the least reactive unit should be chosen. When the recipient control shows hemolysis or agglutination, the crossmatch cannot be interpreted. This is common in patients with hemolytic anemia.

Blood Type

Blood typing is important in preventing A-B mismatch transfusions in cats and preventing sensitization caused by giving DEA 1.1-positive blood to a DEA 1.1-negative

Box 24-5	Crossmatch Incompatibility

0	No agglutination
Trace	Microscopic agglutination
1+	Many small agglutinates admixed with free cells
2+	Large agglutinates mixed with smaller clumps
3+	Many large agglutinates
4+	Single agglutinate, no free cells

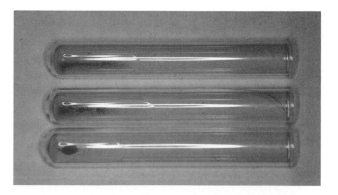

Fig. 24-2 Three tubes demonstrating increasing degrees of crossmatch incompatibility. From top to bottom, the tubes are graded 1+, 2+, and 4+.

dog. A reference laboratory can perform blood typing of dogs and cats, but this is not convenient in emergency situations. Commercially available blood typing cards for feline types A, B, and AB and canine type DEA 1.1 are available. The author has found that sick cats often are typed as AB when the cards are used but when retested in a reference laboratory are actually type A.

VETERINARY HEMOGLOBIN-BASED OXYGEN-CARRYING FLUID (BLOOD SUBSTITUTE)

Previously, a red blood cell transfusion was the only therapy available to increase the oxygen-carrying capacity of the blood. Now another option is available. The Food and Drug Administration has approved a hemoglobin-based oxygen-carrying (HBOC) fluid, Oxyglobin (Biopure Corporation, Cambridge, MA), for use in the dog. Oxyglobin (hemoglobin glutamer-200 [bovine]) is ultrapurified, polymerized hemoglobin of bovine origin (13 g/dL) in a modified Ringer's lactate solution with a physiologic pH (7.8). The hemoglobin polymers range in molecular mass from 65 to 500 kD, with an average of 200 kD. The viscosity is low compared with blood (1.3 and 3.5 centipoise, respectively), and the solution is isosmotic (300 mOsm/kg) with blood. The concentration of methemoglobin, the inactive form of hemoglobin, is 10%. Oxyglobin can be stored at room temperature or refrigerated (2 to 30° C) for up to 3 years. Its intravascular half-life is dose dependent (18 to 43 hours, at a dosage of 10 to 30 mL/kg), as measured in healthy dogs. It is expected that more than 90% of the administered dose will be eliminated from the body in 5 to 7 days after infusion. The oxygen half-saturation pressure (P-50) of Oxyglobin is greater than that of canine blood (38 versus 30 mm Hg, respectively). This increase in P-50 facilitates offloading of oxygen from hemoglobin. The hemoglobin is packaged in the deoxygenated state in an overwrap that is impermeable to oxygen.

Complications of severe anemia result from poor oxygenation of tissues. Restoration of adequate tissue oxygenation typically is achieved by administering a blood transfusion. Improvement in the clinical signs of anemia results from a corresponding increase in hemoglobin concentration, which in turn increases the arterial oxygen content of the blood. The increased oxygen content of the blood supplied by Oxyglobin also relieves the clinical signs of anemia.

Oxyglobin has been tested in a multicenter clinical trial in dogs with moderate to severe anemia (PCV, 6% to 23%). Sixty-four dogs in need of blood transfusion were studied, including those with anemia caused by blood loss (n = 25), hemolysis (n = 30), or ineffective erythropoiesis (n = 9).[69] Thirty dogs were randomized to the Oxyglobin group and 34 dogs to an untreated control group. Dogs in both groups were monitored for a decrease in hemoglobin concentration or deterioration in physical condition at which time they received additional oxygen-carrying support. If additional oxygen-carrying support was needed, Oxyglobin-treated dogs received PRBCs (n = 1), and untreated control dogs received Oxyglobin (n = 19). Treatment success was defined as the lack of need for additional oxygen-carrying support for 24 hours. The success rate in treated dogs (95%) was significantly greater than the success rate in control dogs (32%). This difference between treated and control dogs was significant, regardless of the cause of anemia.

Although Oxyglobin is not approved for use in cats, a retrospective study of its use in 72 cats recently has been published.[20] Oxyglobin was administered to these cats off-label and with owner consent. Anemia caused by blood loss, ineffective erythropoiesis, and hemolysis was the reason for Oxyglobin administration in all but two cats. The dose of Oxyglobin administered varied widely, but the mean ($\pm$ SD) dose per infusion was 14.6 ($\pm$ 13.1) mL/kg at a rate of 4.8 ($\pm$ 6.2) mL/kg/hr. After infusion, the PCV decreased approximately 2% because of the dilutional effect of Oxyglobin, and the hemoglobin concentration increased approximately 1.5 g/dL.

The use of Oxyglobin as an oxygen-carrying solution eliminates some of the pretransfusion testing required with red blood cell transfusions. No reconstitution or preparation is necessary before infusion. Blood typing and crossmatching are not necessary because the red blood cell membrane, which is the major cause of transfusion incompatibility, has been removed during the manufacturing process. Repeated dosing of Oxyglobin was evaluated in the retrospective study of its use in cats. No allergic reactions were reported. A laboratory study of repeated dosing in dogs showed antibodies to Oxyglobin did form, but those antibodies did not decrease binding of oxygen to Oxyglobin and did not result in systemic allergic reactions.[34]

Adverse effects of treatment with Oxyglobin are similar in dogs and cats. After treatment, a transient discoloration (yellow, brown, or red) of the mucous membranes, sclera, urine, and sometimes skin occurs. Overexpansion of the vascular volume may occur, especially in normovolemic animals. Rates of administration greater than 10 mL/kg/hr in anemic, clinically ill dogs sometimes resulted in increased central venous pressure, with or without pulmonary edema or other respiratory signs of circulatory overload. Pleural effusion and pulmonary edema were found commonly in cats given Oxyglobin, but evidence was insufficient to directly link either to the administration of Oxyglobin.[20] In the clinical trial in dogs, vomiting occurred in 35% of the treated dogs. Diarrhea, fever, and death also were seen in approximately 15% of Oxyglobin-treated dogs; however, an association with Oxyglobin or the underlying disease

could not be determined. These findings were most common in dogs with immune-mediated hemolytic anemia that received Oxyglobin.

The presence of Oxyglobin in serum may cause artifactual changes in the results of serum chemistry tests. Interference by Oxyglobin depends on the type of analyzers and reagents used but is not typical of hemolysis.[9,61] Blood samples for analysis should be collected before infusion. A list of valid chemistry tests by analyzer is included in the product labeling. Results of any clinical chemistry test performed on serum containing Oxyglobin should be interpreted with consideration of the validity of the test. In general, all tests using colorimetric techniques are invalid, but other methodologies also show some interference. No interference is seen with hematologic or coagulation parameters except when optical methods are used for measuring prothrombin time and activated partial thromboplastin time. Dipstick measurements (pH, glucose, ketones, protein) of urine are inaccurate when gross discoloration of the urine is present. The urine sediment is not affected.

REFERENCES

1. Allyson K, Abrams-Ogg ACG, Johnstone IB: Room temperature storage and cryopreservation of canine platelet concentrates, *Am J Vet Res* 58:1338-1347, 1997.
2. Auer L, Bell K: Blood transfusion reactions in the cat, *J Am Vet Med Assoc* 180:729-730, 1982.
3. Auer L, Bell K: The AB blood group system in cats, *Anim Blood Groups Biochem Genet* 12:287-297, 1981.
4. Birkenheuer AJ, Levy MG, Stebbins M, et al: Serosurvey of anti-Babesia antibodies in stray dogs and American Pit Bull Terriers and American Staffordshire Terriers from North Carolina, *J Am Anim Hosp Assoc* 39:551-557, 2003.
5. Brownlee L, Wardrop KJ, Sellon RK, et al: Use of a prestorage leukoreduction filter effectively removes leukocytes from canine whole blood while preserving red blood cell viability, *J Vet Intern Med* 14:412-417, 2000.
6. Bucheler J, Cotter SM: Outpatient blood donor program. In Hohenhaus A, editor: *Problems in veterinary medicine*, Philadelphia, 1992, JB Lippincott, pp. 572-582.
7. Buchler J, Cotter SM: Storage of feline and canine whole blood in CPDA-1 and determination of the posttransfusion viability, *J Vet Intern Med* 8:172, 1994.
8. Callan MB, Oakley DA, Shofer FS, et al: Canine red blood cell transfusion practice, *J Am Anim Hosp Assoc* 32:303-311, 1996.
9. Callas DD, Clark TL, Moriera PL, et al: In vitro effects of a novel hemoglobin-based oxygen carrier on the routine chemistry, therapeutic drug, coagulation, hematology, and blood bank assays, *Clin Chem* 43:1744, 1997.
10. Capon SM, Goldfinder D: Acute hemolytic transfusion reaction, a paradigm of the systemic inflammatory response: new insights into pathophysiology and treatment, *Transfusion* 35:513-520, 1995.
11. Casal ML, Jezyk PF, Giger U: Transfer of colostral antibodies from queens to their kittens, *Am J Vet Res* 57:1653-1658, 1996.

12. Ching YNLH, Meyers KM, Brassard JA, et al: Effect of cryoprecipitate and plasma on plasma von Willebrand factor multimeters and bleeding time in Doberman Pinschers with type-I von Willebrand's disease, *Am J Vet Res* 55:102-110, 1994.

13. Clark CH, Woodley CH: The absorption of red blood cells after parenteral injection at various sites, *Am J Vet Res* 10:1062-1066, 1959.

14. Cote CJ, Drop LJ, Daniels AL, et al: Calcium chloride versus calcium gluconate: comparison of ionization and cardiovascular effects in children and dogs, *Anesthesiology* 66:465-470, 1987.

15. Eibert M, Lewis DC: Post transfusion viability of stored canine red blood cells after vacuum facilitated collection, *J Vet Intern Med* 11:143, 1997.

16. Eisenbrandt DL, Smith JE: Evaluation of preservatives and containers for storage of canine blood, *J Am Vet Med Assoc* 163:988-990, 1973.

17. Eisenbrandt DL, Smith JE: Use of biochemical measures to estimate viability of red blood cells in canine blood stored in acid citrate dextrose solution with and without added ascorbic acid, *J Am Vet Med Assoc* 163:984-987, 1973.

18. Freeman MJ, Kirby BM, Panciera DL, et al: Hypotensive shock syndrome associated with acute *Babesia canis* infection in a dog, *J Am Vet Med Assoc* 204;94-96, 1994.

19. Galloway SJ, Jones PD: Transfusion acquired *Yersinia enterocolitica*, *Aust N Z J Med* 16:248-250, 1986.

20. Gibson GR, Callan MB, Hoffman V, et al: Use of a hemoglobin-based oxygen-carrying solution in cats: 72 cases (1998-2000), *J Am Vet Med Assoc* 221:96-102, 2002.

21. Giger U: Feline transfusion medicine. In Hohenhaus A, editor: *Problems in veterinary medicine*, Philadelphia, 1992, JB Lippincott, pp. 600-611.

22. Giger U: Where to get blood donors? *J Am Vet Med Assoc* 202:705-706, 1993 (letter).

23. Giger U, Akol KG: Acute hemolytic transfusion reaction in an Abyssinian cat with blood type B, *J Vet Intern Med* 4:315-316, 1990.

24. Giger U, Bucheler J: Transfusion of type-A and type-B blood to cats, *J Vet Med Assoc* 198:411-418, 1991.

25. Giger U, Bucheler J, Patterson DF: Frequency and inheritance of A and B blood types in feline breeds of the United States, *J Hered* 82:15-20, 1991.

26. Giger U, Gelens CJ, Callan MB, et al: An acute hemolytic transfusion reaction caused by dog erythrocyte antigen 1.1 incompatibility in a previously sensitized dog, *J Am Vet Med Assoc* 206:1358-1362, 1995.

27. Giger U, Gorman NT, Hubler M, et al: Frequencies of feline A and B blood types in Europe, *Anim Genet* 23(suppl 1):17-18, 1993.

28. Giger U, Griot-Wenk M, Bucheler J, et al: Geographical variation of the feline blood type frequencies in the United States, *Feline Pract* 19:22-27, 1991.

29. Goldman M, Roy G, Frechette N, et al: Evaluation of donor skin disinfection methods, *Transfusion* 37:309-312, 1997.

30. Green CE: Blood transfusion therapy: an updated overview, *Proc Am Anim Hosp Assoc* 187-189, 1982.

31. Griot-Wenk ME, Callan MB, Chisholm-Chait A, et al: Blood type AB in the feline AB blood group system, *Am J Vet Res* 57:1438-1442, 1996.

32. Grosjean NL, Vrable RA, Murphy AJ, et al: Seroprevalence of antibodies against *Leishmania* spp among dogs in the United States, *J Am Vet Med Assoc* 222:603-606, 2003.

33. Hale AS: Canine blood groups and their importance in veterinary transfusion medicine, *Vet Clin North Am Small Anim Pract* 25:1323-1332, 1995.

34. Hamilton RG, Kelly N, Gawryl MS, et al: Absence of immunopathology associated with repeated IV administration of bovine Hb-based oxygen carrier in dogs, *Transfusion* 41:219-225, 2001.

35. Henson MS, Kristensen AT, Armstrong PJ, et al: Feline blood component therapy: retrospective study of 246 transfusions, *J Vet Intern Med* 8:169, 1994.

36. Hohenhaus A: Management of the inpatient canine blood donor. In Hohenhaus A, editor: *Problems in veterinary medicine*, Philadelphia, 1992, JB Lippincott, pp. 565-571.

37. Hohenhaus AE, Drusin LM, Garvey MS: *Serratia marcescens* contamination of feline whole blood in a hospital blood bank, *J Am Vet Med Assoc* 210:794-798, 1997.

38. Howard A, Callan B, Sweeny M, et al: Transfusion practices and costs in dogs, *J Am Vet Med Assoc* 210:1697-1701, 1992.

39. http://www.midwestabs.com. Accessed June 25, 2004.

40. http://www.vet.upenn.edu/research/centers/penngen/services/transfusionlab/pabb.html. Accessed June 25, 2004.

41. Hurst TS, Turrentine MA, Johnson GS: Evaluation of microwave-thawed canine plasma for transfusion, *J Am Vet Med Assoc* 190:863-865, 1987.

42. Iserson KV, Huestis DW: Blood warming: current applications and techniques, *Transfusion* 31:558-571, 1991.

43. Jutkowitz LA, Rozanski EA, Moreau JA: Massive transfusion in dogs, *J Am Vet Med Assoc* 220:1664-1669, 2002.

44. Kaufman PM: Management of the feline blood donor. In Hohenhaus A, editor: *Problems in veterinary medicine*, Philadelphia, 1992, JB Lippincott, pp. 555-564.

45. Kerl ME, Hohenhaus AE: Packed red blood cell transfusions in dogs: 131 cases (1989), *J Am Vet Med Assoc* 202:1495-1499, 1993.

46. Killen DA, Grogan EL, Gower RE, et al: Response of canine plasma-ionized calcium and magnesium to the rapid infusion of acid-citrate-dextrose (ACD) solution, *Surgery* 70:736-741, 1971.

47. Killingsworth C: Use of blood and blood components for feline and canine patients, *J Am Vet Med Assoc* 185: 1452-1455, 1984.

48. Klaser DA, Reine NJ, Hohenhaus AE: Red blood cell transfusions in cats: 126 cases (1999) in press, *J Am Vet Med Assoc* 226:920-923, 2005.

49. Kordick DL, Breitschwerdt EB: Relapsing bacteremia after blood transmission of *Bartonella henelae* to cats, *Am J Vet Res* 58:492-497, 1997.

50. Kristensen AT: General principles of small animal blood component administration, *Vet Clin North Am Small Anim Pract* 25:1277-1290, 1995.

51. Lester SJ, Hume JB, Phipps B: *Haemobartonella canis* infection following splenectomy and transfusion, *Can Vet J* 36:444-445, 1995.

52. Levy JK, Crawford PC, Collante WR, et al: Use of adult cat serum to correct failure of passive transfer in kittens, *J Am Vet Med Assoc* 219:1401-1405, 2001.

53. Logan JC, Callan MB, Drew K, et al: Clinical indications for use of fresh frozen plasma in dogs: 74 dogs (October through December 1999), *J Am Vet Med Assoc* 218: 1449-1455, 2001.

54. Lower R: A treatise on the heart on the movement and colour of the blood and on the passage of the chyle into the blood. In Franklin KJ, editor: *Special edition, the classics of medicine library*, Birmingham, AL, 1989, Gryphon Editions, p. xvi.

55. Macintire DK, Boudreaux MK, West GD, et al: *Babesia gibsoni* infection among dogs in the southeastern United States, *J Am Vet Med Assoc* 220:325-329, 2002.

56. Majilton EA, Kelley LL: The blood and plasma bank, *Vet Med* 46:226-232, 1951.

57. Marion RS, Smith JE: Posttransfusion viability of feline erythrocytes stored in acid citrate dextrose solution, *J Am Vet Med Assoc* 183:1459-1460, 1983.

58. Melzer KJ, Wardrop KJ, Hale AS, et al: A hemolytic transfusion reaction due to DEA 4 alloantibodies in a dog, *J Vet Intern Med* 17:931-933, 2003.

59. Meyers KM, Wardrop KJ, Meinkoth J: Canine von Willebrand's disease; pathobiology, diagnosis and short-term treatment, *Comp Cont Ed* 14:13-22, 1992.

60. Mooney SC: Preparation of blood components. In Hohenhaus A, editor: *Problems in veterinary medicine*, Philadelphia, 1992, JB Lippincott, pp. 594-599.

61. Moreira PL, Lansden CC, Clark TL, et al: Effect of Hemopure® on the performance of Ektachem and Hitachi clinical analyzers, *Clin Chem* 43:1790, 1997.

62. National Institutes of Health Consensus conference: Fresh-frozen plasma: indications and risks, *JAMA* 253: 551-553, 1985.

63. Otto CM, Kaufman GM, Crowe DT: Intraosseous infusion of fluids and therapeutics, *Comp Cont Ed* 11:421-430, 1989.

64. Owens S, Oakley D, Marryott K, et al: Transmission of visceral leishmaniasis through blood transfusions from infected English Foxhounds to anemic dogs, *J Am Vet Med Assoc* 219:1081-1088, 2001.

65. Poffenbarger EM, Olson PN, Chandler ML, et al: Use of adult dog serum as a substitute for colostrums in the neonatal dog, *Am J Vet Res* 52:1221-1224, 1991.

66. Porter JA, Canaday WR: Hematologic values in mongrel and Greyhound dogs being screened for research use, *J Am Vet Med Assoc* 159:1603-1606, 1971.

67. Potkay S, Zinn RD: Effects of collection interval, body weight, and season on the hemograms of canine blood donors, *Lab Anim Care* 19:192-197, 1969.

68. Price LS: A method for collecting and storing feline whole blood, *Vet Tech* 7:561-563, 1991.

69. Rentko VT, Wohl J, Murtaugh R, et al: A clinical trial of a hemoglobin based oxygen carrier (HBOC) fluid in the treatment of anemia in dogs, *J Vet Intern Med* 10:177, 1996.

70. Ring J, Messmer K: Incidence and severity of anaphylactoid reactions to colloid volume substitutes, *Lancet* 1:466-468, 1977.

71. Schneider A: Blood components: collection, processing and storage, *Vet Clin North Am Small Anim Pract* 25:1245-1261, 1995.

72. Schneider A: Principles of blood collection and processing. In Feldman BF, Zinkl JG, Jain NC, editors: *Schalms' veterinary hematology*, ed 5, Philadelphia, 2000, Lippincott, Williams & Wilkins, pp. 827-832.

73. Smith CA: Transfusion medicine: the challenge of practical use, *J Am Vet Med Assoc* 198:474-452, 1991.

74. Smith JE: Erythrocytes, *Adv Vet Sci Comp Med* 36:9-55, 1991.

75. Sprague WS, Hackett TB, Johnson JS, et al: Hemochromatosis secondary to repeated blood transfusions in a dog, *Vet Pathol* 40:334-337, 2003.

76. Stegeman JR, Birkenheuer AJ, Kruger JM, et al: Transfusion-associated Babesia gibsoni infection in a dog, *J Am Vet Med Assoc* 222:959-963, 2003.

77. Stiles J, Raffe MR: Hemolysis of canine fresh and stored blood associated with peristaltic pump infusion, *Vet Emerg Crit Care* 1:50-53, 1991.

78. Stokol T, Parry BW: Efficacy of fresh frozen plasma and cryoprecipitate in dogs with von Willebrand's disease or hemophilia A, *J Vet Intern Med* 12:84-92, 1998.

79. Sullivan PS, Evans HL, McDonald TP: Platelet concentration and hemoglobin function in greynounds, *J Am Vet Med Assoc* 205:838-841, 1994.

80. Szama K: Reports of 355 transfusion associated deaths: 1976-1985, *Transfusion* 30:583-590, 1990.

81. Taboada J, Harvey JW, Levy MG, et al: Seroprevalence of babesiosis in greyhounds in Florida, *J Am Vet Med Assoc* 200:47-50, 1992.

82. Turnwald GH, Pichler ME: Blood transfusion in dogs and cats. Part II. Administration, adverse effects and component therapy, *Compend Contin Educ* 7:115-126, 1985.

83. Walker RH, editor: *Technical manual*, ed 11, Bethesda, MD, 1993, American Association of Blood Banks.

84. Wardrop KJ: Canine plasma therapy, *Vet Forum* 14:36-40, 1997.

85. Wardrop KJ, Brooks MB: Stability of hemostatic proteins in canine fresh frozen plasma units, *Vet Clin Pathol* 30:91-95, 2001.

86. Wardrop KJ, Lewis D, Marks S, et al: Posttransfusion purpura in a dog with hemophilia A, *J Vet Intern Med* 11:261-263, 1997.

87. Wardrop KJ, Owen TJ, Meyers KM: Evaluation of an additive solution for preservation of canine red blood cells, *J Vet Intern Med* 8:253-257, 1994.

88. Wardrop KJ, Reine NJ, Birkenheuer A, et al: Consensus Statement on Canine and Feline Blood Donor Screening for Infectious Disease, *J Vet Intern Med* 19:135-142, 2005.

89. Wardrop KJ, Tucker RL, Munai K: Evaluation of canine red blood cells stored in a saline, adenine and glucose solution for 35 days, *J Vet Intern Med* 11:5-8, 1997.

90. Weingart C, Giger U, Kohn B: Whole blood transfusions in 91 cats: a clinical evaluation, *J Feline Med Surg* 6:139-148, 2004.

91. Yaphe W, Giovengo S, Moise NS: Severe cardiomegaly secondary to anemia in a kitten, *J Am Vet Med Assoc* 202:961-964, 1993.

92. Yuile CL, VanZandt TF, Ervin DM, et al: Hemolytic reactions produced in dogs by transfusion of incompatible dog blood and plasma, *Blood* 4:1232-1239, 1948.

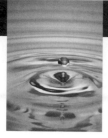

CHAPTER · 25

TOTAL PARENTERAL NUTRITION

Lisa M. Freeman and Daniel L. Chan

HISTORICAL VIEW OF PARENTERAL NUTRITION

Parenteral nutrition has been used routinely in human patients since the late 1960s. However, the use of parenteral nutrition goes as far back as 1656 when Sir Christopher Wren infused wine and beer into dogs using a goose quill and pig bladder.[52] Although there were sporadic reports of the use of intravenous nutrition, such as the intravenous infusion of saline and milk into human cholera patients in 1832, it was not until the mid-1900s that physicians began conducting more organized experiments in providing nutrients via the intravenous route.[52] Elman began administering protein hydrolysates and glucose via peripheral veins in the late 1930s and in 1947 published a book on parenteral alimentation in surgery.[27] Meng and Early began using lipid emulsions in dogs in the 1940s and published an article on parenteral nutrition in dogs in 1949.[52] However, it was in 1968 that physicians from the University of Pennsylvania published the seminal article on parenteral nutrition in dogs.[19] These authors fed six male beagle puppies beginning at 12 weeks of age for a total of 72 to 256 days.[19] The puppies were compared with their littermates that were fed orally during this same time period. The parenterally fed puppies grew at a faster rate and were larger at the end of the study compared with their littermates.[19] In the same publication, Dudrick et al[19] also reported on the results of feeding 30 human patients via total parenteral nutrition (TPN) for 10 to 200 days.

The Dudrick article became the start of a new era in nutritional support for hospitalized patients. After the recognition that people (and dogs) could be fed successfully for relatively long periods via the intravenous route, physicians and researchers proceeded to develop better ways to accomplish this goal. Two issues that were addressed early were developing better methods of central venous access and the formulation of parenteral nutrient admixtures. Once these techniques were further developed, a great deal of attention began to be focused on malnutrition—its prevalence, its detrimental effects, and methods for preventing and treating it. In 1976, Butterworth was the first to report an association between the mortality and morbidity associated with malnutrition in hospitalized patients.[10] Soon, it became widely recognized that hospital malnutrition was a major problem and that it varied among different patient populations. This finding led to the concept of nutritional assessment and its role in overall patient management. In addition, clinical trials were conducted testing the benefits, complications, and timing of parenteral nutrition. In many studies, it has not been shown that routine use of perioperative TPN is justified, and often it is associated with more complications compared with enteral nutrition or no nutrition at all.[7,18,23,51] However, certain patient populations, such as the malnourished, do appear to benefit from parenteral nutrition.[7,23,51] More recently in human medicine, meta-analyses on parenteral nutrition have been conducted to determine specific patient populations in which parenteral nutrition would be most beneficial.[7,23] Currently, research in parenteral nutrition in human medicine is focusing on optimizing the selection of patients who will benefit from parenteral nutrition and improved formulations, such as modified lipid and amino acid solutions.

Although dogs often have been used as models for the study of parenteral nutrition, the clinical use of parenteral nutrition in companion animal species is a relatively new modality of therapy. The first clinical report of the use of parenteral nutrition in companion animals was in 1977.[11] In 1989, Lippert et al[30] reported the use of TPN in seven normal cats for 14 days. In this study, cats were fed at maintenance energy requirements (MERs; calculated as $1.4 \times$ resting energy requirements [RERs]).[30] However, in one group, the calories provided by protein were included in the calculations, whereas in the other group, protein calories were not included.[30] Thus the latter group actually received calories in excess of

MER.[30] The cats that were fed more than MER developed vomiting, oral ulcerations, and hyperglycemia.[30] However, all cats developed anemia, thrombocytopenia, hypertriglyceridemia, villous atrophy, and hepatocellular changes.[30]

In 1993, Lippert et al[31] published the first retrospective study on the use of TPN in clinical patients. This study reported the results of the use of TPN in 72 dogs and 12 cats seen at Michigan State University.[31] The primary indication for TPN in this population was gastrointestinal (primarily small intestinal) disease.[31] The median duration of TPN was 3.8 days, with a range of 1 to 14 days.[31] Thirty-nine mechanical complications occurred, and metabolic complications were common, including hyperglycemia (37%), electrolyte abnormalities (30%), and hyperlipidemia (23%).[31] Cats were significantly more likely to develop hyperglycemia than were dogs.[31] Seven percent of animals developed sepsis (i.e., clinical signs of sepsis in combination with either a positive catheter tip culture or positive blood culture).[31] In this study, both total calories and protein were administered at a higher level than is currently done.[31]

A second retrospective study was published in 1998 from the University of California, Davis.[46] This study reported the results of the use of TPN in 209 dogs.[46] In this study, the main indication for TPN was pancreatitis, and similar to the Lippert study, the median duration of administration was 3.5 days (range, 0.5 to 25 days).[46] One hundred-eighteen mechanical complications occurred, and 37% of the dogs had at least one mechanical complication.[46] Hyperglycemia was the most common metabolic complication, with 32% of dogs evaluated developing this abnormality, but 329 individual metabolic complications occurred in this population of dogs.[46] Seven percent of the animals developed sepsis.[46] The overall complication rate was 0.52 complications per day of TPN.[46]

Two retrospective studies on the use of TPN in cats have been published recently.[16,43] The major reasons for using TPN were pancreatitis in one study and hepatic disease in the second study, and the median duration of TPN administration was 4.8 and 3.7 days, respectively.[16,43] In one study, the 25 of 75 cats with weights measured at both timepoints gained a mean of 0.23 kg, but the median weight did not change in the other study.[16,43] Although the number of mechanical and septic complications was similar between the two studies, 18% of cats in the more recent study became hyperglycemic, compared with 47% in the larger study.[16,43] The overall complication rate was 0.62 per day of TPN in the Pyle study and 0.29 in the Crabb study.[16,43] There also were two interesting findings regarding hyperglycemia from these two studies.[16,43] First, the study from Pyle et al showed that hyperglycemia 24 hours after starting TPN was significantly associated with an increased mortality rate.[43] In this study, cats' energy requirements were calculated by multiplying the resting energy requirements (RER) by an illness factor. In the Crabb et al study, we showed that cats in which the RER was multiplied by an illness factor were more likely to develop hyperglycemia than those in which energy requirements were provided at or below RER.[16] One retrospective study has been published for partial parenteral nutrition (PPN). This study, from Tufts University, reported the results of PPN administration in 80 dogs and 47 cats.[13] The most common indication for PPN was pancreatitis, and the median duration of PPN administration was 3.0 days (range, 0.3 to 8.8 days).[13] Twenty-five mechanical complications occurred, and as in the previous studies, hyperglycemia was the main metabolic complication.[13] In this study, however, hyperglycemia occurred in 13% of dogs and 19% of cats (15% of animals overall).[13] Twenty-four other metabolic complications also occurred, and four septic cases were documented (3%).[13] The complication rate was 0.18 and 0.15 complications per day of PPN for dogs and cats, respectively.[13] One notable feature of this study is that animals that received some enteral nutrition in combination with PPN administration were more likely to survive compared with animals not receiving any enteral nutrition.[13]

To date, these are the most comprehensive published studies on results of parenteral nutrition use in clinical patients (see Table 25-1 for a summary of these studies). However, there are at least two other studies that have been helpful in enhancing the use of parenteral nutrition in dogs. The first is a study by Chandler et al[15] in which an amino acid solution, a dextrose solution, and an electrolyte solution were administered to compare their effects on nitrogen balance. These solutions were individually administered to three healthy dogs via a peripheral vein for 10 hr/day for 4 days.[15] Only the amino acid solution resulted in a positive nitrogen balance, suggesting that in healthy dogs it provided adequate amino acids to prevent breakdown of lean body mass.[15] Finally, Mauldin et al[34] reported a study evaluating parenteral nutrition in healthy dogs. In this study, dogs received intravenous infusions of either non-lactated Ringer's solution or isocaloric solutions containing 0, 1.36, or 2.04 g of amino acids/kg body weight/day with the remaining calories (to meet MER) provided by dextrose and lipid solutions.[34] Dogs received these solutions intravenously for 12 hr/day for 7 days.[34] The first two groups (Ringer's and 0 g/kg amino acids) had negative nitrogen balance, and a regression analysis suggested that intravenous administration of 2.32 g/kg/day of amino acids would result in zero nitrogen balance in a healthy dog of beagle size (i.e., the minimum amount required to prevent catabolism of lean body mass by supplying basal amino acid requirements).[34] These two studies in healthy dogs have been helpful in better understanding the metabolism of parenteral amino acids in this species and

TABLE 25-1 Summary of Five Retrospective Studies on Parenteral Nutrition (PN) in Dogs and Cats

	Lippert	Reuter	Chan	Pyle	Crabb
Years included in study	1985-1989	1988-1995	1994-1999	1994-2001	1991-2003
Dogs included (n)	72	209	80	0	0
Cats included (n)	12	0	47	75	40
Major indication	Gastrointestinal	Pancreatitis	Pancreatitis	Pancreatitis	Hepatic
Duration of PN in days [median (range)]	3.8 (1-14)	3.5 (0.5-25)	3.0 (0.3-8.8)	4.8 (0.5-18.5)	3.7 (0.3-9.5)
Weight change (mean)	+3–4%	+0.2 kg	−0.3 kg	+0.23 kg (n=25)	0.0 kg
Mechanical complications (number)	39	118	25	19	12
Hyperglycemia (%)	37	32	15	47	23
Septic complications (%)	7	7	4	0	0
Total complications (per day of PN)	0.42	0.52	0.16	0.62	0.29
Survival (%)	70	51	73	48	60

will serve as a foundation on which to base future research into the specific requirements of ill and injured animals.

RATIONALE FOR NUTRITIONAL SUPPORT IN HOSPITALIZED ANIMALS

Ill and injured animals undergo a unique metabolic response that puts them at high risk for malnutrition and its subsequent complications. In a healthy animal that receives insufficient calories to meet its needs, the body compensates for this calorie deficit in the short term by first utilizing hepatic glycogen and then by mobilizing amino acids from muscle. Glycogen stores are rapidly depleted, particularly in carnivores such as cats. Although these processes can provide needed energy, they are inefficient energy sources; therefore after several days, the healthy animal adapts by decreasing protein turnover and preferentially using fat. By this process, a healthy animal can survive for a long period without food, provided that adequate water is available. In the ill or injured animal, however, this normal adaptive response to a calorie deficit does not occur, primarily as a result of alterations in the cytokine and hormonal milieu that are associated with the catabolic response. Thus these animals continue to mobilize protein, perpetuating the loss of lean body mass.

The problem with this continued loss of lean body mass is that all of the body's protein is functional tissue, as compared with fat and carbohydrate, both of which have storage depots. In addition, loss of lean body mass negatively impacts wound healing, immune function, strength (both skeletal and respiratory muscle), and ultimately prognosis. Although it has not been demonstrated in companion animals, hospitalized people with weight loss have a worse outcome than those without. A loss of lean body mass in an ill or injured animal will occur, to a certain degree, even if the animal is provided with adequate calories. However, appropriate nutritional support can minimize the amount of lean body mass lost and the sequela of this loss. Therefore the goal of nutritional support in the hospitalized animal should be not only treatment of those that are already malnourished but also minimizing the development of malnutrition in animals at risk.

PATIENT SELECTION

Any route of nutritional support carries some risk of complications, and parenteral nutrition is not an exception. Studies in people have shown that parenteral nutrition in some patient populations actually increases the risk of complications and worsens outcome.[7,18,23,51] Therefore careful patient selection is particularly important in the case of parenteral nutrition. Ideally, one would select only those patients that would benefit from parenteral nutrition, but the appropriate selection criteria are not yet known in people or in companion animals. Most companion animals receive parenteral nutrition for relatively short periods (median, 3 to 4 days), and one must determine whether short-term provision of parenteral nutrition is likely to be beneficial. Occasionally, parenteral nutrition is administered for more prolonged periods, and as always the risk/benefit ratio must be considered. In a previously healthy dog that has been anorectic for 2 to 3 days and in which oral or enteral intake is likely to resume quickly, parenteral nutrition may not be beneficial. However, in a vomiting cat that has not eaten for 1 week at home and is not expected to be eating again soon, parenteral nutrition would be indicated.

The indications for parenteral nutritional support are situations in which an animal cannot voluntarily consume adequate calories and cannot tolerate enteral nutrition.

The specific indications for parenteral nutrition are shown in Box 25-1. Proper patient selection is an important aspect of nutritional assessment because administration of parenteral nutritional support to patients unlikely to benefit from this form of nutrition only subjects them to risk of complications.

NUTRITIONAL ASSESSMENT

In critically ill animals, nutrition often is not considered to be a priority during the early phases of resuscitation, stabilization, and diagnostic testing. However, this population is at high risk for developing malnutrition, and identification of animals that are already malnourished or those that are at high risk for becoming malnourished should be of high importance. Being aware of an animal's nutritional status at admission and of changes that occur during hospitalization will optimize patient care.

It is easy to recognize the classical picture of the starved patient as being malnourished (Fig. 25-1). However, many of our patients have more subtle signs of malnutrition or develop malnutrition while hospitalized because the risk for malnutrition was not recognized early enough to prevent it (Fig. 25-2, A). Even obese animals are at risk for malnutrition (Fig. 25-2, B) because if they lose weight, they will lose lean body mass rather than fat. A quick assessment of nutritional status on each patient can be incorporated into the daily examination of each patient. Nutritional assessment identifies malnourished patients that require nutritional support and also identifies patients at risk for malnutrition in which nutritional support will help prevent malnutrition.[12,38]

For many years, investigators have attempted to develop a single measurement or group of measurements that will identify malnutrition in humans. Unfortunately, few of these have worked well on a clinical basis. Therefore most nutritionists in human and veterinary medicine use a subjective global clinical assessment to identify patients

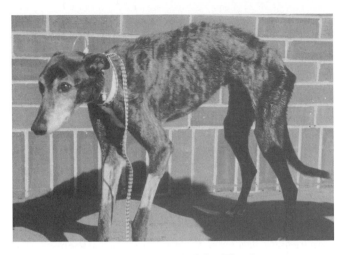

Fig. 25-1 An obviously malnourished dog. This dog requires aggressive nutritional support.

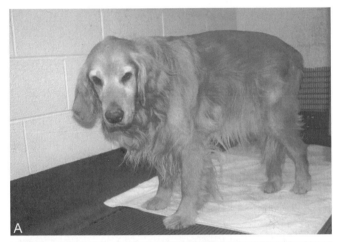

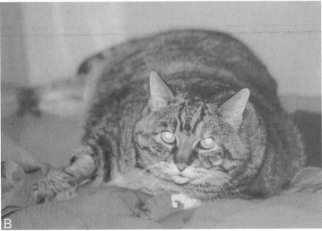

Fig. 25-2 A, Malnutrition can be subtle in the early stages. This dog has been eating reduced amounts of food for 1 week as a result of chronic renal failure. It is not obviously thin but is already exhibiting muscle loss. Appropriate nutritional support can help to minimize further losses. **B,** Even an obese animal can become quickly malnourished in the hospital when ill or injured. If insufficient calories are supplied, the cat will lose weight but it will be functional lean body mass, rather than fat, that is lost.

Box 25-1	Indications for Parenteral Nutrition*

Vomiting
Regurgitation
Acute pancreatitis
Intestinal obstruction
Severe malabsorption
Prolonged ileus
Inability to guard airway

*Whenever possible, enteral nutrition should be used to supplement parenteral nutrition (even if provided at a very low rate) to prevent atrophy of the intestinal tract.

in need of nutritional support (Box 25-2). This assessment includes historical information (e.g., duration of clinical signs, history of weight loss), clinical parameters (e.g., underlying disease, severity of illness, clinical signs, anticipated course of recovery), and laboratory results. Any clinical or laboratory findings that would specifically alter the nutritional plan should be carefully considered. Examples include the presence of congestive heart failure (which would necessitate careful attention to fluid volume), electrolyte abnormalities, hyperglycemia, hypertriglyceridemia, or hepatic encephalopathy. These factors then are incorporated into an overall assessment of the degree of malnutrition or the animal's risk for developing malnutrition. Prevention (or correction) of nutritional deficiencies and imbalances then can be accomplished by providing adequate energy substrates, protein, and micronutrients.

The authors categorize hospitalized animals into three groups: (1) those that are already malnourished (see Fig. 25-1); (2) those that are not malnourished but are at high risk for developing malnutrition (Fig. 25-3); and (3) those that are not malnourished and are at low risk for developing malnutrition (Fig. 25-4). Animals in the first group require prompt nutritional support. Animals in the second group require nutritional support in the first 2 to 3 days of hospitalization, or at the

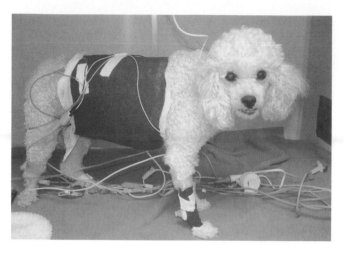

Fig. 25-3 This dog is anorectic and is being treated with an open abdomen for septic peritonitis. Although not yet malnourished, it is at high risk for becoming so because of the lack of nutrient intake and the large protein losses via the abdomen.

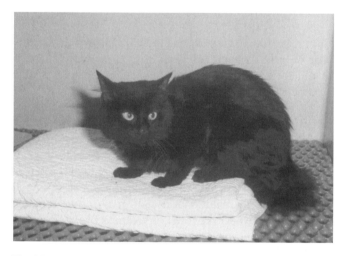

Fig. 25-4 A cat with asthma that is not malnourished and is at low risk for becoming so. This cat does not require immediate nutritional support and can be monitored to ensure adequate food intake. However, if the underlying disease does not resolve quickly or the animal continues to be anorectic, nutritional support may be required.

| **Box 25-2** | **Indicators of Malnutrition in Dogs and Cats** |

Historical Findings
Vomiting
Regurgitation
Chronic diarrhea
Anorexia
Unintended weight loss

Physical Examination Findings
Weight loss (although this may be masked by fluid shifts in the critically ill patient)
Muscle loss
Poor haircoat
Signs of poor wound healing
Coagulopathy
Pale mucous membranes

Laboratory Findings*
Hypoalbuminemia
Lymphopenia
Anemia
Coagulopathies

*These laboratory abnormalities are not specific to malnutrition and generally are not present early in the process of developing malnutrition.

---

time of anesthetizing them for diagnostic or therapeutic procedures, a feeding tube should be placed. Factors that put an animal at high risk for malnutrition include anorexia lasting longer than 3 days (be sure to include the time the animal has been anorectic at home before admission to the hospital), serious underlying disease (e.g., trauma, sepsis, peritonitis, pancreatitis, extensive gastrointestinal surgery), and large protein losses (e.g., protracted vomiting or diarrhea, open abdomen, or large draining wounds). Animals in the third group do not require immediate nutritional support and can be monitored to ensure adequate food intake. However, if the underlying disease does not resolve quickly or the animal continues to be anorectic, nutritional support may be required. Indicators of malnutrition are listed in Box 25-2.

ROUTE OF NUTRITIONAL SUPPORT

Most clinicians have heard the adage, "If the gut works, use it." This approach still holds true, and parenteral nutrition should not be the first consideration in an ill or injured animal. The suitability of the enteral route should always be addressed first because it is the safest, most convenient, most physiologically sound, and least expensive method of nutritional support (see Chapter 26).[53] If only parts of the gastrointestinal tract are functional, further consideration should be given to utilize those functional segments. For example, a dog or cat with severe esophagitis should be considered a candidate for a jejunostomy feeding tube. However, when patients are unable to tolerate any enteral feeding, parenteral nutrition should be considered. Before parenteral nutrition is instituted, however, it is critical that fluid, electrolyte, and acid-base abnormalities are corrected.

PARENTERAL NUTRITION

Parenteral nutrition can be delivered via a central vein (TPN) or a peripheral vein (PPN). TPN, as defined in this chapter, is the provision of all of the animal's calorie and protein requirements (and ideally, all of the micronutrient requirements as well; see section on Other Nutrient Requirements). PPN only supplies part of the animal's energy, protein, and other nutrient requirements.[55] In this chapter, we use the abbreviation PPN to refer to partial parenteral nutrition, which can be supplied through either a peripheral or central vein.

Because TPN will supply all of the animal's calorie and protein requirements, it is often the modality of choice for an animal requiring parenteral nutrition. The disadvantages are that it requires a jugular venous catheter, it is slightly more expensive (typically ~10% to 20% more for a TPN solution compared with a PPN solution for the same-sized animal), and it may be associated with more metabolic complications. PPN may be an alternative to TPN in selected cases (Box 25-3), but it is important to be aware that it will not provide all of the animal's requirements. Both TPN and PPN are typically a combination of dextrose, an amino acid solution, and a lipid solution. However, the concentration of some components (e.g., dextrose) varies depending on whether TPN or PPN is chosen. Table 25-2 compares a PPN and a TPN admixture for a 20-kg dog.

Box 25-3 | **Indications for Partial Parenteral Nutrition (PPN; i.e., providing less than the animal's total calorie, protein, and micronutrient requirements)**

- To maintain nutritional status, rather than replete the malnourished patient. Debilitated patients should get total parenteral nutrition (TPN) or a combination of PPN and enteral nutrition.
- Animals with average nutritional requirements. Those with high requirements (e.g., open abdomen, large draining wound, severe vomiting or diarrhea) should receive TPN.
- When only short-term nutritional support in a nondebilitated patient is anticipated (<5 days).
- To supplement oral or enteral nutrition.*
- When a central vein is not accessible.

*Whenever possible, enteral nutrition should be used to supplement parenteral nutrition (even if provided at a very low rate) to prevent atrophy of the intestinal tract.

FORMULATION OF PARENTERAL NUTRITION REQUIREMENTS
Calorie Requirements

When formulating parenteral nutrition, the first step is to determine the animal's calorie requirements. The patient's RER is the number of calories required for maintaining homeostasis while the animal rests quietly. The RER is calculated using the formula:

TABLE 25-2 Comparison of Partial Parenteral Nutrition (PPN) and Total Parenteral Nutrition (TPN) Formulations for 20-kg Dog with Acute Pancreatitis

	PPN	TPN
5% dextrose (mL)	900	—
50% dextrose (mL)	—	164
8.5% amino acids (mL)	450	312
20% lipid (mL)	77	139
Total mL/day	1427	615
PPN mL/hr	60	26
Maintenance fluid rate (mL/hr)	55	55

$$RER = 70 \times (\text{current body weight in kilograms})^{0.75}$$

This exponential equation will more accurately estimate the animal's true requirements across all body weights. However, for animals weighing between 3 and 25 kg, the following linear formula gives a reasonable approximation of energy needs:

$$RER = 30 \times (\text{current body weight in kilograms}) + 70$$

One should avoid using the linear equation for animals larger than 25 kg because the linear equation will overestimate these animals' energy requirements (Fig. 25-5).

For animals that are underweight, the authors recommend using the animal's current weight for the RER calculation. The goal of parenteral nutrition should not be weight gain, which can be achieved after the animal's underlying disease has been treated and the animal is able to tolerate enteral or oral feedings. Overfeeding for the animal's current weight also increases the risk for metabolic complications (see section on Complications). For animals that are overweight, one should feed an appropriate number of calories to avoid weight loss because seriously ill or injured animals lose lean body mass rather than fat. There are a number of ways to calculate parenteral nutrition requirements in markedly overweight animals (i.e., >25% above ideal body weight). One is to use the animal's current body weight for the RER calculation while carefully monitoring body weight to ensure that the animal does not lose or gain weight. Another option is to use the assumption that 25% of excess weight is lean tissue and the remaining 75% is

metabolically inactive fat (i.e., if a dog's ideal weight is 20 kg and it weighs 30 kg, it has 10 kg of excess weight, 2.5 kg of which is lean tissue and 7.5 kg of which is fat). Therefore one can take the ideal weight plus 25% of the excess weight (to account for the extra lean body mass) as the weight to use for calculation of RER. Using the 30-kg dog and ideal weight of 20 kg from the example above, the adjusted body weight to use for calculation of RER would be 20 kg + (25% × 10 kg) or 20 kg + 2.5 kg = 22.5 kg. Thus the RER for this overweight dog would be 723 kcal/day.

Traditionally, the RER has been multiplied by an illness factor between 1.0 and 2.0 to account for increases in metabolism associated with different conditions and injuries.[1,9,29,33] Recently, there has been less emphasis on these subjective illness factors, and current recommendations are to use more conservative energy estimates to avoid overfeeding.[12,21,44] Overfeeding can result in metabolic and gastrointestinal complications, hepatic dysfunction, and increased carbon dioxide production.[4,5] We have shown in cats receiving TPN that those in which the RER was multiplied by an illness factor were more likely to develop hyperglycemia than those in which energy requirements were provided at or below RER.[16] Maintaining euglycemia has been shown to be highly beneficial in critically ill people.[20,50] Although this benefit has not been documented in companion animals, avoiding hyperglycemia appears prudent. To reduce the risk of hyperglycemia and other complications, the authors use RER as an initial estimate of a critically ill patient's energy requirements. Further adjustments are made based on the animal's response to feeding, body weight, and changes in the underlying condition. Indirect calorimetry can accurately assess the caloric needs of individual patients, but it is rather cumbersome to use in a clinical setting. This technique may be more commonly used in the future, particularly for patients that are difficult to manage on nutritional support. More recently, studies using indirect calorimetry support the hypothesis that the application of illness factors in calculating energy expenditure in clinical patients overestimates energy needs.[42,54] At the current time, the key to successful nutritional support is vigilant monitoring after therapy has been initiated to ensure that provision of calories is adjusted as necessary.

Other Nutrient Requirements

After calorie requirements are determined, one must also address protein requirements. Animals require a nitrogen source and essential amino acids. These are typically provided parenterally by an amino acid solution. Essential fatty acids (linoleic acid in the dog, linoleic and arachidonic acids in the cat) are also required. These are provided by a lipid emulsion; however, fat is not required on a daily basis. Some nutritionists formulate parenteral nutrition without lipids or provide an intermittent infusion of a lipid emulsion when animals remain on parenteral

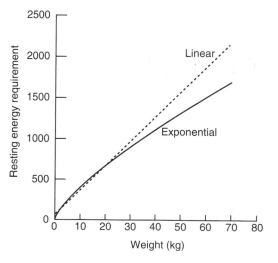

Fig. 25-5 Comparison of resting energy requirements (RERs), as calculated using a linear equation [(30 × body weight) + 70] versus an exponential equation [70(body weight)$^{0.75}$]. Note that the equations yield similar results for animals weighing between 3 and 25 kg. For animals that weigh more than 25 kg, the linear equation overestimates the animal's RER.

nutrition for prolonged periods over which essential fatty acid supplementation would be required.[1,8]

Electrolytes, vitamins, and trace elements also may be added to the parenteral nutrition formulation. Depending on the hospital and the patient, electrolytes can be added individually to the admixture, added as an electrolyte mixture, included as part of the amino acid solution, or left out altogether and managed separately in the animal's crystalloid fluid prescription. Amino acids with or without electrolytes can be included based on clinician preference. Because most animals receive parenteral nutrition for only a short duration, fat-soluble vitamins usually are not limiting, and supplementation with TPN vitamin preparations designed for humans usually is not indicated. The exception is obviously malnourished animals in which supplementation may be desirable. Conversely, because B vitamins are water soluble, they are more likely to become depleted, particularly in anorectic animals. Therefore B vitamins should be routinely supplemented in the parenteral nutrient admixture. Some authors recommend vitamin K supplementation for animals receiving parenteral nutrition because parenteral nutrition preparations are thought to be low in vitamin K. Generally, vitamin K is administered subcutaneously on the first day of TPN and then once weekly. However, vitamin K deficiency is unlikely to occur, particularly when a lipid emulsion is used, and the authors do not routinely supplement vitamin K unless indicated by the animal's underlying disease. Trace elements serve as cofactors in a variety of enzyme systems and can become depleted in malnourished animals or during long-term parenteral nutrition. In people receiving parenteral nutrition, zinc, copper, manganese, and chromium are routinely included in the parenteral nutrient admixture. These are sometimes added to parenteral nutrition preparations for malnourished animals, but in the authors' practice, they are not routinely included.

Other nutritional requirements will depend on the patient's underlying disease, clinical signs, and laboratory test results. Adjustments to the nutritional plan may include sodium restriction for cardiac patients, protein restriction for encephalopathic and end-stage renal failure patients, and fat restriction for patients with hypertriglyceridemia. Finally, there may be certain nutrients that may have benefits when added in amounts above their nutrient requirements. This concept is often called nutritional pharmacology. The addition of immune-modulating substances such as arginine, glutamine, antioxidants, and *n*-3 fatty acids to parenteral nutrition preparations may offer added benefits, but few studies have been conducted in companion animals.[12,37]

PARENTERAL NUTRITION COMPONENTS

Typically, the desired parenteral nutrition formula is calculated, and the components are compounded into a parenteral nutrient admixture. This solution is most often composed of amino acids, dextrose, and lipid along with vitamins and minerals. Information on the various parenteral nutrition components is presented in Table 25-3.

Amino Acids

Amino acid solutions provide a nitrogen source and essential amino acids. Amino acid solutions are available in varying concentrations from 3.5% to 10%. However, the worksheets in this chapter use amounts specific for an 8.5% amino acid solution (the most commonly used). Other concentrations could be used, but the amounts would need to be adjusted accordingly. Most amino acid solutions are available in two formulations: one with electrolytes and one without (see Table 25-3). In the authors' hospital, most animals receive parenteral nutrition using amino acids with electrolytes. However, an amino acid solution without electrolytes is used for patients with electrolyte disturbances, and electrolyte imbalances are corrected separately via other administered intravenous fluids.

The standard amount of protein included in the parenteral formulation is 4 to 5 g/100 kcal for dogs and 6 g/100 kcal for cats (although the optimal concentration for ill and injured dogs and cats has not been determined).[12] This concentration can be reduced for animals with protein intolerance (e.g., those with hepatic encephalopathy or severe renal failure) or increased for those with higher needs (e.g., animals with large draining wounds or hypoalbuminemia).

It is important to note that the essential amino acids provided in these solutions are intended to meet the essential amino acid requirements in people. Currently, no amino acid solutions are made specifically for dogs or cats, and therefore these solutions do not meet all of these species' needs or provide amino acids in the optimal proportions. However, when used for short-term nutritional support, this situation is unlikely to result in clinically relevant deficiencies. This may not be the case for certain amino acids such as taurine, which could become limiting if parenteral nutrition were to be used long term.

Other amino acid products are commercially available for people, including those intended for patients with renal failure, hepatic failure (e.g., high concentrations of branched chain amino acids), and for neonates. Some of these products may meet companion animal needs, but their additional cost usually does not justify their hypothetical benefits.

Dextrose

Dextrose is a component of nearly all parenteral nutrition formulations. In the formulations provided in this chapter, a 5% dextrose solution is used in PPN, whereas a 50% dextrose solution is used in TPN. Different concentrations can be used, but the worksheets would need

TABLE 25-3 Parenteral Nutrition Components

Parenteral Nutrition Components	Trade Name	Osmolarity (mOsm/L)	pH	Na$^+$ (mEq/L)	Cl$^-$ (mEq/L)	K$^+$ (mEq/L)	Mg^{++} (mEq/L)	Ca^{++} (mEq/L)	PO$_4^-$ (mMol/L)	Calories (kcal/L)
8.5% amino acids	Travasol*	890	6.0	—	34	—	—	—	—	340
8.5% amino acids	Aminosyn II†	706	5.8	32	—	—	—	—	—	340
8.5% amino acids with electrolytes	Travasol*	1144	6.0	70	70	60	10	—	30	340
8.5% amino acids with electrolytes	Aminosyn II†	920	5.8	78	86	66	10	—	30	340
5% dextrose	—	252	4.0	—	—	—	—	—	—	170
10% dextrose	—	505	4.0	—	—	—	—	—	—	340
50% dextrose	—	2520	4.0	—	—	—	—	—	—	1700
20% lipid	Intralipid*	268	8.0	—	—	—	—	—	15	2000
20% lipid	Liposyn III†	292	8.3	—	—	—	—	—	—	2000
10% lipid	Intralipid*	260	8.0	—	—	—	—	—	15	1000
10% lipid	Liposyn III†	284	8.3	—	—	—	—	—	—	1000
Commercial Combination Products										
2.75% amino acids/5% dextrose	Clinimix*	525	6.0	—	11	—	—	—	—	280
2.75% amino acids/5% dextrose with electrolytes	Clinimix E*	665	6.0	35	39	30	5	4.5	15	280
3% amino acids/3% glycerin	ProcalAmine‡	735	6.8	35	41	25	5	3	3.5	246
3.5% amino acids/5% dextrose	Nutrimix†	585	5.8	18	—	—	—	—	—	310
3.5% amino acids/5% dextrose with electrolytes	Nutrimix†	616	5.8	41	36.5	13	3	—	3.5	310
4.25% amino acids/5% dextrose	Clinimix*	675	6.0	—	17	—	—	—	—	340

Manufacturers:
*Baxter Healthcare Corporation, Deerfield, IL.
†Abbott Laboratories, North Chicago, IL.
‡B. Braun Medical Inc, Irvine, CA.

to be adjusted accordingly. A 50% dextrose solution provides 1.7 kcal/mL, whereas the 5% solution provides 0.17 kcal/mL. Typically, in TPN, half of the nonprotein calories are provided by dextrose, but the ratio between dextrose and lipid can be adjusted depending on the individual circumstances (e.g., a greater proportion of lipid compared with dextrose would be given to a hyperglycemic animal). In people, the maximal amount of dextrose that can be oxidized is 5 mg/kg/min. In fact, dextrose infusion rates exceeding 4 mg/kg/min have been associated with the development of hyperglycemia in nondiabetic patients.[47] In light of these findings, the authors recommend limiting the amount of dextrose infused during parenteral nutrition to less than 4 mg/kg/min. When formulating parenteral nutrition for diabetic patients, a greater proportion of calories should be provided from amino acids and lipids. Despite adjustments to the formulation, diabetic patients often require adjustment of insulin therapy during parenteral nutritional support.

Lipid

Lipid emulsions are used in parenteral nutrition as an energy source (a 20% solution provides 2 kcal/mL) and as a source of essential fatty acids. Commercial lipid emulsions in the United States are usually based on soybean oil or soybean and safflower oil. They also include egg yolk phospholipids, glycerin, and water. The presence of soybean and safflower oil means that these solutions are composed primarily of n-6 fatty acids. High doses of lipid can cause immunosuppression via granulocyte and reticuloendothelial cell dysfunction.[22,25] In addition to immunologic effects, lipids can have hemodynamic and inflammatory effects, the latter mediated by the more inflammatory eicosanoids produced from n-6 fatty acids. In other countries, different types of lipid emulsions are available that may be preferable to the standard soybean-based emulsions (e.g., n-3 fatty acids, n-9 fatty acids, medium-chain triglycerides, structured lipids), but these are not commercially available in the United States. The authors try to limit the lipid dosage in dogs and cats to 2.0 g/kg/day to avoid the potential for immunosuppression. Animals with hypertriglyceridemia also require lower doses of lipid and may require a TPN formulation without any lipid. Although some dogs with pancreatitis have hypertriglyceridemia and require reduction (or elimination) of the lipid dose, dogs with pancreatitis without hypertriglyceridemia do not need any reduction in the amount of lipid provided from the standard calculation.

Minerals

As previously mentioned, parenteral nutrition can be formulated without any electrolytes or electrolytes can be included, either as a component of an amino acid solution, added individually, or added as a combination of TPN electrolytes (most commonly, a combination of sodium, potassium, calcium, magnesium, chloride, and acetate). The most effective method will depend on the individual hospital and, in some cases, the individual patient. In certain situations, additional potassium or magnesium may be added directly to parenteral nutrition. However, the disadvantage of adding directly to the parenteral nutrient admixture is that if the animal's requirements change during the day (or over a few days if more than 1 day of parenteral nutrition is compounded at one time) and the electrolyte is already in the admixture, the parenteral admixture must be reformulated or the animal will receive a less than optimal electrolyte composition. Adjusting electrolytes separately from the parenteral nutrition allows greater flexibility.

Trace elements are sometimes added to the parenteral nutrient admixture, but the authors only add them for animals that are malnourished or are receiving parenteral nutrition for 5 days or more. The most common trace elements supplemented are zinc, copper, manganese, and chromium, with copper considered the most limiting of these elements. The authors use a commercial trace element product containing (per 5 mL): 4 mg zinc, 1 mg copper, 0.8 mg manganese, and 10 μg chromium at a dosage of 0.2 to 0.3 mL/100 kcal (4 Trace Elements, Abbott Laboratories, North Chicago, IL).

Vitamins

For most hospitalized animals, including a B vitamin complex to the parenteral nutrient admixture is sufficient. Some B vitamins, particularly riboflavin, are light sensitive. Therefore sufficient B vitamin complex should be given such that the riboflavin dose is administered within the first 6 hours of the parenteral nutrition infusion. When using a commercial B vitamin complex containing thiamine, niacin, pyridoxine, pantothenic acid, riboflavin, and cyanocobalamin (B vitamin complex, Veterinary Laboratories, Lenexa, KS), a dosage of 0.2 mL/100 kcal should provide this amount of riboflavin.

For debilitated animals or those that receive parenteral nutrition for prolonged periods, a TPN vitamin complex can be included in the nutrient admixture (Cernevit-12, Baxter Healthcare Corporation, Deerfield, IL). These products typically contain vitamins A, D, E, and C, in addition to the B vitamins.

Although certain medical conditions may result in vitamin K deficiency (e.g., biliary obstruction, hepatic disease), vitamin K is not typically administered intravenously and therefore is not added to the parenteral nutrition admixture. Interestingly, lipid solutions do contain vitamin K, which can be at sufficient concentrations to interfere with warfarin therapy in human patients.[28,32] The amount of vitamin K found in lipid solutions has not been reported to cause anaphylactic reactions in companion animals. When deemed necessary, vitamin K supplementation is administered subcutaneously with dosages appropriate for the medical condition.

Commercial Combination Parenteral Nutrition Products

Although veterinarians have clinically used single nutrient solutions (e.g., amino acids or dextrose alone), these solutions do not provide balanced nutrition and are problematic when used alone (e.g., 50% dextrose is too hyperosmolar to be administered through a peripheral vein, 5% dextrose is too low in calories to be beneficial when administered alone). If 5% dextrose were administered at 66 mL/kg/day to an 11-kg dog, it would provide only 123 kcal/day (<30% of the dog's calorie requirements and no protein). Administering lipid as a single solution can suppress immune function and, like dextrose, provides no protein. The osmolarity of amino acid solutions (1144 mOsm/L) makes them inappropriate for peripheral administration, and if amino acids are provided without sufficient calories, the amino acids will be used for calories rather than protein synthesis.

However, there are a number of combination products commercially available that combine an amino acid source with a calorie source. These are listed in Table 25-3. Because dextrose cannot be sterilized in combination with amino acids, the approach to these products is to use dual-chamber bags in which the two compartments are separate until the seal between them is broken by squeezing the bag and the solutions are mixed (e.g., Clinimix, Baxter Healthcare Corporation; Nutrimix, Abbott Laboratories). In another product (ProcalAmine, B. Braun Medical Inc., Irvine, CA), glycerin, which can be safely sterilized with amino acids, is used as a calorie source along with the amino acids. The advantages of these commercial combination products are their availability and the fact that they require no compounding. These products, when administered at maintenance fluid rates (cats, 50 mL/kg/day; dogs, 66 mL/kg/day) by continuous-rate infusion, provide all of a dog's (and most of a cat's) protein requirements but only 30% to 40% of their energy requirements. In addition, their electrolyte composition varies, but they generally are high in potassium. Therefore they should be used with caution in critically ill patients. The authors typically use these products as a temporary measure for parenteral nutritional support (i.e., overnight or on weekends) or in combination with low-dose enteral nutrition.

COMPOUNDING PARENTERAL NUTRITION

The authors recommend using a parenteral nutrient admixture, which refers to the inclusion of the dextrose, amino acids, and lipids (with or without electrolytes, vitamins, trace elements) in a single bag. The calculations of calorie requirements, as well as the amino acid, lipid, and dextrose components for TPN and PPN, are shown in Boxes 25-4 and 25-5.

Other methods of calculating parenteral nutrition formulations have been described,[29,33,44,45] but the methods listed in this chapter reflect the ones currently used in our hospital. The TPN worksheet produces a parenteral nutrient admixture with an osmolarity greater than 1000 mOsm/L, and it must be administered via a jugular vein. The PPN worksheet produces an admixture with an osmolarity less than 700 mOsm/L, which can be administered via a peripheral vein, provided that a long, nonthrombogenic catheter is used. Calculating the actual osmolarity of the parenteral nutrition admixture can be done using the osmolarity of each component listed in Table 25-3 and the equation listed in Box 25-6. The PPN worksheet is designed for simplicity and not to provide optimal proportions of nutrients based on body weight categories. The rationale for the weight categories is that these calculations will provide PPN at approximately maintenance fluid rates. Animals with metabolic disturbances or those that require volume restriction may require adjustments in the PPN calculations or may require TPN, which allows more flexibility.

Drug-nutrient compatibility is a very critical and very complex issue for parenteral nutrition.[24,39,49] A number of deaths have been reported in people from parenteral nutrition because of precipitation of calcium phosphate in the admixture.[24] At the time of compounding TPN or PPN, some additives can be included using aseptic technique, but others definitely are not compatible. Commonly used drugs that are compatible with parenteral nutrition admixtures include insulin, heparin, and metoclopramide. It is strongly recommended that a pharmacist experienced in parenteral nutrition compounding be consulted before considering adding anything to parenteral nutrition admixtures.

ADMINISTRATION

Catheters

Administration of parenteral nutrition requires a catheter that is placed using aseptic technique (Fig. 25-6). Adherence to aseptic technique is crucial because the skin has been identified as the most common source of catheter-related infections.[2,6,35,41] Long catheters composed of silicone, polyurethane, or tetrafluoroethylene are recommended for use with parenteral nutrition to reduce the risk of thrombophlebitis. Short catheters and catheters composed of polyvinyl chloride or polyethylene should be avoided. The catheter should be "dedicated"—i.e., it should not be used for any other purpose (e.g., administering medications, collecting blood samples, measuring central venous pressure) than administration of parenteral nutrition. If a multilumen catheter is used, a single port should be dedicated to parenteral nutrition.[41] Multilumen catheters are very useful for patients receiving parenteral nutrition because they can remain in place for longer periods compared with normal

Box 25-4 Worksheet for Calculating a Total Parenteral Nutrition Formulation

1. Resting energy requirement (RER)

   $70 \times$ (current body weight in kilograms)$^{0.75}$ = kcal/day or for animals 3-25 kg, can also use:

   $30 \times$ (current body weight in kilograms) + 70 = kcal/day   RER = _____kcal/day

2. Protein requirements

	Canine	Feline
*Standard	4-5 g/100 kcal	6 g/100 kcal
*Decreased requirements (hepatic/renal failure)	2-3 g/100 kcal	3-4 g/100 kcal
*Increased requirements (protein-losing conditions)	6 g/100 kcal	6 g/100 kcal

   (RER ÷ 100) × _____g/100 kcal   = _____g protein required/day (protein required)

3. Volumes of nutrient solutions required each day

   a. 8.5% amino acid solution = 0.085 g protein/mL

   _____g protein required/day ÷ 0.085 g/mL   = _____mL of amino acids/day

   b. Nonprotein calories:

   The calories supplied by protein (4 kcal/g) are subtracted from the RER to get total nonprotein calories needed:

   _____g protein required/day × 4 kcal/g   = _____kcal provided by protein

   RER – kcal provided by protein   = _____nonprotein kcal needed/day

   c. Nonprotein calories are usually provided as a 50:50 mixture of lipid and dextrose. However, if the patient has a preexisting condition (e.g., diabetes, hypertriglyceridemia), this ratio may need to be adjusted:

   *20% lipid solution = 2 kcal/mL

   To supply 50% of nonprotein kcal

   _____lipid kcal required ÷ 2 kcal/mL   = _____mL of lipid

   *50% dextrose solution = 1.7 kcal/mL

   To supply 50% of nonprotein kcal:

   _____dextrose kcal required ÷ 1.7 kcal/mL   = _____mL dextrose

4. Total daily requirements

   _____mL 8.5% amino acid solution

   _____mL 20% lipid solution

   _____mL 50% dextrose solution

   _____mL total volume of TPN solution

5. Administration rate

   Day 1: _____mL/hr

   Day 2: _____mL/hr

   Day 3: _____mL/hr

   *Be sure to adjust the patient's other fluids accordingly!

   *Note: Fluids can be added directly to TPN if desired (at the time of compounding only).

   *The monitoring required will depend on the individual patient. However, at least the following should be measured daily:

   *Heart/respiratory rate

   *Catheter site

   *Attitude

   *Body weight

   *Temperature

   *Glucose, total solids (check hematocrit tubes for lipemia)

   *Electrolytes (especially potassium) should be monitored at least every other day

catheters and provide additional ports for blood sampling and administration of additional intravenous fluids and medications. All catheters should be well secured and wrapped, but the bandage should be changed daily so that the catheter site can be evaluated. This practice will help to identify swelling, erythema, or malpositioning of the catheter. All handling of the catheter and lines should be done using aseptic technique. Appropriate catheter care has been shown to be one of the most effective measures in reducing catheter-related complications.[2,41]

Parenteral Nutrition Solutions

For logistical and economical reasons, more than 1 day's supply of parenteral nutrition usually is compounded at one time. As such, the bag of parenteral nutrition for the current day should be set up for the animal, and the other bags should be stored in a refrigerator until the time of use. No more than a 3-day supply of parenteral nutrition should be compounded and stored at a time. This practice is particularly important in critically ill patients, in which adjustments to the parenteral nutrition admixture may become necessary (e.g., decreasing

Box 25-5 Worksheet for Calculating a Partial Parenteral Nutrition Formulation

1. Resting energy requirement (RER)
   $70 \times$ (current body weight in kilograms)$^{0.75}$ = kcal/day or for animals weighing 3 to 25 kg can also use:
   $30 \times$ (current body weight in kilograms) + 70 = kcal/day   RER = _____kcal/day
2. Partial energy requirement (PER)
   Plan to supply 70% of the animal's RER with PPN:
   PER = RER × 0.70 = _____kcal/day
3. Nutrient composition
   (Note: For animals ≤3 kg, the formulation will provide a fluid rate higher than maintenance fluid requirements. Be sure that the animal can tolerate this volume of fluids.)
   a. Cats and dogs weighing 3-5 kg:
      PER × 0.20 = _____kcal/day from dextrose
      PER × 0.20 = _____kcal/day from protein
      PER × 0.60 = _____kcal/day from lipid
   b. Cats and dogs weighing 6-10 kg:
      PER × 0.25 = _____kcal/day from dextrose
      PER × 0.25 = _____kcal/day from protein
      PER × 0.50 = _____kcal/day from lipid
   c. Dogs weighing 11-30 kg:
      PER × 0.33 = _____kcal/day from dextrose
      PER × 0.33 = _____kcal/day from protein
      PER × 0.33 = _____kcal/day from lipid
   d. Dogs weighing >30 kg:
      PER × 0.50 = _____kcal/day from dextrose
      PER × 0.25 = _____kcal/day from protein
      PER × 0.25 = _____kcal/day from lipid
4. Volumes of nutrient solutions required each day
   a. 5% dextrose solution = 0.17 kcal/mL
      _____kcal from dextrose ÷ 0.17 kcal/mL   = _____mL dextrose/day
   b. 8.5% amino acid solution = 0.085 g/mL = 0.34 kcal/mL
      _____kcal from protein ÷ 0.34 kcal/mL   = _____mL amino acids/day
   c. 20% lipid solution = 2 kcal/mL
      _____kcal from lipid ÷ 2 kcal/mL   = _____mL lipid/day
5. Total daily requirements
   _____mL 5% dextrose solution
   _____mL 8.5% amino acid solution
   _____mL 20% lipid solution
   _____mL total volume of PPN solution
6. Administration rate
   This formulation provides approximately a maintenance fluid rate.
   _____mL/hr PPN solution
   *Be sure to adjust the patient's other intravenous fluids accordingly!
   Notes:
   *Fluids can be added directly to the PPN solution (at the time of compounding only).
   *In some cases, the calculated PPN rate may be greater than maintenance fluid requirements or greater than what the animal can tolerate (e.g., cardiac disease).
   *The monitoring required will depend on the individual patient. However, at least the following should be measured daily:
      *Heart/respiratory rate
      *Catheter site
      *Attitude
      *Body weight
      *Temperature
      *Glucose, total solids (check hematocrit tubes for lipemia)
      *Electrolytes should be monitored at least every other day

Box 25-6   Calculation of Osmolarity of Parenteral Nutrition Admixture

[(mL of amino acids × osmolarity of amino acid solution) + (mL of dextrose × osmolarity of dextrose solution) + (mL of lipid × osmolarity of lipid solution) + (mL of additional fluids × osmolarity of fluids)] ÷ total volume of parenteral nutrition

dextrose or lipid content). Parenteral nutrition admixtures should never be frozen, and any unused portions should be discarded (i.e., not saved for use at a later time or in another patient).

Initiating Parenteral Nutrition

The worksheets in this chapter provide an admixture that is intended to last 24 hours when administered at a constant-rate infusion. Bags of parenteral nutrition admixtures should not be at room temperature for more than 24 hours. The bag should be administered during the 24-hour period via a fluid infusion pump (Fig. 25-7). During this time, the lines should not be disconnected from the bag or the patient (i.e., it should remain a closed system). When taking dogs outside, either the pump should accompany the dog or the bag can be removed from the pump (if this does not disconnect the lines from the bag or the patient) and carried along. In the latter situation, one must be careful to allow the parenteral nutrition to continue to drip slowly (i.e., avoid clamping it off completely but ensure that it is not administered at a faster than desired rate during this time) and keep the drip chamber upright. At the end of each 24-hour period, the infusion should be complete, and the empty bag, along with the lines, can be changed using aseptic technique and a new bag and lines substi-

tuted. In our hospital, all parenteral nutrition is administered through a 1.2-μm in-line filter (extension set with 1.2-μm downstream filter, Baxter Healthcare Corporation), but not all hospitals use these. The filter can help to prevent lipid globules or precipitates (particularly calcium phosphate) from being introduced to the patient.[3,36] Because of the high osmolarity of the TPN solution, it must be administered through a central venous (jugular) catheter. PPN (as formulated using the worksheet in this chapter) can be administered through a peripheral or jugular catheter, but because it is more dilute, it can only provide a portion of the patient's energy requirements.

TPN should be instituted gradually over 48 to 72 hours. Most animals tolerate receiving 50% of total requirements on the first day and 100% on the second day. Animals that have been without food for long periods may require slower introduction (i.e., 33% on the first day, 66% on the second day, and 100% on the third day). PPN does not require gradual introduction and can be initiated at 100% on the first day. It is important to adjust the animal's other intravenous fluids when initiating parenteral nutritional support to avoid fluid volume overload.

Potential Complications

A number of possible complications can be associated with parenteral nutrition, and these generally are grouped

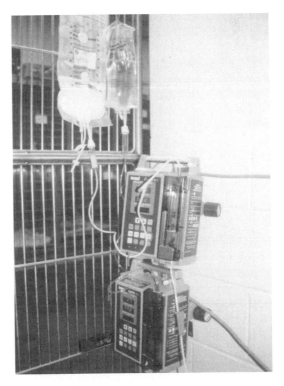

Fig. 25-7 Parenteral nutrition should be infused over a 24-hour period by continuous-rate infusion via a fluid pump.

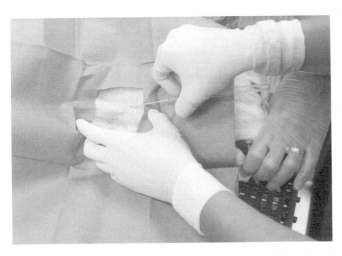

Fig. 25-6 The catheter for parenteral nutrition should be placed with aseptic technique and should be a dedicated catheter.

into one of three categories (Box 25-7). Metabolic complications are the most common, with hyperglycemia typically seen most frequently.[13,31,45] Electrolyte disturbances can develop either after instituting nutritional support or may worsen in animals with preexisting abnormalities. Refeeding syndrome is uncommon in companion animals but can be difficult to manage when it occurs.[26] Refeeding syndrome refers to a potentially fatal complication secondary to nutritional management of severely malnourished patients.[17,40,47] It includes the development of hypophosphatemia with or without hypokalemia, hypomagnesemia, thiamine deficiency, and fluid shifts.[17,48] It can develop when nutritional support, either parenteral or enteral, is initiated in a severely malnourished animal (particularly those that have not eaten for a prolonged period). The glucose provided stimulates insulin secretion that drives extracellular ions (e.g., phosphorus, potassium, magnesium) intracellularly and stimulates protein synthesis. The result may be clinically significant hypophosphatemia, hypokalemia, and hypomagnesemia. The shift to carbohydrate metabolism increases demands for important cofactors such as thiamine, which may already be depleted in malnourished patients, and neurological manifestations of thiamine deficiency may occur.[17,40,48] Congestive heart failure also can occur secondary to fluid shifts. It is important, particularly in animals with prolonged anorexia, to initiate parenteral nutrition slowly, to supplement vitamins (particularly thiamine), and to monitor serum electrolytes for the first 3 to 4 days after initiation.

The most important factor in reducing the risk of mechanical and septic complications is prevention protocols. Careful attention to catheter placement and catheter and line care will reduce the risk of problems. Placement of catheters by experienced personnel has been shown to reduce mechanical and septic complications.[31,41] Elizabethan collars should be used for any animal that shows a propensity to chew lines. Creative solutions may be needed for animals that circle in the cage or are otherwise fractious. Protocols for catheter placement, handling catheters and line with aseptic technique, and maintaining dedicated catheters also are beneficial in minimizing the incidence of sepsis. If clinical evidence of sepsis does develop, conventional recommendations include submission of the parenteral nutrition admixture and the catheter tip for bacteriologic cultures. Often, sepsis develops as a result of the underlying disease rather than being related to parenteral nutrition. However, another indirect link exists between sepsis and parenteral nutrition. An increased risk for bacterial translocation is present because villous atrophy occurs when an animal is fed parenterally (i.e., when the animal is not receiving any nutrients via the enteral route). This factor is another argument for reinstituting oral or enteral nutrition as soon as possible in animals receiving parenteral nutrition.

Box 25-7 — Potential Complications of Parenteral Nutrition

Mechanical
Line breakage
Chewed lines
Disconnected lines
Perivascular infiltration
Catheter occlusion
Phlebitis
Thrombosis

How to Reduce the Risk:
Aseptic placement of catheter
Aseptic handling of catheter and lines
Use Elizabethan collars for animals that try to chew lines
Change bandage and check catheter site daily for swelling, erythema, malpositioning of catheter

Metabolic
Hyperglycemia
Hypoglycemia (most common when discontinuing parenteral nutrition)
Hyper/hypokalemia
Hyper/hypochloremia
Hyper/hyponatremia
Hyper/hypophosphatemia
Hyper/hypomagnesemia
Hyperbilirubinemia
Hyperammonemia
Hypertriglyceridemia
Hypercholesterolemia
Refeeding syndrome (i.e., hypophosphatemia with or without hypokalemia and hypomagnesemia)

How to Reduce the Risk:
Use a conservative estimate (RER) for calculation of calorie requirements
Initiate TPN gradually
Monitor glucose and electrolytes daily

Septic (Clinical Signs of Sepsis in Conjunction with a Positive Catheter Tip or Blood Culture)
How to Reduce the Risk:
Maintain a dedicated catheter
Catheter composed of materials of low thrombogenicity
Placing catheters, handling catheters and lines with aseptic technique
Changing catheters at prescribed time
Monitor body temperature, catheter site, general attitude
If sepsis is suspected, parenteral nutrition solution and catheter tip should be cultured

---

The other critical aspect in reducing the risk of complications is vigilant monitoring. Checking the catheter site daily can identify malpositioning of the catheter and phlebitis or cellulitis early, before serious problems develop. Body weight should be monitored daily in animals receiving parenteral nutrition. Fluid shifts also can explain rapid changes in weight during hospitalization, emphasizing the need for continued nutritional assessment. Use of the RER as the patient's caloric requirement is merely a starting point. The number of calories provided may need to be increased to prevent weight loss or to keep up with the patient's changing needs. To avoid complications with parenteral nutrition, the patient should be monitored carefully and frequently. Body temperature, heart rate, and respiratory rate should be recorded several times a day. Metabolic complications can occur frequently in animals receiving parenteral nutrition, and monitoring is crucial to detect and address them early, if necessary. The clinical situation should dictate the frequency and spectrum of monitoring required because some patients will need more intensive monitoring. Each case is individual, and good clinical judgment is imperative. In animals receiving parenteral nutrition, the authors recommend that general attitude, body weight, temperature, blood glucose concentration, total solids (check the serum for gross lipemia or hemolysis), and serum electrolyte concentrations should be assessed daily or more frequently if indicated. Other variables that may require monitoring include ammonia (for animals that are at risk of developing hepatic encephalopathy), triglycerides (for those with gross lipemia), and bilirubin. The development of metabolic abnormalities usually does not require discontinuation of parenteral nutrition but may require reformulation (e.g., a reduction in the lipid content for animals that develop hypertriglyceridemia). Box 25-7 lists the methods that can be used to reduce the risk of the common complications. Other variables to monitor include gastrointestinal signs and appetite so that enteral nutrition or oral intake can be initiated as soon as possible. Finally, the overall nutritional plan should be reassessed on a regular basis so that it can be adjusted to meet the animal's changing needs. For example, an animal receiving PPN for 3 days may need to be switched to TPN if its underlying disease has not resolved, or a small amount of enteral nutrition can be introduced in conjunction with PPN if tolerated.

Discontinuing Parenteral Nutrition

Transitioning to oral intake or enteral nutrition should be done as soon as possible to avoid the problem of gut atrophy that is associated with lack of oral intake. In veterinary medicine, parenteral nutrition typically is administered for less than 1 week. However, it is important to ensure that the patient is tolerating oral intake or enteral nutrition and is ingesting sufficient amounts (at least 50% of RER) before discontinuing parenteral nutrition. Once the patient is able to eat, it should be offered food regularly to assess its appetite, or a feeding tube should be placed if the animal is anorectic. When the animal is voluntarily consuming or enterally receiving at least 50% of RER, TPN

can be gradually decreased over a period of 4 to 8 hours (while monitoring blood glucose concentration). To accomplish this withdrawal, TPN is administered at half the calculated rate for 4 to 8 hours and then discontinued completely. If TPN is discontinued abruptly, there is a small risk of rebound hypoglycemia. PPN can be discontinued abruptly without this gradual decrease.

How To Obtain Parenteral Nutrition

To compound the parenteral nutrient admixtures (dextrose, amino acid, and lipid) calculated using the TPN and PPN worksheets provided in this chapter, there are a number of different options. One option is an automated compounder, which provides quick and accurate mixing. However, these compounders are expensive and usually are not cost-effective unless parenteral nutrition is used frequently. A second option for compounding parenteral nutrition solutions manually is using a "3-in-1" bag (Empty 3-in-1 mixing container with attached 3-lead transfer set, Abbott Laboratories; All-in-One Container for gravity transfer, Baxter Healthcare Corporation). These bags have three attached leads that can be connected using aseptic technique to bags of dextrose, amino acids, and lipids, respectively. The components then are added to the recipient bag in a closed system by gravity. Like the automated compounder, these bags require a knowledgeable person to perform the compounding, a very clean environment, and good aseptic technique. Many hospitals that do not use parenteral nutrition frequently do not find this method to be time- or cost-effective. Alternatives include making arrangements with a large veterinary referral hospital that compounds parenteral nutrition or with a human hospital in the community. Another solution that has worked very well for many veterinary hospitals is to make arrangements with a human home health care company. These companies compound parenteral nutrition for human patients who often are receiving it for many years in their homes. A formula can be provided to the company, and the solution can be delivered to the veterinary hospital within a short time period. In many cases, this approach works out to be more cost-(and time-) effective than compounding parenteral nutrition in an individual veterinary hospital.

FUTURE GOALS

Parenteral nutrition can now be safely provided to hospitalized dogs and cats, and it is an important part of their optimal care. Future directions in parenteral nutrition research include developing species-specific amino acid solutions rather than being limited to preparations designed for humans, and determining the optimal proportions of nutrients for critically ill animals. Nutritional pharmacology, such as the use of glutamine, n-3 fatty acids, or antioxidants also may prove to be beneficial. One of the most exciting areas of research in human critical care medicine is stricter control of blood glucose concentrations. Critically ill cats respond similarly in terms of glucose regulation to critically ill people, and more careful control of blood glucose concentrations also may have similar benefits in companion animals.[14] Finally, efficacy studies continue to be performed in human medicine to determine the patients most likely to benefit from parenteral nutrition and those most likely to have complications. Similar types of studies are needed in veterinary patients to most effectively use this exciting nutritional support modality and to most successfully care for our hospitalized patients.

REFERENCES

1. Abood SK, Mauterer JV, et al: Nutritional support of hospitalized patients. In Slatter D, editor: *Textbook of small animal surgery*, ed 2, Philadelphia, 1993, WB Saunders, pp. 63-83.
2. Adal KA, Farr BM: Central venous catheter-related infection: a review. *Nutrition* 12:208-213, 1996.
3. Ball PA: Intravenous in-line filters: filtering the evidence, *Curr Opin Clin Nutr Metab Care* 6:319-325, 2003.
4. Barton RG: Nutrition support in critical illness, *Nutr Clin Pract* 9:127-139, 1994.
5. Biffl WL, Moore EE, Haenel JB, et al: Nutritional support of the trauma patient, *Nutrition* 18:960-965, 2002.
6. Bjornson HS, Colley R, Bowen RH, et al: Association between microorganism growth at the catheter insertion site and colonization of the catheter in patients receiving total parenteral nutrition, *Surgery* 92:720-727, 1982.
7. Braunschweig CL, Levy P, Sheean PM, et al: Enteral compared with parenteral nutrition: a meta-analysis, *Am J Clin Nutr* 74: 534-542, 2001.
8. Buffington T, Holloway C, Abood A: Clinical dietetics. In Buffington T, Holloway C, Abood S, editors: *Manual of veterinary dietetics*, St. Louis, 2004, WB Saunders, pp. 49-141.
9. Burkholder WJ: Metabolic rates and nutrient requirements of sick dogs and cats, *J Am Vet Med Assoc* 206:614-618, 1995.
10. Butterworth CE: Skeleton in the hospital closet, *Nutr Today* 9:4, 1976.
11. Carter JM, Freedman AB: Total intravenous feeding in the dog, *J Am Vet Med Assoc* 171:71-76, 1977.
12. Chan DL: Nutritional requirements of the critically ill patient, *Clin Tech Small Anim Pract* 19:1-5, 2004.
13. Chan DL, Freeman LM, Labato MA, et al: Retrospective evaluation of partial parenteral nutrition in dogs and cats, *J Vet Intern Med* 16:440-445, 2002.
14. Chan DL, Freeman LM, Rozanski EA, et al: Alterations in carbohydrate metabolism in critically ill cats, *J Vet Emerg Crit Care* (In Press).
15. Chandler ML, Guilford WG, Maxwell A, et al: A pilot study of protein sparing in healthy dogs using peripheral parenteral nutrition, *Res Vet Sci* 69:47-52, 2000.
16. Crabb SE, Chan DL, Freeman LM: Retrospective evaluation of total parenteral nutrition in cats: 40 cases (1991–2003), *J Vet Emerg Crit Care* (In Press).
17. Crook MA, Hally V, Pantelli JV: The importance of the refeeding syndrome, *Nutrition* 17:632-637, 2001.
18. Detsky AS, Baker JP, O'Rourke K, et al: Perioperative parenteral nutrition: a meta-analysis, *Ann Intern Med* 107:195-203, 1987.
19. Dudrick SJ, Wilmore DW, Vars HM, et al: Long-term total parenteral nutrition with growth, development, and positive nitrogen balance, *Surgery* 64:134-142, 1968.
20. Finney SJ, Zekveld C, Elia A, et al: Glucose control and mortality in critically ill patients, *JAMA* 290:2041-2047, 2003.
21. Freeman LM, Chan DL: Parenteral and enteral nutrition, *Compend Stand Care Emerg Crit Care* 3:1-7, 2001.
22. Hamawy KJ, Moldawer LL, Geogieff M, et al: The effect of lipid emulsions on reticuloendothelial system function in the injured animal, *JPEN J Parenter Enteral Nutr* 9:559-565, 1985.
23. Heyland DK, MacDonald S, Keefe L, et al: Total parenteral nutrition in the critically ill patient: a meta-analysis, *JAMA* 280:2013-2019, 1998.
24. Hill SE, Heldman LS, Goo EDH, et al: Fatal microvascular pulmonary emboli from precipitation of a total nutrient admixture solution, *JPEN J Parenter Enteral Nutr* 20:81-87, 1996.
25. Jarstrand C, Berghem L, Lahnborg G: Human granulocyte and reticuloendothelial system function during Intralipid infusion, *JPEN J Parenter Enteral Nutr* 2:663-670, 1978.
26. Justin RB, Hohenhaus AE: Hypophosphatemia associated with enteral alimentation in cats, *J Vet Intern Med* 9:228-233, 1995.
27. Kinney JM: History of parenteral nutrition, with notes on clinical biology. In Rombeau JL, Rolandell RH, editors: *Clinical nutrition: parenteral nutrition*, Philadelphia, 2001, WB Saunders, pp. 1-20.
28. Lennon C, Davidson KW, Sadowski JA, et al: The vitamin K content of intravenous lipid emulsions, *JPEN J Parenter Enteral Nutr* 17:142-144, 1993.
29. Lippert AC: The metabolic response to injury: enteral and parenteral nutritional support. In Murtaugh RJ, Kaplan PM, editors: *Veterinary emergency and critical care medicine,* St. Louis, 1992, Mosby Yearbook, pp. 593-617.
30. Lippert AC, Faulkner JE, Evans AT, et al: Total parenteral nutrition in clinically normal cats, *J Am Vet Med Assoc* 194: 669-676, 1989.
31. Lippert AC, Fulton RB, Parr AM: A retrospective study of the use of total parenteral nutrition in dogs and cats, *J Vet Intern Med* 7:52-64, 1993.
32. Lutomski DM, Palascak JE, Bower RH: Warfarin resistance associated with intravenous lipid administration, *JPEN J Parenter Enteral Nutr* 11:316-318, 1987.
33. Marks SL: Enteral and parenteral nutritional support. In Ettinger SJ, Feldman ED, editors: *Textbook of veterinary internal medicine*, ed 5, Philadelphia, 2000, WB Saunders pp. 275-283.
34. Mauldin GE, Reynolds AJ, Mauldin GN, et al: Nitrogen balance in clinically normal dogs receiving parenteral nutrition solutions, *Am J Vet Res* 62:912-920, 2001.
35. McGee DC, Gould MK: Preventing complications of central venous catheterization, *N Engl J Med* 348:1123-1133, 2003.
36. McKinnon BT: FDA safety alert: hazards of precipitation associated with parenteral nutrition, *Nutr Clin Pract* 11:59-65, 1996.
37. Michel KE: Interventional nutrition for the critical care patient: optimal diets, *Clin Tech Small Animal Pract* 13:204-210, 1998.
38. Michel KE: Prognostic value of clinical nutritional assessment in canine patients, *J Vet Emerg Crit Care* 3:96-104, 1993.
39. Michel KE, Higgins C: Nutrient-drug interactions in nutritional support, *J Vet Emerg Crit Care* 12:163-168, 2002.

40. Miller CC, Bartges JW: Refeeding syndrome. In Bonagura JD, editor: *Current veterinary therapy XIII,* Philadelphia, 2000, WB Saunders, pp. 87-89.

41. O'Grady NP, Alexander M, Dellinger EP, et al: Guidelines for the prevention of intravascular catheter-related infections, *Infect Control Hosp Epidemiol* 23:759-769, 2002.

42. O'Toole E, Miller CW, Wilson BA, et al: Comparison of the standard predictive equation for calculation of resting energy expenditure with indirect calorimetry in hospitalized and healthy dogs, *J Am Vet Med Assoc* 255:58-64, 2004.

43. Pyle SC, Marks SL, Kass PH: Evaluation of complications and prognostic factors associated with administration of total parenteral nutrition in cats: 75 cases (1994-2001), *J Am Vet Med Assoc* 225:242-250, 2004.

44. Remillard RL: Parenteral nutrition. In DiBartola SP, editor: *Fluid therapy in small animal practice,* ed 2, Philadelphia, 2000, WB Saunders, pp. 465-482.

45. Remillard RL, Armstrong PJ, Davenport DJ: Assisted feeding in hospitalized patients: enteral and parenteral nutrition. In Hand MS, Thatcher CD, Remillard RL, et al, editors: *Small animal clinical nutrition,* ed 3, Philadelphia, 2000, WB Saunders, pp. 351-399.

46. Reuter JD, Marks SL, Rogers QR, et al: Use of total parenteral nutrition in dogs: 209 cases (1988-1995), *J Vet Emerg Crit Care* 8:201-213, 1998.

47. Rosmarin DK, Wardlaw GM, Mirtallo J: Hyperglycemia associated with high, continuous infusion rates of total parenteral nutrition dextrose, *Nutr Clin Pract* 11:151-156, 1996.

48. Solomon SM, Kirby DF: The refeeding syndrome: a review, *JPEN J Parenter Enteral Nutr* 14:90-97, 1990.

49. Trissel LA, Gilbert DL, Martinez JF, et al: Compatibility of medications with 3-in-1 parenteral nutrition admixtures, *JPEN J Parenter Enteral Nutr* 23:67-74, 1999.

50. van den Berghe G, Wouters P, Weekers F, et al: Intensive insulin therapy in the critically ill patients, *N Engl J Med* 8:1359-1367, 2001.

51. Veterans Affairs Total Parenteral Nutrition Cooperative Study Group: Perioperative total parenteral nutrition in surgical patients, *N Engl J Med* 325:525-532, 1991.

52. Vinnars E, Wilmore D: History of parenteral nutrition, *JPEN J Parenter Enteral Nutr* 27:225-231, 2003.

53. Waddell LS, Michel KE: Critical care nutrition: routes of feeding, *Clin Tech Small Anim Pract* 13:197-203, 1998.

54. Walton RS, Wingfield WE, Ogilvie GK: Energy expenditure in 104 postoperative and traumatically injured dogs with indirect calorimetry, *J Vet Emerg Crit Care* 6:71-79, 1998.

55. Zsombor-Murray E, Freeman LM: Peripheral parenteral nutrition, *Compend Contin Educ Pract Vet* 21:512-523, 1999.

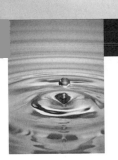

CHAPTER · 26

ENTERAL NUTRITION

Sarah K. Abood, Mary A. McLoughlin, and C.A. Tony Buffington

NUTRITIONAL ASSESSMENT

Identification of patients needing nutritional support requires a thorough history, physical examination, and evaluation of laboratory data. A diet history should be taken to ascertain the quality, total daily intake, and appropriateness of the diet fed (Fig. 26-1). Clients also should be asked about any current drugs the animal may have been prescribed (e.g., corticosteroids, antibiotics, diuretics, cancer chemotherapeutic agents) because these drugs affect nutritional homeostasis. Historical information suggestive of malnutrition includes rapid weight loss (>10% of usual body weight), recent surgery or trauma, and increased nutrient losses from wounds, vomiting, diarrhea, or burns. Infection, trauma, burns, and surgery can increase nutrient needs, whereas prolonged use of antinutrient or catabolic drugs may result in nutrient depletion.

Physical evaluation begins with the assignment of a body condition score,[24] ranging from 1 (cachexic) to 5

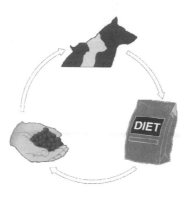

Date:_____

Weight (lb):

Current_____ Usual_____

History taken by:_____

Reason for today's visit:_____

Body condition score (1-5)_____

I. Pet Information

Pet name:_____

Breed:_____   Age:_____

Spayed or neutered? _____

Pet's activity level (type, duration, frequency):_____

Current or past diseases or problems:_____

Current medications:_____

Most recent thyroid level check:_____

How is pet's appetite? _____

Estimated energy needs (see chart):_____

Species:_____

Sex:_____

II. Diet Information

The following descriptions should be sufficiently specific that a member of the practice could go to a store and purchase the food described.

Food Fed (Brand Name; Dry or Canned?)	How Much Is Fed? (What Is the Size of the Cup or Can Used?)	How Often Is the Food Fed? (Is It Fed on a Free-Choice Basis? How Many Meals per Day?)	Calories per Day
Usual			
Recent (since when?)			
		Total calories per day:_____	

What Type of Treats or Table Food Is Fed Each Day? What Is Brand Name of Treat or Special Food?	How Much?	How Often?	Calories Per Day
Pet treats: Size S, M, L, XL			

Rawhides, pig ears, etc.
_____

Table food (be specific):
_____

Breakfast
_____

Lunch
_____

Dinner
_____

Between meals
_____

Food covering medication
_____

Additives to pet food for flavoring (e.g., gravy, broth)
_____

Vitamins or supplements
_____

Total calories per day:_____

III. Owner and Environmental Information
Who feeds the animal?_____
On average, how many hours a day is the pet home
alone?_____
How many adults and children in the household?_____
How many pets in the household?_____
What types of pets?_____
Where is the pet fed?_____
Does the animal have access to other pets'
food?_____
Is there competition for food?_____
Is more than one animal fed out of each feeding dish?_____
Is the animal prone to getting into the trash?_____
Is the animal contained in a yard or does it have access to the neighborhood?_____

How frequently is the animal boarded or in the care of someone else?_____

IV. Current Protein Intake Minimum Requirements
Dogs: 2 g per kilogram (lean body mass)
Cats: 4 g per kilogram (lean body mass)

Protein evaluation
1. Calculate protein needs of animal by multiplying minimum protein requirement by the animal's lean body mass.
2. Using information in dietary history, calculate how much protein the animal is currently taking in per day (most food product keys give protein content in grams per 100 kcal).
3. Evaluate protein status and consider a diet with more protein if needed.
   Pet's minimum protein requirement:_____ g/day
   Current protein intake:_____ g/day
   Action taken:_____
   _____

Comments:_____
_____
_____
_____

Fig. 26-1 Diet history form. (From Buffington T, Holloway C, Abood S: *Manual of veterinary dietetics*, St. Louis, 2004, Elsevier.)

(obese), with 3 being normal (Table 26-1). Other scoring systems have been developed for dogs and cats.[36,37] Underweight and malnourished animals often have a body condition score less than 3 of 5 because of loss of muscle mass and subcutaneous fat. Thin, dry skin, hair that is easily epilated, pressure sores, and poor wound

TABLE 26-1 Body Condition Score

Score	Classification	Description
1	Cachexic	Severely underweight, decreased muscle mass, no subcutaneous fat present, skeleton prominent.
2	Thin	Muscle mass adequate, little subcutaneous fat, skeleton apparent but not prominent.
3	Normal	Muscle mass adequate, ribs not seen but easily felt, obvious waist present when viewed from lateral or dorsoventral aspect.
4	Overweight	Individual ribs and spinous processes of vertebrae palpable only with moderate pressure, obvious fat pads present.
5	Obese	Palpation gives feeling of extensive fat cover over body. Large fat pads, respiratory and/or locomotor compromise.

healing may be seen, indicating the body has redirected its nutrient resources to support visceral protein synthesis at the expense of peripheral tissues.

In patients with a body condition score greater than 3 of 5, the possibility that an "overcoat syndrome" has developed must be considered. Because metabolic changes associated with critical illness cause lean body mass to be broken down more quickly than adipose tissue, the body condition may appear normal when an overcoat of adipose tissue is covering a malnourished animal. These patients usually can be recognized by their poor haircoat quality and abnormal bony prominences of the skull.

Many biochemical and hematologic abnormalities may occur during prolonged anorexia,[40] including hypoalbuminemia, lymphopenia, and anemia, but they are not specific "markers of malnutrition." Serum albumin concentration often is decreased in patients secondary to increased permeability of the vascular endothelium, as well as to decreased synthesis (or increased degradation) rates. Serum albumin concentration also is affected by hydration status and the presence of gastrointestinal, hepatic, or renal disease.[34] Malnutrition, stress, or immunosuppressive drugs may cause lymphopenia. Starvation may interfere with immune competence even when the total lymphocyte count remains within the normal range.[14]

The main objective of nutritional assessment is to identify malnutrition as an independent problem. If not present initially, the animal should be periodically reevaluated during hospitalization to ensure that malnutrition does not develop secondary to an ongoing disease process, drug therapy, inability to eat, inappetence, or food deprivation.[11] Nutritional support should be instituted in malnourished patients and in those for which voluntary food intake is impossible for prolonged periods.[2]

NUTRIENT NEEDS

Dogs and cats that are eating require 50 to 100 mL of water per kilogram of body weight for daily maintenance, depending on environmental temperature, type of food, and amount of activity. Water requirements of normal fasting animals are only 5 to 10 mL/kg body weight/day (10% of the requirement of animals that are eating)[49] because the solute load ingested with the diet and ultimately excreted by the kidneys is reduced.[63]

In sick animals, increased water losses via the urine may occur in some settings (e.g., diabetes mellitus, polyuric renal failure, hyperadrenocorticism, hyperthyroidism). Water also is lost in vomitus, diarrhea, burns, or hemorrhage. Insensible water losses (e.g., respiratory, cutaneous, fecal) may account for 20% to 40% of total water loss,[5] and fluid loss by this route increases in the presence of fever, hyperventilation, hypermetabolism, and burn wounds.

TABLE 26-2 Vitamin and Mineral Requirements (per 1000 kcal) of the Young Growing Dog and Cat

Substance	U.S. Recommended Daily Allowance Children (1-3 yr)	Cats	Dogs
Vitamins			
Vitamin A	1320 IU	670 IU	1011 IU
Vitamin D	400 IU	100 IU	110 IU
Vitamin E	6 IU	6 IU	6.1 IU
Vitamin K	15 IU	20 IU	N/A
Thiamin	0.7 mg	1.0 mg	0.28 mg
Riboflavin	0.8 mg	0.8 mg	0.70 mg
Niacin	9.0 mg	8.0 mg	3.1 mg
Pyridoxine	1.0 mg	0.8 mg	0.3 mg
Folate	50 µg	0.16 mg	56 µg
Vitamin B12	0.7 µg	4.0 µg	7.0 µg
Minerals			
Calcium	800 mg	160 mg	1666 mg
Phosphorus	800 mg	120 mg	1246 mg
Magnesium	80 mg	80 mg	115 mg
Zinc	10 mg	10 mg	10 mg
Iron	10 mg	16 mg	9.1 mg
Iodine	70 µg	70 µg	168 µg

N/A, Not available.

Energy needs of anorexic or injured patients are estimated by summing requirements for basal metabolic functions, activity, and the effects of disease. Basal metabolic rate (the energy required for protein turnover and maintenance of ionic gradients across semipermeable membranes) may be estimated by a variety of methods. In kilocalories per day, basal energy has been estimated by both exponential[3] ($97 \times BW_{kg}^{0.655}$ [Fig. 26-2] or $70 \times BW_{kg}^{0.75}$) and linear ($30 \times BW_{kg} + 70$) equations. All of these equations yield similar results for animals weighing between 15 and 30 kg, but exponential equations are considered more accurate for very small and very large patients.[31]

We estimate the energy needs of our patients by assuming that those resting in a hospital cage have basal energy needs, determined from Fig. 26-2. Although sepsis and burn injuries have been found to increase energy expenditure 25% to 35% in dogs,[61] more recent data suggest that the energy needs of resting critically ill, postoperative, and severely traumatized dogs were not higher than the basal needs of healthy animals.[60] Based on these considerations and the risks associated with overfeeding, we determine initial estimates of energy needs on the basal requirement for the current body weight of the animal. Studies in humans suggest that metabolic rates greater than twice the basal requirement rarely occur, even in severely injured patients. In addition, overestimating nutrient needs increases the risk of the patient for problems associated with overfeeding.

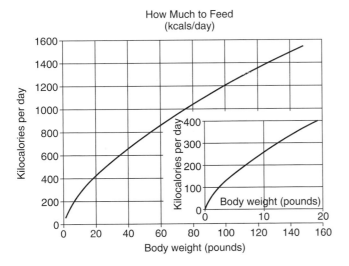

How Much to Feed
(kcals/day)

To meet basal needs: use graph

To meet needs of stress:
1. mild stress   25% increase
2. moderate stress   50% increase
3. severe stress   100% increase

Fig. 26-2 Approximate basal energy needs of dogs and cats. (From Abood SK, Mauterer JV, McLoughlin MA, et al: Nutritional support of hospitalized patients. In Slatter DH, editor: *Textbook of small animal surgery*, ed 2, Philadelphia, 1993, WB Saunders.)

The protein requirements of critically ill patients are not known. The protein requirements of young animals for growth are approximately 17% to 22% of total kilocalories,[51] and we use this guideline as an estimate for patients fed liquid-formula diets containing high-quality protein. Commercial pet foods may have lower protein quality and digestibility. If such diets are fed, higher protein concentrations (25% to 40% of kilocalories) are required. We have used successfully for short periods (<2 weeks) liquid diets containing 17% to 20% of kilocalories as protein in small animal patients with severe chronic renal failure and have not found further restriction to be necessary. Patients with protein-losing diseases (e.g., protein-losing enteropathy or nephropathy) should have their estimated losses replaced. Protein losses by patients with protein-losing nephropathy are small relative to daily needs.[13] In contrast, burned patients may lose clinically relevant amounts of protein and should be provided higher percentages of kilocalories as protein.[42]

Hospitalized patients also require essential fatty acids, minerals, and vitamins. Specific vitamin and mineral needs depend on the type and severity of the underlying disease process. For short-term nutritional supplementation, at least sodium, chloride, potassium, phosphate, calcium, and magnesium should be provided. Provision of supplemental zinc should also be considered, especially in anorexic patients with gastrointestinal disease, where losses may be increased.[62] Zinc also is important because of its role in protein synthesis, immune function, in vitro phagocytic activity, and taste and smell.[48] Liquid enteral diets for nutritional support contain all of the necessary minerals, and additional supplementation probably is not warranted. No studies have specifically evaluated the needs of veterinary patients for these nutrients. At present, provision of vitamins at or near the National Research Council requirements for growth seems reasonable in the absence of any specific contraindication.[45]

APPETITE STIMULATION

The primary objective of nutritional support is to reestablish voluntary food intake. When invasive techniques of nutritional support are necessary, they should only be used until the animal will eat voluntarily. Food must be offered regularly to evaluate appetite; it is impossible to tell whether an animal will eat unless it is "asked." Food intake of hospitalized patients should be measured with a food scale. Electronic scales that weigh to the nearest gram are inexpensive and allow the food and its container to be weighed in and out of the cage.

Dry pet foods contain approximately 350 kcal/8 oz, and canned foods contain approximately 1 kcal/g. To estimate the adequacy of food intake, multiply the caloric density of the food by the amount eaten. If the result is less than two thirds of the goal intake, more intensive nutritional support is necessary.

Nursing techniques to improve and encourage food intake are the simplest methods of nutritional support. If it is possible for owners to bring food from home and feed the patient out of its cage, this practice should be encouraged. Petting and vocal reassurance when food is offered may induce some animals to begin eating again. Warming food to body temperature to enhance aroma or changing the type of food offered may help. If the animal's nasal passages are occluded by exudate, cleaning them with warm water or saline may improve olfaction.

When introducing a new food to ill patients, care should be taken to minimize the possibility of creating a learned aversion. A **learned aversion** is the association of an adverse stimulus with a novel diet, so that when the animal is offered the diet again, it associates the food with feelings of ill health and refuses to eat it. If instituting a particular diet as part of long-term patient treatment, it should not be introduced during hospitalization if at all possible. Introducing the diet when the animal is feeling better, so that it associates a feeling of well-being with the new food, increases the probability of success.

Learned aversions in veterinary patients have not been studied in any systematic way, but they may occur. In fact, such aversions may be one reason some veterinary therapeutic diets are difficult to institute in sick animals. A variety of chemicals have been used to stimulate appetite. Two commonly recommended pharmacologic agents are B vitamins and appetite-stimulating drugs. There is no evidence that administration of any of the individual B vitamins or combinations of them stimulates food intake in sick dogs or cats. Sick animals may have vitamin deficits, but they also have energy and other nutrient deficits that must be addressed simultaneously if nutritional support is to be effective.

Drugs used to stimulate appetite include the benzodiazepine derivatives oxazepam (Serax, Wyeth, Madison, NJ) and diazepam (Valium, Roche, Basel, Switzerland) and the antiserotonergic agent cyproheptadine (Periactin, Merck, Whitehouse Station, NJ).[43] Benzodiazepines are effective appetite stimulants in healthy dogs and cats.[21] No controlled studies are available in veterinary patients for any of these compounds, which appear to be more effective for psychogenic than for pathologic anorexia. Psychogenic, or fear-induced, anorexia is common in hospitalized dogs and cats because of the strange surroundings, the stress of disease and trauma, and the unfamiliar humans caring for them. Administration of 0.2 mg/kg body weight of diazepam intravenously or 2.5 mg/cat/feeding of oxazepam orally has been recommended to stimulate food intake in these settings.[43] The recommended dosage of cyproheptadine for cats is 2 mg orally two to three times daily. Although sometimes effective for psychogenic anorexia, these drugs do not appear to be effective for pathologic, disease-induced anorexia. Moreover, their sedative effects are undesirable in depressed animals, and they are contraindicated in patients with liver disease.[58]

Other drugs, including glucocorticoids (0.25 to 0.5 mg/kg body weight every other day) and the anabolic steroids nandrolone decanoate (5 mg/kg, or maximal dosage of 200 mg/patient/week intramuscularly) and stanozolol (1 to 2 mg twice daily orally or 25 to 50 mg intramuscularly) also have been recommended to stimulate appetite.[43] Megestrol acetate, formally advocated because one of its many side effects is increased appetite, should **not** be given to cats to stimulate food intake because of the risk of induction of diabetes mellitus, hyperlipidemia, adrenal suppression, and mammary neoplasia.[6,52] Although any of these drugs may be effective in isolated patients, none have been tested in controlled trials in veterinary medicine, and none have been demonstrated to be of consistent value.

The greatest danger of pharmacologic appetite stimulation is that its use may give the false impression that adequate nutritional support is being provided. These drugs often stimulate animals to eat small meals immediately,[43] and the clinician may conclude that food intake is adequate. Unless the total quantity of food eaten is measured, however, it cannot be determined whether the animal continues to eat during the remainder of the 24-hour period. Use of these drugs should be restricted to animals in which food intake is being measured because of the inconsistent response to their use and the probability of delay of appropriate nutritional support.

SYRINGE-FEEDING

If all attempts to induce the animal to eat voluntarily fail, it may be syringe-fed for 1 or 2 days. Syringe-feeding provides some nutrition, but the stress imposed on the patient during feeding may limit the effectiveness of this technique. A convenient method of syringe-feeding is to cut off the end of a disposable syringe and cut a core of food from a can of pet food. The syringe plunger is then used to force the food into the animal's mouth.

Patients also may be fed by passing a tube through the mouth or nose into the stomach for each feeding. To pass an orogastric feeding tube,[16,57] first measure the distance from the mouth to the tenth rib, and mark the tube with a piece of tape. Hold the animal's head, insert a mouth gag (a roll of adhesive tape works well), and close the mouth around it. Lubricate the end of the tube with a water-soluble lubricant. Pass the tube through the mouth gag and into the pharynx. Hold the animal's head at the normal angle of articulation to minimize the possibility of endotracheal intubation. When the animal swallows, advance the tube into the esophagus to the depth of the premeasured mark. Using limited restraint and opening the mouth just far enough to introduce the tube minimizes the animal's objection to the procedure.

The equipment required for orogastric intubation of large dogs consists of a double-action rubber bulb connected to the appropriate size and length of red rubber tubing. This type of bulb ensures a continuous forward flow of material. A three-way stopcock connecting a tube from the food container to the feeding tube via a syringe of appropriate size may be used to feed small dogs and cats.

NASOGASTRIC INTUBATION

If the patient is too debilitated to tolerate repeated tube feedings, if feeding must continue for more than 2 or 3 days, or if the disease prevents periodic intubation, a nasogastric tube may be used. Techniques of nasogastric tube intubation are available in the written[1,15,18,25] and video literature[9]; the materials needed for this procedure are listed in Box 26-1. Nasogastric feeding tubes are made in various sizes and lengths, from a variety of materials, and by different manufacturers (Box 26-2). Polyvinyl chloride tubes are inexpensive and work well for intragastric feeding. However, they may harden if left in the stomach for prolonged periods and should be changed approximately every 2 weeks. Polyurethane or silicone tubes are most expensive but are resistant to gastric acid and may be used for prolonged periods. We choose the least expensive tube needed in the largest diameter and longest length that the patient can tolerate comfortably. Large-diameter tubes present less resistance to solution flow, whereas long tubes can be placed into the stomach, secured to the head, and still be attached behind an Elizabethan collar for easy access.

Box 26-1	List of Materials Needed for Nasogastric Tube Placement

1. Nasogastric tube
   a. 5 French, 36″ for cats/small dogs
   b. 8 French, 42″ for dogs >20 lb
   c. 10 French for dogs >75 lb
2. Stylet or guidewire (optional for tubes placed in large dogs)
3. Mineral oil if using stylet or guidewire
4. Topical anesthetic to desensitize nostril
5. KY jelly to lubricate feeding tube
6. Adhesive tape to mark and secure feeding tube
7. Sterile water
8. 6-mL and 12-mL syringes
9. Stethoscope
10. Glue or suture material to secure feeding tube

Box 26-2	Manufacturers of Products for Enteral Nutritional Support

A: Feeding tubes
B: Feeding products
C: Guidewires, placement devices, or placement kits

Abbott Laboratories—Animal Health [A, B, C]
100 Abbott Park Road
Abbott Park, IL 60064-6400
847-937-6100
888-299-7416
http://www.ross.com/productHandbook/devices.asp

Baxter Healthcare (formerly Travenol Labs) [A]
One Baxter Parkway
Deerfield, IL 60015
888-229-0001

C.R. Bard, Inc.
Bard Medical Division [A, C]
8195 Industrial Boulevard
Covington, GA 30014
770-784-6100
800-526-4455

Corpak MedSystems Company [A, B]
100 Chaddick Drive
Wheeling, IL 60090-6006
847-537-4601
800-323-6305
http://www.corpakmedsystems.com/home.asp

Cook Critical Care [A, C]
P.O. Box 489
750 Daniels Way
Bloomington, IN 47402
821-339-2235
800-457-4500

Davol, Inc. [A, C]
100 Sockanossett Crossroad
Cranston, RI 02920
401-463-7000
www.davol.com

Global Veterinary Products (formerly Cook Veterinary Products) [A, C]
19601 West U.S. Highway 12
New Buffalo, MI 49117
269-469-8882
http://www.globalvetproducts.com

Hill's Pet Nutrition [B]
P.O. Box 148
Topeka, KS 66601-0148
800-548-8387
www.hillspet.com

(Continued)

larger dogs because their nasal passages are more tortuous than those of small dogs or cats. One to two drops of mineral oil should be instilled into a feeding tube before introducing the stylet to facilitate easy removal of the stylet after the tube has been passed.

To pass a nasogastric tube, a topical anesthetic is instilled into a nostril (four or five drops of 0.5% proparacaine hydrochloride for cats or 2% lidocaine hydrochloride for dogs). Before passing the tube, measure the distance to the stomach (approximately the caudal margin of the last rib at the level of the costochondral junction), and mark the tube with an adhesive tape "butterfly." With the animal's head held at the normal static angle of articulation to avoid endotracheal intubation, the tube is passed through the nose of the patient by directing it caudomedially, then ventrally and caudally as the nasal planum is pressed upward (Fig. 26-3). Pushing the tip of the nose upward in dogs, as the tube is passed, guides the tube into the ventral meatus.[1] Cats are intubated by passing the tube directly through the ventral meatus without manipulating the nose. In other respects, the technique for cats is similar to that described for dogs.

Once the tube is installed, the stylet (if present) is removed, and the position of the tube in the stomach is confirmed. Placement is assessed by infusion of a small amount of sterile water (3 to 5 mL) through the tube, which should cause the animal to cough or sneeze if the tube is in the respiratory tract. If no reaction occurs, a bolus of air (6 to 12 mL) is injected through the tube while auscultating the cranial abdomen for borborygmus. If uncertainty persists, a lateral thoracic radiograph may be taken after injecting 1 mL of radiopaque dye to confirm the tube's position. Once the position of the tube in the stomach is confirmed, the tape butterfly that was used to mark the distance from the nose to caudal rib is sutured or fixed with cyanoacrylate adhesive (Superglue) just lateral to the nostril (Fig. 26-4). A second butterfly tape tab should be placed and secured to the forehead or lateral maxillary region. An Elizabethan collar is placed to avoid inadvertent tube removal.

For dogs heavier than 10 kg, we use an 8-French (catheter gauge) × 106-cm tube; for smaller dogs and all cats, we use a 5-French × 91-cm tube. Some clinicians prefer 10-French × 106-cm tubes for dogs heavier than 34 kg. A stylet (0.035 cm for 8-French or 10-French feeding tubes) is used to assist passage of the tube into

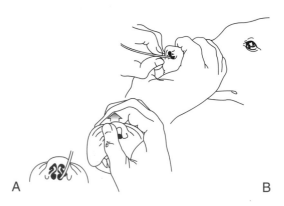

A

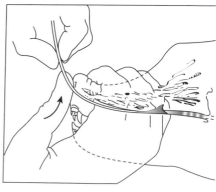

B

Fig. 26-3 Position of head during nasogastric intubations. (From Abood SK, Buffington CA: Improved nasogastric intubation technique for administration of nutritional support in dogs, *J Am Vet Med Assoc* 199:578, 1991.)

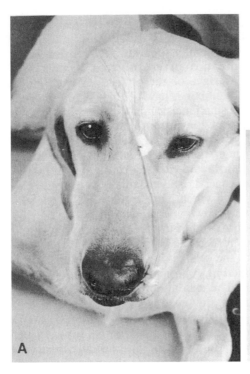
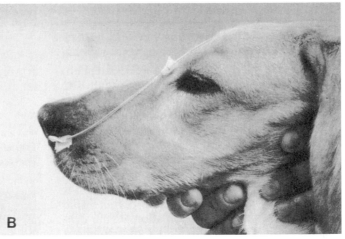

Fig. 26-4 Technique for securing a nasogastric tube. Tube should be secured as close to the nostril as possible. (From Abood SK, Mauterer JV, McLoughlin MA, et al: Nutritional support of hospitalized patients. In Slatter DH, editor: *Textbook of small animal surgery*, ed 2, Philadelphia, 1993, WB Saunders.)

ESOPHAGOSTOMY

The current use of cervical esophagostomy for the placement of a feeding tube in dogs and cats has replaced previously described techniques of pharyngostomy tube placement. Esophagostomy tubes are specifically indicated for patients requiring bypass of the oral cavity or oropharynx as a result of dysphagia, infection, inflammation, neoplasia, fracture, oronasal fistula, surgical procedures, or trauma.[19,50,59] The diameter and length of the esophagostomy tube depend on the size of the patient, type of diet, and personal preference. Silastic tubing or soft red rubber urethral catheters are used commonly as esophagostomy feeding tubes; recommended feeding tube sizes are 12- to 16-French catheters for cats and dogs less than 10 kg and 12- to 20-French catheters for larger dogs. The larger diameter feeding tubes (>14 French) permit feeding of pureed commercial pet foods. The distal end of esophagostomy tubes should **not** be placed through the lower esophageal high-pressure zone into the stomach. Studies have shown that such placement can cause gastroesophageal reflux by disrupting the integrity of this caudal esophageal high-pressure zone.[38,39] Esophageal dysfunction, including abnormal clearing of acid within the distal esophagus, also may occur.[39] In addition, chronic esophageal irritation by refluxed gastric acid may result in esophageal stricture formation. Placing the distal end of the esophagostomy feeding tube in the anterior or mid-thoracic region of the esophagus prevents mechanical disruption of the caudal esophageal high-pressure zone. Secondary peristaltic waves move the food bolus through the remainder of the esophagus into the stomach.

The necessary materials required for this technique are listed in Box 26-3. To place the esophagostomy tube, the patient is anesthetized (with either a short-acting injectable or inhalant anesthetic technique) and placed in right lateral recumbency with the head and neck extended. The hair is clipped from the lateral and ventral

Box 26-3	List of Materials Needed for Esophagostomy Tube Placement

1. Esophagostomy tube (14 French red rubber, silastic, or polyurethane tubing)
2. Injectable or inhalant anesthetic
3. Hair clippers
4. Surgical scrub and alcohol
5. Oral speculum
6. Curved Kelly, right angle, or Carmalt forceps
7. No. 10 (and no. 15) scalpel blades
8. Suture material (3-0) Dermalon

aspects of the neck using the vertical ramus of the mandible, the base of the vertical ear canal, and the caudal edge of the larynx as landmarks. The skin is aseptically prepared for surgery. The mouth is held open by an oral speculum to permit visual examination of the oral cavity and digital palpation of the oropharynx for surgical landmarks and structural abnormalities.

A long curved Carmalt or Mixtner forceps is inserted through the oral cavity and oropharynx into the proximal one third of the esophagus (Fig. 26-5). The instrument is pressed laterally against the esophageal wall to create a visible bulge in the skin along the left lateral aspect of the neck. A 1- to 2-cm incision is made through the skin and subcutaneous tissues directly over the end of the forceps (Fig. 26-6). A no. 15 scalpel blade can be used to make a small incision in the esophageal wall at the tip of the forceps, or gentle pressure can be applied to them to force the tips through the esophageal wall. Care must be taken to avoid the external jugular, linguofacial, and maxillary veins, carotid artery, vagosympathetic trunk, and hypoglossal nerve. The distal end of the feeding tube is grasped by the forceps and drawn through the incision into the oral cavity (Fig. 26-7). A minimum of 10 cm of feeding tube should remain exterior to the skin (Fig. 26-8). The distal end of the feeding tube is gently manipulated into the esophagus by retracting the tongue and extending the end of the tube 180 degrees (Fig. 26-9). The surgeon should palpate the tube to be sure there are no kinks and visually examine the region to confirm that the tube is placed caudal to the pharyngeal region.

Esophagostomy tubes can be maintained for several weeks or months with good nursing care. A small amount of drainage may occur at the incision site; the area should be cleaned and bandaged daily or every other day as needed. Complications associated with esophagostomy feeding tubes may include local infection and swelling or

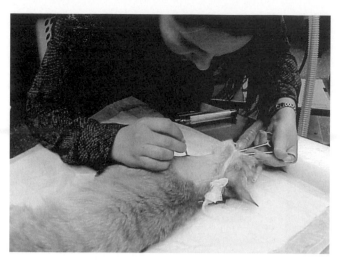

Fig. 26-6 Technique for esophagostomy tube placement. (Photo courtesy of Dr. Andrew Sprecht.)

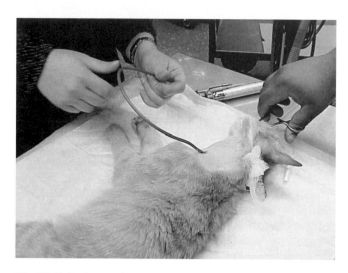

Fig. 26-7 Technique for esophagostomy tube placement. (Photo courtesy of Dr. Andrew Sprecht.)

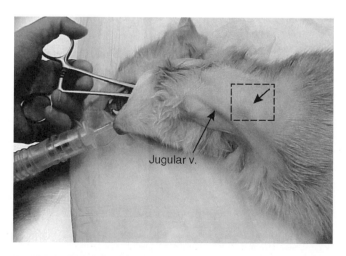

Fig. 26-5 Technique for esophagostomy tube placement. (Photo courtesy of Dr. Andrew Sprecht.)

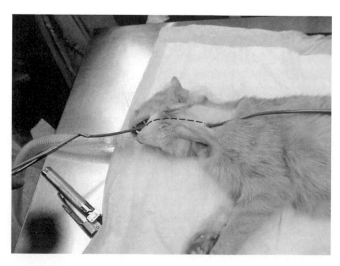

Fig. 26-8 Technique for esophagostomy tube placement. (Photo courtesy of Dr. Andrew Sprecht.)

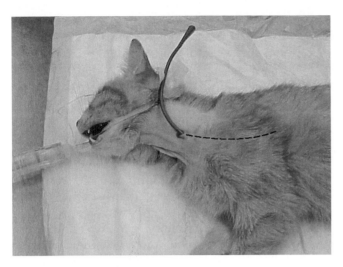

Fig. 26-9 Technique for esophagostomy tube placement. (Photo courtesy of Dr. Andrew Sprecht.)

cellulitis, coughing, and gastroesophageal reflux if the tube is improperly placed; vomiting and aspiration of food if the animal is fed too much food rapidly; esophageal erosion or esophagitis if the tube is too large or left in place too long; and premature displacement or occlusion of the tube if not cared for adequately.[32,41] When tube feeding is no longer necessary, esophagostomy tubes can be removed without sedation and discomfort. The cervical wound is left to heal by second intention.

Esophagostomy feeding tubes offer several advantages over other enterally placed feeding tubes: they require only a single surgical incision to place; they do not require specialized or costly equipment such as an endoscope; they do not require sedation or anesthesia for tube removal; patients tolerate these tubes well; tubes can be left in place for extended periods; and these feeding tubes are easy for clients to manage in the home environment.

SURGICAL GASTROSTOMY

When nutrients cannot be introduced proximal to the stomach in patients with normal gastrointestinal function, gastrostomy tube feeding is an excellent method of temporary or permanent nutritional support.[17,18] Gastrostomy feeding tubes are specifically indicated in patients that are comatose or in those that require bypass of the oral cavity, oral pharynx, larynx, and esophagus as a result of neurologic or neuromuscular diseases, dysphagia, neoplasia, obstruction, inflammation, stricture, or after surgical procedures of the head and neck. Gastrostomy feeding tubes generally are placed through a limited left paracostal laparotomy, which provides excellent exposure to the gastric fundus. They can be placed in conjunction with other abdominal procedures through a ventral midline celiotomy. If an endoscope is available, it may be used to place the gastrostomy tube percutaneously. The patient is anesthetized with a general inhalant anesthetic and placed in right lateral recumbency. Endotracheal intubation is recommended to ensure a patent airway and to prevent aspiration of gastric contents during manipulation of the stomach. The hair is clipped in the left paracostal region from dorsal to ventral midline, and the skin is aseptically prepared for surgery. A 4- to 8-cm curvilinear incision is made in the skin caudal to the last rib and 2 to 4 cm ventral to the paravertebral epaxial muscles.[17]

Care must be taken to ensure that this incision is located ventral enough to enter the peritoneal cavity. The external and internal abdominal oblique and transversus muscles can be separated by blunt dissection or incised with a scalpel blade. The peritoneal cavity is opened, and the greater curvature of the stomach is identified. A small stab incision is made through the abdominal wall, cranial to the celiotomy incision and directly caudal to the last rib or between the last two ribs. The tip of a large-bore, mushroom-tipped Pezzer catheter (14 to 28 French) is passed through this incision into the abdominal cavity. Two stay sutures are placed in the gastric fundus and used to retract the stomach into the celiotomy incision. A relatively avascular area near the greater curvature of the fundic region of the stomach should be chosen, and moistened laparotomy sponges should be used to isolate this region of the stomach for feeding tube placement. Two full-thickness purse-string sutures are placed concentrically through all layers of the gastric wall using a 3-0 synthetic absorbable monofilament suture material. The free ends of the sutures are tagged with forceps. A no. 11 scalpel blade is used to make a small stab incision in the center of the inner purse-string suture. Care must be taken to avoid leakage of gastric contents from this stab incision. The mushroom tip of the catheter is inserted into the gastric lumen, and the inner purse-string suture is gently tightened around the tube and tied, after which the second suture is tightened to minimize leakage around the tube.

The gastrostomy site is secured to the left abdominal wall with approximately four to six synthetic absorbable monofilament sutures placed in a mattress pattern through the seromuscular layer of the stomach and the transversus abdominus muscle of the body wall. The gastropexy suture should be placed as close as possible to the feeding tube. The paracostal incision then is closed in a routine manner. The feeding tube should be capped and fixed to the skin using 3-0 nylon sutures through an adhesive tape butterfly or a 0 nylon antitension suture (Fig. 26-10). The tube then is incorporated into a light abdominal bandage to prevent removal by the patient.

Gastrostomy feeding tubes can be maintained in patients for months with good nursing care. Tubes should remain in place for a minimum of 5 to 7 days, and

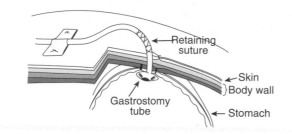

Fig. 26-10 Technique for securing gastrostomy tube. Retaining suture and/or adhesive tape can be used. (Line drawing by Dana Schumacher.)

preferably 14 days, to allow firm adhesions (or a stoma tract) to form between the stomach and peritoneum. Formation of the stoma tract prevents leakage of food or fluid into the peritoneal cavity. If prolonged feeding tube use is indicated, the original mushroom-tipped catheter can be removed and replaced by a low profile tube to improve patient comfort. When the gastrostomy feeding tube is no longer needed, it may be removed with gentle but firm traction and the wound left to heal by second intention.

PERCUTANEOUS ENDOSCOPIC GASTROSTOMY

The patient is anesthetized (with a neuroleptanalgesic or general inhalant anesthetic) and placed in right lateral recumbency. The left paracostal region is clipped, and the skin is aseptically prepared for surgery. An oral speculum is placed in the patient's mouth, and a flexible endoscope, with a biopsy channel, is passed through the mouth and esophagus into the stomach. The stomach is insufflated with air until distension of the left abdominal wall is visible externally. This procedure displaces any abdominal viscera that were located between the stomach and left body wall. The endoscope then is positioned so the illuminated end is located within the stomach directly caudal to the last rib.

A small stab incision is made through the skin at this site. An 18-gauge intravenous cannula with a needle stylet is placed through the skin incision and through the abdominal and gastric walls into the gastric lumen. The endoscope is repositioned within the stomach to visualize and confirm the presence of the cannula. The stylet is removed from the cannula, and the end of a 1-0 or 2-0 piece of suture material is passed through the cannula into the gastric lumen. The length of suture material required can be estimated by measuring from the tip of the animal's nose to the greater trochanter of the femur. The biopsy snare is passed through the biopsy channel of the endoscope and used to grasp the suture material. The biopsy instrument with the suture attached should not be retracted through the biopsy channel of the endoscope. While holding the biopsy snare in a closed posi-

tion to retain the suture material, the entire endoscope is withdrawn from the stomach through the mouth. The cannula then can be removed from the abdominal wall, with care taken not to remove the suture. The suture end exiting from the mouth is passed retrograde through this cannula. An 18-gauge needle is passed through the feeding tube just below the bevel of the catheter, and the suture is passed through the needle and tied securely to the tube (Fig. 26-11).

The gastrostomy tube is stretched and gently manipulated to feed the tapered end into the flared end of the cannula, which guides the feeding tube back through the gastric and abdominal walls. The cannula and feeding tube pass through the mouth, oropharynx, esophagus, and stomach and exit through the gastric and abdominal walls (Fig. 26-12). The cannula is removed, and the gastrostomy tube is gently retracted to pull the internal flange and mushroom tip securely against the gastric

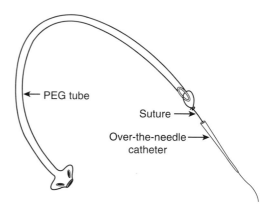

Fig. 26-11 Technique for passing a percutaneous endoscopically guided gastrostomy tube. An 18-gauge needle is passed through the feeding tube just below the bevel of the catheter, and the suture is passed through the needle and tied securely to the tube. (Line drawing by Dana Schumacher.)

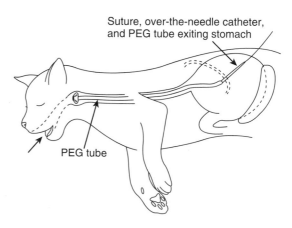

Fig. 26-12 Technique for passing a percutaneous endoscopically guided gastrostomy tube. The cannula and feeding tube pass through the mouth, esophagus, and stomach and exit through the gastric and abdominal walls. (Line drawing by Dana Schumacher.)

mucosa. Replacement of the endoscope into the stomach allows visualization of the positioning of the tube. An external flange can be placed around the feeding tube next to the skin to prevent separation of the stomach from the abdominal wall until a permanent adhesion forms (Fig. 26-13). The remaining end of the tube is capped and fixed to the skin with an antitension suture. A lightweight abdominal bandage or stockinette can be used to protect the exit site from contamination (Fig. 26-14). Complications associated with gastrostomy tubes include leakage around the feeding tube resulting in peritonitis, necrotizing fasciitis, or subcutaneous abscessation.[8,17,18] However, tubes should not be secured very tightly because doing so can cause the same problems secondary to ischemia. Vomiting, regurgitation, gastroesophageal reflux, and aspiration pneumonia also may occur, usually as a consequence of overdistension of the stomach during feeding.

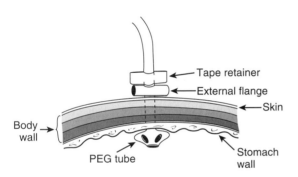

Fig. 26-13 Technique for passing a percutaneous endoscopically guided gastrostomy tube. An external flange can be placed around the feeding tube to prevent separation of the stomach from the abdominal wall. (Line drawing by Dana Schumacher.)

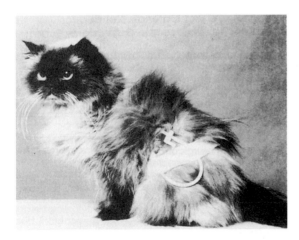

Fig. 26-14 Percutaneous endoscopically guided gastrostomy tube placement: a lightweight bandage or stockinette can be used to protect the tube exit site.

PERCUTANEOUS NONENDOSCOPIC GASTROSTOMY

Methods of blind placement (nonsurgical or nonendoscopic) of gastrostomy tubes in dogs and cats have been reported.[26,44] The technique is similar to that described above for endoscopic gastrostomy tube placement, except that a tube placement device is used instead of an endoscope to guide the suture from the skin through the stomach and esophagus to the oral cavity (Fig. 26-15). Alternative techniques for gastric feeding tube placement were developed for practitioners with limited access to an endoscope and for patients in which abdominal exploration or endoscopy is not indicated as part of case management, yet controlled, postesophageal, nutrition support is indicated. Blind placement of a gastrostomy feeding tube is not indicated for patients with esophageal stricture or other obstruction, primary gastric disease, or gastric outflow obstruction.

Animals may be fed through esophagostomy or gastrostomy tubes soon after they recover from anesthesia. Although the stomach of normal animals serves as a feeding reservoir, prolonged anorexia may decrease gastric capacity or cause gastric atony. Initial feeding volumes of 5 to 10 mL/kg of body weight/feeding (four feedings/day) usually are safe and are increased as tolerance permits. Motility modifiers, such as metoclopramide (0.2 to 0.5 mg/kg orally or subcutaneously, three times a day), may stimulate gastric emptying if atony is present, but the effect is inconsistent. Attempts

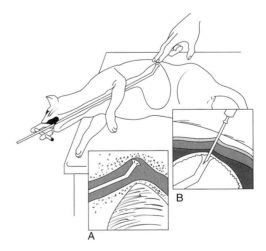

Fig. 26-15 Percutaneous nonendoscopic gastrostomy tube placement. Passage of the placement device with animal in right lateral recumbency. Palpation of the device in the stomach is facilitated by positioning the animal's head over the end of the table and extended. **A,** Tube placement device rotated 90 degrees counterclockwise to pass freely over the base of the heart. **B,** The catheter needle is inserted through the skin into the flared end of the device at a 45-degree angle to parallel the distal end of the device.

to aspirate stomach contents before each feeding should be made. If more than half of the previous meal is recovered, administration of the next meal should be delayed. To avoid occlusion with food or mucus, feeding tubes are flushed with water before and after each feeding and kept securely capped so that water remains in the tube between feedings. The materials required for placement of a percutaneous gastrostomy tube are listed in Box 26-4.

ENTEROSTOMY (DUODENOSTOMY OR JEJUNOSTOMY)

Placement of a feeding tube directly into a segment of the proximal small intestine, such as the descending duodenum or proximal jejunum, using a needle catheter or antimesenteric stab incision has been advocated in small animal patients that cannot be fed more proximally.[22,47,56] Specific indications for use of the enterostomy feeding tubes may include pancreatitis, pancreatic surgery, hepatobiliary surgery, proximal gastrointestinal obstruction, neoplasia, or extensive gastrointestinal surgery. Enterostomy feeding tubes usually are placed during abdominal surgery or through a limited right paracostal approach when prompt return to food intake is doubtful. Small 5-French or 8-French red rubber urethral catheters or silastic infant feeding tubes are typically used. Regardless of the surgical approach, it is essential that enterostomy feeding tubes pass through the right

body wall and enter the small intestine at the level of the descending duodenum or the proximal loop of the jejunum to maximize the absorptive surface of the remaining small intestine. The segment of descending duodenum or proximal loop of jejunum selected for enterostomy tube placement is isolated from the peritoneal cavity with moistened laparotomy sponges. A purse-string suture is placed along the antimesenteric border using a 4-0 synthetic monofilament suture material. A full-thickness stab incision is made through the center of the purse-string using a no. 11 scalpel blade. The distal tip of the enterostomy feeding tube is inserted through the stab incision and advanced aborally approximately 12 to 24 cm. The purse-string suture is tightened around the enterostomy feeding tube, and the enterostomy site is secured to the adjacent right body wall with an interlocking box suture technique using 3-0 or 4-0 synthetic monofilament suture material.[20] Enterostomy feeding tubes should be secured to the skin using an antitension technique and should remain in place long enough (7 to 10 days) to allow adhesion formation. Complications associated with enterostomy feeding tubes include hemorrhage, cellulitis, infection, and leakage around the catheter into the peritoneal cavity or subcutaneous tissues if the tube is not properly installed; premature tube displacement; and colic and diarrhea if patients are not fed properly.[20,22,56] When the tube is no longer necessary, it is removed without sedation by gentle traction.

Some patients are not candidates for enteral nutritional support. Animals that are vomiting uncontrollably or have intractable diarrhea, those with adynamic ileus of the small intestine, intestinal obstruction, or severe mucosal disease, and those that cannot guard their respiratory tract should be fed parenterally (see Chapter 25). Nutritional support also is not indicated for patients with grave prognoses. Although the lives of these patients may be prolonged briefly by intensive nutritional intervention, the quality of life rarely is improved.

Box 26-4	**List of Materials Needed for Percutaneous Endoscopic Gastrostomy Tube Placement**

1. Endoscope
2. Endoscope grasping forceps
3. Bard urological catheter or polyurethane percutaneous endoscopic gastrostomy tube with collapsible bumper
4. 14-gauge peripheral or indwelling catheter or open-end, tom cat catheter
5. Three-way stopcock
6. Braunamid suture (Vetafill) 2-0; approximately 2 ft
7. No. 11 surgical blade
8. 20-gauge, 1-in needles
9. Rubber tubing (1.5 in long)
10. 1-in-wide adhesive tape; approximately 6 in long
11. Scissors
12. Hemostats
13. Bandage material optional; Vet wrap, stockingette, cast padding, or Kling

---

DIETS

Enteral diets for nutritional support should be palatable, easily digested, readily assimilated, efficiently utilized with a minimum of metabolic waste products, and easy to deliver. Box 26-5 presents criteria for selection of an appropriate diet.[53] The ideal oral food for anorexic animals should be so well tolerated by the gastrointestinal mucosa that it can be administered to patients with gastritis, enteritis, or colitis without producing additional irritation. The choice of an appropriate diet for a given patient depends on the route chosen and any disease-related nutrient modifications. Injured or diseased animals should not lose weight while being fed the diet at the recommended dosage. Patients with orogastric or gastrostomy tubes can be fed by measured amounts of an appropriate canned

Box 26-5   Criteria for Selection of Liquid Enteral Diets

A. Categories of enteral diets
  i. Polymeric—Intact macronutrients (protein, fat, carbohydrate) for use in patients with normal or near-normal gastrointestinal function (caloric density is ~1 kcal/mL)
    1. High fat (>50% of kcal)—Caloric density is about 1.5 kcal/mL; use for high energy needs, volume restriction, or diarrhea caused by high (>50% of kcal) carbohydrate products
    2. Fiber containing—Improved feces consistency over high-carbohydrate diets
  ii. Defined-formula diets—Diets specifically modified for use in patients with impaired organ function
    1. Impaired gastrointestinal function (including anorexia for >2 weeks); contains peptides, medium-chain triglyceride, and glucose polymers versus intact macronutrient sources; may cause diarrhea
    2. Impaired liver function—High branched chain/aromatic amino acid content
    3. Impaired kidney function—Supplemented with β-ketoacids of some essential amino acids
    4. "Stress"—High branched chain amino acid content, high caloric density (>1 kcal/mL) efficacy disputed
B. Energy
  i. Total kilocalories
    1. Restricted (<1 kcal/mL) because of obesity or uncontrollable hyperglycemia (rare)
    2. Increased (>1 kcal/mL) because of disease-induced increases in requirements; severe trauma, burns, sepsis, hyperthyroidism
  ii. Carbohydrate
    1. Increased (>50% of kcal) because of diarrhea (high-carbohydrate feedings) or increased energy needs
    2. Decreased (<30% of kcal) because of prolonged anorexia, fat maldigestion, or fat malabsorption
  iii. Triglycerides—long-chain or medium-chain. Long chain for patients with adequate pancreatic and intestinal function; medium chain for patients with severely impaired pancreatic or liver function
C. Protein
  i. Total intake
    1. Restricted (<18% of kcal) because of impaired liver or kidney function
    2. Increased (>22% of kcal) because of increased losses via intestinal tract, draining wounds, trauma
D. Form of diets
  i. Intact—Patients with adequate pancreatic and intestinal function
  ii. Hydrolyzed—Patients unable to tolerate intact protein
E. Specific amino acids for cats
  i. Arginine—recommend 2.5 mg/kcal/day; human enteral formulas should be supplemented with 1 mg/kcal
  ii. Taurine—not necessary for short-term feeding; for long-term feeding the requirement is 0.1 mg/kcal/day
F. Electrolytes—Sodium, potassium, chloride at about 40 mEq/L have been adequate; should be adjusted based on laboratory determinations
G. Minerals and vitamins—Follow National Research Council recommendations in absence of specific information to the contrary
H. Osmolality
  i. Hypoalbuminemia: 250-650 mOsm/kg, depending on severity

food pureed with water in a blender to the desired consistency.

Numerous commercial products are available for enteral support, most falling into one of two groups. The first group includes polymeric diets for use in patients with nearly normal gastrointestinal function. These products contain casein, soy, or egg albumin as protein; medium- or long-chain triglycerides as fat; glucose polymers as carbohydrate; and vitamins and minerals. Nutrients are provided in high molecular weight forms to maintain osmolality at approximately 350 mOsm/kg. These products also are low in lactose and residue.

Defined-formula diets, the other major group, are those modified to accommodate disease-associated limitations on nutrient intake. Peptide and "elemental" diets essentially are predigested forms of the polymeric diets.

Protein is present in the form of peptides or amino acids, and carbohydrates as oligosaccharides or monosaccharides. These products usually are low in fat, and many have a portion of the fat present as medium-chain triglyceride oil to enhance absorption. The osmolality of these solutions may be higher (450 to 850 mOsm/L) than meal replacement formulas because of the inclusion of small molecular weight nutrients. These diets have been recommended for patients with abnormal gastrointestinal function (e.g., severe inflammatory bowel disease or pancreatic insufficiency).[35] Other defined diets have been marketed for impaired hepatic, renal, and respiratory function and for stress. The efficacy of these formulas has not yet been completely established.[53,55]

A third class of enteral product is the feeding module. These products are concentrated sources of one nutrient (i.e., protein, fat, or carbohydrate). Modules may be added to increase specific nutrient concentrations or to reduce required volumes. They also may increase the osmolality of the formulation. In the past, when using a human enteral product, we supplemented diets containing 17% of the kilocalories as protein, with 5 g of protein powder (ProMod, Abbott Labs, Abbott Park, IL) per 8-oz diet for all cats with normal protein needs and for dogs with increased protein needs. Commercial nutritional products for humans are available at large public and hospital pharmacies, or manufacturers may be contacted for local availability. A local nutrition support service dietician also may be of help; these professionals may have nutritional products and delivery apparatus available and possess extensive training and experience in nutritional support.

Table 26-3 presents the nutrient compositions of the liquid enteral products currently used in the Critical Care Unit at Michigan State University and in the Small Animal Intensive Care Unit at The Ohio State University. Other than CliniCare Feline (Abbott Laboratories, Abbott Park, IL), no human enteral product contains adequate arginine for cats. Signs compatible with arginine deficiency have been reported after prolonged feeding of enteral diets designed for humans and those designed specifically for cats. In the absence of data to support other recommendations, we add 1 mg arginine/kcal (~200 to 300 mg/cat/day) to human enteral liquid diets fed to cats. Arginine (as the hydrochloride salt) is readily available at health food stores and at many pharmacies.

RATE AND VOLUME OF FEEDING

Approach the calculated goal for nutrients and fluids over approximately 48 hours to avoid vomiting, abdominal distension or signs of colic, and diarrhea (Box 26-6). Slow rates of administration, particularly in animals that have been inappetent for prolonged periods, avoid the problems of diarrhea and cramping and maximize the uptake of nutrients. Bolus feeding instructions are outlined in Box 26-7. Reservoirs and delivery tubes for feeding solutions are available from a number of manufacturers. Reservoirs containing a 12-hour supply of diet solution can be hung and allowed to drip in by gravity. Using a fluid therapy burette or a gavage set attached to a baby bottle minimizes the possibility of "overdosing" the patient with an excessive volume of feeding solution.

If the animal has been anorexic for more than 72 hours, the volume of the first "meal" (bolus feeding) should be reduced by one half to prevent emesis. In most instances, the second dose can be increased to the total calculated dose, unless anorexia has been prolonged. Most anorexic patients begin voluntary food consump-

tion after the second or third dose. If fluid losses are present, they can be replaced by administration of additional water along with the diet.

PROBLEMS

Mechanical, gastrointestinal, and metabolic problems can occur with enteral tube feeding. Mechanical problems relate to placement and maintenance of the tube, as well as clogged or blocked tubes. Tubes can become clogged if pills are crushed and forced into the tube, if food is not adequately flushed out of the tube after bolus feeding, or if the tube is not capped to leave a column of water in the tube. Flushing clogged tubes with a variety of solutions (cranberry juice and cola beverages have been recommended in the past) may be irrational if the pK_a of the clogging material is not considered.[10] Another potential problem that should be considered is drug incompatibility with enteral feeding formulas. Potassium chloride elixir is the most commonly reported incompatibility, causing formula precipitation and blocked tubes.[4] Tube clogging is best prevented by prohibiting its use for the administration of nonliquid materials and by properly flushing and capping it after each use.

Most of the gastrointestinal problems caused by enteral feeding are caused by excessively rapid administration of the solution or feeding solutions of high osmolality (>600 mOsm). Solutions entering the duodenum too quickly can cause vomiting, cramps, and diarrhea by overwhelming the normal neural and endocrine control mechanisms of the gastrointestinal tract.[12] Hyperosmolar solutions cause rapid fluid and electrolyte influx into the gut lumen, leading to abdominal distension and cramping. These problems can be managed by reducing the feeding rate or solution concentration or by feeding diets that delay gastric emptying. Fiber-enriched enteral products marketed for human patients are designed to normalize gastrointestinal transit times, but there is little evidence to suggest that these products minimize or reduce diarrhea in tube-fed patients.[55]

Cold feeding solutions are thought to be a major cause of diarrhea, but research available to support this conclusion is inconclusive. We have not observed problems with diets fed at room temperature and recommend that diets stored in a refrigerator be brought to room temperature before being tube fed or offered for oral consumption. Bacterial contamination of formulas during reconstitution and administration also can cause diarrhea[7]; diets should be handled carefully and not allowed to remain in the feeding tube system for more than 24 hours.[28]

Patient problems that may result in gastrointestinal intolerance to feeding include protein malnutrition, hypoalbuminemia from any cause, fat malabsorption, and associated gastrointestinal disorders. Hypoalbuminemia

TABLE 26-3 Nutrient Composition of Veterinary Liquid Enteral Products

Product	kcal/8-oz can (g)	kcal/mL	mOsm/kg	Protein (g)	Protein Source	Fat (g)	Fat Source
CliniCare Canine/Feline	237 (1)	1	310	8.2 g/100 kcal	Casein, whey protein	5.1 g/100 kcal	Soybean oil, chicken fat
CliniCare Feline Renal	237 (1)	1	235	6.3 g/100 kcal	Casein, whey protein	6.7 g/100 kcal	Soybean oil, chicken fat

Product	Carbohydrate (g)	Carbohydrate Source	Fiber (g)	Fiber Source	Na^+ % Dry Matter	Na^+ (mg)	K^+ % Dry Matter
CliniCare Canine/Feline	6.8 g/100 kcal	Corn maltodextrin	0.05 g/100 kcal		0.37	84 mg/100 kcal	0.73
CliniCare Feline Renal	5.9 g/100 kcal	Corn maltodextrin	0.05 g/100 kcal		0.30	62 mg/100 kcal	0.60

Product	K^+ (mg)	Ca^{2+} % Dry Matter	Ca^{2+} (mg)	P_i (mg)	Mg^{2+} (mg)	Manufacturer	Comments
CliniCare Canine/Feline	124 mg/100 kcal	0.65	147 mg/100 kcal	126 mg/100 kcal	11.50 mg/100 kcal	Abbott Labs	
CliniCare Feline Renal	168 mg/100 kcal	0.60	124 mg/100 kcal	103 mg/100 kcal	9.30 mg/100 kcal	Abbott Labs	

Box 26-6	Recommended Rates and Volumes for Enteral Feeding

A. General guidelines
   i. Determine basal energy expenditure (BEE) caloric needs from Fig. 26-2
   ii. For formulas containing 1.5 kcal/mL, divide energy needs by 1.5 to get volume needed to feed
   iii. Increase feeding rate and volume only as patient tolerance allows
B. Bolus feeding
   i. Day 1: first feeding should be water only
   ii. Day 1: subsequent feedings delivered at $0.25 \times$ BEE caloric goal
   iii. Day 2: feedings delivered at $0.5 \times$ BEE caloric goal
   iv. Day 3: feedings delivered at $0.75 \times$ BEE caloric goal
   v. Feeding rate and volume can be increased as patient tolerance allows
C. Continuous feeding (hourly rate)
   i. Day 1: provide water only for first 6-12 hr; rate $= 0.5 \times$ BEE/24 hr
   ii. Day 1: provide enteral diet for second 12 hr; rate $= 0.5 \times$ BEE/24 hr
   iii. Day 2: delivery rate of enteral diet should be $0.75 \times$ BEE/24 hr
   iv. Day 3: delivery rate of enteral diet should be $100 \times$ BEE/24 hr
   v. Feeding rate and volume can be increased as patient tolerance allows

Box 26-7	Bolus Feeding Instructions (To Be Done at Each Feeding)

1. Auscultate abdomen for gut sounds. Aspirate gently on tube; measure and record any residual fluids, then replace fluid through tube. If more than half the volume previously fed is removed, do not feed animal at this time (wait until next scheduled feeding).
2. Inject 3-5 mL water through tube; this produces coughing if the tube is in the respiratory tract.
3. When satisfied the animal can be fed, resume feeding schedule. If necessary, place the animal in sternal or right lateral recumbency. Solution should be warm, at least room temperature, and should be fed slowly. Bolus feed for several minutes to assess the patient's tolerance, and monitor for vomiting or aspiration.

IF THE ANIMAL VOMITS, STOP FEEDING.
4. After feeding, flush the tube with 3-5 mL warm water, and replace cap or cover, leaving the tube full of water.
5. Observe the animal for discomfort, colic, or diarrhea for the next few minutes.
6. Record each feeding, and document any problems.
7. Nothing is to be administered via the tube except the feeding solution without the permission of the clinician.

can lead to malabsorption and diarrhea because the intravascular osmotic pressure required for nutrient uptake is greatly reduced.[27] Pancreatic disease, biliary obstruction, ileitis, bacterial overgrowth, gastric surgery, and intestinal resection all can lead to varying degrees of fat malabsorption. Many medical disorders are associated with diarrhea,[33] including enteric infections, malabsorption syndromes, gastroenteritis, mucosal defects, diabetes mellitus, carcinoid syndromes, hyperthyroidism, and immunodeficiency states.

The most important cause of diarrhea in tube-fed human patients is concomitant antibiotic or drug use because it is the most difficult factor to change. Development of diarrhea often results in discontinuation of tube feedings in an attempt to reduce the diarrhea that nursing staff and clinicians associate with liquid feedings. The problem may in fact be the antibiotic used. By altering the normal gastrointestinal flora, antibiotic usage also can change the fatty acid composition of gut contents, which may adversely affect sodium and water absorption by the colon. Intestinal bacteria also may ferment undigested nutrients, forming organic acids, hydrogen and carbon dioxide gas, and ultimately causing diarrhea.

Many antibiotics and drugs have been associated with diarrhea, including penicillins, aminoglycosides, cephalosporins, chloramphenicol, clindamycin, aminophylline, cimetidine, potassium chloride, digoxin, and magnesium-containing antacids.[30] The oral suspensions of some antibiotics, electrolytes, and other medications are hyperosmolar, suggesting that these drugs may play a role in the pathogenesis of diarrhea.[46] A study investigating the cause of diarrhea in tube-fed patients found that medicinal elixirs containing theophylline, as well as liquid preparations of acetaminophen, codeine, cimetidine, isoniazid, and vitamins, all contained sorbitol. Although commonly added to improve the palatability of some medications, sorbitol is also known to have an osmotic effect in sensitive individuals and should be considered a potential cause of diarrhea in patients receiving enteral diets.[23]

Metabolic problems include rapid absorption of high-carbohydrate solutions, which could result in hyperglycemia, osmotic diuresis, and ultimately nonketotic, hyperosmolar coma. This constellation of findings is referred to as the refeeding syndrome,[54] but we do not routinely observe this complication. Metabolism of glucose also results in the production of CO_2 and metabolic water; excess CO_2 production can further compromise patients with pulmonary disease. If metabolic water is retained, it can contribute to hyponatremia and edema. Most of these complications can be avoided by acclimatization of the patient to the feeding solution, slow rates of administration, and not overfeeding. Additional monitoring and potential supplementation of electrolytes such as potassium, magnesium, calcium, and phosphate may be required in critically ill patients. Urine or blood glucose concentrations should be monitored at regular intervals if hyperglycemia is suspected. Hyperglycemia can be managed by reducing nutrient flows or by giving insulin as discussed in Chapter 25. Until there is more documentation (i.e., controlled studies) in the veterinary literature, evidence-based guidelines for enteral feeding in adult human patients[29,55] should be reviewed by practitioners and their staff interested in providing nutritional support to veterinary patients.

REFERENCES

1. Abood SK, Buffington CA: Improved nasogastric intubation technique for administration of nutritional support in dogs, *J Am Vet Med Assoc* 199:577-579, 1991.
2. Abood SK, Mauterer JV, McLoughlin MA, et al: Nutritional support of hospitalized patients. In Slatter DH, editor: *Textbook of small animal surgery*, ed 2, Philadelphia, 1993, WB Saunders.
3. Abrams JT: The nutrition of the dog. In Rechcigl M, editor: *CRC handbook series in nutrition and food. Section G: diets, culture, media, and food supplements*, Boca Raton, FL, 1977, CRC Press, pp. 1-27.
4. Altman E, Cutee AJ: Compatibility of enteral products with commonly employed drug additives, *Nutr Supp Serv* 4:8-17, 1984.
5. Anderson RS: Water balance in the dog and cat, *J Small Anim Pract* 23:588-598, 1982.
6. Bauer JE: Hyperlipidemias. In Ettinger SJ, Feldman EC, editor: *Textbook of veterinary internal medicine*, ed 5, Philadelphia, 2000, WB Saunders.
7. Belknap DC, Davidson U, Flournoy DJ: Microorganisms and diarrhea in enterally fed intensive care unit patients, *J Parenter Enteral Nutr* 14:622-628, 1990.
8. Bright RM: Percutaneous tube gastrostomy. In Bojrab MJ, editor: *Current techniques in small animal surgery*, ed 2, Philadelphia, 1990, Lea and Febiger.
9. Buffington CA: Nutritional support of the hospitalized patient. Video Forum Small Anim Clin 1(4), 1989.
10. Buffington CA, Blaisdell J: Effect of citrate solutions on enteral formula clot formation, *J Parenter Enteral Nutr* 13:14S, 1989.
11. Butterworth CE Jr: The skeleton in the hospital closet, *Nutr Today* 9:4-8, 1974.
12. Cataldi-Betcher EC, Seltzer MH, Slocum BA et al: Complications occurring during enteral nutrition support: a prospective study. *J Parenter Enteral Nutr* 7:546-552, 1983.
13. Center SA, Wilkinson E, Smith CA, et al: 24-Hour urine protein/creatinine ratio in dogs with protein losing nephropathies, *J Am Vet Med Assoc* 187:820-824, 1985.
14. Chandra RK, Scrimshaw NS: Immuno-competence in nutritional assessment, *Am J Clin Nutr* 33:2694-2697, 1980.
15. Clark CH: Fluid therapy. In Catcott EF, editor: *Feline medicine and surgery*, ed 2, Santa Barbara, CA, 1975, American Veterinary Publications, pp. 601-609.
16. Collette WL, Merriweather WF: Oral alimentation of cats, *Vet Med Small Anim Clin* 59:839-845, 1964.
17. Crane SW: Placement and maintenance of a temporary feeding tube gastrostomy in the dog and cat, *Comp Cont Ed Vet Pract* 10:770-780, 1980.
18. Crowe DT: Enteral nutrition for the critically ill or injured patient: Part II, *Comp Cont Ed Vet Pract* 8:719-730, 1986.
19. Crowe DT: Methods of enteral feeding in the seriously ill or injured patient: Part 1, *J Vet Emerg Crit Care* 3:1-6,1985.
20. Daye RM, Huber ML, Henderson RA: Interlocking box jejunostomy: a new technique for enteral feeding, *J Am Anim Hosp Assoc* 35:129-134, 1999.
21. Della-Fera MA, Baile CA, McLaughlin CL: Feeding elicited by benzodiazepine-like chemicals in puppies and cats: structure-activity relationships, *Pharmacol Biochem Behav* 12:195-200, 1980.
22. DeNovo RE, Churchill J, Faudskar L, et al: Limited approach to the right flank for placement of a duodenostomy tube, *J Am Anim Hosp Assoc* 37:193-199, 2001.
23. Edes TE, Walk BE, Austin JL: Diarrhea in tube-fed patients: feeding formulas not necessarily the cause, *Am J Med* 88:91-93, 1990.
24. Edney ATB, Smith PM: Study of obesity in dogs visiting veterinary practices in the United Kingdom, *Vet Rec* 118:391-396, 1986.
25. Ford RB: Nasogastric intubation in the cat, *Comp Cont Ann Health Tech* 1:29-33, 1980.
26. Fulton RB Jr, Dennis JS. Blind percutaneous placement of a gastrostomy tube for nutritional support in dogs and cats, *J Am Vet Med Assoc* 201:697-700, 1992.
27. Gottschlich MM, Warden GD, Michel M, et al: Diarrhea in tube-fed burn patients: incidence, etiology, nutritional impact, and prevention, *J Parenter Enteral Nutr* 12:338-345, 1988.
28. Grunow JE, Christenson JW, Moutos D: Contamination of enteral nutrition systems during prolonged intermittent use, *J Parenter Enteral Nutr* 13:23-25, 1989.
29. Guidelines for the Use of Parenteral and Enteral Nutrition in Adult and Pediatric Patients, *J Parenter Enteral Nutr* 26S:1SA-6SA, 2002.
30. Hayes-Johnson V: Tube feeding complications: causes, prevention, therapy, *Nutr Supp Serv* 6:17-24, 1988.
31. Hill RC, Scott KR: Energy requirements and body surface area of cats and dogs, *J Am Vet Med Assoc* 225:689-694, 2004.
32. Ireland LM, Hohenhaus AE, Broussard JD, et al: A comparison of owner management and complications in 67 cats with esophagostomy and percutaneous endoscopic gastrostomy feeding tubes, *J Am Anim Hosp Assoc* 39:241-246, 2003.
33. Jergens AE: Diarrhea. In Ettinger SJ, Feldman EC, editors: *Textbook of veterinary internal medicine*, Philadelphia, 1995, WB Saunders.
34. Kaneko JJ: Serum proteins and the dysproteinemias. In Kaneko JJ, editor: *Clinical biochemistry of the domestic animals*, ed 4, New York, 1989, Academic Press, pp. 142-165.35. Koretz RL, Meyer JH: Elemental diets-facts and fantasies, *Gastroenterology* 78:393-410, 1980.
36. Laflamme DP, Kealy RD, Schmidt DA: Estimation of body fat by body condition score, *J Vet Intern Med* 8:154, 1994.
37. Laflamme DP, Kuhlman G, Lawler DF, et al: Obesity management in dogs, *J Vet Clin Nutr* 1:59-65, 1994.
38. Lantz GC: Pharyngostomy tube placement. In Bojrab MJ, editor: *Current techniques in small animal surgery*, ed 2, Philadelphia, 1990, Lea and Febiger.

39. Lantz GC, Cantwell HD, Van Vleet JF, et al: Pharyngostomy tube induced esophagitis in the dog: an experimental study, *J Am Vet Med Assoc* 19:207-212, 1983.

40. Levenson SM, editor: *Nutritional assessment—present status, future directions, and prospects.* Report of the Second Ross Conference in Medical Research, Ross Laboratories, Columbus, OH, 1981.

41. Levine PB, Smallwood LJ, Buback JL: Esophagostomy tubes as a method of nutritional management in cats: a retrospective study, *J Am Anim Hosp Assoc* 33:405-410, 1997.

42. Long CL, Schaffel N, Geiger JW, et al: Metabolic response to injury and illness: estimation of energy and protein needs from indirect calorimetry and nitrogen balance, *J Parenter Enteral Nutr* 3:452-456, 1979.

43. Macy DW, Ralston SL: Cause and control of decreased appetite. In Kirk RW, editor: *Current veterinary therapy X,* Philadelphia, 1989, WB Saunders, pp. 18-24.

44. Mauterer JV, Abood SK, Buffington CA, et al: New technique and management guidelines for percutaneous nonendoscopic tube gastrostomy, *J Am Vet Med Assoc* 205:574-579, 1994.

45. National Research Council: *Nutrient requirements of the dog and cat,* Washington DC, 2003, National Academies.

46. Niemiec PW Jr, Vanderveen TW, Morrison JI, et al: Gastrointestinal disorders caused by medications and electrolyte solution osmolality during enteral nutrition, *J Parenter Enteral Nutr* 7:387-389, 1983.

47. Orton EC: Needle catheter jejunostomy. In Bojrab MJ, editor: *Current techniques in small animal surgery,* ed 2, Philadelphia, 1990, Lea and Febiger.

48. Prasad A: *Zinc in human nutrition,* Boca Raton, FL, 1979, CRC Press.

49. Prentiss PG, Wolf AV, Eddy HE: Hydropenia in the cat and dog: ability of the cat to meet its water requirements solely from a diet of meat or fish, *Am J Physiol* 196:626-632, 1959.

50. Rawlings CA: Percutaneous placements of a midcervical esophagostomy tube: new technique and representative cases, *J Am Anim Hosp Assoc* 29:526-530, 1993.

51. Schaeffer MC, Rogers QR, Morris JG: Protein in the nutrition of dogs and cats. In Burger IH, Rivers JPW, editors: *Nutrition of the dog and cat,* Cambridge, 1989, Cambridge University Press, pp. 159-205.

52. Sherding RG: Diseases of the small bowel. In Ettinger SJ, editor: *Textbook of veterinary internal medicine,* ed 3, Philadelphia, 1989, WB Saunders.

53. Silk DBA: The continuing journey towards the optimization of enteral nutrition 1978-2000—The Nutricia Research Foundation Award acceptance lecture, *Clin Nutr* 20:5, 2001.

54. Solomon S, Kirby DF: The refeeding syndrome: a review, *J Parenter Enteral Nutr* 14:90-97, 1990.

55. Stroud M, Duncan H, Nightingale J: Guidelines for enteral feeding in adult hospital patients, *Gut* 52(suppl VII):vii1-vii12, 2003.

56. Swann HM, Sweet DC, Holt DE, et al: Placement of a low-profile duodenostomy and jejunostomy device in five dogs, *J Small Anim Pract* 39:191-194, 1998.

57. Teeter SM, Collins DR: Intragastric intubation of small animals, *Vet Med Small Anim Clin* 61:1067-1076, 1966.

58. Tyler JW: Hepatoencephalopathy. Part II. Pathophysiology and treatment, *Comp Cont Ed Vet Pract* 12:1260-1270, 1990.

59. Von Werthern CJ, Wess G: A new technique for insertion of esophagostomy tubes in cats, *J Am Anim Hosp Assoc* 37:140-144, 2001.

60. Walton RS, Wingfield WE, Ogilvie GK, et al: Energy expenditure in 104 postoperative and traumatically injured dogs with indirect calorimetry, *J Vet Emerg Crit Care* 6:71-79, 1996.

61. Wolfe RR, Durkot MJ, Wolfe MH: Effect of thermal injury on energy metabolism, substrate kinetics, and hormonal concentrations, *Circ Shock* 9:383-394, 1982.

62. Wolman 5L, Anderson GH, Marless EB, et al: Zinc in total parenteral nutrition: requirements and metabolic effects, *Gastroenterology* 76:458-467, 1979.

63. Ziegler EE, Fomon SJ: Fluid intake, renal solute load, and water balance in infancy, *J Pediatr* 78:561-568, 1971.

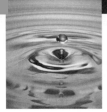

CHAPTER · 27

FLUID THERAPY WITH MACROMOLECULAR PLASMA VOLUME EXPANDERS

Dez Hughes and Amanda K. Boag

"Those who fill our professional ranks are habitually conservative. This salutary mental attitude expresses itself peculiarly in our communal relations; namely, when a new idea appears which is more or less subversive to old notions and practices, he who originates the idea must strike sledge hammer blows in order to secure even a momentary attention. This must then be followed by a long, patient, propaganda and advertising until in the grand finale, the public, indifferent at first, is aroused, proceeds to discuss, and finally accepts the iconoclastic proposal as a long-accepted fact of its own invention and asks wonderingly, "Why such a bother? What after all is new about this? We knew it long ago!"
—Howard A. Kelly, MD. Electrosurgery in gynaecology, Ann Surg 93:323, 1931.

In the late nineteenth century, Ernest Starling proposed the concept that the balance between hydrostatic and osmotic pressure gradients between the intravascular and interstitial fluid compartments governed transvascular fluid exchange.[130] A hydrostatic pressure gradient in excess of the osmotic gradient at the arterial end of the capillary bed results in a net transudation of fluid into the interstitium. At the venous end of the capillary bed, plasma proteins (which do not normally pass out of the blood vessels) exert an osmotic force in excess of the hydrostatic gradient, resulting in a net fluid flux into vessels. More than a century of research has confirmed that Starling's hypothesis provides the foundation for microvascular fluid exchange but also has revealed that the anatomy and physiology of the microvasculature, interstitium, and lymphatic system are much more complex. Consequently, a much deeper understanding of transvascular fluid dynamics is necessary for a logical and rational approach to intravenous therapy with fluids containing macromolecules. This chapter assumes the reader is familiar with the information given in Chapter 1 explaining the fluid compartments of the body and the mechanisms of water and solute flow among compartments. Although this chapter discusses the anatomy, physiology, and biophysics of transvascular fluid dynamics in some depth, comprehensive reviews and texts are available on the subject for a more complete discussion of solute and solvent exchange among the microvasculature, interstitium, and lymphatics.[5,109,133] The main aim of this chapter is to address the complexities and controversies of colloid therapy while avoiding the tendency toward bias apparent in many articles dealing with the crystalloid-colloid controversy. A deeper appreciation of the relevant issues should ensure a more rational approach when deciding whether colloid therapy is appropriate. The present chapter is exhaustive in its dealing with some issues but not all-inclusive, and the reader also is referred to several reviews of colloid fluid therapy available in the veterinary* and human medical literature.[48,86,111]

THE MICROVASCULAR BARRIER

In simple terms, the healthy microvascular barrier is a capillary wall that is relatively impermeable to protein. In addition to the endothelial cell and the capillary basement membrane, a luminal surface layer (the glycocalyx) and the interstitial matrix also contribute to the selective permeability of the microvascular barrier.[5,109,155] The glycocalyx coats the luminal aspect of the endothelial cell and is composed of proteins, glycoproteins, and glycolipids that modify the permeability of the microvessel by occupying spaces within the wall or via electrostatic attraction or repulsion.[80] Plasma proteins, especially albumin and orosomucoid, are thought to contribute significantly to maintaining the selective permeability of the endothelium.[40-42,64,85]

On a morphological basis, capillary walls may be continuous, fenestrated, or discontinuous.[104,137] Continuous capillaries, which are found in the majority of tissues and

---

*References 32,72,82,117-119,128.

organs of the body, are so called because the wall is composed of a continuous endothelial cell and basement membrane. They are freely permeable to water and small solutes such as sodium but are relatively impermeable to macromolecules. The passage of smaller plasma proteins, such as albumin (molecular radius of 3.5 nm), is restricted less than the passage of larger plasma proteins. Fenestrated capillaries have a continuous basement membrane with regions that are only covered by thin endothelial diaphragms or are entirely devoid of endothelium. They are found in tissues characterized by large fluxes of water and small solutes such as the glomerulus and the intestine. Interestingly, the permeability of fenestrated capillaries to macromolecules is similar to that of continuous capillaries. This feature has been shown to be a result of a net negative charge of the basement membrane.[12,127] Discontinuous capillaries are found in the liver, spleen, bone marrow, and some glands. They have gaps up to 1 μm between endothelial cells with no basement membrane and are therefore freely permeable to protein.

The permeability of the microvascular barrier has been explained by the presence of pores of differing sizes.[94] These pore sizes often are extrapolated from experimental data regarding fluid and solute fluxes and do not always correlate with morphological studies such as electron microscopy, implying that they represent functional rather than anatomical entities. The majority of experimental data suggest two effective pore sizes in the microvascular barrier in most tissues, with a high frequency of small pores that restrict efflux of macromolecules and a low frequency of large ones through which macromolecules can pass freely.[109]

Rather than being a free fluid space, the interstitium represents a dynamic environment that may contribute to the permeability characteristics of the microvascular barrier and modify the flow of fluid and macromolecules from the blood vessels to the lymphatics.[5,10,11] The interstitium is composed of a collagen framework that contains a gel phase of glycosaminoglycans (of which hyaluronan is the most common), along with protein macromolecules and electrolytes in solution. The relative proportions of these constituents differ widely among organs and tissues, resulting in variations in the permeability and mechanical properties of the interstitium. Glycosaminoglycans are extremely long chains of repeating disaccharide subunits wound into random coils and entangled with each other and the collagen framework. They have molecular weights of the order of 10^7, and each molecule bears many thousand anionic moieties.[5] This interstitial structure has been suggested to mechanically oppose distention (i.e., edema formation) and resists contraction during dehydration because of repulsion between the anionic moieties.[61] The interstitial matrix itself is differentially permeable to macromolecules, and a colloid osmotic gradient also can exist from the perimicrovascular space across the interstitium. Although the collagen network and many of the glycosaminoglycans are fixed in the interstitium, hyaluronan may be mobilized and removed via lymphatic drainage, thereby altering the permeability of the interstitium.[5]

TRANSVASCULAR FLUID DYNAMICS

Although not stated implicitly in his seminal article, Starling's hypothesis subsequently was formalized to state simply that the hydrostatic pressure gradient between the capillary and the interstitium ($P_c - P_i$) is equal to the osmotic pressure gradient between the plasma and the interstitium ($\pi_p - \pi_i$). This expression can be expanded to describe fluid flux (J_v) across the microvascular barrier:

Fluid flow = hydrostatic gradient − osmotic gradient

or

$$J_v = (P_c - P_i) - (\pi_p - \pi_i)$$

For a solute to exert its full osmotic pressure across a membrane, the membrane must be impermeable to the solute. If the membrane is partially permeable to the solute molecule, the equilibrium concentration gradient is lower, and the solute exerts only part of its potential osmotic pressure. The realization that the microvasculature was only partially impermeable to smaller macromolecules led to the inclusion of the reflection coefficient (σ) in the fluid flux equation.[134]

$$J_v = (P_c - P_i) - \sigma (\pi_p - \pi_i)$$

In descriptive terms, the reflection coefficient is the fraction of the total potential osmotic pressure exerted by the solute in question. Conceptually, one also can consider it as the fraction of the solute molecules reflected from the microvascular barrier. If a membrane is completely impermeable, no solute molecules pass through, the concentration gradient is maximal, and the solute exerts its full osmotic pressure (i.e., the reflection coefficient = 1). If the membrane is completely permeable to the solute in question, it passes through freely, no concentration difference exists, and no osmotic pressure can be exerted (i.e., the reflection coefficient = 0).

Further research showed that fluid flow from vessels differed among tissues depending on the surface area of the capillary beds in the organ and the hydraulic conductance (i.e., the ease of fluid flow) through the microvascular barrier. To account for this variability, the fluid flux equation is modified by the filtration coefficient (K_{fc}). This term simply implies that fluid flow is equal to a fraction of the effective hydrostatic and osmotic pressure gradients.

$$J_v = K_{fc} \left[(P_c - P_i) - \sigma (\pi_p - \pi_i) \right]$$

Each different constituent of plasma may differ in its rate of efflux from a vessel depending on such factors as its molecular radius, shape, and charge, and the permeability of the microvascular barrier to the constituent in question. The two major groups of molecules with respect to transvascular fluid flux are termed the solvent phase and the solute phase, and expressions were developed to predict the egress of both major groups of molecules from the microvasculature.[71,79,93,98] The solvent phase includes water and those molecules that are not significantly impeded in their passage through the microvascular barrier, whereas the solute flux equation describes the passage of molecules that do not flow freely from the vasculature.

The solvent flow equation remains the same as the previous expression of fluid flow except that the filtration coefficient is subdivided into the hydraulic conductance (L_p) and the membrane surface area (S), and the hydrostatic and osmotic gradients are expressed as ΔP and $\Delta \pi$, respectively:

$$J_v = L_p S \left(\Delta P - \sigma \Delta \pi \right)$$

The two major mechanisms of solute flow through the microvascular barrier are convection (i.e., carriage in a bulk flow of fluid) and diffusion (i.e., random motion resulting in net movement of molecules from an area of high concentration to an area of lower concentration).[109] An analogy to illustrate the two mechanisms would be a wave breaking on a beach. Some of the sodium molecules in the wave will be moving away from the beach by diffusion; however, the forward convective flow of the wave carries them in the opposite direction.

The solute flow equation (which is the most relevant expression with respect to intravenous therapy with fluids containing macromolecules) states simply that the rate of solute flux (J_s) is equal to the sum of the convective flow and the diffusional movement.

$$\text{Solute flow } (J_s) = \text{convective flow} + \text{diffusion}$$

Convective flow is equal to the product of fluid flow (J_v), the fractional permeability of the membrane ($1 - \sigma$), and the mean intramembrane solute concentration, $\bar{C}$. Diffusion is equal to the product of the solute permeability (P), the surface area of the microvascular barrier (S), and the solute concentration gradient across the membrane (ΔC). Therefore the expression representing macromolecular flux becomes:

$$J_s = J_v (1 - \sigma) \bar{C} + PS \Delta C$$

Solute flow = convective flow + diffusion

At normal lymph flow rates, convection has been estimated to account for approximately 30% of the total flux of albumin into lymph.[105] An important point that warrants further emphasis is that the rate of solute efflux is dependent on the rate of solvent efflux. Any condition that increases the rate of fluid flow across a membrane can increase the extravasation of macromolecules. Hence, intravenous fluid therapy with crystalloid or colloid can increase albumin loss into the interstitium.[106]

These mathematical expressions give the impression of a constant hydrostatic pressure gradient acting across a single membrane of static and uniform conductivity and permeability (homoporous), with filtration opposed by an osmotic pressure resulting from a single impermeant solute, the plasma "protein." In fact, the hydrostatic pressure and osmotic pressure gradients vary among different tissues and at different levels of the capillary bed within the same tissue.[103,135,138] The total osmotic gradient is a summation of all the impermeant solutes present within plasma, which all have unique reflection coefficients and efflux rates.[135] Furthermore, the surface area of the capillary bed may change depending on precapillary sphincter activity, and the permeability of the microvascular barrier also can vary physiologically and in disease states.[8,61,96,155,156]

NORMAL STARLING FORCES AND THE TISSUE SAFETY FACTORS

PLASMA COLLOID OSMOTIC PRESSURE

Although in popular usage colloid often is interpreted as referring to a macromolecule that cannot pass through a membrane, the strict definition refers to the dispersion in a gas, liquid, or solid medium of atoms or molecules that resist sedimentation, diffusion, and filtration. This definition is in contradistinction to crystalloids, which are freely diffusible. Oncotic pressure is defined as the osmotic pressure exerted by colloids in solution (hence it is redundant to use the phrase colloid oncotic pressure). Proteins in plasma are truly in solution, but they closely resemble a colloid solution and thus are referred to and treated as such. The osmotic pressure exerted by the naturally occurring colloids in plasma is higher than that calculated for an ideal solution in vitro. One of the main reasons for this discrepancy is that negatively charged proteins (such as albumin, which has a net negative charge of 17 at physiological pH) retain cations within the intravascular space by electrostatic attraction (termed the Donnan effect).[61] These cations contribute to the effective plasma protein osmotic pressure because osmotic pressure is proportional to the number of molecules present rather than their size. Therefore colloid osmotic pressure (COP) would be the most correct term when referring to the osmotic pressure exerted by plasma proteins and their associated electrolyte molecules. For comparison, the oncotic pressure exerted by an albumin solution of 7 g/dL is 19.8 mm Hg, the in vivo COP is 28 mm Hg, and the total osmotic pressure of all plasma solutes is 5400 mm Hg.[61]

By virtue of its relatively high concentration in the vascular space, albumin usually accounts for 60% to 70% of the plasma COP with globulins making up the remainder.[91,146,153] Interestingly, the variation in COP in dogs may be because of more differences in globulin concentration than in albumin concentration.[55,91] Red blood cells and platelets do not contribute significantly to plasma COP.[100] Serum albumin concentration is determined by the relative rates of synthesis, degradation, and loss from the body and its distribution between the intravascular and interstitial spaces. Albumin synthesis, which is unique to the liver, appears to be regulated, at least in part, by the hepatic plasma COP.[47,99,112] Increases of plasma COP independent of albumin concentration, such as in hyperglobulinemia, are associated with decreased serum albumin concentration.[18,113,114] The main site of albumin degradation is uncertain, but the reticuloendothelial system has been suggested. Equations have been derived to estimate plasma COP from plasma protein concentrations,[91,139] but direct measurement is more accurate.[7,25,139,153] COPs measured in normal dogs and cats are given in Table 27-1.[39,91,161]

INTERSTITIAL COLLOID OSMOTIC PRESSURE

Capillaries are permeable to protein, despite the fact that the microvascular barrier greatly restricts macromolecular flux. Of the total quantity of albumin present in the body, 40% is intravascular and 60% is extravascular.[115] Furthermore, all of the albumin present in plasma circulates through the interstitium every 24 hours.[97] The interstitial COP varies from tissue to tissue depending on such factors as the permeability of the capillary wall to protein, the rate of transvascular solvent flow, the retention of protein in the interstitial matrix, and the rate of lymphatic clearance of protein. The microvascular barrier of skeletal muscle or subcutaneous tissue is relatively

impermeable to protein, whereas the pulmonary capillary endothelium is more permeable with a reflection coefficient to albumin of approximately 0.5 to 0.64.[96] Consequently, the normal protein concentration in lymph from skin or skeletal muscle is approximately 50% that of plasma compared with 65% in pulmonary lymph.[96] Hyaluronan and its associated cations also may contribute to interstitial COP.[5] Because of the volume occupied by the interstitial matrix, interstitial albumin is distributed in a volume that is less than the total interstitial volume. This phenomenon is called the volume exclusion effect, and the "excluded volume" with respect to albumin may be as high as one half to two thirds of the total interstitial volume.[13,95,152] Consequently, in a normally hydrated interstitium, much less protein is required to exert a given osmotic pressure, and relatively smaller volumes of extravasated fluid result in greater decrements in interstitial COP. This effect maintains the intravascular-to-extravascular COP gradient in early edema formation. Conversely, when interstitial volume is overexpanded by fluid in edematous states, a dramatic increase occurs in the volume available for albumin sequestration.[61] The increase in interstitial COP that occurs with dehydration acts to restrict mobilization of interstitial fluid.[66]

INTRAVASCULAR HYDROSTATIC PRESSURE

Intravascular hydrostatic pressure is the main force that determines fluid egress from the vasculature. It may vary in different tissues and at different levels within each capillary bed. The normal hydrostatic pressure in the capillary bed is controlled by local myogenic, neurogenic, and humoral modulation of the arterial and venous resistances. Precapillary arteriolar constriction may reduce flow, and therefore hydrostatic pressure, through a capillary bed or shunt, flows away from that bed, resulting in changes in the total surface area available for transvascular fluid movement. The hydrostatic pressure within a blood vessel at any particular site depends in part on where resistance to flow occurs, with hydrostatic pressures decreasing most across the areas of major resistance. In most tissues, the majority of resistance has been attributed to small arterioles, but experimental studies of the lung suggest that a significant pressure decrease may occur across the capillary bed itself.[15,16,124]

INTERSTITIAL HYDROSTATIC PRESSURE

As with all the other Starling forces, normal interstitial pressure also varies among tissues. Interestingly, in many tissues the resting pressure is slightly negative (subatmospheric), tending to favor rather than oppose fluid filtration from the microvasculature.[154] This finding has been postulated to be the result of the molecular structure of the interstitial matrix, such that with normal hydration the biomechanical stresses on the molecules and the

TABLE 27-1 Colloid Osmotic Pressure in Normal Cats and Dogs

Species	Colloid Osmotic Pressure Mean ± SD (mm Hg)	Reference Number
Canine (plasma)	20.8 ± 1.8	161
Canine (plasma)	17.5 ± 3.0	91
Canine (whole blood)	19.9 ± 2.1	39
Feline (plasma)	19.8 ± 2.4	161
Feline (whole blood)	24.7 ± 3.7	39

repulsion among like electrostatic charges act to expand the interstitium.[5] In encapsulated organs, such as the kidney, normal interstitial pressures are positive. Interstitial pressures can change depending on the functional state of the organ. For example, interstitial pressures in the nonabsorbing intestine are negative to slightly positive, whereas intestinal interstitial pressures are positive in the absorptive state.[60] As mentioned before, the molecular structure of the interstitium mechanically opposes distention. Conventionally, it is said that one third of the total body water is found in the extracellular space and that the interstitium constitutes three fourths of the extracellular space. These figures are averages for the whole body, and the relative sizes of the intravascular and interstitial spaces vary among tissues. Tissues vary in their capacity to accommodate interstitial fluid depending on the size of the interstitial space relative to the total volume of the tissue and the nature of the interstitial matrix itself, especially its distensibility. The distensibility of an organ or tissue is termed its compliance, and depending on the nature of the tissue, the compliance of the interstitium may vary widely. Extreme examples would be tendon (which is relatively noncompliant) and loose subcutaneous connective tissue (which is relatively distensible). The peribronchial accumulation of edema fluid in the lungs is likely the result of the higher compliance of this region of the pulmonary interstitium.

An extremely important concept related to the interstitial hydrostatic pressure is that of stress relaxation. In a normally hydrated animal, the interstitium in most tissues is relatively noncompliant. Small increases in volume caused by increased fluid extravasation result in large changes in interstitial hydrostatic pressure that act to oppose further extravasation of fluid and increase lymphatic drainage pressure—two of the tissue safety factors described later.[62,136] As the interstitium becomes gradually more distended, it opposes distension until a critical point is reached (suggested to correspond to the disordering of the interstitial matrix). Abruptly, the resistance to distension decreases (i.e., compliance increases), and fluid then can accumulate without a corresponding protective increase in interstitial pressure and lymph flow. At this point, the distended interstitium no longer opposes the movement of fluid and protein, resulting in increased extravasation and self-perpetuation of the edemagenic process. Furthermore, the greatly increased interstitial space provides a large volume for protein sequestration.

TISSUE SAFETY FACTORS

From the previous discussion, it should be apparent that there are three main ways in which accumulation of fluid in the interstitium can be avoided. First, extravasation of fluid into a relatively nondistensible interstitium results in an increased interstitial hydrostatic pressure that opposes further extravasation. Second, after extravasation of low-protein fluid, interstitial COP decreases

because of dilution and washout of protein, thereby maintaining or even enhancing the COP gradient between the intravascular space and interstitium. Third, because the perimicrovascular interstitium is not compliant, increased interstitial fluid results in an increased driving pressure for lymphatic drainage. These alterations in Starling forces that act to limit interstitial fluid accumulation have been termed the tissue safety factors.[62,136] Their relative importance varies depending on the characteristics of the tissue.[5,28] In a tissue that is relatively nondistensible (e.g., tendon), an increase in interstitial pressure may be the most important means by which to counteract filtration. In a tissue with moderate distensibility and with a relatively impermeable microvascular barrier (e.g., skin), the decrease in interstitial COP assumes more importance in protecting against interstitial fluid accumulation. In a distensible tissue that is quite permeable to protein (e.g., lungs), increased lymph flow appears to be the most important safeguard against interstitial edema.[158]

PHARMACOKINETICS AND PHARMACODYNAMICS OF MACROMOLECULAR PLASMA VOLUME EXPANDERS

Transvascular fluid dynamics are extremely complex. The balance of the hydrostatic and osmotic pressure gradients between the intravascular and interstitial fluid compartments forms the basis for microvascular fluid exchange. However, this simple concept is belied by the great heterogeneity in Starling forces and transvascular fluid dynamics that exists among and within tissues in both healthy and diseased states. The relative importance of the different tissue safety factors also varies among tissues, and the potential for self-regulation of transvascular fluid fluxes often is underestimated. When considering fluid therapy with macromolecular volume expanders, a great deal of emphasis has been placed on the manipulation of individual Starling forces (such as intravascular COP) in isolation rather than addressing the system in its entirety. Maintenance of intravascular volume depends on an intricate and dynamic interaction between the intravascular and interstitial Starling forces and the structure and function of the microvascular barrier, interstitium, and lymphatic system. Infusion of intravenous fluids can change all of the Starling forces, modify the permeability of the microvascular barrier, change the volume and composition of the interstitium, and increase lymphatic flow. Furthermore, the magnitude and relative significance of these changes vary among and within tissues. Consequently, it is a gross and potentially dangerous oversimplification to view the body as the homogenous sum of its individual parts when contemplating intravenous fluid therapy. From a clinical standpoint, the differences between the lungs and the systemic circulation are of the utmost importance. For example, in a dog with systemic inflammatory response syndrome and aspiration pneumonia causing pulmonary edema by means of increased microvascular permeability, colloid therapy may be effective in limiting subcutaneous edema at the expense of worsening pulmonary fluid extravasation.

Despite this great heterogeneity, the concept that net fluid extravasation depends on the balance between intravascular COP and capillary hydrostatic pressure forms the basis for intravenous colloid therapy.[54,63,77,151] By virtue of their larger molecular size, and in the absence of an increase in microvascular permeability, colloid molecules are retained within the vasculature to a greater degree than are crystalloids. Consequently, smaller volumes of colloid result in greater plasma volume expansion compared with crystalloid,[46,125,126] and crystalloid is expected to leak into the interstitium to a greater degree than colloid and cause more interstitial edema.[24] One hour after infusion of a crystalloid solution, as little as 10% of the infused volume may remain in the intravascular space.[126] Some evidence indicates that tissue perfusion is better after volume expansion with colloids than with crystalloids, even when resuscitation is titrated to physiological endpoints.[53]

Many factors influence the volume and duration of intravascular expansion associated with artificial colloids, including the species of animal, dose, specific colloid formulation, preinfusion intravascular volume status, and the microvascular permeability. These factors may explain the great variability in intravascular persistence and volume expansion in published studies. Artificial colloids are polydisperse, that is, they contain molecules of different molecular weight. In contrast, in a monodisperse colloid, such as albumin, molecules are all the same size. The artificial colloids have extremely complex pharmacokinetics in part because of this large range of molecular sizes.[73] The smaller molecules pass rapidly into the urine and interstitium, whereas the larger molecules remain in circulation and gradually are hydrolyzed by amylase or removed by the monocyte phagocytic system.[140] This initial rapid excretion of small, osmotically active molecules followed by gradual elimination of large molecules results in an exponential decline in intravascular expansion. Manufacturer data sheets are misleading because they imply that a major proportion of the volume expansion lasts for 24 to 36 hours. Estimates of the degree of initial plasma volume expansion for hetastarch (HES) and dextran 70 vary from 70% to 170% of the infused volume.[57,67,76,78,106] This decreases to approximately 50% of the infused volume after 6 hours. Volume expansion with hydroxyethyl starch declines gradually from 60% to 40% of the infused volume during the next 12 to 18 hours, whereas with dextran 70 it decreases gradually from 40% to 20% of

the infused volume.[140] In dogs with hypoalbuminemia of varying causes receiving hydroxyethyl starch, COP was not significantly different from baseline 12 hours after infusion.[89] In the authors' experience, the duration of volume expansion with artificial colloids can be even shorter, especially with capillary leak syndromes. This relatively short duration of action and the high cost of artificial colloids have led some authors to question the cost-effectiveness of colloid infusions in veterinary patients.[150]

The duration of action of colloids may be expressed in terms of plasma colloid concentrations, plasma COP measurements, or degree of volume expansion. The initial volume of intravascular expansion is the result of the COP of the infused colloid, which is determined by the number of molecules, not their size. This concept is extremely important because the distribution of molecular weights is narrowed after intravenous infusion.[49,50] The smaller molecules that are responsible for a large part of the COP and intravascular volume expansion are extravasated or excreted within hours. The concentration (i.e., mass per unit volume) still is high, but COP is relatively low, and hence COP and degree of volume expansion tend to decrease faster than does the plasma concentration of colloid. Data from an experimental study of euvolemic human volunteers given twice the usual dose of a high molecular weight form of hydroxyethyl starch may therefore have little bearing on the effects of commercially available HES in a dog with systemic inflammatory response syndrome in hypodynamic septic shock.

The osmotic effect of macromolecules is because of their number rather than their size. Consequently, if more than 50% of the molecules leak into the interstitium, a net reduction in intravascular volume could occur as water leaves the intravascular space with colloid. Therefore the difficulty is how to determine the magnitude of increase in permeability (i.e., the size of the "gaps" in the microvascular barrier). Although experimental techniques exist to detect an increase in microvascular permeability,[14,22] they currently are not applicable in a clinical setting. A growing body of evidence suggests that hydroxyethyl starches can mitigate increases of microvascular permeability in several capillary leak states.[29,92,159] The optimal molecular weight for this effect seems to be between 100 and 300 kDa.[160] Unfortunately, relatively few artificial colloid products with molecules in this size range are available in the United States. For example, only 35% of the molecules in HES fall within this optimal size range.[159] European formulations of pentastarch contain more molecules in the optimal molecular size range.

Given the many factors involved in the efficacy and persistence of colloid therapy and the heterogeneous nature of the patient population in which they are used, it is crucial to carefully assess the need for colloidal therapy and the clinical response of the patient. Colloid therapy is not a panacea; rather it represents one more group of drugs with specific indications, contraindications, benefits, and risks. The treatment of critically ill human patients with colloid solutions recently has been questioned in several meta-analyses of randomized clinical trials in human patients.[4,17,30,121,148] Despite the limitations of randomized clinical trials and meta-analyses,[110] all showed a trend toward increased mortality when colloids were used to resuscitate human trauma patients. Subdivision of the patients in one study[148] demonstrated that in trauma patients there was a 12.3% difference in mortality rate in favor of crystalloid therapy, and when data from studies that used nontrauma patients were pooled, there was a 7.8% difference in mortality rate in favor of colloid treatment. The only meta-analysis designed a priori to investigate resuscitation after trauma showed a lower mortality rate associated with the use of crystalloid fluids.[30]

The artificial colloids used most commonly worldwide fall into three major groups: the hydroxyethyl starch derivatives, the dextrans, and the gelatins. The hydroxyethyl starches are synthesized by partial hydrolysis of amylopectin (the branched form of plant starch), the dextrans from a macromolecular polysaccharide produced from bacterial fermentation of sucrose, and the gelatins from hydrolysis of bovine collagen followed either by succinylation or linkage to urea. The preparations used most commonly in the United States are hydroxyethyl starch preparations (HES) and dextran 70, both of which are available as 6% (6 g/dL) solutions in 0.9% saline. Several gelatin-based products are available in Europe (Haemaccel, Intervet UK Ltd., Milton Keynes, UK; Gelofusine, B. Braun Melsungen AG, Melsungen, Germany).

During manufacturing, the parent mixtures are separated into fractions by molecular weight. The hydroxyethyl starches have a much wider range of molecular weights than does dextran 70, and the distribution of molecular weights in the available preparations of hydroxyethyl starch often is underestimated. The package insert for Hespan states that 80% of molecules fall between 2 and 2500 kDa; however, this statement also means that 20% fall outside of this range. An independent analysis found that 85% of Hespan consisted of molecules smaller than 300 kDa, 50% consisted of molecules smaller than 100 kDa, and molecular masses ranged up to 5000 kDa.[159] Hydroxyethyl starch with a weight average molecular mass of 100 to 300 kDa seems to provide the best compromise between colloid osmotic volume expansion and duration of action.[35] Furthermore, this size distribution has less effect on coagulation[143] and is the best size for reducing the increases in permeability present in patients with vascular leak states.[159]

To reduce intravascular hydrolysis of hydroxyethyl starch by amylase, the amylopectin is hydroxyethylated at carbons 2, 3, and 6 of the constituent glucose molecules. The number of hydroxyethyl groups per glucose unit is defined as the molar substitution ratio, and the pattern of substitution varies depending on the synthetic process. Substitution at the carbon 2 position is more effective in reducing intravascular hydrolysis than hydroxyethylation at the other positions.[145] Therefore hydroxyethyl starches are characterized by their weight average molecular weight, substitution ratio, and C-2/C-6 hydroxyethylation ratio.[142] HES, for example, has an average molecular weight of 450,000 and a substitution ratio of 0.7 and therefore is referred to as HES 450/0.7. Two forms of high molecular weight hydroxyethyl starch are available in the United States, HES 450/0.7 (Hespan, DuPont Pharmaceuticals, Wilmington, DE) and Hextend (Abbott Laboratories, North Chicago, IL), which has a weight average molecular weight of 670 kDa, a molar substitution of 0.75, and a high C-2/C-6 ratio. In Europe, several hydroxyethyl starch products are available with smaller average molecular weights, including pentastarch (HES 200/0.5) and HES 130/0.4 (Voluven, Fresenius Kabi). These products have been developed to maximize volume expansion effects while minimizing the risk of adverse effects on the hemostatic system by reducing the number of large molecules.

The recommended dosage for both hydroxyethyl starch and dextran is 20 mL/kg/day. Although higher dosages have been used without apparent adverse effects,[89,129] the deleterious effects on coagulation occur at and above this dosage. A dosage of 20 mL/kg represents one quarter of a dog's blood volume, and if repeated doses are required to maintain perfusion, the underlying reason should be pursued aggressively. The hydroxyethyl starches are the most expensive intravenous colloid solutions available. Colloid solutions contain no bacteriostat and therefore are intended for single-dose usage.

Albumin, obtained from purified human plasma, has been used to provide colloid support in human medicine for many years. Albumin most commonly is given to small animal patients as stored or fresh frozen plasma, stored whole blood, or fresh whole blood. However, human serum albumin has been increasingly used in small animal patients. Albumin has a molecular weight of approximately 69,000 and a molecular radius of 3.5 nm. It is a monodisperse colloid (i.e., all albumin molecules are the same size). In addition to its role in maintaining plasma COP, it carries a wide range of substances such as bilirubin, fatty acids, metals and other ions, hormones, and drugs.[116] Albumin equilibrates with the interstitial space more rapidly and to a greater extent than artificial colloids, and relatively large volumes must be given to achieve a sustained increase in plasma COP. Administration of 25% human albumin solution to a heterogeneous population of critically ill dogs was associated with effective increases in serum albumin concentration, refractometric total solids, and COP with relatively few adverse effects.[27] In human medicine, a large trial comparing fluid resuscitation of critical patients with either saline or albumin found no significant differences between the groups in a number of variables, including 28-day outcome.[52] The authors of the study concluded that decisions about which fluid to use should be based on clinician preference, possible adverse effects, and cost. When considering chronic albumin supplementation, as opposed to acute volume expansion, the amount of albumin required can be estimated using an equation that corrects for the expected volume of distribution across the intravascular and interstitial spaces[65]:

$$\text{Albumin deficit (g)} = 10 \times [\text{desired albumin (g/dL)} - \text{patient albumin (g/dL)}] \times \text{body weight (kg)} \times 0.3$$

To increase the serum albumin concentration from 1.5 g/dL to 2.5 g/dL in a 20-kg dog:

$$\text{Albumin deficit} = 10 \times (2.5 - 1.5) \times 20 \times 0.3 = 60 \text{ g}$$

This amount is equivalent to 2 L of plasma or 4 L of fresh whole blood and does not take into account ongoing losses! Hence, administration of albumin in plasma is an inefficient means of providing colloid support. In the authors' experience, human serum albumin can be effective in some dogs with hypoproteinemia or vasculitis, but efficacy can be extremely variable among patients.

COLLOID THERAPY IN PULMONARY DISEASE

The majority of pulmonary diseases result in accumulation of excess fluid in the interstitium alone or in the interstitium and alveoli. This increase in extravascular lung water is synonymous with pulmonary edema. The lung is relatively resistant to the edemagenic effects of hypoproteinemia,[157] and the two most important mechanisms by which pulmonary edema occurs are an increase in pulmonary hydrostatic pressure and an increase in pulmonary microvascular permeability.[132] High-pressure edema may occur secondary to left-sided heart failure or volume overload, whereas increased permeability edema may be caused by pneumonia, sepsis, toxic lung injury, or pancreatitis. In some clinical settings, the pathogenesis of pulmonary edema may be unclear or include both components (e.g., neurogenic and reexpansion edema).

The pulmonary endothelium is relatively permeable to protein compared with other tissues, and albumin[147] and HES[75] equilibrate more rapidly with the interstitial space even in normal lung. Consequently, the effective COP gradient that can be generated between the intravascular space and the pulmonary interstitium is lower than that in other tissues. Therefore the lung must rely more on increased lymph flow than interstitial COP dilution to protect against pulmonary edema.[132] Certain types of lung injury, such as pneumonia or chemical injury, further increase the permeability of the capillary endothelium to protein. When one considers the Starling equation, it becomes obvious that the capillary hydrostatic pressure becomes the major determinant of edema formation. Smaller increases in capillary hydrostatic pressure result in much greater fluid extravasation than occur when the endothelium remains intact. This finding clearly explains clinical and experimental studies that show that colloid therapy significantly worsens pulmonary edema caused by increased microvascular permeability.[68] If the alveolar epithelium also is damaged, interstitial edema can rapidly progress to alveolar flooding.

Absorption of water, solutes, and protein occurs via different mechanisms and at vastly different rates. Resorption of sodium-containing alveolar fluid occurs mainly via active transport by the alveolar epithelium, most likely via a sodium-potassium pump with glucose cotransport, which β-adrenergic agonists stimulate.[1] Fluid absorption occurs against the colloid osmotic gradient, which increases as fluid is reabsorbed and protein remains behind. Protein is cleared from the alveoli at a very slow rate,[83] which is one of the reasons for the protracted resolution often seen with edema caused by increased permeability.

Colloid therapy may worsen pulmonary edema if the increase in endothelial permeability is such that the majority of colloid molecules can pass through the pulmonary capillary endothelium.[69] This is particularly true if a significant increase in pulmonary capillary pressure occurs simultaneously, as is more likely with colloid infusion. Considering the extremely slow clearance of macromolecules from the alveolar space, this increase in edema may be life threatening. Conversely, if the increase in permeability is insufficient to allow loss of colloid into the interstitium, prudent colloid therapy can reduce extravascular lung water. Therefore it is important to critically evaluate the patient's response to a test infusion of colloid. An increase in COP should be titrated to avoid an increase in extravascular lung water, pulmonary capillary wedge pressure, or, at worst, a decrease in arterial oxygen concentration. When using colloids in the patient with a systemic vascular leak state, and in the absence of hemorrhage, failure to retain colloid in the intravascular space for an appropriate time period suggests that extravascular leakage of colloid is worsening, not helping, hypovolemia and edema. If arterial oxygenation worsens after colloid therapy in an animal with pulmonary edema caused by altered permeability, one must consider the possibility that the colloid is contributing to the pulmonary edema.

The use of colloids in patients with high-pressure pulmonary edema is controversial because of their greater propensity for volume overload and because existing therapies for heart failure are so effective. Therefore colloid therapy should be used with extreme caution to avoid increases in pulmonary capillary hydrostatic pressure. Colloid support in the patient with left-sided heart failure should only be used in a critical care environment with invasive monitoring capabilities. Increased left atrial pressure secondary to left-sided heart failure results in increased pulmonary capillary pressure and increased fluid extravasation into the pulmonary interstitium.[63] Lymph flow in the lung increases to protect against interstitial fluid accumulation,[157] but as extravasation increases, fluid begins to accumulate in the interstitium. In the alveoli, where gas exchange occurs, the capillary endothelial cell is closely apposed to the alveolar epithelial cell, and the perimicrovascular interstitium is relatively noncompliant. In contrast, the peribronchovascular interstitial tissue is more compliant, and fluid tends to accumulate as peribronchovascular edema cuffs, thereby protecting gas exchange.[33,34] Eventually, edema fluid distends all parts of the pulmonary interstitium and ultimately fills the airspaces of the lung. Current theory suggests that because the alveolar membrane is so impermeable to solutes, alveolar filling does not occur by fluid flow through the epithelium, but rather fluid spills into the airspaces at the junction of the alveolar and airway epithelia.[131] In the absence of increases in permeability, maintenance of intravascular COP via colloid administration can be protective against cardiogenic pulmonary edema.[151] Furosemide also increases COP, and, contrary to popular belief, it does not appear to reduce plasma volume.[43,123] Because of the opposing effects of intravascular hydrostatic pressure and COP, monitoring the gradient between pulmonary artery occlusion pressure and COP has been suggested in the management of pulmonary edema.[43,101,102]

CHRONIC HYPOPROTEINEMIA

The effective COP acting to retain fluid within the intravascular space is the net difference between the intravascular COP and interstitial COP. As intravascular COP decreases, fluid with a lower COP passes from the vasculature and dilutes the interstitial protein concentration such that interstitial COP also decreases. Consequently, the gradient between intravascular and interstitial COP is preserved. This effect means that a low plasma COP per se does not necessitate colloid therapy in the absence of clinical signs such as hypovolemia or edema. Indeed, people with a hereditary form of complete albumin deficiency have plasma COP that still is half of normal because of increased globulin concentrations, and affected individuals exhibit minimal peripheral edema.[9,44] There also appear to be no serious clinical signs in an autosomal recessive hereditary albumin deficiency in rats.[90] Interestingly, affected rats have marked hypercholesterolemia.

In the authors' clinical experience and in experimental studies,[157] animals with severe hypoproteinemia (COP, <11 mm Hg) may exhibit peripheral edema but rarely develop pulmonary edema. In dogs with hypoalbuminemia, hydroxyethyl starch has been shown to result in clinical improvement of peripheral edema or ascites.[129] The role of albumin in maintaining the selective permeability of the microvascular barrier to macromolecules[41,85] provides a rationale for the prophylactic use of albumin or artificial colloid. However, it is most important to diagnose and treat the underlying cause of the hypoproteinemia rather than administer palliative colloid therapy. Furthermore, if large ongoing losses are present, colloid support may not be effective.[89]

TREATMENT COMPLICATIONS AND ADVERSE EFFECTS

The debate about whether artificial colloids cause abnormalities in coagulation is largely superfluous because all of the commonly used artificial colloids can cause abnormal coagulation. The important question is whether these coagulopathies are clinically relevant. Despite many studies supporting a lack of clinically relevant bleeding, there also is a large amount of clinical and experimental evidence documenting serious, potentially life-threatening bleeding after administration of hydroxyethyl starch and dextran.[6,19,37,141,149] This apparently conflicting evidence implies that coagulation abnormalities are clinically relevant only in some cases. The effects on coagulation appear to be directly related to the intravascular concentration of artificial colloid.[141] Higher plasma concentrations of colloid may occur after larger doses, repeated administration, or reduced intravascular degradation. Large colloid molecules have a greater effect on coagulation than do small colloid molecules.[143] With repeated administration, the small colloid molecules constantly are excreted, and the relative concentration of larger molecules increases. This fact explains why many studies reporting clinically relevant bleeding refer to patients who received repeated doses of colloid over a period of days.

The exact mechanism of action by which coagulation is affected still is not fully understood. The most repeatable findings are reductions in factor VIII and von Willebrand's factor greater than those expected by dilution and weakened clot formation.[1-3,58,59,70] As a result of these findings, it seems reasonable to supplement clotting factors in animals at risk by use of fresh frozen plasma. In addition, desmopressin has been shown to increase factor VIII:C activity after hydroxyethyl starch infusion and should be considered as adjunctive therapy along with fresh frozen plasma administration.[36] Colloid molecules may impair the action of endothelial adhesion molecules, thereby reducing endothelial release of von Willebrand's factor.[31] This observation also raises the possibility that colloid-induced reduction in adhesion molecule interaction may reduce neutrophil adhesion in sepsis[31] and explain the higher neutrophil counts observed after dextran 70 infusion in endotoxic shock.[88]

Colloids are retained within the vascular system to a greater extent than are crystalloids, and there is a greater likelihood of absolute or relative volume overload with injudicious administration of colloids. Most clinicians are more familiar with crystalloid than with colloid infusion rates, and a helpful method to ensure a safe colloid infusion rate is to estimate the equivalent crystalloid infusion rate. Approximately 20% to 25% of crystalloid remains within the intravascular space 1 hour after infusion compared with 100% of the volume of infused colloid. Therefore multiplying the colloid infusion rate by four allows one to conceptualize the volume expansion effects of the colloid in terms of an equivalent crystalloid volume. Although this approach can be helpful in limiting excessive infusion rates, animals with cardiac or pulmonary disease or oliguria warrant direct monitoring of central venous pressure.

The low molecular weight dextrans such as dextran 40 have been reported to cause acute renal failure.[51,81] Glomerular filtration of a high concentration of small dextran molecules is postulated to cause obstruction of the renal tubules or osmotic nephrosis.[51,81] Colloids should be used with caution in patients with oliguric or anuric renal failure because the kidneys are the major routes of excretion for all artificial colloids. Nevertheless, colloids likely provide the most effective means of intravascular volume expansion in patients with capillary leak syndrome and oliguria resulting from hypovolemia and hypotension.

Anaphylactic or anaphylactoid reactions have been reported with use of dextrans, hydroxyethyl starches, and gelatins,[107] but the incidence of serious complications is extremely low.[108] Hydroxyethyl starch was associated with pruritus in up to 33% of patients treated with long-term infusions.[56] Deposits of hydroxyethyl starch in cutaneous nerves[84] and histiocytic skin infiltrates[38] were thought to be responsible. Interestingly, pruritus also has been reported after infusion of lactated Ringer's solution.[21] Several studies have raised concerns about the potential effects of plasma substitutes on reticuloendothelial function.[122] Decreased concentrations of the opsonic plasma factor fibronectin have been reported with use of hydroxyethyl starch[144] and gelatins.[23]

LABORATORY TESTS AND INTERPRETATION, CLINICAL EVALUATION, AND MONITORING

Refractometry does not accurately reflect the concentration or the osmotic effect of synthetic colloids.[26] The forms of hydroxyethyl starch and dextran 70 available in the United States both yield refractometric total solids

(TS) readings of 4.5 g/dL. As plasma volume is replaced by artificial colloid, the measured refractometric concentration of TS approaches that of the artificial colloid. Consequently, administering artificial colloid to an animal with an initial TS concentration greater than 4.5 g/dL reduces the measured TS, whereas administering artificial colloids to an animal with an initial refractometric TS concentration less than 4.5 g/dL increases the measured TS toward 4.5 g/dL. However, addition of either of these colloid preparations (in an amount corresponding to a 22-mL/kg dose in a patient) to a 2.5% solution of human serum albumin (initial TS concentration, <2.5 g/dL) led to minimal increases in the refractometric TS concentration despite an increase in measured COP.[26] As more artificial colloid was added to the albumin solution, the TS concentration did increase, but the amount of colloid necessary to cause this change would be unlikely to be used clinically.

The in vivo situation is more complicated because of other effects such as extravasation, excretion of colloid, and fluid shifts into the vascular space after administration. In clinical practice, virtually all patients with preinfusion TS concentrations of 5 g/dL experience a decrease in TS concentration after colloid administration. Conversely, increases in TS after colloid administration are uncommon, regardless of the starting TS concentration. The clinician should anticipate the dilutional effect caused by intravascular volume expansion that occurs with colloid infusion. Failure to recognize the potential decrease in TS as a result of dilution of the colloid itself could cause the clinician to misinterpret the decrease as an indication for more colloid. Unfortunately, assays for the determination of serum colloid concentrations are not readily available. Consequently, therapy with artificial colloids is best monitored by direct measurement of COP using a membrane osmometer or indirectly by assessing the cardiovascular response to infusion. More objective measures of hemodilution (e.g., serum albumin concentration) almost invariably decrease after colloid infusion. In addition to serum albumin concentration, packed cell volume, platelet count, and serum potassium concentration seem to be most affected. After administration of HES, serum amylase activity may be increased 200% to 250% of normal because of its binding to HES and decreased excretion.[20,74,87] Artificial colloids are excreted primarily by the kidneys, and urine specific gravity measured after colloid administration should be interpreted with caution. Hydroxyethyl starch also can produce predictable but potentially misleading results in blood typing and crossmatching.[45]

REFERENCES

1. Aberg M, Arfors KE, Bergentz SE: Effect of dextran on factor VIII and thrombus stability in humans. Significance of varying infusion rates, *Acta Chir Scand* 143:417, 1977.

2. Aberg M, Hedner U, Bergentz SE: Effect of dextran 70 on factor VIII and platelet function in von Willebrand's disease, *Thromb Res* 12:629, 1978.

3. Aberg M, Hedner U, Bergentz SE: Effect of dextran on factor VIII (antihemophilic factor) and platelet function, *Ann Surg* 189:243, 1979.

4. Alderson P, Schierhout G, Burns I, et al: Colloids versus crystalloids for fluid resuscitation in critically ill patients (Cochrane review). In *The Cochrane library, issue 3*, Chichester, UK, 2004, John Wiley & Sons, Ltd.

5. Aukland K, Reed RK: Interstitial-lymphatic mechanisms in the control of extracellular fluid volume, *Physiol Rev* 73:1, 1993.

6. Baldassarre S, Vincent JL: Coagulopathy induced by hydroxyethyl starch, *Anesth Analg* 84:451, 1997.

7. Barclay SA, Bennett ED: The direct measurement of colloid osmotic pressure is superior to colloid osmotic pressure derived from albumin or total protein, *Intensive Care Med* 13:114, 1987.

8. Bates DO, Curry FE: Vascular endothelial growth factor increases hydraulic conductivity of isolated perfused microvessels, *Am J Physiol* 271:H2520, 1996.

9. Bennhold H: Volume regulation and renal function in analbuminemia, *Lancet* 2:1169, 1960.

10. Bent-Hansen L: Initial plasma disappearance and tissue uptake of 131I-albumin in normal rabbits, *Microvasc Res* 41:345, 1991.

11. Bent-Hansen L: Whole body capillary exchange of albumin, *Acta Physiol Scand Suppl* 603:5, 1991.

12. Bent-Hansen L, Feldt-Rasmussen B, Kverneland A, et al: Plasma disappearance of glycated and non-glycated albumin in type 1 (insulin-dependent) diabetes mellitus: evidence for charge dependent alterations of the plasma to lymph pathway, *Diabetologia* 36:361, 1993.

13. Bert JL, Mathieson JM, Pearce RH: The exclusion of human serum albumin by human dermal collagenous fibres and within human dermis, *Biochem J* 201:395, 1982.

14. Berthezene Y, Vexler V, Jerome H et al: Differentiation of capillary leak and hydrostatic pulmonary edema with a macromolecular MR imaging contrast agent, *Radiology* 181:773, 1991.

15. Bhattacharya J, Nanjo S, Staub NC: Factors affecting lung microvascular pressure, *Ann NY Acad Sci* 384:107, 1982.

16. Bhattacharya S, Glucksberg MR, Bhattacharya J: Measurement of lung microvascular pressure in the intact anesthetized rabbit by the micropuncture technique, *Circ Res* 64:167, 1989.

17. Bisonni RS, Holtgrave DR, Lawler F, et al: Colloids versus crystalloids in fluid resuscitation: an analysis of randomized controlled trials, *J Fam Pract* 32:387, 1991.

18. Bjorneboe M, Schwartz M: Investigations concerning the changes in serum proteins during immunization: the cause of hypoalbuminemia with high gamma globulin levels, *J Exp Med* 110:259, 1959.

19. Boldt J, Knothe C, Zickmann B, et al: Influence of different intravascular volume therapies on platelet function in patients undergoing cardiopulmonary bypass, *Anesth Analg* 76:1185, 1993.

20. Boon JC, Jesch F, Ring J, et al: Intravascular persistence of hydroxyethyl starch in man, *Eur Surg Res* 8:497, 1976.

21. Bothner U, Georgieff M, Vogt NH: Assessment of the safety and tolerance of 6% hydroxyethyl starch (200/0.5) solution: a randomized, controlled epidemiology study, *Anesth Analg* 86:850, 1998.

22. Brigham KL, Harris TR, Owen PJ: [14C]urea and [14C]sucrose as permeability indicators in histamine pulmonary edema, *J Appl Physiol* 43:99, 1977.

23. Brodin B, Hesselvik F, von Schenck H: Decrease of plasma fibronectin concentration following infusion of a gelatin-based plasma substitute in man, *Scand J Clin Lab Invest* 44:529, 1984.

24. Brown RH, Zerhouni EA, Mitzner W: Visualization of airway obstruction in vivo during pulmonary vascular engorgement and edema, *J Appl Physiol* 78:1070, 1995.

25. Brown SA, Dusza K, Boehmer J: Comparison of measured and calculated values for colloid osmotic pressure in hospitalized animals, *Am J Vet Res* 55:910, 1994.

26. Bumpus SE, Haskins SC, Kass PH: Effect of synthetic colloids on refractometric readings of total solids, *J Vet Emerg Crit Care* 8:21, 1998.

27. Chan DL, Rozanski EA, Freeman LM, et al: Retrospective evaluation of human albumin use in critically ill dogs, *J Vet Emerg Crit Care* 14:S8, 2004.

28. Chen HI, Granger HJ, Taylor AE: Interaction of capillary, interstitial, and lymphatic forces in the canine hindpaw, *Circ Res* 39:245, 1976.

29. Chi OZ, Lu X, Wei HM, et al: Hydroxyethyl starch solution attenuates blood-brain barrier disruption caused by intracarotid injection of hyperosmolar mannitol in rats, *Anesth Analg* 83:336, 1996.

30. Choi PT, Yip G, Quinonez MD, et al: Crystalloids vs colloids in fluid resuscitation: a systematic review, *Crit Care Med* 27:200, 1999.

31. Collis RE, Collins PW, Gutteridge CN, et al: The effect of hydroxyethyl starch and other plasma volume substitutes on endothelial cell activation; an in vitro study, *Intensive Care Med* 20:37, 1994.

32. Concannon KT: Colloid oncotic pressure and the clinical use of colloidal solutions, *J Vet Emerg Crit Care* 3:49, 1993.

33. Conhaim RL, Lai-Fook SJ, Eaton A: Sequence of interstitial liquid accumulation in liquid-inflated sheep lung lobes, *J Appl Physiol* 66:2659, 1989.

34. Conhaim RL, Lai-Fook SJ, Staub NC: Sequence of perivascular liquid accumulation in liquid-inflated dog lung lobes, *J Appl Physiol* 60:513, 1986.

35. Conhaim RL, Rosenfeld DJ, Schreiber MA, et al: Effects of intravenous pentafraction on lung and soft tissue liquid exchange in hypoproteinemic sheep, *Am J Physiol* 265:H1536, 1993.

36. Conroy JM, Fishman RL, Reeves ST, et al: The effects of desmopressin and 6% hydroxyethyl starch on factor VIII:C, *Anesth Analg* 83:804, 1996.

37. Cope JT, Banks D, Mauney MC, et al: Intraoperative hetastarch infusion impairs hemostasis after cardiac operations, *Ann Thorac Surg* 63:78, 1997.

38. Cox NH, Popple AW: Persistent erythema and pruritus, with a confluent histiocytic skin infiltrate, following the use of a hydroxyethylstarch plasma expander, *Br J Dermatol* 134:353, 1996.

39. Culp AM, Clay ME, Baylor IA, et al: Colloid osmotic pressure (COP) and total solids (TS) measurement in normal dogs and cats (abstract). Fourth International Emergency and Critical Care Symposium, San Antonio, TX, 1994, pp. 705.

40. Curry FE: Effect of albumin on the structure of the molecular filter at the capillary wall, *Fed Proc* 44:2610, 1985.

41. Curry FE, Michel CC, Phillips ME: Effect of albumin on the osmotic pressure exerted by myoglobin across capillary walls in frog mesentery, *J Physiol* 387:69, 1987.

42. Curry FE, Rutledge JC, Lenz JF: Modulation of microvessel wall charge by plasma glycoprotein orosomucoid, *Am J Physiol* 257:H1354, 1989.

43. da Luz P, Shubin H, Weil MH, et al: Pulmonary edema related to changes in colloid osmotic and pulmonary artery wedge pressure in patients after acute myocardial infarction, *Circulation* 51:350, 1975.

44. Dammacco F, Miglietta A, D'Addabbo A, et al: Analbuminemia: report of a case and review of the literature, *Vox Sang* 39:153, 1980.

45. Daniels MJ, Strauss RG, Smith-Floss AM: Effects of hydroxyethyl starch on erythrocyte typing and blood cross-matching, *Transfusion* 22:226, 1982.

46. Dawidson IJ, Willms C, Sandor ZF, et al: Lactated Ringer's solution versus 3% albumin for resuscitation of a lethal intestinal ischemic shock in rats, *Crit Care Med* 18:60, 1990.

47. Dich J, Hansen SE, Thieden HID: Effect of albumin concentration and colloid osmotic pressure on albumin synthesis in the perfused rat liver, *Acta Physiol Scand* 89:352, 1973.

48. Falk JL, Rackow EC, Weil MH: Colloid and crystalloid fluid resuscitation. In Shoemaker WC, Ayres S, editors: *Textbook of critical care*, Philadelphia, 1989, WB Saunders.

49. Farrow SP, Hall M, Ricketts CR: Changes in the molecular composition of circulating hydroxyethyl starch, *Br J Pharmacol* 38:725, 1970.

50. Ferber HP, Nitsch E, Forster H: Studies on hydroxyethyl starch. Part II: Changes of the molecular weight distribution for hydroxyethyl starch types 450/0.7, 450/0.5, 450/0.3, 300/0.4, 200/0.7, 200/0.5, and 200/0.1 after infusion in serum and urine of volunteers, *Arzneimittelforschung* 35:615, 1985.

51. Ferraboli R, Malheiro PS, Abdulkader RC, et al: Anuric acute renal failure caused by dextran 40 administration, *Ren Fail* 19:303, 1997.

52. Finfer S, Bellomo R, Boyce N, et al: A comparison of albumin and saline for fluid resuscitation in the intensive care unit, *N Engl J Med* 350:2247, 2004.

53. Funk W, Baldinger V: Microcirculatory perfusion during volume therapy. A comparative study using crystalloid or colloid in awake animals, *Anesthesiology* 82:975, 1995.

54. Gaar KAJ, Taylor AE, Owens LJ, et al: Effect of capillary pressure and plasma protein on development of pulmonary edema, *Am J Physiol* 213:79, 1967.

55. Gabel JC, Scott RL, Adair TH, et al: Errors in calculated oncotic pressure of dog plasma, *Am J Physiol* 239:H810-H812, 1980.

56. Gall H, Schultz KD, Boehncke WH, et al: Clinical and pathophysiological aspects of hydroxyethyl starch-induced pruritus: evaluation of 96 cases, *Dermatology* 192:222, 1996.

57. Gollub S, Kangwalklai K, Schaefer C: Treatment of experimental hemorrhage with colloid-crystalloid mixtures, *J Surg Res* 9:311, 1969.

58. Gollub S, Schaefer C: Structural alteration in canine fibrin produced by colloid plasma expanders, *Surg Gynecol Obstet* 127:783, 1968.

59. Gollub S, Schaefer C, Squitieri A: The bleeding tendency associated with plasma expanders, *Surg Gynecol Obstet* 124:1203-1211, 1967.

60. Granger DN, Barrowman JA: Gastrointestinal and liver edema. In Staub NC, Taylor AE, editors: *Edema,* New York, 1984, Raven Press.

61. Granger HJ, Laine GA, Barnes GE, et al: Dynamics and control of transmicrovascular fluid exchange. In Staub NC, Taylor AE, editors: *Edema,* New York, 1984, Raven Press.

62. Guyton AC, Granger HJ, Taylor AE: Interstitial fluid pressure, *Physiol Rev* 51:527, 1971.

63. Guyton AC, Lindsay NW: Effect of elevated left atrial pressure and decreased plasma protein concentration on the development of pulmonary edema, *Circ Res* 7:649, 1959.

64. Haraldsson B, Rippe B: Orosomucoid as one of the serum components contributing to normal capillary permselectivity in rat skeletal muscle, *Acta Physiol Scand* 129:127, 1987.

65. Hardin TC, Page CP, Schwesinger WH: Rapid replacement of serum albumin in patients receiving total parenteral nutrition, *Surg Gynecol Obstet* 163:359, 1986.

66. Heir S, Wiig H: Subcutaneous interstitial fluid colloid osmotic pressure in dehydrated rats, *Acta Physiol Scand* 133:365, 1988.

67. Hempel V, Metzger G, Unseld H, et al: The influence of hydroxyethyl starch solutions on circulation and on kidney function in hypovolaemic patients, *Anaesthesist* 24:198, 1975.

68. Holcroft JW, Trunkey DD, Carpenter MA: Extravasation of albumin in tissues of normal and septic baboons and sheep, *J Surg Res* 26:341, 1979.

69. Holcroft JW, Trunkey DD, Carpenter MA: Sepsis in the baboon: factors affecting resuscitation and pulmonary edema in animals resuscitated with Ringer's lactate versus Plasmanate, *J Trauma* 17:600, 1977.

70. Jones PA, Tomasic M, Gentry PA: Oncotic, hemodilutional, and hemostatic effects of isotonic saline and hydroxyethyl starch solutions in clinically normal ponies, *Am J Vet Res* 58:541, 1997.

71. Kedem O, Katchalsky A: Thermodynamic analysis of the permeability of biological membranes to non-electrolytes, *Biochim Biophys Acta* 27:229, 1958.

72. Kirby R, Rudloff E: The critical need for colloids: maintaining fluid balance, *Comp Cont Ed Pract Vet* 19:705, 1997.

73. Klotz U, Kroemer H: Clinical pharmacokinetic considerations in the use of plasma expanders, *Clin Pharmacokinet* 12:123, 1987.

74. Kohler H, Kirch W, Horstmann HJ: Hydroxyethyl starch-induced macroamylasemia, *Int J Clin Pharmacol Biopharm* 15:428, 1977.

75. Korent VA, Conhaim RL, McGrath AM, et al: Molecular distribution of hetastarch in plasma and lung lymph of unanesthetized sheep, *Am J Respir Crit Care Med* 155:1302, 1997.

76. Korttila K, Grohn P, Gordin A, et al: Effect of hydroxyethyl starch and dextran on plasma volume and blood hemostasis and coagulation, *J Clin Pharmacol* 24:273, 1984.

77. Kramer GC, Harms BA, Bodai BI, et al: Effects of hypoproteinemia and increased vascular pressure on lung fluid balance in sheep, *J Appl Physiol* 55:1514, 1983.

78. Lamke LO, Liljedahl SO: Plasma volume changes after infusion of various plasma expanders, *Resuscitation* 5:93, 1976.

79. Landis EM, Pappenheimer JR: Exchange of substances through the capillary walls. In Hamilton WF, Dow P, editors: *Handbook of physiology,* vol 2, Baltimore, 1963, Williams and Wilkins.

80. Luft JH: The structure and properties of the cell surface coat, *Int Rev Cytol* 45:291, 1976.

81. Mailloux L, Swartz CD, Capizzi R, et al: Acute renal failure after administration of low-molecular weight dextran, *N Engl J Med* 277:1113, 1967.

82. Mathews KA: The various types of parenteral fluids and their indications, *Vet Clin North Am Small Anim Pract* 28:483, 1998.

83. Matthay MA, Berthiaume Y, Staub NC: Long-term clearance of liquid and protein from the lungs of unanesthetized sheep, *J Appl Physiol* 59:928, 1985.

84. Metze D, Reimann S, Szepfalusi Z, et al: Persistent pruritus after hydroxyethyl starch infusion therapy: a result of long-term storage in cutaneous nerves, *Br J Dermatol* 136:553, 1997.

85. Michel CC, Phillips ME, Turner MR: The effects of native and modified bovine serum albumin on the permeability of frog mesenteric capillaries, *J Physiol* 360:333, 1985.

86. Mishler JM: Synthetic plasma volume expanders: their pharmacology, safety, and clinical efficacy, *Clin Haematol* 13:75, 1984.

87. Mishler JM, Durr HK: Macroamylasaemia following the infusion of low molecular weight-hydroxyethyl starch in man, *Eur Surg Res* 11:217, 1979.

88. Modig J: Beneficial effects of dextran 70 versus Ringer's acetate on pulmonary function, hemodynamics and survival in a porcine endotoxin shock model, *Resuscitation* 16:1, 1988.

89. Moore LE, Garvey MS: The effect of hetastarch on serum colloid oncotic pressure in hypoalbuminemic dogs, *J Vet Intern Med* 10:300, 1996.

90. Nagase S, Shimamune K, Shumiya S: Albumin-deficient rat mutant, *Science* 205:590, 1979.

91. Navar PD, Narar LG: Relationship between colloid osmotic pressure and plasma protein concentration in the dog, *Am J Physiol* 233:H295-H298, 1977.

92. Oz MC, FitzPatrick MF, Zikria BA, et al: Attenuation of microvascular permeability dysfunction in postischemic striated muscle by hydroxyethyl starch, *Microvasc Res* 50:71, 1995.

93. Pappenheimer JR: Passage of molecules through capillary walls, *Physiol Rev* 33:387, 1953.

94. Pappenheimer JR, Renkin EM, Borrero LM: Filtration, diffusion and molecular sieving through peripheral capillary membranes. A contribution to the pore theory of capillary permeability, *Am J Physiol* 167:13, 1951.

95. Parker JC, Falgout HJ, Grimbert FA, et al: The effect of increased vascular pressure on albumin-excluded volume and lymph flow in the dog lung, *Circ Res* 47:866, 1980.

96. Parker JC, Perry MA, Taylor AE: Permeability of the microvascular barrier. In Staub NC, Taylor AE, editors: *Edema*, New York, 1984, Raven Press.

97. Parving HH, Rasmussen SM: Transcapillary escape rate of albumin and plasma volume in short- and long-term juvenile diabetics, *Scand J Clin Lab Invest* 32:81, 1973.

98. Patlak CS, Goldstein DA, Hoffman JF: The flow of solute and solvent across a two membrane system, *J Theor Biol* 5:426, 1963.

99. Pietrangelo A, Panduro A, Chowdhury JR, et al: Albumin gene expression is down-regulated by albumin or macromolecule infusion in the rat, *J Clin Invest* 89:1755, 1992.

100. Prather JW, Gaar KA, Guyton AC: Direct continuous recording of plasma colloid osmotic pressure of whole blood, *J Appl Physiol* 24:602, 1968.

101. Rackow EC, Fein IA, Leppo J: Colloid osmotic pressure as a prognostic indicator of pulmonary edema and mortality in the critically ill, *Chest* 72:709, 1977.

102. Rackow EC, Fein IA, Siegel J: The relationship of the colloid osmotic-pulmonary artery wedge pressure gradient to pulmonary edema and mortality in critically ill patients, *Chest* 82:433, 1982.

103. Renkin EM: B.W. Zweifach Award lecture: regulation of the microcirculation, *Microvasc Res* 30:251, 1985.

104. Renkin EM: Multiple pathways of capillary permeability, *Circ Res* 41:735, 1977.

105. Renkin EM, Joyner WL, Sloop CH, et al: Influence of venous pressure on plasma-lymph transport in the dog's paw: convective and dissipative mechanisms, *Microvasc Res* 14:191, 1977.

106. Rieger A: Blood volume and plasma protein. 3. Changes in blood volume and plasma proteins after bleeding and immediate substitution with Macrodex, Rheomacrodex and Physiogel in the splenectomized dog, *Acta Chir Scand Suppl* 379:22, 1967.

107. Ring J: Anaphylactoid reactions to plasma substitutes, *Int Anesthesiol Clin* 23:67, 1985.

108. Ring J, Messmer K: Incidence and severity of anaphylactoid reactions to colloid volume substitutes, *Lancet* 1:466, 1977.

109. Rippe B, Haraldsson B: Transport of macromolecules across microvascular walls: the two pore theory, *Physiol Rev* 74:163, 1994.

110. Rizoli SB: Crystalloids and colloids in trauma resuscitation: a brief overview of the current debate, *J Trauma* 54:S82, 2003.

111. Roberts JS, Bratton SL: Colloid volume expanders. Problems, pitfalls and possibilities, *Drugs* 55:621, 1998.

112. Rothschild MA, Oratz M, Evans C, et al: Alterations in albumin metabolism following serum and albumin infusions, *J Clin Invest* 43:1874, 1964.

113. Rothschild MA, Oratz M, Franklin EC, et al: The effect of hypergammaglobulinemia on albumin metabolism in hyperimmunized rabbits studied with albumin I131, *J Clin Invest* 41:1564, 1962.

114. Rothschild MA, Oratz M, Mongelli J, et al: Albumin metabolism in rabbits during gamma globulin infusions, *J Lab Clin Med* 66:733, 1965.

115. Rothschild MA, Oratz M, Schreiber SS: Extravascular albumin, *N Engl J Med* 301:497, 1979.

116. Rothschild MA, Oratz M, Schreiber SS: Serum albumin, *Hepatology* 8:385-401, 1988.

117. Rudloff E, Kirby R: Fluid therapy. Crystalloids and colloids, *Vet Clin North Am Small Anim Pract* 28:297, 1998.

118. Rudloff E, Kirby R: The critical need for colloids: administering colloids effectively, *Comp Cont Ed Pract Vet* 20:27, 1998.

119. Rudloff E, Kirby R: The critical need for colloids: selecting the right colloid, *Comp Cont Ed Pract Vet* 19:811, 1997.

120. Sakuma T, Okaniwa G, Nakada T, et al: Alveolar fluid clearance in the resected human lung, *Am J Respir Crit Care Med* 150:305, 1994.

121. Schierhout G, Roberts I: Fluid resuscitation with colloid or crystalloid solutions in critically ill patients: a systematic review of randomised trials, *BMJ* 316:961, 1998.

122. Schildt B, Bouveng R, Sollenberg M: Plasma substitute induced impairment of the reticuloendothelial system function, *Acta Chir Scand* 141:7, 1975.

123. Schuster CJ, Weil MH, Besso J, et al: Blood volume following diuresis induced by furosemide, *Am J Med* 76:585, 1984.

124. Shepard JM, Gropper MA, Nicolaysen G, et al: Lung microvascular pressure profile measured by micropuncture in anesthetized dogs, *J Appl Physiol* 64:874, 1988.

125. Shoemaker WC: Comparison of the relative effectiveness of whole blood transfusions and various types of fluid therapy in resuscitation, *Crit Care Med* 4:71, 1976.

126. Shoemaker WC, Schluchter M, Hopkins JA, et al: Comparison of the relative effectiveness of colloids and

crystalloids in emergency resuscitation, *Am J Surg* 142:73, 1981.

127. Simionescu M, Simionescu N, Palade GE: Preferential distribution of anionic sites on the basement membrane and the abluminal aspect of the endothelium in fenestrated capillaries, *J Cell Biol* 95:425, 1982.

128. Smiley LE: The use of hetastarch for plasma expansion, *Probl Vet Med* 4:652, 1992.

129. Smiley LE, Garvey MS: The use of hetastarch as adjunct therapy in 26 dogs with hypoalbuminemia: a phase two clinical trial, *J Vet Intern Med* 8:195, 1994.

130. Starling EH: On the absorption of fluid from the connective tissue spaces, *J Physiol (Lond)* 19:312, 1896.

131. Staub NC: Alveolar flooding and clearance, *Am Rev Respir Dis* 127:S44, 1983.

132. Staub NC: Pulmonary edema. In Staub NC, Taylor AE, editors: *Edema*, New York, 1984, Raven Press.

133. Staub NC, Taylor AE: *Edema*, New York, 1984, Raven Press.

134. Staverman AJ: Non-equilibrium thermodynamics of membrane processes, *Trans Faraday Soc* 48:176, 1952.

135. Taylor AE: Capillary fluid filtration: Starling forces and lymph flow, *Circ Res* 49:557, 1981.

136. Taylor AE: The lymphatic edema safety factor: the role of edema dependent lymphatic factors (EDLF), *Lymphology* 23:111, 1990.

137. Taylor AE, Granger DN: Exchange of macromolecules across the microcirculation. In Renkin EM, Michel CC, editors: *Handbook of physiology: microcirculation*, Bethesda, 1985, American Physiological Society.

138. Taylor AE, Moore T, Khimenko P: Microcirculatory exchange of fluid and protein and development of the third space. In Zikria BA, Oz MO, Carlson RW, editors: *Reperfusion injuries and clinical capillary leak syndrome*, Armonk, 1994, Futura Publishing Company.

139. Thomas LA, Brown SA: Relationship between colloid osmotic pressure and plasma protein concentration in cattle, horses, dogs, and cats, *Am J Vet Res* 53:2241, 1992.

140. Thompson WL, Fukushima T, Rutherford RB, et al: Intravascular persistence, tissue storage, and excretion of hydroxyethyl starch, *Surg Gynecol Obstet* 131:965, 1970.

141. Treib J, Haass A, Pindur G: Coagulation disorders caused by hydroxyethyl starch, *Thromb Haemost* 78:974, 1997.

142. Treib J, Haass A, Pindur G, et al: A more differentiated classification of hydroxyethyl starches is necessary, *Intensive Care Med* 23:709, 1997.

143. Treib J, Haass A, Pindur G, et al: Avoiding an impairment of factor VIII:C by using hydroxyethyl starch with a low in vivo molecular weight, *Anesth Analg* 84:1391, 1997.

144. Treib J, Haass A, Pindur G, et al: Decrease of fibronectin following repeated infusion of highly substituted hydroxyethyl starch, *Infusionsther Transfusionsmed* 23:71, 1996.

145. Treib J, Haass A, Pindur G, et al: HES 200/0.5 is not HES 200/0.5. Influence of the C2/C6 hydroxyethylation ratio of hydroxyethyl starch (HES) on hemorheology, coagulation and elimination kinetics, *Thromb Haemost* 74:1452, 1995.

146. Tullis JL: Albumin. 1. Background and use, *JAMA* 237:355-360, 1977.

147. Vaughan TRJ, Erdmann AJ, Brigham KL, et al: Equilibration of intravascular albumin with lung lymph in unanesthetized sheep, *Lymphology* 12:217, 1979.

148. Velanovich V: Crystalloid versus colloid fluid resuscitation: a meta-analysis of mortality, *Surgery* 105:65, 1989.

149. Villarino ME, Gordon SM, Valdon C, et al: A cluster of severe postoperative bleeding following open heart surgery, *Infect Control Hosp Epidemiol* 13:282, 1992.

150. Wall PL, Nelson LM, Guthmiller LA: Cost effectiveness of use of a solution of 6% dextran 70 in young calves with severe diarrhea, *J Am Vet Med Assoc* 209:1715, 1996.

151. Wareing TH, Gruber MA, Brigham KL, et al: Increased plasma oncotic pressure inhibits pulmonary fluid transport when pulmonary pressures are elevated, *J Surg Res* 46:29, 1989.

152. Weiderhelm CA, Black LL: Osmotic interaction of plasma proteins with interstitial macromolecules, *Am J Physiol* 231:638, 1976.

153. Weisberg HF: Osmotic pressure of the serum proteins, *Ann Clin Lab Sci* 8:155-164, 1978.

154. Wiig H, Reed RK: Volume-pressure relationship (compliance) of interstitium in dog skin and muscle, *Am J Physiol* 253:H291, 1987.

155. Wissig SL, Charonis AS: Capillary ultrastructure. In Staub NC, Taylor AE, editors: *Edema*, New York, 1984, Raven Press.156. Yuan Y, Granger HJ, Zawieja DC, et al: Flow modulates coronary venular permeability by a nitric oxide-related mechanism, *Am J Physiol* 263:H641-H646, 1992.

157. Zarins CK, Rice CL, Peters RM, et al: Lymph and pulmonary response to isobaric reduction in plasma oncotic pressure in baboons, *Circ Res* 43:925, 1978.

158. Zarins CK, Rice CL, Smith DE, et al: Role of lymphatics in preventing hypooncotic pulmonary edema, *Surg Forum* 27:257, 1976.

159. Zikria BA: A biophysical approach: sealing of capillary leak by intravenous biodegradable macromolecules. In Zikria BA, Oz MO, Carlson RW, editors: *Reperfusion injuries and clinical capillary leak syndrome*, Armonk, NY, 1994, Futura Publishing Company.

160. Zikria BA, King TC, Stanford J, et al: A biophysical approach to capillary permeability, *Surgery* 105:625, 1989.

161. Zweifach BW, Intaglietta M: Measurement of blood plasma colloid osmotic pressure. II. Comparative study of different species, *Microvasc Res* 3:83, 1971.

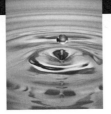

PERITONEAL DIALYSIS

Linda A. Ross and Mary Anna Labato

PERITONEAL DIALYSIS

Dialysis is the process by which water and solutes move between two compartments that are separated by a semi-permeable membrane. In peritoneal dialysis (PD), the two compartments consist of blood in the peritoneal capillaries and fluid (dialysate) instilled into the peritoneal cavity; the peritoneum serves as the semipermeable membrane. The primary indication for PD in animals is for renal failure to correct the resulting water, solute, and acid-base abnormalities and to remove uremic toxins.

BIOLOGY OF THE PERITONEAL MEMBRANE

The peritoneum is the serosal membrane that lines the abdominal cavity. The portion that covers the viscera and other intraabdominal structures is known as the visceral peritoneum, and that which lines the abdominal cavity is known as the parietal peritoneum. In humans, the surface area of the peritoneum is approximately the same as the body surface area (1 to 2 m^2), and the visceral peritoneum accounts for approximately 80% of the total.[9] Peritoneal surface area is proportionately larger in comparison to body surface area in infants and children,[10] suggesting that this difference would also be true for dogs and cats.

Anatomically, the peritoneum consists of the mesothelium and underlying interstitial tissue (Fig. 28-1). The mesothelium consists of a simple squamous epithelial-like monolayer supported by a basement membrane. The mesothelial cells have many apical microvilli that increase the functional surface area of the membrane. In humans, the basement membrane contains type IV collagen, proteoglycans, and glycoproteins. The interstitium is a layer of connective tissue below the basement membrane. Found within the connective tissue are extracellular matrix molecules, including collagen, fibronectin, and elastin. This layer has a gel-like character because of the presence of various proteoglycans. Blood vessels are located at various distances from the mesothelial surface and can be found throughout the connective tissue layer. Lymphatics also are found in this layer, most commonly in the subdiaphragmatic peritoneum. These lymphatics drain primarily via stomata in the diaphragmatic peritoneum.[9,45] The role of lymphatics in fluid and solute exchange from the peritoneum is poorly understood because of the difficulty in directly measuring lymph flow. Lymph flow is affected more by gravity than is blood flow through vessels, and therefore the upright posture of humans versus the quadruped stance of animals may mean that the role of peritoneal lymphatics differs between species.

The most important function of the peritoneal membrane is to provide a protective, lubricating surface for the abdominal organs. Mesothelial cells secrete glycosaminoglycans including hyaluronic acid, proteoglycans such as decorin and biglycan, and phosphatidylcholine-containing lamellar bodies.[45] However, recent research has shown that mesothelial cells play a role in a number of other processes, including antigen presentation, control of inflammation, tissue repair, coagulation, and fibrinolysis.[12,31] Interestingly, the role of the mesothelium in fluid and solute transport is controversial. Some studies suggest that mesothelial cells can play an active role in fluid and solute transport. Plasmalemmal vesicles may mediate transport across mesothelial cells.[28,45] Mesothelial cells also may affect blood flow through peritoneal capillaries by secretion of various vasoactive substances, including nitric oxide and endothelin.[45] However, it is generally believed that the mesothelium does not represent a significant barrier to water transport. Most studies indicate that transport across the mesothelium occurs primarily by passive diffusion through intercellular clefts in response to differences in osmotic and fluid pressures,[45] and others have shown that damage to or removal of the mesothelium has no effect on water transport across the peritoneal membrane.[23] Still other studies have shown differences in permeability of different regions of the mesothelium, with visceral mesothelium being more permeable than parietal mesothelium.[10]

The anatomic structures that appear to play the most important role in fluid and solute transport are the walls of the capillaries and the extracellular matrix located in the

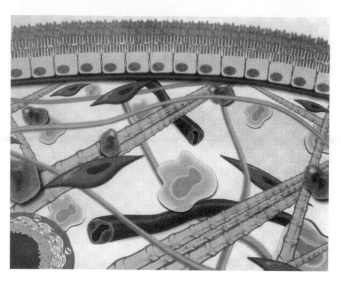

Fig. 28-1 Diagrammatic representation of the peritoneal membrane. (From Nagy JA, Jackman RW: *Dialysis and transplantation: a companion to Brenner & Rector's The Kidney,* Philadelphia, 2000, WB Saunders, p. 110.)

submesothelial cell connective tissue.[22,23,58] Peritoneal capillaries are composed primarily of nonfenestrated endothelial cells supported by a basement membrane. Endothelial cells contain aquaporins, which are 20-kDa cellular membrane proteins that are responsible for water transport. Intercellular clefts between endothelial cells also play a role in solute transport.[32]

Although the anatomic surface area of the peritoneum is large, the effective surface area—that area involved in fluid and solute movement—is considerably smaller. This discordance is because transport of water and solutes is primarily dependent on the surface area of peritoneal capillaries, rather than the mesothelium.[3,9,32]

FLUID AND SOLUTE TRANSPORT

The mechanisms by which fluids and solutes are transported across the peritoneal membrane involve several physical processes, including diffusion, convection, and ultrafiltration. Diffusion can be defined as the tendency for solutes to disperse within the available space.[10] Solutes move by osmosis from a space with a higher concentration of that solute to one with a lower concentration. When this movement occurs across a semipermeable membrane, the rate of diffusion is governed by the permeability of the membrane, the available surface area for diffusion, and the concentration of solute on either side of the membrane. Diffusion is most rapid when the two solutions have markedly different solute concentrations, and the rate of movement of solute slows as the concentrations become more equal. Diffusion continues until the solutions on either side of the semipermeable membrane are of equal solute concentration.

Ultrafiltration is the movement of water across a semipermeable membrane caused by differences in osmolality or hydrostatic pressure in the two solutions. In PD, ultrafiltration is accomplished by instilling fluid into the peritoneal cavity that is of higher osmolality than that of plasma. Water then will move from plasma circulating in the peritoneal capillaries, across the endothelium and the peritoneum, and enter the peritoneal space. Ultrafiltration frequently is desired when performing PD in animals with renal failure because they often are overhydrated as a result of fluid therapy.

Convection occurs when solutes are carried along with the bulk flow of water during ultrafiltration. This movement can occur even when the concentrations of solute on either side of the semipermeable membrane would not promote diffusion of the solute. This effect does not play an important role in PD; it is more important in hemodialysis, where this process can be mechanically manipulated (see Chapter 29).

A variety of mathematical models have been proposed over the years to account for movement of water and solutes across the peritoneum. The three-pore model appears to best describe peritoneal transport.[3,21,58] Large pores, greater than 150 Å in diameter, allow the transport of macromolecules. They are present in only small numbers, accounting for 5% to 7% of the total pore surface area. Small pores, 20 to 25 Å in diameter, allow the passage of low molecular weight substances such as urea, creatinine, and glucose. It is believed that the clefts between capillary endothelial cells function as small pores and are present in large numbers, representing more than 90% of the pore surface area. Ultrasmall pores, 3 to 5 Å in diameter, allow the passage of only water. These ultrasmall pores are believed to be molecular water channels called aquaporins. Aquaporins are a family of transmembrane polypeptides that permit water transport across the cellular membrane in response to an osmotic gradient.[48,55] Aquaporin 1 appears to be the channel that is involved in water transport across the peritoneum. However, the location and amount of aquaporin 1 are not yet well understood. Aquaporin 1 appears to be constitutively expressed in peritoneal capillary endothelium[48,49,55] but recently has been found to also be expressed in peritoneal mesothelial cells.[36,47,55] Aquaporin expression in mesothelial cells can be induced by exposure of the cells to hyperosmotic solutions.[47]

It has also been postulated that the location and the number of peritoneal capillaries affect the rate of transport of fluid and solutes.[9,37,52] Those capillaries that are located farther from the mesothelium would participate less in the transport process.

In PD, diffusion is responsible for the transfer of urea, creatinine, and other small solutes from the compartment in which they are present in high concentration (plasma in peritoneal capillaries) to that in which they have low or no concentration (dialysate). Because the rate of diffusion depends on the osmotic gradient between the two solutions, movement of uremic solutes into dialysate by diffusion occurs most rapidly at the start of a dwell cycle. The rate of removal of a substance by diffusion is not only related to osmotic gradients but also to the size of the molecule and to the area available for diffusion. Urea has a relatively low molecular weight of 60 and diffuses more rapidly than creatinine, which has a molecular weight of 113. Larger molecules such as albumin (MW 69,000) are dependent on diffusion through larger pores, and the rate is comparably slower (Fig. 28-2).

The rate of ultrafiltration of water during PD is dependent on the osmotic gradient between peritoneal capillary plasma and dialysate, as well as the effective peritoneal surface area and capillary blood flow. In addition, the movement of charged solutes (especially sodium) by convection across the peritoneal membrane does not occur in direct proportion to their concentration in blood. This effect is termed sieving and occurs because there is a greater barrier to solute than water movement across the peritoneum. Sieving coefficients for different solutes vary with charge and molecular weight.[9,32] As a result of sieving, the rate of decrease in solute concentration gradient gradually slows with longer dwell times. In humans, different patients have different characteristics of the peritoneal membrane, resulting in different coefficients. People treated with chronic PD undergo testing to determine the rate of ultrafiltration and solute clearance. One such test measures the rate at which creatinine appears in the dialysate compared with its concentration in plasma. The reason

for performing such tests is that humans who are treated with chronic peritoneal dialysis have or develop changes in the peritoneal membrane that affect the rate at which solutes are transported. In low solute transporters, the osmotic gradient between plasma and dialysate remains high for a longer period, and therefore there is a high rate of ultrafiltration of water into dialysate. In high transporters, there is more efficient removal of urea, creatinine, and other uremic substances, but ultrafiltration is less efficient. In average transporters, the rates of solute and water movement are intermediate between the above two types.[10,32,46] There is no such corresponding information available for clinical use in dogs and cats. Although such information would be useful in formulating an accurate dialysis prescription, its benefit in the treatment of acute disease is likely less important than for chronic disease.

INDICATIONS FOR PERITONEAL DIALYSIS

The primary indication for PD in animals is for the treatment of acute renal failure. This includes oliguric or anuric renal failure, acute polyuric renal failure with severe uremia that is unresponsive to fluid therapy, and postrenal uremia resulting from ureteral obstruction or a rupture in the urinary collecting system. Although PD is less efficient than hemodialysis in correcting uremia and water and solute abnormalities, it still has a number of therapeutic advantages (Box 28-1). The decreased efficacy may be beneficial in treating cats and small dogs, in which rapid water and electrolyte shifts can result in serious clinical consequences. The equipment and supplies used for PD are easily obtained, and the technique for performing PD, although labor intensive, is not difficult. This makes PD a useful therapeutic modality for private practices, especially those located in areas distant from hemodialysis facilities.

Although acute renal failure is the most common indication for PD, it is not the only one. PD can be utilized for treatment of toxicities in which the offending toxin can be removed by diffusion across the peritoneal

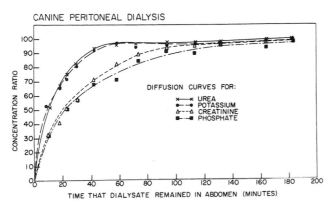

Fig. 28-2 Equilibrium for urea, potassium, creatinine, and phosphate during peritoneal dialysis in dogs. Urea and potassium diffused rapidly and reached 85% of equilibrium in 40 minutes, whereas creatinine and phosphate were only 65% equilibrated. The flattening shapes of diffusion curves indicate that equilibration periods (dwell times) of 40 minutes or less were most efficient. (From Kirk RW: *Current veterinary therapy VII*, Philadelphia, 1980, WB Saunders, p. 1107.)

Box 28-1	**Comparison of Clinical Use of Hemodialysis and Peritoneal Dialysis**

Hemodialysis
- More efficacious in altering water and solute balance
- Requires expensive equipment and supplies
- Requires a high level of technological expertise

Peritoneal Dialysis
- More efficacious in removing uremic middle molecules
- Technologically simple
- Labor intensive

membrane. Such toxins include ethylene glycol, ethanol, and barbiturates. Severe metabolic disturbances, such as hypercalcemia, hyperkalemia, hepatic encephalopathy, and resistant metabolic acidosis, also can be corrected with PD. PD with hypertonic dialysate can be used to remove excess body water in animals with life-threatening fluid overload, such as may occur with heart failure. There are other disorders in which peritoneal lavage, using solutions and techniques very similar to those for PD, may be beneficial. These include hypothermia, hyperthermia resulting from heat stroke, and pancreatitis (Box 28-2).[19]

There are few published reports on the clinical use of PD in the treatment of renal failure in animals.[*] Although most described improvement in renal function during dialysis, overall survival remained poor. In one study of 27 dogs and cats, 24% improved and were discharged from the hospital.[17] However, 11 of 21 of the animals with acute renal failure suffered from ethylene glycol intoxication, which is known to result in a mortality rate approaching 100%.[25,63] A recent study of PD for the treatment of leptospirosis in dogs reported a survival rate of 80%.[43] The success of PD must be compared with the overall survival rate of animals with acute renal failure treated with other means because animals undergoing dialysis traditionally have been those with the most severe renal failure. The survival rate of dogs with leptospirosis treated with fluids and antibiotics has been reported to be 59% to 85%.[1,29,51] In a study of 99 dogs with acute renal failure, 43% were discharged from the hospital. Of these, 24% were left with residual renal dysfunction, and only 19% had return to normal renal function.[63] In another report of 80 dogs with acute renal

failure, only 20% survived to discharge; 44% of the dogs had ethylene glycol intoxication.[25] It may be that the survival of animals with acute renal failure treated with PD is more dependent on the underlying cause of disease than the technique.

PD could theoretically be used for the long-term management of animals with chronic renal failure. However, technical problems with catheter flow and complications such as infection make chronic PD difficult. Few such cases have been reported.[11,17,54,57,62]

CONTRAINDICATIONS TO PERITONEAL DIALYSIS

There are few situations in which PD is absolutely contraindicated. In humans, these include peritoneal adhesions that prevent fluid distribution throughout the abdominal cavity and pleuroperitoneal leaks that would result in pleural effusion and respiratory compromise. Although adhesions are common in humans, especially those that have had abdominal surgery,[12] they are not often seen in dogs and cats. Diaphragmatic or pericardiodiaphragmatic hernias are seen in animals and could result in respiratory or cardiac dysfunction. That said, pleural dialysis has been described in two dogs with acute renal failure.[56] Relative contraindications for PD include recent thoracic or abdominal surgery, inguinal or abdominal hernias, and severe hypercatabolic states, such as those seen with cutaneous burns or skin denudation. Animals with recent abdominal surgery, especially gastrointestinal surgery, are at risk for dehiscence and infection during PD because of the increased abdominal pressure and potential fluid leakage through the incision site. Similarly, progressive herniation may occur as the result of increased intraabdominal pressure. Concomitant catabolic diseases contribute to the hypoalbuminemia that can occur during PD.

PROTOCOL FOR PERITONEAL DIALYSIS

CATHETER TYPES AND PLACEMENT

The key to successful PD is the catheter and its placement. An ideal catheter allows efficient inflow and outflow, is biocompatible, resists infection of both the peritoneum and subcutaneous tunnel, and retards leakage at the peritoneal exit site.[15] One of the most common causes of catheter failure in small animals is catheter obstruction by omentum, resulting in failure to drain dialysate from the abdomen. There are many catheter designs available (see Box 28-3), and most are modifications of a fenestrated silicone tube with Dacron (INVISTA, Wichita, KS) cuffs applied to promote fibrous attachments at the peritoneal and cutaneous exit sites (Fig. 28-3). Simple tube catheters with stylets can be placed percutaneously in conscious animals using local

---

Box 28-2	Indications for Acute Peritoneal Dialysis

Oliguric or anuric acute renal failure
Acute renal failure associated with nonresponsive uremia
Postrenal failure
   Ureteral obstruction
   Rupture in urine collecting system
Removal of dialyzable toxins
   Ethylene glycol
   Ethanol
   Barbiturates
Volume overload
Hypercalcemia
Hyperkalemia
Hypothermia
Hyperthermia caused by heatstroke
Pancreatitis

---

[*]*References 8,17,26,30,34,43,61.*

anesthetics in an emergency situation.[18,19,50] A percutaneous cystotomy tube catheter (Stamey percutaneous suprapubic catheter set, Cook, Spencer, IN) also has been used successfully for acute short-term PD (Fig. 28-4). The Tenckhoff catheter, developed in 1968, is a straight soft silastic tube fenestrated at the distal end and furnished with two Dacron velour cuffs.[60] Because of the high rate of omental entrapment, surgical omentectomies are advocated when using this catheter in animals in which more than 3 days of dialysis is anticipated.[11,18,19] PD for acute renal failure should be performed for a minimum of 48 to 72 hours, but the animal's condition often necessitates a longer period of treatment.

An alternative catheter style called the fluted-T (Ash Advantage peritoneal dialysis catheter, Medigroup, Aurora, IL) has produced good results in dogs (Fig. 28-5). In one study, 17 dogs had fluted-T catheters placed by peritoneoscope and were dialyzed daily. Only four catheters had outflow failure that occurred 7 to 18 days after placement. The remaining catheters functioned for the entire study period of 60 days.[6,59] In the same study, Tenckhoff catheters in the dogs were obstructed by omentum 2 to 4 days after placement.

The flutes are designed to offer minimal resistance to influx and efflux of fluid while preventing omental adhesion. The design of this catheter prevents outward migration. There is diminished hydraulic resistance during inflow and outflow because most of the dialysate flow pathways are around the catheter rather than within it. There is more complete drainage of the peritoneum through the limbs of the catheter, which are directed both cranially and caudally in the abdomen. Any residual omentum appears to have more difficulty attaching to the slots in the catheter than to the small holes in more traditional catheters. This silicone catheter has two Dacron cuffs that when implanted in the rectus muscle and subcutaneous layers become anchored by ingrowth of fibroblasts.[6,59] The fluted aspect of the catheter is placed against the parietal peritoneum and oriented in a cranial to caudal plane. The catheter is flexible and designed to temporarily fold at the crosspiece to facilitate insertion. The fluted aspect of the catheter is 30 cm in length but can be cut to a shorter length for small patients. In humans, it is placed in a paramedian location, with the long aspect directed toward the inguinal ring. A subcutaneous tunnel is directed laterally for placement of the superficial cuff and the exit site of the catheter.[7] A similar approach is used in both dogs and cats. Alternatives to the fluted-T catheter are the 15-French Blake surgical drain[2] (Johnson and Johnson, Arlington, TX), the Swan Neck straight or curled Missouri catheter (Kendall Healthcare, Mansfield, MA) (Fig. 28-6) and the 10-cm-length PD catheter, coaxial design (Global Veterinary Products, New Buffalo, MI) (Fig. 28-7). These catheters are placed surgically. Although not specifically designed for PD, the Blake

---

Box 28-3   Suppliers of Peritoneal Dialysis Catheters

Medigroup, Inc.
505 Weston Ridge Drive
Naperville, IL 60563-3932
800-323-5389
630-428-4148 (fax)
www.medigroupinc.com

Ash Advantage Peritoneal Catheter
Adult, standard
Flex-Neck Peritoneal Catheter
Coiled Adult Standard and Large

Kendall Healthcare/Kendall Vascular
15 Hampshire Street
Mansfield, MA 02048
800-962-9888
www.kendallhq.com
A variety of peritoneal dialysis catheters

Medcomp
1499 Delp Drive
Harleyville, PA 19438
215-256-4201
www.medcompnet.com
Straight and curled, one and two cuff peritoneal dialysis catheters

Cook Surgical
P.O. Box 489
750 Daniels Way
Bloomington, IN 47402-0489
812-339-2235
800-457-4500
www.cooksurgical.com
Acute and chronic peritoneal dialysis catheters, Tenckhoff and Spiral

Global Veterinary Products, Inc.
19601 West U.S. Highway 12
New Buffalo, MI 49117
269-469-8882
269-469-9940 (fax)
www.globalvetproducts.com
Acute peritoneal dialysis catheter, coaxial design

Cook Urological Incorporated
1100 West Morgan Street
P.O. Box 227
Spencer, IN 47460
812-829-4891
800-457-4448
812-829-2022 (fax)
www.cookurological.com
Stamey percutaneous suprapubic catheter

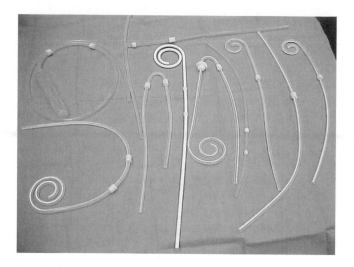

Fig. 28-3 A collection of straight (Tenckhoff) and spiral fenestrated silicone peritoneal dialysis catheters.

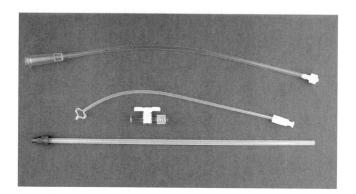

Fig. 28-4 A Stamey percutaneous suprapubic catheter. May be used as a short-term peritoneal dialysis catheter (Cook Catheters, Spencer, IN).

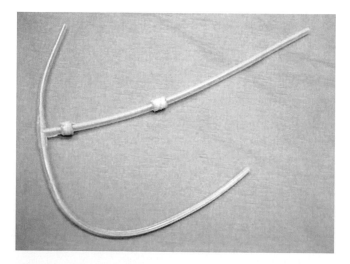

Fig. 28-5 T-style fluted peritoneal dialysis catheter with folding crosspiece. Fluted design prevents omental obstruction (Ash Advantage Peritoneal Catheter, Medigroup, Inc, Aurora, IL).

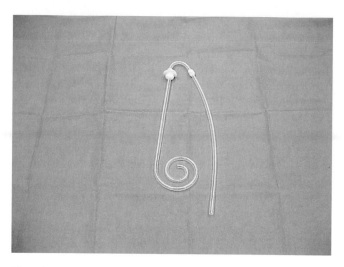

Fig. 28-6 A surgically implantable catheter design. An omentectomy is required for optimal use (Curl Cath Missouri Peritoneal Dialysis Catheter, Kendall Healthcare, Mansfield, MA).

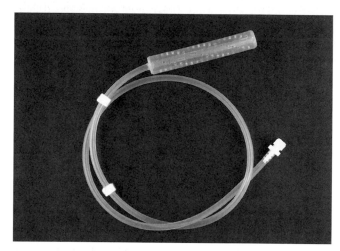

Fig. 28-7 A surgically implantable catheter design. An omentectomy is required for optimal use. (The coaxial design by Global Veterinary Products, Spencer, IN.)

drain functions in a manner similar to the fluted-T catheter and has been utilized for PD in human infants.[19]

Depending on the catheter selected, there are three placement methods: laparoscopically (with a spiral catheter guide), blind (guidewire or trocar), and dissective (surgical).[4,16] In veterinary medicine, in the emergency situation, a simple catheter that is placed percutaneously for short-term use often is chosen. After a catheter has been selected, the animal is placed in dorsal recumbency, and the abdomen is shaved and scrubbed for a surgical procedure. It is essential that the animal be draped and aseptic technique maintained to prevent contamination of the peritoneal catheter system. The simple tube catheters are placed by trocar. Using aseptic technique, the catheter (over the trocar) is inserted through a stab incision 3 to 5 cm lateral to the umbilicus oriented toward the pelvis (Fig. 28-8).[19,50] The trocar is tunneled subcutaneously for several centimeters before being inserted through the abdominal muscles into the abdomen. The catheter then is threaded over the trocar until fully in the abdomen.[19] The subcutaneous tunnel ideally should create a snug fit, but a purse-string suture should be placed to secure the catheter, and a tape butterfly can be added to secure the catheter to the skin on the lateral abdomen. Sutures have been reported to promote tunnel infections in human patients; therefore for long-term use it is recommended that a catheter with Dacron cuffs be used and no purse-string suture placed. If a cuffed catheter is to be used, the cuffs should be soaked in sterile saline before placement to remove air and facilitate fibroblast cuff invasion.[5,19] The inner cuff is placed in the rectus muscle, and the other cuff is placed in the subcutaneous tunnel. A tight

subcutaneous tunnel with fibrous ingrowth into the cuff decreases the incidence of dialysate leak.[35,40]

When it is believed PD will be performed for longer than 24 hours, a surgically placed catheter should be utilized. Although some catheters such as the fluted-T or the Quinton Swan Neck curled catheter have been designed to be placed either via laparoscope or blind trocarization in human medicine, it is preferable to place these catheters surgically in dogs and cats. Omentectomy is necessary to provide adequate exchanges for long durations. The curled tip catheter or the tip of the Missouri catheter should be positioned in the inguinal area. The subcutaneous tunnel should be such that there is a gentle bend in the catheter that does not kink and that exits caudally and off midline by 3 to 5 cm (Fig. 28-9).

Initially, large volumes of dialysate should be avoided to minimize excess intraabdominal pressure, which can promote leaks and retard healing of exit sites.[15,27,39] It is recommended that one quarter to one half of the

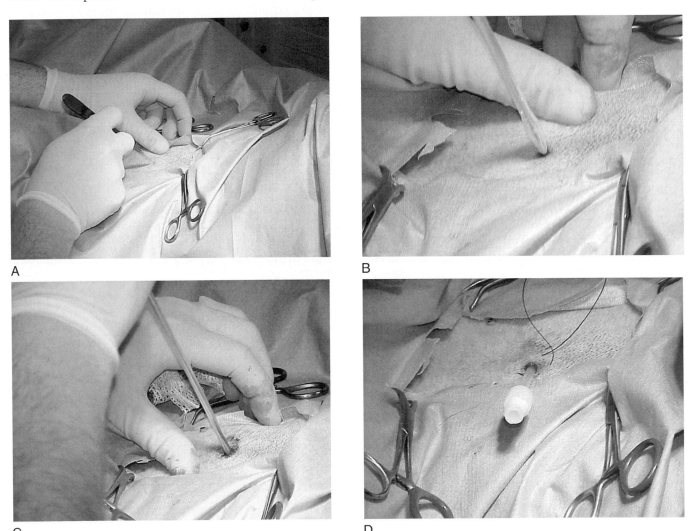

Fig. 28-8 Placement of a percutaneous dialysis catheter. **A,** A stab incision made 3 cm lateral to the umbilicus. **B,** The catheter with trocar is inserted through the stab incision. **C,** Once inserted the catheter and trocar are directed toward the pelvis. **D,** Once the catheter is fully inserted the trocar is removed.

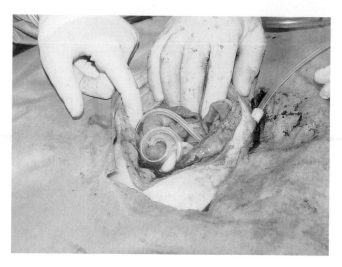

Fig. 28-9 A surgically placed catheter following omentectomy.

calculated prescription volume for the first 24 hours be infused at the start of dialysis exchanges. The catheter should be attached to a sterile closed exchange system and carefully bandaged into position with dry sterile dressings. The use of topical antibiotic ointments is not recommended because of the potential to cause maceration of the exit site tissues and fibroblast inhibition. Minimizing catheter movement during the invasion of fibroblasts into the cuffs is crucial for minimizing exit site leaks and infections. After placement of the dialysis catheter, the tail of the catheter tubing is connected to a transfer tubing set, which previously has been attached to and primed with a prewarmed bag of dialysate. Strict sterile technique should be maintained throughout all manipulations. Connections should be protected with povidone-iodine connection shields or chlorhexidine-soaked sponges.

DIALYSATE SOLUTIONS

The biocompatibility of a PD solution can be defined as the ability of a solution formulation to permit long-term dialysis without any clinically relevant changes in the functional characteristics of the peritoneum and is of paramount importance not only in maintaining the health of the membrane but also in permitting PD to be a successful long-term therapy. Solution components can affect leukocyte, mesothelial cell, endothelial cell, and fibroblast function, resulting in alterations in cytokine, chemokine, and growth factor networks, up-regulation of proinflammatory and profibrotic pathways, impaired peritoneal host defense, and the induction of carbonyl and oxidative stress.[14] Such perturbations of normal physiology have been proposed as causative factors contributing to changes in peritoneal structure, such as peritoneal fibrosis, sclerosis, and vasculopathy, and changes in peritoneal function including increased solute permeability and ultrafiltration failure.[14]

The ideal solution for PD should not be unduly hypertonic, should not impair host defenses, and should not damage the peritoneal membrane. It should be bicarbonate-based with normal pH. It should be sterilized in a manner that does not promote generation of glucose degradation products (GDPs). Most existing glucose-based solutions are lactate-based, have low pH and high tonicity, contain GDPs, and glycosylate the peritoneal membrane.

Commercially prepared dialysate solutions containing various concentrations of dextrose are available. Dialysis for removal of solutes generally is performed using 1.5% dextrose. Dialysates containing 2.5% and 4.25% dextrose are used in moderate to severely overhydrated patients. Dialysate solutions are buffered, slightly hyperosmolar crystalloid solutions designed to pull fluid, potassium, urea, and phosphate from the plasma into the dialysate while providing diffusible buffer and other needed compounds such as magnesium and calcium.[38]

Hypertonic dextrose-containing dialysate solutions are effective for minimizing edema in overhydrated patients and for enhancing ultrafiltration (removal of water) in all patients. Hypertonic dextrose appears to favor capillary vasodilatation and promotes solute drag. A 1.5% dextrose dialysate is used in dehydrated or normovolemic patients. The 2.5% and 4.25% dialysates should be used in mildly to severely overhydrated patients. Intermittent use of a 4.25% dialysate solution may increase the efficiency of dialysis in all patients.[38] Heparin (250 to 1000 U/L) should be added to the dialysate for the first few days after catheter placement to help prevent occlusion of the catheter by fibrin deposition. This heparin is minimally absorbed by the patient's circulation and is unlikely to prolong clotting times.[15,19,39] The recommended infusion volume for small animals is 7 to 20 mL/kg for the first 24 hours and then 30 to 40 mL/kg. The dialysate should be warmed to 38° C to improve permeability of the peritoneum. The dialysate line should be placed in a fluid warmer to help maintain this temperature.

Adding dextrose to lactated Ringer's solution can make a suitable dialysate solution. Osmolality should closely approximate that of the patient, and the dextrose concentration should be at least 1.5%. Adding 30 mL of 50% glucose to 1 L of lactated Ringer's solution will result in a 1.5% dextrose solution.

Glucose itself is harmful to the peritoneum. The glucose concentration of dialysate solutions is high. The tissues of the peritoneal membrane are continuously exposed to glucose concentrations that are clearly in the diabetic range. These concentrations of glucose are toxic to the mesothelium. Glucose activates the polyol pathway and the secretion of transforming growth factor-β1 (TGF-β1), monocyte chemoattractant protein-1 (MCP-1), and fibronectin. In vitro data suggest that glucose is involved in the development of peritoneal fibrosis.[64] Glucose is likely to be involved in the development of peritoneal neoangiogenesis. The clinical importance of this finding is that it leads to enlargement of the peritoneal vascular surface area, resulting in loss of the osmotic gradient, which ultimately impairs ultrafiltration.[64] A third mechanism by which glucose can damage the peritoneal tissue is by inducing nonenzymatic glycosylation of tissue proteins, which leads to the formation of advanced glycosylation end products (AGEs). The deposition of AGEs in the vascular wall also leads to ultrafiltration failure.[64]

GDPs are formed during the heat sterilization process of dialysate solutions. GDPs consist of aldehydes such as formaldehyde and dicarbonyl products such as glyoxal and methylglyoxal. GDPs may affect the peritoneal membrane by three mechanisms. They are toxic to fibroblasts. Methylglyoxal enhances the production of vascular endothelial growth factor (VEGF). Finally, GDPs trigger the formation of AGEs at a much faster rate than glucose.[64]

Thus standard glucose-based PD solutions have long-term detrimental effects on the peritoneum because of the presence of high concentrations of lactate, glucose, GDPs, and low pH, which may result in diminished defense mechanisms and ultrafiltration failure.[64] However, for short-term use in veterinary medicine, no adverse effects have been recognized.

Until recently, there have been few practical alternatives to glucose. Now polyglucose (icodextrin) (Extrarenal, Baxter Healthcare Corporation, Deerfield, IL) is available. Icodextrin (7.5% polyglucose) is a mixture of high molecular weight, water-soluble glucose polymers isolated by fractionation of hydrolyzed cornstarch. Icodextrin is a glucose polymer of MW 16,800 and osmolality of 285 mOsm/kg. No diffusion into the blood occurs, and the colloid osmotic gradient and ultrafiltration are maintained as the dwell proceeds. Ultrafiltration occurs by colloid osmosis via small pores. Minimal ultrafiltration occurs via ultrapores, through which glucose mainly acts, and consequently there is no sodium sieving. Icodextrin is absorbed via lymphatics and metabolized to maltose. No toxicity has been identified. However, a number of adverse effects have been reported with icodextrin use (e.g., sterile peritonitis, peritoneal mononucleosis, antibody formation). In humans undergoing chronic ambulatory PD, icodextrin is utilized during the long dwell periods.[42,44,64] Icodextrin's role in veterinary PD has yet to be investigated.

Bicarbonate-based solutions are being developed to increase solution biocompatibility and thus protect the peritoneal membrane. Their formulation also reduces infusion pain. These solutions require use of a double chamber bag to separate bicarbonate from calcium. A 1.1% amino acid solution now is available in many countries to supplement protein intake and treat or prevent malnutrition.[20,64] One exchange of the 1.1% amino acid solution per day has been shown to improve nitrogen balance and biochemical markers of nutrition in malnourished continuous ambulatory PD patients.[33]

DELIVERY TECHNIQUE

Aseptic technique during delivery of dialysate is essential to minimize the risk of peritonitis (Box 28-4). Hands should be thoroughly washed and sterile gloves used while changing the dialysate bags or lines because the most common cause of peritonitis is contamination of the bag spike.[11,19] Routine use of a face mask while doing bag exchanges and catheter maintenance has been shown to be unnecessary as long as proper hand care is maintained.[24] Every line connection should be covered with a povidone-iodine connection shield or chlorhexidine-soaked dressings covered with sterile gauze. All injection ports should be scrubbed with chlorhexidine and alcohol before injections, and the use of multiple-dose vials (e.g., heparin or potassium chloride) for dialysate supplements should be avoided to decrease the risk of introducing microorganisms.

Although dialysis can be performed with a straight-line transfer set, use of a closed, flush system has been associated with lower infection rates.[11,41] The closed "Y" system allows the lines to be flushed free of possible bacterial contamination before each dialysate infusion without opening the system to outside air.

THE EXCHANGE PROCEDURE

For the first 24 to 48 hours after catheter placement, exchange volumes should be one quarter to one half the

---

Box 28-4 | **Guidelines for Preventing Infection During Peritoneal Dialysis**

1. Wash hands before beginning. Wear sterile gloves when changing bags or handling lines. Work in a clean environment.
2. Use povidone-iodine connection shields or chlorhexidine-soaked dressings covered with sterile gauze over all line connections.
3. Scrub injection ports for 2 minutes before injections, or allow chlorhexidine to sit on injection ports and medication bottles for 5 minutes before use.
4. Avoid multiple dose vials for dialysate additives.
5. Adjust dialysate prescription to prevent exit site leaks.
6. Minimize catheter movement at cutaneous exit site. Wash the area with chlorhexidine scrub, and dry with sterile gauze once daily. Dry sterile bandages are recommended at catheter exit site from body wall.
7. Examine dialysate for cloudiness before and after each exchange.
8. Provide adequate nutritional support to the patient by enteral or parenteral routes.

calculated ideal volume to assess the degree of abdominal distention, the effect on respiratory function, and the potential for dialysate leakage. After the first 24 hours, the dialysate is infused at a dosage of 30 to 40 mL/kg during a 10-minute period.[11,13,35,53] The dialysate is allowed to remain in the peritoneal cavity for 30 to 40 minutes (dwell time) and then is drained into a collection bag by gravity during a 20- to 30-minute period. A 90% to 100% recovery of dialysate is expected. This process is repeated continually, and the dialysate formula and dwell times are adjusted every 12 to 24 hours according to the animal's need.

A Y-set tubing with a fresh dialysate bag and a drainage container attached to either segment is connected to the catheter tubing or transfer set (Fig. 28-10). First, a small amount of fresh dialysate is flushed into the drainage bag, and then the peritoneal cavity is drained, so that any contaminants introduced during the connection procedures are flushed into the drainage bag and not into the peritoneal cavity. After drainage, the fresh dialysate is infused. This "drain first–infuse later" principle has markedly decreased the incidence of peritonitis in humans on PD as compared with the "infuse first–drain later" principle used in the straight single-spiked system.[5,35]

The exchange technique for severe uremia should follow the protocol described below:

1. The dialysate should remain in the abdomen for 30 to 40 minutes.
2. Dialysis cycles should be repeated every 1 to 2 hours until the animal is clinically improved and blood urea nitrogen (BUN) and serum creatinine concentrations have decreased.
3. This initial intensive dialysis typically continues for 24 to 48 hours. DO NOT attempt to bring BUN and

serum creatinine concentrations into the normal range. A reasonable target is a BUN concentration of 60 to 100 mg/dL and a serum creatinine concentration of 4.0 to 6.0 mg/dL.

4. The animal then can be changed to the chronic dialysis cycle.

The chronic dialysis protocol includes the following:

1. Dialysate should remain in the abdomen for 3 to 6 hours.
2. Three to four exchanges per day are performed. The dialysate should remain in the abdomen during these extended exchange periods.
3. Rate of infusion can be rapid in most cases without problems. If the animal shows signs of discomfort during infusion, check that the solution temperature is not too hot or too cold. Also slow the rate of infusion.

The frequency of the dialysis exchanges and the duration of the dwell time are adjusted for each animal's individual needs. The goal of PD for an animal with renal failure is to remove enough urea to maintain the BUN concentration at 70 mg/dL.[19,53] The amount of solute transferred across the peritoneal membrane is determined by the concentration gradient for each solute. If there is a need to increase the removal of large molecules such as creatinine, the dwell time for each exchange is extended.

Dialysis should be continued until renal function has normalized or is adequate to maintain the patient without dialysis as determined by urine output, stabilization of laboratory values, and clinical signs. Gradual reduction of the number of exchanges and having "rest" periods are recommended. This intermittent PD should be done during a 3- to 4-day period, with continual reevaluation of the patient's clinical state. If the animal receiving aggressive, well-managed continual PD has not improved according to biochemical parameters or uremic signs after several days, chronic PD, chronic hemodialysis, renal transplantation, or euthanasia should be considered.

MONITORING

Careful records of the dialysate volume infused and recovered during each exchange period should be maintained (Fig. 28-11). Less fluid may be recovered from the abdomen than was delivered for the first few exchanges. As dialysis proceeds, outflow should approximate or exceed inflow if the patient is adequately hydrated.

In the acute setting, body weight and hydration status should be monitored frequently, with body weight recorded consistently (i.e., either with or without dialysate in the abdomen). Measurement of central venous pressure (CVP) through a jugular catheter is a

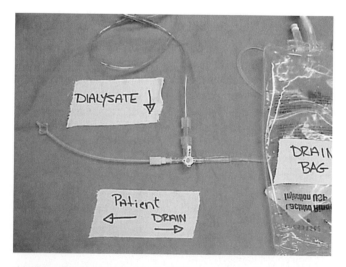

Fig. 28-10 The "Y-set" system. Dialysate bag upper left and the collecting bag at the bottom right of the photo. The connecting tubing to the patient is to the left.

Peritoneal Dialysis Flow Sheet

Exchange #	Inflow Time	Dwell Time	Outflow Time	Dialysate Volume In	Dialysate Volume Out	Net Balance of Dialysate Only	IV Fluids In	Urine Out	Total Fluids In	Total Fluids Out	Fluid Differences, Comments
1	8-8:20pm	8:20-8:40	8:40-9pm	200ml	180ml	-20/-20	20ml	1cc	220ml (220)	181ml (229)	+39ml (Fluid balance + in animal)
2	9-9:20	9:20-9:40	9:40-10	200ml	229ml	+29/+9	20ml	0cc	440 (220)	410ml (230)	+30ml

Fig. 28-11 Flow chart used at the author's institution for monitoring dialysate and fluid volumes.

relatively sensitive method for detecting overhydration and should be performed every 4 hours. Determination of packed cell volume (PCV) and total protein should be performed at least twice daily (Box 28-5). Serum electrolyte concentrations and other blood chemistries including BUN, creatinine, albumin, and acid-base should be assessed initially every 8 to 12 hours and then daily (Fig. 28-12).[35]

A number of metabolic aberrations may occur in patients on PD, including alterations in serum sodium, potassium, magnesium, and glucose concentrations as well as changes in acid-base status. Frequent monitoring and adjustment in dialysate and supplemental parenteral fluid composition may be necessary.

In cases of acute renal failure, the objectives of PD are to reduce azotemia, resolve the clinical signs of uremia, and to help correct fluid, electrolyte, and acid-base imbalances until the animal's renal function can recover sufficiently. Conversion of the anuric or oliguric state to a polyuric state and stabilization or improvement of azotemia are the primary indications for discontinuation of PD.

COMPLICATIONS

Complications are common with PD, but they are manageable if recognized early (Box 28-6). The most common complications include catheter flow problems, exit site leaks, hypoalbuminemia, peritonitis, pleural effusion, dyspnea resulting from increased abdominal pressure, changes in hydration status, and electrolyte abnormalities.

Catheter flow obstruction by fibrin and omentum leading to dialysate retention are common problems when catheters are placed percutaneously.[13,35] In one study, 30% of dogs undergoing PD developed such obstructions.[17] Careful catheter placement and management are important preventative steps. Heparinized saline flushes of the catheter for the first few days may decrease the occurrence

Box 28-5	Guidelines for Monitoring the Animal Undergoing Peritoneal Dialysis

1. Weigh the animal twice daily before dialysate infusion.
2. Check central venous pressure (CVP) every 4 to 6 hours.
3. Check systemic arterial blood pressure every 6 to 8 hours.
4. Check body temperature every 6 to 8 hours.
5. Record heart rate and respiratory rate every 2 hours. Note if there is respiratory difficulty with dialysate infusion.
6. Perform adequate peritoneal catheter exit site care, and evaluate for exit site infection daily.
7. Evaluate serum urea nitrogen (BUN), creatinine, electrolyte, albumin, and venous blood gas analysis once to twice daily depending on severity of azotemia. Evaluate serum magnesium every 3 days.
8. Record or weigh the amount of dialysate infused and recovered with each exchange.

of omentum wrapping around the catheter.[19] If a clot in the catheter is suspected, a high-pressure saline flush or the addition of 15,000 U of urokinase to the catheter for 3 hours may dislodge clots.[5] Decreasing volumes of dialysate during outflow or abdominal pain on dialysate inflow are evidence of omental entrapment. If omental entrapment occurs, catheters can be repositioned or replaced to correct this problem. For this reason, it is strongly recommended that catheters be surgically placed and an omentectomy performed if use of the PD catheter is anticipated for longer than 48 hours.

Protein losses can be clinically important with PD. Losses may increase dramatically (50% to 100%) when peritonitis is present. Hypoalbuminemia was the most common complication in a review of PD cases in dogs and cats, and 41% of the animals were affected.[17] Hypoalbuminemia may be the result of low dietary protein intake, gastrointestinal or renal protein loss, loss in the dialysate itself, uremic catabolism, and concurrent diseases. Usually, the animal can maintain normal serum protein concentrations if nutritional intake is adequate. However, anorexia and vomiting are common in uremic patients, and adequate enteral nutrition may be difficult

PERITONEAL DIALYSIS FLOW SHEET

Date Parameters	Day 1	Day 2	Day 3	Day 4	Day 5	Day 6	Day 7	Day 8
Wt. TID (same scale)								
Creat & BUN BID								
Na/Cl/K+ BID								
PCV / TS / BG BID								
Fluid character								
Fluid cytology SID								
CVP TID								
BP BID								
Blood Gas SID								
Profile EOD								
CBC EOD								
Urine output q 4 hrs								

Fig. 28-12 Flow chart used at the author's institution to monitor dialysis patient's laboratory values.

Box 28-6 Potential Complications of Peritoneal Dialysis

Catheter related
  Catheter obstruction
  Exit site and tunnel infection
  Leakage of dialysate
Peritonitis
  Diagnosis is based on at least two of the three
following criteria:
    Cloudy dialysate effluent
    Detection of >100 inflammatory cells/mL or
      organisms in Gram stain or cultures
    Clinical signs of peritonitis
Acute pleural effusion
Hypoalbuminemia
Electrolyte disorders

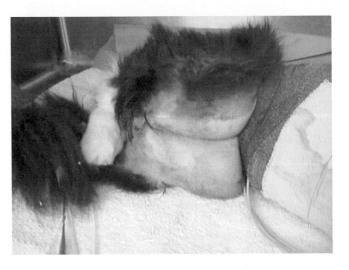

Fig. 28-13 Example of subcutaneous leakage after dialysis exchange.

to maintain. Supportive measures to maintain positive nitrogen balance often must be utilized. Nutritional support includes feeding tubes, partial parenteral nutrition, total parenteral nutrition, and a new technique of PD utilizing 1.1% amino acid solutions.[19,33] Gastrostomy and jejunostomy tubes are contraindicated during PD because of increased risk of infection and abdominal wall exit site dialysate leaks.

The prevalence of peritonitis (22%) in veterinary patients on PD is higher than that reported for humans.[17] The most common source of peritonitis is contamination of the bag spike or tubing by the handler, but intestinal, hematogenous, and exit site sources of infection do occur. To minimize exit site sources of infection, it is important to recognize pericatheter leaks.[19] Peritonitis is diagnosed when two of the following three criteria are recognized: (1) cloudy dialysate effluent, (2) greater than 100 inflammatory cells/μL of effluent or positive culture results, and (3) clinical signs of peritonitis.[19] Because *Staphylococcus* spp. is the most common organism, cephalosporins administered systemically and intraperitoneally are recommended empirically. In a recent study at the authors' institution, peritonitis was not identified in any of the PD cases reviewed during a 4-year period.[43]

Acute pleural effusion is an uncommon complication and usually occurs early in the course of treatment. A common PD complication at the authors' institution is overhydration of the patient. If the patient is gaining weight, the CVP is increasing, or the effluent recovered is not at least 90% of the dialysate infused, the prescription should be changed to ultrafiltration with more concentrated dextrose (2.5% or 4.25%) solutions. The most frequent complication at the authors' institution is dialysate leakage into the subcutaneous tissue (Fig. 28-13). This complication is managed by having the surgeon closely appose the abdominal incision (simple interrupted suture pattern only), starting the initial exchange volumes at one quarter of the calculated infusion amount, and if leakage does occur, intermittently wrapping the limbs to promote mobilization of the edema.

Dialysis dysequilibrium is a rare complication characterized by dementia, seizures, or death. Dysequilibrium may occur during early exchanges, especially in patients with extreme azotemia, acidosis, hypernatremia, or hyperglycemia. Rapid removal of urea and other small solutes apparently causes influx of water into brain cells and neurological dysfunction.[17,19] If evidence of dysequilibrium occurs, the dialysate prescription should be adjusted to remove urea and small solutes at a slower rate (i.e., fewer exchanges or longer dwell times).

CONCLUSION

PD is a realistic option for veterinary patients with acute nonresponsive renal failure or dialyzable toxin exposure. The protocol requires careful intraperitoneal catheter placement and care, aggressive exchange prescriptions, and careful monitoring for complications. Veterinarians should recognize that PD is an extremely effective tool in human medicine and should consider it as a treatment modality in an acute critical care setting.

The future role of PD in veterinary medicine may be as alternative management therapy for end-stage renal failure when hemodialysis and transplantation are not options. As advanced renal replacement therapy becomes a more common treatment modality, we may find chronic ambulatory PD is the next area to emerge. In some patients, chronic hemodialysis is not a viable option because of poor vascular access, other underlying diseases, the size of the animal, or unavailability of a hemodialysis center. Continuous ambulatory PD may serve as a treatment option for these patients. Cats that are not transplant candidates and are too small for hemodialysis are ideal candidates for chronic ambulatory PD. The active lifestyles of most dogs traditionally have made PD challenging for them. However, with a dedicated owner, chronic ambulatory PD may serve a role in renal replacement therapy. Typically, the patient is maintained in the hospital while the dialysis prescription is formulated, the incision heals, and the animal becomes accustomed to the dialysis process. Long-term care at home with outpatient visits is a goal for the future. Success will necessitate active cooperation among the owner, veterinarian, and technical staff. Long-term maintenance of low-profile gastrostomy tubes and low-profile cystostomy tubes has become commonplace. The challenge of maintaining a chronic ambulatory PD catheter will require developing and establishing excellent aseptic technique, daily bandage changes, and early recognition of any signs of infection. Investigational use of intradialytic amino acid solution and alternatives to traditional dialysate solutions will become areas of investigation in veterinary PD as more chronic dialysis is performed.

REFERENCES

1. Adin CA, Cowgill LD: Treatment and outcome of dogs with leptospirosis: 36 cases (1990-1998), *J Am Vet Med Assoc* 216:371, 2000.
2. Alexander JW, Aerni SE: Comparison of fluted silicone and polyvinyl chloride drains for closed suction drainage following cholecystectomy, University of Cincinnati and Johnson and Johnson Products Inc., 1984.
3. Anglani F, Forino M, Del Prete D, et al: Molecular biology of the peritoneal membrane; in between morphology and function, *Contrib Nephrol* 131:61, 2001.
4. Ash SR: *Techniques of peritoneal access placement, short courses in the clinical practice of nephrology,* Boston, 1993, p. 27. from the Proceedings of the ASN annual meeting.
5. Ash SR, Carr DJ, Diaz-Buxo JA: Peritoneal access devices: hydraulic function and biocompatiblity. In Nissenson A, editor: *Clinical dialysis,* Stanford, 1995, Appleton and Long, pp. 212-236.
6. Ash SR, Janle EM: T-fluted peritoneal dialysis catheter, *Adv Perit Dial* 9:223, 1993.
7. Ash Advantage Peritoneal Catheter: *Implantation instructions using a modified y-tec peritoneoscopic procedure,* Aurora, IL, 1996, Medigroup Inc.
8. Avellini G, Fruganti G, Morettini B, et al: Peritoneal dialysis in the treatment of canine leptospirosis, *Atti della Societa Italiana Delle Scienze Veterinairie* 27:377, 1973.
9. Blake PG, Daugirdas JT: Physiology of peritoneal dialysis. In Daugirdas JT, Blake PG, Ing TS, editors: *Handbook of dialysis,* ed 3, Philadelphia, 2001, Lippincott, Williams & Wilkins, pp. 281-296.
10. Burkhart JM: Peritoneal dialysis. In Brenner BM, editor: *The kidney,* ed 6, Philadelphia, 2000, WB Saunders, pp. 2454-2517.
11. Carter LJ, Wingfield WE, Allen TE: Clinical experience with peritoneal dialysis in small animals, *Compend Cont Educ Pract Vet* 11:1335, 1989.
12. Chegini N: Peritoneal molecular environment, adhesion formation and clinical implication, *Front Biosci* 7:91, 2002.
13. Christie BA, Bjorling DE: Kidneys. In Slatter D, editor: *Textbook of small animal surgery,* ed 2, Philadelphia, 1993, WB Saunders, pp. 1439-1440.
14. Cooker LA, Holmes CJ, Hoff CM: Biocompatibility of icodextrin, *Kidney Int* 62:S34, 2002.
15. Cowgill LD: Application of peritoneal dialysis and hemodialysis in the management of renal failure. In Osborne CA, editor: *Canine and feline nephrology and urology,* Baltimore, 1995, Lea and Febiger, p. 573.
16. Crabtree JH, Fishman A: Laparoscopic implantation of swan neck presternal peritoneal dialysis catheters, *J Laparoendosc Adv Surg Tech A* 13:131, 2003.
17. Crisp MS, Chew DJ, DiBartola SP, et al: Peritoneal dialysis in dogs and cats: 27 cases (1976-1987), *J Am Vet Med Assoc* 195:1262, 1989.
18. Dzyban LA, Labato MA, Ross LA: CVT update: peritoneal dialysis. In Bonagura JD, editor: *Kirk's current veterinary therapy XIII,* Philadelphia, 2000, WB Saunders.
19. Dzyban LA, Labato MA, Ross LA, et al: Peritoneal dialysis: a tool in veterinary critical care, *J Vet Emerg Crit Care* 10:91, 2000.
20. Feriani M, Passlich-Deetjen J, Jaeckle-Meyer I, et al: Individualized bicarbonate concentrations in the peritoneal dialysis fluid to optimize acid-base status in CAPD patients, *Nephrol Dial Transplant* 19:195, 2004.
21. Flessner JF: The peritoneal dialysis system: importance of each component, *Perit Dial Int* 17:S91, 1997.
22. Flessner MF: Peritoneal transport physiology: insights from basic research, *J Am Soc Nephrol* 2:122, 1991.
23. Flessner M, Henegar J, Bigler S, et al: Is the peritoneum a significant transport barrier in peritoneal dialysis? *Perit Dial Int* 23:542, 2003.
24. Figueiredo AE, de Figueiredo CE, d'Avila DO: Peritonitis prevention in CAPD: to mask or not? *Perit Dial Int* 20:354, 2000.
25. Forrester SD, McMillan NS, Ward DL: Retrospective evaluation of acute renal failure in dogs, *J Vet Intern Med* 16:354, 2002 (abstract).
26. Fox LE, Grauer GF, Dubielzig RR, et al: Reversal of ethylene glycol-induced nephrotoxicosis in a dog, *J Am Vet Med Assoc* 191:1433, 1987.
27. Goldrach I, Mariano M: One-step peritoneal catheter replacement in children, *Adv Perit Dial* 9:325, 1993.
28. Gottloib L, Shostak A: Endocytosis and transcytosis of albumin gold through mice peritoneal mesothelium, *Kidney Int* 47:1274, 1995.
29. Harkin KR, Gartrell CL: Canine leptospirosis in New Jersey and Michigan: 17 cases (1990-1995), *J Am Anim Hosp Assoc* 32:495, 1996.
30. Jackson RF: The use of peritoneal dialysis in the treatment of uremia in dogs, *Vet Rec* 76:1481, 1964.
31. Jörres A: PD: a biological membrane and a non-biological fluid, *Contrib Nephrol* 140:1, 2003.
32. Khanna R: Peritoneal transport: clinical implications. In *Dialysis and transplantation,* Philadelphia, 2000, WB Saunders, pp. 129-143.
33. Kopple JD, Bernard D, Messana J, et al: Treatment of malnourished CAPD patients with an amino acid based dialysate, *Kidney Int* 47:1148, 1995.
34. Kirk RW: Peritoneal lavage in uremia in dogs, *J Am Vet Med Assoc* 131:101, 1957.
35. Labato MA: Peritoneal dialysis in emergency and critical care medicine, *Clin Tech Small Anim Pract* 15:126, 2000.
36. Lai KN, Li FK, Lan HY, et al: Expression of aquaporin-1 in human peritoneal mesothelial cells and its upregulation by glucose in vitro, *J Am Soc Nephrol* 12:1036, 2001.
37. Lameire N, Mortier S, DeVriese A: Peritoneal microcirculation, *Contrib Nephrol* 140:56, 2003.

38. Lane IF, Carter LJ: Peritoneal dialysis and hemodialysis. In Wingfield W. editor: *Veterinary emergency medicine secrets,* Philadelphia, 1997, Hanley and Belfus, p. 350.

39. Lane IF, Carter LJ, Lappin MR: Peritoneal dialysis: an update on methods and usefulness. In Bonagura JD, editor: *Kirk's current veterinary therapy XI,* Philadelphia, 1992, WB Saunders, pp. 865-870.

40. Langston C: Advanced renal therapies: options when standard treatments are not enough, *Vet Med* 98:999, 2003.

41. Maiorca R, Cancarini G: Experiences with the Y-system, *Contemp Issue Nephrol Perit Dial* 22:167-190, 1990.

42. Martin J, Sansone G, Cirugeda A, et al: Severe peritoneal mononucleosis associated with icodextrin use in continuous ambulatory peritoneal dialysis, *Adv Perit Dial* 19:191, 2003.

43. Beckel N, O'Toole T, Rozanski E, et al: Peritoneal dialysis in the management of acute renal failure in five dogs with leptospirosis, *J Vet Emerg Crit Care* 15(3): 201-205, 2005.

44. Moberly JB, Mujais S, Gehr T, et al: Pharmacokinetics of icodextrin in peritoneal dialysis patients, *Kidney Int* 62:S23, 2002.

45. Nagy JA, Jackman RW: Peritoneal membrane biology. In *Dialysis and transplantation,* Philadelphia, 2000, WB Saunders, pp. 109-128.

46. Oreopoulos DG, Rao PS: Assessing peritoneal ultrafiltration, solute transport, and volume status. In Daugirdas JT, Blake PG, Ing TS, editors: *Handbook of dialysis,* ed 3, Philadelphia, 2001, Lippincott, Williams & Wilkins, pp. 361-372.

47. Ota T, Kuwahara M, Fan S, et al: Expression of aquaporin-1 in the peritoneal tissues: localization and regulation by hyperosmolality, *Perit Dial Int* 22:307, 2002.

48. Pannekeet MM, Krediet RT: Water channels in the peritoneum, *Perit Dial Int* 16:255, 1996.

49. Pannekeet MM, Mulder JB, Weening JJ, et al: Demonstration of aquaporin–CHIP in peritoneal tissue of uremic and CAPD patients, *Perit Dial Int* 16:S54, 1996.

50. Parker HR: Peritoneal dialysis and hemofiltration. In Bovee K, editor: *Canine nephrology,* New York, 1984, Harwal, pp. 723-744.

51. Rentko VT, Clark N, Ross LA, et al: Canine leptospirosis: a retrospective study of 17 cases, *J Vet Intern Med* 6:235, 1992.

52. Ronco C, Feriani M, Chiaramonte S: Peritoneal blood flow: does it matter? *Perit Dial Int* 16:S70, 1996.

53. Ross LA: Peritoneal dialysis. In Morgan RV, editor: *Handbook of small animal practice,* New York, 1988, Churchill Livingstone, pp. 585-588.

54. Rubin J, Jones Q, Quillen E, et al: A model of long-term peritoneal dialysis in the dog, *Nephron* 35:259, 1983.

55. Schoenicke G, Diamant R, Donner A, et al: Histochemical distribution and expression of aquaporin 1 in the peritoneum of patients undergoing peritoneal dialysis: relation peritoneal transport, *Am J Kidney Dis* 44:146, 2004.

56. Shahar R, Holmberg DL: Pleural dialysis in the management of acute renal failure in two dogs, *J Am Vet Med Assoc* 187:952, 1985.

57. Simmons EE, Lockard BS, Moncrief JW, et al: Experience with continuous ambulatory peritoneal dialysis and maintenance of a surgically anephric dog, *Southwest Vet* 33:129, 1980.

58. Stelin G, Rippe B: A phenomenological interpretation of the variation in dialysate volume with dwell time in CAPD, *Kidney Int* 35:1234, 1989.

59. Stone RW: A protocol for peritoneal dialysis, *J Vet Crit Care* 8:2, 1985.

60. Thornhill JA: Peritoneal dialysis: applications in acute and chronic end-stage kidney disease in the dog and cat, Proceedings of the 15th ACVIM Forum, Lake Buena Vista, FL, 1997, p. 31.

61. Thornhill JA, Ash SR, Dhein CR, et al: Peritoneal dialysis with the Purdue column disc catheter, *Minn Vet* 20:27, 1980.

62. Thornhill JA, Hartman J, Boon GD, et al: Support of an anephric dog for 54 days with ambulatory peritoneal dialysis and a newly designed peritoneal catheter, *Am J Vet Res* 45:161, 1984.

63. Vaden SL, Levine J, Breitschwerdt EB: A retrospective case control of acute renal failure in 99 dogs, *J Vet Intern Med* 11:58, 1997.

64. Vardham A, Zweers MM, Gokal R, et al: A solutions portfolio approach to peritoneal dialysis, *Kidney Int* 64:S114, 2003.

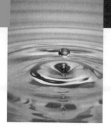

HEMODIALYSIS

Larry D. Cowgill and Thierry Francey

emodialysis is an extracorporeal renal replacement therapy used to manage the biochemical and fluid disorders of uremia. Hemodialysis was first performed in experimental dogs in 1913[1] and has evolved to become the foundation for the management of chronic kidney disease in human patients for more than 30 years.[126] The clinical use of hemodialysis has been described in dogs for nearly this same period, but only in the past 10 years has it transitioned from clinical obscurity to mainstream for the management of acute uremia in dogs and cats.[29,31,49,81] Since 1990 there has been a steady progression of technological advancements and clinical experience with extracorporeal techniques in dogs and cats. These factors have reinforced the safety and efficacy of dialytic procedures and solidified the role of hemodialysis as the standard of advanced care for uremic animals.

The major application of hemodialysis in all species is the supportive management of uremia (Box 29-1). No collection of conventional therapies can reproduce its efficacy for correction of the cumulative biochemical, acid-base, endocrine, and fluid disorders of this syndrome. Acute uremia is the most common indication for hemodialysis in dogs and cats, but the indefinite use of intermittent hemodialysis in animals with chronic kidney disease is equally indicated.[29-31,49,81] Finite periods of hemodialysis are commonly prescribed as part of the preoperative management for animals awaiting renal transplantation. Postoperatively, hemodialysis is used for delayed graft function, acute rejection, technical complications, or pyelonephritis to stabilize the animal until the episode has resolved. Hemodialysis can be used to clear toxins and toxic metabolites from animals after accidental poisoning or drug overdosage.[153]

PHYSICAL PRINCIPLES OF HEMODIALYSIS

Hemodialysis alters the composition of blood by exposing it indirectly to a contrived solution, the dialysate, across a semipermeable membrane. Solute and fluid exchange occurs by diffusion or convection, and the magnitude of the exchange is predicated on physical characteristics of the solute and ultrastructure of the porous membrane. Water and low molecular weight solutes (<500 daltons) can pass readily through the membrane pores, but the movement of larger solutes, plasma proteins, and the cellular components of blood is limited by pore size.

Diffusive dialysis occurs by the thermal motion of molecules in solution causing their random encounter with the membrane and transfer through pores of appropriate size. These random events are proportional to the concentration of the solute and result in its net transfer from the solution at higher concentration to the solution at lower concentration until the concentrations become equal and filtration equilibrium is achieved. At filtration equilibrium, the driving force for diffusion stops, and there is no further net change in composition of the respective solutions despite ongoing bidirectional exchanges between them. The rate of diffusion for each solute is determined by its concentration gradient and respective kinetic energy in solution and the permeability characteristics of the membrane. Molecular weight is the main determinant of the kinetic motion of a solute and its rate of diffusion under physiologic conditions. Small solutes such as urea (60 daltons) diffuse faster than larger solutes such as creatinine (113 daltons), and its plasma concentration decreases faster than that of larger solutes during the course of dialysis.[34,100] The permeability of a membrane is determined by its thickness, its effective surface area, and the number, size, and shape of its pores or diffusion channels.

Convective transport of solutes across dialysis membranes is associated with the process of ultrafiltration, in which water is driven through the membrane by hydrostatic pressure gradients. Diffusible solutes dissolved in the water are swept through the membrane by solvent drag.[34] Unlike diffusive transport, convective transport does not require a concentration gradient across the membrane and does not alter diffusive gradients or serum concentrations. The transmembrane hydrostatic pressure gradient between

Box 29-1 Indications for Dialytic Therapy in Animals

Acute Uremia
1. Anuria
2. Failure of fluid administration or diuretic therapy to initiate an adequate diuresis
3. Failure of conventional therapy to control the azotemia, biochemical, or clinical manifestations of acute uremia
4. Life-threatening fluid overload
5. Life-threatening electrolyte (hyperkalemia, hypernatremia, hyponatremia) or acid-base disturbances
6. Severe azotemia–BUN > 100 mg/dL; serum creatinine > 10 mg/dL
7. Clinical course refractory to conservative therapy for 12 to 24 hours
8. Delayed graft function following renal transplantation

Chronic Kidney Disease
1. Preoperative conditioning for renal transplantation
2. Indefinite intermittent renal replacement therapy
3. Recovery from acute decompensation of chronic kidney disease
4. Finite renal replacement therapy for client transition to irreversible disease status

Miscellaneous
1. Severe overhydration, pulmonary edema, congestive heart failure
2. Acute poisoning/drug overdose

the blood and dialysate compartments, the hydraulic permeability, and the surface area of the membrane determine the rate of ultrafiltration and solute transfer. During hemodialysis, a dialysate-directed transmembrane pressure gradient (dialysate pressure < blood-side pressure) is generated to initiate and control the rate of ultrafiltration. Independent changes in the dialysate- and blood-side pressures can influence the rate of ultrafiltration by altering the transmembrane pressure. The hydraulic permeability of a dialyzer is determined by physical features of the membrane (e.g., composition, thickness, pore size) and is rated by its ultrafiltration coefficient, K_{uf}, defined as milliliters of fluid transferred per hour per mm Hg of transmembrane pressure. Hemodialyzers are qualified as low flux or high flux according to their K_{uf}. A minimal transmembrane pressure of 25 mm Hg is required for ultrafiltration to offset the oncotic pressure of plasma proteins, which favors fluid reabsorption and opposes ultrafiltration.[100] Convective transport can contribute to total solute removal, especially for large solutes with limited diffusibility. However, for standard hemodialysis, ultrafiltration primarily is targeted at fluid removal, and convective clearance contributes less

than 5% to total solute removal. Convective clearance techniques are exploited further in the process of hemofiltration where solute removal occurs entirely by ultrafiltration with replacement of desired solutes and fluid with a prefilter or postfilter reinfusion solution. Hemodiafiltration and continuous renal replacement techniques represent hybrid treatment modalities combining both diffusive dialysis and large-volume ultrafiltration to achieve solute and fluid removal.[14]

UREMIC TOXICITY AND ADEQUACY OF HEMODIALYSIS

The uremic syndrome is the clinical manifestation of the cumulative metabolic disturbances resulting from renal failure.[18,149] These alterations have been viewed classically as a state of progressive retention of a broad spectrum of solutes, which are not cleared by the diseased kidneys, the so-called uremic toxins. Many of the systemic manifestations of uremia are consistent with a state of endogenous intoxication,[16] but no unique solute has been shown to account for the stereotypical clinical signs associated with uremia.[18,105] The concept of uremic toxicity is supported further by the clinical improvement observed after removal of small molecular weight solutes in uremic subjects who are treated with hemodialysis.[40,89] Water also should be considered a uremic toxin because its retention has severe clinical consequences, including pulmonary edema, cardiovascular overload, and death. However, the complete spectrum of potential uremic toxins is much wider and includes most molecules under the glomerular sieving limit, those cleared by tubular secretion and renal metabolism, and a variety of molecules that undergo progressive, irreversible, nonenzymatic modification (e.g., glycosylation, carbamylation, lipoxidation).*

Many uremic signs result from endocrine and metabolic derangements that cannot be viewed as a classic toxicity. Similarly, nutritional and fluid deficiencies are important clinical features of the uremic syndrome in all species.[20] Recent clinical evidence also supports a role for inflammation as a major contributor to the pathophysiology of uremia.[47,73-75,103]

The uremic syndrome must now be viewed more broadly as a toxic, metabolic, endocrine, and inflammatory disorder with diverse systemic manifestations. This global understanding is required to guide a comprehensive therapeutic approach to uremic animals. Hemodialysis serves to improve only the toxic component of this complex syndrome by the preferential removal of some small molecular weight solutes closely linked to the clinical expression of renal failure.[147]

*References 63,65,99,146,147,150.

UREMIC TOXINS: THE ROLE OF UREA

Uremic toxins are broadly classified based on their molecular size as small (MW, <500 daltons), middle (500 to 15,000 daltons), and large molecular weight solutes (>15,000 daltons).[146] The protein binding affinity of each substance further defines its dialytic clearance, and its volume of distribution determines its compartmentalization and accessibility for dialytic removal.[19,82] Only a few molecules have demonstrated intrinsic toxicity that mimics or reproduces particular aspects of the uremic syndrome. Other retained solutes, like urea, have minimal inherent toxicity but serve as markers for the retention of similar but unidentified solutes with greater clinical significance.[40,148]

Small molecular weight toxins have been considered the most important retained solutes because many manifestations of uremia can be corrected with their removal from the body by conventional dialysis.[147] Extensive prospective analysis in human patients with renal failure confirms significant outcome benefits associated with the extent of low-molecular-weight–solute removal (dialysis dose).[61,64,89,104,108] However, uremic toxicity is more complex than can be explained by retained small molecular weight solutes and involves retention of middle molecules and modified proteins that are poorly removed by dialysis.[26]

There is an empirical link between the appearance of uremic signs and the accumulation of nitrogenous end products of protein (amino acid) oxidation. Urea is a small molecular weight (60 daltons) nitrogenous metabolite whose plasma concentration exceeds that of all other uremic solutes. It contributes minimally to the clinical manifestations of uremia[57,71] but has remained fundamentally associated with the uremic syndrome because of its abundance and its central position in the metabolism of dietary and endogenous nitrogen, which correlate clearly with the clinical expression of uremia.[40] No single nitrogenous solute (including urea) has been shown to explain the major consequences of the uremic syndrome. Azotemia must be viewed as a marker for the collective appearance of numerous nitrogenous compounds, protein carbamylation, redirected metabolic pathways, or other small molecular weight solutes coupled to nitrogen metabolism.

Removal of urea and other (unidentified) small molecular weight solutes by hemodialysis has a proven correlation with clinical improvement and decreased morbidity and mortality of renal failure. Consequently, urea has been designated the surrogate index for all putative low molecular weight uremic toxins that remain unidentified or unmeasured.[40,67] Reduction of urea appearance and the extrarenal removal of urea are used to prescribe the therapy for uremia and to monitor the efficiency and adequacy of these therapies.[101] This designation is both rational and problematic. Urea is uncharged, present in high concentrations, readily detected, and easily diffuses across all body fluid compartments and the dialysis membrane. As such, it serves as an excellent solute to document dialyzer performance and whole body clearance of low molecular weight solutes. However, these unique features and its minimal uremic toxicity question whether it appropriately or accurately reflects the dialytic behavior of other solutes with more profound uremic toxicity and thus may overrepresent removal of these solutes.[148,151]

Dietary protein intake directly influences the generation rate of urea, and residual renal function influences its removal from the body. Thus serum urea concentration is poised to reflect both renal function and nutritional adequacy. The individual contributions of urea generation and removal cannot be differentiated by routine urea measurement, but perturbations of the steady state induced by dialysis allow kinetic dissection of these independent parameters in patients undergoing hemodialysis.[39,120] The kinetics of urea generation and removal have become the bellwether of the adequacy of dialysis delivery and nutritional status in uremic subjects.[101] Urea kinetic analysis predicts only the effect of dialysis on removal of small molecular weight solutes, but it has been shown to correlate with morbidity and mortality outcomes in humans with end-stage renal disease (ESRD).[64,67,89,104]

A variety of mathematical models have been developed to characterize the kinetics of urea during dialysis.[39,55,120,128,136] Of these, the fractional clearance of the urea distribution volume (Kt/V) has become the standard measure of the dose of dialysis delivered during a dialysis session.[101] From the same analysis, the generation rate of urea (G) can be derived to estimate the protein catabolic rate (PCR) of the patient as a measure of the adequacy of dietary protein intake.[39,54,76,77]

DIALYSIS ADEQUACY

The optimal outcome for animals with acute renal failure (ARF) is survival for sufficient time for recovery of renal function, but secondary goals may vary qualitatively depending on the nature of the underlying disease. An optimal outcome should promote physiologic and metabolic stability to optimize the conditions for recovery and an acceptable quality of life while avoiding secondary injury to the recovering kidneys.[45,53] As an outcome, survival is predicated on the diverse nature of the underlying etiology and delivered therapy, such that outcome assessment by survival alone may be disassociated from recovery of renal function or adequate delivery of dialysis.[52,107] Consequently, more sensitive and predictive outcome measures should be considered for assessment of dialysis adequacy, including recovery of renal function, improvement of the systemic manifestations of uremia, and reduction of complications attending uremia or its therapy per se.[17]

Survival still is the optimal outcome for animals with chronic ESRD because there is no prospect for recovery of renal function. The major outcome of dialysis adequacy must focus on quality of life, metabolic stability, and nutritional adequacy. Realistic expectations for the quality-of-life outcomes of animals treated with hemodialysis vary depending on age, chronicity, comorbid diseases, and residual renal function. Appropriate markers for dialysis adequacy include length of survival, owners' perceived quality of life (e.g., activity, social interaction, appetite), improvement of physiologic and biochemical variables, and prevalence of complications related to dialysis procedures or uremia.

For both acute and chronic dialysis, survival as an adequacy marker may be strongly influenced by the diverse nature of the underlying disease and the adequacy of adjunctive medical therapy, making its specificity for the dialytic intervention difficult to differentiate. Despite these constraints, the dose of dialysis (Kt/V) has been shown to be associated independently with survival as an outcome in humans with ESRD,[64,89,104,108] and it is likely to be linked similarly to the success of dialysis in animals. The empirical use of proven standards of dialysis adequacy and clinical experience in humans may serve well as first approximations for appropriate veterinary standards,[29,49] but large-scale application and evaluation are necessary to better understand the dialytic needs of dogs and cats with severe renal failure.

QUANTIFICATION OF HEMODIALYSIS AND UREA KINETIC MODELING

The dose and efficacy of hemodialysis can be expressed in a variety of ways with differing degrees of complexity. Predialysis and immediate postdialysis concentrations of routine chemistries (e.g., blood urea nitrogen [BUN], creatinine, phosphorus, bicarbonate, electrolytes) are the simplest expression of efficacy and can be applied similarly to their use in conventional therapy.[39] However, uremic toxicity and patient well-being are not necessarily predicted by the highest or lowest concentration of presumed toxins or solutes.[56] The mean exposure to uremic toxins over time is considered a more realistic determinant of well-being in dialysis patients and is expressed for urea as time-averaged concentration (TAC).[84,89,96,138] TAC is calculated as the area under the BUN profile (curve) divided by the duration of the dialysis cycle (Fig. 29-1; Appendix, Eq. 1).[39,76,87,104]

Urea and creatinine reduction ratios (URR and CrRR, respectively) are calculated from the predialysis and postdialysis plasma concentrations of urea and creatinine and are used routinely to evaluate the intensity of

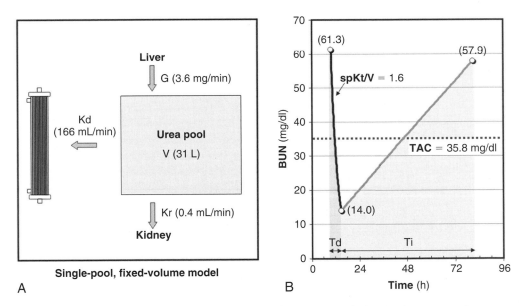

Fig. 29-1 A, Single-pool, fixed-volume kinetic model of the urea metabolism and representative modeled kinetic parameters determined in a 33-kg dog on intermittent maintenance hemodialysis consuming approximately 56 g of dietary protein. Urea is generated in the liver as the major end product of protein metabolism. The urea generation rate, G (mg urea/min), determines the accumulation of urea in the urea pool with a volume, V (L). Its removal from the urea pool is determined by the continuous residual renal clearance, Kr (mL/min), and intermittently by hemodialysis via the urea clearance of the dialyzer, Kd (mL/min).

B, Graphic illustration of a three-point BUN profile (before and after hemodialysis values in parentheses) that can be fitted to the single-pool model in the right panel. With direct measurement of renal and dialyzer urea clearances (Kr, Appendix, Eq. 6 and Kd, Appendix, Eq. 5, respectively), kinetic modeling allows computation the urea generation rate (G, Appendix, Eq. 9), the urea distribution volume (V, Appendix, Eq. 10), and the time-average concentration of BUN (TAC, Appendix, Eq. 1). The dose of dialysis expressed as the fractional clearance of the urea distribution volume using single-pool kinetics (spKt/V, Appendix, Eq. 11) also can be calculated. Td is the duration of dialysis, and Ti is the duration of the interdialytic interval. AUC is the area under the BUN versus time curve and can be estimated using a trapezoidal method or, ideally, calculated by fitting the changes in BUN to the kinetic model.

therapy (Appendix, Eqs. 2 and 3).* Reduction ratios are convenient for clinical assessment but do not account for all aspects of urea transfer. Analogous to dosing medications as the amount of drug (milligram) administered, the dose of hemodialysis can be described in simplest terms as the amount of solute (urea or other solutes) effectively removed from the animal.[12] Solute removal can be computed from either blood-side (Appendix, Eq. 4) or dialysate-side measurements.

For more precision, intradialytic and interdialytic changes in urea can be modeled similarly to pharmacokinetic profiles used to describe drug metabolism.[39,120,154] Urea kinetic modeling (UKM) is fundamental to understanding all aspects of prescribing, monitoring, and quality assurance of hemodialysis procedures and must be familiar to all practitioners of this therapeutic modality. With urea kinetic modeling, the mutually independent influences of dialysis, residual renal function (Kr), nutrition, and catabolism on the concentration of urea during or between the dialysis sessions can be assessed. This kinetic approach to urea metabolism yields the fractional clearance of urea (Kt/V, equivalent to dialysis dose), urea generation rate (G), PCR, and volume of distribution of urea (V) that are otherwise beyond clinical assessment. These parameters of nitrogen metabolism have become standards for the assessment of dialysis delivery and patient management.[67,76,101] With UKM, an animal with a low predialysis BUN can be clearly distinguished as either well dialyzed (high dialysis delivery), recovering (increased residual renal clearance), or malnourished (low urea generation rate or PCR). Conversely, underdialysis, worsening renal function, or high catabolic rate can be determined as the cause of a high predialysis BUN.

The simplest kinetic model is the single-pool, fixed-volume system, in which the entire volume of distribution of urea (total body water) is presumed to behave as a single pool with no change in volume during or between the dialysis treatments (see Fig. 29-1).[39,120,122] The kinetic variables characterizing this system are V, G, and the total urea clearance (K) (see Fig. 29-1). Total urea clearance, K, is the sum of the residual renal function (Kr) and the clearance of the dialyzer (Kd) (Appendix, Eq. 5).[155]

The relationships between G, V, and K (illustrated in Fig. 29-1) can be described mathematically such that the mathematical description of each variable is defined in terms of the other two (Appendix, Eqs. 8 through 10). When one of the variables (G, V, or K) is known, the others can be resolved by simultaneous iterative solution of the equations to yield a unique value for the known residual renal clearance (Kr) and the measured changes in BUN during and after the treatment.[39] These computations are easily performed with readily available software (Mistebar Hemodialysis Kinetic Modeling, Mistebar Computer

Consultants Inc., Las Cruces, NM; Hypertension, Dialysis, and Clinical Nephrology, www.hdcn.com) or can be programmed into routine spreadsheet applications.

The simplified single-pool, fixed-volume model presumes conditions not generally valid in clinical settings and loses accuracy if total body water (TBW) changes during or between treatments. The model also loses accuracy with high efficiency treatments of short duration, when the urea distribution volume does not behave as a single homogenous pool. Delayed diffusion from the intracellular compartment or differences in diffusion among discrete fluid compartments (e.g., skin, muscle, gut) with different perfusion and transference characteristics creates a solute disequilibrium between compartments that results in a postdialysis rebound phenomenon.[109,123] These deviations from the assumptions for single-pool, fixed-volume kinetics can be dispelled by measurement of postdialysis urea between 30 and 60 minutes after the end of the dialysis treatment rather than immediately postdialysis. At this time, intercompartmental shifts (or rebound) have reestablished solute equilibrium, and the plasma concentration reflects the true equilibrated concentration of urea across all body compartments.[127,137]

The more mathematically complex double-pool[121] or noncompartmental kinetic modeling methods (Fig. 29-2) and algorithms that account for these compartmental deviations can be performed using additional intradialytic or interdialytic BUN measurements and appropriate software.[39,59] Hemodialysis treatments incorporating ultrafiltration require use of variable-volume kinetic models to account for the additional urea removed by convection and the changes in urea distribution.

The dose of dialysis also can be defined in these derived kinetic terms as the amount of clearance provided by the hemodialyzer during the dialysis session. Using the modeled or measured clearance (K, mL/min) and the time of dialysis (T_d, minutes), the dose of dialysis can be defined as $K \times T_d$ or the volume of blood cleared of urea during the treatment (mL). This value can be indexed further to the urea distribution volume (V, mL) to compare treatment efficacy among patients of different body sizes. This expression is analogous to conventional dosing of drugs as mg/kg body weight. The value obtained with this kinetic expression, Kt/V (Appendix, Eq. 11), is unitless and represents the fractional clearance of the urea distribution volume.[39,132] Kt/V has become the international reference for dialysis dosing and delivery.[101] Kt/V is further classified according to the type of kinetic model used for its calculation as single-pool (sp), double-pool (dp), or equilibrated (e) Kt/V. The limitations of the single-pool model preclude consideration of solute diffusion from rebound after dialysis, and spKt/V overestimates the true dose of dialysis and the actual amount of urea removed during the treatment. Alternative expressions of urea kinetics mini-

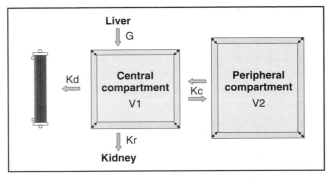

Double-pool variable-volume model

Fig. 29-2 Graphic illustration of the double-pool variable-volume kinetic model of the urea metabolism during high efficiency hemodialysis. In this model, the urea generation rate (G), the renal clearance (Kr), and the dialyzer clearance (Kd) are the major determinants of urea content in the central compartment (volume V1). An additional peripheral compartment (volume V2) continuously exchanges solutes and water with the central pool. The bidirectional rate constant for urea transference between the two pools is indicated by Kc. When Kc = 1, urea diffuses freely between the compartments and the system reverts to a single-pool model. A lower Kc implies a slower diffusional component into and out of the peripheral compartment. If the peripheral compartment remains unaccounted for, single-pool kinetic modeling results in a lower apparent V, a more rapid decrease of the urea concentration in the central pool, a greater postdialysis rebound, and overestimation of the dose of dialysis, Kt/V. Anatomically, the two compartments can represent the extracellular and intracellular spaces, respectively, or body areas with different perfusion characteristics.

mize many of these limitations of single-pool estimates. The double-pool variable volume kinetic model, dpKt/V, accounts for intercompartmental solute diffusion during and after the completion of hemodialysis and is regarded as the gold standard for dialysis dose. Alternatively, single-pool kinetic calculations using equilibrated BUN (30 or 60 minutes postdialysis) instead of immediate postdialysis BUN (eKt/V) provide an adequate estimate of dpKt/V but can be calculated more readily.

Recent incorporation of ionic dialysance modules in delivery systems permits the automated performance of bloodless on-line kinetic modeling for each dialysis treatment as an alternative to these blood-derived techniques. Dialysance of a dialyzer is a measure of solute mass transfer from blood to dialysate when the solute is present in both the blood and dialysate.[154] The clearance of a solute is equal to its dialysance when the solute is present only in the blood and absent in the dialysate. Ionic dialysance is a measure of the transfer characteristics of all dialyzable ions that contribute to plasma conductivity. The collective dialysance of small molecular weight ions is considered equivalent to the dialysance of urea, and

consequently ionic dialysance can be used as a reasonable surrogate for urea dialysance. For conventional single-pass hemodialysis circuits in which the dialysate contains no urea, urea dialysance becomes equal to urea clearance, and ionic dialysance becomes an acceptable predictor of the dialyzer urea clearance, $Kd_{(urea)}$, and the delivered dialysis dose ($Kd_{(urea)} \times T_d$), where T_d is treatment time. Ionic dialysance can be measured without blood sampling, sequentially, and in real-time by measurement of dialysate conductivity at the inlet and outlet ports of the dialyzer in response to changes in dialysate conductivity programmed by the delivery system.* Ionic dialysance can be measured repeatedly during the dialysis treatment and provides serial estimates of the delivered clearance ($K_d \times T_d$). When ionic dialysance is indexed to the urea distribution volume, V, it yields the ionic Kt/V as a measure of the dialysis dose. The availability and simplicity of ionic dialysance to predict dialysis delivery at every treatment should promote a better understanding of the kinetics of dialytic therapy and the efficacy of the dialysis prescriptions.

Routine animal hemodialysis is provided intermittently three times weekly based on the human convention. As for humans, this schedule represents a compromise between clinical benefits, time constraints, and financial burden. However, recent experience in human patients with daily dialysis schedules has demonstrated marked clinical benefits with increased dialysis frequency.[62,84] Because of the first order kinetics of diffusion, dialysis becomes more efficient as the frequency of dialysis increases.[38] Critical analysis of varying dialysis schedules has shown that the total weekly dose calculated as the sum of the individual treatments is not equivalent among dialysis schedules with differing frequencies. Daily treatment schedules have equivalent clinical outcomes to traditional thrice-weekly hemodialysis schedules even if delivered at a lower total weekly dose. For example, six treatments per week each at a Kt/V of 1.0 are more efficient than three conventional treatments per week each with a Kt/V of 2.0. To reconcile these differences, the concept of standard Kt/V (stdKt/V) has been proposed to compensate for the differences in efficiency when comparing schedules with different intermittence.[55,56] Standard Kt/V is an hypothetical continuous urea clearance that would achieve a constant blood urea concentration identical to the average predialysis urea concentration for all intermittent treatments throughout the week. This theoretical concept allows comparison among dialysis schedules with different dialysis times and intervals, including the extreme case of continuous therapy.

A dialysis schedule with three 4-hour treatments per week with a single-pool Kt/V of 2.0 per treatment is

*References 43,44,57,78,111,112.

equivalent to a stdKt/V of 2.7. Increasing the schedule to six 2-hour (Kt/V, 1.0) treatments per week with the same total 12 hours of weekly dialysis substantially increases the amount of dialysis delivered to a stdKt/V of 3.9 (Appendix, Eq. 12). Equivalent efficacy to the thrice-weekly schedule (stdKt/V, 2.7) could be obtained with even shorter treatments of 70 minutes per session when provided six times weekly for a total weekly dialysis time of 7 hours instead of 12 hours. Although a reduction of the individual treatment time is possible according to this analogy, this recommendation would not be clinically prudent.[42] Conversely, decreasing the frequency of dialysis to two treatments per week would require extension of each treatment to almost 24 hours to achieve an equivalent stdKt/V. These quantitative predictions illustrate the marked benefit to increased frequency of therapy and are in accordance with recent clinical observations that it is difficult to compensate for decreased frequency of therapy with longer treatment times.[143]

As an alternative to sdtKt/V, the intermittent kinetics of hemodialysis can be converted to a continuous equivalent clearance (EKR).[21,155] This concept is more intuitive for most clinicians in that the relative contribution of dialysis can be compared directly with that of residual renal function and with other intermittent or continuous dialytic therapies (Appendix, Eq. 7). Total patient clearance (renal clearance, Kr, and dialyzer clearance, EKR) is expressed in the familiar terms of clearance, similar to glomerular filtration rate, and the resulting total clearance can be used to predict the expected uremic morbidity, similarly to patients with earlier stages of chronic kidney disease.

A prerequisite for the validity of most urea kinetic modeling algorithms is the presumption of steady-state urea metabolism—constant food intake (quality and quantity), constant endogenous nitrogen metabolism and catabolism, stable body weight, and a regular dialysis schedule.[39] These conditions rarely exist in a clinical setting, but classic double-pool and equilibrated and EKR analyses appear valid under these conditions in human patients if careful attention is paid to the accuracy of all input variables.[22,72]

The effect of dose of dialysis on outcome has been demonstrated in humans with ESRD in several large-scale clinical studies.[*] The dose of dialysis that is adequate to manage dogs and cats with ESRD needs to be established using appropriate tools for treatment quantification. However, until these parameters are established, routine application of UKM extends the therapeutic insights of dialysis delivery far beyond reliance on routine chemistry tests and clearly benefits the assessment and clinical management of uremic animals. Kinetic modeling and quantitation of dialysis dose

are important tools for quality assurance of dialytic therapy in animals; however, they are not therapeutic goals per se.[155] The provision of dialysis at a yet-to-be-defined minimal dose is only one of the requirements of adequacy; management of uremic animals necessitates an individually tailored global approach to the animal.

USE OF HEMODIALYSIS TO CORRECT UREMIA

The major benefit of dialytic therapy is the transient elimination of innumerable and unspecified solutes and fluid retained during renal failure that would otherwise be cleared by healthy kidneys. The benefits of dialysis to improve the patient's solute and fluid abnormalities are transient. With cessation of dialysis, the concentrations of urea and all toxic solutes increase immediately until a new steady state is achieved or until the next dialysis session (Fig. 29-3). Urea has become designated the surrogate index for all putative small molecular weight uremic toxins, and reduction of urea appearance and extrarenal removal of urea are used both to prescribe and to monitor the efficiency and adequacy of dialytic therapy.[*]

The diffusive removal of urea and other small molecular weight solutes is exceptionally efficient in animals because of their small size (volume) relative to the surface area and clearance capabilities of the hemodialyzer. Theoretically, most solute and fluid abnormalities attending uremia could be corrected temporarily with a single hemodialysis session, but risks associated with excursions in the solute and fluid content of the patient dictate the practical rate at which they can be altered. The change in solute concentration (e.g., urea) during dialysis is influenced by the size of the animal and the interactive parameters defining the dialysis prescription (see Appendix, Eq. 8). The intensity of dialysis can be adjusted by altering blood flow rate (Qb), dialysate flow rate (Qd), clearance of the hemodialyzer (Kd), rate of ultrafiltration (UF), or length of the dialysis session (T_d) to accommodate the size and therapeutic needs of the animal. After dialysis, BUN increases in proportion to urea generation from dietary nitrogen and endogenous protein catabolism (G) and inversely with residual renal function (Kr) (see Figs. 29-1 through 29-3). Higher dietary protein intake, increased catabolism, and lower residual renal function will produce a steeper increase and higher steady-state concentration of urea after dialysis unless interrupted by an intervening dialysis treatment before achieving steady state. The peak predialysis urea and time-averaged urea concentrations and the exposure to urea and other uremic toxins will be lower the more frequently and effectively a patient is dialyzed.[38,39,41,55,155]

---

*References 24,46,60,64,89,104,108.

*References 39,40,46,61,89,101,104.

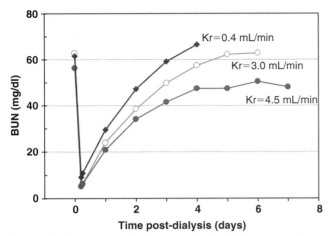

Fig. 29-3 Changes in BUN during and after 5-hour hemodialysis treatments in a 33-kg dog presented for acute antifreeze poisoning at varying degrees of equivalent urea clearance. The eKt/V (~2.9 per session) for the dialysis treatments was identical for each level of urea clearance, yet the rate of increase and the equilibrated BUN concentration after stopping dialysis increased inversely with residual urea clearance.

The hemodialysis session is defined by the dialysis prescription that must be formulated with an understanding of the alterations of body fluid volume and composition that are subject to dialytic correction and the physiologic, hematologic, and biochemical status of the patient before dialysis (Box 29-2). Patient assessment should include (1) the degree of azotemia, (2) the hemodynamic stability and predisposition to hypotension and hypovolemia (i.e., body weight, estimated blood volume, blood pressure, volemic status), (3) hematocrit and total plasma solids, (4) electrolyte and acid-base abnormalities, (5) oxygenation capacity, and (6) bleeding potential. The prescription must be individualized for each patient and every dialysis session by selecting the dialytic options that best achieve the solute removal and ultrafiltration goals of the session. Specific factors regulating these processes are prescribed independently and are outlined in Box 29-3. Hemodialysis prescriptions for animals have been derived empirically with little attempt to justify or standardize dialysis therapy, but as the art of animal dialysis advances, dialysis prescriptions should be based on a solid understanding of the physical and physiological principles governing dialysis, clinical aspects of uremia, and the results of outcomes-directed clinical investigation.

HEMODIALYSIS PRESCRIPTION FOR ACUTE UREMIA

The rapid accumulation of uremic toxins in animals with acute uremia exceeds the rate of metabolic adaptations to these toxins that are possible in animals with progressive kidney disease. Therapeutic priorities are to resolve

---

Box 29-2 **Clinical Considerations Influencing the Hemodialysis Prescription**

1. Magnitude of the azotemia and retained uremic toxins
2. Electrolyte and mineral disorders: sodium, potassium, chloride, bicarbonate calcium, magnesium, and phosphate
3. Acid-base imbalances and depleted or deficient solutes: bicarbonate, calcium, glucose
4. Exogenous intoxications (e.g., ethylene glycol)
5. Excesses or deficits in fluid volume
6. Physiologic disturbances: blood pressure, body temperature, oxygenation, change in body weight
7. Coagulation status
8. Medications and comorbid clinical conditions
9. Dialysis treatment history

Box 29-3 **Hemodialysis Prescription Parameters**

1. Selection of the hemodialyzer (surface area, bundle volume, solute and ultrafiltration characteristics, hemocompatibility, and biocompatibility)
2. Blood flow rate (Qb)
3. Dialysis time (Td)
4. Dialysate composition and/or modeling
5. Dialysate flow rate and direction (Qd)
6. Treatment schedule
7. Access connection (induced recirculation)
8. Degree and method of anticoagulation
9. Ancillary medications

---

the hyperkalemia, profound azotemia, fluid imbalance, and metabolic acidosis, and to remove persisting nephrotoxins. However, therapeutic restraint is necessary to prevent overtreatment when the risks of dialysis disequilibrium syndrome are high. Dialysis goals for initial treatments in animals with acute uremia also differ considerably from the goals for later dialysis treatments.

Hemodialyzers

Selection of the hemodialyzer is based primarily on its contribution to the extracorporeal volume and secondarily on its diffusive, convective, and biocompatibility properties according to guidelines in Table 29-1. The smallest neonatal hemodialyzer currently used has a 0.2 M^2 surface area and an 18-mL blood volume compartment (100 HG, Gambro Renal Products, Lakewood, CO). This dialyzer is selected for cats and dogs weighing less than 6 kg because of these physical characteristics

TABLE 29-1 Recommended Extracorporeal Volumes and Characteristics of Hemodialyzers Used for Hemodialysis in Dogs and Cats

	Body Weight	Dialyzer Volume	Total Extracorporeal Volume	% BV
Cats, dogs	< 6 kg	< 20 mL	< 60 mL	13-40
Cats	> 6 kg	< 30 mL	< 70 mL	< 23
Dogs	6-12 kg	< 45 mL	< 90 mL	9-19
Dogs	12-20 kg	< 80 mL	100-160 mL	6-17
Dogs	20-30 kg	<120 mL	150-200 mL	6-13
Dogs	> 30 kg	> 80 mL	150-250 mL	6-10

Dialyzer	Kd_{urea} (mL/min)	Kd_{creat} (mL/min)	Kd_{phos} (mL/min)	Kd_{B12} (mL/min)	Kuf (mL/hr/mm Hg)	Area (M^2)	Volume (mL)
Conventional Dialyzer:							
100HG[a]	82	69	61	19	2	0.22	18
F3[b]	125	95	50	20	1.7	0.4	28
F4[b]	155	128	78	32	2.8	0.7	42
High-Efficiency Dialyzer							
500HG[a]	182	164	151	64	8.3	1.1	58
F8[b]	186	172	138	76	7.5	1.8	110
Medium-Flux Dialyzer							
F40[b]	165	140	138	75	20	0.7	42
F80 M[b]	190	177	170	110	27	1.8	110
High-Flux Dialyzer:							
F160 NR[b]	194	181	178	128	45	1.5	84
F200 NR[b]	195	191	183	148	56	2	112
Polyflux140H[a]	193	181	174	128	60	1.4	94
Polyflux170H[a]	196	186	180	137	70	1.7	115

In vitro clearances @ Qb, 200 mL/min; Qd, 500 mL/min; UF, 0 mL/hr.
[a]*Gambro Renal Products, CO.*
[b]*Fresenius Medical Care, North America.*
All conventions as defined in the text.

despite its cellulose-based Hemophan[7] membrane. For cats and dogs weighing more than 6 kg, a dialyzer with a surface area between 0.2 and 0.4 M^2 and a priming volume less than 30 mL generally is tolerated. A synthetic hollow fiber dialyzer (neonatal or pediatric) with a surface area between 0.4 and 0.8 M^2 and a priming volume less than 45 mL is appropriate for use in dogs weighing between 6 and 12 kg body weight. Dialyzers with surface areas up to 1.5 M^2 and priming volumes up to 80 mL can be used on dogs between 12 and 20 kg body weight. Larger dialyzers with surface areas greater than 2.0 M^2 and priming volumes greater than 100 mL can be used in dogs weighing more than 30 kg.

A dialyzer with a smaller surface area (0.2 and 0.5 M^2) than recommended may be chosen preferentially in dogs of all sizes for initial hemodialysis treatments when the BUN concentration is greater than 200 mg/dL to reduce the intensity of the treatment and risk of dialysis disequilibrium. Solute removal follows first order kinetics, and animals with marked azotemia (BUN, >250 mg/dL) will experience quantitatively greater urea removal per unit of time and blood flow than those with lesser degrees of azotemia. For patients with severe azotemia, selection of a conventional dialyzer with a lower urea clearance may be more appropriate and safer than use of a high-efficiency device.

Treatment Intensity

Initial dialysis treatments are purposefully less intense and performed with treatment times and blood flow rates substantially lower than those used for later treatments. At low blood flow rates, urea extraction across the dialyzer approaches 100%, and urea clearance (Kd_{urea}, in mL/min) is approximately equal to extracorporeal blood flow (Q_b, in mL/min). For high-efficiency dialyzers used for maintenance treatments, solute removal again is governed primarily by blood flow through the dialyzer until blood flow exceeds 200 mL/min.[34] At faster blood flow rates, the relationship flattens, and urea clearance will be influenced by membrane characteristics and dialysate flow in addition to Qb. The flow dependency of dialysis at these extremes of treatment requirement and the conformational uniformity of animals (especially cats) establish the total volume of blood passed through the dialyzer during the treatment ($Qb \times T_d$) as a reasonable estimate of the intensity of the treatment as predicted by the URR (Figs. 29-4 and 29-5).[29,49,81] Thus total blood processed can be used as an operational parameter to guide delivery of the desired URR for differing degrees of uremia and for each phase of management (Table 29-2).

Dialysis Time

Once the appropriate URR is defined for the treatment, the approximate volume of blood requiring dialytic processing and appropriate combinations of blood flow rate and dialysis time can be derived. Short dialysis treatments of 60 to 120 minutes had been advocated for animals with severe azotemia, but this approach may predispose inadvertently to the prescription of fast blood flow rates that decrease BUN too rapidly.[29,31] Short treatments usually produce inadequate URR outcomes that delay progress to resolve the azotemia. A patient

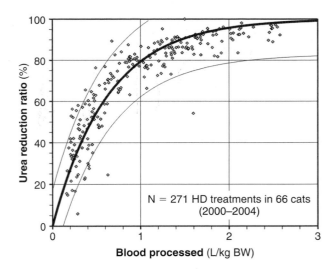

Fig. 29-5 Prediction of dialysis treatment intensity (urea reduction ratio [URR]) as a function of the volume of blood processed in 66 cats undergoing hemodialysis. Other conventions are as described for Fig. 29-4. The closer correlation ($r^2 = 0.85$) between volume of blood processed and URR in cats compared with dogs is probably because of the more uniform body shape and sizes in this species.

with an initial BUN concentration of 250 mg/dL treated for 120 minutes to yield a URR of 0.2 (0.1 URR/hr, postdialysis BUN, 200 mg/dL) may rebound with a BUN approaching 250 mg/dL by the next treatment. The subsequent treatment will be constrained by the same concerns for rapid urea reduction and dialysis disequilibrium as the initial treatment because no progress was made to resolve the azotemia. A more

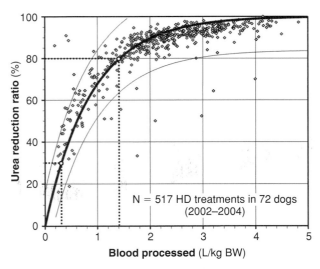

Fig. 29-4 Predicition of dialysis treatment intensity (urea reduction ratio [URR]) as a function of the volume of blood processed in 72 dogs undergoing hemodialysis. URR was computed from predialysis and postdialysis BUN concentration (Appendix, Eq. 2). The volume of blood processed ($Qb \times Td$) was indexed to body weight to compare dogs of different sizes. The relation (modeled as URR = $1-e^{-a \cdot (Qb \cdot Td/BW)}$, $r^2 = 0.69$) is displayed as a thick solid line with its 95% confidence interval (CI; thin lines). To achieve a low-efficiency treatment with URR equal to 30%, a volume of 0.3 L of blood/kg body weight must be processed during the treatment (e.g., 6 L in a 20-kg dog). The variation in resulting URR (95% CI, 15% to 45%) underscores the necessity for close monitoring of the delivered (and not prescribed) dose of dialysis for each treatment. Similarly, a URR of 80% is obtained with 1.4 L (95% CI, 0.9 to 2.9) of blood processed per kg body weight (e.g., 28 L in a 20-kg dog).

TABLE 29-2   Treatment Intensity Prescription

Initial Treatment

BUN < 200 mg/dL	URR < 0.5 @ no greater than 0.1 URR/hr
200-300 mg/dL	URR 0.5-0.3 @ no greater than 0.1 URR/hr
>300 mg/dL	URR ≤ 0.3 @ no greater than 0.05-0.07 URR/hr

Second Treatment

BUN < 200 mg/dL	URR 0.6-0.7 @ 0.12-0.15 URR/hr
200-300 mg/dL	URR 0.6-0.4 @ 0.12-0.1 URR/hr
>300 mg/dL	URR ≤ 0.4 @ no greater than 0.05-0.1 URR/hr

Third and Subsequent Treatments

BUN < 150 mg/dL	URR > 0.8 @ > 0.15 URR/hr
150-300 mg/dL	URR 0.5-0.6 @ 0.15-0.1 URR/hr
>300 mg/dL	URR 0.5-0.6 @ < 0.1 URR/hr

effective approach for initial treatments is to prescribe extended-slow dialysis to target a URR between 0.3 and 0.5 over 4 to 6 hours. Once the predialysis BUN is less than 150 mg/dL, dialysis time can be maintained or increased in both dogs and cats concurrent with faster blood flow rates to achieve URRs greater than 0.8.

The hourly URR can be used as an additional guide to determine the appropriate length for the treatment. An excessive rate of urea reduction is more likely to cause intradialysis complications than the absolute decrease in BUN.[81] The risk of dialysis disequilibrium syndrome can be minimized by adherence to the hourly URR recommendations as indexed to the degree of azotemia in Table 29-2. With these guidelines, the appropriate treatment time is readily determined by dividing the URR goal for the treatment by the designated hourly URR. Animals become more tolerant of rapid urea shifts as their azotemia is reduced and as the number of dialysis treatments is increased; more aggressive hourly URR goals can be prescribed beyond the initial two to three treatments. It should be recalled that URR is determined cumulatively over the entire dialysis treatment, but the absolute change in serum urea and osmolality will be higher during the first hours of treatment than during subsequent hours. Hourly URR recommendations could exceed safe rates of urea removal if the animal is extremely azotemic, the URR treatment goal is too high, or the treatment time is short and exposes the animal to risks of disequilibrium.

Extended-slow dialysis treatments also facilitate removal of large volumes of fluid that would cause volume contraction and hypotension during shorter treatments. Dialysis time also should be a consideration for the differential rates of solute removal during dialysis. Treatment efficiency generally is indexed to urea transfer, which is faster than that of other uremic solutes (e.g., potassium, phosphate, creatinine) that are less diffusable or compartmentalized and poorly transferable. Longer treatments enhance removal of these secluded solutes that do not behave like urea.

Extracorporeal Blood Flow

Blood flow is a major determinant of treatment intensity and becomes defined in sequence as the URR goal, required volume of processed blood, and treatment time are decided. For a 20-kg dog presenting with acute uremia and a BUN of 295 mg/dL, the desired URR would be 0.3 for the first treatment. The requisite treatment volume would be 0.3 L/kg or 6 L of total treatment (see Table 29-2; Fig. 29-4). Appropriate combinations of dialysis time and blood flow rate can be computed to achieve the 6-L goal. For a 180-minute dialysis treatment (0.1 URR/hr), the required Q_b would be 33 mL/min (1.7 mL/kg/min), whereas for a 240-minute treatment (0.075 URR/hr), the required Q_b would be 25 mL/min (1.25 mL/kg/min).

Without URR-derived estimates for Q_b, blood flow must be determined empirically to provide adequate and safe treatments. For animals with BUN concentrations greater than 300 mg/dL, the blood flow rate should be limited to 1 to 1.5 mL/kg/min or less to prevent overly rapid treatment. If the BUN concentration is between 150 and 300 mg/dL, blood flow for initial treatments should be limited to 1.5 to 2.0 mL/kg/min. By the third and subsequent treatments, the BUN usually is less than 150 mg/dL, and blood flow can be increased cautiously to 5 mL/kg/min. For high-efficiency maintenance treatments, blood flow rates between 10 and 20 mL/kg/min or the maximal flow achieved by the vascular access can be used.

For severely uremic cats or small dogs with BUN concentrations greater than 250 mg/dL, it may be necessary to extend the treatment time to greater than 5 hours while providing exceptionally slow blood flow rates and urea clearance rates to deliver a sufficiently gradual treatment (<0.1 URR/hr). In some cases, it may not be possible to adjust either the treatment time or the pump speed sufficiently to deliver a treatment that is slow enough to safely correct the azotemia. For these circumstances, it is useful to alternate periods of active dialysis with deliberate intervals of bypass in which dialysate flow and diffusion are stopped. A plausible recommendation is to alternate 20 to 30 minutes of dialysis with 20 to 30 minutes of bypass. This procedure is very effective when the blood flow rate (pump speed) cannot be reduced sufficiently for a standard dialysis treatment. The bypass intervals prolong the time required to achieve the URR goal and decrease the delivered hourly URR. Ultrafiltration continues during the bypass, facilitating fluid removal during the extended treatment time. Blood flow can be increased during the bypass intervals to minimize clotting in the extracorporeal circuit without the risk of excessive dialysis.

Dialysate Composition

Dialysate composition and its temperature and flow rate are active components of the dialysis prescription. Dialysate is formulated to maximize the elimination of uremic toxins, prevent depletion of normal blood solutes, replenish depleted solutes, and prevent physiologic and metabolic perturbations during and after the dialysis sessions. Conventional dialysate formulations for dogs and cats include sodium, approximately 145 mmol/L (dogs), 150 mmol/L (cats); potassium, 0.0 to 3.0 mmol/L; bicarbonate, 25 to 35 mmol/L; chloride, approximately 113 mmol/L (dogs), approximately 117 mmol/L (cats); calcium, 1.5 mmol/L; magnesium, 1.0 mmol/L; and dextrose, 200 mg/dL, which are produced from standard dialysate concentrates. Dialysate flow conventionally is 500 mL/min but can be decreased to reduce solute clearance during initial treatments or increased to maximize efficiency of maintenance treatments. For practical purposes, however, there is little additional solute clearance until dialysate flow exceeds twice the countercurrent blood flow rate.[133] Similarly, urea extraction across the dialyzer is nearly complete at the blood flow rates used during initial treatments. As such, it is not practical (or possible on most delivery systems) to reduce dialysate flow sufficiently to decrease dialysis efficiency.

Rapid solute removal exposes the patient to nonphysiologic osmotic changes and fluid shifts that can cause osmotic disequilibrium between the vasculature, the interstitium, and cells, resulting in a shift of fluid out of the vasculature and signs of hypovolemia, hypotension, cramping, nausea, vomiting, and dialysis disequilibrium syndrome. The patient may experience additional hypovolemia, hypotension, and poor catheter performance when ultrafiltration is superimposed. These signs are especially likely to develop early in the treatment when solute removal is quantitatively greatest. To offset these physiologic trends, the sodium composition of the dialysate can be modeled (or profiled) so that dialysate sodium is adjusted systematically during the treatment to counteract solute disequilibrium, promote vascular refilling, and lessen or prevent these adverse signs.[50,141] Dialysate sodium can be programmed to change in stepped or linear adjustments from hypernatric (155 to 160 mmol/L) during the initial stages of the dialysis treatment to isonatric or hyponatric (150 to 140 mmol/L) at the termination of the treatment. During the hypernatric phase of the profile, the sodium gradient from dialysate to plasma causes sodium loading and expansion of the extracellular fluid (ECF) during this critical time when the extracorporeal circuit has filled, ultrafiltration has started, and solute removal is greatest.

The efficacy of sodium profiling has not been validated in animals but appears beneficial in human patients predisposed to hypotension or intradialytic discomfort.[6,27,130,138,141] A modeled dialysate with a sodium concentration of 155 mmol/L for the initial 20% to 25% of the treatment, 150 mmol/L for the next 40% of the treatment, and 145 mmol/L for the remainder of the treatment has been is used for small dogs that are not hypertensive and predisposed to hypovolemia.[29,49] For cats, sodium modeling using the respective sodium concentrations of 160 mmol/L, 155 mmol/L, and 150 mmol/L appears to prevent hypotension in the face of the large extracorporeal volume required for hemodialysis in cats. The effects of sodium modeling on intravascular volume are illustrated in Fig. 29-6 in which expansion (refilling) of blood volume coincides with the application of a high-to-low dialysate profile in a dog receiving ultrafiltration concurrently.

Modeling dialysate sodium from isonatric or hyponatric to hypernatric (dogs: 145 mmol/L for the initial 20% to 25% of the treatment, 150 mmol/L for the next 40% of the treatment, and 155 mmol/L for the remainder

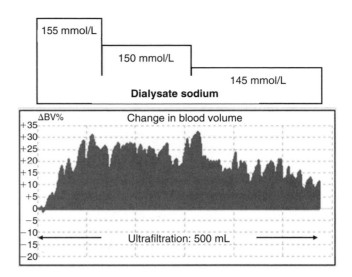

Fig. 29-6 Relative percent changes in blood volume (ΔBV%) assessed by an in-line blood volume monitor in response to stepped sodium profiling and simultaneous ultrafiltration during hemodialysis in an uremic dog. The concentration and duration of each dialysate sodium step are indicated by the bars at the top of the figure. The sodium profiling supports a positive blood volume during the simultaneous ultrafiltration.

of the treatment; cats: 150 mmol/L, 155 mmol/L, and 160 mmol/L, respectively) has been used to help protect severely azotemic animals from the neurologic effects of dialysis disequilibrium. This sodium profile promotes osmotic (sodium) loading of the ECF in the later stages of treatment when urea disequilibrium can cause osmotic fluid shifts into the intracellular fluid, exacerbating cerebral edema and increasing intracranial pressure. This profile has been derived empirically but appears to offer a margin of protection in animals with BUN concentrations greater than 200 mg/dL. Conceptually, the low-to-high dialysate profile could increase the osmolality of the ECF by 20 mOsm/kg (approximately equivalent to the osmotic effects of 60 mg/dL of urea disequilibrium) and could add an effective osmotic buffer to inhibit fluid shifts into cells (Fig. 29-7).

Sodium profiling will alter the patient's sodium balance if the cumulative sodium transfer is not neutral. A positive sodium balance is expected with the low-to-high profile and is accepted as a transient disturbance to protect the patient from dialysis disequilibrium. If, however, the profile consistently promotes sodium accumulation, the patient may develop untoward complications including postdialysis thirst, interdialysis weight gain, hyperkalemia, and hypertension. Routine high sodium dialysate profiles should be prescribed with care to anuric or severely uremic animals because they might exaggerate potassium rebound and increase interdialytic serum potassium concentrations.[35] Severe hypertension has been seen in animals in association with prolonged use of high sodium

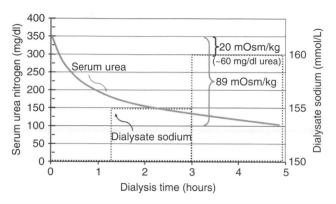

Fig. 29-7 Hypothetical plot of the changes in serum urea nitrogen and dialysate sodium concentration during a dialysis treatment employing low-to-high sodium profiling from 150 to 160 mmol/L. The 20 mOsm/kg (Na + Cl) change in serum osmolality resulting from the sodium modeling could help offset, in part, the 89-mOsm/kg change in serum osmolality resulting from the dialytic change in urea of 250 mg/dL during the treatment. The osmotic buffer provided by dialysate sodium profiling is equivalent to approximately 60 mg/dL change in blood urea nitrogen.

dialysate profiling. The profile must be adjusted to produce neutral sodium balance, or an isonatric dialysate should be used if these signs are recognized.

A standard dialysate potassium concentration of 3 mmol/L can be used for most animals with acute or chronic renal failure. Serum potassium concentration may not be corrected adequately if a standard dialysate is used in animals with severe hyperkalemia during short dialysis sessions or during treatments using slow blood flow rates. Similarly, the potassium load in animals treated medically for severe hyperkalemia before dialysis may be sequestered in cells and not accessible for dialytic removal during short dialysis treatments. For these conditions, a dialysate containing 0 mmol/L of potassium has been recommended.[29,31,49] Evidence in human patients suggests large dialysis gradients or rapid changes in serum potassium concentration can alter the intracellular/extracellular potassium ratio and resting cell membrane potential and increase the risk for ventricular arrhythmias.[86,114,115] The appearance of ventricular arrhythmias during the treatment may warrant changing to a dialysate containing potassium. The bulk of body potassium is compartmentalized in intracellular pools, and its transfer to ECF may lag behind its rate of removal by the dialyzer, causing transient hypokalemia at the end of the treatment.[116] A rebound of the hyperkalemia occurs within hours as a result of delayed transfer from intracellular pools and extends to the next dialysis treatment. Daily dialysis may be required until the bulk of the potassium load is corrected. Animals with profound electrocardiographic abnormalities resulting from hyperkalemia may demonstrate complete reversal of these signs within minutes of initiating hemodialysis with a

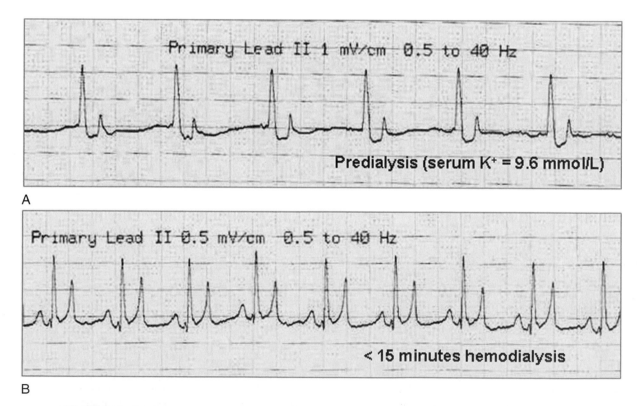

Fig. 29-8 A, Predialysis electrocardiogram (ECG) from a uremic dog with a serum potassium concentration of 9.6 mmol/L and evident cardiotoxicity. **B,** ECG from the same animal within 15 minutes of starting hemodialysis with a 0 mmol/L potassium dialysate. The improvement in the ECG was independent of changes in the peripherial potassium concentration.

dialysate containing 0 mmol/L potassium (Fig. 29-8). The mechanism promoting this rapid reversal of the cardiotoxicity is not known but illustrates the efficacy of hemodialysis to provide both immediate and prolonged resolution to this life-threatening complication of uremia.

Buffer Formulation

Hydrogen ions are present at too low a concentration for the acid burden to be disposed of by dialysis alone. Alternatively, the acid load can be buffered by base equivalents supplied in the dialysate. The buffer (acetate or bicarbonate) is formulated to a concentration higher than that of plasma to cause accrual of new buffer by the patient and replenish the deficits caused by the production and retention of metabolic acids. The amount of base transferred depends on the dialysate buffer concentration, choice of dialyzer, the blood and dialysate flow rates, and the transcellular distribution of hydrogen ions during the dialysis session.[48]

High-flux and high-efficiency dialysis procedures require a bicarbonate-based dialysate that has replaced virtually all use of acetate as a source of base equivalents in both human and animal dialysis. The rapid or excessive accumulation of acetate during high-efficiency dialysis may exceed its metabolism in skeletal muscle and liver. Acetate accumulation produces a toxicity that includes peripheral vasodilatation, hypotension, and hypoxemia, and its use cannot be recommended in small animals.[33,66,152]

Many delivery systems can proportion dialysate bicarbonate concentration from 20 to 40 mmol/L. Use of a low dialysate bicarbonate concentration (25 mmol/L) has been suggested for animals with severe metabolic acidosis (serum bicarbonate, <12 mmol/L) on the premise that a higher bicarbonate concentration may correct serum bicarbonate concentration too rapidly, increase cerebrospinal fluid (CSF) Pco_2, decrease CSF pH, and precipitate paradoxical cerebral acidosis, cerebral edema, and dialysis disequilibrium syndrome.[8,10,29] In practice, it is very difficult to alter serum bicarbonate concentration during short treatments at low blood flow rates even with high dialysate bicarbonate concentrations.[48] Under these conditions, dialysate bicarbonate can be set to 30 mmol/L with little likelihood of neurologic complications. It should be decreased promptly if the animal shows signs of tachypnea, restlessness, stupor, blindness, or other clinical evidence of impending dialysis disequilibrium syndrome. Dialysate bicarbonate concentration should be set more cautiously at 20 to 25 mmol/L for intensive dialytic treatment in animals with severe metabolic acidosis associated with nonazotemic diseases such as antifreeze intoxication. A low dialysate bicarbonate concentration also should be selected for treatment of animals with metabolic or respiratory alkalosis. Inappropriate selection of a standard or high dialysate bicarbonate could worsen the alkalemia. For maintenance hemodialysis treatments, a dialysate bicarbonate concentration of 30 mmol/L will produce a postdialysis serum bicarbonate concentration of approximately 23 mmol/L after 4 or 5 hours of dialysis. A dialysate concentration of 35 to 40 mmol/L yields greater accrual of buffer but often is associated with relentless panting during the treatment.

Dialysate Additions

Hyperphosphatemia is a common feature of acute and chronic uremia,[30,113] and for both conditions the dialysate is formulated to contain no phosphate so as to facilitate removal of the phosphate load. The dialysance of phosphate is less than that for either urea or creatinine. Additionally, the interstitial and intracellular pools of phosphate are large, compartmentalized, and poorly exchangeable with the serum pool; therefore the amount of phosphate eliminated during a dialysis treatment may be small compared with the overall phosphate load.[96] Serum phosphate concentration usually is not corrected during short and less intensive treatments, but it can be normalized or transient hypophosphatemia can develop with treatments longer than 4 or 5 hours. In uremic animals, postdialysis hypophosphatemia rebounds rapidly after treatment without development of clinical signs. In contrast, persistent hypophosphatemia and the risks of hemolysis, decreased oxygen delivery, or central nervous system (CNS) and neuromuscular disturbances can occur in animals with normal predialysis serum phosphate concentration that are dialyzed with a standard dialysate. For these conditions (i.e., hemodialysis for toxin or fluid removal), the dialysate can be adjusted to near physiologic phosphate concentrations by addition of a neutral sodium phosphate solution (Fleet Enema, Fleet Brand Pharmaceuticals, C. B. Fleet Company, Inc., Lynchberg, VA) to the dialysate concentrate. The amount of phosphate additive required will vary depending on the proportioning ratio of the delivery system, but 16 mL of Fleet Enema solution per liter of concentrate solution produces a dialysate phosphate concentration that is approximately 2 mg/dL when proportioned roughly at 1:40.

Absolute alcohol is an important additive to bicarbonate-based dialysate for the treatment of acute ethylene glycol or methanol intoxications.[25] Alcohol is added directly to the acid concentrate in sufficient volume to produce an enriched dialysate with a proportioned concentration of approximately 0.1% ethanol.[102] The ethanol diffuses from the dialysate into the patient to maintain a constant blood alcohol concentration sufficient to competitively inhibit alcohol dehydrogenase and minimize further metabolism of the ethylene glycol while it is being dialyzed from the patient.

Dialysate Temperature

Dialysate temperature rarely is regarded as a functional component of the dialysis prescription and is generally set as close as possible to the normal temperature of the animal. Dialysis machines manufactured for human patients usually are configured with a high temperature limit at 38° C, which is the lower temperature reference for normal dogs and cats. Even at 38° C, the hypothermia often seen in animals with severe azotemia will be corrected, and most hypothermic patients will warm to approximately this temperature. Some euthermic animals develop chills with a dialysate temperature of 38° C as a result of cooling of the blood in the extracorporeal circuit before it returns to the animal. These signs can be controlled with heated blankets or heat lamps.

Dialysate temperature also can influence the hemodynamic stability of patients predisposed to hypotension during hemodialysis.[85,86,91,92,130] A dialysate set to normal body temperature can cause heat accumulation in the animal and subsequently increase core body temperature. When animals are undergoing ultrafiltration, even subtle increases in body temperature can augment the development of hypotension. This hemodynamic response is initiated by cutaneous vasoconstriction induced by ultrafiltration-associated hypovolemia and decreased dissipation of the accumulated heat. At a critical increase in core body temperature, a thermal homeostatic reflex is triggered, causing peripheral vasodilatation, decreased peripheral vascular resistance, and symptomatic hypotension.[86,91,92,119,130] Finite increases in body temperature can be documented in animals during routine hemodialysis treatments, but they may be protected inadvertently from this hemodynamic sequence by the default temperature limits of the machine (i.e., those set for human body temperature). Recent studies in human patients have demonstrated that hemodynamic tolerance is better preserved in dialysis treatments in which the patient maintains isothermic balance.[91,92] To obviate these events, rectal temperature should be monitored in patients undergoing ultrafiltration and in those predisposed to hypotension. If core temperature increases, dialysate temperature should be adjusted to maintain core temperature constant throughout the treatment.[110] For animals predisposed to hypotension during dialysis, decreasing the dialysate temperature by 1° to 2.5° C could induce peripheral vasoconstriction and increase vascular resistance and cardiac contractility and improve oxygenation during the treatment. Some dialysis delivery systems have integrated biofeedback systems with input blood temperature sensors to detect increases in blood temperature in the arterial blood line that could exacerbate hypotensive or vasodilatory events. The effector system dissipates increased heat through programmed alterations in dialysate temperature to decrease the temperature in the returning blood to maintain an isothermal core body temperature throughout the dialysis session.[85,91,110,124]

Heparin

The patient must be anticoagulated to prevent clotting in the extracorporeal circuit. Heparin is used universally but has variable and unpredictable effects in each animal that require frequent assessment of coagulation time.

Automated activated clotting time (ACT) is used most commonly to prescribe and monitor heparin requirements, but other coagulation measures also could be utilized. The degree of anticoagulation and heparin requirement vary with individual characteristics of the animal and its underlying disease, choice of hemodialyzer, predialysis hematocrit, extracorporeal blood flow rate, predialysis ACT, rate of ultrafiltration, and the patient's risks for bleeding (e.g., recent surgery, hyphema, gastric ulceration, predisposition for CNS hemorrhage). A heparin loading dosage of 10 to 25 U/kg intravenously (cats) to 50 U/kg intravenously (dogs) is standard for most animals and will establish an ACT in the target range of 150 to 180 seconds before starting treatment. Thereafter, a continuous infusion of 20 to 50 U/hr (cats) or 50 to 100 U/kg/hr (dogs) is provided to maintain the ACT in the target range. The hourly heparin dose is adjusted or intermittent boluses of heparin are administered based on sequential ACT measurements performed every 30 to 60 minutes to maintain the desired ACT. The target ACT is increased to more than 180 seconds if the animal has a propensity to clot the extracorporeal circuit. It is set to the bottom of the target range if there is a risk of bleeding. Hemodialysis can be performed without anticoagulation in animals in which the risks for bleeding are great, but these sessions are very demanding and predispose to clotting and blood loss in the extracorporeal circuit.

HEMODIALYSIS PRESCRIPTION FOR CHRONIC KIDNEY DISEASE

Experience with long-term intermittent hemodialysis for animals with chronic kidney disease is meager compared with that for acute uremia, yet hemodialysis is clearly indicated, is effective, and affords a good quality of life. Many of the considerations used to prescribe acute hemodialysis are equally valid for chronic dialytic therapy. Adequacy standards for animals with chronic renal failure await future definition, but intensive hemodialysis provided every 2 to 3 days can augment residual renal function and the medical management of ESRD. As animals are supported beyond their fated life expectancy with dialysis, the spectrum and severity of clinical signs referable to renal failure increase. Collectively, chronic malnutrition, fluid overload, hyperkalemia, hyperparathyroidism, metabolic bone disease, refractory hypertension, progressive anemia, infection, and drug interactions and toxicities replace concerns of hypothermia, hypovolemia, and dialysis disequilibrium syndrome so prevalent in patients with acute uremia.

The dialysis prescription for chronic kidney disease is targeted to reduce the azotemia maximally during each session. Animals starting hemodialysis with severe ESRD or decompensated chronic renal failure should be approached similarly as those with acute uremia until the predialysis BUN is less than 100 mg/dL. Thereafter, high-efficiency dialysis schedules are well tolerated.

Dialysis prescriptions for chronic uremia should promote a predialysis BUN less than 90 mg/dL, a postdialysis BUN less than 10 mg/dL, and a time-averaged BUN less than 50 mg/dL. Targeted spKt/V should be greater than 2.0 to provide an equivalent renal clearance (EKR) of at least 10% of normal renal function. The choice of dialyzer and dialysate composition generally are similar to those for maintenance treatments in animals with acute uremia. Blood flow rate can be increased cautiously to 15 to 25 mL/kg/min or the performance limits of the vascular access, and dialysis time lengthened to 240 minutes (cats) or 300 minutes (dogs) or more for improved urea and solute removal. The temptation to reduce dialysis time with the opportunity to use higher efficiency dialyzers and faster blood and dialysate flow rates should be avoided. Longer treatment times may appear to have limited additional efficiency for urea removal, but many solutes, including creatinine, phosphate, potassium, and middle molecular weight solutes, have different kinetic profiles and are slower to dialyze or have delayed transference from cellular or sequestered compartments.[41] Effective clearance of these solutes requires longer treatments than would be adequate for urea removal.

Three treatments per week is a traditional schedule for human patients with end-stage chronic kidney disease and is used for animal patients with serum creatinine concentrations greater than 8 mg/dL. A twice-weekly dialysis schedule has been used for animals with serum creatinine concentrations between 5 mg/dL and 8 mg/dL before starting dialysis therapy, but a twice-weekly schedule likely represents the minimum recommendation that will be beneficial. Even highly efficient individual treatments performed intermittently twice weekly provide only small contributions to the weekly solute clearance required for therapeutic adequacy. There are finite limits on the efficacy of individual dialysis treatments to improve the time-averaged solute concentrations of a patient. Solute generation and rebound are ongoing and unopposed by dialysis during the interdialytic period; they contribute substantially to the cumulative solute retention occurring throughout the week and become more significant as the interdialysis interval lengthens.[41] The limitations of dialysis can only be improved with more frequent rather than more intensive dialysis schedules that impart greater efficiency to this intermittent clearance technique.[38,41,142] A twice-weekly dialysis schedule only will be effective if the patient has sufficient residual renal function (i.e., a continuous clearance) to offset the effects of solute accumulation in the interdialysis interval to maintain predialysis azotemia and TAC within therapeutic guidelines (see Fig. 29-3).

Chronic maintenance hemodialysis is an indefinite therapeutic commitment, and efforts must be taken to avoid long-term complications of hemodialysis that are not as evident during shorter-term treatments. Maintenance of the vascular access is paramount, and rigorous attention must be paid to ensure that minor exit site infections are resolved and that the catheter is protected from physical damage or movement within the subcutaneous tunnel. Animals supported with chronic hemodialysis still must be given standard medical therapy to manage the nutritional deficiencies, anemia, mineral disturbances, acidosis, and hypertension associated with end-stage renal failure.[49,113] Prolonged survival unmasks features of chronic renal failure rarely identified in animal patients managed only with medical therapy. Hyperkalemia, fluid retention, renal osteodystrophy, hypercalcemia, and refractory hypertension become consistent clinical features and therapeutic challenges.

SUPPORT FOR RENAL TRANSPLANTATION

Renal transplantation is becoming more widely available for both dogs and cats with renal failure when other options for treatment are exhausted and there is no likelihood for recovery of renal function.[2,4,15] Hemodialysis frequently is used as a bridge to renal transplantation to resolve the uremia and metabolic disturbances contributing to the risks of anesthesia and surgery. Hemodialysis expands the pool of animals acceptable for renal transplantation that otherwise would be considered unsuitable and unlikely to survive because of the severity of their uremia.[29,30] Finite periods of dialytic support may be used for animals with acute uremia in which transplantation is considered to provide the most favorable long-term or most cost-effective outcome. The hemodialysis prescription for animals awaiting renal transplantation is predicated on the severity of the uremia and attendant signs as described for acute and chronic kidney disease, but the course of dialysis should be as short as possible to minimize development of complications that would jeopardize the success or opportunity for transplantation. Any infection associated with dialysis procedures could delay indefinitely or preclude transplantation. Repeated administration of blood products may sensitize the recipient, making it incompatible with potential donor animals. After transplantation, hemodialysis frequently is used to manage acute uremia precipitated by delayed graft function, surgical complications, acute rejection, or pyelonephritis.

USE OF HEMODIALYSIS TO CORRECT DISORDERS OF FLUID BALANCE

Animals with oliguric or anuric ARF have insufficient excretory function to effectively eliminate administered fluids and become predisposed to life-threatening fluid accumulation.[30] Similarly, polyuric animals with severe chronic kidney disease accumulate orally administered fluids associated with tube feeding and parenteral fluids used to supplement hydration or to manage episodes of decompensation. In both circumstances, hypervolemia and circulatory overload develop with variable clinical expression as chemosis, pleural effusion, peripheral or pulmonary edema, congestive heart failure, and hypertension. Once established, overhydration may not resolve with cessation of fluid delivery or diuretic administration, leaving no conventional means to manage these clinical disorders. Restoration of fluid balance is an important indication for hemodialysis and a consistent component of the dialysis prescription.

During hemodialysis, fluid can be extracted from the patient across the dialysis membrane by ultrafiltration. Decisions as to the volume and rate of fluid that can be removed safely must be made for each dialysis session. The ultrafiltration prescription is based on clinical assessment of the degree of overhydration using blood pressure; presence of edema, ascites, or pleural effusion; pulmonary congestion; and the deviation of the predialysis weight from the animal's ideal dry body weight. Ideal dry body weight is a progressively derived value determined as the body weight at which additional fluid removal would produce hypotension or signs of hypovolemia.[68,69] Ideal dry weight usually is predicted from recent historical weight measurements before the onset of illness, or it is estimated from evaluation of postdialysis body weight when blood pressure was controlled or there was no demonstrated fluid accumulation. Ideal dry weight should not be considered a static parameter but should be redefined regularly to compensate for ongoing changes in the animal's lean body mass and body fat. Failure to update the targeted ideal dry weight can cause excessive ultrafiltration and hypovolemia or progressive overhydration as the patient gains or loses nonfluid mass, respectively.[68] Progressive deviation from dry weight also can be recognized by routine assessment of body condition score or by body composition analysis using bioimpedance spectroscopy.[28,29,94,98]

The rate and volume of ultrafiltration achieved is contingent on the hemodynamic stability of the animal. All available hemodialyzers have sufficient ultrafiltration performance to remove fluid from the vascular space faster than its rate of redistribution (refill) from the interstitium and intracellular compartments. This potential imbalance can subject animals to hypovolemia, hypotension, and circulatory collapse if ultrafiltration is not prescribed and monitored carefully. The process of ultrafiltration is precisely regulated by ultrafiltration controllers designed into the delivery systems, but small errors or deviations in the tolerance of these systems can cause unscheduled volume losses in small animals during the course of a dialysis session. Slow rates of ultrafiltration between 5 and 10 mL/kg/hr generally are tolerated by dogs and cats, but faster rates must be prescribed cautiously and adjusted according to the animal's vital signs and blood pressure or by use of fluid monitoring equipment (e.g., in-line blood volume monitor, venous oxygen saturation, continuous weight, bioimpedance

spectroscopy).[*] In-line blood volume monitors are especially useful to assess the efficacy and the safety of ultrafiltration (Fig. 29-9).[36,37,139,140]

A lack of change in blood volume during ultrafiltration indicates the rate of fluid removal from the vasculature is precisely matched by a refilling volume from extravascular reservoirs containing the fluid load. If blood volume does not decrease after starting ultrafiltration, the fluid removal rate may not be maximized, and faster rates could be attempted to increase the efficiency

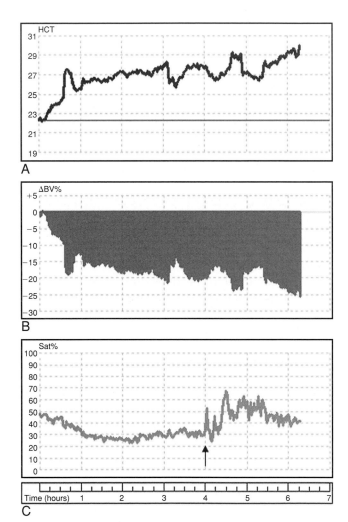

Fig. 29-9 Change in hematocrit (HCT, **A**), relative blood volume (ΔBV%, **B**), and venous oxygen saturation (Sat%, **C**) assessed by an in-line monitor in a dog with acute uremia during hemodialysis and continuous ultrafiltration. The figure illustrates the decreases in relative blood volume and venous oxygen saturation associated with hypovolemia induced by ultrafiltration. The late increase in oxygen saturation reflects the supplemental administration of oxygen (arrow).

*References 29,49,68,70,80,97,125,156,157.

of fluid removal. As vascular refill rate lags behind ultrafiltration rate, the relative change in blood volume becomes negative in proportion to the disparity in these respective transfer rates. The change in blood volume will stabilize when the driving force for vascular refilling again matches ultrafiltration at the contracted but steady-state blood volume. Moderate fluid loads can be removed at a steady 5% to 8% decrease in relative blood volume without overt clinical consequences. More intensive ultrafiltration at a stable 10% to 12% decrease in blood volume is tolerated by some animals with readily transferable fluid loads, but greater decreases in blood volume are likely to lead to clinically evident hypovolemia. The rate of change in blood volume helps to predict the capacity of an individual animal to surrender its fluid burden and attain dry weight.[69] Steep changes in relative blood volume at greater than 10% per hour (especially at the initiation of the treatment) indicate that the ultrafiltration rate is too rapid, and the decrease in blood volume is unlikely to plateau at a safe level (see Fig. 29-9). If ultrafiltration is stopped transiently, a rapid positively directed change in blood volume indicates the fluid load has not been corrected completely, whereas no change suggests the fluid load has been resolved and the animal is at dry weight. A positive change in blood volume may be seen when dialysate sodium is greater than the animal's serum sodium concentration or after administration of intravenous or oral fluids or mannitol (see Fig. 29-6).

Animals often tolerate ultrafiltration better at the beginning of the treatment than at the end, and the rate of fluid removal can be profiled to achieve greater fluid losses at the beginning and scaled back later in the session to achieve the same treatment goal. Sodium profiling can be used to offset the hypovolemic and hypotensive effects of aggressive ultrafiltration and maximize fluid removal. Sodium loading during the hypernatric stages of the modeling profile expands intravascular volume and facilitates redistribution of fluid from the interstitium and intracellular compartments (see Fig. 29-6). Progressive hypovolemia from excessive ultrafiltration is detectable with in-line blood volume monitors well before development of hemodynamic signs, permitting adjustment of the ultrafiltration rate to avert hemodynamic complications.[36] Changes in blood pressure and heart rate are rarely sensitive or early predictors of hypovolemia under these conditions.

A decrease in venous oxygen saturation also is a sensitive indicator of progressive or sudden changes in cardiac output secondary to hypovolemia and can foreshadow an impeding hypotensive episode. Venous oxygen saturation can be monitored continuously with an in-line hematocrit monitor or even visibly observed as a darkening of the desaturated blood in the extracorporeal circuit (see Fig. 29-9).[139] Any decrease in venous oxygen saturation should prompt immediate assessment of the patient and potentially warrants adjustments to ultrafiltration.

Ultrafiltration and diffusive solute removal are independent processes controlled by separate functions of the delivery system. Animals with life-threatening fluid overload and severe azotemia are at risk for excessive solute removal and dialysis disequilibrium syndrome if the dialysis treatment is extended to safely resolve the overhydration. Conversely, they remain at risk of dying if the overhydration is not corrected when dialysis is curtailed for safe solute removal. Both of these contrasting dialysis requirements and risks can be managed safely by prescribing periods of **ultrafiltration without hemodialysis** throughout the treatment or by scheduling independent periods of ultrafiltration before or after the azotemia has been treated to an appropriate URR. During ultrafiltration without dialysis, the machine is placed in bypass mode to stop dialysate flow to the dialyzer (and diffusive solute removal) while blood flow and transmembrane pressure gradients are maintained to continue ultrafiltration. This technique permits slower and more complete fluid removal without producing unsafe rates of diffusive hemodialysis. Isolated ultrafiltration also is used in nonuremic humans to treat fluid congestion associated with heart failure and pulmonary edema refractory to diuretics.[5,93,118,129] Resolution of the fluid load from patients with congestive heart failure improves hemodynamic function, clinical well-being, pulmonary function, drug dependency, and exercise capacity.[5,93,129] Similar indications exist in animals, and this aspect of extracorporeal therapy should be evaluated further. Ultrafiltration requirements for individual treatments should be increased to offset the volume of administered blood products, drugs, and alimentation solutions. Ultrafiltration becomes especially important in oliguric animals with no excretory capacity and no tolerance for additional volume loads. The volume of essential fluid-containing therapies should be balanced by an equivalent or proportional volume of fluid removal during the dialysis session to accomodate a portion or all of the anticipated fluid input. The net balance of fluid removed at the end of the dialysis treatment is influenced by the volume of the priming solution administered at the beginning of the treatment and the amount of rinseback fluid used at the end to return blood to the animal. Air can be used as a rinseback medium to displace the extracorporeal blood rather than fluid to maximize net fluid removal.

With routine hemodialysis techniques, ultrafiltration contributes marginally to solute removal by convective transfer. Convective solute removal does not change the plasma concentration of solutes as they traverse the membrane in the bulk fluid flow because the transfer occurs at their respective concentrations in plasma water. Dialysis dose assessments predicted by URR, simple urea kinetic models, and measurement of postdialysis serum urea concentrations will underestimate true dialysis dose because of failure to account for convective dialysis.[39]

USE OF HEMODIALYSIS TO CORRECT ELECTROLYTE IMBALANCES

Uremic animals experience a wide spectrum of electrolyte imbalances. These imbalances are to be expected because the kidneys are responsible for homeostasis of body electrolytes. Hyperkalemia is the most common and life-threatening electrolyte imbalance encountered in animals with either acute or chronic uremia and can cause severe cardiovascular instability and death. The toxicity of potassium is intensified by acidosis, hypocalcemia, and hyponatremia that may coexist with uremia. Hyperkalemia is a consistent complication of acute uremia intensifying with the severity of the azotemia and presence of oligoanuria.[30] Hyperkalemia rarely is seen in animals with chronic kidney disease,[113] but predialysis serum potassium concentrations between 6 and 10 mmol/L are seen as a persisting problem in approximately 75% of dogs maintained on chronic intermittent hemodialysis for longer than 2 weeks.[106] The hyperkalemia is associated with varying degrees of hyponatremia and metabolic acidosis, and its prevalence is associated with the duration of dialytic support, degree of azotemia, ultrafiltration requirements, and the intensity of dialysis. The hyperkalemia often is difficult to manage and can represent a persistent and life-threatening risk. The cause remains unknown but could involve dialysis-induced disruptions of potassium or cell volume regulation, excesses in dietary potassium load, or altered potassium regulation associated with severe chronic uremia.[106] In contrast to medical treatments for hyperkalemia, which merely shift extracellular potassium to intracellular pools or antagonize its neuromuscular toxicity, hemodialysis eliminates excessive potassium loads from both extracellular and intracellular pools.[114] Correction of hyperkalemia with dialysis is transient, and after dialysis is stopped, there is variable rebound of potassium from poorly equilibrated extracellular and intracellular compartments. Guidelines for the dialytic management of hyperkalemia are discussed above under Acute Uremia.

The dialysate sodium concentration can be proportioned to concentrations ranging from 125 to 160 mmol/L. It also can be programmed to change in user-defined patterns throughout the dialysis session to achieve specific treatment goals or to correct predialysis dysnatremias. Hyponatremia caused by sodium losses from excessive vomiting, diarrhea, diuretic administration, parenteral sodium-free fluid administration, or oral water can be corrected by programming the dialysate sodium concentration to increase in stepped increments or continuous gradients to the desired postdialysis concentration. Hypernatremia caused by excessive bicarbonate or hypertonic saline administration may be difficult or inappropriate to correct with additional fluid administration but can be resolved easily by adjusting the dialysate sodium concentration in progressive or incremented steps to concentrations less than the serum sodium concentration until the desired concentration is achieved. The rate of correction can be regulated precisely without the uncertainty of the interim concentration or overcorrection. Excessive isonatric loads of sodium can be eliminated by ultrafiltration without simultaneous changes in serum sodium concentration. With the exception of minor Gibbs-Donnan effects, the ultrafiltrate is formed with the same sodium concentration as present in plasma water. Consequently, large sodium loads can be eliminated without perturbations in sodium concentration or the risk of inducing sodium disequilibrium that may trigger an undesirable redistribution of fluid and electrolytes from intracellular stores.[35,115]

USE OF HEMODIALYSIS IN ACUTE INTOXICATIONS

Elimination of toxins and support for the consequences of the intoxication are important but overshadowed applications of hemodialysis. This use of hemodialysis is especially important if there has been a delay in medical management, there is limited endogenous clearance of the toxin or its metabolites, or there is no specific antidote for the toxicant. Hemodialysis can be used to eliminate toxins from the body before they promote cellular damage or are converted to more toxic metabolites. The dialytic removal of exogenous toxins is governed by the same molecular characteristics that define diffusive clearance of endogenous toxins. Molecular size, concentration in ECF, distribution volume, degree of protein binding, and lipid solubility significantly influence the potential for a toxin's elimination.[23,153] Toxins or drugs with low molecular weights (<1500 daltons), small volumes of distribution, and minimal protein binding are excellent candidates for diffusive and convective clearance. A small volume of distribution predicts that the toxin is restricted to the extracellular space and is readily accessible for extracorporeal clearance. A toxin with a large distribution volume is likely to be concentrated in tissues and will have minimal transference or availability in plasma for removal. Only the free fraction of protein-bound toxins can be dialyzed, and toxins or drugs that are highly protein bound are not good candidates for dialytic removal. Ethylene glycol has a molecular weight of 62 daltons, negligible protein binding, and a volume of distribution equivalent to total body water (0.5 to 0.8 L/kg) and consequently is an excellent candidate for dialytic removal. With timely application, it can be removed effectively from the body before its enzymatic oxidation to more toxic metabolites, including glycoaldehyde, glycolate, glyoxylate, and oxalate.[23,117] Toxins that are highly bound to serum proteins, including diazepam, salicylates, nonsteroidal antiinflammatory drugs (NSAIDs), and tricyclic antidepressants, are dialyzed less effectively, but dialysis may still be a therapeutic option. Rebound of the toxin or drug from peripheral tissues or cellular compartments to plasma may limit the efficacy of dialysis to resolve the poisoning. If redistribution of the toxin from extravascular pools is much slower than its dialytic removal, the animal may become reintoxicated within hours after dialysis with slowed reequilibration of the toxin into blood. For these sequestered toxins, the length and frequency of dialysis may need to be increased to facilitate their whole body elimination.

Hemoperfusion is an alternative blood purification procedure in which whole blood is exposed directly to sorbent materials with the capacity to selectively or nonselectively bind molecules of defined chemical composition. Hemoperfusion using activated charcoals, ion-exchange resins, and nonionic macroporous resins has been used historically in human patients for the elimination of toxic solutes after acute poisoning or overmedication and provides an attractive adjunct to hemodialysis as a means of blood purification.[23,153] Hemoperfusion is a small but defined niche in medical therapeutics and represents a novel and important frontier in veterinary medicine with the increasing availability of extracorporeal therapies. Hemoperfusion is especially effective at eliminating high molecular weight, protein-bound, or lipid-soluble toxins or drugs, which are cleared poorly, if at all, by hemodialysis. Typical toxins include barbiturates, salicylates, NSAIDs, antimicrobials, antidepressants, and chemotherapeutics. Specific toxic indications include mushroom poisoning (amanitin toxins and phalloidin), herbicides, and insecticides. The combination of hemodialysis for small solute removal and hemoperfusion for removal of larger, protein-bound, or lipid-soluble molecules provides opportunity for a greater spectrum of blood purification in animal poisonings (Fig. 29-10).[51]

Hemodialysis is indicated for the treatment of poisoning or drug overdosage with ethylene glycol, methanol, ethanol, salicylate, lithium, phenobarbital, acetaminophen, theophylline, aminoglycosides, tricyclic antidepressants, and possibly metaldehyde.[153] Hemodialysis secondarily corrects the acid-base and electrolyte abnormalities and the azotemia that accompany some intoxications (e.g., ethylene glycol, salicylate). Hemodialysis should be initiated once conventional treatments are deemed ineffective and continued until the concentration of the toxin has decreased to an acceptable level and the clinical toxicity has disappeared. Dialysis treatments should be continued for prolonged periods for toxins with delayed toxicity (i.e., paraquat) and low blood concentrations.

Ethylene glycol (antifreeze poisoning) is one of the most common intoxications encountered in companion animal practice.[29,30,49,81,144] Clinical signs develop within minutes and progress variably from lethargy, nausea, vomiting, dehydration, agitation, and depression to convulsions, coma, and death. Severe metabolic acidosis and hypocalcemia are seen with significant exposure, and in

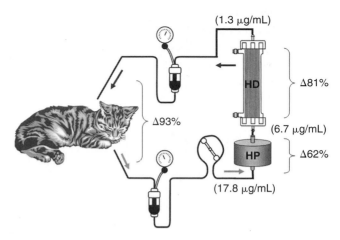

Fig. 29-10 Combined hemoperfusion (HP) and hemodialysis (HD) for the treatment of enrofloxacin overdose in a uremic cat. A neonatal extracorporeal circuit was modified to include a 50-mL Clark biocompatible HP system (Clark Research and Development Inc., Folsom, LA) activated charcoal cartridge upstream to a Cobe 100HG hemodialyzer (Gambro Renal Products, Lakewood, CO). This combined blood purification technique resulted in a marked decrease in the blood enrofloxacin concentration (numbers in parentheses) through the extracorporeal circuit: from 17.8 to 6.7 µg/mL (Δ62%) across the HP cartridge and from 6.7 to 1.3 µg/mL (Δ81%) across the hemodialyzer and 93% reduction across both devices at 10 minutes of treatment. Combined HD/HP provided a safe and effective additional route of clearance for enrofloxacin in this cat with renal compromise.

later stages of the intoxication (12 to 24 hours), hypertension, cardiopulmonary failure, and acute oliguric renal failure dominate the clinical presentation. Ethylene glycol concentrations are highly variable and significantly higher in nonazotemic compared with azotemic dogs presented for antifreeze poisoning (Fig. 29-11).[117] Serum ethylene glycol and glycolic acid concentrations may persist for days at toxic concentrations in azotemic or anuric animals despite therapy with alcohol or 4-methylpyrazole. These inhibitors of alcohol dehydrogenase merely delay the enzymatic conversion of ethylene glycol, and their efficacy relies on the potential for renal elimination of both the toxin and its metabolites.

The goals for hemodialysis are to eliminate the ethylene glycol and its metabolites from the animal as quickly as possible and to correct the accompanying fluid, electrolyte, and acid-base disturbances and attending uremia. For suspected poisonings, hemodialysis should be initiated immediately to ensure rapid elimination of the toxin regardless of previous administration of antidotal therapy or the absence of clinical signs. If the animal needs to be transported, an initial dose of ethanol or 4-methylpyrazole should be administered, and existing

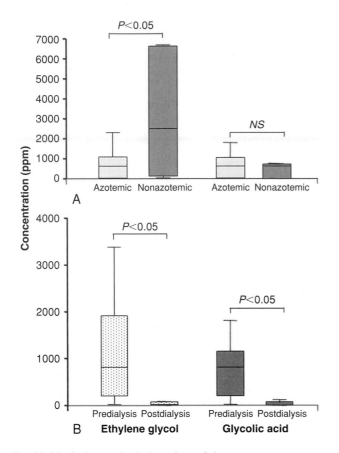

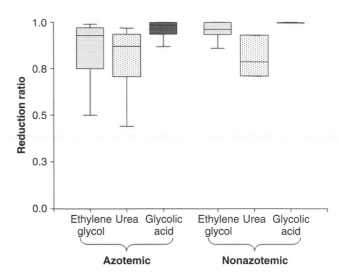

Fig. 29-11 A, Box and whisker plots of the serum concentrations for ethylene glycol (*left*) and glycolic acid (*right*) in azotemic (*light boxes*; n = 20) and nonazotemic (*dark boxes*; n = 6) dogs presenting for hemodialysis. **B,** Box and whisker plots of the change in serum ethylene glycol (*left*) and glycolic acid (*right*) concentrations before and following hemodialysis in 26 azotemic and nonazotemic dogs poisoned with antifreeze.[123]

Fig. 29-12 Box and whisker plots demonstrating the reduction ratios for ethylene glycol (*light boxes*), urea (*stippled boxes*), and glycolic acid (*dark boxes*) in azotemic (n = 20) and nonazotemic (n = 6) dogs. These observations demonstrate that both ethylene glycol and glycolic acid have removal kinetics similar to those for urea, and urea reduction ratio can serve as a convenient surrogate to predict removal of these toxins with hemodialysis.

dehydration and metabolic acidosis should be corrected.[31,144] It generally is possible to eliminate 90% to 95% or more of the toxin with a single intensive dialysis treatment (see Fig. 29-11).[30,117] However, uncertainty arises in predicting the necessary amount of dialysis to deliver when toxicological results are not readily available to confirm toxin removal during the treatment. Urea (MW, 60 daltons) is similar in molecular size and distribution volume to ethylene glycol (MW, 62 daltons) and can serve as an index for changes in ethylene glycol clearance similar to its surrogate role for removal of small molecular weight uremic toxins. The URR also can be used to predict ethylene glycol reduction and the depurated blood volume required to achieve the removal goal (Fig. 29-12).[117] To achieve a 90% ethylene glycol reduction during the course of treatment, it is necessary to select treatment parameters that would promote the same URR for that patient.

For nonazotemic animals, 90% to 100% of the toxin should be removed during the first dialysis treatment.

A second treatment is provided if delivery is incomplete during the first session and for possible rebound of ethylene glycol after treatment. Vascular access with a temporary dialysis catheter generally provides adequate blood flow. The highest efficiency hemodialyzer compatible with the extracorporeal volume requirement of the animal should be used to maximize diffusive removal of the toxins. Blood flow rates between 15 and 25 mL/kg/min or faster are tolerated. A standard dialysate flow between 500 and 600 mL/min is used but can be increased if the blood flow rate is greater than 200 mL/min. A dialysate formulated with 3 or 4 mmol/L potassium, 30 to 35 mmol/L bicarbonate, and a physiologic sodium concentration is appropriate unless specific electrolyte, acid-base, or hemodynamic disorders are present. A neutral sodium phosphate solution should be added to the dialysate concentrate to prevent hypophosphatemia (see Dialysate Additives above). Ultrafiltration can be used in animals with pulmonary edema or congestive heart failure secondary to the toxin or fluid administration. However, ultrafiltration is minimally effective for pulmonary effusions arising from respiratory distress syndrome or uremic pneumonitis associated with antifreeze poisoning. Simultaneous fluid administration and balanced ultrafiltration can increase convective toxin removal, but the benefits generally are small.

In uremic animals, the goals for toxin removal are constrained by requirements to prevent dialysis disequilibrium syndrome, and dialysis must be delivered carefully to accommodate all of the patient's needs. A temporary hemodialysis catheter generally is placed to expedite the initial treatment, but it is replaced with a permanent tunneled catheter after 2 weeks if additional dialysis is required. If the BUN concentration is less than 125 mg/dL, an intensive treatment as used in nonuremic animals is suitable. For animals with BUN concentrations greater than 150 mg/dL, more than one treatment may be required to remove the toxins adequately. The dialysis prescription should be targeted for a 60% to 100% ethylene glycol reduction but carefully tailored to the requirement for acute uremia with hourly URR targets appropriate for the degree of azotemia (see Table 29-2). For severely uremic animals, safe urea reduction and greater toxin removal are achieved when dialysis is provided slowly over 6 to 12 hours or more and designed to produce a URR of 0.05 to 0.1/hr. The remainder of the dialysis prescription should be formulated to specific complications accompanying the uremia, fluid volume status, acid-base and electrolyte disturbances, and hemodynamic stability. Mannitol (Mannitol Injection USP, Abbott Laboratories, North Chicago, IL) should be administered at 0.5 to 1.0 g/kg intravenously 45 to 60 minutes after starting dialysis and maintained with a constant-rate infusion at 1 to 2 mg/kg/min in both mild and severely azotemic animals to prevent manifestations of dialysis disequilibrium syndrome. For both nonazotemic and azotemic animals, absolute ethanol should be added to the dialysate concentrate to achieve a serum ethanol concentration of 0.1% in an effort to inhibit ongoing metabolism of ethylene glycol to its toxic metabolites during the extended hours of dialysis when it is being removed (see Dialysate Additives above).

COMPLICATIONS OF HEMODIALYSIS

The clinical and procedural complications associated with hemodialysis in humans and animals have been reviewed.[29,49,126] The most serious complications include those associated with the interaction of the patient with the dialysis machinery, vascular access, hemodynamic stability, and solute disequilibrium. Hemodialysis is a technically complex therapy applied to patients with profound physiologic and metabolic derangements. Therapeutic complications can be anticipated from both the technical aspects of the process, the dynamic oscillations of solute and fluid homeostasis, exposure to nonbiological materials and sources of contamination, and toxicities associated with medical therapies. Often it is difficult to distinguish whether adverse events are caused by the severity of the uremia per se or the intensity of its treatment. The frequency and intensity of complications related to homeostatic excursions early in dialysis diminish as the patient adapts to the procedures and the uremia is controlled, but they may be replaced with more subtle homeostatic imbalances imposed chronically.

Technical complications associated with hemodialysis procedures are uncommon because of the advances in technology, intrinsic safeguards, internal systems, and patient monitors designed into modern dialysis delivery systems. Transcutaneous venous catheters remain the most probable angioaccess for animal dialysis, but they represent the most predictable, problematic, and serious source of dialysis-related complications. Access complications are beyond the scope of the present discussion and have been reviewed recently.[49]

Hypotension is an anticipated but generally transient and manageable complication of hemodialysis. Blood pressure should be monitored at 15- to 30-minute intervals throughout the dialysis session. The susceptibility to hypotensive events is influenced by body size, hydration status, the severity of the uremia, the presence of concurrent cardiac disease or comorbid conditions (e.g., hemorrhage, anemia, sepsis, pancreatitis), and current medications (e.g., antihypertensives, diuretics). For cats and small dogs, the volume of the extracorporeal circuit may exceed 20% of intravascular volume and cause hypovolemia as the circuit is filled. The rapid removal of plasma solutes in the early stages of a dialysis treatment decreases intravascular volume and opposes refilling of fluid from the extravascular space. Excessive or rapid ultrafiltration of fluid from the vascular compartment faster than it can be replenished from extravascular reserves is the most frequent cause of hypovolemia and transient hypotension. Dialysis-induced hypotension usually responds quickly to modest fluid supplementation, which transiently refills vascular volume while fluid from the extravascular space is mobilized. Administration of small volumes of synthetic colloid solutions often is more effective at maintaining blood pressure, blood volume, and ongoing ultrafiltration with less net fluid administration.

Dialysis disequilibrium syndrome is a serious neurologic manifestation induced by rapid dialysis of animals with severe azotemia. The pathogenesis of dialysis disequilibrium syndrome is not completely understood but culminates with development of cerebral edema and the potential for herniation of the brainstem. The disproportionate removal of solutes (mostly urea) from ECF relative to intracellular fluid in the brain imposes an osmotic pressure causing influx of water into brain cells, cerebral edema, and an increase in intracranial pressure.[126,134,135] Paradoxical cerebral acidosis caused by rapid correction of severe metabolic acidosis and large transmembrane bicarbonate gradients also has been suggested to impose osmotic gradients by induction of idiogenic osmoles within the brain, causing further brain swelling.[7-11]

Dialysis disequilibrium is most serious in cats and small dogs during initial dialysis treatments when the degree of azotemia and metabolic acidosis is greatest. Clinical signs such as tremors, restlessness, disorientation, vocalization, amaurosis, seizures, and coma may develop during the dialysis session or up to 24 hours after dialysis. If not recognized and managed properly, the syndrome may progress from subtle neurologic alterations to seizures, coma, and death from respiratory arrest from compression of the brainstem by herniation of the cerebellum.[29] In dogs, dialysis disequilibrium syndrome is generally insidious and commences with restlessness and vocalization before the onset of seizures or coma and affords ample opportunity to intervene at an early stage. In cats, the development of serious or fatal manifestations frequently is more acute and without warning.

Treatment of dialysis disequilibrium requires immediate attention, slowing or discontinuing the hemodialysis treatment, and intravenous administration of hypertonic (20% to 25%) mannitol (0.5 to 1.0 g/kg intravenously) to increase plasma osmolality and dissipate the osmotic gradient. Diazepam (Diazepam Injection, USP, Schein Pharmaceutical, Inc., Norham Park, NJ) is used as required to control seizures. Animals with preexisting CNS disease, BUN concentrations greater than 200 mg/dL, severe metabolic acidosis, or body weights less than 5 kg are at highest risk. For high-risk animals, the efficiency of the dialysis treatment should be reduced purposefully by interspacing periods of dialysis with periods of bypass and decreasing the dialysate bicarbonate to better match that of the patient (see Hemodialysis Prescription for Acute Uremia, above). Mannitol can be administered prophylactically at 0.5 to 1.0 g/kg intravenously after the initial 20% to 25% of the dialysis treatment and also at the end of the treatment to reduce delayed onset of signs. Mild signs usually dissipate immediately with mannitol administration, whereas severe signs may require several doses and 24 to 48 hours of supportive care before resolution. Respiratory arrest from cerebral edema and brainstem compression requires ventilatory support until the edema resolves but carries a poor prognosis for recovery.

OUTCOME AND PROGNOSIS

The ultimate treatment outcome for hemodialysis is recovery of renal function in animals with acute uremia and indefinite survival for those with chronic kidney disease. Dogs have been supported on chronic intermittent hemodialysis as long as 1.5 years, but complications related to vascular access and anemia management often curtail dialytic support beyond 6 months. Regional availability and financial and time constraints further limit utilization of hemodialysis for management of either acute or chronic uremia. For acute uremia, renal recovery is not predicated primarily on dialysis per se, but rather the etiology, extent of damage, comorbid diseases, multiple organ involvement, and availability of diagnostic and therapeutic services. There is little documentation in the veterinary literature to accurately predict the importance of these independent variables, and the validity of the dialysis prescription remains mostly based on anecdotal experience.

A retrospective case-control study of 99 dogs with ARF treated conventionally reported a mortality of nearly 60%, with only 44% of the surviving dogs recovering normal renal function.[145] Survival for 29 dogs with hospital-acquired ARF was reported as 38%, with age and initial urine production significantly predicting mortality.[13] Compared with these surveys of animals managed with conventional medical therapy, a retrospective study of 36 dogs treated for leptospirosis-induced ARF documented equivalent survival outcomes of greater than 80%, both for animals with severe uremia and expected to die before dialytic intervention and for those with milder presentations that were medically managed.[3] A recent review of 138 dogs with severe acute uremia requiring hemodialysis after failure to respond to conventional medical management identified an overall survival rate of nearly 40% for the entire 12-year period of review and 50% survival during the last 6 years of evaluation (86 dogs).[52] For most surviving dogs, renal function recovered substantially by the time of discharge, and progression to chronic renal failure was observed rarely. Survival from infectious (80%) and hemodynamic and metabolic etiologies (40%) was more favorable than survival from toxic causes (20%).

Early observations in cats with severe ARF treated with hemodialysis demonstrated partial or complete recovery of renal function and survival in 60% (9 of 15), although some of these cats required renal transplantation.[81] More recently, a retrospective review of 119 cats treated with hemodialysis for severe acute uremia identified a survival rate of 52%, with better outcomes documented in cats with ureteral obstruction (75%) than in those with infectious (60%) or toxic etiologies (20%).[107] In all studies involving hemodialysis as part of the therapy in dogs and cats, the magnitude of azotemia at presentation did not predict the potential for survival.

Overall, these observations illustrate that hemodialysis has a vital role in the therapeutic stratification of dogs and cats with severe acute uremia that remain nonresponsive to conventional medical therapy. Hemodialysis improves survival for animals with acute uremia beyond what would be expected with conventional management of the same animals. Clinical evidence and experience in human patients suggest a role for earlier intervention with renal replacement to avoid the morbidity of uremia and to promote better metabolic stability and recovery.[95]

REFERENCES

1. Abel JJ, Rowntree LC, Turner BB: On the removal of diffusible substances from the circulating blood by means of dialysis, *Trans Assoc Am Physiol* 28:41, 1913.
2. Adin CA: Screening criteria for feline renal transplant recipients and donors, *Clin Tech Small Anim Pract* 17:184-189, 2002.
3. Adin CA, Cowgill LD: Treatment and outcome of dogs with leptospirosis: 36 cases (1990-1998), *J Am Vet Med Assoc* 216:371-375, 2000.

4. Adin CA, Gregory CR, Kyles AE, et al: Diagnostic predictors of complications and survival after renal transplantation in cats, *Vet Surg* 30:515-521, 2001.

5. Agostoni PG, Marenzi GC: Sustained benefit from ultrafiltration in moderate congestive heart failure, *Cardiology* 96:183-189, 2001.

6. Al-Hilali N, Al-Humoud HM, Ninan VT, et al: Profiled hemodialysis reduces intradialytic symptoms, *Transplant Proc* 36:1827-1828, 2004.

7. Arieff AI: More on the dialysis disequilibrium syndrome, *West J Med* 151:74-76, 1989.

8. Arieff AI: Dialysis disequilibrium syndrome: current concepts on pathogenesis and prevention, *Kidney Int* 45:629-635, 1994.

9. Arieff AI, Guisado R, Massry SG, et al: Central nervous system pH in uremia and the effects of hemodialysis, *J Clin Invest* 58:306-311, 1976.

10. Arieff AI, Lazarowitz VC, Guisado R: Experimental dialysis disequilibrium syndrome: prevention with glycerol, *Kidney Int* 14:270-278, 1978.

11. Arieff AI, Mahoney CA: Pathogenesis of dialysis encephalopathy, *Neurobehav Toxicol Teratol* 5:641-644, 1983.

12. Bankhead MM, Toto RD, Star RA: Accuracy of urea removal estimated by kinetic models, *Kidney Int* 48:785-793, 1995.

13. Behrend EN, Grauer GF, Mani I, et al: Hospital-acquired acute renal failure in dogs: 29 cases (1983-1992), *J Am Vet Med Assoc* 208:537-541, 1996.

14. Bellomo R, Ronco C: Continuous haemofiltration in the intensive care unit, *Crit Care* 4:339-345, 2000.

15. Bernsteen L, Gregory CR, Kyles AE, et al: Renal transplantation in cats, *Clin Tech Small Anim Pract* 15:40-45, 2000.

16. Biasioli S, D'Andrea G, Feriani M, et al: Uremic encephalopathy: an updating, *Clin Nephrol* 25:57-63, 1986.

17. Blake PG: Adequacy of dialysis revisited, *Kidney Int* 63:1587-1599, 2003.

18. Boure T, Vanholder R: Biochemical and clinical evidence for uremic toxicity, *Artif Organs* 28:248-253, 2004.

19. Brunet P, Dou L, Cerini C, et al: Protein-bound uremic retention solutes, *Adv Ren Replace Ther* 10:310-320, 2003.

20. Carvalho KT, Silva MI, Bregman R: Nutritional profile of patients with chronic renal failure, *J Ren Nutr* 14:97-100, 2004.

21. Casino FG, Lopez T: The equivalent renal urea clearance: a new parameter to assess dialysis dose, *Nephrol Dial Transplant* 11:1574-1581, 1996.

22. Casino FG, Marshall MR: Simple and accurate quantification of dialysis in acute renal failure patients during either urea non-steady state or treatment with irregular or continuous schedules, *Nephrol Dial Transplant* 19:1454-1466, 2004.

23. Chang IJ, Fischach BV, Sile S, et al: Extracorporeal treatment of poisoning. In Brenner BM, editors: *Brenner and Rector's the kidney*. Philadelphia, 2004, WB Saunders, pp. 2733-2757.

24. Charra B, Calemard E, Ruffet M, et al: Survival as an index of adequacy of dialysis, *Kidney Int* 41:1286-1291, 1992.

25. Chow MT, Di Silvestro VA, Yung CY, et al: Treatment of acute methanol intoxication with hemodialysis using an ethanol-enriched, bicarbonate-based dialysate, *Am J Kidney Dis* 30:568-570, 1997.

26. Clark W, Winchester J: Middle molecules and small molecular weight proteins in ESRD: properties and strategies for their removal, *Adv Ren Replace Ther* 10:270-278, 2003.

27. Coli L, Ursino M, Donati G, et al: Clinical application of sodium profiling in the treatment of intradialytic hypotension, *Int J Artif Organs* 26:715-722, 2003.

28. Cooper BA, Aslani A, Ryan M, et al: Comparing different methods of assessing body composition in end-stage renal failure, *Kidney Int* 58:408-416, 2000.

29. Cowgill LD, Elliott DA: Hemodialysis. In DiBartola SP, editors: *Fluid therapy in small animal practice*, Philadelphia, 2000, WB Saunders, pp. 528-547.

30. Cowgill LD, Francey T: Acute uremia. In Ettinger SJ, Feldman EC, editors: *Textbook of veterinary internal medicine: diseases of the dog and cat*, Philadelphia, 2004, WB Saunders, pp. 1731-1751.

31. Cowgill LD, Langston CE: Role of hemodialysis in the management of dogs and cats with renal failure, *Vet Clin North Am Small Anim Pract* 26:1347-1378, 1996.

32. Daugirdas JT: The post:pre-dialysis plasma urea nitrogen ratio to estimate K.t/V and NPCR: mathematical modeling, *Int J Artif Organs* 12:411-419, 1989.

33. Daugirdas JT: Dialysis hypotension: a hemodynamic analysis, *Kidney Int* 39:233-246, 1991.

34. Daugirdas JT, Van Stone JC: Physiologic principles and urea kinetic modeling. In Daugirdas JT, Blake PG, Ing TS, editors: *Handbook of dialysis*, Philadelphia, 2001, Lippincott Williams & Wilkins, pp. 15-45.

35. De Nicola L, Bellizzi V, Minutolo R, et al: Effect of dialysate sodium concentration on interdialytic increase of potassium, *J Am Soc Nephrol* 11:2337-2343, 2000.

36. De Vries JP, Donker AJ, De Vries PM: Prevention of hypovolemia-induced hypotension during hemodialysis by means of an optical reflection method, *Int J Artif Organs* 17:209-214, 1994.

37. de Vries JP, Kouw PM, van der Meer NJ, et al: Non-invasive monitoring of blood volume during hemodialysis: its relation with post-dialytic dry weight, *Kidney Int* 44:851-854, 1993.

38. Depner T: Benefits of more frequent dialysis: lower TAC at the same Kt/V, *Nephrol Dial Transplant* 13:20-24, 1998.

39. Depner TA: *Prescribing hemodialysis: a guide to urea modeling*. Boston, 1990, Kluwer Academic Publishers.

40. Depner TA: Uremic toxicity: urea and beyond, *Semin Dial* 14:246-251, 2001.

41. Depner TA, Bhat A: Quantifying daily hemodialysis, *Semin Dial* 17:79-84, 2004.

42. Depner TA, Gotch FA, Port FK, et al: How will the results of the HEMO study impact dialysis practice? *Semin Dial* 16:8-21, 2003.

43. Di Filippo S, Manzoni C, Andrulli S, et al: How to determine ionic dialysance for the online assessment of delivered dialysis dose, *Kidney Int* 59:774-782, 2001.

44. Di Filippo S, Manzoni C, Andrulli S, et al: Ionic dialysance allows an adequate estimate of urea distribution volume in hemodialysis patients, *Kidney Int* 66:786-791, 2004.

45. DuBose TD Jr, Warnock DG, Mehta RL, et al: Acute renal failure in the 21st century: recommendations for management and outcomes assessment, *Am J Kidney Dis* 29:793-799, 1997.

46. Eknoyan G, Beck GJ, Cheung AK, et al: Effect of dialysis dose and membrane flux in maintenance hemodialysis, *N Engl J Med* 347:2010-2019, 2002.

47. Eustace JA, Astor B, Muntner PM, et al: Prevalence of acidosis and inflammation and their association with low serum albumin in chronic kidney disease, *Kidney Int* 65:1031-1040, 2004.

48. Feriani M: Behaviour of acid-base control with different dialysis schedules, *Nephrol Dial Transplant* 13(suppl 6):62-65, 1998.

49. Fischer JR, Pantaleo V, Francey T, et al: Veterinary hemodialysis: advances in management and technology, *Vet Clin North Am Small Anim Pract* 34:935-967, vi-vii, 2004.

50. Flanigan MJ: Role of sodium in hemodialysis, *Kidney Int Suppl* 76:S72-78, 2000.
51. Francey T, Benitah N, Pantaleo V, et al: Use of combined hemoperfusion and hemodialysis in accidental enrofloxacin overdose, *2004 ACVIM Forum Proceedings* 18:441-442, 2004.
52. Francey T, Cowgill LD: Use of hemodialysis for the management of ARF in the dog: 124 cases (1990-2001), *J Vet Intern Med* 16:352, 2002.
53. Friedman AN, Jaber BL: Dialysis adequacy in patients with acute renal failure, *Curr Opin Nephrol Hypertens* 8:695-700, 1999.
54. Goldstein DJ, Frederico CB: The effect of urea kinetic modeling on the nutrition management of hemodialysis patients, *J Am Diet Assoc* 87:474-479, 1987.
55. Gotch FA: Evolution of the single-pool urea kinetic model, *Semin Dial* 14:252-256, 2001.
56. Gotch FA: Is Kt/V urea a satisfactory measure for dosing the newer dialysis regimens? *Semin Dial* 14:15-17, 2001.
57. Gotch FA, Panlilio FM, Buyaki RA, et al: Mechanisms determining the ratio of conductivity clearance to urea clearance, *Kidney Int Suppl* S3-S24, 2004.
58. Grollman EF, Grollman A: Toxicity of urea and its role in the pathogenesis of uremia, *J Clin Invest* 38:749-754, 1959.
59. Guh JY, Yang CY, Yang JM, et al: Prediction of equilibrated postdialysis BUN by an artificial neural network in high-efficiency hemodialysis, *Am J Kidney Dis* 31:638-646, 1998.
60. Hakim RM, Breyer J, Ismail N, et al: Effects of dose of dialysis on morbidity and mortality, *Am J Kidney Dis* 23:661-669, 1994.
61. Hakim RM, Depner TA, Parker TF 3rd: Adequacy of hemodialysis, *Am J Kidney Dis* 20:107-123, 1992.
62. Heidenheim AP, Muirhead N, Moist L, et al: Patient quality of life on quotidian hemodialysis, *Am J Kidney Dis* 42:36-41, 2003.
63. Heiene R, Vulliet PR, Williams RL, et al: Use of capillary electrophoresis to quantitate carbamylated hemoglobin concentrations in dogs with renal failure, *Am J Vet Res* 62:1302-1306, 2001.
64. Held PJ, Port FK, Wolfe RA, et al: The dose of hemodialysis and patient mortality, *Kidney Int* 50:550-556, 1996.
65. Henle T, Miyata T: Advanced glycation end products in uremia, *Adv Ren Replace Ther* 10:321-331, 2003.
66. Henrich WL: Hemodynamic instability during hemodialysis, *Kidney Int* 30:605-612, 1986.
67. Ikizler TA, Schulman G: Adequacy of dialysis, *Kidney Int Suppl* 62:S96-100, 1997.
68. Ishibe S, Peixoto AJ: Methods of assessment of volume status and intercompartmental fluid shifts in hemodialysis patients: implications in clinical practice, *Semin Dial* 17:37-43, 2004.
69. Jaeger JQ, Mehta RL: Assessment of dry weight in hemodialysis: an overview, *J Am Soc Nephrol* 10:392-403, 1999.
70. Jaffrin MY, Fenech M, de Fremont JF, et al: Continuous monitoring of plasma, interstitial, and intracellular fluid volumes in dialyzed patients by bioimpedance and hematocrit measurements, *ASAIO J* 48:326-333, 2002.
71. Johnson WJ, Hagge WW, Wagoner RD, et al: Effects of urea loading in patients with far-advanced renal failure, *Mayo Clin Proc* 47:21-29, 1972.
72. Kanagasundaram NS, Greene T, Larive AB, et al: Prescribing an equilibrated intermittent hemodialysis dose in intensive care unit acute renal failure, *Kidney Int* 64:2298-2310, 2003.
73. Kaysen GA: The microinflammatory state in uremia: causes and potential consequences, *J Am Soc Nephrol* 12:1549-1557, 2001.
74. Kaysen GA: Role of inflammation and its treatment in ESRD patients, *Blood Purif* 20:70-80, 2002.
75. Kaysen GA, Kumar V: Inflammation in ESRD: causes and potential consequences, *J Ren Nutr* 13:158-160, 2003.
76. Kloppenburg WD, Stegeman CA, Hooyschuur M, et al: Assessing dialysis adequacy and dietary intake in the individual hemodialysis patient, *Kidney Int* 55:1961-1969, 1999.
77. Kosanovich JM, Dumler F, Horst M, et al: Use of urea kinetics in the nutritional care of the acutely ill patient, *J Parenter Enteral Nutr* 9:165-169, 1985.
78. Kuhlmann U, Goldau R, Samadi N, et al: Accuracy and safety of online clearance monitoring based on conductivity variation, *Nephrol Dial Transplant* 16:1053-1058, 2001.
79. Laird NM, Berkey CS, Lowrie EG: Modeling success or failure of dialysis therapy: the National Cooperative Dialysis Study, *Kidney Int Suppl* Apr:S101-106, 1983.
80. Lambie SH, McIntyre CW: Developments in online monitoring of haemodialysis patients: towards global assessment of dialysis adequacy, *Curr Opin Nephrol Hypertens* 12:633-638, 2003.
81. Langston CE, Cowgill LD, Spano JA: Applications and outcome of hemodialysis in cats: a review of 29 cases, *J Vet Intern Med* 11:348-355, 1997.
82. Lesaffer G, De Smet R, D'Heuvaert T, et al: Comparative kinetics of the uremic toxin p-cresol versus creatinine in rats with and without renal failure, *Kidney Int* 64:1365-1373, 2003.
83. Levine J, Bernard DB: The role of urea kinetic modeling, TACurea, and Kt/V in achieving optimal dialysis: a critical reappraisal, *Am J Kidney Dis* 15:285-301, 1990.
84. Lindsay RM, Leitch R, Heidenheim AP, et al: The London Daily/Nocturnal Hemodialysis Study—study design, morbidity, and mortality results, *Am J Kidney Dis* 42:5-12, 2003.
85. Locatelli F, Buoncristiani U, Canaud B, et al: Haemodialysis with on-line monitoring equipment: tools or toys? *Nephrol Dial Transplant* 20:22-33, 2005.
86. Locatelli F, Covic A, Chazot C, et al: Optimal composition of the dialysate, with emphasis on its influence on blood pressure, *Nephrol Dial Transplant* 19:785-796, 2004.
87. Lopot F, Valek A: Time-averaged concentration–time-averaged deviation: a new concept in mathematical assessment of dialysis adequacy, *Nephrol Dial Transplant* 3:846-848, 1988.
88. Lowrie E, Lew N: The urea reduction ratio (URR): a simple method for evaluating hemodialysis treatment, *Contemp Dial Nephrol* 12:11-20, 1991.
89. Lowrie EG, Laird NM, Parker TF, et al: Effect of the hemodialysis prescription of patient morbidity: report from the National Cooperative Dialysis Study, *N Engl J Med* 305:1176-1181, 1981.
90. Lowrie EG, Teehan BP: Principles of prescribing dialysis therapy: implementing recommendations from the National Cooperative Dialysis Study, *Kidney Int Suppl* Apr:S113-122, 1983.
91. Maggiore Q: Isothermic dialysis for hypotension-prone patients, *Semin Dial* 15:187-190, 2002.
92. Maggiore Q, Pizzarelli F, Santoro A, et al: The effects of control of thermal balance on vascular stability in hemodialysis patients: results of the European randomized clinical trial, *Am J Kidney Dis* 40:280-290, 2002.
93. Marenzi G, Lauri G, Grazi M, et al: Circulatory response to fluid overload removal by extracorporeal ultrafiltration in refractory congestive heart failure, *J Am Coll Cardiol* 38:963-968, 2001.

94. Mawby DI, Bartges JW, DAvignon A, et al: Comparison of various methods for estimating body fat in dogs, *J Am Anim Hosp Assoc* 40:109-114, 2004.

95. Mehta RL, McDonald B, Gabbai FB, et al: A randomized clinical trial of continuous versus intermittent dialysis for acute renal failure, *Kidney Int* 60:1154-1163, 2001.

96. Messa P, Gropuzzo M, Cleva M, et al: Behaviour of phosphate removal with different dialysis schedules, *Nephrol Dial Transplant* 13(suppl 6):43-48, 1998.

97. Michael M, Brewer ED, Goldstein SL: Blood volume monitoring to achieve target weight in pediatric hemodialysis patients, *Pediatr Nephrol* 19:432-437, 2004.

98. Michel KE, Sorenmo K, Shofer FS: Evaluation of body condition and weight loss in dogs presented to a veterinary oncology service, *J Vet Intern Med* 18:692-695, 2004.

99. Miyata T, Saito A, Kurokawa K, et al: Advanced glycation and lipoxidation end products: reactive carbonyl compounds-related uraemic toxicity, *Nephrol Dial Transplant* 16(suppl 4):8-11, 2001.

100. Mujais SK, Schmidt B: Operating characteristics of hollow-fiber dialyzers. In Nissensen AR, Fine RN, Gentile DE, editors: *Clinical dialysis,* Norwalk, CT, 1995, Appleton & Lange, pp. 77-92.

101. NKF: I. NKF-K/DOQI Clinical Practice Guidelines for Hemodialysis Adequacy: update 2000, *Am J Kidney Dis* 37:S7-S64, 2001.

102. Noghnogh AA, Reid RW, Nawab ZM, et al: Preparation of ethanol-enriched, bicarbonate-based hemodialysates, *Artif Organs* 23:208-209, 1999.

103. Oberg BP, McMenamin E, Lucas FL, et al: Increased prevalence of oxidant stress and inflammation in patients with moderate to severe chronic kidney disease, *Kidney Int* 65:1009-1016, 2004.

104. Owen WF Jr, Lew NL, Liu Y, et al: The urea reduction ratio and serum albumin concentration as predictors of mortality in patients undergoing hemodialysis, *N Engl J Med* 329:1001-1006, 1993.

105. Palmer CA: Neurologic manifestations of renal disease, *Neurol Clin* 20:23-34, v, 2002.

106. Pantaleo V, Francey T, Cowgill LD: Analysis of hyperkalemia in dogs on chronic hemodialysis, *ACVIM Forum 2005,* Baltimore, MD, 2005.

107. Pantaleo V, Francey T, Fischer JR, et al: Application of hemodialysis for the management of acute uremia in cats: 119 cases (1993-2003), *J Vet Intern Med* 18:418, 2004.

108. Parker TF 3rd, Husni L, Huang W, et al: Survival of hemodialysis patients in the United States is improved with a greater quantity of dialysis, *Am J Kidney Dis* 23:670-680, 1994.

109. Pedrini LA, Zereik S, Rasmy S: Causes, kinetics and clinical implications of post-hemodialysis urea rebound, *Kidney Int* 34:817-824, 1988.

110. Pergola PE, Habiba NM, Johnson JM: Body temperature regulation during hemodialysis in long-term patients: is it time to change dialysate temperature prescription? *Am J Kidney Dis* 44:155-165, 2004.

111. Petitclerc T: Festschrift for Professor Claude Jacobs. Recent developments in conductivity monitoring of haemodialysis session, *Nephrol Dial Transplant* 14:2607-2613, 1999.

112. Polaschegg HD: Automatic, noninvasive intradialytic clearance measurement, *Int J Artif Organs* 16:185-191, 1993.

113. Polzin DJ, Osborne CA, Ross S: Chronic kidney disease. In Ettinger SJ, Feldman EC, editors: *Textbook of veterinary internal medicine,* Philadelphia, 2004, WB Saunders, pp. 1756-1776.

114. Redaelli B: Electrolyte modelling in haemodialysis–potassium, *Nephrol Dial Transplant* 11(suppl 2):39-41, 1996.

115. Redaelli B: Hydroelectrolytic equilibrium change in dialysis, *J Nephrol* 14(suppl 4):S7-11, 2001.

116. Redaelli B, Bonoldi G, Di Filippo G, et al: Behaviour of potassium removal in different dialytic schedules, *Nephrol Dial Transplant* 13(suppl 6):35-38, 1998.

117. Rollings CE, Francey T, Cowgill LD: Use of hemodialysis in uremic and non-uremic dogs with ethylene glycol toxicity, *J Vet Intern Med* 18:416, 2004.

118. Ronco C, Ricci Z, Brendolan A, et al: Ultrafiltration in patients with hypervolemia and congestive heart failure, *Blood Purif* 22:150-163, 2004.

119. Rosales LM, Schneditz D, Morris AT, et al: Isothermic hemodialysis and ultrafiltration, *Am J Kidney Dis* 36:353-361, 2000.

120. Sargent JA, Gotch FA: Mathematic modeling of dialysis therapy, *Kidney Int Suppl* 10:S2-10, 1980.

121. Sargent JA, Gotch FA: Principles and biophysics of dialysis. In Maher JF, editor: *Replacement of renal function by dialysis: a textbook of dialysis,* Boston, 1989, Kluwer Academic Publishers, pp. 87-143.

122. Sargent JA, Lowrie EG: Which mathematical model to study uremic toxicity? National Cooperative Dialysis Study, *Clin Nephrol* 17:303-314, 1982.

123. Schneditz D, Daugirdas JT: Compartment effects in hemodialysis, *Semin Dial* 14:271-277, 2001.

124. Schneditz D, Ronco C, Levin N: Temperature control by the blood temperature monitor, *Semin Dial* 16:477-482, 2003.

125. Schroeder KL, Sallustio JE, Ross EA: Continuous haematocrit monitoring during intradialytic hypotension: precipitous decline in plasma refill rates, *Nephrol Dial Transplant* 19:652-656, 2004.

126. Schulman G, Himmelfarb J: Hemodialysis. In Brenner BM, editor: *Brenner & Rector's the kidney,* Philadelphia, 2004, WB Saunders, pp. 2564-2624.

127. Shackman R, Chisholm GD, Holden AJ, et al: Urea distribution in the body after haemodialysis, *BMJ* 5301:355-358, 1962.

128. Sharma A, Espinosa P, Bell L, et al: Multicompartment urea kinetics in well-dialyzed children, *Kidney Int* 58:2138-2146, 2000.

129. Sheppard R, Panyon J, Pohwani AL, et al: Intermittent outpatient ultrafiltration for the treatment of severe refractory congestive heart failure, *J Card Fail* 10:380-383, 2004.

130. Sherman RA: Modifying the dialysis prescription to reduce intradialytic hypotension, *Am J Kidney Dis* 38:S18-25, 2001.

131. Sherman RA, Cody RP, Rogers ME, et al: Accuracy of the urea reduction ratio in predicting dialysis delivery, *Kidney Int* 47:319-321, 1995.

132. Shinaberger JH: Quantitation of dialysis: historical perspective, *Semin Dial* 14:238-245, 2001.

133. Sigdell JE, Tersteegen B: Clearance of a dialyzer under varying operating conditions, *Artif Organs* 10:219-225, 1986.

134. Silver SM, DeSimone JA Jr, Smith DA, et al: Dialysis disequilibrium syndrome (DDS) in the rat: role of the "reverse urea effect," *Kidney Int* 42:161-166, 1992.

135. Silver SM, Sterns RH, Halperin ML: Brain swelling after dialysis: old urea or new osmoles? *Am J Kidney Dis* 28:1-13, 1996.

136. Smye SW, Hydon PE, Will E: An analysis of the single-pool urea kinetic model and estimation of errors, *Phys Med Biol* 38:115-122, 1993.

137. Smye SW, Tattersall JE, Will EJ: Modeling the postdialysis rebound: the reconciliation of current formulas, *ASAIO J* 45:562-567, 1999.

138. Song JH, Park GH, Lee SY, et al: Effect of sodium balance and the combination of ultrafiltration profile during sodium profiling hemodialysis on the maintenance of the quality of dialysis and sodium and fluid balances, *J Am Soc Nephrol* 16:237-246, 2005.

139. Steuer RR, Bell DA, Barrett LL: Optical measurement of hematocrit and other biological constituents in renal therapy, *Adv Ren Replace Ther* 6:217-224, 1999.

140. Steuer RR, Harris DH, Weiss RL, et al: Evaluation of a noninvasive hematocrit monitor: a new technology, *Am Clin Lab* 10:20-22, 1991.

141. Stiller S, Bonnie-Schorn E, Grassmann A, et al.: A critical review of sodium profiling for hemodialysis. *Semin Dial* 14:337-347, 2001.

142. Suri R, Depner TA, Blake PG, et al: Adequacy of quotidian hemodialysis, *Am J Kidney Dis* 42:42-48, 2003.

143. Suri RS, Depner T, Lindsay RM: Dialysis prescription and dose monitoring in frequent hemodialysis, *Contrib Nephrol* 145:75-88, 2004.

144. Thrall M: Advances in therapy for antifreeze poisoning, *Calif Vet* 52:18-22, 1998.

145. Vaden SL, Levine J, Breitschwerdt EB: A retrospective case-control of acute renal failure in 99 dogs, *J Vet Intern Med* 11:58-64, 1997.

146. Vanholder R, De Smet R, Glorieux G, et al: Review on uremic toxins: classification, concentration, and interindividual variability, *Kidney Int* 63:1934-1943, 2003.

147. Vanholder R, Glorieux G, De Smet R, et al: Low water-soluble uremic toxins, *Adv Ren Replace Ther* 10:257-269, 2003.

148. Vanholder R, Glorieux G, De Smet R, et al: New insights in uremic toxins, *Kidney Int* 63:S6-10, 2003.

149. Vanholder R, Winchester J: Introduction: uremic toxins, *Adv Ren Replace Ther* 10:256, 2003.

150. Vanholder RC, Glorieux GL: An overview of uremic toxicity, *Hemodial Int* 7:156-161, 2003.

151. Vanholder RC, Glorieux GL, De Smet RV: Uremic toxins: removal with different therapies, *Hemodial Int* 7:162-167, 2003.

152. Vinay P, Cardoso M, Tejedor A, et al: Acetate metabolism during hemodialysis: metabolic considerations, *Am J Nephrol* 7:337-354, 1987.

153. Winchester JF: Dialysis and hemoperfusion in poisoning, *Adv Ren Replace Ther* 9:26-30, 2002.

154. Wolf AV, Remp DG, Kiley JE, et al: Artificial kidney function; kinetics of hemodialysis, *J Clin Invest* 30:1062-1070, 1951.

155. Yeun JY, Depner TA: Complications related to inadequate delivered dose: recognition and management in acute and chronic dialysis. In Lameire N, Mehta RL, editors: *Complications of dialysis*, New York, 2000, Marcel Dekker, Inc., pp. 89-115.

156. Zhu F, Kuhlmann MK, Sarkar S, et al: Adjustment of dry weight in hemodialysis patients using intradialytic continuous multifrequency bioimpedance of the calf, *Int J Artif Organs* 27:104-109, 2004.

157. Zhu F, Sarkar S, Kaitwatcharachai C, et al: Methods and reproducibility of measurement of resistivity in the calf using regional bioimpedance analysis, *Blood Purif* 21:131-136, 2003.

APPENDIX

MATHEMATICAL EQUATIONS USED FOR DIALYSIS QUANTIFICATION

Equation 1: Time-averaged urea concentration

$$\textbf{TAC} = \frac{\text{AUC}}{(T_d + T_i)}$$

Abbreviations: TAC, time-averaged urea concentration (mg/dL); AUC, area under the BUN-time profile curve (mg/dL × min); T_d, time on dialysis (min); T_i, duration of the interdialytic interval (min).

Equation 2: Urea reduction ratio

$$URR(\%) = \frac{\text{preBUN} - \text{postBUN}}{\text{preBUN}} \times 100$$

or

$$URR(\%) = \left(1 - \frac{\text{postBUN}}{\text{preBUN}}\right) \times 100$$

Equation 3: Creatinine reduction ratio

$$CrRR(\%) = \frac{\text{preCrea} - \text{postCrea}}{\text{preCrea}} \times 100$$

or

$$CrRR(\%) = \left(1 - \frac{\text{postCrea}}{\text{preCrea}}\right) \times 100$$

Abbreviations: URR, urea reduction ratio (%); CrRR, creatinine reduction ratio (%); pre, predialysis; post, postdialysis; BUN, blood urea nitrogen concentration (mg/dL); Crea, creatinine concentration (mg/dL).

Equation 4: Total urea removal

$$\text{Total Urea Removal} = [\text{preBUN} \cdot \text{preV}] - [\text{postBUN} \cdot \text{postV}]$$

Abbreviations: BUN, blood urea nitrogen concentration (mg/mL); pre, predialysis; post, postdialysis; V, volume of distribution of urea (mL) often estimated as 58% of body weight, but the frequent perturbations of fluid metabolism seen in uremic animals severely limit the accuracy of this prediction.

Equation 5: Hemodialyze urea clearance

$$Kd = Q_b \cdot \frac{BUN_{in} - BUN_{out}}{BUN_{in}}$$

Abbreviations: Kd, hemodialyzer urea clearance (mL/min); Qb, blood flow rate through the hemodialyzer (mL/min); BUN_{in}, BUN concentration at the dialyzer inlet (mg/dL); BUN_{out}, BUN concentration in the dialyzer outlet (mg/dL).

Equation 6: Residual renal clearance

$$Kr = \frac{U_{urea} \cdot V}{BUN}$$

Abbreviations: Kr, residual renal clearance for urea (mL/min); U_{urea}, urinary urea nitrogen concentration (mg/dL); V, urine flow rate (mL/min); BUN, blood urea nitrogen concentration (mg/dL).

Equation 7: Continuous equivalent of intermittent clearance

$$EKR = G/TAC$$

Abbreviations: EKR, continuous equivalent of urea clearance (mL/min); G, urea generation rate (mg/min); TAC, time-averaged BUN concentration (mg/mL).

Equations 8-12: Kinetics of urea using a single-pool fixed volume model and resulting dose of dialysis: intradialytic and interdialytic BUN concentration (Eq. 8), urea generation rate (Eq. 9), and urea distribution volume (Eq. 10). In equation 8, the interdialytic BUN con-

centration is obtained by setting Kd as 0. The solution of equations 9 and 10 requires iterative simultaneous calculations as G is a function of V and reciprocally. The transformation of the dose of dialysis in standard Kt/V (Eq. 12) allows comparison of different dialysis schedules and modalities.

Equation 8: BUN concentration at time t

$$C_t = Co \cdot e^{-(Kr + Kd) t/V} + \frac{G \cdot \left[1 - \bar{e}^{(Kr + Kd) t/V} \right]}{K_r + K_d}$$

Equation 9: Urea generation rate

$$G = Kr \cdot \left[\frac{C_3 - C_2 \cdot e^{-Kr \, Ti/V}}{1 - e^{-Kr \, Ti/V}} \right]$$

Equation 10: Volume of distribution of urea

$$V = \frac{(K_r + K_d) \cdot T_d}{\ln \left[\dfrac{G - C_1 (K_d + K_r)}{G - C_2 (K_d + K_r)} \right]}$$

Equation 11: Single-pool Kt/V

$$spKt/V = K_d \cdot T_d / V$$

Equation 12: Standard Kt/V

$$StdKt/V = \frac{10080 \cdot (1 - e^{-Kt/V})}{T_d \cdot \left[\dfrac{(1 - c^{-Kt/V})}{Kt/V} + \dfrac{10080}{N \cdot T_d} - 1 \right]}$$

Abbreviations: C_t, BUN concentration at time t (mg/mL), where t = 0 at the beginning of the interval analyzed, t = 1 predialysis, t = 2 postdialysis, t = 3 predialysis for the next session; Kr, residual renal urea clearance (mL/min); Kd, dialyzer urea clearance (mL/min); T_d, duration of the dialysis session (min); T_i, duration of the interdialytic interval (min); V, urea distribution volume (mL); G, urea generation rate (mg/min); spKt/V, single-pool Kt/V; stdKt/V, standard

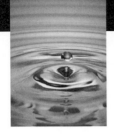

INDEX

A

ABCs of resuscitation, 547–548
Abdominal compartment syndrome, 398
Abdominal effusion. *See* Ascites
Abdominocentesis, 398
ACD (acid citrate dextrose), 573, 573t
ACE inhibitors. *See* Angiotensin-converting enzyme (ACE) inhibitors
Acepromazine
  for congestive heart failure, 503
  side effects of, 402
Acetate, in fluid solutions, 334, 384, 407, 408f
Acetated polyionic solutions
  compatibility with intravenous drugs, 397t
  complications of, 384
  in perioperative management, 407, 408f
Acetazolamide, and metabolic acidosis, 257
Acetoacetate, as organic anion, 317
N-Acetylcysteine, for renal failure, 531
Acetylsalicylic acid, and salicylate intoxication, 261, 304
Acid
  defined, 229
  gastric secretion of, 421, 421f
  nonvolatile (fixed), 229, 235
  nonvolatile, weak, in acid-base disorders. *See* $[A_{tot}]$
  volatile, 229, 235–236
Acid citrate dextrose (ACD), 573, 573t
Acid load, acute, response to, 252–253, 252f
Acid-base balance
  acidity in, 229
  bicarbonate–carbonic acid system in, 233–234, 284, 285
  body buffers in, 234–235, 235f, 235t, 239
  buffering in, 230–232, 232f, 232t
  chloride and, 81–83
  external hydrogen ion balance in, 244
  isohydric principle in, 232–233
  law of mass action in, 230
  pH in, 229–230, 230f, 231t
  potassium and, 94–95, 101–102, 248–249

Acid-base balance *(Continued)*
  renal regulation of, 244–248, 245–246f, 248f, 249f
  whole-body regulation in, 244
Acid-base disorders, 229–249.
    See also Acidosis; Alkalosis
  anion gap in. *See* Anion gap (AG)
  blood gas measurement in, 237–243, 239f
    interpretation of, 241–242, 272
    normal values, 240–241, 241t
    sample collection and handling, 239–240
  compensatory responses in, 236t, 237, 237t, 297t, 298t
    metabolic, 288–290, 289b, 292–293, 298–299
    in mixed acid-base disorders, 297–299, 297t
    respiratory, 252, 270, 271f, 297–298
  in congestive heart failure, 502
  in diabetic ketoacidosis, 482–483
  diarrhea and, 428
  hypoperfusion and, 382–383
  in liver disease, 454–457, 455t, 456f, 458–459f
    treatment of, 467–468
  metabolic. *See* Metabolic acidosis; Metabolic alkalosis
  mixed. *See* Mixed acid-base disorders
  nontraditional approach to. *See* Strong ion approach
  perioperative management of, 396–397
  primary, 236, 236t
  in renal failure, 525
  respiratory. *See* Respiratory acidosis; Respiratory alkalosis
  simple vs. mixed, 236–237
  terminology for, 236
  vomiting and, 427
Acid-base status, evaluation of, 241–244, 299–301, 300b, 302f, 303t. *See also* Anion gap (AG); Base excess (BE); Strong ion difference (SID)
Acidemia
  defined, 236, 297
  effects of, 253, 291

Acidity, 229, 247
Acidosis. *See also* Metabolic acidosis; Respiratory acidosis
  defined, 236, 297
  dilutional, 258, 316–317, 316b, 317f
  lactic. *See* Lactic acidosis
  mechanisms of, 312f
    $[A_{tot}]$ changes in, 313b, 314
    P_{CO_2} in, 311
    strong ion difference changes in, 314t, 316–317, 316b, 317f
  membrane excitability and, 92
  organic, 316b, 317, 317f
  renal tubular. *See* Renal tubular acidosis
  uremic, 262–263, 306, 317
Acromegaly
  and hyperphosphatemia, 203
  polydipsia/polyuria in, 72t
ACTH (adrenocorticotropic hormone), levels of, in portosystemic shunting, 450
Action potential, development of, 92
Activity coefficient, 229
Acute intrinsic renal failure (AIRF).
    See Renal failure, acute (ARF)
Addison's disease. *See* Hypoadrenocorticism
Additive solutions, in fluid therapy, 332, 334t
  label for, 338f
Adenocarcinoma, anal sac, and hypercalcemia, 151–152, 151f, 152f
ADH. *See* Antidiuretic hormone (ADH, vasopressin)
b-Adrenergic blockers
  for congestive heart failure, 498t, 504–505
  and hyperkalemia, 115
Adrenocorticotropic hormone (ACTH), levels of, in portosystemic shunting, 450
AG. *See* Anion gap (AG)
Aging, perioperative management and, 399, 415
Air embolism, 369, 578
AIRF (acute intrinsic renal failure).
    See Renal failure, acute (ARF)
Albumin
  for ascites, 469–470
  as blood buffer, 235, 312, 313–314

Page numbers followed by f indicate figures; t, tables; b, boxes